Imaging the Aging Brain

Imaging the Aging Brain

EDITED BY

William Jagust, MD
Helen Wills Neuroscience Institute
University of California
Berkeley, CA

Mark D'Esposito, MD
Helen Wills Neuroscience Institute
University of California
Berkeley, CA

OXFORD
UNIVERSITY PRESS

2009

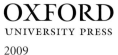

OXFORD
UNIVERSITY PRESS

Oxford University Press, Inc., publishes works that further
Oxford University's objective of excellence
in research, scholarship, and education.

Oxford   New York
Auckland   Cape Town   Dar es Salaam   Hong Kong   Karachi
Kuala Lumpur   Madrid   Melbourne   Mexico City   Nairobi
New Delhi   Shanghai   Taipei   Toronto

With offices in
Argentina   Austria   Brazil   Chile   Czech Republic   France   Greece
Guatemala   Hungary   Italy   Japan   Poland   Portugal   Singapore
South Korea   Switzerland   Thailand   Turkey   Ukraine   Vietnam

Published by Oxford University Press, Inc.
198 Madison Avenue, New York, New York 10016

www.oup.com

Library of Congress Cataloging-in-Publication Data
Imaging the aging brain / edited by William Jagust, Mark D'Esposito.
     p.   ;   cm.
  Includes bibliographical references and index.
  ISBN: 978-0-19-532887-5 (alk. paper)
  1. Geriatric neurology.   2. Brain—Imaging.   3. Alzheimer's
  disease—Imaging.   4. Brain—Aging.   I. Jagust,
  William.   II. D'Esposito, Mark.
  [DNLM: 1. Brain—physiopathology.   2. Diagnostic Imaging—methods.
  3. Aging—physiology.   4. Dementia—physiopathology.
  WL 141 I3156 2009]
  RC346.I43 2009
  618.97′68—dc22
                                                      2008052716

1   3   5   7   9   8   6   4   2

Printed in China
on acid-free paper

To Robyn
— William Jagust

To Judy, Zoe, and Zack
— Mark D'Esposito

Preface

Understanding the mechanisms of normal brain function is intimately involved with understanding its dysfunction. While molecular approaches have yielded major insights into many age-related diseases, other ways of understanding the brain play an equally important role. This is particularly true in brain aging, a situation in which no single molecule or even groups of molecules can explain an entire phenomenon. Brain aging has come to be defined as a heterogeneous process that affects some systems and spares others. Furthermore, these patterns of involvement vary from individual to individual. While there are no doubt underlying molecular mechanisms that define both vulnerability and damage, our current state of knowledge is so rudimentary that we are still defining phenotypes, behavior, longitudinal change and thereby focusing gradually on potential molecular targets. But we have a long way to go.

In this situation, it has occurred to many people that brain imaging has a great deal to offer. The past decade has seen an incredible explosion of interest in brain imaging as it is applied to aging and disease. Clearly, as described in Chapter 1, this has much to do with fundamental advances in technology and the diffusion of this technology into the research community. But there are also fundamental reasons, based on the types of information that imaging can bring to bear, that this technology is so appealing. It is interesting to think about how broad brain imaging is in terms of traditional areas of biology: it spans biochemistry (or neurochemistry), neuroanatomy, and neurophysiology. These different levels of analysis can be brought to bear at relatively high spatial and temporal resolution (changes in sub-hippocampal brain activity occurring in milliseconds) or low spatial and temporal resolution (whole brain volume atrophy occurring in years). These measurements can resolve system-level processes, sub-system component processes, or whole brain measures.

This volume is meant to provide the reader with a representative sample of the questions, methods, and technologies that a number of leading laboratories have applied to the study of brain aging. We believe that it is a timely compendium in view of the growing interest in the field, and the large number of new investigators who have been drawn to the study of aging using imaging technologies in recent years. The information is meant to provide a context in which to interpret the rapid and accelerating pace of new findings that may be hard to fully appreciate without the relevant background. As such, we think this book will be especially interesting to newcomers to the field of brain aging but we also hope it becomes a landmark in defining the current state of our knowledge for those working in the field.

As such, we have endeavored to span problems that could be considered both basic and applied. Basic science sections are concerned with laying out the patterns of brain changes seen in different brain systems—both anatomical and chemical—and in defining underlying mechanisms of compensation, change, and vulnerability. The Clinical sections are more focused on the detection of decline and prediction of disease, but as a reader will soon see, questions of disease and normal aging are no longer as easy to separate as they once might have been (if they ever truly were). We hope that readers who work in applied fields will explore the basic chapters, and that basic scientists will read through the clinical sections. Too often, the approaches of one group have been ignorant of the concepts and methods of the other.

There is no doubt that one of the major forces at work in shaping the book has been the importance and interest in Alzheimer's disease (AD), the most common cause of age-related cognitive decline and dementia. This is not only a result of the enormous public health concern about this disease but also because many of the problems in relating age-related change to AD have become tractable with the advent of new imaging approaches. But we would like to stress that this book is not meant to be an exploration of the diagnosis or early prediction of AD. Changes in brain structure, biochemistry, and function are far more heterogeneous and, as a reader of Chapter 3 will quickly determine, aging without AD has significant molecular and structural consequences. The importance of degeneration of frontal and subcortical systems, the importance of brain dopamine, and the importance of vascular disease are other themes that are repeated throughout the book. These may interact with AD, but they are also clearly separate and can be differentiated with imaging.

The process of preparing this book was very enjoyable for the editors. We were able to interact with colleagues in conceptualizing the contributions, and we learned a great deal by reading and editing the chapters. These research groups are all at the forefront of the use of imaging technologies, and have lead the way in the application of imaging to problems of the aging brain. We think that the thoughtful and encyclopedic contributions will be informative and maybe even inspirational to all of us.

William Jagust
Mark D'Esposito
Berkeley, CA

Contents

Contributors

Lars Bäckman, PhD
Aging Research Center
Karolinska Institutet
Stockholm, Sweden

António J. Bastos-Leite, MD, PhD
Department of Medical Imaging
University of Oporto, Portugal
Image Analysis Center and Alzheimer Center
VU University Medical Center
Amsterdam, The Netherlands

Susan Y. Bookheimer, PhD
Joaquin Fuster Professor of Cognitive Neuroscience
Center for Cognitive Neuroscience
Dept. of Psychiatry and Biobehavioral Sciences
Brain Research Institute
Los Angeles, CA

Miroslaw Brys, MD, PhD
Center for Brain Health
New York University School of Medicine
New York, NY

Fabienne Collette, PhD
Cyclotron Research Centre
University of Liège
Liège, Belgium

Charles DeCarli, MD
Alzheimer's Disease Center
Imaging of Dementia and Aging (IDeA) Laboratory
Department of Neurology and
Center for Neuroscience
University of California at Davis
Davis, CA

Mony J. de Leon, EdD
Director, Center for Brain Health
Department of Psychiatry
New York University Medical Center
New York, NY

Susan De Santi, PhD
Center for Brain Health
New York University Medical Center
New York, NY

Mark D'Esposito, MD
Helen Wills Neuroscience Institute
University of California
Berkeley, CA

Dara L. Dickstein, PhD
Department of Neuroscience
Kastor Neurobiology of Aging Laboratories
Alzheimer's Disease Research Center
Mount Sinai School of Medicine
New York, NY

Gaëtan Garraux, MD, PhD
Cyclotron Research Centre
University of Liège
Liège, Belgium

Adam H. Gazzaley, MD, PhD
Director, Neuroscience Imaging Center
University of California, San Francisco
San Francisco CA

Lidia Glodzik-Sobanska, MD, PhD
Center for Brain Health
Departments of Orthopedic Surgery and
    Psychiatry
New York University Medical Center
New York, NY

Cheryl L. Grady, PhD
Rotman Research Institute at Baycrest
University of Toronto
Toronto, Ontario, Canada

Harald Hampel, MD
Department of Psychiatry, School of Medicine
Trinity College Institute of Neuroscience
University of Dublin, Trinity Center for Health
    Sciences
Dublin, Ireland

Hauke R. Heekeren, MD, PhD
Neurocognition of Decision Making Group
Max Planck Institute for Human Development
Affective Neuroscience & Psychology of Emotion
Cluster of Excellence "Languages of Emotion"
Freie Universität Berlin
Berlin, Germany

Karl Herholz, MD
Professor in Clinical Neuroscience
Director, Wolfson Molecular Imaging Centre
Biomedical Imaging Institute
University of Manchester
Manchester, England

Patrick R. Hof, MD
Department of Neuroscience
Kastor Neurobiology of Aging Laboratories
Alzheimer's Disease Research Center
Mount Sinai School of Medicine
New York, NY

Clifford R. Jack, Jr., MD
Department of Radiology
Mayo Clinic
Rochester, MN

William Jagust, MD
Helen Wills Neuroscience Institute
University of California
Berkeley, CA

Frank Jessen, MD
Department of Psychiatry
Rheinische-Friedrich-Wilhelm University Bonn
Bonn, Germany

Sidonie T. Jones
Taub Institute for Research on Alzheimer's Disease and the
    Aging Brain
Department of Neurology and Department of
    Pathology
Center for Neurobiology and Behavior
Columbia University College of Physicians and Surgeons
New York, NY

Jeffrey Kaye, MD
Layton Aging and Alzheimer's Disease Center
Oregon Center for Aging and Technology
Departments of Neurology and Biomedical
    Engineering
Oregon Health and Science University
Portland Veterans Affairs Medical Center
Portland, OR

Kristen M. Kennedy, PhD
Center for BrainHealth
School of Behavioral and Brain Sciences
University of Texas at Dallas
Dallas, TX

William E. Klunk, MD, PhD
Departments of Psychiatry and Neurology
Co-Director Alzheimer's Disease Research Center
University of Pittsburgh School of Medicine
Pittsburgh, PA

Jessica B. S. Langbaum, PhD
Banner Alzheimer's Institute
Arizona Alzheimer's Consortium
Phoenix, AZ

Shu-Chen Li, PhD
Center for Lifespan Psychology
Max Planck Institute for Human Development
Berlin, Germany

Yi Li, MD
Center for Brain Health
New York University School of Medicine
New York, NY

Ulman Lindenberger, PhD
Center for Lifespan Psychology
Max Planck Institut
Berlin, Germany

Chester A. Mathis, PhD
Departments of Radiology, Pharmacology, and Pharmaceutical
    Sciences
Director of the Positron Emission Tomography Facility
University of Pittsburgh School of Medicine
Pittsburgh, PA

Adriane Mayda,
Alzheimer's Disease Center
Imaging of Dementia and Aging (IDeA) Laboratory
Department of Neurology and
Center for Neuroscience
University of California at Davis
Davis, CA

Rachel Mistur, MS
Center for Brain Health
New York University School of Medicine
New York, NY

John H. Morrison, PhD
Department of Neuroscience
Kastor Neurobiology of Aging Laboratories
Mount Sinai School of Medicine
New York, NY

Lisa Mosconi, PhD
Center for Brain Health
New York University School of Medicine
New York, NY

Lars Nyberg, PhD
Department of Integrative Medical Biology
University of Umeå, Sweden
Umeå, Sweden

Naftali Raz, PhD
Institute of Gerontology and Department of
    Psychology
Wayne State University
Detroit, MI

Eric M. Reiman, MD
Banner Alzheimer's Institute
Translational Genomics Research Institute
Department of Psychiatry, University of
    Arizona
Arizona Alzheimer's Consortium
Phoenix, AZ

Henry Rusinek, PhD
Department of Radiology
New York University Medical Center
New York, NY

Eric Salmon, MD, PhD
Cyclotron Research Centre
University of Liège
Liège, Belgium

Philip Scheltens, MD, PhD
Department of Neurology and Alzheimer Center
VU University Medical Center
Amsterdam, The Netherlands

Scott A. Small, MD
Taub Institute for Research on Alzheimer's Disease and the
  Aging Brain
Department of Neurology and Department of Pathology
Center for Neurobiology and Behavior
Columbia University College of Physicians and Surgeons
New York, NY

Reisa Sperling, MD
Memory Disorders Unit, Brigham and Women's Hospital
Alzheimer's Disease Research Center, Massachusetts General
  Hospital
Harvard Medical School
Boston, MA

Yaakov Stern, PhD
Cognitive Neuroscience Division of the Taub Institute
Departments of Neurology and Psychiatry

Columbia University College of Physicians and
  Surgeons
New York, NY

Remigiusz Switalski, MD
Center for Brain Health
New York School of Medicine
New York, NY

Arthur W. Toga, PhD
Laboratory of Neuro Imaging (LONI)
Department of Neurology
David Geffen School of Medicine
University of California Los Angeles
Los Angeles, CA

Wai Tsui, MS
Center for Brain Health
New York University Medical Center
New York, NY

John Darrell Van Horn, PhD
Laboratory of Neuro Imaging (LONI)
Department of Neurology
David Geffen School of Medicine
University of California Los Angeles
Los Angeles, CA

Mitsuhiro Yoshita, MD, PhD
Department of Neurology and Neurobiology of Aging
Kanazawa University Graduate School of Medical
  Science
Kanazawa, Japan

Imaging the Aging Brain

1

Introduction: Still More Questions than Answers

William Jagust and Mark D'Esposito

What are the Major Questions that Imaging Can Resolve?

Understanding how the brain ages has been a major goal of translational and basic neuroscience for many decades. Yet, only within the past few years has an exciting series of conceptual and technological advances in molecular biology, clinical medicine, cognitive neuroscience, and brain imaging propelled this field to a level that is beginning to make this goal a possibility. Thus, while the focus of this book is brain imaging, our ability to apply new imaging technologies has been enhanced by developments extrinsic to the imaging field. In particular, these advances involve more sophisticated methods of clinical characterization and analysis of human cognition, and the definition of molecular and cellular mechanisms underlying changes in the aging brain. Imaging the brain to comprehend the fundamental processes of aging has therefore become a truly multidisciplinary effort that must involve molecular neuroscientists, clinicians, cognitive neuroscientists, and imaging scientists. A goal of this chapter is to define how basic and clinical insights, along with appropriate developments in imaging technology, have enabled us to begin to ask the important questions. In addition, however, we must point out how limitations in concepts, knowledge, methods, and techniques still pose barriers to the study of brain aging.

Perhaps because of this conjunction of fortunate scientific developments, brain imaging has undergone a transformation and renaissance within the past decade. Several particular features are worth noting as major advances in the field. First, the imaging technologies themselves have become widely available. Magnetic resonance imaging (MRI) has proliferated, allowing structural and, in many cases, functional imaging of the brain to be conducted in a wide range of institutions previously excluded from "high tech" scientific inquiry. Most academic medical centers today are capable of structural and functional MRI (fMRI) research, and colleges and universities without medical schools, as well as privately run imaging centers, are performing MR studies. Positron emission tomography (PET), once the domain of a few well-endowed centers with access to cyclotrons and physicists, has diffused into the community largely because of the commercial availability of longer-lived PET nuclides like Fluorine-18, which is used in glucose metabolic imaging with [18F]Fluorodeoxyglucose (FDG) in oncology. This radiotracer, along with other potential [18F] imaging agents, can be synthesized in regional centers, transported to local hospitals and academic centers, and used to study brain function and biochemistry. At this point,

many institutions have the ability to perform structural MRI, fMRI, and PET studies of the brain, in addition to the already widely available techniques of single photon emission computed technology (SPECT) and electrophysiological methods like electroencephalograms (EEG) and event-related potentials.

Second, a key ingredient of brain imaging—image analysis—has also reached a level of maturity characterized by easily accessible software for data analysis. Many of these programs are freely available on the Internet, well-documented with online manuals and user groups, run on multiple platforms, and generally accepted by the community so that publications using these techniques are well-understood. While the use of any individual analysis package has limitations that depend on the context (discussed further in the next chapter), the strength and weaknesses of different approaches to data analysis are openly and transparently debated by users with extensive knowledge and experience.

Third, while there is still disagreement in clinical circles on how to diagnose and characterize various sorts of age- and disease-related cognitive decline, there is now greater agreement on terminology and definitions. Not that long ago, clinicians debated whether the diagnosis of Alzheimer's Disease (AD) was really possible during life. Now, commonly accepted diagnostic criteria have been shown to have reasonably high sensitivity and specificity (Knopman et al., 2001). A proliferation of terms describing age-related memory loss, including benign senescent forgetfulness and age-associated memory impairment, has largely been replaced by the concept of mild cognitive impairment (MCI) (Flicker, Ferris, and Reisberg, 1991; Petersen et al., 1999). While MCI does not solve all the problems related to the subtle cognitive changes observed during aging, nor does it clearly define boundaries between "normal" age-related memory loss and disease (see below), it provides nosological agreement that had previously been lacking. Finally, a host of other diagnostic criteria for dementing illnesses, such as dementia with Lewy bodies (DLB) (McKeith et al., 2005), frontotemporal lobar degeneration (Neary et al., 1998) and vascular dementia (Chui et al., 1992; Roman et al., 1993), while still limited in their degree of validation, nevertheless provide common definitions that have undoubtedly improved the description and recruitment of research subjects.

Fourth, while the discoveries in molecular and cellular neuroscience are obviously not a topic for this book, they have major implications for our understanding of normal and diseased brain function that bear on aging and imaging. The elucidation of the molecular pathology of AD, for example, offers promise for the development of "disease modifying" therapeutic approaches that might halt, or even reverse, its progression (Roberson and Mucke, 2006). In this setting, early diagnosis and therapeutic monitoring (discussed in many chapters in the second half of this book) have become a major goal of brain imaging. Cellular changes associated with brain aging, such as alterations in synaptic structure and function (see Chapter 3), have provided insights into regional susceptibility to disease and concepts of brain and cognitive reserve and compensation (see Chapters 6 and 7). Insights into how genetic influences affect brain structure and function provide models for both early detection of disease and biochemical influences on age-related decline (Chapters 9 and 20). These are only a few of the ways in which molecular and cellular neuroscience have affected the types of questions that can now be addressed with imaging, and have provided renewed motivation for understanding the neural mechanisms underlying age-related brain and cognitive changes.

Finally, many of these developments have combined with the fields of neuropsychology and cognitive neuroscience to give rise to a reasonably coherent and mechanistic "cognitive neuroscience of aging." While there are still many problems, both conceptual and methodological, the ability to characterize cognitive functions more precisely, and to relate these functions to underlying brain mechanisms, has helped define how disease and age together and separately may produce dysfunction. This book is not particularly directed towards the cognitive neuroscience of aging, as previous books have done an excellent job in this regard (e.g., Cabeza, Nyberg, and Park, 2005). However, the ability to relate behavior in domains like episodic memory, semantic memory, and working memory to underlying mechanisms by carefully examining both behavior and brain correlates has provided powerful ways of studying age-related change.

In essence, this introduction states the obvious—the timing for a review of how brain imaging can inform the study of brain aging is right, given the state of the field. The themes of this book include both basic and applied topics, issues related to both normal aging and disease, and issues that transcend any particular technology. We have generally avoided a technique-based approach in favor of a "problem-based" approach, since many questions can be answered with more than one method (although, in some cases, methods are separated because the topics are so large and methods so different). In the following sections, we will review what we consider to be the main conceptual challenges in the field, while in the next chapter we will review the main technical challenges. Not surprisingly, there are more questions than answers.

Brain Aging or Brain Disease?

A major question in the study of brain aging is the boundary between age and disease. This is a complex problem that involves both conceptual and methodological issues. The problem is compounded by the fact that different disciplines may be highly focused on different concepts and techniques, so that scientists involved in the study of aging may neglect the presence of preclinical dementia, while those involved in the study of diseases of aging may view all cognitive decline as incipient disease.

The field of gerontology has grappled with these issues on a conceptual front for decades. Initial advances strove to differentiate disease-related change from age-related change in an effort to define "normal aging," while further effort has attempted to differentiate "usual" from "successful" aging (Rowe and Kahn, 1987), or aging that is at least "above average" in some respects. With regard to separating age and disease, many have suggested that aging is not simply defined by the aggregation of disease, and that factors related to the passage of time, the presence of systemic vulnerabilities, and the accumulation of damage mediated by processes that are largely stochastic provide ways of understanding age-related change as distinct from known diseases. However, it is also becoming increasingly apparent that many diseases exist in mild or preclinical forms, so dichotomizing a disease process as "present" or "absent" may not reflect the reality of something that occurs on a biological continuum. As will subsequently be seen, this effort at disentangling normal aging from disease, while conceptually difficult, may in fact be a largely methodological issue.

The arguments about what constitutes normal aging are influenced by data showing both considerable variability in performance among older individuals, as well as the observation that most age-related data sets contain older individuals with minimal to no significant loss of performance (Lupien and Wan, 2004). These individuals characterized as "aging successfully" likely differ from individuals who follow more typical or average age-related trajectories in many ways. In this setting, then, it is reasonable to try to identify many different mediators of both decline and preserved function. It is likely, of course, that individuals vary along the many continua that include preclinical disease, time-related but disease-independent processes we call "aging," and something that we may refer to as "optimal" or "successful" aging. Indeed, the latter point—cognitive and molecular mechanisms, as well as environmental associations, that preserve or even enhance brain function in aging—have been poorly addressed. Together, factors that lead to different aging outcomes must include factors that are related to both disease and optimal function.

The study of brain aging has often been dominated by the study of Alzheimer's Disease (AD), the most common cause of dementia in adults that has assumed enormous scientific and public health importance. While the study of cognitive aging may utilize cohorts of "healthy" older adults, a number of recent observations suggest that all of these individuals may not truly be disease-free. For example, it is clear that AD has a protracted prodrome, during which symptoms are subtle or absent, and that many cognitively intact individuals have Alzheimer neuropathology (Davis, et al., 1999; Bennett, et al., 2006). Studies of normal age-related cognitive decline thus may be recruiting some participants with early, subclinical AD, as evidenced in one study in which a high proportion of normal individuals with age-associated memory impairment developed dementia when followed longitudinally (Goldman and Morris, 2001). Thus, while one can conceptually differentiate aging and disease, methodological ability has been limited. As our methods for detecting disease in earlier forms become better, the conditions left after these subtle disease-related processes are excluded will be defined as "normal" aging.

One promising approach, therefore, to at least answering questions about what is "normal" aging is the recent ability to both improve the cognitive characterization of subjects and to improve the imaging characterization of subjects through the use of MR and amyloid imaging. For example, in Chapters 10 and 14, authors review how changes in brain structure that might reflect early AD and the deposition of beta-amyloid—the protein strongly associated with AD—can now be imaged with MR and PET, respectively, to better characterize cognitively normal individuals. Differentiating cognitive processes in individuals with and without these biomarkers may help us separate at least some age-related from disease-related processes so that individuals without these biomarkers at least represent those who have successfully aged while avoiding AD.

Another major advance has been the gradual understanding that age-related decline, rather than reflecting a single unitary process, is likely an interplay of many different processes, some of which can be described as disease-related and others that cannot (Buckner, 2004; Hedden and Gabrieli, 2004). Thus, while it has been suggested that much age-related cognitive decline might be due to AD (Brayne and Calloway, 1988), or to another single factor such as a non-pathological decline in information-processing resources (Salthouse and Ferrer-Caja, 2003), a unitary factor underlying all age related cognitive decline fails to account for the multiple etiological pathways that have slowly been revealed. These include not only early AD, but factors related to cerebrovascular disease (Breteler and Claus, 1994; Raz, Rodrigue, and Acker, 2003; Petkov et al., 2004), changes in neurotransmitter systems like dopamine (Volkow et al., 1996; Backman et al., 2000), endocrine function (McEwen, 2002; Eberling et al., 2003; Rasgon et al., 2005), and a host of lifestyle and environmental stressors and protective factors, many of which appear to operate on brain systems that are independent of any single disease (Lupien et al., 1998; Raz et al., 1998; Seeman et al., 2001; Gustafson et al., 2004). While these factors have been heuristically defined as largely influencing either the medial temporal or prefrontal-subcortical memory and executive systems (Buckner, 2004), their effects are regionally and cognitively complex and likely to interact.

While it therefore seems likely that a single factor, such as preclinical AD, cannot account for the myriad systems affected by age, it is also interesting to note that many of the subtle age-related processes bear passing resemblance to other known diseases in sub-clinical or preclinical forms. For example, changes in the dopamine system seen in aging (and further discussed in Chapter 5) may, to some extent, resemble Parkinson's disease both pharmacologically and behaviorally (Fearnley and Lees, 1991; Ross et al., 2004), while changes in frontal lobe/executive systems reflect damage that may occur consequent to cerebrovascular disease (Raz, Rodrigue, and Acker, 2003). Thus, it appears likely that age-related brain changes reflect a full spectrum of different mechanisms—early or preclinical disease, time-dependent processes that are not specifically disease-related (such as endocrine alterations), and subtle manifestations of processes that, at least superficially, resemble known diseases at least by virtue of sharing pathways of damage.

Thus, a major question facing those interested in brain aging is not simply the differentiation of aging from disease, nor is it the differentiation between usual and successful aging. Instead, the question has become how to identify the mechanisms and pathways through which disease, normal aging, and successful aging occur and interact. This book offers hints of what these pathways may be and how to detect them, in chapters related to the systems affected by brain aging, the roles of compensation and reserve, the influence of genes, and the ability to detect early, and preclinical manifestations of AD. We feel that it is likely that over the coming years, distinctions between what is normal aging and what is disease will be answered by a series of advances that permit us to measure biomarkers of subtle disease in older people, track these changes over time, and relate both their presence and absence to specific changes in behavior and cognitive processes.

Extrinsic Factors Affect the Application of Imaging Technology

As noted above, for the most part we have endeavored to construct this book to avoid technology-based approaches in favor of addressing key questions or problems in the field. However, technology is important in several respects. First, of course, is the fact that all technology is limited and we must strive to understand these limitations. As new abilities to image brain function, structure, and biochemistry become available, it is tempting to accept the results enthusiastically. But as the next chapter points out, technical factors limit conclusions that can be drawn and, in some cases, it is likely that these limitations may not become fully apparent until years after a technology is introduced.

Another key factor that must be considered is cost, but cost and utility are inextricably linked. The cost/benefit equation for a research tool, for example, is driven by a variety of factors that may be irrelevant for a clinical tool. If a given technology is the only way we can study a problem, it will likely be deployed in the lab—but if it provides no information of direct benefit to people, it will not likely be applied clinically. Let us again turn to the question of the diagnosis or prediction of AD as an illustrative example.

Decades of research have shown associations between patterns of glucose metabolism using FDG-PET and AD, as many studies have shown associations between hippocampal atrophy on MRI and AD. These studies have included clinical-imaging pathological results demonstrating reasonable pathological specificity for the imaging findings (Hoffman et al., 2000; Silverman et al., 2001; Gosche et al., 2002; Jack et al., 2002; Jagust et al., 2007), and many studies have also found that these techniques have the ability to detect preclinical or presymptomatic AD (Small et al., 1995; Fox, Warrington, and Rossor, 1999; Jack et al., 1999; Chetelat et al., 2003; Reiman et al., 2004; Jagust et al., 2006). Yet, current diagnostic guidelines do not recommend either technique to diagnose AD, either preclinically or even in the presence of manifest disease (Knopman et al., 2001), and it is unusual for these techniques to be employed in this clinical situation. While there are likely many reasons for this state of affairs, including the limitations of existing studies, a major limitation has, of course, been the lack of effective AD therapies. In this sense then, the most important factor driving patient-oriented imaging research on age-related cognitive decline are is the advances in molecular therapeutics that offer hope for the treatment of age-related cognitive disorders. Thus, developments entirely extrinsic to the world of brain imaging are the greatest drivers of clinical imaging research right now. If effective AD treatments become available, early detection will be important and imaging is likely to play a major clinical role. Without these treatment advances, the necessity of early diagnosis is questionable.

The issue of competing technologies, however, is also crucial to understanding the role of brain imaging in both the research and clinical arenas. Again, with regard to the diagnosis of AD, many other approaches besides imaging are promising. These range from simple cognitive examinations that may have predictive power (DeCarli et al., 2004; Galvin et al., 2005) to proteomic methods (Graff-Radford et al., 2007; Ray et al., 2007; Sundelof et al., 2008). While these techniques are also largely unvalidated, the importance of a brain-imaging modality to diagnose or predict AD must eventually be judged, not only by whether or not effective treatments are available, but by whether a cheaper and simpler test produces similar results. From a strictly research perspective, there is no argument about whether a blood test relying on proteomic methods could replace a PET or fMRI scan—they measure different things that are likely to be complementary. A full understanding of brain aging will probably require this sort of multidimensional understanding. But as a clinical tool, one can clearly replace the other. Thus, it is important to consider the precise role of a technique in defining its utility.

In a related way, it is important to understand how different imaging technologies provide different types of information—anatomic, physiological, and biochemical, for example. Which technique is "better" is often the wrong issue. While it is true that different techniques may offer similar predictive or diagnostic abilities (and therefore ought to be compared with one another), it is more often the case that information is complementary. For example, PET and MRI differ significantly in their temporal and spatial resolution. Again, whether complementary information is worthwhile depends on the clinical cost and benefit—or, in the research arena, the novelty and importance of the data that can be collected. Yet at this stage, it appears likely that combining different imaging modalities offers considerable promise for understanding the aging process during which changes occur in so many different dimensions.

The strength of imaging technologies, therefore, may not simply reside in the ability to define the presence or absence of a certain disease state. While this is definitely an important issue, it is also a question that may legitimately be answered by a variety of techniques. Imaging does offer the exclusive ability to localize the brain regions affected by a process, and potentially draw mechanistic inferences about how this process occurs and produces symptoms. This is the sort of information that does not appear likely to be supplanted by other approaches in the foreseeable future.

The Promise of Multimodal Approaches

A major characteristic of the progress of brain imaging over the past decade is the current maturity of a number of different approaches that yield different sorts of complementary information. Structural MRI, functional MRI, and PET imaging provide different types of data that illuminate different aspects of what was once known as anatomy, physiology, and biochemistry. Combining these techniques, discussed to some extent in many chapters in this book, offers considerable promise for understanding mechanisms of age-related cognitive decline.

As one example, we can again revisit the question of preclinical AD to ask how beta-amyloid affects brain function and structure. The ability to combine PET measurements for the detection of preclinical amyloid deposition (Chapter 14) with fMRI measurements of cognitive function (Chapter 18) may permit us to begin to understand how beta-amyloid affects certain brain systems and spares others. As discussed in Chapter 11, combining PET measures with other biomarkers may provide ways of diagnosing the disease earlier—this approach has already proven to be productive when amyloid imaging is combined with CSF measurement of beta-amyloid (Fagan et al., 2006).

The combination of molecular or functional imaging with structural imaging has already been important in investigating how brain atrophy affects measurement (see Chapter 2), and defining how atrophy and function interact in predicting disease progression (Meltzer et al., 1999; Johnson et al., 2000; Dickerson et al., 2004). Definition of where and over what time course biochemical changes such as amyloid deposition affect brain atrophy will now be possible. This approach is already beginning to yield interesting results in the study of AD (Jack et al., 2008) and is discussed in Chapter 12.

Finally, relating a host of neurochemical changes to functional changes is an area that is just beginning to be investigated. It has been clear for a while that the ability to measure basic pharmacological properties of a neural system, such as dopamine with PET, offers us links between behavior and neurochemistry (Volkow et al., 1998; Cools et al., 2008). However, pharmacology can also be related to brain activity during cognitive tasks with fMRI or PET by either directly measuring neurotransmitter function (Carbon et al., 2004), or by pharmacological manipulation during an fMRI procedure (Kimberg et al., 2001). Combining measures of brain structure, function, and biochemistry offers ways to attack the complex multivariate problem of brain aging.

The Wide Spectrum of Age-related Diseases

Much of the previous discussion has involved the differentiation of normal age-related processes from the most common age-related cognitive disorder, AD. However, there are a host of other diseases, many of which may also exist in preclinical or asymptomatic forms, that are likely to play a role in age-related cognitive decline. This poses two sorts of problems. The obvious problem of course, is the development of technologies for the detection and quantification of these other disease processes in ways that permit the mapping of change over time beginning with subtle evidence. The second problem is inherent in all multifactorial, complex conditions. There are so many different processes, some of which may share pathways or mechanisms, that the ability to define how these interact with one another to cause decline is a daunting problem.

As one example, it is clear from a variety of approaches—clinical, epidemiological, cognitive, and imaging—that cerebrovascular disease has an effect on age-related cognitive decline (Hofman et al., 1997; DeCarli et al., 2001; Nordahl et al., 2005). Reasonably good imaging biomarkers for cerebrovascular disease are available, particularly MRI scans that appear to be capable of detecting both clear cerebral infarction and milder, subclinical forms of ischemic damage to white matter (Breteler et al., 1994; Pullicino et al., 1995). However, even with such a biomarker, there are limitations to our understanding of how vascular disease interacts with other processes that occur in brain aging. For example, it now appears that there is considerable interaction between cerebrovascular disease and AD in producing brain atrophy (Jagust et al., 2008), that topographic differences in the location of white matter disease may be significant (DeCarli et al., 2005), and that some subtle changes in white matter can probably only be detected with new techniques like diffusion tensor imaging (DTI) (Medina et al., 2006; Huang, Friedland, and Auchus, 2007). Furthermore, specific alterations in white matter tracts that play major mechanistic roles in cognition, such as the perforant pathway and the cingulum bundle (Kalus et al., 2006; Zhang et al., 2007), can now be detected. The simple question of whether or not cerebrovascular disease is present or absent has now been expanded to a complex question of how severe the vascular disease is, what specific white matter pathways are affected, and how vascular disease interacts with other disorders. This becomes a complex problem of defining mechanistic pathways to cognitive decline. However, our ability to measure this sort of change, even in very mild degrees and specific brain regions provides us with the possibility of selecting individuals for study who have no evidence of cerebrovascular disease at all. Further excluding those with any evidence of Alzheimer pathology begins to create the possibility of studying some form of aging less likely to be associated with known disease.

This same situation is apparent in a variety of other conditions that we can now begin to detect with improved imaging technologies. This includes age-related changes in many different neurotransmitter systems, such as dopamine (Backman et al., 2000), acetylcholine (Kuhl et al., 1999; Podruchny et al., 2003), and serotonin

(Moller, Jakobsen, and Gjedde, 2007), to name a few. While in some cases evidence shows that subtle changes might reflect preclinical disease, such as Parkinson's disease (Adams et al., 2005), in many situations reductions in neurotransmitter function are unrelated to any specific disease process. Therefore, the ability to define how these neurotransmitter changes interact with both cognition and regional brain activation offers other ways to define age-related cognitive alterations. Our ability to measure so many different processes allows for far better characterization of our research subjects, but also creates a complex multivariable problem for defining relationships between the aging brain and cognition.

Cognitive Neuroscience of Aging

Studying the neural mechanisms that underlie the cognitive decline in aging has been greatly enhanced by new brain imaging technologies. Although psychologists have carefully described the cognitive changes that occur with aging for many years, neuroscientists have begun to link these cognitive changes to changes in neural systems over the last decade. New data from fMRIs, in particular, has led to tremendous insight and new theoretical models regarding the neural mechanisms underlying cognitive aging. These studies go beyond the typical clinical study of aging by using sophisticated cognitive methods developed in experimental psychology (rather than behavioral paradigms developed for diagnostic purposes) to precisely define the processing deficits in individuals as they age. Chapters in this volume by Stern and Grady highlight this approach. The addition of other imaging methods (such as DTI) and the combining of fMRI data with data from other modalities (such as PET) will provide even greater insight into cognitive aging. Overall, the outlook is quite promising for making significant gains in our knowledge of the aging brain. As mentioned, however, all such studies that attempt to link the brain to behavior must be considered in the context of the limitations of the methods being utilized. This issue will be discussed in great detail in Chapter 2.

Studies that seek to understand the neural basis of so-called "normal" aging can also be another means in which one can attempt to differentiate aging from disease. For example, it is evident from almost all imaging studies of cognitive aging that there is tremendous individual variability within older individuals when compared to a cohort of younger individuals. This variability, which includes some individuals that perform as well as younger individuals, provides an opportunity to study the neural mechanisms underlying compensation and protection. Functional MRI studies have demonstrated quite distinct patterns of brain activity in these two groups, which have provided insight regarding how the aging brain adapts to "normal" or "abnormal" changes with time. These issues are discussed in Chapters 4, 6, and 7. Furthermore, if such studies begin to examine the relationship between "normal" aging and disease by examining other factors (e.g., amyloid, white matter disease), even more information can be obtained regarding the spectrums of aging and disease. These studies have been rare to date, but are likely to appear in the literature in the near future.

Experimental Design Limits Inferences from Imaging Studies

While many contributors to this book note the strengths and existing limitations of the current state of knowledge, it is also important to be aware that just as advances in nonimaging fields affect the success of imaging, they also are important in understanding the limitations of current knowledge. For example, the strength and weaknesses of existing approaches to the study of brain aging are crucially dependent on how we select and follow subjects using a variety of nonimaging modalities. These design issues must be carefully addressed to move the field of imaging and aging forward.

There is a growing understanding that we have over-relied on cross-sectional as opposed to longitudinal studies. Some conclusions about how age is related to cognitive decline thus may rely on cross-sectional comparisons of groups with very low (young individuals) risks compared to the very high (older individuals) risks of early or preclinical AD. Large cohort studies may screen those with dementia or even mild cognitive impairment, but this of course can leave samples contaminated with participants with still milder AD symptoms. The ability to follow individuals over time for signs of decline, and the ability to track the nature of this decline, offers greater promise for differentiating those with disease from those without.

While the reasons for reliance on cross-sectional studies are clear—longitudinal studies take more time, cost more, and have methodological problems of their own, such as subject attrition—the problems related to cohort or secular effects are well-known to plague cross-sectional approaches (Flynn, 1987; Schaie, Willis, and Pennak, 2005). These problems have real significance for imaging studies. Thus, while cross-sectional studies of atrophy in aging highlight effects in the prefrontal cortex, longitudinal studies indicate that atrophy is likely to be more pervasive (Raz et al., 1997; Raz et al., 2004) (reviewed in Chapter 4). In this situation, longitudinal studies detect more change than cross-sectional studies. Of course, a major problem with longitudinal studies in the imaging field also involves technological change—scanner upgrades are the simplest example—that seriously complicate such studies. However, approaches to these problems are being developed and they appear to be tractable, even if complex (Mueller et al., 2005). A key issue in longitudinal studies is also the length of follow-up, since time constants for age- or disease-related change may be slow and different from one another. For example, defining patients with MCI as "converters" or "stable," based on whether or not they develop AD over a period of observation, may yield very different results depending on how long an individual is followed. It is possible also that the only difference between a benign or malignant form of age-related memory loss is the rate of decline. These differences may be clinically meaningful (if an individual declines so slowly that there is no appreciable disability during life) or biologically meaningful (if different rates of decline are caused by different processes). In either case, only long-term observation is likely to be able to differentiate such pathways.

Subject recruitment and description are methodological aspects of imaging studies that bear heavily on study outcomes, and yet are not always clearly addressed or described. While it is true that classification and description of subjects has come a long way in the past decade, there are still problems, and these particularly plague "normal aging" studies. The problem is exacerbated since we do not understand all the factors involved, so subject description is key. We can agree relatively well on what might constitute AD or even MCI; it is not so clear what constitutes a normal older person—neither "normal" nor "old" are fully agreed upon. Studies that compare individuals in their 6th decade to those in their 2nd may, in fact, be aging studies, but are likely to be investigating different phenomena than those enrolling people over the age of 85 (Kawas and Corrada, 2006; Whittle et al., 2007). More difficult, however, is the question of how to define normal—as already noted, this is a question that can be answered by excluding individuals with a host of different diseases (such as stroke, cardiovascular disease, diabetes, etc.). However, this approach can also produce a group of subjects that have been called "supernormals," who are certainly not representative of the population of normal older people, and are clearly not statistically normal. The converse approach would include a wider range of individuals that are statistically normal and thus suffer from the usual age-related diseases. There is no correct solution to this problem—highly screened subjects may provide a way to investigate the more "pure" effects of age-related processes on the brain but are not likely to be easily generalized, while a broader sample of individuals may be more easily generalized but mechanistically complex. These issues are only the tip of the iceberg, as questions related to where and how subjects are recruited (by responding to advertisements, by coming to clinics, by epidemiological sampling, etc.) are likely to bear on whether they have subclinical disease, comorbid conditions, and high or low baseline functioning, to name just a few characteristics. These are extremely important in relating imaging measures to behavior or change over time. The only solution to these problems appears to be careful description of subjects and precise characterization of brain structure, function, and biochemistry.

Another methodological issue is the use of prospective or retrospective designs in imaging research—particularly applicable to studies that endeavor to predict who will decline or develop dementia. While many investigators recruit subjects, test them at baseline, and use baseline measures to predict outcomes, the majority of such studies are not really prospective. The reason for this is that imaging parameters are usually defined after the outcome is known. That is, groups of individuals who decline are compared to individuals who did not decline, and regional differences in brain structure or function in baseline scans are reported. While such studies advance the field, they are not truly prospective in comparison to studies in which *a priori* decisions are made about what precise image characteristics (such as a specific size "cutoff" for a brain volume or metabolic measure) will predict decline, allowing us to truly compute test performance characteristics in a prospective fashion.

Finally, when we describe "normal" as opposed to pathological aging we must rely to some extent on definitions of pathology, and here also there is lack of certainty. It is amply clear that the pathological diagnosis of AD is not straightforward, with several different efforts at categorizing this process culminating in the probabilistic NIA-Reagan Institute criteria (Khachaturian, 1985; Mirra et al., 1991; N.I.A., 1997). Whether a given individual is pathologically characterized as having AD or not depends on which criteria are used (Bennett et al., 2006). Furthermore, the significance of differences between levels of certainty (i.e., high and intermediate) are not clear, as individuals may be demented or not with different levels of pathology. At this point, it seems that the best we can do is note the presence and severity of AD pathology and try to understand why it exerts effects in some individuals and not others.

The Future

As noted, some of the biggest questions in the field of cognitive aging now seem as if they are becoming tractable through improvements in technique. Longitudinal studies using a host of imaging biomarkers offer the promise of differentiating pathways of decline that are related to the common problem of AD from pathways that may not. The ability to probe the cognitive changes that occur in

AD and in older individuals who are free from AD by using carefully designed cognitive experiments and fMRI may permit us to understand how the disease exerts effects, and also how individuals may respond to and even overcome these effects. These are big steps in the cognitive neuroscience of aging.

While there may never be full agreement on what constitutes "normal" or even "aging," the limitations to our understanding are becoming clarified, and more careful description and definition of cognitive status, subject selection criteria, and the use of longitudinal and truly prospective designs will help the situation. If the goal of aging studies is to understand mechanisms—for example, a basic science approach—then we now have tools at our disposal to begin to look at such mechanisms. If the goal is clinical—to predict who might benefit from treatment or to monitor treatment—we also have promising techniques for that.

Thus, as imaging and other technologies develop, questions about what is normal or disease may indeed become secondary in comparison to our ability to understand mechanisms of cognitive change or stability. If, for example, deposition of beta-amyloid explains a significant component of normal age-related memory loss, we are slowly moving to the point where we can understand that. Alternatively, if individuals without beta-amyloid deposition show substantial cognitive decline, the ability to follow such individuals longitudinally with techniques such as fMRI and structural MRI may permit us to understand how these changes occur.

It seems then that rather than argue about what constitutes normal aging, we can begin to address some key important questions with the tools and techniques described in this volume. These questions include:

1. How much age-related cognitive decline is related to subclinical AD?
2. What is the role of cerebrovascular disease in age-related cognitive decline?
3. What cognitive systems and processes are affected in older people who have neither manifest nor subclinical age-related disease?
4. How do different age-related diseases interact to affect cognitive systems and behavior?
5. How much can we predict about a given individual's cognitive trajectory—and can we predict disease before it manifests?
6. How do neurochemical changes affect functional activity and behavior?
7. Can we alter the trajectory of cognitive decline with interventions?

The ability to tackle these questions is slowly developing largely because of innovative ways of imaging the human brain, and by thoughtfully combining brain imaging with other productive neuroscience techniques. The next decade should be another exciting one for those involved in these studies.

References

Adams, J. R., van Netten, H., Schulzer, M., Mak, E., McKenzie, J., Strongosky, A., Sossi, V., et al. (2005). PET in LRRK2 mutations: Comparison to sporadic Parkinson's disease and evidence for presymptomatic compensation. *Brain*, 128: 2777–2785.

Backman, L., Ginovart, N., Dixon, R. A., Wahlin, T. B., Wahlin, A., Halldin, C., and Farde, L. (2000). Age-related cognitive deficits mediated by changes in the striatal dopamine system. *American Journal of Psychiatry*, 157: 635–637.

Bennett, D. A., Schneider, J. A., Arvanitakis, Z., Kelly, J. F., Aggarwal, N. T., Shah, R. C., and Wilson, R. S. (2006). Neuropathology of older persons without cognitive impairment from two community-based studies. *Neurology*, 66: 1837–1844.

Brayne, C. and Calloway, P. (1988). Normal ageing, impaired cognitive function, and Senile Dementia of the Alzheimer's type: A Continuum? *Lancet*, 1: 1265–1267.

Breteler, M. M. and Claus, J. J. (1994). Cardiovascular disease and distribution of cognitive function in elderly people: The Roterdam study. *British Medical Journal*, 308: 1604–1608.

Breteler, M. M. B., van Swieten, J. C., Bots, M. L., Grobbee, D. E., Claus, J. J., van den Hout, J. H. W., van Harskamp, F., et al. (1994). Cerebral white matter lesions, vascular risk factors, and cognitive function in a population-based study: The Rotterdam study. *Neurology*, 44: 1246–1252.

Buckner, R. L. (2004). Memory and executive function in aging and AD: Multiple factors that cause decline and reserve factors that compensate. *Neuron*, 44: 195–208.

Cabeza, R., Nyberg, L., and Park, D. (2005). *Cognitive Neuroscience of Aging*. New York: Oxford University Press.

Carbon, M., Ma, Y., Barnes, A., Dhawan, V., Chaly, T., Ghilardi, M. F., and Eidelberg, D. (2004). Caudate nucleus: Influence of dopaminergic input on sequence learning and brain activation in Parkinsonism. *Neuroimage*, 21: 1497–1507.

Chetelat, G., Desgranges, B., De La Sayette, V., Viader, F., Eustache, F., and Baron, J. C. (2003). Mild cognitive impairment: Can FDG-PET predict who is to rapidly convert to Alzheimer's Disease? *Neurology*, 60: 1374–1377.

Chui, H. C., Victoroff, J. I., Margolin, D. I., Jagust, W. J., Shankle, W. R., and Katzman, R. (1992). Criteria for the diagnosis of Ischemic vascular dementia proposed by the state of California Alzheimer Disease diagnostic and treatment centers. *Neurology*, 42: 473–480.

Cools, R., Gibbs, S. E., Miyakawa, A., Jagust, W., and D'Esposito, M. (2008). Working memory capacity predicts dopamine synthesis capacity in the human striatum. *Journal of Neuroscience*, 28: 1208–1212.

Davis, D. G., Schmitt, F. A., Wekstein, D. R., and Markesbery, W. R. (1999). Alzheimer neuropathologic alterations in aged cognitively normal subjects. *Journal of Neuropathology and Experimental Neurology*, 58: 376–388.

DeCarli, C., Fletcher, E., Ramey, V., Harvey, D., and Jagust, W. J. (2005). Anatomical Mapping of White Matter Hyperintensities (WMH): Exploring the relationships between periventricular WMH, deep WMH, and total WMH burden. *Stroke*, 36: 50–55.

DeCarli, C., Miller, B. L., Swan, G. E., Reed, T., Wolf, P. A., and Carmelli, D. (2001). Cerebrovascular and brain morphologic correlates of mild cognitive impairment in the National Heart, Lung, and Blood Institute Twin Study. *Archives of Neurology*, 58: 643–647.

DeCarli, C., Mungas, D., Harvey, D., Reed, B., Weiner, M., Chui, H., and Jagust, W. (2004). Memory impairment, but not cerebrovascular disease, predicts progression of MCI to dementia. *Neurology*, 63: 220–227.

Dickerson, B. C., Salat, D. H., Bates, J. F., Atiya, M., Killiany, R. J., Greve, D. N., et al. (2004). Medial temporal lobe function and structure in mild cognitive impairment. *Annals of Neurology*, 56: 27–35.

Eberling, J. L., Wu, C., Haan, M. N., Mungas, D., Buonocore, M., and Jagust, W. J. (2003). Preliminary evidence that estrogen protects against age-related hippocampal atrophy. *Neurobiology of Aging*, 24: 725–732.

Fagan, A. M., Mintun, M. A., Mach, R. H., Lee, S. Y., Dence, C. S., Shah, A. R., LaRossa, G. N., et al. (2006). Inverse relation between in vivo amyloid imaging load and cerebrospinal fluid Abeta42 in humans. *Annals of Neurology*, 59: 512–519.

Fearnley, J. M. and Lees, A. J. (1991). Aging and Parkinson's disease: Substantia nigra regional selectivity. *Brain*, 114: 2283–2301.

Flicker, C., Ferris, S. H., and Reisberg, B. (1991). Mild cognitive impairment in the elderly: Predictors of dementia. *Neurology*, 41: 1006–1009.

Flynn, J. R. (1987). Massive IQ gains in 14 nations: What IQ tests really measure. *Psychological Bulletin*, 101: 171–191.

Fox, N. C., Warrington, E. K., and Rossor, M. N. (1999). Serial magnetic resonance imaging of cerebral atrophy in preclinical Alzheimer's Disease. *Lancet*, 353: 2125.

Galvin, J. E., Powlishta, K. K., Wilkins, K., McKeel, D. W., Jr., Xiong, C., Grant, E., et al. (2005). Predictors of preclinical Alzheimer Disease and dementia: A clinicopathologic study. *Archives of Neurology*, 62: 758–765.

Goldman, W. P. and Morris, J. C. (2001). Evidence that age-associated memory impairment is not a normal variant of aging. *Alzheimer Disease and Associated Disorders*, 15: 72–79.

Gosche, K. M., Mortimer, J. A., Smith, C. D., Markesbery, W. R., and Snowdon, D. A. (2002). Hippocampal volume as an index of Alzheimer neuropathology: Findings from the nun study. *Neurology*, 58: 1476–1482.

Graff-Radford, N. R., Crook, J. E., Lucas, J., Boeve, B. F., Knopman, D. S., Ivnik, R. J., Smith, G. E., Younkin, L. H., Petersen, R. C., and Younkin, S. G. (2007). Association of low plasma Abeta42/Abeta40 ratios with increased imminent risk for mild cognitive impairment and Alzheimer Disease. *Archives of Neurology*, 64: 354–362.

Gustafson, D., Lissner, L., Bengtsson, C., Bjorkelund, C., and Skoog, I. (2004). A 24-year follow-up of body mass index and cerebral atrophy. *Neurology*, 63: 1876–1881.

Hedden, T. and Gabrieli, J. D. E. (2004). Insights into the ageing mind: A view from cognitive neuroscience. *Nature Reviews Neuroscience*, 5: 87–96.

Hoffman, J. M., Welsh-Bohmer, K. A., Hanson, M., Crain, B., Hulette, C., Earl, N., et al. (2000). FDG PET Imaging in patients with pathologically verified dementia. *Journal of Nuclear Medicine*, 41: 1920–1928.

Hofman, A., Ott, A., Breteler, M. M., Bots, M. L., Slooter, A. J. C., van Harskamp, F., et al. (1997). Atherosclerosis, apolipoprotein E, and prevalence of dementia and Alzheimer's Disease in the Rotterdam study. *Lancet*, 349: 151–154.

Huang, J., Friedland, R. P., and Auchus, A. P. (2007). Diffusion tensor imaging of normal-appearing white matter in mild cognitive impairment and early Alzheimer Disease: Preliminary evidence of axonal degeneration in the temporal lobe. *American Journal of Neuroradiology*, 28: 1943–1948.

Jack, C. R., Dickson, D. W., Parisi, J. E., Xu, Y. C., Cha, R. H., O'Brien, P. C., et al. (2002). Antemortem MRI findings correlate with hippocampal neuropathology in typical aging and dementia. *Neurology*, 58: 750–757.

Jack, C. R., Jr., Lowe, V. J., Senjem, M. L., Weigand, S. D., Kemp, B. J., Shiung, M. M., Knopman, D. S., et al. (2008). 11C PiB and structural MRI provide complementary information in imaging of Alzheimer's Disease and amnestic mild cognitive impairment. *Brain*, 131: 665–680.

Jack, C. R., Petersen, R. C., Xu, Y. C., O'Brien, P. C., Smith, G. E., Ivnik, R. J., et al. (1999). Prediction of AD with MRI-based hippocampal volume in mild cognitive impairment. *Neurology*, 52: 1397–1403.

Jagust, W., Gitcho, A., Sun, F., Kuczynski, B., Mungas, D., and Haan, M. (2006). Brain imaging evidence of preclinical Alzheimer's Disease in normal aging. *Annals of Neurology*, 59: 673–681.

Jagust, W., Reed, B., Mungas, D., Ellis, W., and Decarli, C. (2007). What does fluorodeoxyglucose PET imaging add to a clinical diagnosis of dementia? *Neurology*, 69: 871–877.

Jagust, W. J., Zheng, L., Harvey, D. J., Mack, W. J., Vinters, H. V., Weiner, M. W., et al. (2008). Neuropathological basis of Magnetic Resonance Images in aging and dementia. *Annals of Neurology*, 63: 72–80.

Johnson, S. C., Saykin, A. J., Baxter, L. C., Flashman, L. A., Santulli, R. B., McAllister, T. W., et al. (2000). The relationship between fMRI activation and cerebral atrophy: Comparison of normal aging and Alzheimer Disease. *Neuroimage*, 11: 179–187.

Kalus, P., Slotboom, J., Gallinat, J., Mahlberg, R., Cattapan-Ludewig, K., Wiest, R., et al. (2006). Examining the gateway to the limbic system with diffusion tensor imaging: The perforant pathway in Dementia. *Neuroimage*, 30: 713–720.

Kawas, C. H. and Corrada, M. M. (2006). Alzheimer's and dementia in the oldest-old: A century of challenges. *Current Alzheimer Research*, 3: 411–419.

Khachaturian, Z. (1985). Diagnosis of Alzheimer's Disease. *Archives of Neurology*, 42: 1097–1105.

Kimberg, D. Y., Aguirre, G. K., Lease, J., and D'Esposito, M. (2001). Cortical effects of Bromocriptine, a D-2 dopamine receptor agonist, in human subjects, revealed by fMRI. *Human Brain Mapping*, 12: 246–257.

Knopman, D. S., DeKosky, S. T., Cummings, J. L., Chui, H., Corey-Bloom, J., Relkin, N., et al. (2001). Practice parameter: Diagnosis of Dementia (an evidence-based review). Report of the quality standards subcommittee of the American Academy of Neurology. *Neurology*, 56: 1143–1153.

Kuhl, D. E., Koeppe, R. A., Minoshima, S., Snyder, S. E., Ficaro, E. P., Foster, N. L., et al. (1999). In vivo mapping of cerebral acetylcholinesterase activity in aging and Alzheimer's Disease. *Neurology*, 52: 691–699.

Lupien, S. J., de Leon, M., de Santi, S., Convit, A., Tarshish, C., Nair, N. P., et al. (1998). Cortisol levels during human aging predict hippocampal atrophy and memory deficits. *Nature Neuroscience*, 1: 69–73.

Lupien, S. J. and Wan, N. (2004). Successful ageing: From cell to self. *Philosophical Transactions of Royal Society of London*, 359: 1413–1426.

McEwen, B. S. (2002). Sex, stress and the hippocampus: Allostasis, allostatic load and the aging process. *Neurobiology of Aging*, 23: 921–939.

McKeith, I. G., Dickson, D. W., Lowe, J., Emre, M., O'Brien, J. T., Feldman, H., et al. (2005). Diagnosis and management of dementia with Lewy bodies: Third report of the DLB consortium. *Neurology*, 65: 1863–1872.

Medina, D., DeToledo-Morrell, L., Urresta, F., Gabrieli, J. D., Moseley, M., Fleischman, D., et al. (2006). White matter changes in mild cognitive impairment and AD: A diffusion tensor imaging study. *Neurobiology of Aging*, 27: 663–672.

Meltzer, C. C., Kinahan, P. E., Greer, P. J., Nichols, T. E., Comtat, C., Cantwell, M. N., et al. (1999). Comparative evaluation of MR-based partial-volume correction schemes for PET. *Journal of Nuclear Medicine*, 40: 2053–2065.

Mirra, S. S., Heyman, A., McKeel, D., Sumi, S. M., Crain, B. J., Brownlee, L. M., et al. (1991). The Consortium to Establish a Registry for Alzheimer's Disease (CERAD): Part II. Standardization of the neuropathologic assessment of Alzheimer's Disease. *Neurology*, 41: 479–486.

Moller, M., Jakobsen, S., and Gjedde, A. (2007). Parametric and regional maps of free serotonin 5HT1A receptor sites in human brain as function of age in healthy humans. *Neuropsychopharmacology*, 32: 1707–1714.

Mueller, S. G., Weiner, M. W., Thal, L. J., Petersen, R. C., Jack, C. R., Jagust, W., et al. (2005). Ways toward an early diagnosis in Alzheimer's Disease: The Alzheimer's Disease Neuroimaging Initiative (ADNI). *Alzheimer's and Dementia*, 1: 55–66.

N.I.A and Reagan Institute Working Group on Diagnostic Criteria for the Neuropathological Assessment of Alzheimer's Disease (1997). Consensus recommendations for the postmortem diagnosis of Alzheimer's Disease. *Neurobiology of Aging*, 18: S1–S2.

Neary, D., Snowden, J. S., Gustafson, L., Passant, U., Stuss, D., Black, S., et al. (1998). Frontotemporal lobar degeneration: A consensus on clinical diagnostic criteria. *Neurology*, 51: 1546–1554.

Nordahl, C. W., Ranganath, C., Yonelinas, A. P., DeCarli, C., Reed, B. R., and Jagust, W. J. (2005). Different mechanisms of episodic memory failure in mild cognitive impairment. *Neuropsychologia*, 43: 1688–1697.

Petersen, R. C., Smith, G. E., Waring, S. C., Ivnik, R. J., Tangalos, E. G., and Kokmen, E. (1999). Mild cognitive impairment: Clinical characterization and outcome. *Archives of Neurology*, 56: 303–308.

Petkov, C. I., Wu, C. C., Eberling, J. L., Mungas, D., Zrelak, P. A., Yonelinas, A. P., et al. (2004). Correlates of memory function in community-dwelling elderly: The importance of white matter hyperintensities. *Journal of the International Neuropsychological Society*, 10: 371–381.

Podruchny, T. A., Connolly, C., Bokde, A., Herscovitch, P., Eckelman, W. C., Kiesewetter, D. O., et al. (2003). In vivo muscarinic 2 receptor imaging in cognitively normal young and older volunteers. *Synapse*, 48: 39–44.

Pullicino, P. M., Miller, L. L., Alexandrov, A. V., and Ostrow, P. T. (1995). Infraputaminal 'lacunes'. Clinical and pathological correlations. *Stroke*, 26: 1598–1602.

Rasgon, N. L., Silverman, D., Siddarth, P., Miller, K., Ercoli, L. M., Elman, S., et al. (2005). Estrogen use and brain metabolic change in postmenopausal women. *Neurobiology of Aging*, 26: 229–235.

Ray, S., Britschgi, M., Herbert, C., Takeda-Uchimura, Y., Boxer, A., Blennow, K., Friedman, L. F., et al. (2007). Classification and prediction of clinical Alzheimer's diagnosis based on plasma signaling proteins. *Nature Medicine*, 13: 1359–1362.

Raz, N., Gunning, F. M., Head, D., Dupuis, J. H., McQuain, J., Briggs, S. D., et al. (1997). Selective aging of the human cerebral cortex observed in vivo: Differential vulnerability of the prefrontal gray matter. *Cerebral Cortex*, 7: 268–282.

Raz, N., Gunning-Dixon, F. M., Head, D., Dupuis, J. H., and Acker, J. D. (1998). Neuroanatomical correlates of cognitive aging: Evidence from structural magnetic resonance imaging. *Neuropsychology*, 12: 95–114.

Raz, N., Rodrigue, K. M., and Acker, J. D. (2003). Hypertension and the brain: Vulnerability of the prefrontal regions and executive functions. *Behavioral Neuroscience*, 117: 1169–1180.

Raz, N., Rodrigue, K. M., Head, D., Kennedy, K. M., and Acker, J. D. (2004). Differential aging of the medial temporal lobe: A study of a five-year change. *Neurology*, 62: 433–438.

Reiman, E. M., Chen, K., Alexander, G. E., Caselli, R. J., Bandy, D., Osborne, D., et al. (2004). Functional brain abnormalities in young adults at genetic risk for late-onset Alzheimer's dementia. *Proceedings of the National Academy of Sciences of the USA*, 101: 284–289.

Roberson, E. D. and Mucke, L. (2006). 100 Years and counting: Prospects for defeating Alzheimer's Disease. *Science*, 314: 781–784.

Roman, G. C., Tatemichi, T. K., Erkinjuntti, T., Cummings, J. L., Masdeu, J. C., Garcia, J. H., et al. (1993). Vascular dementia: Diagnostic criteria for research studies. Report of the NINDS-AIREN International Workshop. *Neurology*, 43: 250–260.

Ross, G. W., Petrovitch, H., Abbott, R. D., Nelson, J., Markesbery, W., Davis, D., et al. (2004). Parkinsonian signs and substantia nigra neuron density in decendents elders without PD. *Annals of Neurology*, 56: 532–539.

Rowe, J. W. and Kahn, R. L. (1987). Human aging: Usual and successful. *Science*, 237: 143–149.

Salthouse, T. A. and Ferrer-Caja, E. (2003). What needs to be explained to account for age-related effects on multiple cognitive variables? *Psychology of Aging*, 18: 91–110.

Schaie, K. W., Willis, S. L., and Pennak, S. (2005). An historical framework for cohort differences in intelligence. *Research in Human Development*, 2: 43–67.

Seeman, T. E., McEwen, B. S., Rowe, J. W., and Singer, B. H. (2001). Allostatic load as a marker of cumulative biological risk: MacArthur studies of successful aging. *Proceedings of the National Academy of Sciences of the USA*, 98: 4770–4775.

Silverman, D. H., Small, G. W., Chang, C. Y., Lu, C. S., Kung De Aburto, M. A., Chen, W., et al. (2001). Positron emission tomography in evaluation of dementia: Regional brain metabolism and long-term outcome. *Journal of the American Medical Association*, 286: 2120–2127.

Small, G. W., Mazziotta, J. C., Collins, M. T., Baxter, L. R., Phelps, M. E., Mandelkern, M. A., et al. (1995). Apolipoprotein E type 4 allele and cerebral glucose metabolism in relatives at risk for familial Alzheimer's Disease. *Journal of the American Medical Association*, 273: 942–947.

Sundelof, J., Giedraitis, V., Irizarry, M. C., Sundstrom, J., Ingelsson, E., Ronnemaa, E., et al. (2008). Plasma {beta} Amyloid and the risk of Alzheimer Disease and dementia in elderly men: A prospective, population-based cohort study. *Archives of Neurology*, 65: 256–263.

Volkow, N. D., Ding, Y. S., Fowler, J. S., Wang, G. J., Logan, J., Gatley, S. J., et al. (1996). Dopamine transporters decrease with age. *J Nuclear Medicine*, 37: 554–559.

Volkow, N. D., Gur, R. C., Wang, G. J., Fowler, J. S., Moberg, P. J., Ding, Y. S., et al. (1998). Association between decline in brain dopamine activity with age and cognitive and motor impairment in healthy individuals. *American Journal of Psychiatry*, 155: 344–349.

Whittle, C., Corrada, M. M., Dick, M., Ziegler, R., Kahle-Wrobleski, K., Paganini-Hill, A., et al. (2007). Neuropsychological data in nondemented oldest old: the 90+ Study. *Journal of Clinical and Experimental Neuropsychology*, 29: 290–299.

Zhang, Y., Schuff, N., Jahng, G. H., Bayne, W., Mori, S., Schad, L., et al. (2007). Diffusion tensor imaging of cingulum fibers in mild cognitive impairment and Alzheimer Disease. *Neurology*, 68: 13–19.

2

Methodological and Conceptual Issues in the Study of the Aging Brain

Mark D'Esposito, William Jagust, and Adam Gazzaley

Introduction

The emergence of functional neuroimaging technology, such as positron emission tomography (PET) and functional MRI (fMRI) and their associated analytical methods, has ushered a new stage into the study of the aging brain, allowing us to gain a unique appreciation of the complexity of brain and cognitive aging (Cabeza, 2002; Gazzaley and D'Esposito, 2003; Grady, 2000; Reuter-Lorenz, 2002). Complementing these functional neuroimaging methods, more traditional structural imaging methods with CT or MRI have evolved into newer volumetric techniques (Salat, Kaye, and Janowsky, 2001; Tisserand et al., 2002), which also provide an opportunity for investigating age-related regional cortical or subcortical changes (and links to specific cognitive deficits) (Sullivan et al., 2002; Tisserand et al., 2000; Ylikoski et al., 2000). Although the application of new imaging methods is exciting and promising, it is important to be cautious given its increasing availability. We must critically examine these methods and the potential for misinterpretation of results and overstatement of conclusions that might occur as a result of applying these methods to the aging brain. In this chapter, therefore, we will discuss methodological and conceptual issues that affect the interpretation of imaging data with specific regard to the study of brain aging.

Issues in Functional Magnetic Resonance Imaging

The Physiological Basis of the BOLD Signal

An important consideration when interpreting changes in the blood-oxygenation level-dependent (BOLD) signal is that it is not a direct reflection of neural activity, but rather reflects local changes in cerebral blood flow. Specifically, the BOLD signal is the ratio of diamagnetic oxyhemoglobin (which in relative terms, raises the BOLD signal) to paramagnetic deoxyhemoglobin, which reduces the BOLD signal (Thulborn et al., 1982; Turner et al., 1991). Neural activity leads to a change in this ratio by influencing several factors: cerebral blood flow (CBF), cerebral blood volume (CBV), and the cerebral metabolic rate of oxygen consumption ($CMRO_2$) (Buxton and Frank, 1997). Neural activity induces mediators that are still being characterized (Bonvento, Sibson, and Pellerin, 2002; Lindauer et al., 1999) to generate a local hemodynamic response that increases the CBF and CBV, resulting in an elevation in the supply of oxyhemoglobin within a local region of brain tissue. The process by which neural activity influences the hemodynamic properties of the surrounding vasculature is known as *neurovascular coupling*. Neural activity also raises local metabolic demands that, in turn, result in an increase in the $CMRO_2$ and a resultant elevation in the level of deoxyhemoglobin. Although all of these factors increase in response to neural activity, the magnitude of the CBF increase far exceeds the $CMRO_2$ increase (Fox and Raichle, 1986; Fox et al., 1988). This results in an excess of oxyhemoglobin localized to the activation site, an imbalance that is then detected as an increase in the BOLD signal. Thus, under most conditions, neural activity results in a positive BOLD signal that is primarily a reflection of increased local CBF.

When comparing changes in BOLD signal within the brain of an individual during the performance of different cognitive tasks, and making conclusions regarding changes in neural activity and the pattern of activity, numerous assumptions are made regarding the steps that comprise neurovascular coupling (stimulus → neural activity → hemodynamic response → BOLD signal), and the regional variability of the metabolic and vascular parameters influencing the BOLD signal. This in itself is an area of intensive research and debate (Mechelli, Price, and Friston, 2001; Miller et al., 2001; Rees et al., 1997). These confounding factors are further amplified when compared between individuals within a population and even more so when compared across groups of different populations. This concern is especially relevant to studies involving an aging population in which structural changes in cerebral vasculature, such as local vascular compromise, or diffuse vascular disease, can alter the vascular response to neural activity. For example, a vascular disparity in the absence of a difference in neural activity may alter the neurovascular coupling, and thus affect a component of the hemodynamic response to neural activity, such as the CBF. This will, in turn, alter the influx of oxyhemoglobin into the region, thus modifying the BOLD signal and resulting in the potential misinterpretation of a signal change as a difference in neural activity. It is clear that an evaluation of BOLD signal differences in the aging population is dependent upon an understanding of alterations in the aging neurovascular system, including vascular pathology, changes in vascular reactivity, and cerebral blood flow. Although this chapter focuses on vascular changes and its impact on the BOLD signal, it should be recognized that any change in the levels of any of the mediators of the neuro-vascular response (including neurotransmitters) during aging and disease are important considerations (see D'Esposito, Deouell, and Gazzaley, 2003 for further discussion of this issue).

The Aging Neurovascular System and its Influence on the BOLD Signal

Extensive research on the aging neurovascular system has revealed that it undergoes significant changes in multiple domains in a continuum throughout the human lifespan, probably as early as the fourth decade (for review see Farkas and Luiten, 2001). These changes affect the vascular ultrastructure, the resting CBF, and the vascular reactivity of the vessels in older brains.

Ultrastructure

The compromise to the ultrastructural integrity of the cerebral vasculature in aging is largely the result of arteriosclerotic changes, principally fibrohyaline thickening of the vessel wall (Furuta et al., 1991), smooth muscle cell necrosis (Masawa et al., 1994), and thickening of the basement membrane (Nagasawa et al., 1979) that gradually increases with age. Although sclerotic changes correlate with the degree of hypertension (Furuta et al., 1991), age itself appears to be an independent risk factor (Knox et al., 1980; Masawa et al., 1994). It is a general consensus that these changes result in a decrease in the elasticity and compliancy of affected vessels, which include the capillaries, the larger arterioles, and cerebral arteries (for a review see Kalaria, 1996). Venous alterations that accompany aging, known as periventricular venous collagenosis (PVC), have also been observed in 65% of subjects over 60 years old, and in severe cases can completely occlude veins (Moody et al., 1997). In addition to ultrastructural changes of the vessels, there is also an increase in the tortuosity of some vessels with aging (see Figure 2.1)—most notably in the arteriole-venous-capillary bed (Fang, 1976)—as well as changes in the density of capillaries and arterioles (Abernethy et al., 1993) that have not been observed

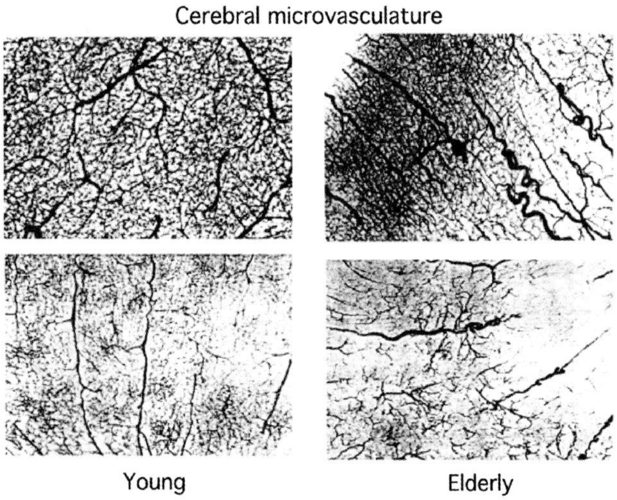

Cerebral microvasculature

Young   Elderly

Figure 2–1 Ultrastructural changes observed in the cerebral microvasculature of elderly individuals as compared to younger individuals (Fang, 1976). Note abnormal "coiling and looping" (upper-right panel) and "twists and turns" or "windings" (lower-right panel) in arteries and venules from elderly individuals.

in venules (Sonntag et al., 1997). Finally, both age and specific disease processes such as Alzheimer's disease may result in vascular deposition of amyloid that may affect cerebrovascular structure and function (Benarroch, 2007).

The presence of diverse pathological changes that differentially affect the various components of the vascular system of the brain may influence the interpretation of age-related BOLD signal changes when comparing results between age groups, as well between studies using different strength magnets and different pulse sequences. Stronger magnets—such as 4 Tesla systems—are more sensitive to influences from capillaries (Menon et al., 1995) compared to weaker magnets that are influenced more by the magnetic properties of blood within venules and draining veins (Gati et al., 1997). In addition, gradient-echo echo-planar imaging (EPI) generates a significant portion of its signal from large veins with contributions from capillaries (Song, Fichtenholtz, and Woldorff, 2002), whereas spin-echo EPI exhibits a higher degree of spatial resolution and a greater contribution from smaller vessels (Norris et al., 2002).

Resting Cerebral Blood Flow (CBF)

Vascular pathology may also have a large impact on BOLD signal interpretations secondary to its influence on baseline CBF and vascular reactivity (Kawamura et al., 1993; Kuwabara et al., 1996). The primary techniques that have been used to determine the presence of changes in the resting CBF in the microvasculature of the cortex are PET, SPECT, and gas-inhalation contrast CT. However, more recently an MRI technique called arterial spin labeling (ASL) has been developed that allows the determination of CBF with high anatomic resolution (Detre and Alsop, 1999; Wolf and Detre, 2007). Multiple studies using PET, SPECT, CT, and MRI have compared resting CBF between old and young groups, as well as CBF changes with age as a continuum, and have observed that aging is associated with a significant decrease in resting CBF in cortical and subcortical parenchyma (Ances et al., 2008; Bentourkia et al., 2000; Biagi et al., 2007; Kawamura et al., 1993; Reich and Rusinek, 1989; Restom et al., 2007; Schultz et al., 1999). Similar findings have also been reported for blood flow in large cerebral arteries, such as decreases in blood flow velocity in the middle, posterior, and anterior cerebral arteries with advancing age (Krejza et al., 1999).

Measurement of the resting CBF is an important but usually unaddressed issue when interpreting BOLD signal changes. The BOLD signal is not an absolute value, but rather a value that represents a relative ratio of oxy- vs. deoxyhemoglobin concentration. An assumption that the baseline CBF is the same between two populations, when in actuality it is not, may lead to incorrect conclusions when forming direct comparisons between those populations. An additional note of caution is that the baseline CBF may not only be influenced by age, but also by different physiological states. For instance, fluctuating carbon dioxide (CO_2) levels, such as those influenced by the rate of breathing, have been shown to affect the BOLD signal baseline and alter the magnitude of the BOLD response to visual stimulation (Cohen, Ugurbil, and Kim, 2002).

Vascular Reactivity

In addition to a decline in resting CBF in aging, there also seems to be an age-associated decrease in the vascular reactivity of cerebral vessels to various chemical modulators, including the concentration of CO_2. This is particularly relevant to our discussion of the BOLD signal, since a local change in CO_2 associated with increased metabolism is believed to be one of the chemical mediators responsible for neurovascular coupling. Two techniques frequently used to assess vascular reactivity is the induction of hypercapnia by breath-holding or inhalation of high CO_2 gas, which results in increased CBF; and the induction of hypocapnia with hyperventilation, which results in decreased CBF. Decreased vascular responsiveness to hypercapnia has been observed in aged rats (Tamaki et al., 1995) and humans with and without risk factors for atherosclerosis (Yamamoto et al., 1980). In another study of elderly subjects, regional CBF (rCBF) changes monitored with PET revealed a significant deficit in the total vascular response from a hypocapnic to a hypercapnic state in comparison to young adults (Ito et al., 2002). Of significant importance in the interpretation of regional BOLD changes is an assessment of age-related changes in vascular reactivity across different brain regions. A study comparing the resting and stimulus-evoked rCBF in rats revealed that basal forebrain stimulation elicited ipsilateral increases in CBF in both the parietal and frontal cortex of young rats, but only the frontal cortex of the aged rats. (Linville and Arneric, 1991). Regional variability in vascular factors is clearly an important issue for functional imaging studies of cognitive aging since many hypotheses are likely to include comparisons between different neural systems.

Photic stimulation is a robust cortical stimulator, and when coupled with transcranial Doppler sonography of cerebral blood flow velocities, it has been used to detect alterations in neurovascular coupling in a number of different conditions (Diehl et al., 1998; Urban et al., 1995). Using this technique, Niehaus et al. (2001) reported an age-related reduction in blood-flow velocity in the posterior cerebral artery in response to photic stimulation. This change, however, cannot be attributed with certainty to an alteration of neurovascular coupling because a change in neural activity was not ruled out.

The exact mechanisms of age-related changes in resting CBF and vascular reactivity have not been completely elucidated, although it is often suggested that it is secondary to the increased stiffness and lack of compliance of the aging vasculature. Several studies on rats have concluded that the decline in vasoreactivity may be the result of impaired vasodilatory mechanisms, as determined by a significantly reduced degree of vasodilation in older rats in response to cerebrospinal fluid perfusion of vasodilators adenosine (Jiang et al., 1992), acetylcholine, and bradykinin (Mayhan et al., 1990). Regardless of the mechanism of these changes, it is clear that their presence should invoke a high degree of caution in researchers who attempt to directly compare the magnitude of BOLD signal changes between two age groups.

Cerebral Metabolic Rate of Oxygen Consumption (CMRO$_2$)

The importance of identifying age-related changes in cerebral oxygen metabolism and studying its influence on the BOLD signal should not be underestimated. The BOLD signal is not solely dependent on the level of oxyhemoglobin as regulated by CBF, but also the level of deoxyhemoglobin, which is largely influenced by $CMRO_2$. As mentioned previously, although the hemodynamic effects on the BOLD signal appear to be dominant, increasing neural activity results in increased $CMRO_2$, leading to increased levels of deoxyhemoglobin and a significant decrease in the BOLD signal (Schwarzbauer and Heinke, 1999).

An effect of aging on $CMRO_2$ has been appreciated for some time now. Two PET studies have revealed a significantly lower resting $CMRO_2$ in cortical and subcortical regions of older subjects compared with younger subjects, which actually exceeded age-related changes in CBF (Takada et al., 1992; Yamaguchi et al., 1986). A recent study that measured BOLD, CBF, and $CMRO_2$ in younger and older subjects revealed that, during a visual activation task, the magnitude of the BOLD response was significantly lower for the older group compared to the younger group despite similar fractional changes in the CBF and $CMRO_2$ responses. The weaker BOLD response for the older group was thought to be due to a reduction in baseline CBF in older subjects (Ances et al., 2008).

The Influence of Age-associated Co-morbidities on the BOLD Signal

Aging is frequently associated with co-morbidities such as diabetes, hypertension, and hyperlipidemia, all of which may affect the BOLD signal by affecting CBF and neurovascular coupling (Claus et al., 1998). The importance of screening older patients for these commonly associated conditions has unfortunately been underemphasized in functional neuroimaging studies of cognitive aging. In addition to the independent influences of these conditions on vascular physiology, they are also risk factors for cerebrovascular disease and arteriosclerosis (Shantaram, 1999). Cerebrovascular disease is a prevalent finding in older populations and, aside from clinically significant stroke, it can also result in clinically silent small vessel disease, large vessel disease, and lacunar infarcts, all of which have been shown to alter CBF, neurovascular coupling or the BOLD signal. Although any of these pathologies may be present without the subjects or researcher's knowledge, they are not routinely screened for prior to fMRI studies on older populations.

Leukoariosis

White matter lucencies on CT (leukoariosis), or hyperintensities on MRI scans, are common findings in older patients, often found without other evidence of vascular disease but also often associated with large-vessel atherosclerosis (Bots et al., 1993) and hypertension (Dufouil et al., 2001). Most, but not all, areas of lucency are believed to be associated with small vessel disease, and microscopic evaluation of these regions reveals arteriolar hyalinization and arteriosclerotic changes (Fazekas et al., 1993; George et al., 1986), and pathological correlation with vascular disease (Jagust et al., 2008). The severity of leukoariosis has been shown to directly correlate with a reduction in CBF (Hatazawa et al., 1997), cerebral perfusion within the white matter areas (Kawamura et al., 1993; Kobari, Meyer, and Ichijo, 1990; Marstrand et al., 2002), and a decreased cerebrovascular response to hypercapnia (Kuwabara et al., 1996) and acetazolamide (Marstrand et al., 2002). In a recent study, the effect of white matter hyperintensities (WMH) on BOLD activation was studied in cognitively normal healthy individuals performing a working memory task (Nordahl et al., 2006). Results showed that increases in global as well as regional prefrontal cortical WMH volume (as measured by structural MRI) were associated with decreases in BOLD fMRI PFC activity. This study highlights the importance of using imaging in aging studies to differentiate the potential pathological influence of WMH from true age-related changes.

Strokes

In addition to clinically silent small-vessel disease, older subjects may also have had small strokes that were never clinically recognized. There has been limited research to investigate whether structural lesions secondary to stroke might influence the BOLD signal in a manner unrelated to changes in neural activity. Despite this lack of research, there have been multiple fMRI studies that have made statements regarding functional reorganization in stroke populations (Cao et al., 1999; Feydy et al., 2002; Small et al., 2002; Thirumala, Hier, and Patel, 2002; Thulborn, Carpenter, and Just, 1999). Ignoring these issues can lead to gross misinterpretations, as there is probably no other study population in which the potential confounding effects of changes in neurovascular coupling on interpretations of BOLD signal changes is more apparent than in the stroke population.

An fMRI study by Pineiro et al. (2002) addressed the issue of the influence of vascular factors on the BOLD signal in a symptomatic stroke population. They analyzed the time course of the BOLD hemodynamic response function (HRF) in the sensorimotor cortex of patients with an isolated subcortical lacunar stroke, compared to a group of age-matched controls. They found a decrease in the rate of rise and the maximal BOLD HRF to a finger- or hand-tapping task in both the sensorimotor cortex of the hemisphere affected by the stroke and the unaffected hemisphere (see Figure 2.2a). The authors suggested that given the widespread changes of these BOLD signal differences, the change was unlikely a direct consequence of the subcortical lacunar stroke, but rather a manifestation of pre-existing diffuse vascular pathology. Furthermore, the assumption was made that the BOLD change was secondary to an alteration in the CBF, since the other contributing factors to the HRF, the CBV, and $CMRO_2$ were unlikely to be different between the two groups.

Given that changes in vascular parameters will alter the BOLD signal, we believe it is necessary to carefully screen structural MRIs in all older subjects for leukoariosis (or lacunar infarcts) that may

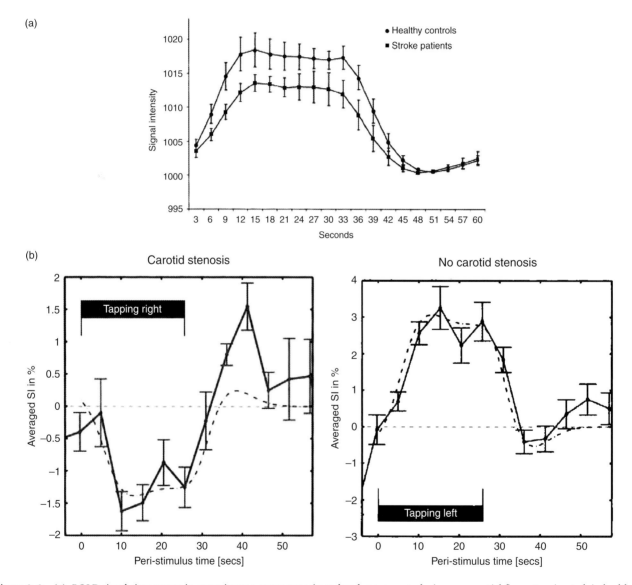

Figure 2–2   (**a**). BOLD signal-time course in sensorimotor cortex opposite to hand movements during a sequential finger-tapping task in healthy controls (•) and stroke patients (■). This data demonstrates a decreased BOLD response in stroke patients. (Adapted from Pineiro et al., 2002.) (**b**). BOLD signal-time course during a tapping task in a single patient from motor cortex on the same side as carotid stenosis (left panel) and no carotid stenosis (right panel). The fit (dotted line) and the averaged BOLD response (solid line) is shown. Activation on the side of carotid stenosis revealed an abnormal negative BOLD response lasting for the whole period of finger tapping, whereas the BOLD response on the side without carotid stenosis was normal. (Adapted from Rother et al., 2002.)

be clinically silent. Unfortunately, most fMRI protocols do not collect images with appropriate pulse sequences for detecting white matter lesions (i.e., T2 weighted). It is also critical to obtain a comprehensive medical and neurological history when looking for the history of possible transient ischemic attacks or stroke. Again, most subjects in cognitive-aging fMRI studies are not screened by neurologists, who have the expertise to determine if the subject has had a vascular event in their past—which may not necessarily be detected by routine screening questionnaires.

Extracranial Disease

In addition to screening for the presence of small vessel disease and lacunar strokes, future fMRI studies of aging should also consider the use of Doppler ultrasound and magnetic resonance angiography in evaluating the extracranial vasculature for the presence of significant occlusion. A recent fMRI study concluded that severe extracranial carotid stenosis in a patient without MRI evidence of an infarct, led to neurovascular uncoupling that presented as a negative BOLD signal response during a motor task (Rother et al., 2002) (see Figure 2.2b). Furthermore, this negative BOLD response occurred in only the affected hemisphere, and correlated with a severely impaired hemodynamic response to hypercapnia isolated to that hemisphere. Given that abnormal neural activity in a patient with normal motor performance was unlikely, the finding was interpreted as a local activity-driven increase in deoxyhemoglobin, secondary to oxygen consumption, in the absence of an accompanying increase in CBF. Although this is a rather extreme example of the effect of impaired autoregulation on the BOLD response, it serves as an important illustration that extracranial vascular disease can impair this process and alter the BOLD response.

Medications

Aside from the presence and influence of pathological processes, most patients are prescribed medications for the prevention or treatment of these conditions. Few studies strictly screen subjects for the use of all medications, including estrogen replacement therapy and common nonprescription drugs such as nonsteroidal anti-inflammatory drugs (e.g., aspirin) that inhibit the cycloxygenase pathway of arachidonic acid and may alter neurovascular coupling and thus the BOLD signal independent of the pathological influence. There are very few studies that have investigated the effect of medications on CBF (e.g., Bednar and Gross, 1999; Bell et al., 2005; Miller et al., 1997; Nobler, Olvet, and Sackeim, 2002) or the BOLD signal (Neele et al., 2001; Pariente et al., 2001). As groups of older patients with diseases are studied, this sort of control data will be increasingly important. The necessity of increasing our understanding of the effects of medications such as aspirin and hypertensive and hyperlipidemic medications on the BOLD signal will continue to escalate. We also need to be cognizant of, and control for, the potential effects of frequently used substances such as caffeine and nicotine on the BOLD signal, which may have independent vascular effects and/or effects on neural activity (e.g., Bednar and Gross, 1999; Bell et al., 2005; Dager and Friedman, 2000; Jacobsen et al., 2002; Laurienti et al., 2002; Miller et al., 1997; Mulderink et al., 2002; Nobler, Olvet, and Sackeim, 2002; Stein et al., 1998).

Hemodynamic Response Characteristics Determined by BOLD fMRI

Several researchers have recognized the potential for confounding results using BOLD fMRI to study cognitive aging, and have designed fMRI experiments to study this issue. One method has been to study the spatial and temporal characteristics of the BOLD HRF during a stimulation that is expected to result in equivalent neural activity in young and old subjects, such as a simple motor task (Aizenstein et al., 2004; Buckner et al., 2000; D'Esposito et al., 1999; Hesselmann et al., 2001; Mattay et al., 2002; Taoka et al., 1998; Tekes et al., 2005) or a simple visual stimulation task (Ances et al., 2008; Buckner et al., 2000; Handwerker et al., 2007; Huettel, Singerman, and McCarthy, 2001; Ross et al., 1997). A summary of the findings of these studies is presented in Table 2.1. If there are changes in the HRF in response to a task that is assumed to induce no age-related change in neural activity, then an alteration in another contributor to the HRF can be attributed, such as a change in CBF or neurovascular coupling. The limitation of these fMRI studies is that the absence of an age-related change in neural activity is an assumption that is not directly recorded, and it is possible that motor and sensory processes are affected by aging (Lindenberger and Baltes, 1994).

Our laboratory compared the HRF characteristics in the sensorimotor cortex of young and older subjects in response to a simple motor reaction-time task (D'Esposito et al., 1999). The provisional assumption was made that there was identical neural activity between the two populations based on physiological findings of equivalent movement-related electrical potentials in subjects under similar conditions (Cunnington et al., 1997). Thus, we presumed that any changes that we observed in BOLD fMRI signal between young and older individuals in motor cortex would be due to vascular (and not neural) activity changes in normal aging. Several important similarities and differences were observed between age groups. Although there was no significant difference in the shape of the hemodynamic response curve or peak amplitude of the signal, we found a significantly decreased signal-to-noise ratio in the BOLD signal in older individuals as compared to young individuals. This was attributed to a greater level of noise in the older individuals. We also observed a decrease in the spatial extent of the BOLD signal in older individuals compared to younger individuals in sensorimotor cortex (i.e., the median number of suprathreshold voxels). Aizenstein et al. (Aizenstein et al., 2004) proposed an additional explanation for BOLD signal decreases found in normal aging. They noted that more negative BOLD responses in older individuals can decrease the mean magnitude of the positive BOLD responses. These findings suggest that there is some property of the coupling between neural activity and BOLD signal that changes with age.

Several other studies have also investigated the HRF characteristics in response to simple motor tasks and have reached similar conclusions (Buckner et al., 2000; Hesselmann et al., 2001; Taoka et al., 1998; Tekes et al., 2005), while one study revealed disparate findings (Mattay et al., 2002). Taoka et al. found an age-associated time lag in the BOLD signal in reaching half maximum in the precentral gyrus between the start and end of a 10 s hand-grasping task. They proposed that this lag may be attributable to arteriolar changes such as vascular stiffening. Hesselman et al. (2001) observed a decrease in both the signal amplitude and the number of activated voxels with age during a finger-tapping task, and suggested the possibility of a deterioration of neurovascular coupling or an impairment of vascular supply.

Other studies have analyzed the HRF characteristics in the visual cortex in response to simple visual stimuli. A study by Buckner et al. (2000) revealed the presence of an age-associated, regional difference in the BOLD signal between the motor and visual cortex. Hemodynamic response characteristics were examined in young and older adults as they viewed a large-field

Table 2–1 Functional MRI studies of the BOLD hemodynamic response in aging.

Study	Age	Stimulus/ Task	Cortical Area Examined	Spatial Extent	Peak Amplitude	Form of HRF	Other Findings
Ross et al. (1997)	Y: 24 (20–36) O: 71 (57–84)	Flashlight	Visual	↔	↓	NA	
Taoka et al. (1998)	All: (20–76)	Hand Grasp	Motor	NA	NA	↑ Rise Time ↔ Return to Baseline	
D'Esposito, Zarahn, Aguirre, and Rypma (1999)	Y: 22.9 (18–32) O: 71.3 (61–82)	Button Press	Sensorimotor	↓	↔	↔	↑ noise
Buckner, Snyder, Sanders, Raichle, and Morris (2000)	y: 21.1 (18–24) o: 74.9 (66–89)	Button Press / Checkerboard	Sensorimotor / Visual	↓ / ↓	↔ / ↓	NA	↔ summation
Huettel, Singerman, and McCarthy (2001)	Y: 23 (18–32) O: 66 (57–76)	Checkerboard	Visual	↓	↔	↔ Rise Time Peaked Earlier	↔ Refractoriness ↑ Noise
(esselmann et al. (2001)	All: (20-83)	Finger-Thumb Opposition	Sensorimotor	↓	↓	NA	
Mattay et al. (2002)	Y: 30 (24–34) O: 59 (50-74)	Button Press	Sensorimotor	↑	↑	NA	↑ Extent and Amplitude in Multiple Regions
Aizenstein et al. (2004)	Y: 24.2 O: 67.2	Button Press	Visual, Motor	NA	↔	More Sustained Response	↑ Negative Voxels
Tekes et al. (2005)	Y: 29 (26–33) O: 75 (69-85)	Visuomotor	Visual, Motor	NA	↓	NA	
Handwerker et al. (2007)	Y: 24 (18–36) O: 64 (51-78)	Button Press:saccade / Checkerboard	Sensorimotor / Visual	↓ / ↓	↔ / ↓	Delayed time to peak in M1 and V1	

- All results are changes observed in the older age group relative to the younger group.
- ↔ = no change; NA = not analyzed

flickering checkerboard. They were also instructed to press a key upon stimulus presentation so that motor cortex responses could be examined simultaneously. They recorded a decrease in BOLD signal amplitude in the visual cortex in concordance with the findings of Ross et al. (1997) on a flashlight stimulation task, and no change in the BOLD signal amplitude in the motor cortex—a finding consistent with our own results from the motor cortex (D'Esposito et al., 1999). The authors proposed that these findings might represent a regional difference in the deterioration of neurovascular coupling with age, but they also concede that the findings in the visual cortex might very well be a correlate of regionally reduced neural activity. Another study addressing the characteristics of a visually evoked HRF to checkerboard stimuli found a decrease in spatial extent, similar amplitudes, and increased noise levels in the older visual cortex (Huettel et al., 2001). These findings were consistent with our observations in the motor cortex (D'Esposito et al., 1999) and questions the presence of regional variability.

There are other aspects of the BOLD signal that have been studied in young adults, such as refractoriness and summation, which have also been analyzed in the aging brain. Refractoriness refers to the finding of an attenuated HRF amplitude evoked by a second stimulus that is spaced closely (1–2 sec) to the first stimulus. The degree of attenuation of the amplitude correlates with the length of the interval between the paired stimuli (Huettel and McCarthy, 2000). Summation is the property by which a paired group of stimuli will summate in a roughly linear fashion when presented at intervals of 5–6 sec or greater (Miezin et al., 2000). It was determined that there was no age-related effect on the refractoriness (Huettel, Singerman, and McCarthy, 2001) or the ability of the HRF to summate (Buckner et al., 2000). These are encouraging findings for continued use of event-related fMRI designs in the study of aging. If even in the setting of decreased signal or increase noise, the relationship of the coupling is similar between young and old adults, it bodes well for our ability to study within-group interactions, as we will discuss below.

Implications for BOLD fMRI Design, Analysis and Interpretation

The presence of alterations in vascular ultrastructure, resting CBF, vascular responsiveness, and BOLD HRF characteristics associated with aging leads to limitations in conclusions about the link between neural activity and behavior derived from directly comparing the BOLD response between populations of young and old adults. Such comparisons assume that the absolute levels of hemodynamic response and the baseline CBF are the same between the two study groups and, as we have discussed, there is considerable evidence to question this assumption. The design, analysis, and interpretation of BOLD experiments aimed at the study of age- related changes in neural activity must consider these relationships.

The vascular pathology described in this chapter is a very common feature in the aging brain, and it is possible that age-related cognitive changes might exist on the basis of such vascular changes. We are therefore not recommending the exclusion of all subjects with significant vascular changes from aging investigations. Rather, we stress the necessity in identifying vascular changes in all older subjects (i.e., T2 sequences and breath-holding trials) and consider this data when interpreting fMRI data and behavioral changes.

Logan et al. (2002) formed direct comparisons between BOLD signal levels from young and old study groups in a memory paradigm. They state that by "using younger adults' mean regional activity levels as a baseline, under-recruitment was defined as less activity in older adults compared to younger adults." They proceeded to determine that there was a main effect of age in decreasing the BOLD signal amplitude in certain frontal regions. Such an effect is often interpreted as under-recruitment of neural systems. As already mentioned, decreased age-related BOLD signal could be due to an age-related decrease in neurovascular reactivity, or a decrease in the baseline CBF, and not a decrease in neural activity. However, Logan et al. also identified new areas of significant BOLD activity in older subjects that were not present in young adults, as well as regions that did not seem to change from the young adult baseline. Thus, the overall finding of a network of brain regions—where some brain regions exhibit decreased age-related activity, some increased age-related activity, and some exhibited no change between old and young groups—is unlikely to be accounted for by a global change in neurovascular coupling in the aging brain. Also, the finding of the recruitment of brain regions in older individuals that are not recruited in younger individuals during a particular cognitive task cannot likely be accounted for by age-related changes in neurovascular coupling.

In studies where only under-recruitment is observed (Jonides et al., 2000) the possible interpretation that the change is due to vascular causes, and not neural changes is unavoidable. However, there are several approaches that may address this potential confound. For example, we have proposed that greater levels of noise per voxel in sensorimotor cortex in the aging brain will lead to erroneous inferences when comparing younger and older adults based on statistical maps that rely on scaling of signal components by noise. However, if the magnitude of voxel-wise, task-related signals is not different between age groups, then one approach may be to analyze the signal component of fMRI data separately from the noise component. For example, in Rypma and D'Esposito (2000), we investigated age-related differences in prefrontal neural activity with random-effects tests of age-differences in the mean parameter estimates (i.e., the beta values derived from the least-squares solution of a linear model of the dependent data) that characterized the fMRI signal during each task component. These parameter estimates were *not* scaled by the model error term (which would typically be used to obtain t-statistics for each voxel). This method avoided the use of the noise component of an fMRI signal.

Another possible approach to account for the differences in the global hemodynamics between young and old individuals may be to establish a baseline within each subject or within each group. For example, each subject could perform a simple sensorimotor or visual task, as described in previous studies characterizing the HRF, to assess the signal and noise characteristics of each individual or group. Some authors (e.g., Jonides et al., 2000) have suggested that normalizing the global signal to a common scale may reduce the possibility of confounds due to vascular factors.

Another approach is to develop a normalization method that adjusts the data for any non-neural variation regardless of its source. Hypercapnia, which is an increase in blood PCO_2, can be achieved with a breath-holding task that can be used to normalize the BOLD signal for vascular differences (Bandettini and Wong, 1997; Cohen et al., 2004; Handwerker et al., 2007; Riecker et al., 2003). During hypercapnia, CBF increases diffusely, resulting in an increase in the ratio of oxygenated hemoglobin to deoxygenated hemoglobin, and thus causing a robust, global increase in the BOLD signal (Handwerker et al., 2007; Kwong et al., 1995;

Li et al., 1999). Unlike increases in BOLD signal due to neural activity, which are relatively localized around the site of neural activity, the increases in BOLD signal magnitude are global. Since neural activity and hypercapnia both increase BOLD through a CBF increase, the BOLD signal changes from each should be similarly affected by variations in vascular mechanics. In an implementation of this procedure (Handwerker et al., 2007), it was shown that decreases in the magnitude of activation in V1 in older subjects were still present after signal variability during a hypercapnia task. Thus, assuming the hypercapnia task accounted for all vascular variability, then the observed BOLD signal decrease in V1 in older subjects likely had neural origins.

Instead of testing for the main effects of age for a particular behavioral condition, an excellent approach is to test for age by behavioral condition interactions, as was done in an fMRI study comparing the BOLD signal in young and old adults on a memory task (Mitchell et al., 2000). The authors did not attempt to identify overall differences in levels of neural activation between young and older adults (i.e., main effect of age), but rather differences in the relative performance of young and older adults on working memory trials that required combining different types of information together (i.e., object and spatial features) vs. working memory trials that required remembering only a single feature (i.e., an age by condition interaction – Figure 2.3a). Thus, this analysis was designed to identify areas that were differentially active between young and older adults in the combination condition relative to the single feature condition. The results revealed that the BOLD signal associated with the combination condition relative to the single feature condition was increased only in the young group and not in the old group. Because the study design employed an internal control, these results are more likely to be due to an age-related change in neural activity during binding than the result of a hemodynamic change.

The use of event-related fMRI designs, where the BOLD signal corresponding to particular stages of processing within a trial can be detected, also allows for the additional option to test for age by condition interactions. For example, Rypma and D'Esposito (2000) found decreased activation in older adults only during the retrieval stage of a delayed response task and not during the encoding or maintenance stages. Again, finding age-related changes in one processing stage during a cognitive task and not another cannot be accounted for by vascular changes between age groups.

Finally, another potential powerful design option that helps alleviate the possible confounds of experiments designed only to investigate the main effects of age, is to investigate age-related changes within a behavioral condition that is varied parametrically (e.g., monotonic increases in memory load – Figure 2.3b). Correlating changes in BOLD signal with changes in behavioral measures will also help to increase the chances that observed age-related differences are true correlates of changes in neural activity. For example, Rypma and D'Esposito (2000) found that better behavioral performance was associated with less prefrontal cortex activation in young individuals and increased prefrontal cortex activation in older individuals. Additionally, Stebbins et al. (2002) reported changes in the extent of the BOLD signal in the frontal cortex that was significantly associated with performance on behavioral tests of declarative and working memory. It is less likely that a BOLD signal change that was solely reflecting an alteration in CBF or neurovascular coupling, and not a change in neural activity, would correlate with a change of behavioral performance.

Analytical methods, such as the newly applied multivariate methods, may also help to circumvent some of these issues and allow us to investigate age-related changes in regional interactions. These methods are used to characterize network patterns of BOLD signal correlations between brain regions within the context of defined anatomical circuits (Cabeza et al., 1997; McIntosh, 1999; Rissman, Gazzaley, and D'Esposito, 2004; Sun, Miller, and D'Esposito, 2004). The determination of the *functional* or *effective connectivity* within a given subject could then be extended to the population where comparisons should show a reduced contribution of vascular changes.

By studying age by behavioral condition interactions, all of the analysis options we have discussed will reduce the possibility that non-neural changes (such as a global decrease in CBF or vascular responsiveness) account for BOLD signal changes between age groups. However, the success of all of these options in accurately describing changes in neural activity rely upon assumptions of limited regional variability in vascular change and preserved linearity of neurovascular coupling with aging. It is encouraging that the processes of summation and refractoriness of the HRF seem to be age-independent, and that similar HRF characteristics have been observed in both the motor and visual cortex, although this was not a consistent finding. Clearly, more studies need to be performed specifically addressing linearity and regional variability of vascular changes during aging.

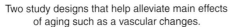

Two study designs that help alleviate main effects of aging such as a vascular changes.

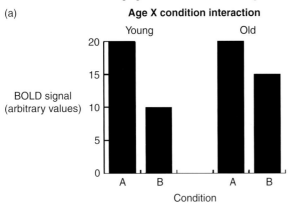

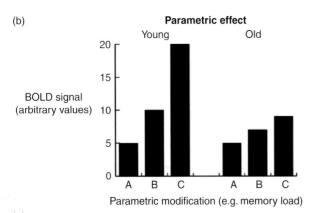

Figure 2–3 Two experimental designs that improve the inferences drawn from BOLD fMRI cognitive aging studies that age-related changes are due to neural and not vascular effects.

Issues in Molecular Brain Imaging

While the preceding sections amply demonstrate how cerebrovascular physiology and structure can have profound effects on the BOLD signal in fMRI experiments, changes in gross neuroanatomy are also an important component of brain aging. Some of these structural alterations—such as stroke and leukoariaosis—have effects on cerebrovascular function that have already been discussed in relation to effects on the BOLD signal. However, a major age-associated change, brain atrophy, can also have substantial effect on the measurement of brain function and chemistry with PET or SPECT that may, if not carefully managed, produce spurious results. Brain atrophy may exert its effects in several different ways, but in essence, these problems derive either from interactions between instrument resolution and atrophy (the partial volume effect) or from effects on spatial normalization of images during analysis.

Brain Atrophy and the "Partial Volume Effect"

All modern three-dimensional (3D) brain-imaging techniques take advantage of similar principles in defining the distribution of a signal of some sort within a volume. With fMRI, this usually represents the change in BOLD signal occurring within a brain region or a group of voxels. For nuclear medicine techniques like PET, the signal represents radioactive emissions from decaying radionuclides attached to tracers that are distributed in the brain and similarly mapped to a region or group of voxels. In both cases, the actual composition of the tissue will have an effect on the ability of the imaging technique to detect the true amount of signal produced.

This situation is perhaps easiest to understand for PET when one considers a tracer that is taken up by the cerebral cortex but not CSF or white matter. If a group of voxels (or region of interest, ROI) in subject A contains 100% cortex, but a similar ROI in subject B contains 50% cortex and 50% CSF, subject B will appear to have reduced tracer uptake when, in reality, the subject may have identical uptake of the tracer but simply less cortex. This problem is complex, as it occurs in three dimensions and also involves contamination of the ROI by any tracer that is taken up by voxels outside the ROI (a "spillover" effect)—for example, if the tracer is taken up by white matter. PET measurements of physiological and biochemical processes have been known to suffer from this partial volume effect for many years, and while improved instrument resolution has mitigated it, it remains an important consideration in studies of aging and diseases of aging in which atrophy predominates.

The partial volume problem may not appear to be as significant in fMRI studies since the BOLD technique makes use of a within-subject comparison design using a baseline and stimulated condition, or two different cognitive tasks. In the course of this comparison, the degree of atrophy will not change from the first to the second scan (although subject movement can introduce a major limitation in this assumption). Just as atrophy affects the PET signal, however, it can affect the BOLD signal, since this signal is also primarily generated in the cortex and different amounts of cortex in different subjects may produce differences in BOLD response. Thus, differences in BOLD signal between young and old subjects could simply reflect the different amounts of cortex available for activation. The partial volume effect could be related to a number of issues discussed previously, including changes in resting CBF (which would appear diminished as a result of partial

volume effects) and changes in the hemodynamic response function (which might show alterations in magnitude, shape, or extent).

These effects have been carefully analyzed by a number of investigators, and some methodological approaches are available to deal with them. With regard to PET scanning, for example, it did not take very long once voxel-based techniques for mapping the 3D distribution of brain atrophy appeared for investigators to realize that the image of regional cortical atrophy on an MRI looked very much like the image of regional cortical hypometabolism on PET in a number of age-related degenerative diseases (see Figure 2.4). Many studies have shown patterns of atrophy that, to various degrees, replicate patterns of cerebral hypometabolism in these disorders (Barch et al., 1999; Chetelat et al., 2008; Karas et al., 2003). However, when one examines the relationships closely, it is clear that reductions of glucose metabolism are not entirely explained by brain atrophy. Methods for "correction" of PET images generally make use of contemporary MRI measures of brain atrophy that are smoothed to the resolution of the PET scanner, permitting investigators to calculate the true concentration of tracer by calculating the correct amount of relevant brain tissue in the ROI. These techniques may take into consideration either effects from CSF, or effects from CSF and white matter (Meltzer et al., 1990, 1999; Quarantelli et al., 2004; Videen et al., 1988), although the latter approach is highly sensitive to errors of misregistration of MRI and PET datasets and segmentation of the MRI. When using this approach, age-related reductions in a variety of physiological or biochemical processes may reduce or even vanish, although changes related to degenerative disease are usually not as strongly affected (Chawluk et al., 1987; Ibáñez et al., 1998; Meltzer et al., 1996, 2000; Rosa-Neto et al., 2007; Yanase et al., 2005). In fact, the correction of images for partial volume effects may reveal increases in tracer binding in disease conditions that might otherwise be missed (Truchot et al., 2007)—a particular concern in evaluating tracers that would be expected to increase in atrophy-related disorders, as is the case with amyloid imaging agents in Alzheimer's disease (see Figure 2.5).

With regard to fMRI scanning, corrections and management of the partial volume approaches have not been as well-studied, although atrophy may underlie changes in the HRF. In one study of normal aging and AD patients employing a semantic decision task, Johnson et al. (2000) found that while there was no relationship between atrophy and activation in the controls, greater activation

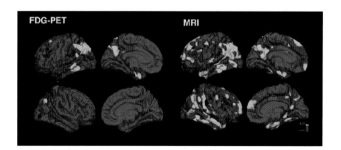

Figure 2–4 This shows a contrast between a group of patients with Alzheimer's disease and normal controls using FDG-PET measures of glucose metabolism (left) and MRI measures of cortical thickness (right). There is extensive overlap between regional atrophy and hypometabolism, particularly in parietal and temporal cortex and precuneus/posterior cingulate cortex suggesting that some of the metabolic effects might be due to atrophy.

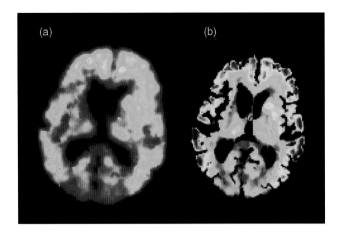

Figure 2–5 These are PET images taken using the amyloid ligand [11C] PIB. Image (**a**) shows raw counts obtained at the scanner resolution, while Image (**b**) has been atrophy corrected using a brain mask to elevate count rates that include CSF partial volume effects. This atrophy correction significantly raises the amount of PIB uptake seen in the image.

was associated with more atrophy in AD. While the authors raised the possibility that this represented functional compensation for structural change, they also noted that a host of methodological problems might be responsible for the findings. Many other studies have examined brain activation in aging, mild cognitive impairment, and dementia, and many report reductions in brain activation in those with MCI and AD (Daselaar et al., 2003; Machulda et al., 2003; Small et al., 1999; Sperling et al., 2003). Yet, since it is known that aging, and especially MCI and AD, produce both global brain atrophy and regionally-predominant atrophy in medial temporal lobes, it is also important to examine interactions between atrophy and activation. In one study, for example, Dickerson et al. (2004) found associations between hippocampal activation and memory and between hippocampal volume and memory in MCI patients. Adjusting the activations for volume did not change the effect, despite the fact that more clinical impairment was associated with smaller hippocampal volume and greater activation. It is thus clear that the relationships between activation, cortical atrophy, or volume and performance are complex and may vary differently with aging and disease, but interactions between these variables require careful analysis.

Atrophy and Stereotaxic Normalization

Brain atrophy, in addition to affecting the detection of signals in the brain, may also have effects on the ability to spatially normalize functional images. The topic of spatial normalization of images is complex and is reviewed in more detail in Chapter 22, however issues of normalization in relationship to studies of brain aging often cause confusion. This is especially so because the issue of detecting signal changes in a group of individuals is affected by both the partial volume effect and effects of spatial transformation. The essential problem, again, is conceptually straightforward. Spatial normalization is performed to transform images into a standard space so that signals can be averaged across subjects—a process that is aided by spatial smoothing that compensates to some extent for intersubject differences in anatomy (e.g., Friston et al., 1996; Woods, et al., 1998; Ashburner and Friston, 1999). However, because the aging brain may be characterized by relatively severe morphological change, it remains possible that this

approach is inadequate and may not always produce images that truly superimpose identical brain regions across subjects. This problem has been studied with regard to both PET and fMRI techniques.

The problem appears to be particularly relevant to the detection of functional change in medial temporal lobe structures. For example, Mosconi et al. (2005) noted that despite a large number of FDG-PET studies that reported reductions in cortical metabolism in AD, very few reported reductions in hippocampal glucose metabolism, despite the known pathological predilection for this structure. They provided compelling evidence that the use of standard brain templates (such as the MNI template implemented in SPM) limits the detection of hippocampal changes, while the use of a native-space ROI definition or a masking procedure optimized the detection of change. A very similar approach was used in an fMRI study of MCI patients (Sandstrom et al., 2006) in which a correlation was detected between the degree of hippocampal atrophy and fMRI activation when a template-based approach was used, but not when a native-space ROI analysis was used. This suggests that spatial normalization alters the averaged fMRI signal in ways that are related to atrophy. The problem is not restricted to disease. In a study of hippocampal activation in normal older people, individual-subject native space analyses revealed heterogeneous activations that went undetected when spatially averaged (Vandenbroucke et al., 2004). Other studies have examined spatial normalization itself in this regard, and found problems with normalization of the hippocampus that is related both to the degree of atrophy and to the sorts of normalization templates that are utilized (Krishnan et al., 2006; Sun et al., 2007). While the majority of published work has evaluated this problem with respect to the hippocampus and associated medial temporal lobe structures, it remains likely that anatomic change can affect many different brain regions. Both the detection of changes in BOLD signal and glucose metabolism and the failure to detect such changes need to be carefully considered in light of this methodological concern when studying the aging brain.

"Atrophy Correction" and When it Should be Applied

The issue of "atrophy correction" is neither technically nor conceptually straightforward. While there are ways of manipulating images to reduce partial volume effects, these manipulations can also be a source of additional experimental error. Partial volume corrections do not solve the problems involved in spatial normalization and vice versa.

The problem is compounded because even if completely adequate solutions were available, the problem is to some extent an ultrastructural one. For example, it is reasonably clear that one of the reasons brain glucose metabolism is reduced in aging is because of atrophy. However, if one considers the physiology and anatomy of these changes, it is likely that reductions in metabolism are due to diminished synaptic activity (Rocher et al., 2003). Synaptic changes in aging, particularly reductions in spine length, volume, and number, are well-recognized and may, in fact, be the predominant ultrastructural age-related alteration (see Chapter 3). Indeed, while both metabolism and perfusion change with age and age-related neurodegenerative disorders, the case that these changes reflect anything other than these sorts of ultrastructural events (i.e., primary disturbances in enzymes or regulators of blood flow and metabolism) remains unestablished despite decades of research. Thus, on a fundamental level, whether one corrects for atrophy or not, changes in brain structure may drive many functional changes that have been described in aging.

Finally, it may not always be wise or necessary to perform atrophy related corrections, especially for partial volume effects. If the goal of the use of some of these imaging techniques is purely clinical—such as diagnostic—then all the available information should be used. In this case, the atrophy effects may, in fact, contribute to the utility of a technique by essentially magnifying group differences. Of course, in situations where the goal is to understand basic biological processes, atrophy is more of a problem that must be dealt with.

The problem of "correcting" for the atrophy-related spatial distortions occurring in the process of normalization of scans is more complex. Different approaches to spatial normalization—including probabilistic atlas techniques and ROI definition, along with group-specific templates—may minimize this problem to some extent (Fischl et al., 2002; Kochunov et al., 2001; see also Chapter 22). Approaches that covary volumetric measurements of brain regions with atlas-obtained measurements may also provide insight into the role that atrophy may play. Finally, convergent evidence from studies employing both atlas-based and native-space analyses will be required to convincingly demonstrate that the normalization process is not affecting results.

Conclusions

The continued use of functional and molecular brain imaging has the potential to revolutionize our understanding of the neural basis of cognitive aging. The high spatial resolution of fMRI, coupled with its ability to assess correlates of neural activity while subjects are performing cognitive tasks, make its role invaluable. The ability to track a multitude of biochemical processes with PET provides a powerful way of relating structure, function, and chemistry. However, caution must be taken to avoid misinterpreting the results of these studies. BOLD signal usually reflects the influence of neural activity on cerebral blood flow and, therefore, age-related changes in resting cerebral blood flow or neurovascular coupling may influence our ability to attribute BOLD signal changes to alterations in neural activity. Until new methods are developed to more closely link functional imaging to neural activity, care must be taken in all levels of study design, analysis, and interpretation to maximize our ability to continue to contribute valuable insights to the literature on the neural mechanisms of cognitive aging. Similarly, the problems related to brain atrophy introduce significant methodological concerns in the interpretation of molecular images that can only be partially overcome. While technical solutions to all of these problems are constantly being developed, the field of brain aging will benefit most with attention to these concerns and to a search for convergent evidence that transcends both particular study designs and methodological boundaries.

References

Abernethy, W. B., Bell, M. A., Morris, M., and Moody, D. M. (1993). Microvascular density of the human paraventricular nucleus decreases with aging but not hypertension. *Experimental Neurology*, 121(2): 270–274.

Aizenstein, H. J., Clark, K. A., Butters, M. A., Cochran, J., Stenger, V. A., Meltzer, C. C., et al. (2004). The BOLD hemodynamic response in healthy aging. *Journal of Cognitive Neuroscience*, 16(5): 786–793.

Ances, B. M., Liang, C. L., Leontiev, O., Perthen, J. E., Fleisher, A. S., Lansing, A. E., et al. (2008). Effects of aging on cerebral blood flow, oxygen metabolism, and blood oxygenation level dependent responses to visual stimulation. *Human Brain Mapping*, 30(4): 1120–1132.

Ashburner, J. and Friston, K. J. (1999). Nonlinear spatial normalization using basis functions. *Human Brain Mapping*, 7(4): 254–266.

Bandettini, P. A. and Wong, E. C. (1997). A Hypercapnia-based normalization method for improved spatial localization of human brain activation with fMRI. *NMR Biomedicine*, 10(4–5): 197–203.

Barch, D. M., Sabb, F. W., Carter, C. S., Braver, T. S., Noll, D. C., and Cohen, J. D. (1999). Overt verbal responding during fMRI scanning: Empirical investigations of problems and potential solutions. *Neuroimage*, 10(6): 642–657.

Bednar, M. M. and Gross, C. E. (1999). Aspirin reduces experimental cerebral blood flow in vivo. *Neurological Research*, 21(5): 488–490.

Bell, E. C., Willson, M. C., Wilman, A. H., Dave, S., and Silverstone, P. H. (2005). Differential effects of chronic lithium and valproate on brain activation in healthy volunteers. *Human Psychopharmacology*, 20(6): 415–424.

Benarroch, E. (2007). Neurovascular unit dysfunction: A vascular component of Alzheimer disease? *Neurology*, 68: 1730–1732.

Bentourkia, M., Bol, A., Ivanoiu, A., Labar, D., Sibomana, M., Coppens, A., et al. (2000). Comparison of regional cerebral blood flow and glucose metabolism in the normal brain: Effect of aging. *Journal of Neurological Science*, 181(1–2), 19–28.

Biagi, L., Abbruzzese, A., Bianchi, M. C., Alsop, D. C., Del Guerra, A., and Tosetti, M. (2007). Age dependence of cerebral perfusion assessed by magnetic resonance continuous arterial spin labeling. *Journal of Magnetic Resonance Imaging*, 25(4): 696–702.

Bonvento, G., Sibson, N., and Pellerin, L. (2002). Does glutamate image your thoughts? *Trends Neuroscience*, 25(7): 359–364.

Bots, M. L., van Swieten, J. C., Breteler, M. M., de Jong, P. T., van Gijn, J., Hofman, A., et al. (1993). Cerebral white matter lesions and atherosclerosis in the Rotterdam study. *Lancet*, 341(8855): 1232–1237.

Buckner, R. L., Snyder, A. Z., Sanders, A. L., Raichle, M. E., and Morris, J. C. (2000). Functional brain imaging of young, nondemented, and demented older adults. *Journal of Cognitive Neuroscience*, 12 (Suppl 2): 24–34.

Buxton, R. B. and Frank, L. R. (1997). A model for the coupling between cerebral blood flow and oxygen metabolism during neural stimulation. *Journal of Cerebral Blood Flow Metabolism*, 17(1): 64–72.

Cabeza, R. (2002). Hemispheric asymmetry reduction in older adults: The HAROLD model. *Psychological Aging*, 17(1): 85–100.

Cabeza, R., McIntosh, A. R., Tulving, E., Nyberg, L., and Grady, C. L. (1997). Age-related differences in effective neural connectivity during encoding and recall. *Neuroreport*, 8(16): 3479–3483.

Cao, Y., Vikingstad, E. M., George, K. P., Johnson, A. F., and Welch, K. M. (1999). Cortical language activation in stroke patients recovering from aphasia with functional MRI. *Stroke*, 30(11): 2331–2340.

Chawluk, J. B., Alavi, A., Dann, R., Hurtig, H. I., Bais, S., Kushner, M. J., et al. (1987). Positron emission tomography in aging and dementia: Effect of cerebral atrophy. *Journal of Nuclear Medicine*, 28(4): 431–437.

Chetelat, G., Desgranges, B., Landeau, B., Mezenge, F., Poline, J. B., de la Sayette, V., et al. (2008). Direct voxel-based comparison between grey matter hypometabolism and atrophy in Alzheimer's disease. *Brain*, 131(Pt 1): 60–71.

Claus, J. J., Breteler, M. M., Hasan, D., Krenning, E. P., Bots, M. L., Grobbee, D. E., et al. (1998). Regional cerebral blood flow and cerebrovascular risk factors in the elderly population. *Neurobiological Aging*, 19(1): 57–64.

Cohen, E. R., Rostrup, E., Sidaros, K., Lund, T. E., Paulson, O. B., Ugurbil, K., et al. (2004). Hypercapnic normalization of BOLD fMRI: Comparison across field strengths and pulse sequences. *Neuroimage*, 23(2): 613–624.

Cohen, E. R., Ugurbil, K., and Kim, S. G. (2002). Effect of basal conditions on the magnitude and dynamics of the blood oxygenation level-dependent fMRI response. *Journal of Cerebral Blood Flow Metabolism*, 22(9): 1042–1053.

Cunnington, R., Iansek, R., Johnson, K. A., and Bradshaw, J. L. (1997). Movement-related potentials in parkinson's disease: Motor imagery and movement preparation. *Brain*, 120 (Pt 8): 1339–1353.

D'Esposito, M., Deouell, L., Gazzaley, A. (2003). Alterations in the BOLD. fMRI signal with ageing and disease: A challenge for neuro imaging. *Nature Reviews Neuroscience*, 4(11): 863–872.

D'Esposito, M., Zarahn, E., Aguirre, G. K., and Rypma, B. (1999). The effect of normal aging on the coupling of neural activity to the bold hemodynamic response. *Neuroimage*, 10(1): 6–14.

Dager, S. R. and Friedman, S. D. (2000). Brain imaging and the effects of Caffeine and Nicotine. *Annals of Medicine*, 32(9): 592–599.

Daselaar, S. M., Veltman, D. J., Rombouts, S. A., Raaijmakers, J. G., and Jonker, C. (2003). Deep processing activates the medial temporal lobe in young but not in old adults. *Neurobiological Aging*, 24(7); 1005–1011.

Detre, J. A. and Alsop, D. C. (1999). Perfusion magnetic resonance imaging with continuous arterial spin labeling: Methods And clinical applications in the Central Nervous System. *European Journal of Radiology*, 30(2): 115–124.

Dickerson, B. C., Salat, D. H., Bates, J. F., Atiya, M., Killiany, R. J., Greve, D. N., et al. (2004). Medial temporal lobe function and structure in mild cognitive impairment. *Annals of Neurology*, 56(1): 27–35.

Diehl, B., Stodieck, S. R., Diehl, R. R., and Ringelstein, E. B. (1998). The photic driving EEG response and photoreactive cerebral blood flow in the posterior cerebral artery in controls and in patients with epilepsy. *Electroencephalography and Clinical Neurophysiology*, 107(1): 8–12.

Dufouil, C., de Kersaint-Gilly, A., Besancon, V., Levy, C., Auffray, E., Brunnereau, L., et al. (2001). Longitudinal study of blood pressure and white matter hyperintensities: The EVA MRI cohort. *Neurology*, 56(7): 921–926.

Fang, H. C. H. (1976). Observations on aging characteristics of cerebral blood vessels, Macroscopic and microscopic features. In: S. Gerson and R. D. Terry (ed.), *Neurobiology of Aging* (pp.155–156). NY: Raven.

Farkas, E. and Luiten, P. G. (2001). Cerebral microvascular pathology in aging and Alzheimer's disease. *Progress in Neurobiology*, 64(6): 575–611.

Fazekas, F., Kleinert, R., Offenbacher, H., Schmidt, R., Kleinert, G., Payer, F., et al. (1993). Pathologic correlates of incidental MRI white matter signal hyperintensities. *Neurology*, 43(9): 1683–1689.

Feydy, A., Carlier, R., Roby-Brami, A., Bussel, B., Cazalis, F., Pierot, L., et al. (2002). Longitudinal study of motor recovery after stroke: recruitment and focusing of brain activation. *Stroke*, 33(6): 1610–1617.

Fischl, B., Salat, D. H., Busa, E., Albert, M., Dieterich, M., Haselgrove, C., et al. (2002). Whole brain segmentation: automated labeling of neuroanatomical structures in the human brain. *Neuron*, 33(3): 341–355.

Fox, P. T. and Raichle, M. E. 1986. Focal physiological uncoupling of cerebral blood flow and oxidative metabolism during somatosensory stimulation in human subjects. *Proceedings of the National Academy of Sciences of the USA*, 83(4): 1140–1144.

Fox, P. T., Raichle, M. E., Mintun, M. A., and Dence, C. (1988). Nonoxidative glucose consumption during focal physiologic neural activity. *Science*, 241(4864); 462–464.

Friston, K., Williams, S., Howard, R., Frackowiak, R., and Turner, R. (1996). Movement-related effects in fMRI time-series. *Magnetic Resonance in Medicine*, 35: 346–355.

Furuta, A., Ishii, N., Nishihara, Y., and Horie, A. (1991). Medullary arteries in aging and dementia. *Stroke*, 22(4): 442–446.

Gati, J. S., Menon, R. S., Ugurbil, K., and Rutt, B. K. (1997). Experimental determination of the BOLD field strength dependence in vessels and tissue. *Magnetic Resonance Medicine*, 38(2): 296–302.

Gazzaley, A. and D'Esposito, M. (2003). The contribution of functional brain imaging to our understanding of cognitive aging. Science's SAGE KE, http://sageke.sciencemag.org/cgi/content/full/sageke;2003/4/pe2, 29 Jan 2003.

George, A. E., de Leon, M. J., Gentes, C. I., Miller, J., London, E., Budzilovich, G. N., et al. (1986). Leukoencephalopathy in normal and pathologic aging:

1. CT of brain lucencies. *American Journal of Neuroradiology*, 7(4), 561–566.

Grady, C. L. (2000). Functional brain imaging and age-related changes in cognition. *Biological Psychology*, 54(1–3): 259–281.

Handwerker, D. A., Gazzaley, A., Inglis, B. A., and D'Esposito, M. (2007). Reducing vascular variability of fMRI data across aging populations using a breathholding task. *Human Brain Mapping*, 28(9): 846–859.

Hatazawa, J., Shimosegawa, E., Satoh, T., Toyoshima, H., and Okudera, T. (1997). Subcortical hypoperfusion associated with asymptomatic white matter lesions on magnetic resonance imaging. *Stroke*, 28(10): 1944–1947.

Hesselmann, V., Zaro Weber, O., Wedekind, C., Krings, T., Schulte, O., Kugel, H., et al. (2001). Age related signal decrease in functional magnetic resonance imaging during motor stimulation in humans. *Neuroscience Letters*, 308(3): 141–144.

Huettel, S. A. and McCarthy, G. (2000). Evidence for a refractory period in the hemodynamic response to visual stimuli as measured by MRI. *Neuroimage*, 11(5 Pt 1): 547–553.

Huettel, S. A., Singerman, J. D., and McCarthy, G. (2001). The effects of aging upon the hemodynamic response measured by functional MRI. *Neuroimage*, 13(1): 161–175.

Ibáñez, V., Pietrini, P., Alexander, G. E., Furey, M. L., Teichberg, D., Rajapakse, J. C., et al. (1998). Regional glucose metabolic abnormalities are not the result of atrophy in Alzheimer's disease. *Neurology*, 50: 1585–1593.

Ito, H., Kanno, I., Ibaraki, M., and Hatazawa, J. (2002). Effect of aging on cerebral vascular response to Paco2 changes in humans as measured by positron emission tomography. *Journal of Cerebral Blood Flow Metabolism*, 22(8): 997–1003.

Jacobsen, L. K., Gore, J. C., Skudlarski, P., Lacadie, C. M., Jatlow, P., and Krystal, J. H. (2002). Impact of intravenous nicotine on BOLD signal response to photic stimulation. *Magnetic Resonance Imaging*, 20(2): 141–145.

Jagust, W. J., Zheng, L., Harvey, D. J., Mack, W. J., Vinters, H. V., Weiner, M. W., et al. (2008). Neuropathological basis of magnetic resonance images in aging and dementia. *Annals of Neurology*, 63(1): 72–80.

Jiang, H. X., Chen, P. C., Sobin, S. S., and Giannotta, S. L. (1992). Age related alterations in the response of the Pial arterioles to adenosine in the rat. *Mechanisms of Ageing and Development*, 65(2–3): 257–276.

Johnson, S. C., Saykin, A. J., Baxter, L. C., Flashman, L. A., Santulli, R. B., McAllister, T. W., et al. (2000). The relationship between fMRI activation and cerebral atrophy: comparison of normal aging and Alzheimer disease. *Neuroimage*, 11(3): 179–187.

Jonides, J., Marshuetz, C., Smith, E. E., Reuter-Lorenz, P. A., Koeppe, R. A., and Hartley, A. (2000). Age differences in behavior and PET activation reveal differences in interference resolution in verbal working memory. *Journal of Cognitive Neuroscience*, 12(1): 188–196.

Kalaria, R. N. (1996). Cerebral vessels in ageing and Alzheimer's disease. *Pharmacological Therapy*, 72(3): 193–214.

Karas, G. B., Burton, E. J., Rombouts, S. A., van Schijndel, R. A., O'Brien, J. T., Scheltens, P., et al. (2003). A comprehensive study of gray matter loss in patients with Alzheimer's disease using optimized voxel-based morphometry. *Neuroimage*, 18(4): 895–907.

Kawamura, J., Terayama, Y., Takashima, S., Obara, K., Pavol, M. A., Meyer, J. S., et al. (1993). Leuko-Araiosis and cerebral perfusion in normal aging. *Experimental Aging Research*, 19(3): 225–240.

Knox, C. A., Yates, R. D., Chen, I., and Klara, P. M. (1980). Effects of aging on the structural and permeability characteristics of cerebrovasculature in normotensive and hypertensive strains of rats. *Acta Neuropathologica (Berl)*, 51(1): 1–13.

Kobari, M., Meyer, J. S., and Ichijo, M. (1990). Leuko-Araiosis, cerebral atrophy, and cerebral perfusion in normal aging. *Archives of Neurology*, 47(2): 161–165.

Kochunov, P., Lancaster, J. L., Thompson, P., Woods, R., Mazziotta, J., Hardies, J., et al. (2001). Regional spatial normalization: Toward an optimal target. *Journal of Computer Assisted Tomography*, 25(5): 805–816.

Krejza, J., Mariak, Z., Walecki, J., Szydlik, P., Lewko, J., and Ustymowicz, A. (1999). Transcranial color doppler sonography of basal cerebral arteries in 182 healthy subjects: Age and sex variability and normal reference values for blood flow parameters. *American Journal of Roentgenology*, 172(1): 213–218.

Krishnan, S., Slavin, M. J., Tran, T. T., Doraiswamy, P. M., and Petrella, J. R. (2006). Accuracy of spatial normalization of the hippocampus: Implications for fMRI research in memory disorders. *Neuroimage*, 31(2): 560–571.

Kuwabara, Y., Ichiya, Y., Sasaki, M., Yoshida, T., Fukumura, T., Masuda, K., et al. (1996). Cerebral blood flow and vascular response to hypercapnia in hypertensive patients with leukoaraiosis. *Annals of Nuclear Medicine*, 10(3): 293–298.

Kwong, K. K., Wanke, I., Donahue, K. M., Davis, T. L., and Rosen, B. R. (1995). EPI imaging of global increase of brain MR signal with breath-hold preceded by breathing O2. *Magnetic Resonance Medicine*, 33(3): 448–452.

Laurienti, P. J., Field, A. S., Burdette, J. H., Maldjian, J. A., Yen, Y. F., and Moody, D. M. (2002). Dietary caffeine consumption modulates fMRI measures. *Neuroimage*, 17(2): 751–757.

Li, T. Q., Kastrup, A., Takahashi, A. M., and Moseley, M. E. (1999). Functional MRI of human brain during breath holding by BOLD and FAIR techniques. *Neuroimage*, 9(2): 243–249.

Lindauer, U., Megow, D., Matsuda, H., and Dirnagl, U. (1999). Nitric oxide: A modulator, but not a mediator, of neurovascular coupling in rat somatosensory cortex. *American Journal of Physiology*, 277(2 Pt 2): H799–811.

Lindenberger, U. and Baltes, P. B. (1994). Sensory functioning and intelligence in old age: A strong connection. *Psychology and Aging*, 9(3): 339–355.

Linville, D. G. and Arneric, S. P. (1991). Cortical cerebral blood flow governed by the basal forebrain: Age-related impairments. *Neurobiology of Aging*, 12(5): 503–510.

Logan, J. M., Sanders, A. L., Snyder, A. Z., Morris, J. C., and Buckner, R. L. (2002). Under-recruitment and nonselective recruitment: Dissociable neural mechanisms associated with aging. *Neuron*, 33(5): 827–840.

Machulda, M. M., Ward, H. A., Borowski, B., Gunter, J. L., Cha, R. H., O'Brien, P. C., et al. (2003). Comparison of memory fMRI response among normal, MCI, and Alzheimer's patients. *Neurology*, 61(4): 500–506.

Marstrand, J. R., Garde, E., Rostrup, E., Ring, P., Rosenbaum, S., Mortensen, E. L., et al. (2002). Cerebral perfusion and cerebrovascular reactivity are reduced in white matter hyperintensities. *Stroke*, 33(4): 972–976.

Masawa, N., Yoshida, Y., Yamada, T., Joshita, T., Sato, S., and Mihara, B. (1994). Morphometry of structural preservation of tunica media in aged and hypertensive human intracerebral arteries. *Stroke*, 25(1): 122–127.

Mattay, V. S., Fera, F., Tessitore, A., Hariri, A. R., Das, S., Callicott, J. H., et al. (2002). Neurophysiological correlates of age-related changes in human motor function. *Neurology*, 58(4): 630–635.

Mayhan, W. G., Faraci, F. M., Baumbach, G. L., and Heistad, D. D. (1990). Effects of aging on responses of cerebral arterioles. *American Journal of Physiology*, 258(4 Pt 2): H1138–1143.

McIntosh, A. R. (1999). Mapping cognition to the brain through neural interactions. *Memory*, 7(5–6): 523–548.

Mechelli, A., Price, C. J., and Friston, K. J. (2001). Nonlinear coupling between evoked rCBF and BOLD signals: A simulation study of hemodynamic responses. *Neuroimage*, 14(4): 862–872.

Meltzer, C. C., Cantwell, M. N., Greer, P. J., Ben-Eliezer, D., Smith, G., Frank, G., et al. (2000). Does cerebral blood flow decline in healthy aging? A PET study with partial-volume correction. *Journal of Nuclear Medicine*, 41(11): 1842–1848.

Meltzer, C. C., Kinahan, P. E., Greer, P. J., Nichols, T. E., Comtat, C., Cantwell, M. N., et al. (1999). Comparative evaluation of MR-based partial-volume correction schemes for PET. *Journal of Nuclear Medicine*, 40(12): 2053–2065.

Meltzer, C. C., Leal, J. P., Mayberg, H. S., Wagner, H. N., and Frost, J. J. (1990). Correction of PET data for partial volume effects in human cerebral cortex by MR imaging. *Journal of Computer Assisted Tomography*, 14: 561–570.

Meltzer, C. C., Zubieta, J. K., Brandt, J., Tune, L. E., Mayberg, H. S., and Frost, J. J. (1996). Regional hypometabolism in Alzheimer's disease as measured by positron emission tomography after correction for effects of partial volume averaging. *Neurology*, 47: 454–461.

Menon, R. S., Ogawa, S., Hu, X., Strupp, J. P., Anderson, P., and Ugurbil, K. (1995). BOLD based functional MRI at 4 Tesla includes a capillary bed contribution: Echo-planar imaging correlates with previous optical imaging using intrinsic signals. *Magnetic Resonance in Medicine*, 33(3): 453–459.

Miezin, F. M., Maccotta, L., Ollinger, J. M., Petersen, S. E., and Buckner, R. L. (2000). Characterizing the hemodynamic response: Effects of presentation rate, sampling procedure, and the possibility of ordering brain activity based on relative timing. *Neuroimage*, 11(6 Pt 1): 735–759.

Miller, D. D., Andreasen, N. C., O'Leary, D. S., Rezai, K., Watkins, G. L., Ponto, L. L., et al. (1997). Effect of antipsychotics on regional cerebral blood flow measured with positron emission tomography. *Neuropsychopharmacology*, 17(4): 230–240.

Miller, K. L., Luh, W. M., Liu, T. T., Martinez, A., Obata, T., Wong, E. C., et al. (2001). Nonlinear temporal dynamics of the cerebral blood flow response. *Human Brain Mapping*, 13(1): 1–12.

Mitchell, K. J., Johnson, M. K., Raye, C. L., and D'Esposito, M. (2000). fMRI evidence of age-related hippocampal dysfunction in feature binding in working memory. *Cognitive Brain Research*, 10(1–2): 197–206.

Moody, D. M., Brown, W. R., Challa, V. R., Ghazi-Birry, H. S., and Reboussin, D. M. (1997). Cerebral microvascular alterations in aging, leukoaraiosis, and Alzheimer's disease. *Annals of the New York Academy of Sciences*, 826: 103–116.

Mosconi, L., Tsui, W. H., De Santi, S., Li, J., Rusinek, H., Convit, A., et al. (2005). Reduced hippocampal metabolism in MCI and AD: Automated FDG-PET image analysis. *Neurology*, 64(11): 1860–1867.

Mulderink, T. A., Gitelman, D. R., Mesulam, M. M., and Parrish, T. B. (2002). On the use of caffeine as a contrast booster for BOLD fMRI studies. *Neuroimage*, 15(1): 37–44.

Nagasawa, S., Handa, H., Okumura, A., Naruo, Y., Moritake, K., and Hayashi, K. (1979). Mechanical properties of human cerebral arteries. Part 1: Effects of age and vascular smooth muscle activation. *Surgical Neurology*, 12(4): 297–304.

Neele, S. J., Rombouts, S. A., Bierlaagh, M. A., Barkhof, F., Scheltens, P., and Netelenbos, J. C. (2001). Raloxifene affects brain activation patterns in postmenopausal women during visual encoding. *Journal of Clinical Endocrinology & Metabolism*, 86(3): 1422–1424.

Niehaus, L., Lehmann, R., Roricht, S., and Meyer, B. U. (2001). Age-related reduction in visually evoked cerebral blood flow responses. *Neurobiological Aging*, 22(1): 35–38.

Nobler, M. S., Olvet, K. R., and Sackeim, H. A. (2002). Effects of medications on cerebral blood flow in late-life depression. *Current Psychiatry Reports*, 4(1): 51–58.

Nordahl, C. W., Ranganath, C., Yonelinas, A. P., Decarli, C., Fletcher, E., and Jagust, W. J. (2006). White matter changes compromise prefrontal cortex function in healthy elderly individuals. *Journal of Cognitive Neuroscience*, 18(3): 418–429.

Norris, D. G., Zysset, S., Mildner, T., and Wiggins, C. J. (2002). An investigation of the value of spin-echo-based fMRI using a Stroop color-word matching task and EPI at 3 T. *Neuroimage*, 15(3): 719–726.

Pariente, J., Loubinoux, I., Carel, C., Albucher, J. F., Leger, A., Manelfe, C., et al. (2001). Fluoxetine modulates motor performance and cerebral activation of patients recovering from stroke. *Annals of Neurology*, 50(6): 718–729.

Pineiro, R., Pendlebury, S., Johansen-Berg, H., and Matthews, P. M. (2002). Altered hemodynamic responses in patients after subcortical stroke measured by functional MRI. *Stroke*, 33(1): 103–109.

Quarantelli, M., Berkouk, K., Prinster, A., Landeau, B., Svarer, C., Balkay, L., et al. (2004). Integrated software for the analysis of brain PET/SPECT studies with partial-volume-effect correction. *Journal of Nuclear Medicine*, 45(2): 192–201.

Rees, G., Howseman, A., Josephs, O., Frith, C. D., Friston, K. J., Frackowiak, R. S., et al. (1997). Characterizing the relationship between BOLD contrast and regional cerebral blood flow measurements by varying the stimulus presentation rate. *Neuroimage*, 6(4): 270–278.

Reich, T. and Rusinek, H. (1989). Cerebral cortical and white matter reactivity to carbon dioxide. *Stroke; a Journal of Cerebral Circulation*, 20(4): 453–457.

Restom, K., Bangen, K. J., Bondi, M. W., Perthen, J. E., and Liu, T. T. (2007). Cerebral blood flow and BOLD responses to a memory encoding task: A comparison between healthy young and elderly adults. *Neuroimage*, 37(2): 430–439.

Reuter-Lorenz, P. (2002). New visions of the aging mind and brain. *Trends in Cognitive Sciences*, 6(9): 394.

Riecker, A., Grodd, W., Klose, U., Schulz, J. B., Groschel, K., Erb, M., et al. (2003). Relation between regional functional MRI activation and vascular reactivity to carbon dioxide during normal aging. *Journal of Cerebral Blood Flow Metabolism*, 23(5): 565–573.

Rissman, J., Gazzaley, A., and D'Esposito, M. (2004). Measuring functional connectivity during distinct stages of a cognitive task. *Neuroimage*, 23(2): 752–763.

Rocher, A. B., Chapon, F., Blaizot, X., Baron, J. C., and Chavoix, C. (2003). Resting-state brain glucose utilization as measured by PET is directly related to regional synaptophysin levels: A study in baboons. *Neuroimage*, 20(3): 1894–1898.

Rosa-Neto, P., Benkelfat, C., Sakai, Y., Leyton, M., Morais, J. A., and Diksic, M. (2007). Brain regional alpha-[11C]methyl-L-tryptophan trapping, used as an index of 5-HT synthesis, in healthy adults: absence of an age effect. *European Journal of Nuclear Medicine and Molecular Imaging*, 34(8): 1254–1264.

Ross, M. H., Yurgelun-Todd, D. A., Renshaw, P. F., Maas, L. C., Mendelson, J. H., Mello, N. K., et al. (1997). Age-related reduction in functional MRI response to photic stimulation. *Neurology*, 48(1): 173–176.

Rother, J., Knab, R., Hamzei, F., Fiehler, J., Reichenbach, J. R., Buchel, C., et al. (2002). Negative dip in BOLD fMRI is caused by blood flow–oxygen consumption uncoupling in humans. *Neuroimage*, 15(1): 98–102.

Rypma, B. and D'Esposito, M. (2000). Isolating the neural mechanisms of age-related changes in human working memory. *Nature Neuroscience*, 3(5): 509–515.

Salat, D. H., Kaye, J. A., and Janowsky, J. S. (2001). Selective preservation and degeneration within the prefrontal cortex in aging and Alzheimer disease. *Archives of Neurology*, 58(9): 1403–1408.

Sandstrom, C. K., Krishnan, S., Slavin, M. J., Tran, T. T., Doraiswamy, P. M., and Petrella, J. R. (2006). Hippocampal atrophy confounds template-based functional MR imaging measures of hippocampal activation in patients with mild cognitive impairment. *American Journal of Neuroradiology*, 27(8): 1622–1627.

Schultz, S. K., O'Leary, D. S., Boles Ponto, L. L., Watkins, G. L., Hichwa, R. D., and Andreasen, N. C. (1999). Age-related changes in regional cerebral blood flow among young to mid-life adults. *Neuroreport*, 10(12): 2493–2496.

Schwarzbauer, C. and Heinke, W. (1999). Investigating the dependence of BOLD contrast on oxidative metabolism. *Magnetic Resonance in Medicine*, 41(3): 537–543.

Shantaram, V. (1999). Pathogenesis of atherosclerosis in diabetes and hypertension. *Clinical and Experimental Hypertension*, 21(1–2): 69–77.

Small, S. A., Perera, G. M., DeLaPaz, R., Mayeux, R., and Stern, Y. (1999). Differential regional dysfunction of the hippocampal formation among elderly with memory decline and Alzheimer's disease. *Annals of Neurology*, 45: 466–472.

Small, S. L., Hlustik, P., Noll, D. C., Genovese, C., and Solodkin, A. (2002). Cerebellar hemispheric activation ipsilateral to the paretic hand correlates with functional recovery after stroke. *Brain*, 125(Pt 7): 1544–1557.

Song, A. W., Fichtenholtz, H., and Woldorff, M. (2002). BOLD signal compartmentalization based on the apparent diffusion coefficient. *Magnetic Resonance Imaging*, 20(7): 521–525.

Sonntag, W. E., Lynch, C. D., Cooney, P. T., and Hutchins, P. M. (1997). Decreases in cerebral microvasculature with age are associated with the decline in growth hormone and insulin-like growth factor 1. *Endocrinology*, 138(8): 3515–3520.

Sperling, R. A., Bates, J. F., Chua, E. F., Cocchiarella, A. J., Rentz, D. M., Rosen, B. R., et al. (2003). fMRI studies of associative encoding in young and elderly controls and mild Alzheimer's disease. *Journal of Neurology, Neurosurgery & Psychiatry*, 74(1): 44 50.

Stebbins, G. T., Carrillo, M. C., Dorfman, J., Dirksen, C., Desmond, J. E., Turner, D. A., et al. (2002). Aging effects on memory encoding in the frontal lobes. *Psychology of Aging*, 17(1): 44–55.

Stein, E. A., Pankiewicz, J., Harsch, H. H., Cho, J. K., Fuller, S. A., Hoffmann, R. G., et al. (1998). Nicotine-induced limbic cortical activation in the human brain: a functional MRI study. *American Journal of Psychiatry*, 155(8): 1009–1015.

Sullivan, E. V., Pfefferbaum, A., Adalsteinsson, E., Swan, G. E., and Carmelli, D. (2002). Differential rates of regional brain change in callosal and ventricular size: A 4-year longitudinal MRI study of elderly men. *Cerebral Cortex*, 12(4): 438–445.

Sun, F. T., Miller, L. M., and D'Esposito, M. (2004). Measuring interregional functional connectivity using coherence and partial coherence analyses of fMRI data. *Neuroimage*, 21(2): 647–658.

Sun, F. T., Schriber, R. A., Greenia, J. M., He, J., Gitcho, A., and Jagust, W. J. (2007). Automated template-based PET region of interest analyses in the aging brain. *Neuroimage*, 34(2): 608–617.

Takada, H., Nagata, K., Hirata, Y., Satoh, Y., Watahiki, Y., Sugawara, J., et al. (1992). Age-related decline of cerebral oxygen metabolism in normal population detected with positron emission tomography. *Neurological Research*, 14(2 Suppl): 128–131.

Tamaki, K., Nakai, M., Yokota, T., and Ogata, J. (1995). Effects of aging and chronic hypertension on cerebral blood flow and cerebrovascular CO2 reactivity in the rat. *Gerontology*, 41(1): 11–17.

Taoka, T., Iwasaki, S., Uchida, H., Fukusumi, A., Nakagawa, H., Kichikawa, K., et al. (1998). Age correlation of the time lag in signal change on EPI-fMRI. *Journal of Computer Assisted Tomography*, 22(4): 514–517.

Tekes, A., Mohamed, M. A., Browner, N. M., Calhoun, V. D., and Yousem, D. M. (2005). Effect of age on visuomotor functional MR imaging. *Academic Radiology*, 12(6): 739–745.

Thirumala, P., Hier, D. B., and Patel, P. (2002). Motor recovery after stroke: Lessons from functional brain imaging. *Neurological Research*, 24(5): 453–458.

Thulborn, K. R., Carpenter, P. A., and Just, M. A. (1999). Plasticity of language-related brain function during recovery from stroke. *Stroke*, 30(4): 749–754.

Thulborn, K. R., Waterton, J. C., Matthews, P. M., and Radda, G. K. (1982). Oxygenation dependence of the transverse relaxation time of water protons in whole blood at high field. *Biochimica Biophysica Acta*, 714(2): 265–270.

Tisserand, D., Pruessner, J., Sanz Arigita, E., van Boxtel, M., Evans, A., Jolles, J., et al. (2002). Regional frontal cortical volumes decrease differentially in aging: An MRI study to compare volumetric approaches and voxel-based morphometry. *Neuroimage*, 17(2): 657.

Tisserand, D. J., Visser, P. J., van Boxtel, M. P., and Jolles, J. (2000). The relation between global and limbic brain volumes on MRI and cognitive performance in healthy individuals across the age range. *Neurobiological Aging*, 21(4): 569–576.

Truchot, L., Costes, S. N., Zimmer, L., Laurent, B., Le Bars, D., Thomas-Anterion, C., et al. (2007). Up-regulation of hippocampal serotonin metabolism in mild cognitive impairment. *Neurology*, 69(10): 1012–1017.

Turner, R., Le Bihan, D., Moonen, C. T., Despres, D., and Frank, J. (1991). Echo-planar time course MRI of cat brain oxygenation changes. *Magnetic Resonance in Medicine*, 22(1): 159–166.

Urban, P. P., Allardt, A., Tettenborn, B., Hopf, H. C., Pfennigsdorf, S., and Lieb, W. (1995). Photoreactive flow changes in the posterior cerebral artery in control subjects and patients with occipital lobe infarction. *Stroke*, 26(10): 1817–1819.

Vandenbroucke, M. W., Goekoop, R., Duschek, E. J., Netelenbos, J. C., Kuijer, J. P., Barkhof, F., et al. (2004). Interindividual differences of medial temporal lobe activation during encoding in an elderly population studied by fMRI. *Neuroimage*, 21(1): 173–180.

Videen, T. O., Perlmutter, J. S., Mintun, M. A., and Raichle, M. E. (1988). Regional correction of positron emission tomography data for the effects of cerebral atrophy. *Journal of Cerebral Blood Flow Metabolism*, 8, 662–670.

Wolf, R. L. and Detre, J. A. (2007). Clinical neuroimaging using arterial spin-labeled perfusion magnetic resonance imaging. *Neurotherapeutics*, 4(3): 346–359.

Woods, R. P., Grafton, S. T., Holmes, C. J., Cherry, S. R., and Mazziotta, J. C. (1998). Automated image registration: I. General methods and intrasubject, intramodality validation. *Journal of Computer Assisted Tomography*, 22(1): 139–152.

Yamaguchi, T., Kanno, I., Uemura, K., Shishido, F., Inugami, A., Ogawa, T., et al. (1986). Reduction in regional cerebral metabolic rate of oxygen during human aging. *Stroke*, 17(6): 1220–1228.

Yamamoto, M., Meyer, J. S., Sakai, F., and Yamaguchi, F. (1980). Aging and cerebral vasodilator responses to hypercarbia: Responses in normal aging and in persons with risk factors for stroke. *Archives of Neurology*, 37(8): 489–496.

Yanase, D., Matsunari, I., Yajima, K., Chen, W., Fujikawa, A., Nishimura, S., et al. (2005). Brain FDG PET study of normal aging in Japanese: Effect of atrophy correction. *European Journal of Nuclear Medicine and Molecular Imaging*, 32(7): 794–805.

Ylikoski, R., Salonen, O., Mantyla, R., Ylikoski, A., Keskivaara, P., Leskela, M., et al. (2000). Hippocampal and temporal lobe atrophy and age-related decline in memory. *Acta Neurologica Scandinavica*, 101(4): 273–278.

3

Neuropathology of Aging

Dara L. Dickstein, John H. Morrison, and Patrick R. Hof

Brain complexity is reflected in the intricacy of its structural makeup. The mammalian brain, independent of its size, is not structurally simple and undergoes many morphological modifications during the aging process. Despite the advancements in our understanding of the molecular genetics and pathology of aging and neurodegeneration, it is still difficult to resolve the regional and neuronal vulnerability that occurs. However, recent progress in cellular and molecular research, neuroimaging, and brain mapping techniques offers extraordinary power to understand this complexity, providing genetic, environmental, and spatially detailed information on the extent and trajectory of neuroanatomical and pathological changes that are occurring. Cortical microcircuits have the ability to reorganize functionally in response to a variety of cues, both intrinsic and extrinsic. Many neuropathological studies have demonstrated that shrinkage of the brain, neuronal loss, loss or regression of dendrites and dendritic spines, alterations in neurotransmitter receptors, and the presence of specific intracellular and extracellular protein aggregates are common age-related findings. However, the distribution of such alterations varies significantly between different brain regions and different types of neurons. Two key principles of aging with respect to morphological alterations will be discussed: the occurrence of age-related memory impairment without neuronal loss; and the loss of synaptic connections in neurodegenerative diseases due to the loss of selectively vulnerable neurons.

Neuropathological Changes During Normal Aging

During normal aging, neuropathological and molecular changes and their resulting cognitive manifestations vary from subtle to severe. While these changes appear to overlap those that occur in Alzheimer's disease (AD), they are two distinct and separate processes. The differences between the two processes are both quantitative and a matter of definition. Patterns of neuronal degeneration and neuronal loss differ between the two and define the shift from neuronal dysfunction, as seen in normal aging, to deterioration and cell death in AD. The neuronal systems that are most vulnerable in aging are those in the neocortex, the basal forebrain and the brainstem monoaminergic systems (Morrison and Hof, 1997, 2002). There are many macroscopic and microscopic changes that occur in the aging brain. Brain weight declines by approximately 2%–3% per decade after age 50, and is accelerated as one ages (Drachman, 2006). Brain volume is also severely affected. It is estimated that after 50 years of age, frontal lobe volume decreases by about 12%, and temporal lobe volume decreases by 9%, while other regions such as the parietal and occipital lobe show little to no atrophy (DeCarli et al., 2005) (see also chapter 4). Annual shrinkage rates in brain volumes are calculated to be on average 0.32% for total brain volume, with hippocampal and temporal atrophy averaging 0.68% and 0.82%, respectively (Scahill et al., 2003). Interestingly, minimal neuronal loss, if any, occurs despite the decline in volume.

Morphological Alterations During Aging

It was originally thought that cognitive decline during normal aging was due to neuronal loss. However, stereological studies have demonstrated minimal neuronal loss in cortical and hippocampal regions during normal aging (Bussière et al., 2003b; Gazzaley et al., 1997; Hof et al., 2003; West et al., 1994, 2004) suggesting that the age-related impairments that occur during normal aging and AD are due to distinct pathological processes. These processes involve irregularities in dendritic arborization and in spine length, volume, distribution, number, and morphology. Neuronal dendrites are instrumental in the receiving and consolidating of neuronal input and the regulation of synaptic plasticity. Therefore, it is not surprising that there are many refined molecular cascades that are involved in the control of dendritic development and growth (Nguyen et al., 2004). In the cortex, the extent of a neuron's dendritic arborization is an important determinant of the cell's synaptic properties and affects how incoming information is integrated and processed. Throughout development, the dendritic arbor is highly dynamic; continually forming new branches and maintaining existing ones (Jan and Jan, 2003), with shape and branching patterns varying among both neuronal classes and individual cells in each class (Samsonovich and Ascoli, 2006). Dendrites are rarely longer than 1–2 mm with a diameter that is proportional to the diameter of the cell body (Chen and Wolpaw, 1994; Ulfhake and Kellerth, 1981). Any fluctuations in dendritic size in one given portion of a neuron are counterbalanced by the remaining dendrites in the same cell, suggesting a morphological homeostasis of dendritic arborization (Samsonovich and Ascoli, 2006).

During aging, many subtle changes in dendritic morphology occur and are associated with impairment in cognitive function (for review, see Morrison and Hof, 2002, and Hof and Morrison, 2004). Many studies have demonstrated age-related regression in the dendritic arbors and the dendritic spines of pyramidal neurons located in the prefrontal, superior temporal, and precentral cortices in humans (de Brabander, Kramers, and Uylings, 1998; Nakamura et al., 1985; Scheibel et al., 1975), in non-human primates (Peters, Sethares, and Moss, 1998), and in aged canines (Mervis, 1978). An early study by Cupp and Uemura (1980) examined Golgi-stained sections from the prefrontal region of young and old rhesus monkeys and concluded that entire branches or segments were lost from apical dendrites with aging. Nakamura et al. (1985) also reported similar results in the motor cortex. They found a significant decline with age in the number of dendrites of pyramidal cells in the motor cortex. More extensive electron microscopic examination of branching parameters in areas 46 (Peters, Sethares, and Moss, 1998) and 17 (Peters, Moss, and Sethares, 2001) in rhesus monkeys showed a substantial loss of branches from apical tufts of pyramidal cells. In a study by de Brabander et al. (1998), analysis of basal dendritic branching patterns of pyramidal cells in the human prefrontal cortex revealed a decrease in total dendritic length, total number of dendritic segments, and terminal dendritic length with age. Further analysis of total dendritic length, mean segment length, and segment number of pyramidal cells from areas 10 and 18 of human cortex found a 9%–11% decrease in total dendritic length (Jacobs et al., 1997, 2001). More recent investigations in nonhuman primates have also examined the state of neurons during aging. Neurons with long corticocortical projections from parietal and temporal regions to area 46 were targeted. Retrograde tract-tracing of these cortical pyramidal neurons filled with the dye Lucifer Yellow revealed age-related changes in the complexity of the apical dendrites in old compared to young monkeys. A minor difference in the length of dendritic segments in old animals was observed; however, this outcome was not statistically significant (Page et al., 2002). Duan et al. (2003) extended these findings and found regressive dendritic changes in apical dendrites in aged macaque monkeys compared to young animals. Sholl analysis of apical dendritic arbors revealed a reduction in the number of dendrites extending to 140 μm and 180 μm from the neuronal somata. Furthermore, significant age-related decreases in dendritic length and segment numbers were observed at the second branch order for apical dendrites (Figure 3.1). Studies in mice also demonstrate changes in dendritic arborization with age. Senescence-accelerated mice (SAMs), which are established models of aging (Takeda et al., 1991), display a gradual retraction

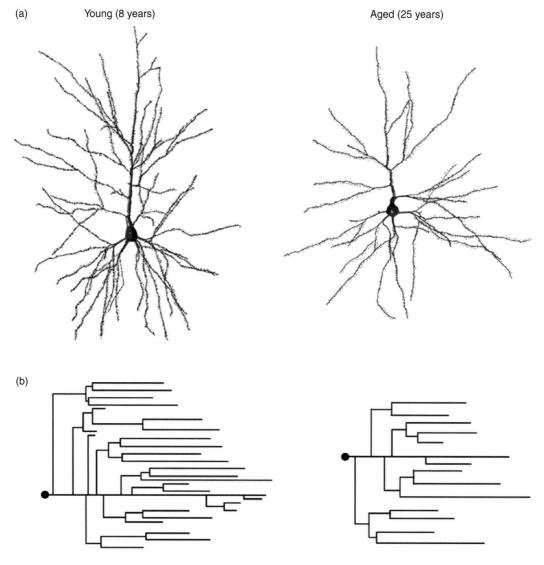

(a)   Young (8 years)   Aged (25 years)

(b)

Figure 3–1   Dendritic morphological aberrations in neocortical pyramidal neurons from young and aged rhesus monkeys. Panel (a) shows examples of a retrogradely traced neuron from young and aged monkeys, filled with Lucifer Yellow, and reconstructed in three dimensions. Panel (b) depicts dendrograms of apical dendrites from young and aged monkeys. Note the decrease in the number of dendritic branches as well as in branching complexity in aged animals compared to young animals. (Adapted from Duan et al., 2003.)

of apical dendrites with relative preservation of overall complexity (Shimada et al., 2006). There was a 45% decrease in total apical dendrite length and a decline in stem thickness. In contrast, no age-related changes were observed in basal dendrites. Immunohistochemical analysis of microtubule-associated protein 2 (MAP2), a dendritic marker, revealed a reduction in the immunoreactivity of MAP2 in the anterior and posterior cortex of aged SAMP10 mice, indicating that dendritic retraction was not limited to layers II/III pyramidal cells, but rather affects other layers as well (Shimada et al., 2006).

Dendritic Spine Changes during Aging

Although a dendrite is adjacent to many axons and other dendrites, functional connectivity occurs at specialized sites called synapses. The most common sites of synapses are dendritic spines. Dendritic spines are specialized membrane compartments that protrude from the dendritic shaft of a neuron. Spines typically have a volume ranging from less than 0.01 to 0.8 μm^3 and an average length of 0.5–2 μm (reviewed in Harris, 1999; Harris and Kater, 1994). Their morphology varies from stubby "neckless" spines, to mushroom shaped and long thin spines. It is estimated that the human brain contains more than 10^{13} dendritic spines (Nimchinsky et al., 2002). The linear density of spines on a mature neuron ranges between 1 and 10 spines per μm of dendritic length; however, spine density is not homogeneous throughout the dendritic tree, but increases at each order (Sorra and Harris, 2000). There is also a variation across cortical areas. Spine densities on basal dendrites in the prefrontal pole and orbitofrontal cortex of primates are generally higher than in neurons of the primary visual and somatosensory cortices (Elston, 2000; Jacobs et al., 2001).

Along with the dendritic alterations that occur during aging, changes in dendritic spines are also evident. Changes in spine length, volume, distribution, number, and morphology have been shown to have detrimental effects. Spine loss has been reported in humans (de Brabander et al., 1998; Nakamura et al., 1985; Scheibel et al., 1975), nonhuman primates (Peters, Sethares, and Moss, 1998) and aged canines (Mervis, 1978). Studies from young and old rhesus monkeys demonstrated a 25% decrease in spines from pyramidal cells in the prefrontal cortex in aged compared to young animals (Cupp and Uemura, 1980). Data from layer I neurons of the prefrontal cortex and the primary visual cortex of aged monkeys have reported a 40%–55% reduction in the number of synapses with age (Peters, Moss, and Sethares, 2001; Peters, Sethares, and Moss, 1998). These data have been corroborated by recent studies by Page et al. (2002) and Duan et al. (2003), who examined the differences in apical versus basal spine densities and changes in spine density along the length of the dendrite. Pyramidal cells from area 46 of aged macaque monkeys demonstrated significant loss of dendritic spines along all levels of dendrites. The total number of spines decreased by 28%–37% in the basal and apical dendrites of aged animals compared to young animals, while spine densities per μm of dendrite decreased by approximately 23% (Page et al., 2002). When examining spine loss along the dendrites it was found that there was an estimated 43% spine loss on proximal apical dendrites, whereas basal dendritic loss was estimated at 27% and occurred primarily on distal branches. Overall, there was a 25% reduction in both apical and basal dendrites in aged animals compared to controls (Duan et al., 2003). Similarly, studies by Jacobs et al. (1997, 2001) in human pyramidal cells from areas 10 and 18 found a 50% decrease in spine density. These observations together suggest that rather mild, yet significant, alterations in the morphologic integrity of select populations of cortical pyramidal cells are likely to be related to the cognitive impairment commonly seen in the course of aging. They point to the demise of a highly specific set of connections that are at higher risk during the natural course of aging, and as such represent key targets for preventive therapeutic interventions.

Age-Related Shifts in Glutamate Receptors

There is a strong link between dendritic changes and the postsynaptic effects of neurotransmitters. Neuronal alterations that occur during aging have a profound effect on the distribution of neurofilament proteins and can affect the dopaminergic and glutamatergic neurotransmitter systems. Changes to these systems render neurons vulnerable to impaired transmission, leading to disruptions in corticocortical pathways, such as those affected during aging and AD (Bussière et al., 2003a; Gazzaley et al., 1996; Hof et al., 1990, 2002; Morrison and Hof, 1997). Several studies have demonstrated an age-related shift in the expression of neurofilament protein (Hof et al., 1990; Vickers et al., 1993, 1994). Data from tract-tracing studies have demonstrated that the neurons of origin of long association corticocortical pathways, such as those connecting the superior temporal cortex and the prefrontal cortex, are particularly enriched in neurofilament protein (Hof et al., 1990, 1995; Morrison and Hof, 1997). The increase of neurofilament protein in these neurons is thought to make them more prone to the formation of neurofibrillary tangles (NFTs), thus rendering these pathways more vulnerable to dysfunction and degeneration.

The age-related changes in dendritic arborization and spine density described above can also affect the distribution of specific glutamate receptors. Glutamate is the major neurotransmitter in corticocortical systems and plays a crucial role in calcium-dependent processes. It had been established in macaque and patas monkeys that during aging, neurons furnishing short and long corticocortical projections significantly downregulate the expression of glutamate receptors: in particular, the ionotropic alpha-amino-3-hydroxy-5-methylisoxazole-4-propionic acid (AMPA) receptor, the glutamate receptor 2 (GluR2), and the N-methyl-D-aspartate receptor subunit 1 (NMDAR1) (Hof et al., 2002). GluR2 expression was decreased to a greater extent in the prefrontal cortex compared to other areas, such as the temporal cortex; whereas significant reductions in NMDAR1 occurred primarily in the long corticocortical projections from the superior temporal cortex (Hof et al., 2002). Furthermore, in aged macaque monkeys, NMDAR1 levels decrease specifically and consistently in the outer molecular layer of the dentate gyrus (Gazzaley et al., 1996). Aged monkeys exhibited a decrease in the fluorescence intensity of NMDAR1 in the outer molecular layer of the dentate gyrus compared to the inner molecular layer (Figure 3.2). This region receives input from the entorhinal cortex and is a region with particular vulnerability in aging and AD. Similar findings have been observed in aged humans. In the cholinergic basal forebrain of elderly humans, GluR2/3 appears to undergo an age-related downregulation (Ikonomovic and Armstrong, 1996; Ikonomovic et al., 2000; Mufson et al., 2003). These data suggest that the intradendritic parcellation of a neurotransmitter receptor is modifiable in an age-related and circuit-specific manner, and that such changes may provide a substrate for age-related memory impairment (Hof et al., 2002).

Age-Related Changes in Synaptic Transmission in the Macaque Monkey Prefrontal Cortex

Structural changes in aging neurons likely affect their electrophysiological properties. Studies of synaptic transmission demonstrate a significant decrease in excitatory synaptic transmission in the

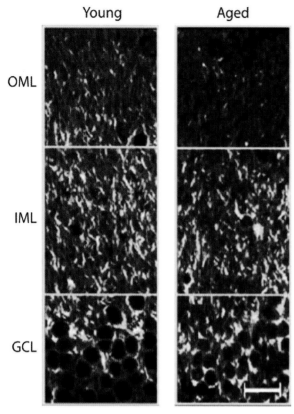

Figure 3–2   NMDAR1 expression decreases in the outer molecular layer (OML) of the dentate gyrus of aged monkeys. Immunolabeling of NMDAR1 in an aged monkey demonstrates a decrease in the immunofluorescence intensity within the OML compared to the IML. Moreover, the aged group had an overal decrease in NMDA1 fluorescence intensity compared to the young group. Localization of NMDAR1 immunofluorescence displayed as glow-scale pseudocolored CLSM images. The lower intensity signal is orange-red and higher intensities are displayed as yellow-white. Scale bar = 25 μm. (Adapted from Gazzaley et al., 1996.)

monkey prefrontal cortex, manifested as a reduction in the frequency of spontaneous excitatory postsynaptic currents (PSCs), the postsynaptic neuronal response to action potential-dependent and action potential-independent release of glutamate from presynaptic sites (Figure 3.3) (Luebke et al., 2004). The mechanisms underlying this reduction in spontaneous excitatory PSCs are unclear, although such synaptic changes may be the consequence of reduced postsynaptic structural and molecular substrates such as dendritic spines and glutamate receptors in aging (Duan et al., 2003; Hof et al., 2002; Jacobs et al., 1997; Page et al., 2002).

Another possible mechanism is an age-related decrease in the frequency of action potential firing in excitatory prefrontal cortex neurons, leading to decreased glutamate release and lower synaptic response frequency. This explanation is less compelling, considering that no changes in resting membrane potential or increases in action potential firing rates have been reported in prefrontal cortex layers II/III neurons from aged macaque monkeys (Chang et al., 2005). However, a lesser excitability and release of glutamate from other excitatory neurons projecting onto layers II/III pyramidal cells cannot be ruled out.

Whereas the overall level of excitatory input to pyramidal cells in the macaque prefrontal cortex decreases in aging, the postsynaptic non-NMDA glutamate receptors, although present in lower numbers (Hof et al., 2002), may be functionally intact. This view is supported by the fact that the amplitude distribution of miniature excitatory PSCs does not differ in neurons between old and young monkeys (Luebke et al., 2004). The kinetics of PSCs also reflect the distribution or composition of receptor subunits, and as such, alterations in the subunits likely result in alterations in the PSCs kinetics (Angulo et al., 1997; Geiger et al., 1995; Swanson, Kamboj, and Cull-Candy, 1997). The recent observation that the rise and decay times of the currents do not differ also suggests that glutamatergic non-NMDA receptors are not functionally altered in layers II/III pyramidal cells of the aging macaque prefrontal cortex (Luebke et al., 2004).

Further investigations in aged macaque monkey prefrontal cortex have shown that in contrast to excitatory transmission, a

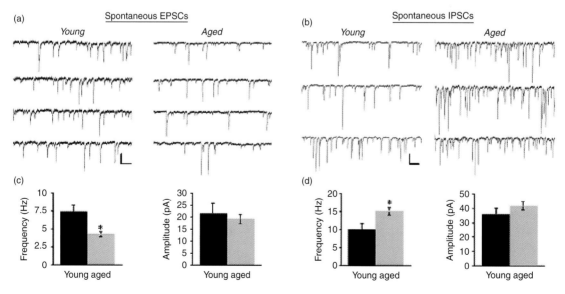

Figure 3–3   Decreased frequency of excitatory and increased frequency of inhibitory PSCs in layers II/III pyramidal cells from aged monkeys. (a) Representative traces of spontaneous excitatory PSCs obtained from cells from young (left) and aged (right) monkeys. (b) Representative traces of spontaneous inhibitory PSCs obtained from cells from young (left) and aged (right) monkeys. (c) Bar graphs showing the mean spontaneous EPSC frequency and amplitude values for young compared to aged pyramidal cells. (d) Bar graphs showing the mean spontaneous EPSC frequency and amplitude values for young vs. aged pyramidal cells. A and B Scale bar = 50 pA, 200 ms.

significant increase occurs in the level of inhibitory synaptic input to layers II/III pyramidal neurons, resulting in an increase in the frequency of spontaneous inhibitory PSCs (Luebke et al., 2004). Such increase in spontaneous inhibitory PSC frequency is likely the consequence of an increase in the action potential-dependent release of GABA from presynaptic interneurons, but this awaits confirmation from systematic investigations of GABAergic interneuron populations in old macaques. Notably, the amplitude and kinetics of inhibitory miniature PSCs is comparable in neurons from old and young macaques, suggesting that GABA$_A$ receptor function is not altered in the postsynaptic pyramidal neurons (Luebke et al., 2004).

Single and multiple unit recordings of prefrontal cortex pyramidal neurons in awake, behaving monkeys have shown that they exhibit increases and decreases in firing frequencies during different epochs of a working memory task. Because the sustained firing pattern of prefrontal cortex neurons reflects information encoding during the execution of a memory task, age-related alterations in firing patterns may be related to functional deficits with repercussions on cognitive performance. As an example of such functional changes, visual cortical neurons in aged monkeys display increased spontaneous AP firing rates in vivo, that are associated with degradation of stimulus selectivity (Leventhal et al., 2003). Similarly, a significant increase in AP firing rates was reported recently in layers II/III pyramidal neurons in the prefrontal cortex of aged macaque monkeys (Chang et al., 2005). Interestingly, these authors found that in the old animals, the firing rate exhibited a U-shaped relationship with performance on working memory tasks, the monkeys with very low and very high firing rates performing poorly and those exhibiting intermediate firing rates (which were still much higher than in young monkeys) performing well. This is consistent with the notion of a shift in optimal firing rate to higher frequencies in aging, which may reflect a compensatory response to failure in action potential (AP) conduction (Rosene, 2003) secondary to the myelin dystrophy known to occur in the macaque monkey prefrontal cortex during aging (Peters, 2002; Peters, Moss, and Sethares, 2001; Peters, Sethares, and Moss, 1998).

Neuropathological Changes during Alzheimer's Disease

AD Overview

AD is a progressive neurodegenerative disease of the central nervous system and accounts for approximately 80% of all dementia cases in the elderly (Terry, 2006). The pathological hallmarks of AD are extracellular senile plaques, composed of amyloid β (Aβ); and neurofibrillary tangles (NFTs), composed of hyperphosphorylated tau protein. During normal aging, plaques can be found in the neocortical, hippocampal, and entorhinal regions of cognitively normal elderly people, while NFTs can be found in the medial temporal areas. Despite the presence of these few plaques and NFTs, there does not seem to be a significant effect on cognition (Arriagada, Marzloff, and Hyman, 1992b; Goldman et al., 2001; Kazee and Johnson, 1998; Price et al., 1991). In addition, Hof and colleagues (1992) found that in spite of recognizable AD-like pathology, aging individuals may have enough of a neuronal reserve and may use different processing strategies to compensate for the cellular damage related to this degree of pathology (Grady et al., 2003; Hof et al., 1992). In contrast, in AD there are significantly more plaques and NFTs found throughout the brain, accompanied

by significant neuronal death and synapse loss in certain cortical regions and layers (Morrison and Hof, 1997). Memory loss, both semantic and episodic, reflects changes, both neurochemical and structural, in specific brain regions.

Hippocampal and Neocortical Pathology in AD

While it was previously thought that age-related memory loss is associated with neuronal death, quantitative stereologic methods have shown that neuronal death is limited in normal aging; however, there is considerable neuronal loss in AD (West, 1993; West et al., 1994). Unlike in normal aging where neurons become smaller with age, neurons are extensively lost from the neocortical and entorhinal regions in the AD brain with neuron loss reaching roughly 30% (Terry et al., 1981). Neuronal loss in the hippocampus is also evident, with an average cell loss of 68% in the CA1 region of AD patients compared to age-matched controls (West et al., 1994). Interestingly, it is in these regions that NFTs are first found to accumulate (Braak and Braak, 1997). Once established there, NFTs then appear in the inferior and lateral temporal, then parietal, occipital, and finally frontal cortices (Apostolova and Thompson, 2007). In the hippocampal region, NFTs are first seen in layers II and IV of the entorhinal cortex, then in the CA1 and subiculum, and finally in the CA3 (Hyman et al., 1984; Schonheit, Zarski, and Ohm, 2004), with greater structural atrophy in CA1 compared to CA3 (Apostolova et al., 2006; Braak and Braak, 1997). Amyloid plaques, in contrast, originate in the lateral temporal cortex and then appear in the inferior temporal, parietal, occipital, and frontal association cortices (Braak and Braak, 1990; Apostolova and Thompson, 2007). The decrease in volume observed in AD is reflected by significant neuron and synapse loss in the aforementioned regions (Hof et al., 2003; Hof and Morrison, 2004; Morrison and Hof, 1997, 2002; Price et al., 2001; West et al., 1994, 2004). This would indicate that the circuits that are most vulnerable to degeneration are the perforant path, which connects the entorhinal cortex with the dentate gyrus, and the long corticocortical projections that link association cortices such as the inferior temporal cortex and the prefrontal cortex (Morrison and Hof, 2002).

Volume loss is evident in the early stages of mild cognitive impairment (MCI) and can progress to severe atrophy in the late stages of AD. Region of interest analysis of MRI images from control and affected individuals has revealed significant changes in specific, defined brain regions. In normal aging, hippocampal atrophy, as determined by magnetic resonance imaging (MRI), occurs at an estimated rate of ~1.6%–1.7% annually. In MCI and AD, atrophy rates are significantly higher at 2.8%–3.7 % and 3.5%–4%, respectively (Jack et al., 1998, 2000) (see chapter 12). Similarly, in the entorhinal cortex, normal aging atrophy is approximately 1.7% annually, whereas in AD, atrophy rates are as high as 7% (Du et al., 2004). There is also evidence for volume loss in the white matter regions, with the greatest reductions occurring in the prefrontal cortex and anterior corpus callosum (Burke and Barnes, 2006; Hedden and Gabrieli, 2004). Diffusion tensor imaging (DTI) of white matter regions in aged brains indicate that there is a correlation between the reduction of white matter and changes in executive function, short-term recall, and processing speed (Gunning-Dixon and Raz, 2000).

Neurofilament Protein as a Marker for Neuronal Vulnerability in AD

While there is extensive neuronal pathology in AD, only a certain population of neurons and circuits are affected. The most vulnerable cells appear to be pyramidal neurons in the neocortex, in particular the corticocortically projecting cells (Hof et al., 1995; Nimchinsky et al., 1996). Vulnerable neurons have a distinct neurochemical phenotype, particularly with respect to cytoskeletal proteins such as tau and neurofilament. Studies in both humans and monkeys have demonstrated that certain subsets of pyramidal neurons in the neocortex are enriched with nonphosphorylated neurofilament protein (NPNFP) (Campbell and Morrison, 1989; Hof et al., 1990; Hof and Morrison, 1995). The distribution of NPNFP in these cells is restricted to the perikaryon and dendrites with the highest immunoreactivity concentrated in the cell body (Campbell and Morrison, 1989).

Interestingly, cells which are enriched with NPNFP have a high susceptibility for NFT formation (Bussière et al., 2003a; Hof and Morrison, 2004) (Figure 3.4). The distribution of NPNFP is of significant importance since it is present in the cellular networks that are implicated in many aspects of cognition and affected in AD (Goldman-Rakic, 1988). A study in the macaque monkey has shown that 90%–100% of the long association corticocortical projecting neurons, which are involved in prefrontal and temporal circuits, are enriched in NPNFP (Hof et al., 1995). Moreover, in humans, the laminar distribution of NPNFP in the visual association, prefrontal, and anterior cingulate cortices is similar to the distribution of NFT; and layers that have high NFT density no longer have many NPNFP-immunoreactive neurons (Hof et al., 1990). The presence of NPNFP can be correlated with clinical assessment as reflected in the Clinical Dementia Rating Scale (CDR). A CDR rating of 0.5 reflects mild cognitive impairment (MCI), CDR 1 reflects probable AD, CDR 2 is mild AD, CDR 3 is moderate AD, and CDR 5 is severe AD (Hof et al., 2003). A quantitative analysis of NPNFP-immunoreactive neurons with and without abnormally phosphorylated tau in layers III and V of area 9 in humans found that NPNFP-containing cells are observed as early as CDR 0.5 and increase with increasing CDR. Tau accumulation in this subset of cells can be seen in CDR 2 cases, and by CDR 3 almost all NPNFP+tau-containing neurons are in a degenerative state, whereas non-NPNFP-expressing neurons remain much less affected even with well-established AD (Bussière et al., 2003a).

AD, Amyloid Beta and Dendritic Complexity

There is substantial evidence suggesting that synapse loss observed in AD occurs early during the pathogenesis of the disease and is closely associated with disease severity. The robust numbers of plaques and NFTs present in AD brains have significant detrimental effect on neuronal circuitry, neuronal morphology, and synaptic capabilities. It has been suggested that the amyloid precursor protein (APP) and APP cleavage products play a crucial role in neuroprotection, interneuronal connections, and synaptic plasticity (Seabrook et al., 1999), and appear to be located in neuronal structures, including synaptic compartments (Schubert et al., 1991; Shigematsu, McGeer, and McGeer 1992). In AD, the accumulation of Aß, in particular the oligomeric forms of Aß, mediate neurotoxic effects including interrupting synaptic transmission, synaptic plasticity, and disrupting neuronal connectivity (Raymond, Ireland, and Abraham, 2003; Wang et al., 2002). Alterations in neuronal morphology and trajectory may cause disruption in neuronal signaling and function and are thought to ultimately contribute to the neuronal loss observed in AD (Knowles et al., 1999). It is established that there is significant neuronal loss in various brain regions in AD. This loss is accompanied by an approximate 45% decline in neocortical synapses (Terry et al., 1991). Studies in humans have demonstrated that neurons in AD undergo morphological alterations. Knowles et al. (1998) examined the effect of amyloid plaques on neuronal processes in humans by measuring mean curvature, length, and width distribution of dendritic projections. After examining over 5000 dendrites from 10 AD cases and five controls, it was found that dendrites were extremely dysmorphic in AD, with an increased curvature and curvilinear length. This was true for dendrites that traversed plaques, as well as those that were in close proximity to plaques (Knowles, Gomez-Isla, and Hyman, 1998). Similar results are seen in the acoustic cortex in AD brains. Neuronal loss, including loss of Cajal-Retzius cell, was observed in layer I. Morphological analysis of dendrites and dendritic spines in layers III and V revealed substantial alterations in dendritic arborization and a loss of dendritic spines in AD brains compared to controls (Baloyannis et al., 2007). Ultrastructural examination of spines showed that spines exhibited pathological abnormalities

(a)

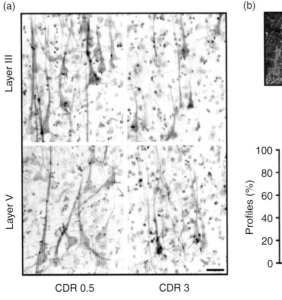

CDR 0.5   CDR 3

(b)

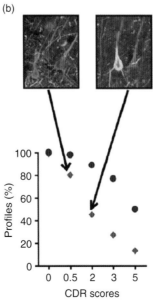

Figure 3–4 Selective neuronal vulnerability in AD. Panel (a) shows examples of nonphosphorylated neurofilament protein (NPNFP) containing pyramidal neurons. More NPNFP-immunoreactive neurons (brown) are present in the clinical dementia rating score (CDR 0.5) than in the CDR3 case. Panel (b) shows the distribution of NPNFP (red) and abnormally phosphorylated Tau (green) in layer III of affected individuals. More NPNFP-/tau-immunoreactive neurons are seen with increased disease severity. The proportion of surviving neurons can be assessed from stereologic analysis The neurons that do not express NPNFP epitopes are less affected in AD (blue dots) than neurons that do (red diamonds). Scale bar = 50 μm. (Adapted from Bussière et al., 2003a, b; Hof and Morrison, 2004.).

ranging from the accumulation in multivesicular bodies, vacuolization of the endoplasmic reticulum, and a reduction in the size of the spine apparatus (Baloyannis et al., 2007). Electron microscopy studies investigating synaptic loss and its relation to the stage of AD

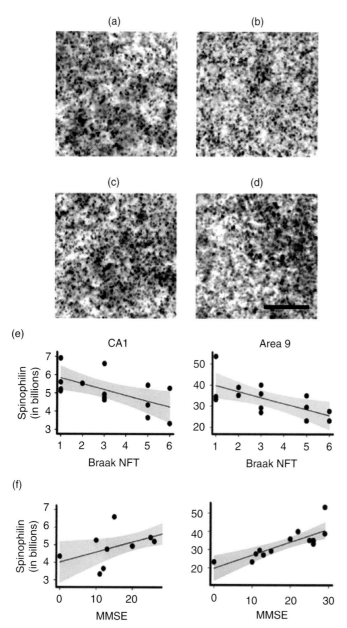

Figure 3–5 Decrease in spinophilin–immunoreactive puncta vs. Braak NFT staging and Mini-Mental State Examination scores in CA1 field and area 9. Panels a–d represent photomicrographs of spinophilin-immunoreactive puncta (100 × magnification). Spines not visualized at their optimal focal plane appear blurred.
(a) spinophilin-immunoreactive puncta in CA1 (CDR 0);
(b) spinophilin-immunoreactive puncta in CA1 (CDR 3);
(c) spinophilin-immunoreactive puncta in CA3 (CDR 0); and
(d) spinophilin immunoreactivity in CA3 section (CDR 3). Scale bar = 20 μm. E and F indicate regression lines with 95% confidence intervals of spinophilin-immunoreactive puncta (billions). Note the significant negative association between Braak NFT staging and total spinophilin-immunoreactive puncta in both the CA1 field and area 9 and the negative relationship between clinical indices. (Adapted from Akram et al., 2007.)

found that there was significant synaptic loss in the brains of patients with early onset AD compared to MCI and nondemented individuals. The loss of synapses also correlated with the Mimi-Mental State Exam (MMSE) score and other cognitive tests. Although there was a greater reduction in synapse numbers in MCI subjects than in nondemented subjects, it was not significant (Scheff et al., 2006). Other groups have corroborated these data and found a significant reduction in spine density as well as a decrease in overall dendritic area in AD patients when compared to age-matched controls (Einstein et al., 1994; Ferrer et al., 1990; Moolman et al., 2004). Recently, Akram and colleagues (2007), used stereologic assessment to estimate spine density in the hippocampus areas 9 and 18 in affected individuals with varying degrees of cognitive decline. They found that there was a significant decrease in spinophilin-reactive puncta which correlated to both Braak NTF staging and clinical severity, but not to Aβ accumulation. In addition, the total number of spinophilin-immunoreactive puncta in CA1 and area 9 were significantly related to MMSE scores, having a strong negative impact on cognition (Akram et al., 2007) (Figure 3.5).

3.5 Dendritic Complexity and Transgenic Mouse Models

Many investigators have examined the effect of Aβ on the type and frequencies of dendritic and synaptic abnormalities in the various transgenic mouse models of AD. These studies use transgenic mice containing varying forms of the mutant human APP and presenilin proteins. Whereas many of these transgenic mice do not exhibit neuronal loss, a few mouse strains (APP[23] and APP[751]/PS-1[M146L]) have been shown to have significant age-related neuronal loss in brain regions containing Aß aggregates (Calhoun et al., 1998; Schmitz et al., 2004). Moreover, neuronal loss was evident in regions which were distant from plaques, suggesting a putative role for intracellular Aß or soluble Aß in neurodegeneration (Schmitz et al., 2004). This phenomenon of neuronal degeneration in the absence of Aß plaques has also been observed in other presenilin 1 mutant mice, PS1[L286V] and PS1[H163R], where accelerated neuronal loss was observed in the frontal cortex and hippocampus. Interestingly, these animals showed signs of intracellular Aß in the aforementioned brain regions (Chui et al., 1999). Nonetheless, in most of these mouse models, the presence of elevated levels of soluble Aβ has been shown to lead to deficits in cognition, as well as reduction of long-term potentiation before plaque formation.

In the context of morphological abnormalities exerted by the extracellular Aß aggregates, neurons which are in close proximity to (10–40 μm), or passing through, Aß plaques undergo spine loss, shaft atrophy, bending, and develop axonal varicosities (Grutzendler et al., 2007; Le et al., 2001; Spires et al., 2005; Tsai et al., 2004). Other abnormalities, such as curvature of dendritic processes, decrease in dendritic density, abruptly terminated dendrite endings, and sprouting, are also evident. Segments farther than 40 μm from Aß plaques appeared unaffected (Grutzendler et al., 2007; Knowles, Gomez-Isla, and Hyman 1998; Tsai et al., 2004). In PSAPP mice, dendritic spine density and shaft diameter decreased by approximately 40% and 20%, respectively. Moreover, 34% of dendrites passing through plaques exhibit single or multiple sharp bends compared to dendrites further away (Grutzendler et al., 2007). In APP/PS1 and J20 mice, swollen bulbous, dystrophic neurites were seen along with a 36% reduction in the number of spines (Moolman et al., 2004). Other mouse models, including Tg2576, PDAPP, PDGF-APP, and APP[V717F] mice, also demonstrated a reduction of spine density in neurons in the CA1 and dentate gyrus of the hippocampus and in the somatosensory cortex (Games et al., 1995; Hsia et al., 1999; Jacobsen et al., 2006; Lanz, Carter, and Merchan, 2003; Mucke et al., 2000; Spires et al., 2005; Wu et al., 2004). Interestingly, while changes in spine density occurred in the presence of Aß aggregates, in some cases the reduction in spine density was independent of the manifestation of fibrillar Aß plaques and increased with age. A more extensive study by Rutten et al. (2005) in APP[751]/PS-1[M146L] mice supported previous studies indicating a reduction in synaptic boutons. They also reported that transgenic animals had larger presynaptic boutons while in close proximity to Aß plaques, as well as a decrease in volume compared to wild-type controls (Rutten et al., 2005). These data suggest that Aβ deposits and the surrounding microenvironment are toxic to neurons, leading to the alteration of dendrites, the elimination of spines, and the disruption of neuronal circuits in AD.

Recently, Alpár and colleagues (2006b) examined more global morphological changes in layer II/III pyramidal cells of the primary somatosensory cortex in the Tg2576 mouse model. No changes were observed in basal dendritic arbors; however, many unambiguous changes were found in the apical dendrites. Total length, surface area, and volume of basal dendrites were the same in Tg2576 mice and controls. There were no variations in the branching patterns of basal dendrites and no change in the number of dendritic endings or in dendritic density. In contrast, apical arbors were shorter in length and less branched than controls and exhibited an increase in diameter in the proximal dendritic segments and a reduction in the distal; however, the total surface area and total volume did not change significantly. Spine density was reduced in both apical and basal arbors along the entire course of the dendrite (Alpár et al., 2006b). It is unclear if the actions of mutated human APP (hAPP) or the elevated Aß levels contribute to the morphological aberrations observed. To address this, many studies in APP null mice and mice expressing nonmutated APP have been performed. In APP null mice, there was a reduction in dendritic length and branching (Perez et al., 1997; Seabrook et al., 1999). In contrast, mice expressing nonmutated hAPP exhibited no overall difference in dendritic length. Interestingly, there was a significant increase in the total surface area and volume of basal dendrites in transgenic mice compared to controls (Alpár et al., 2006a). Whereas there was a shortening of third- and fourth-order branching, the average diameter of second-, third-, and fourth-order segments was larger in hAPP mice than in controls.

It should be noted that in the majority of the studies discussed above, changes in cellular morphology and synaptic density were identified once there was established pathology. Few studies have addressed the development of changes, at the cellular level, prior to visible pathology. High-resolution magnetic resonance microscopy has shown that in PDAPP mice there was a 12.3% reduction in hippocampal volume in Tg2576 mice compared to controls prior to amyloid deposition (Redwine et al., 2003). Moreover, volume estimates in the dentate gyrus demonstrated a 28% volume deficit. This volume loss persisted in transgenic mice, while control mice exhibited an increase in hippocampal volume with age (Redwine et al., 2003).

Tau and Dendritic Complexity

The mechanism of Tau-mediated neuronal death in AD remains elusive. The abnormal phosphorylation of Tau is considered one of the earliest signs of neuronal degeneration and precedes NFT formation and plaque aggregation. It is the hyperphosphorylation of tau that leads to the disengagement of tau from microtubules, which can then have detrimental effects on cellular morphology

and anterograde axonal transport of essential molecules and organelles to the synapse (Ballatore, Lee, and Trojanowski, 2007; Roy et al., 2005). The formation of NFTs is thought to be a multistep process beginning with the detachment of tau from microtubules due to an increased rate in phosphorylation and/or a decreased rate of dephosphorylation. The free, unbound tau can then undergo misfolding and can become more prone to aggregation into paired helical filaments which can then further aggregate into NFTs (Ballatore, Lee, and Trojanowski, 2007). The distribution of NFTs in AD can become widespread and can be found in the hippocampus, neocortex, and limbic neurons, and moves from the axon to somatodendritic compartments (Delacourte and Buée, 2000; Yankner, Lu, and Loerch, 2007). Furthermore, the distribution and number of NFT deposits correlates with neuronal loss, synapse loss, and the degree of cognitive impairment observed in AD (Arriagada et al., 1992a; Braak and Braak, 1991; Terry et al., 1991).

Many studies in a wide variety of mouse models have demonstrated neuronal loss and synaptic deficiency in the presence of NFTs. It is important to note that the transgenic mice harboring only tau mutations develop NFTs and related tau abnormalities and mimic human tauopathies; however, they do not develop Aβ pathology. Transgenic mice harboring the P103L tau mutation (JNPL3) exhibit motor and behavioral deficits, with age- and gene-dose-dependent development of NFT and neuronal loss as early as 6.5 months in hemizygous mice and 4.5 months in homozygous mice (Lewis et al., 2000). In another mouse model expressing the P301L mutation (rTg(tau(P301L))4510), under a different promoter than the JNPL3 mouse, NFT pathology was observed in the neocortex, hippocampus, and limbic structures with increasing age. Significant memory deficits were also evident and were accompanied by gross forebrain atrophy and a prominent loss of neurons, most strikingly in CA1 (Ramsden et al., 2005).

Whereas many studies have investigated the presence of tau pathology and changes in cognition, few studies have investigated the effect of NFTs on dendrites, dendritic spines, and synaptic plasticity. In a recent report utilizing organotypic hippocampal slice cultures infected with Sindbis virus containing an EGFP-Tau construct, it was found that while there was a loss of individual neurons over time, spine density and spine morphology were essentially the same as in controls (Shahani et al., 2006). In contrast, another group transfected tau into mature hippocampal neurons and found that there was an improper distribution of tau into the somatodendritic compartment with concomitant degeneration of synapses, as seen by the disappearance of spines and of presynaptic markers, bassoon and piccolo, and postsynaptic markers such as PSD95, neuroligin, AMPA, and NMDA receptor (NMDAR) subunits (Thies and Mandelkow, 2007).

Recently, a triple transgenic mouse containing $PS1_{M146V}$, APP_{Swe}, and tau_{P301L} transgenes was generated which exhibits both Aβ and tau pathology. Basal synaptic transmission and long-term potentiation were assessed, and it was demonstrated that the triple transgenic mice exhibited significant impairment in synaptic capabilities compared to control littermates as early as 6 months of age (Oddo et al., 2003). Studies utilizing a transgenic mouse model that expresses all 6 isoforms of human tau, but not mutant tau (Andorfer et al., 2003), have also been undertaken. These mice exhibit tau pathology in the neocortex and hippocampus, along with overt neuronal loss in patterns similar to that occurring in NFTs in human tauopathies (Andorfer et al., 2003, 2005). Preliminary data examining dendritic arbors and dendritic spine density demonstrated a reduction in the total number of spines (~35%) as well as a decrease in spine density, which became more severe with age. While it appears that tau can have detrimental effects on synaptic dysfunction, more research using mutant tau transgenic mice needs to be completed.

Other Dementias

Dementia with Lewy bodies (DLB) is the second most common dementia and is characterized by progressive cognitive decline, early onset hallucinations, and delusions, Parkinsonism, and fluctuating course (McKeith et al., 1996). The pathological hallmarks for DLB are synuclein-rich, concentric, intracytoplasmic neuronal deposits referred to as Lewy bodies. Neocortical Lewy bodies are found in approximately 20%–35% of all dementias (Ferman and Boeve, 2007). Many of the regions affected in DLB are also affected in AD; thus it is difficult to distinguish and diagnose one from the other. Lewy bodies can be found throughout various brain regions, including the dorsal motor nucleus of the vagus, locus coeruleus, midbrain tegmentun, hypothalamus, basal forebrain, amygdala, and temporal cortex (Ferman and Boeve, 2007). In contrast to AD, DLB has little cortical atrophy and is primarily localized to the midbrain with some preservation of the hippocampus, inferior temporal, and orbitofrontal cortices (Ballmaier et al., 2004). Recent voxel-based morphometry analyses are able to discern distinct cortical atrophy that occurs in DLB. It has been shown that there is a discrete amount of gray matter loss in cholinergic-rich regions of the nucleus basalis of Meynert in the basal forebrain and dorsal midbrain (Whitwell et al., 2007). A recent Golgi study in human brains from DLB patients showed a decrease in dendritic length and spine density on medium spiny neurons in the dorsolateral prefrontal and lateral orbitofrontal circuits compared to age-matched controls and those with AD (Zaja-Milatovic et al., 2006). In another study examining the brains of individuals with Parkinson's disease with dementia, it was found that there was significant loss of noradrenergic neurons in the locus coeruleus compared to individuals with Parkinson's only and age-matched controls. There was also a substantial loss of dendritic branches and dendritic spines (Baloyannis, Costa, and Baloyannis, 2006). As with AD, more research needs to be done in order to unravel the morphological changes that occur during the pathological process. This would aid in the diagnosis of DLB from AD and also in the development of possible therapeutic interventions.

The Relationship Between Neural and Endocrine Senescence

Estrogens and Aging

A difficult challenge in brain aging research is to determine the relationships between neural senescence and the aging of other systems. Reproductive senescence is of particular interest since there are significant gender differences in the aging brain with greater changes in brain structure, function, and metabolism between females and males. The role of estrogens in controlling the reproductive axis at the level of the hypothalamus is well characterized (Fink, 1986). However, estrogens also affect the nervous system in many ways by impacting synaptic communication in brain regions involved in cognitive function, such as the hippocampus, and as a result can influence verbal fluency, verbal memory tests, performance on spatial tasks, fine motor skills, and symptoms of various neurodegenerative diseases (Kimura, 1992; Markou, Duka, and Prelevic, 2005; Morrison and Hof, 1997). Murphy et al. (1996) have demonstrated that age-related loss of

neurons in the hippocampus and parietal lobes was significantly greater in females than males. Interestingly, these regions are essential for cognitive function, and it is well known that women have a higher age-related risk of AD and have a greater disease severity than men (Markou, Duka, and Prelevic, 2005). Recently, comparative MRI imaging of postmenopausal women who were receiving estrogen replacement therapy and those who were not revealed that women receiving estrogen had significantly smaller ventricles and greater white matter volumes compared to nonusers (Ha, Xu, and Janowsky, 2007). These results were corroborated by voxel-based morphometry analysis of postmenopausal women, which demonstrated that postmenopausal women who had hormone replacement had sparing of gray matter throughout the cortex, smaller ventricles, and more white matter compared to postmenopausal non-hormone users (Erickson et al., 2005). These studies suggest that estrogen is neuroprotective and can aid in white matter preservation; however, the underlying mechanism is still unknown.

Estrogens act via two intracellular receptors: estrogen receptor α (ERα) and estrogen receptor β (ERβ). The expression and distribution of these receptors are quite different. ERα is moderately to highly expressed in the pituitary, kidney, and adrenal gland, with limited expression in the brain (Kuiper et al., 1997; Shughrue, Scrimo, and Merchenthaler, 2000). It has been demonstrated that ERα is present in the cortex and basal forebrain (Shughrue, Lane, and Merchenthaler, 1997), as well as in CA1 spines and synapses, and that its expression decreases with age (Adams et al., 2002; Milner et al., 2001). ERβ, in contrast, is highly expressed in the ovaries, uterus, and brain regions such as the hippocampus, neocortex, cerebellum, amygdala, and hypothalamus (Kuiper et al., 1997, 1998; Shughrue, Scrimo, and Merchenthaler, 2000). This region-specific expression of ERα and ERβ may be important in determining the physiological responses of neuronal populations to estrogen, or lack thereof, in normal and pathological aging processes.

Estrogen also has an impact on synaptic activity. Woolley and colleagues (Woolley et al., 1990) showed that dendritic spine density in CA1 pyramidal cells is sensitive to fluctuating estrogen levels in young animals. Moreover, experimentally-induced estrogen depletion studies in rats showed that there was a decrease in spine density in rat CA1 pyramidal cells (Woolley et al., 1990; Woolley and McEwen, 1992), while replacement with estradiol reversed this effect (Woolley and McEwen, 1993). This effect is important, since the changes in estrogen appear to affect a brain region involved in cognitive processing. Interestingly, estrogen replacement in aged rats failed to increase spine density in CA1 compared to rats that did not receive estrogen (Adams et al., 2001). This can have significant consequences in regards to aging where estrogen levels change and hippocampal-dependent functions decline (Morrison and Hof, 2007).

Nonhuman Primate Studies

Recently, nonhuman primate studies have been undertaken that examined the effect of estrogen on synaptic plasticity and aging by experimentally inducing estrogen depletion and replacement. The data from these studies are consistent with the findings in young rats; however, in contrast to aged rats, aged monkeys were just as responsive to estrogen as young monkeys. Ovariectomy (OVX) results in a profound loss of spines in the CA1 region (Leranth, Shanabrough, and Redmond, 2002) and the prefrontal cortex (Tang et al., 2004). Evidence suggests that there is a substantially greater cognitive benefit of estrogen treatment in aged monkeys that underwent OVX compared to young adults, particularly on tests emphasizing the integrity of the dorsolateral prefrontal cortex (Lacreuse, 2006). OVX young African green monkeys and ovariectomized young and aged female rhesus monkeys had an increase in spine density in CA1 after treatment with 17β-estradiol (Hao et al., 2003; Leranth, Shanabrough, and Redmond, 2002). In addition, layer I pyramidal neurons in the dorsal prefrontal cortex also displayed an estrogen-induced increase in spine density (Tang et al., 2004) as well as enhancement of cholinergic and monoaminergic inputs (Kritzer and Kohama, 1999; Tinkler, Tobin, and Voytko, 2004). Further in-depth analysis on the morphology of spines in 17β-estradiol-treated ovariectomized young and aged monkeys revealed an increase in small thin spines (Hao et al., 2006). This suggests that 17β-estradiol promoted a shift in spine motility, NMDA receptor-mediated activity, and learning. These data support a behavioral study by Rapp and colleagues (Rapp, Morrison, and Roberts, 2003) in which aged female monkeys were overiectomized and treated with a cyclical regimen of estradiol or vehicle. Here it was shown that estrogen-treated monkeys had enhanced performance on both a hippocampal dependant task, delayed nonmatching to sample, and on a delayed response prefrontal dependant task sensitive to age (Rapp, Morrison, and Roberts, 2003). Hao et al. (2007) extended the analysis of estrogen's influence on cognition and neuronal morphology in ovariectomized aged and young adult monkeys treated equivalently with the same cyclical estradiol regimen. The data collected revealed that in young adult animals, treatment with estradiol did not enhance cognitive performance relative to vehicle control groups, but did result in an increase in spine density with a higher complement of small, thin, spines in layer III pyramidal neurons. Aged ovariectomized monkeys, that did not receive estradiol, exhibited a decrease in dendritic length and number of branches, as well as a decrease in spine density with a pronounced lack of long, thin spines. This effect was partially recovered in estradiol-treated aged ovariectomized monkeys, returning spine density to levels of vehicle-treated young adults (Hao et al., 2007). These data demonstrate the effect of estrogen on cognition and aging and suggest the use of estrogen as a therapeutic for reversal of age-related memory loss.

Conclusion

The transition from circumscribed memory impairment to the dramatic loss of cognitive abilities that accompanies AD requires progressive development of neocortical pathology. Neuroimaging techniques offer remarkable power to understand normal and pathological brain aging by providing spatially detailed information on the extent and trajectory of pathology as it develops into disease. During normal aging, changes in dendritic and synaptic integrity, and not overt neuronal loss, are evident and render otherwise intact circuits vulnerable to compromised communication and thus cognitive impairment. In AD, however, cognitive decline can be attributed to neuronal loss, as well as alteration in dendritic and synaptic plasticity, caused by the presence of amyloid plaques and NFTs. Although many studies have begun to elucidate the mechanistic relationships between synaptic integrity and age-associated cognitive impairment, there is still much that remains unknown. Through linking human neuropathology with data from various experimental animal models, correlations have emerged between the distribution of cellular pathological changes, neurochemical characteristics of vulnerable cells, and at-risk

cortical circuits. Understanding these mechanisms will help determine when and how dendrites contribute to the brain's capacity for memory, perception, and action, and aid in the development of new therapeutic avenues to prevent or cure cognitive impairment.

Acknowledgements

We thank W.G.M. Janssen, B. Wicinski, J. Hao, S. Wearne, J. Luebke, and members of the Hof and Morrison laboratories, who have been involved in our studies of brain aging, for their support. This work was supported by NIH grants AG02219, AG05138, AG06647, and AG016765.

References

Adams, M. M., Fink, S. E., Shah, R. A., Janssen, W. G., Hayashi, S., Milner, T. A. et al. (2002). Estrogen and aging affect the subcellular distribution of estrogen receptor-alpha in the hippocampus of female rats. *Journal of Neuroscience*, 22: 3608–3614.

Adams, M. M., Smith, T. D., Moga, D., Gallagher, M., Wang, Y., Wolfe, B. B. et al. (2001). Hippocampal dependent learning ability correlates with N-methyl-D-aspartate (NMDA) receptor levels in CA3 neurons of young and aged rats. *Journal of Comparative Neurology*, 432: 230–243.

Akram, A., Christoffel, D., Rocher, A. B., Bouras, C., Kovari, E., Perl, D. P. et al. (2007). Stereologic estimates of total spinophilin-immunoreactive spine number in area 9 and the CA1 field: Relationship with the progression of Alzheimer's disease. *Neurobiology of Aging*, 29: 1296–1307.

Alpar, A., Ueberham, U., Bruckner, M. K., Arendt, T., and Gartner, U. (2006a). The expression of wild-type human amyloid precursor protein affects the dendritic phenotype of neocortical pyramidal neurons in transgenic mice. *International Journal of Developmental Neuroscience*, 24: 133–40.

Alpar, A., Ueberham, U., Bruckner, M. K., Seeger, G., Arendt, T., and Gartner, U. (2006b). Different dendrite and dendritic spine alterations in basal and apical arbors in mutant human amyloid precursor protein transgenic mice. *Brain Research*, 1099: 189–198.

Andorfer, C., Acker, C. M., Kress, Y., Hof, P. R., Duff, K., and Davies, P. (2005). Cell-cycle reentry and cell death in transgenic mice expressing nonmutant human tau isoforms. *Journal of Neuroscience*, 25: 5446–5454.

Andorfer, C., Kress, Y., Espinoza, M., de Silva, R., Tucker, K. L., Barde, Y. A. et al. (2003). Hyperphosphorylation and aggregation of tau in mice expressing normal human tau isoforms. *Journal of Neurochemistry*, 86: 582–590.

Angulo, M. C., Lambolez, B., Audinat, E., Hestrin, S., and Rossier, J. (1997). Subunit composition, kinetic, and permeation properties of AMPA receptors in single neocortical nonpyramidal cells. *Journal of Neuroscience*, 17: 6685–6696.

Apostolova, L. G., Dinov, I. D., Dutton, R. A., Hayashi, K. M., Toga, A. W., Cummings, J. L. et al. (2006). 3D comparison of hippocampal atrophy in amnestic mild cognitive impairment and Alzheimer's disease. *Brain*, 129: 2867–2873.

Apostolova, L. G. and Thompson, P. M. (2007). Brain mapping as a tool to study neurodegeneration. *Neurotherapeutics*, 4: 387–400.

Arriagada, P. V., Growdon, J. H., Hedley-Whyte, E. T., and Hyman, B. T. (1992a). Neurofibrillary tangles but not senile plaques parallel duration and severity of Alzheimer's disease. *Neurology*, 42: 631–639.

Arriagada, P. V., Marzloff, K., and Hyman, B. T. (1992b). Distribution of Alzheimer-type pathologic changes in nondemented elderly individuals matches the pattern in Alzheimer's disease. *Neurology*, 42: 1681–1688.

Ballatore, C., Lee, V. M., and Trojanowski, J. Q. (2007). Tau-mediated neurodegeneration in Alzheimer's disease and related disorders. *Nature Reviews Neuroscience*, 8: 663–672.

Ballmaier, M., O'Brien, J. T., Burton, E. J., Thompson, P. M., Rex, D. E., Narr, K. L. et al. (2004). Comparing gray matter loss profiles between dementia with Lewy bodies and Alzheimer's disease using cortical pattern matching: diagnosis and gender effects. *Neuroimage*, 23: 325–335.

Baloyannis, S. J., Costa, V., and Baloyannis, I. S. (2006). Morphological alterations of the synapses in the locus coeruleus in Parkinson's disease. *Journal of Neurological Sciences*, 248: 35–41.

Baloyannis, S. J., Costa, V., Mauroudis, I., Psaroulis, D., Manolides, S. L., and Manolides, L. S. (2007). Dendritic and spinal pathology in the acoustic cortex in Alzheimer's disease: morphological and morphometric estimation by Golgi technique and electron microscopy. *Acta Otolaryngologica*, 127: 351–354.

Braak, H. and Braak, E. (1990). Alzheimer's disease: striatal amyloid deposits and neurofibrillary changes. *Journal of Neuropathology and Experimental Neurology*, 49: 215–224.

Braak, H. and Braak, E. (1991). Neuropathological stageing of Alzheimer-related changes. *Acta Neuropathologica*, 82: 239–259.

Braak, H. and Braak, E. (1997). Diagnostic criteria for neuropathologic assessment of Alzheimer's disease. *Neurobiology of Aging*, 18: S85–S88.

Burke, S. N. and Barnes, C. A. (2006). Neural plasticity in the ageing brain. *Nature Reviews Neuroscience*, 7: 30–40.

Bussière, T., Giannakopoulos, P., Bouras, C., Perl, D. P., Morrison, J. H., and Hof, P. R. (2003a). Progressive degeneration of nonphosphorylated neurofilament protein-enriched pyramidal neurons predicts cognitive impairment in Alzheimer's disease: Stereologic analysis of prefrontal cortex area 9. *Journal of Comparative Neurology*, 463: 281–302.

Bussière, T., Gold, G., Kövari, E., Giannakopoulos, P., Bouras, C., Perl, D. P. et al. (2003b). Stereologic analysis of neurofibrillary tangle formation in prefrontal cortex area 9 in aging and Alzheimer's disease. *Neuroscience*, 117: 577–592.

Calhoun, M. E., Wiederhold, K. H., Abramowski, D., Phinney, A. L., Probst, A., Sturchler-Pierrat, C. et al. (1998). Neuron loss in APP transgenic mice. *Nature*, 395: 755–756.

Campbell, M. J. and Morrison, J. H. (1989). Monoclonal antibody to neurofilament protein (SMI-32) labels a subpopulation of pyramidal neurons in the human and monkey neocortex. *Journal of Comparative Neurology*, 282: 191–205.

Chang, Y. M., Rosene, D. L., Killiany, R. J., Mangiamele, L. A., and Luebke, J. I. (2005). Increased action potential firing rates of layer 2/3 pyramidal cells in the prefrontal cortex are significantly related to cognitive performance in aged monkeys. *Cerebral Cortex*, 15: 409–418.

Chen, X. Y. and Wolpaw, J. R. (1994). Triceps surae motoneuron morphology in the rat: a quantitative light microscopic study. *Journal of Comparative Neurology*, 343: 143–157.

Chui, D. H., Tanahashi, H., Ozawa, K., Ikeda, S., Checler, F., Ueda, O. et al. (1999). Transgenic mice with Alzheimer presenilin 1 mutations show accelerated neurodegeneration without amyloid plaque formation. *Nature Medicine*, 5: 560–564.

Cupp, C. J. and Uemura, E. (1980). Age-related changes in prefrontal cortex of Macaca mulatta: quantitative analysis of dendritic branching patterns. *Experimental Neurology*, 69: 143–163.

de Brabander, J. M., Kramers, R. J., and Uylings, H. B. (1998). Layer-specific dendritic regression of pyramidal cells with ageing in the human prefrontal cortex. *European Journal of Neuroscience*, 10: 1261–1269.

DeCarli, C., Massaro, J., Harvey, D., Hald, J., Tullberg, M., Au, R. et al. (2005). Measures of brain morphology and infarction in the framingham heart study: Establishing what is normal. *Neurobiology of Aging*, 26: 491–510.

Delacourte, A. and Buée, L. (2000). Tau pathology: A marker of neurodegenerative disorders. *Current Opinion in Neurology*, 13: 371–376.

Drachman, D. A. (2006). Aging of the brain, entropy, and Alzheimer disease. *Neurology*, 67: 1340–1352.

Du, A. T., Schuff, N., Kramer, J. H., Ganzer, S., Zhu, X. P., Jagust, W. J. et al. (2004). Higher atrophy rate of entorhinal cortex than hippocampus in AD. *Neurology*, 62: 422–427.

Duan, H., Wearne, S. L., Rocher, A. B., Macedo, A., Morrison, J. H., and Hof, P. R. (2003). Age-related dendritic and spine changes in corticocortically projecting neurons in macaque monkeys. *Cerebral Cortex*, 13: 950–961.

Einstein, G., Buranosky, R., and Crain, B. J. (1994). Dendritic pathology of granule cells in Alzheimer's disease is unrelated to neuritic plaques. *Journal of Neuroscience*, 14: 5077–5088.

Elston, G. N. (2000). Pyramidal cells of the frontal lobe: All the more spinous to think with. *Journal of Neuroscience*, 20: RC95.

Erickson, K. I., Colcombe, S. J., Raz, N., Korol, D. L., Scalf, P., Webb, A. et al., (2005). Selective sparing of brain tissue in postmenopausal women receiving hormone replacement therapy. *Neurobiology of Aging*, 26: 1205–1213.

Ferman, T. J. and Boeve, B. F. (2007). Dementia with Lewy bodies. Neurologic Clinics, 25, 741–760, vii.

Ferrer, I., Guionnet, N., Cruz-Sanchez, F., and Tuñon, T. (1990). Neuronal alterations in patients with dementia: A Golgi study on biopsy samples. *Neuroscience Letters*, 114: 11–16.

Fink, G. (1986). The endocrine control of ovulation. *Scientific Progress*, 70: 403–423.

Games, D., Adams, D., Alessandrini, R., Barbour, R., Berthelette, P., Blackwell, C. et al. (1995). Alzheimer-type neuropathology in transgenic mice over-expressing V717F beta-amyloid precursor protein. *Nature*, 373: 523–527.

Gazzaley, A. H., Siegel, S. J., Kordower, J. H., Mufson, E. J., and Morrison, J. H. (1996). Circuit-specific alterations of N-methyl-D-aspartate receptor subunit 1 in the dentate gyrus of aged monkeys. *Proceedings of the National Academy of Sciences of the USA*, 93, 3121–3125.

Gazzaley, A. H., Thakker, M. M., Hof, P. R., and Morrison, J. H. (1997). Preserved number of entorhinal cortex layer II neurons in aged macaque monkeys. *Neurobiology of Aging*, 18: 549–553.

Geiger, J. R., Melcher, T., Koh, D. S., Sakmann, B., Seeburg, P. H., Jonas, P. et al. (1995). Relative abundance of subunit mRNAs determines gating and Ca2+ permeability of AMPA receptors in principal neurons and interneurons in rat CNS. *Neuron*, 15: 193–204.

Goldman, W. P., Price, J. L., Storandt, M., Grant, E. A., McKeel, D. W., Jr., Rubin, E. H. et al. (2001). Absence of cognitive impairment or decline in preclinical Alzheimer's disease. *Neurology*, 56: 361–367.

Goldman-Rakic, P. S. (1988). Topography of cognition: Parallel distributed networks in primate association cortex. *Annual Review Neuroscience*, 11: 137–156.

Grady, C. L., McIntosh, A. R., Beig, S., Keightley, M. L., Burian, H., and Black, S. E. (2003). Evidence from functional neuroimaging of a compensatory prefrontal network in Alzheimer's disease. *Journal of Neuroscience*, 23: 986–993.

Grutzendler, J., Helmin, K., Tsai, J., and Gan, W. B. (2007). Various dendritic abnormalities are associated with fibrillar amyloid deposits in Alzheimer's disease. *Annals of the New York Academy of Sciences*, 1097: 30–39.

Gunning-Dixon, F. M. and Raz, N. (2000). The cognitive correlates of white matter abnormalities in normal aging: A quantitative review. *Neuropsychology*, 14: 224–232.

Ha, D. M., Xu, J., and Janowsky, J. S. (2007). Preliminary evidence that long-term estrogen use reduces white matter loss in aging. *Neurobiology of Aging*, 28: 1936–1940.

Hao, J., Janssen, W. G., Tang, Y., Roberts, J. A., McKay, H., Lasley, B. et al. (2003). Estrogen increases the number of spinophilin-immunoreactive spines in the hippocampus of young and aged female rhesus monkeys. *Journal of Comparative Neurology*, 465, 540–550.

Hao, J., Rapp, P. R., Leffler, A. E., Leffler, S. R., Janssen, W. G., Lou, W. et al. (2006). Estrogen alters spine number and morphology in prefrontal cortex of aged female rhesus monkeys. *Journal of Neuroscience*, 26: 2571–2578.

Hao, J., Rapp, P. R., Janssen, W. G., Lou, W., Lasley, B. L., Hof, P. R., and Morrison, J. H. (2007). Interactive effects of age and estrogen on cognition and pyramidal neurons in monkey prefrontal cortex. *Proceedings of the National Academy of Sciences of the USA*, 104, 11465–11470.

Harris, K. M. (1999). Structure, development, and plasticity of dendritic spines. *Current Opinion on Neurobiology*, 9: 343–348.

Harris, K. M. and Kater, S. B. (1994). Dendritic spines: Cellular specializations imparting both stability and flexibility to synaptic function. *Annual Reviews of Neuroscience*, 17: 341–371.

Hedden, T. and Gabrieli, J. D. (2004). Insights into the ageing mind: a view from cognitive neuroscience. *Nature Reviews of Neuroscience*, 5: 87–96.

Hof, P. R., Bierer, L. M., Perl, D. P., Delacourte, A., Buée, L., Bouras, C., et al. (1992). Evidence for early vulnerability of the medial and inferior aspects of the temporal lobe in an 82-year-old patient with preclinical signs of dementia. Regional and laminar distribution of neurofibrillary tangles and senile plaques. *Archives of Neurology*, 49: 946–953.

Hof, P. R., Bussière, T., Gold, G., Kövari, E., Giannakopoulos, P., Bouras, C. et al. (2003). Stereologic evidence for persistence of viable neurons in layer

II of the entorhinal cortex and the CA1 field in Alzheimer disease. *Journal of Neuropathology and Experimental Neurology*, 62: 55–67.

Hof, P. R., Cox, K., and Morrison, J. H. (1990). Quantitative analysis of a vulnerable subset of pyramidal neurons in Alzheimer's disease: I. Superior frontal and inferior temporal cortex. *Journal of Comparative Neurology*, 301: 44–54.

Hof, P. R., Duan, H., Page, T. L., Einstein, M., Wicinski, B., He, Y., et al. (2002). Age-related changes in GluR2 and NMDAR1 glutamate receptor subunit protein immunoreactivity in corticocortically projecting neurons in macaque and patas monkeys. *Brain Research*, 928: 175–186.

Hof, P. R. and Morrison, J. H. (1995). Neurofilament protein defines regional patterns of cortical organization in the macaque monkey visual system: a quantitative immunohistochemical analysis. *Journal of Comparative Neurology*, 352: 161–186.

Hof, P. R. and Morrison, J. H. (2004). The aging brain: morphomolecular senescence of cortical circuits. *Trends of Neuroscience*, 27: 607–613.

Hof, P. R., Nimchinsky, E. A., and Morrison, J. H. (1995). Neurochemical phenotype of corticocortical connections in the macaque monkey: Quantitative analysis of a subset of neurofilament protein-immunoreactive projection neurons in frontal, parietal, temporal, and cingulate cortices. *Journal of Comparative Neurology*, 362: 109–133.

Hsia, A. Y., Masliah, E., McConlogue, L., Yu, G. Q., Tatsuno, G., Hu, K. et al. (1999). Plaque-independent disruption of neural circuits in Alzheimer's disease mouse models. *Proceedings of the National Academy of Sciences of the USA*, 96: 3228–3233.

Hyman, B. T., Van Hoesen, G. W., Damasio, A. R., and Barnes, C. L. (1984). Alzheimer's disease: cell-specific pathology isolates the hippocampal formation. *Science*, 225: 1168–1170.

Ikonomovic, M. D. and Armstrong, D. M. (1996). Distribution of AMPA receptor subunits in the nucleus basalis of Meynert in aged humans: Implications for selective neuronal degeneration. *Brain Research*, 716: 229–232.

Ikonomovic, M. D., Nocera, R., Mizukami, K., and Armstrong, D. M. (2000). Age-related loss of the AMPA receptor subunits GluR2/3 in the human nucleus basalis of Meynert. *Experimental Neurology*, 166: 363–375.

Jack, C. R., Jr., Petersen, R. C., Xu, Y., O'Brien, P. C., Smith, G. E., Ivnik, R. J. et al. (1998). Rate of medial temporal lobe atrophy in typical aging and Alzheimer's disease. *Neurology*, 51: 993–999.

Jack, C. R., Jr., Petersen, R. C., Xu, Y., O'Brien, P. C., Smith, G. E., Ivnik, R. J. et al. (2000). Rates of hippocampal atrophy correlate with change in clinical status in aging and AD. *Neurology*, 55: 484–489.

Jacobs, B., Driscoll, L., and Schall, M. (1997). Life-span dendritic and spine changes in areas 10 and 18 of human cortex: a quantitative Golgi study. *Journal of Comparative Neurology*, 386: 661–680.

Jacobs, B., Schall, M., Prather, M., Kapler, E., Driscoll, L., Baca, S. et al. (2001). Regional dendritic and spine variation in human cerebral cortex: a quantitative golgi study. *Cerebral Cortex*, 11: 558–571.

Jacobsen, J. S., Wu, C. C., Redwine, J. M., Comery, T. A., Arias, R., Bowlby, M. et al. (2006). Early-onset behavioral and synaptic deficits in a mouse model of Alzheimer's disease. *Proceedings of the National Academy of Sciences of the USA*, 103: 5161–5166.

Jan, Y. N. and Jan, L. Y. (2003). The control of dendrite development. *Neuron*, 40: 229–242.

Kazee, A. M. and Johnson, E. M. (1998). Alzheimer's disease pathology in non-demented elderly. *Journal of Alzheimers Disease*, 1: 81–89.

Kimura, D. (1992). Sex differences in the brain. *Scientific American*, 267: 118–125.

Knowles, R. B., Gomez-Isla, T., and Hyman, B. T. (1998). Abeta associated neuropil changes: correlation with neuronal loss and dementia. *Journal of Neuropathology Experimental Neurology*, 57: 1122–1130.

Knowles, R. B., Wyart, C., Buldyrev, S. V., Cruz, L., Urbanc, B., Hasselmo, M. E., et al., (1999). Plaque-induced neurite abnormalities: Implications for disruption of neural networks in Alzheimer's disease. *Proceedings of the National Academy of Sciences of the USA*, 96: 5274–5279.

Kritzer, M. F. and Kohama, S. G. (1999). Ovarian hormones differentially influence immunoreactivity for dopamine beta-hydroxylase, choline acetyltransferase, and serotonin in the dorsolateral prefrontal cortex of adult rhesus monkeys. *Journal of Comparative Neurology*, 409: 438–451.

Kuiper, G. G., Carlsson, B., Grandien, K., Enmark, E., Haggblad, J., Nilsson, S. et al. (1997). Comparison of the ligand binding specificity and transcript tissue distribution of estrogen receptors alpha and beta. *Endocrinology*, 138: 863–870.

Kuiper, G. G., Shughrue, P. J., Merchenthaler, I., and Gustafsson, J. A. (1998). The estrogen receptor beta subtype: a novel mediator of estrogen action in neuroendocrine systems. *Front Neuroendocrinology*, 19: 253–286.

Lacreuse, A. (2006). Effects of ovarian hormones on cognitive function in nonhuman primates. *Neuroscience*, 138: 859–867.

Lanz, T. A., Carter, D. B., and Merchant, K. M. (2003). Dendritic spine loss in the hippocampus of young PDAPP and Tg2576 mice and its prevention by the ApoE2 genotype. *Neurobiology of Disease*, 13: 246–253.

Le, R., Cruz, L., Urbanc, B., Knowles, R. B., Hsiao-Ashe, K., Duff, K. et al. (2001). Plaque-induced abnormalities in neurite geometry in transgenic models of Alzheimer disease: implications for neural system disruption. *Journal of Neuropathology and Experimental Neurology*, 60: 753–758.

Leranth, C., Shanabrough, M., and Redmond, D. E., Jr. (2002). Gonadal hormones are responsible for maintaining the integrity of spine synapses in the CA1 hippocampal subfield of female nonhuman primates. *Journal of Comparative Neurology*, 447: 34–42.

Leventhal, A. G., Wang, Y., Pu, M., Zhou, Y., and Ma, Y. (2003). GABA and its agonists improved visual cortical function in senescent monkeys. *Science*, 300: 812–815.

Lewis, J., McGowan, E., Rockwood, J., Melrose, H., Nacharaju, P., Van Slegtenhorst, M. et al. (2000). Neurofibrillary tangles, amyotrophy and progressive motor disturbance in mice expressing mutant (P301L) tau protein. *Nature Genetics*, 25: 402–405.

Luebke, J. I., Chang, Y. M., Moore, T. L., and Rosene, D. L. (2004). Normal aging results in decreased synaptic excitation and increased synaptic inhibition of layer 2/3 pyramidal cells in the monkey prefrontal cortex. *Neuroscience*, 125: 277–288.

Markou, A., Duka, T., and Prelevic, G. M. (2005). Estrogens and brain function. *Hormones (Athens)*, 4: 9–17.

McKeith, I. G., Galasko, D., Kosaka, K., Perry, E. K., Dickson, D. W., Hansen, L. A. et al. (1996). Consensus guidelines for the clinical and pathologic diagnosis of dementia with Lewy bodies (DLB): report of the consortium on DLB international workshop. *Neurology*, 47: 1113–1124.

Mervis, R. (1978). Structural alterations in neurons of aged canine neocortex: A Golgi study. *Experimental Neurology*, 62: 417–432.

Milner, T. A., McEwen, B. S., Hayashi, S., Li, C. J., Reagan, L. P., and Alves, S. E. (2001). Ultrastructural evidence that hippocampal alpha estrogen receptors are located at extranuclear sites. *Journal of Comparative Neurology*, 429: 355–371.

Moolman, D. L., Vitolo, O. V., Vonsattel, J. P., and Shelanski, M. L. (2004). Dendrite and dendritic spine alterations in Alzheimer models. *Journal of Neurocytology*, 33: 377–387.

Morrison, J. H. and Hof, P. R. (1997). Life and death of neurons in the aging brain. *Science*, 278: 412–419.

Morrison, J. H. and Hof, P. R. (2002). Selective vulnerability of corticocortical and hippocampal circuits in aging and Alzheimer's disease. *Progress in Brain Research*, 136: 467–486.

Morrison, J. H. and Hof, P. R. (2007). Life and death of neurons in the aging cerebral cortex. *International Review of Neurobiology*, 81: 41–57.

Mucke, L., Masliah, E., Yu, G. Q., Mallory, M., Rockenstein, E. M., Tatsuno, G. et al. (2000). High-level neuronal expression of abeta 1-42 in wild-type human amyloid protein precursor transgenic mice: synaptotoxicity without plaque formation. *Journal of Neuroscience*, 20: 4050–4058.

Mufson, E. J., Ginsberg, S. D., Ikonomovic, M. D., and DeKosky, S. T. (2003). Human cholinergic basal forebrain: Chemoanatomy and neurologic dysfunction. *Journal of Chemical Neuroanatomy*, 26: 233–242.

Murphy, D. G., DeCarli, C., McIntosh, A. R., Daly, E., Mentis, M. J., Pietrini, P. et al. (1996). Sex differences in human brain morphometry and metabolism: an in vivo quantitative magnetic resonance imaging and positron emission tomography study on the effect of aging. *Archives of General Psychiatry*, 53: 585–594.

Nakamura, S., Akiguchi, I., Kameyama, M., and Mizuno, N. (1985). Age-related changes of pyramidal cell basal dendrites in layers III and V of human motor cortex: a quantitative Golgi study. *Acta Neuropathologica*, 65: 281–284.

Nguyen, M. D., Shu, T., Sanada, K., Lariviere, R. C., Tseng, H. C., Park, S. K. et al. (2004). A NUDEL-dependent mechanism of neurofilament assembly regulates the integrity of CNS neurons. *Nature Cell Biology*, 6: 595–608.

Nimchinsky, E. A., Hof, P. R., Young, W. G., and Morrison, J. H. (1996). Neurochemical, morphologic, and laminar characterization of cortical projection neurons in the cingulate motor areas of the macaque monkey. *Journal of Comparative Neurology*, 374: 136–160.

Nimchinsky, E. A., Sabatini, B. L., and Svoboda, K. (2002). Structure and function of dendritic spines. *Annual Reviews of Physiology*, 64: 313–353.

Oddo, S., Caccamo, A., Shepherd, J. D., Murphy, M. P., Golde, T. E., Kayed, R. et al. (2003). Triple-transgenic model of Alzheimer's disease with plaques and tangles: intracellular Abeta and synaptic dysfunction. *Neuron*, 39: 409–421.

Page, T. L., Einstein, M., Duan, H., He, Y., Flores, T., Rolshud, D. et al. (2002). Morphological alterations in neurons forming corticocortical projections in the neocortex of aged Patas monkeys. *Neuroscience Letters*, 317: 37–41.

Perez, R. G., Zheng, H., Van der Ploeg, L. H., and Koo, E. H. (1997). The beta-amyloid precursor protein of Alzheimer's disease enhances neuron viability and modulates neuronal polarity. *Journal of Neuroscience*, 17: 9407–9414.

Peters, A. (2002). The effects of normal aging on myelin and nerve fibers: A review. *Journal of Neurocytology*, 31: 581–593.

Peters, A., Moss, M. B., and Sethares, C. (2001). The effects of aging on layer 1 of primary visual cortex in the rhesus monkey. *Cerebral Cortex*, 11: 93–103.

Peters, A., Sethares, C., and Moss, M. B. (1998). The effects of aging on layer 1 in area 46 of prefrontal cortex in the rhesus monkey. *Cerebral Cortex*, 8: 671–684.

Price, J. L., Davis, P. B., Morris, J. C., and White, D. L. (1991). The distribution of tangles, plaques and related immunohistochemical markers in healthy aging and Alzheimer's disease. *Neurobiology of Aging*, 12: 295–312.

Price, J. L., Ko, A. I., Wade, M. J., Tsou, S. K., McKeel, D. W., and Morris, J. C. (2001). Neuron number in the entorhinal cortex and CA1 in preclinical Alzheimer disease. *Archives of Neurology*, 58: 1395–1402.

Ramsden, M., Kotilinek, L., Forster, C., Paulson, J., McGowan, E., SantaCruz, K. et al. (2005). Age-dependent neurofibrillary tangle formation, neuron loss, and memory impairment in a mouse model of human tauopathy (P301L). *Journal of Neuroscience*, 25: 10637–10647.

Rapp, P. R., Morrison, J. H., and Roberts, J. A. (2003). Cyclic estrogen replacement improves cognitive function in aged ovariectomized rhesus monkeys. *Journal of Neuroscience*, 23: 5708–5714.

Raymond, C. R., Ireland, D. R., and Abraham, W. C. (2003). NMDA receptor regulation by amyloid-beta does not account for its inhibition of LTP in rat hippocampus. *Brain Research*, 968: 263–272.

Redwine, J. M., Kosofsky, B., Jacobs, R. E., Games, D., Reilly, J. F., Morrison, J. H. et al. (2003). Dentate gyrus volume is reduced before onset of plaque formation in PDAPP mice: A magnetic resonance microscopy and stereologic analysis. *Proceedings of the National Academy of Sciences of the USA*, 100: 1381–1386.

Rosene, D. L., Mangiamele L. A., Sandell, and J. H., Peters, A. (2003). Anatomical and physiological properties of the corpus callosum in the gaed rhesus monkey. *Society for Neuroscience Abstract*, 6: 735–737.

Roy, S., Zhang, B., Lee, V. M., and Trojanowski, J. Q. (2005). Axonal transport defects: A common theme in neurodegenerative diseases. *Acta Neuropathologica (Berl)*, 109: 5–13.

Rutten, B. P., Van der Kolk, N. M., Schafer, S., van Zandvoort, M. A., Bayer, T. A., Steinbusch, H. W. et al. (2005). Age-related loss of synaptophysin immunoreactive presynaptic boutons within the hippocampus of APP751SL, PS1M146L, and APP751SL/PS1M146L transgenic mice. *AmericanJournal of Pathology*, 167: 161–173.

Samsonovich, A. V. and Ascoli, G. A. (2006). Morphological homeostasis in cortical dendrites. *Proceedings of the National Academy of Sciences of the USA*, 103: 1569–1574.

Scahill, R. I., Frost, C., Jenkins, R., Whitwell, J. L., Rossor, M. N., and Fox, N. C. (2003). A longitudinal study of brain volume changes in normal aging using serial registered magnetic resonance imaging. *Archives of Neurology*, 60: 989–994.

Scheff, S. W., Price, D. A., Schmitt, F. A., and Mufson, E. J. (2006). Hippocampal synaptic loss in early Alzheimer's disease and mild cognitive impairment. *Neurobiology of Aging*, 27: 1372–1384.

Scheibel, M. E., Lindsay, R. D., Tomiyasu, U., and Scheibel, A. B. (1975). Progressive dendritic changes in aging human cortex. *Experimental Neurology*, 47: 392–403.

Schmitz, C., Rutten, B. P., Pielen, A., Schafer, S., Wirths, O., Tremp, G. et al. (2004). Hippocampal neuron loss exceeds amyloid plaque load in a transgenic mouse model of Alzheimer's disease. *American Journal of Pathology*, 164: 1495–1502.

Schonheit, B., Zarski, R., and Ohm, T. G. (2004). Spatial and temporal relationships between plaques and tangles in Alzheimer-pathology.*Neurobiology of Aging*, 25: 697–711.

Schubert, W., Prior, R., Weidemann, A., Dircksen, H., Multhaup, G., Masters, C. L. et al. (1991). Localization of Alzheimer beta A4 amyloid precursor protein at central and peripheral synaptic sites. *Brain Research*, 563: 184–194.

Seabrook, G. R., Smith, D. W., Bowery, B. J., Easter, A., Reynolds, T., Fitzjohn, S. M. et al. (1999). Mechanisms contributing to the deficits in hippocampal synaptic plasticity in mice lacking amyloid precursor protein. *Neuropharmacology*, 38: 349–359.

Shahani, N., Subramaniam, S., Wolf, T., Tackenberg, C., and Brandt, R. (2006). Tau aggregation and progressive neuronal degeneration in the absence of changes in spine density and morphology after targeted expression of Alzheimer's disease-relevant tau constructs in organotypic hippocampal slices. *Journal of Neuroscience*, 26: 6103–6114.

Shigematsu, K., McGeer, P. L., and McGeer, E. G. (1992). Localization of amyloid precursor protein in selective postsynaptic densities of rat cortical neurons. *Brain Research*, 592: 353–357.

Shimada, A., Tsuzuki, M., Keino, H., Satoh, M., Chiba, Y., Saitoh, Y. et al. (2006). Apical vulnerability to dendritic retraction in prefrontal neurones of ageing SAMP10 mouse: a model of cerebral degeneration. *Neuropathology and Applied Neurobiology*, 32: 1–14.

Shughrue, P. J., Lane, M. V., and Merchenthaler, I. (1997). Comparative distribution of estrogen receptor-alpha and -beta mRNA in the rat central nervous system. *Journal of Comparative Neurology*, 388: 507–525.

Shughrue, P. J., Scrimo, P. J., and Merchenthaler, I. (2000). Estrogen binding and estrogen receptor characterization (ERalpha and ERbeta) in the cholinergic neurons of the rat basal forebrain. *Neuroscience*, 96: 41–49.

Sorra, K. E. and Harris, K. M. (2000). Overview on the structure, composition, function, development, and plasticity of hippocampal dendritic spines. *Hippocampus*, 10: 501–511.

Spires, T. L., Meyer-Luehmann, M., Stern, E. A., McLean, P. J., Skoch, J., Nguyen, P. T. et al. (2005). Dendritic spine abnormalities in amyloid precursor protein transgenic mice demonstrated by gene transfer and intravital multiphoton microscopy. *Journal of Neuroscience*, 25: 7278–7287.

Swanson, G. T., Kamboj, S. K., and Cull-Candy, S. G. (1997). Single-channel properties of recombinant AMPA receptors depend on RNA editing, splice variation, and subunit composition. *Journal of Neuroscience*, 17: 58–69.

Takeda, T., Hosokawa, M., and Higuchi, K. (1991). Senescence-accelerated mouse (SAM): a novel murine model of accelerated senescence. *Journal of American Geriatrics Society*, 39: 911–919.

Tang, Y., Janssen, W. G., Hao, J., Roberts, J. A., McKay, H., Lasley, B. et al. (2004). Estrogen replacement increases spinophilin-immunoreactive spine number in the prefrontal cortex of female rhesus monkeys. *Cerebral Cortex*, 14: 215–223.

Terry, R. D. (2006). Alzheimer's disease and the aging brain. *Journal of Geriatrics Psychiatry and Neurolgoy*, 19: 125–128.

Terry, R. D., Masliah, E., Salmon, D. P., Butters, N., DeTeresa, R., Hill, R., et al. (1991). Physical basis of cognitive alterations in Alzheimer's disease: synapse loss is the major correlate of cognitive impairment. *Annals of Neurology*, 30: 572–580.

Terry, R. D., Peck, A., DeTeresa, R., Schechter, R., and Horoupian, D. S. (1981). Some morphometric aspects of the brain in senile dementia of the Alzheimer type. *Annals of Neurology*, 10: 184–192.

Thies, E. and Mandelkow, E. M. (2007). Missorting of tau in neurons causes degeneration of synapses that can be rescued by the kinase MARK2/Par-1. *Journal of Neuroscience*, 27: 2896–2907.

Tinkler, G. P., Tobin, J. R., and Voytko, M. L. (2004). Effects of two years of estrogen loss or replacement on nucleus basalis cholinergic neurons and cholinergic fibers to the dorsolateral prefrontal and inferior parietal cortex of monkeys. *Journal of Comparative Neurology*, 469: 507–521.

Tsai, J., Grutzendler, J., Duff, K., and Gan, W. B. (2004). Fibrillar amyloid deposition leads to local synaptic abnormalities and breakage of neuronal branches. *Nature Neuroscience*, 7: 1181–1183.

Ulfhake, B. and Kellerth, J. O. (1981). A quantitative light microscopic study of the dendrites of cat spinal alpha-motoneurons after intracellular staining with horseradish peroxidase. *Journal of Comparative Neurology*, 202: 571–583.

Vickers, J. C., Huntley, G. W., Edwards, A. M., Moran, T., Rogers, S. W., Heinemann, S. F. et al. (1993). Quantitative localization of AMPA/kainate and kainate glutamate receptor subunit immunoreactivity in neurochemically identified subpopulations of neurons in the prefrontal cortex of the macaque monkey. *Journal of Neuroscience*, 13: 2982–2992.

Vickers, J. C., Riederer, B. M., Marugg, R. A., Buee-Scherrer, V., Buee, L., Delacourte, A. et al. (1994). Alterations in neurofilament protein immunoreactivity in human hippocampal neurons related to normal aging and Alzheimer's disease. *Neuroscience*, 62: 1–13.

Wang, H. W., Pasternak, J. F., Kuo, H., Ristic, H., Lambert, M. P., Chromy, B. et al. (2002). Soluble oligomers of beta amyloid (1-42) inhibit long-term potentiation but not long-term depression in rat dentate gyrus. *Brain Research*, 924: 133–140.

West, M. J. (1993). New stereological methods for counting neurons. *Neurobiology of Aging*, 14: 275–285.

West, M. J., Coleman, P. D., Flood, D. G., and Troncoso, J. C. (1994). Differences in the pattern of hippocampal neuronal loss in normal ageing and Alzheimer's disease. *Lancet*, 344: 769–772.

West, M. J., Kawas, C. H., Stewart, W. F., Rudow, G. L., and Troncoso, J. C. (2004). Hippocampal neurons in pre-clinical Alzheimer's disease. *Neurobiology of Aging*, 25: 1205–1212.

Whitwell, J. L., Weigand, S. D., Shiung, M. M., Boeve, B. F., Ferman, T. J., Smith, G. E. et al. (2007). Focal atrophy in dementia with Lewy bodies on MRI: a distinct pattern from Alzheimer's disease. *Brain*, 130: 708–719.

Woolley, C. S., Gould, E., Frankfurt, M., and McEwen, B. S. (1990). Naturally occurring fluctuation in dendritic spine density on adult hippocampal pyramidal neurons. *Journal of Neuroscience*, 10: 4035–4039.

Woolley, C. S. and McEwen, B. S. (1992). Estradiol mediates fluctuation in hippocampal synapse density during the estrous cycle in the adult rat. *Journal of Neuroscience*, 12: 2549–2554.

Woolley, C. S. and McEwen, B. S. (1993). Roles of estradiol and progesterone in regulation of hippocampal dendritic spine density during the estrous cycle in the rat. *Journal of Comparative Neurology*, 336: 293–306.

Wu, C. C., Chawla, F., Games, D., Rydel, R. E., Freedman, S., Schenk, D. et al. (2004). Selective vulnerability of dentate granule cells prior to amyloid deposition in PDAPP mice: digital morphometric analyses. *Proceedings of the National Academy of Sciences of the USA*, 101: 7141–7146.

Yankner, B. A., Lu, T., and Loerch, P. (2007). The aging brain. *Annual Reviews Pathology*, 3: 41–66.

Zaja–Milatovic, S., Keene, C. D., Montine, K. S., Leverenz, J. B., Tsuang, D., and Montine, T. J. (2006). Selective dendritic degeneration of medium spiny neurons in dementia with Lewy bodies. *Neurology*, 66: 1591–1593.

Part I

Basic Science

4

A Systems Approach to the Aging Brain: Neuroanatomic Changes, Their Modifiers, and Cognitive Correlates

Naftali Raz and Kristen M. Kennedy

Bear with my weakness; my old brain is troubled.
William Shakespeare, The Tempest, Act IV, Scene I

Abstract

Success in diagnosing and treating age-related brain disease depends on understanding normative and optimal aging, and noninvasive neuroimaging is a vital tool in advancing toward that goal. Studies of the brains of healthy adults reveal uneven, differential shrinkage of the parenchyma and expansion of the ventricular system, with the prefrontal cortices evidencing the largest magnitude of age-related differences, and the tertiary association (prefrontal and parietal) cortices, the neostriatum, and the cerebellum showing the greatest rate of shrinkage. Although findings vary across samples, reduced regional brain volumes and steeper longitudinal declines are usually associated with lower cognitive performance in specific domains. The observed pattern of differential brain aging is significantly modified by negative and positive factors. Although negative effects of vascular risk factors are apparent in the regions deemed most vulnerable to aging, the positive modifying influence of aerobic fitness is clearest in the same age-sensitive areas. Genetic variation may have a significant impact on age-related changes in brain and cognition, although the sparsity of evidence precludes evaluating the true magnitude of the effect of specific polymorphisms. In addition to (and in conjunction with) aerobic fitness, antihypertensive treatment and hormone replacement therapy (in women) may alleviate negative effects of aging on brain structure.

Introduction

All living systems change with time and aging is as much an integral part of their developmental trajectory as is maturation. However, the trajectories that connect the initial and the final moments of life vary across species and among individuals. The reasons for such

variability are not clearly understood, and it is not easy to gauge how much of the individual differences in aging can be ascribed to its normal physiological course and how much is attributable to beneficial and pathological effects that constitute one's life history and are included with one's genetic endowment. In this chapter, we will attempt to summarize the current state of knowledge regarding adult development and aging of the central nervous system, and more specifically the brain. Although informed by investigations of animal models and postmortem human material, our narrative is focused on the in vivo studies of human brain aging, its cognitive correlates, and the pathological as well as therapeutic factors that alter the course of brain aging in a predictable way. Our main premise is that if the objective is alleviating the negative and accentuating the positive extremes of the normal aging process, it is imperative to understand the physiological and pathological underpinnings of that variability and its relation to cognition and behavior.

In the past hundred years, aging of the human brain attracted the attention of neuroanatomists and neuropathologists, and postmortem (PM) studies revealed many gross and microanatomical characteristics of the aging brain (for a detailed account of postmortem neuropathology of aging see Dickstein, Morrison and Hof Chapter 3 in this volume). Gross anatomic investigations noted age-related reduction in brain weight and volume, ventricular and sulcal enlargement, reduction in the bulk and quality of the white matter (e.g., see Kaes [1907] for meticulous neuroanatomical work and Kemper [1994] for a comprehensive review of the topic). A series of elegant studies in primates revealed significant age-related alterations in the structure of the myelin sheath (Marner et al., 2003; Peters and Sethares, 2002). Loss and shrinkage of neurons, albeit not pervasive and global, is also observed (Haug, 1985). Neuroanatomical and neurophysiological studies demonstrate age-related differences in the basic cellular structure and function of the organism (Brunk and Terman, 2002; Lenaz et al., 2002).

Thus, the postmortem investigations have demonstrated that aging affects the brain at virtually every level, and histological studies of postmortem material remain a valuable exploratory tool of modern neurogerontology.

Nonetheless, for all the advantages afforded by the precise microanalyses, PM studies have several significant disadvantages. Although the PM tissue collected from sources with good quality control show excellent protein stability and RNA quality (Stan et al., 2006), the degree to which ante-mortem hypoxia, hyper-pyrexia, and ischemia affect the results of most studies is unknown. Moreover, PM studies are inherently incapable of addressing several fundamental questions, such as how the brain is changing over time, what the neuroanatomical picture of optimal (as opposed to common) aging would be, and what cognitive consequences the observed changes entail.

Structural Brain Aging: Volumetric Findings

Cross-Sectional Studies of Age-Related Differences in Brain Volumes

Although the cumulative results of more than two decades of cross-sectional studies of age differences in regional brain volumes may be variable and at times contradictory, they converge onto several general trends. According to the neuroimaging volumetric literature (for detailed reviews see Raz, 2000, 2004; Raz and Rodrigue, 2006), the prefrontal cortices emerge as the most vulnerable region of the aging brain, whereas sensory (e.g., primary visual) cortices and lower regions of the central nervous system (CNS) such as the ventral pons show little, if any, aging-related variability. In some regions of the brain, such as the hippocampus, temporal and parietal lobes, the volume declines seem to accelerate with age as nonlinear trends observed in several samples suggest (Cohen et al., 2006a; DeCarli et al., 2005; Jernigan et al., 2001; Lupien et al., 2007; Raz et al., 2004b). In the entorhinal cortex, age-related differences in volume are observed only in the later part of the lifespan (see Raz [2004] for a review and Miyahira et al, [2004] as well as Siwak-Tapp et al. [2008] for findings in canines). Studies that assessed cortical thickness and sulcal depth rather than regional volumes report a similar pattern of age-related differences (Kochunov et al., 2005; Nesvåg et al. 2008; Salat et al., 2004), although in a notable exception, at least one study reported a significant negative correlation between age and thickness of the pericalcarine cortex as well (Salat et al., 2004).

Assessing volume differences in the brain is not an easy task. It requires many hours of tedious work by highly trained personnel. To alleviate the difficulties of manual measurement, semi-automated methods that use whole-brain data to estimate local differences in gray matter "density" or, with an appropriate correction, "volume," have been introduced in the past decade (e.g., voxel-based morphometry, VBM; Ashburner and Friston, 2000). VBM and related methods have several advantages over manual morphometry: perfect repeatability, no requirement of complex decision making on the part of highly trained operators, and examination of the whole brain, not just selected regions of interest (ROIs). However, the disadvantages become apparent when the issues of validity are considered. In VBM, the brain tissue is automatically segmented into gray matter, white matter, and cerebral spinal fluid (CSF), and errors of segmentation are possible when the image is less than perfect and contains artifacts. What a knowledgeable human operator would dismiss as an artifactual variation in intensity and a mere nuisance is treated by a segmentation algorithm as a legitimate difference in tissue density. To compensate for significant individual differences in brain geometry, the images are normalized, i.e., fitted into a standard or study-specific template. In the process, the images are filtered, and as a result, while gaining signal-to-noise ratio, they lose resolution, sometimes by a factor of 10^3. Reduction of resolution and improvement in the signal-to-noise ratio may result in increased sensitivity to global group differences at the expense of variability in small structures (Bookstein, 2001; Crum et al., 2003; Davatzikos, 2004). Refining the methods of data acquisition and tailoring sequences for visualizing and assessing specific structures may improve the validity of automated methods (van der Kouwe et al., 2008).

Although VBM and similar methods produced results that are broadly consistent with those of manual morphometry (e.g., Good et al., 2001; see also Raz and Rodrigue [2006] for a review), several comparisons between semi-automated and manual methods indicate those methods are not interchangeable (e.g., Allen et al., 2005; Cardenas et al., 2003; Dorion et al., 2001; Douaud et al., 2006; Good et al., 2002; Gong et al., 2005; Kennedy et al., 2008a; Tisserand et al., 2002). One striking feature of those comparisons is that VBM analyses are more likely than the manual measures to find larger age differences in the regions bordering CSF such as the insula, the cingulate gyri, and the superior temporal and superior parietal cortex, i.e., regions that show minor though significant age-related differences in volumetric studies (Kennedy et al., 2008a; Raz, 2004).

A comparative study of VBM and manual volumetry has suggested that statistically defined peak values of modulated density produced by VBM may indicate stronger age differences than manual measures do, and they may identify age effects in a different set of regions (Kennedy et al., 2008a). Whether the larger age effects reflect true differences in the aging brain structure, or stem from exaggeration of local partial volume artifacts at the border of CSF and parenchyma or gray and white matter is unclear. It is important to note that when VBM-derived measures are aggregated over anatomically defined regions (i.e., ROI masks) the pattern of age differences was more similar to that produced by the manual measures (Kennedy et al., 2008a). Semi-automated VBM methods may be more likely to report nonlinearities in age-volume relationships (Kennedy et al., 2008a; Walhovd et al., 2005a). There are no neurobiological reasons why a specific cluster of voxels is age-dependent whereas its neighbor, within the cytoarchitectonically identical area, is not. Moreover, statistically, the fact that "red pixels" on color-coded maps of the gray matter differences in local densities significantly differ from zero does not mean that they also significantly differ from "orange" or even "yellow" pixels on the same map of age difference, a problem highlighted previously in regards to fMRI activation maps (Jernigan et al., 2003). In the context of the outlined concerns, it is important to note that when voxel-based analysis provides information that is biologically interpretable, it may open new windows to understanding of the neuroanatomy of aging. For example, a recent study of older adults revealed amplified age-related differences in the hippocampal regions that have long been suspected of excessive vulnerability to ischemia (i.e., CA1 field) in conjunction with age-related differences in hippocampal volume revealed by manual volumetry (Xu et al., 2008).

In sum, the magnitude and location of age-related differences in the brain volume may depend on the method of measurement. Whereas VBM may be a useful first-pass approach to the analysis of a large set of brains, findings from automated procedures should not be treated without question as replications of manual studies.

Automated first-pass analyses should be followed by manual measures in the regions identified as the candidates for age-related differences, and in the regions that can be missed due to the method limitations, especially in the locations with intricate geometry and high risk of artifacts (e.g., entorhinal cortex). In addition, voxel-based methods may add to current knowledge by providing information about regional differences within structures that are difficult to demarcate on the basis of external landmarks. Although development of new methods more sensitive to local geometry of the brain parenchyma appears to add neuroanatomic validity to semi-automated morphology (for more details see Van Horn and Toga, Chapter 21 in this volume) a well-trained human operator guided by top-down knowledge of neuroanatomy will proably remain an instrument of choice in cases of analysis of less-than-perfect and artifact-ridden images

Longitudinal Studies of Brain Volume Change in Adulthood

Thus far, the discussion of age-related differences in brain volumes has been limited to cross-sectional studies. Such studies indeed represent the most popular way of estimating age effects. However, the cross-sectional design has major limitations. Although ideally, cross-sectional investigations should yield estimates of age-related change, this is rarely the case. Cross-sectional studies provide a snapshot of individual variability and in doing so they confound individual differences in brain and cognition, which are brought into the study from years of previous development, with age-related variance. Thus, findings from cross-sectional investigations should be interpreted with caution, taking into account the problem of variance commonality among multiple variables, which is impossible to sort out without introducing the time dimension (Kraemer et al., 2000; Lindenberger and Pötter, 1998). Granted, the longitudinal approach has its own share of problems such as "3M"—the mobility, morbidity, and mortality of the participants (Raz, 2004). Nonetheless, the results of longitudinal studies, unlike those of cross-sectional investigations, can be interpreted as an indication of true change or the lack thereof, within the limits of generalizability predicated on the nature of the sample. Indeed, longitudinal studies of brain volume show that for some regions, cross-sectional estimates are quite accurate, whereas for others they are wide off the mark (e.g., Raz et al., 2005).

One of the most frequently used indices of brain health is the volume of the cerebral ventricles, and in many longitudinal studies this is the only neuroanatomical measure. The volume of the cerebral ventricles reflects many diverse alterations in the volume and pressure of the CSF, and represents a summary measure of change in the whole CNS. The extant studies of ventricular enlargement are consistent in showing significant age-related declines, which proceed at an average pace of almost 3% per year. Moreover, the annual rate of ventricular expansion increases with age, exceeding 4% per annum in the 6th and 7th decades of life (Carmichael et al., 2007; Raz, 2004). Even in healthy adults, ventricular expansion over a 5-year period may be visible with the naked eye, as illustrated in Figure 4.1.

In contrast to ventricular size, the total brain size changes at a significantly slower pace (Raz, 2004). This discrepancy may be rooted in the fact that the boundaries of the fluid-filled system of connected CSF cavities (ventricles, cisterns, etc.) are not fixed because they are defined by the bulk of surrounding tissue. Thus, ventricular expansion occurs in response to loss of brain tissue anywhere in the CNS, and barring significant pathological changes in CSF production and drainage, loss of tissue in multiple locations

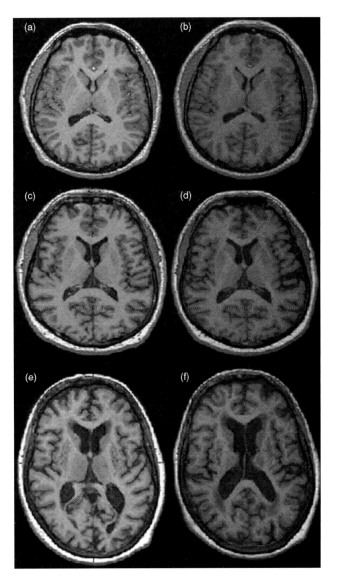

Figure 4–1 Ventriculomegaly is a hallmark of the aging brain reflecting nonspecific, total expansion of CSF and contraction of brain parenchyma. The images were acquired five years apart. (a) Young adult age 24 and (b) the same person, age 29 years; (c) a middle-aged adult at age 46 and (d) the same person at the age of 51; (e) an older adult age 75 and (f) the same person at the age of 80. Notice that even in healthy middle- and older-aged adults, ventricular expansion is evident across 5 years.

adds up to fluid expansion to fill the newly created space. Hence, specificity of ventricular size as an index of brain health is low but its sensitivity is high. In contrast, differential and localized changes in the brain parenchyma coexist with localized preservation (or even enlargement), and the total brain volume may represent an averaged net change.

Longitudinal studies that examined distinct brain regions reveal significant local differences in shrinkage rates. Association cortices, such as prefrontal and inferior parietal, tend to show the greatest rate of change, with temporal cortex following closely behind, and occipital (especially primary visual) cortex showing no or minimally significant changes (Pfefferbaum et al., 1998; Raz et al., 2005; Resnick et al., 2003). Note that in contrast to cross-sectional studies, longitudinal investigations tend to show significant decline in parietal volume, a region that is marked with significant individual variability (Raz et al., 2005).

Because the decline of the medial temporal structures (the hippocampus and the entorhinal cortex) is believed to be a harbinger of Alzheimer's disease (AD, see chapters 10, 12 for a detailed discussion), they have been measured in several longitudinal samples. These investigations reveal significant shrinkage of the hippocampus (HC), usually, though not always, with a nonlinear, age-accelerated trend (Jack et al., 2000; Liu et al., 2003; Raz et al., 2004a, 2005; Rusinek et al., 2003). The implication of that trend is that restricting samples to persons of advanced age would increase the likelihood of finding hippocampal shrinkage that may be missed in investigations of younger adults.

This expectation is illustrated by the current literature on the volume of the entorhinal cortex. To date, most of the longitudinal studies of the entorhinal cortex have been conducted on samples of older adults, and their results indicate significant shrinkage comparable to that of the hippocampus (Cardenas et al., 2003; Du et al., 2003; Jack et al., 2007). By comparison, in a sample covering a wide age range, entorhinal shrinkage is significantly smaller than decline in hippocampal volume and becomes evident only in some individuals at the sixth and seventh decade of life (Raz et al., 2004a, 2005). When it occurs, entorhinal shrinkage is more likely to happen in persons with lower cognitive aptitude (Raz et al., 2008) and may fortell impending cognitive decline (Dickerson et al., 2001; Tapiola et al., 2008).

A few other key structures deemed age-sensitive in cross-sectional studies were investigated in very few longitudinal studies. Longitudinal investigations found significant shrinkage of the caudate nuclei in a sample of healthy adults of a wide age range (Raz et al., 2003a, 2005), while slower shrinkage was observed in the putamen and globus pallidus (Raz et al., 2003a). Substantial longitudinal shrinkage of the cerebellum that exceeded the rate estimated from cross-sectional data has been observed in samples with adequate age range (Raz et al., 2003b, 2005), whereas shrinkage of the pons is minimal as predicted by cross-sectional studies (Raz et al., 2003b). Apparently, when individual differences are controlled, the caudate nucleus and the cerebellum emerge as the leading candidates for the dubious honor of the most vulnerable regions of the aging brain.

The degree to which the observed age-related changes and differences reflect the normal aging picture is unknown. Some studies in nonhuman primates reported that by contrast to humans there is little or no neuronal loss (e.g., Keuker, Luiten, and Fuchs, 2003), although such a conclusion frequently reflects the lack of statistical power. For example, "conservation of neuron number" in rhesus monkey entorhinal cortex corresponds to an age effect of $d = 0.6$ standard deviation in the most vulnerable layer II, with a smaller effect of $d = 0.28$ in layer III (Merrill, Roberts, and Tuszynski, 2000). In some samples and for some types of cells, the age effects are so dramatic that no statistical analyses are necessary to reveal them (Smith et al., 1999). There are significant individual and interstrain differences in brain structure even among animals that are bred and reared under standard and controlled conditions (e.g., Chen et al., 2005). Although those differences may be not as large as among humans, it would take more than eight animals to show effects that are not visible to the naked eye.

In vivo neuroimaging studies of nonhuman primates will shed more light on the notion of greater preservation and lesser declines in the animals protected from virtually all pathogens associated with even the most optimal human existence. Such studies are associated with significant logistic effort and expenses.

Nonetheless, in a recent investigation of 19 rhesus monkeys, the pattern of aging derived from a VBM analysis was quite similar to the one observed in human studies (Alexander et al., 2008). Dorsolateral and orbital frontal regions evidenced the largest negative effect of age; smaller or none were observed for occipital, parietal cortices as well as globus pallidus. Contrary to human studies, including a small-sample study from the same group (Alexander et al., 2006), the cerebellum was also relatively intact (Alexander et al., 2008).

The dearth of MRI studies on normal aging animals and the virtual absence of combined MRI-histology studies precludes inferences about the validity of MRI evidence for mammalian aging in general. As a rule, as almost all primate studies do, the combined imaging-histological investigations have such low statistical power that when they essentially replicate effects reported in human studies (e.g., a correlation between age and HC volume $r = -0.32$, Shamy et al., [2006]), they cannot demonstrate their statistical significance.

One comparative cross-sectional study stands out, as it combines stereology, in vivo neuromorphometry (MRI) and metabolic (magnetic resonance spectroscopy, MRS) assessment with multiple behavioral tests in a sample of rats within a typical adult life span (Driscoll et al., 2006). In that study, lower hippocampal cell density and smaller hippocampal volumes were observed in old animals compared to the young and middle-aged. Notably, presence of immature neurons (adult neurogenesis) predicted both larger HC volumes and better performance on the HC-sensitive tasks. The link between learning, environmental enrichment, and neurogenesis in rodents has been suggested before (Drapeau et al., 2003, 2007; Kempermann, Gast, and Gage, 2002, but see Merrill et al., 2003). Studies in rodents indicate that hippocampal neurogenesis is significantly reduced with age (Kuhn, Dickinson-Anson, and Gage, 1996), but can be brought to the young-age levels by environmental manipulations (Cameron and McKay, 1999; Kempermann, Kuhn, and Gage, 1998). Thus, neurogenesis and other plasticity-related phenomena may emerge as an important process shaping mammalian brain aging (Burke and Barnes, 2006). Currently it is impossible to assess neurogenesis in vivo and to directly measure neural plasticity in humans, although one study on terminally ill persons supports the claims of adult neurogenesis in the dentate gyrus (Eriksson et al., 1998). Moreover, the rates of neurogenesis vary dramatically across and within rodent species (Kempermann, Kuhn, and Gage, 1997), and the researchers are still struggling to establish reliable methods of assessing neurogenesis across various brain areas and various species (Gould, 2007). Thus, the implications of brain plasticity observed in rodents for human aging are still unclear.

If cross-sectional comparative studies combining imaging and histology are rare, a longitudinal one is truly unique. One such study of a typical rodent revealed neither age-related regional shrinkage, nor ventricular enlargement over the entire lifespan (Sullivan et al., 2006a). The study showed a steady increase of the corpus callosum area, as well as volumes of the hippocampus and the cerebellum in two samples of rats. Although cerebellar volume leveled off toward the end of the life span, it did not decline. There are several caveats in interpreting these findings. First, the sample was very small and, although no strong trends were observed, it is unclear whether the observed age trajectories reflect the state of affairs in the population. Second, a rodent model of aging, with all its usefulness, still may not account for some specific features of the primate brain. Third, age-related changes could still happen in the regions not sampled in that study.

In sum, cross-sectional and longitudinal studies of neuroanatomical aging indicate a substantial age-accelerated expansion of CSF-filled cavities, mild shrinkage of the cerebral parenchyma, and a pattern of differential regional changes. Association cortices (e.g., prefrontal and inferior parietal), the neostriatum, the hippocampus and the cerebellum appear more sensitive to aging than do the primary sensory cortices, entorhinal cortex, the paleostriatum, and the pons. Little is known what neurobiological changes are reflected in the apparent shrinkage observed on the MR images. Given the ethical impossibilities, comparative studies, especially in primates (for an account of cross-species studies focused on AD see Chapter 8), are of critical importance in that area of research. However, such studies must adhere to the design standards applicable to the human studies, especially those ensuring adequate statistical power.

Age-related differences and changes in the white matter. Unlike most of the regional cortical volumes, the gross volume of the white matter shows a nonlinear relationship with calendar age (Bartzokis, 2004; Walhovd et al., 2005a). It increases from childhood to young adulthood, remains stable throughout middle age, and exhibits linear decline in the late years. Thus, the results of a particular study depend on the age range of the subjects. Observations on the developing brain reveal steady increases in white matter volume (see Lenroot and Giedd, 2006 for a review); studies with a significant proportion of older participants are likely to find decline in white matter volume (e.g., Ikram et al., 2008), whereas those that examine the whole adult age range find little if any age differences in that cerebral compartment (e.g., Raz et al., 1997, 2004c). Notably, complexity of the white matter structure, as indexed by fractal dimensionality, is lower in older adults even in the absence of gross volume differences (Zhang et al., 2007), a finding that is in accord with age-related reduction of structural complexity observed in cytoarchitectonic studies (Dickstein et al., 2007). It is unknown how microstructural complexity decline is related to loss of tissue volume, and the relation between the two, especially with regards to temporal precedence, needs to be examined. However, the magnitude of cross-sectional age differences and longitudinal shrinkage in a specific brain region is associated with the ontogenetic status of the region with respect to myelination as described by Flechsig (1901). This relationship, first noted in Raz (2000), is depicted in Figure 4.2. In fact, myelination precedence order accounts for 36% of the variance in magnitude of age-differences in volume and 38% of volume shrinkage.

One of the most commonly used indicators of white matter health is the burden of white matter hyperintensities (WMH) observed on T2-weighted MRI scans, illustrated in Figure 4.3 (for a more detailed account see Chapter 17 in this volume). What appear as WMH on the MRI are localized and circumscribed areas of extreme reduction in white matter density. Most WMH are of pathological origin and are believed to reflect hypoperfusion (Fernando et al., 2006; Holland et al., 2008), microbleeds, and infarcts (De Leeuw, De Groot, and Breteler, 2001). A larger, irregularly shaped WMH may represent "silent" lacunar infarcts that are found in up to 28% of asymptomatic and ostensibly healthy older adults (Vermeer, Longstreth, and Koudstaal, 2007), and are associated with other signs of brain aging such as reduction of cortical metabolism, especially in the prefrontal regions (Reed et al., 2004; Tullberg et al., 2004).

Age differences in WMH mirror the pattern of age-related differences in the white matter volume. As expected for healthy

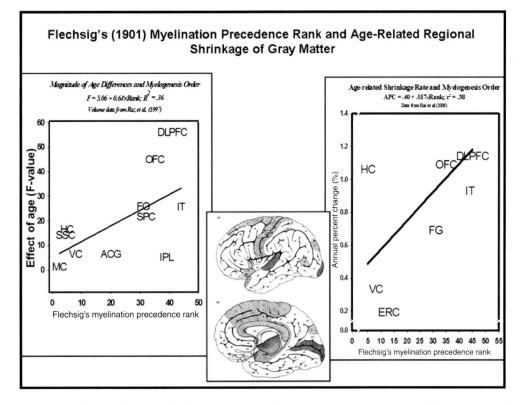

Figure 4–2 Flechsig's (1901) order of regional myelination precedence predicts the magnitude of age-related differences (adapted from Raz et al., 1997) and annual rate of shrinkage (adapted from Raz et al., 2005) in the regional gray matter. In the left graph, the effect size is indexed by the F statistic for the age effect on regional volumes, adjusted for sex and height. In the right panel, the effect is annualized percent change in volume.

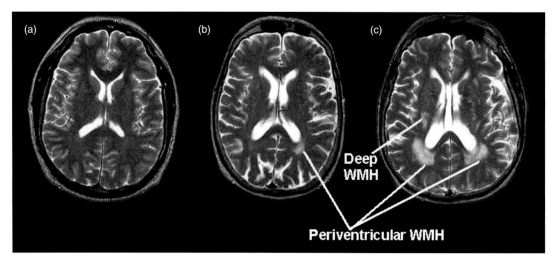

Figure 4–3   Individual differences in the burden of white matter hyperintensities (WMH) observed on T2-weighted MR images. (a) 24-year-old man; (b) 80-year-old man; (c) 79-year-old man. Note the lack of WMH in the young man and the relatively mild periventricular WMH in the 80-year-old man compared with moderate deep and periventricular WMH in a 79-year-old man. All persons are normotensive and have no known neurological or psychiatric conditions.

white matter in the process of adequate myelination, WMH of any kind are extremely rare in young and middle-aged adults. Their prevalence and size increase with time. Risk for WMH that represent silent infarctions increases exponentially with age, and such WMH are significantly more frequent in persons with vascular risk factors (Vermeer, Longstreth, and Koudstaal, 2007). Anti-hypertensive treatment, while significantly reducing the risk for WMH and slowing their progression, does not eliminate them completely (Dufouil et al., 2001, 2005; Raz et al., 2003c, 2007), although there are no sufficient data about possible differential effects of various antihypertensive medications. Some studies suggest that WMH are more prevalent in the frontal regions than elsewhere in the brain (Fazekas et al., 2005; Raz et al., 2003c, 2007; Tullberg et al., 2004; Yoshita et al., 2006). The relatively light posterior WMH burden may progressively expand with increase in cardiovascular risk and increased probability of neurodegenerative disease (Artero et al., 2004; Yoshita et al., 2006). In initially asymptomatic persons it is the parietal rather than frontal WMH burden that increases in the long run, as they manifest cerebrovascular disease (Raz et al., 2007).

Recently, examination of microbleeds visible on T2*-weighted images has been proposed as a useful and sensitive tool for assessing cerebrovascular health and related white matter integrity. A comprehensive review of the extant literature on cerebral microbleeds yielded only four studies of healthy older adults. The prevalence of microbleeds in healthy adults was 5%, compared to about 26% in patients with AD, 45% in persons with miscellaneous vascular risk factors, and up to 70% of persons who have suffered a stroke (Cordonnier, Al-Shahi Salman, and Wardlaw, 2007). The review also showed that hypertension conveys a fourfold increase in risk for microbleeds, and diabetes doubles it. A more recent study of a population sample of (mostly hypertensive) older adults revealed age-related progression in microbleed prevalence (Vernooij et al., 2008a). For now, however, analysis of microbleeds does not yet have the same degree of quantification as does the more established WMH burden analysis, and low prevalence of identifiable microbleeds in healthy adults makes it a less than optimal candidate index for an aging brain study. The latter may change, however, with a wider use of medium- and high-field magnets and

application of MRI sequences optimized for detection of microbleed-induced inhomogeneities (Vernooij et al., 2008b).

Whereas WMH is a reflection of pathological changes at the gross level, diffusion tensor imaging (DTI) and diffusion weighted imaging (DWI) are sensitive enough to examine age-related changes in the microstructure of the white matter (see Moseley, 2002 and Sullivan and Pfefferbaum; 2006c for reviews). Examples of these diffusion images are illustrated in Figure 4.4. Water content and relative contributions of different water fractions in the brain tissue not only determine MRI appearance, but may reveal pathological processes in normally appearing white matter (e.g., Laule et al., 2004). DTI capitalizes on the ability of water diffusion to create local measurable inhomogeneity of the magnetic field (Basser, Mattiello, and Le Bihan, 1994; Merboldt, Hanicke, and Frahm, 1985). It is designed to measure directional properties of diffusion and allow inference of the directionality of the fibers that are characterized by a high degree of diffusion anisotropy. Notably, the white and the gray matter have comparable diffusivity, which is determined by multiple factors, such as the presence of cell membranes as barriers to diffusion, and variations in viscosity of the cellular environment. In contrast, the anisotropy of the intact white matter, in which a layer of myelin represents a formidable barrier to diffusion, is higher than that of the gray matter by an order of magnitude (Pierpaoli et al., 1996). Although multiple indices may be computed from DTI data, the most widely used are apparent diffusion coefficient (ADC) and fractional anisotropy (FA), illustrated in Figures 4.4b and 4.4c, respectively. The former is a computed diffusion coefficient in a given voxel and it can be summed or averaged across any given region. The second index, FA, is a dimensionless indicator of the relative ease of diffusion along each principal direction. Hence, in an intact myelinated fiber, the anisotropy is high (reflected as areas of brighter signal in Figure 4.4c) because it is much easier for water to diffuse along the fiber than across. DTI has only recently been applied to the study of a limited number of regions in the aging brain (see Mosely, 2002, Sullivan and Pfefferbaum, 2003, and Sullivan and Pfefferbaum, 2006c for reviews).

In the DTI literature on aging, there is still no consensus as to the relative utility of various indices of white matter integrity.

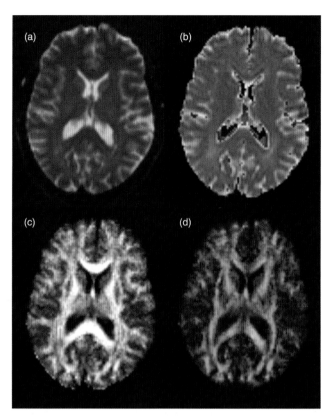

Figure 4–4 Example of DTI scans and maps commonly used for analysis. (a) *b*0-weighted image from DTI scan; (b) apparent diffusion coefficient (ADC) map computed from the DTI scan; (c) fractional anisotropy (FA) map computed from the diffusion tensor; (d) color-coded directional fractional anisotropy map. Notice that in this map, voxels assigned to red represent leftward to rightward fibers (e.g., commissural bundles such as the genu and splenium of the corpus callosum), green voxels represent fibers running anterior-posterior (e.g., most association pathways), and blue voxels represent ascending-descending (ventral-dorsal) fibers (e.g., projection pathways).

Extant studies have often been limited to either few regions of interest measured or large sections of the whole brain. Some of these studies relied on histogram analyses of the ADC maps of the whole brain white matter compartment (Benedetti et al., 2006; Chun et al., 2000; Nusbaum, et al., 2001; Rovaris et al., 2003) and provide no information relevant to regional, anatomically specific age differences. Other studies used specific ROI analyses that examined regional FA and/or ADC coefficients. However, many of these regional studies suffer from questionable reliability, with most studies failing to report computed reliability of the ROIs drawn or placed on the scans. Without knowledge of regional reliability, it is difficult to fully interpret the results. Differences in selection of ROIs across studies also make evaluation of this literature difficult. The most frequently investigated white matter ROIs are the corpus callosum and frontal white matter. Other regions included internal capsule, thalamus, temporal, parietal, and occipital white matter, and the basal ganglia. A handful of studies examined cerebellar hemispheres, peduncles, and the pons. In the extant literature, the number of ROIs per study ranges from one to 16. Further, samples sizes of these studies are relatively small, ranging from 18 to 294 subjects, with the median $N = 38$. Some samples contain only women or only men, mix left- and right-handers, or compare small extreme groups of young and old adults.

The literature on diffusion-based assessment of the white matter and aging consists entirely of cross-sectional studies. It shows that advanced age is associated with reduced white-matter integrity in the whole brain, and, according to some studies, particularly in the anterior white matter (Charlton et al., 2006; Head et al., 2004; Hugenschmidt et al., 2008; Kochunov et al., 2007; Lehmbeck et al., 2006; Sullivan and Pfefferbaum, 2006c). There appear to be no consistent differences in white matter integrity between men and women (Abe et al., 2002; Chepuri et al., 2002; Helenius et al., 2002; Ota et al., 2006; Sullivan et al., 2001; Zhang et al., 2005) or between the left and right hemispheres (Abe et al., 2002; Furutani et al., 2005; Helenius et al., 2002; Zhang et al., 2005); and it remains unclear whether the observed trend is linear or accelerates with age (Charlton et al., 2006; Engelter et al., 2000; Kennedy and Raz, submitted; O'Sullivan et al., 2001; Naganawa et al., 2003). In a lifespan sample of corpus callosum anisotropy, a significantly nonlinear trend was observed in the genu and the total corpus callosum, with FA increasing until the third decade of life, leveling off for about a decade, and then taking a downward course (McLaughlin et al., 2007). Notably, the variability appeared substantially larger in the callosal FA of the older third of the sample. In another study that examined multiple regions of white matter, only the prefrontal FA exhibited a nonlinear trajectory. However, several regions evidenced an accelerated rate of change in diffusivity, including the splenium (but not the genu) of the corpus callosum, the anterior and posterior limbs of the internal capsule, and the superior/posterior parietal white matter (Kennedy and Raz, submitted).

Most studies replicate reduced FA and increased ADC in the broadly defined cerebral regions such as centrum semiovale, corona radiata, pericallosal frontal and parietal areas, and periventricular regions (Bhagat and Beaulieu 2004; Chun et al., 2000; Deary et al., 2006; Furutani et al., 2005; Huang, Ling, and Liu 2006; Nusbaum et al., 2001; Pfefferbaum et al., 2000; Pfefferbaum and Sullivan 2003; Salat et al., 2005; Shenken et al., 2003, 2005; Sullivan et al., 2001; Zhang et al., 2005). However, lack of anatomical specificity make these comparisons difficult to interpret. The findings are less consistent in other regions of the brain. For example, whereas age-related differences in anisotropy among the limbs of the internal capsule have been shown in some studies, no consistent pattern can be discerned (Abe et al., 2002; Bhagat and Beaulieu, 2004; Furutani et al., 2005; Huang, Ling, and Liu, 2006; Hugenschmidt et al., 2007; Kennedy and Raz, submitted; Madden et al., 2004; Nusbaum et al., 2001; Salat et al., 2005; Zhang et al., 2005). In one sample, lobar white matter displayed almost identical age differences in frontal, parietal, and temporal lobes, whereas occipital white matter showed a null effect of age (Grieve et al., 2007), thus conforming to the observed pattern of age differences in cortical regions (Raz and Rodrigue, 2006). Notably, the regional load of WMH correlates with decreased FA and increased regional diffusivity in regions that appear normal on WMH-sensitive MRI sequences (Taylor et al., 2007a). Thus, it is possible that diffusion-based indices of white-matter integrity can reveal early signs of deterioration. That proposition can be tested only in a longitudinal study, yet to be conducted.

The most consistent age-related difference found across studies appears to be reduction in white matter tract integrity in the anterior regions of the brain, especially the genu and body of the corpus callosum and pericallosal frontal white matter (Ardekani et al., 2007; Grieve et al., 2007; Head et al., 2004; Hugenschmidt et al., 2007; Kochunov et al., 2007; Madden et al., 2007; O'Sullivan et al., 2001; Pfefferbaum et al., 2005; Salat et al., 2005; Sullivan and

Pfefferbaum, 2006b; Sullivan et al., 2001); although a recent study found occipital anisotropy and diffusivity effects on par with the age-related differences in the prefrontal white matter (Kennedy and Raz, submitted). Most studies also show little or no reduction in the splenium anisotropy (Abe et al., 2002; Bhagat and Beaulieu, 2004; Chepuri et al., 2002; Head et al., 2004; Hugenschmidt et al., 2007; Ota et al., 2006; Pfefferbaum et al., 2000, 2005; Pfefferbaum and Sullivan, 2003; Salat et al., 2005; Sullivan et al., 2006b). However, Kennedy and Raz (submitted) recently found that not only did the splenium evidence the highest FA and lowest ADC of all the regions examined, but it also displayed a stronger age effect than the genu and most other regions measured. This discrepancy among studies may reflect the more inferior portion of the splenium that was measured, as it is known histologically to be highly age-sensitive (Aboitiz et al., 1996). Interestingly, although there is no evidence of consistent regional differences in diffusivity or anisotropy across the white matter of younger adults, in a sample of 83-year-olds frontal white matter showed a significantly reduced FA and elevated diffusivity, in accord with the suggested anterior-posterior gradient (Deary et al., 2006). This can be taken as limited and circumstantial evidence confirming excessive vulnerability of the frontal regions to aging.

Surprisingly, only one study examined age-related differences in the fornix, a major myelinated tract between the hippocampus and the mammillary bodies that plays an important role in episodic memory performance (Aggleton and Brown 1999). In that study, significant age-related differences in all diffusion parameters of the fornix were noted, whereas no age effect on the cingulum fibers was observed (Stadlbauer et al., 2008a). The estimated number of fibers in the fornix showed the strongest negative correlation with age ($r = -0.79$), thus suggesting that in future studies this index may become a measure of choice. With recent advances in DTI-based fiber tracking methods, more specific investigation of differential aging of white matter becomes possible. In a small sample of young and older adults, the number of frontal connecting fibers (in the anterior corpus callosum) was disproportionately reduced in the older group (Sullivan et al., 2006b). Comparison of the diffusion characteristics in specific fiber tracts suggests selective reduction in white matter integrity in the association but not the projection fibers (Stadlbauer et al., 2008b).

It is unclear whether alterations in white matter microstructure as indexed by FA precede shrinkage, follow it, or are just associated with it. When averaged across the whole brain, FA values correlate significantly and positively with cortical thickness and negatively with WMH load (Kochunov et al., 2007). Significant associations between regional FA values and local volumes derived from modulated VBM were also reported (Hugenschmidt et al., 2008). In that study, VBM-derived volumes of regional white matter showed weaker and less widespread associations with age than did the index of anisotropy. That apparent difference was interpreted as an indication of microstructural change preceding the macro volume changes in the white matter. Regional measures of FA and ADC also correlated significantly with manual volumetry measures in both adjacent gray and white matter volumes, and with the volumes of connected regions in the opposite hemisphere (Kennedy and Raz, 2007). However, only longitudinal studies with multiple waves of measurement can verify this speculation, and at the time of this writing no such studies were available.

Animal models have yielded contradictory results with regards to age effect on the microstructure of the white matter. In aging primates, a pattern of decline on par with human white matter aging has been observed, specifically in the genu of the corpus callosum, superior longitudinal fasciculus, and the cingulum, but no difference in the posterior internal capsule, (Makris et al., 2007). In rats, significant reduction of ADC was observed with age (Heiland et al., 2002), whereas in mice no age-related differences in whole-brain ADC were noted (Rau et al., 2006). Those studies examined the whole-brain (gray and white matter) diffusion properties. Such an approach may be fruitful in studying diffuse and poorly differentiated degenerative processes, but in a phenomenon with demonstrable heterochronicity such as aging, whole-brain histograms are not particularly informative.

Another index of white matter integrity believed to be specifically sensitive to the loss of myelin is magnetization transfer ratio (MTR). Like DTI, magnetization transfer (MT) imaging uses differences in behavior of bound and free water to examine differences in brain tissue (Mehta, Pike, and Enzmann, 1996). In MT imaging, two identical scans are acquired, with one of them being preceded by an off-resonance radio-frequency pulse. The pulse saturates the protons bound to large molecules such as myelin, and the signal in the free water pool is reduced by transferring the restricted pool's saturation. Thus, in comparison to the baseline (no pulse) image, contrast in a magnetization transfer (pulsed) image can be produced: the lowest signal intensity is associated with the mobile water and the highest with the bound or restricted water mainly in the myelinated axons. Experimental studies of ex vivo and in vivo white matter suggest that MTR is a reasonably specific measure of myelin integrity (Wozniak and Lim, 2006).

MTR and DTI approaches do not provide overlapping indices of white matter integrity. Ex vivo high-field MRI demonstrated that myelin content and axonal density correlated strongly with MTR and diffusion anisotropy (FA), but only weakly with the ADC (Mottershead et al., 2003). Mean diffusivity and fractional anisotropy do not reflect the same properties of the white matter as they correlate negatively, with the range of values of FA being quite wide, and that of ADC rather narrow. In abnormal white matter, i.e., WMH, the correlation between the two is reasonably high (Bastin et al., 2007; Taylor et al., 2007a). Thus, in a normal brain, diffusion of intracellular water is tightly controlled, and significant deviation from that range of values indicates pathological disruption of the membranes, and in the case of the white matter, a breach of myelin integrity. In comparison to DTI, MTR is more sensitive to gliosis (Kimura et al., 1996), mechanical axonal injury (Gareau et al., 2000), and Wallerian degeneration (Lexa, Grossman, and Rosenquist, 1994) of myelinated axons.

Like DTI, the MT-derived indices show deterioration of white matter in older adults (Rovaris et al., 2003; but see Mehta, Pike, and Enzmann, 1995), and there is some evidence that MT differences increase with age (Ge et al., 2002). Assessments of MTR in normally appearing and pathological white matter provided converging evidence of the anterior-to-posterior gradient of brain aging: the mean MTR of the frontal periventricular WMH was lower than that of the occipital WMH (Spilt et al., 2006). Notably, MTR usefulness is not restricted to white matter. It shows gray matter abnormalities in older persons with WMH, even when gross volume differences are absent (Mezzapesa et al., 2003). In healthy elderly persons, MTR is significantly more homogenous than in their cognitively impaired peers (van der Flier et al., 2002), but smaller and less homogenous than in young adults (Hofman et al., 1999). However, with the exception of one sample (Silver et al., 1997), MT imaging studies of the aging brain have thus far addressed only global white matter differences, and yielded little information about regional variability in white matter integrity and possible differential vulnerability of specific brain regions to aging.

In one study, however, a trend for greater age-related reduction of MTR in the frontal white matter was reported (Silver et al., 1997).

Of all noninvasive neuroimaging approaches reviewed here, the diffusion-based ones are characterized by probably the most dynamic state of development. New, exciting techniques promise to deliver assessment of white matter integrity along specific fiber tracks. Until recently, the biological underpinnings of MRI-based tractography were unclear. However, two recent studies have demonstrated the validity of diffusion-based fiber-tracking techniques by comparing their results to those of traditional autoradiography and histology (Dauguet et al., 2007; Schmahmann et al., 2007). It would also be interesting to see that approach applied to validating MRI appearance of age-related changes. Thus, future investigations of human brain aging may reveal new information on the integrity of specific white matter tracts beyond age differences in coarse indices of integrity such as FA.

Cognitive Correlates of Brain Aging

Under the basic assumption that the brain is a physical substrate of behavior, it seems highly plausible that age-related differences in brain structure (regional volumes and white matter integrity) should be associated with differences in cognitive performance. Such plausibility notwithstanding, the reality is more complicated. To date, the research of structure-cognition relationships in healthy persons has yielded modest effects and many contradictory findings (see Gunning-Dixon and Raz, 2000; Raz, 2000; Van Petten, 2004 for reviews).

The difficulty of finding reliable structure-function associations stems from multiple sources. First, the very notion that structural MRI reflects valid neurobiological differences caused by physiological aging is problematic, as discussed above. Because it is unclear what exactly is reflected by measured changes and differences in regional volumes, the relationship between volume and cognitive performance, even when observed, is difficult to interpret. Thus, if smaller volume means atrophy and loss of valuable neural elements, then it should predict poorer performance on cognitive tests. However, if increased regional volume reflects pathological processes, such as gliosis or failure to dispose of the unnecessary elements of the neural networks, then decreased volume is expected to go with better cognitive status. A more likely scenario is a multifactorial equilibrium of brain processes that are like vectors in a multiple forces system pulling in different directions, with their summed influences representing the state of the system. Depending on the prevalent forces, such equilibrium shifts toward a specific direction that is associated with better or worse cognitive performance. Because most age-related pathologies are characterized by atrophy, the results are clearer in the studies of Alzheimer's disease or Parkinson disease patients, although some notable exceptions do occur. In some pathological conditions, such as Down syndrome, enlargement of specific regions (e.g., the parahippocampal gyrus) was associated with greater cognitive deficits (Raz et al., 1995). In samples composed of healthier and younger persons, other factors determine the local brain volumes and may overshadow the effects of atrophy on cognition. For example, genetic predispositions to have larger brain structures or to possess qualities that are advantageous for performance on cognitive tasks (see discussion below) may serve as powerful modifiers of structure-function relationships.

When it comes to examining the relations between brain structure and cognition, the controversy is not only about whether "bigger is better," but also about specificity of associations between volume and the cognitive functions, and the notions of brain localization and cognitive specialization. A venerable and still highly influential view dating back to Spearman's (1904) seminal work holds that general intelligence is the source of individual differences in cognition. In the context of cognitive aging, such a "generalist" or "globalist" position is represented by the body of research that points at reduction in speed of processing as the paramount and probably singular reason for age-related declines in cognition (Verhaeghen and Salthouse, 1997). Other analyses indicate that a single factor solution does not account for the observed age-related variability in cognitive performance as well as the solution containing at least two factors, such as fluid and crystallized abilities (McArdle et al., 2002).

The literature on structural correlates of cognitive aging can be interpreted as supporting both views. Some of the findings favor the "globalist" view. A significant proportion of age-related differences in complex cognitive skills can be explained by global reduction in cortical volume (Walhovd et al., 2005b). In many studies, performance in specific cognitive domains (e.g., executive functions) correlate with global indices of brain health, such as WMH burden (see Gunning-Dixon and Raz [2000] for a review of the earlier work and also: Au et al., 2006; Leaper et al., 2001; Söderlund et al., 2006; Tullberg et al., 2004; van der Flier et al., 2005). When scores from the specific cognitive tests are distilled into a g factor they correlate with the total volume of gray and white matter, and controlling for g eliminates the associations between brain volume and cognitive scores (e.g., Staff et al., 2006). Little support emerges in favor of the globalist view, as the evidence of association between speed of processing and brain volume is meager. However, the total white matter volume and WMH load were shown to predict increased variability of reaction time (RT), independently of age, even when RT per se was unrelated to the brain indices (Bunce et al., 2007; Walhovd and Fjell, 2007). On the other hand, in a large sample of older adults, greater cross-sectional corpus callosum (CC) area was linked to faster RT, whereas RT variability was unrelated to CC size (Anstey et al., 2007).

The "globalist" argument does not hold very well against the evidence from studies that have targeted dissociations among specific cognitive skills and specific brain regions. For example, there is limited support for the notion that better preserved executive functions and fluid reasoning abilities are associated with larger prefrontal volumes (Gong et al., 2005; Gunning-Dixon and Raz, 2003; Head et al., 2008; Paul et al., 2007; Raz et al., 1998; Schretlen et al., 2000; Zimmerman et al., 2006), larger prefrontal white matter volumes (Brickman et al., 2006), and smaller frontal WMH load (Gunning-Dixon and Raz, 2003). One study reported that older adults who performed very well on age-sensitive executive function tests had significantly thicker cortex in a circumscribed set of loci, including orbitofrontal, inferior temporal, and insular cortices, as well as the posterior cingulate gyrus and the cuneus (Fjell et al., 2006). The finding of the posterior cingulate involvement is especially interesting in light of its hypothesized role in the early stages of AD (Buckner, 2004). In one study of older adults, declines in performance on a fluid intelligence test (Cattell Culture Fair Intelligence Test) were associated with loss of whole brain volume (Rabbitt et al., 2008), but when various ROIs were evaluated, another sample revealed a specific link between shrinkage of the entorhinal cortex and declines on the same test (Raz et al., 2008).

In investigating neuroanatomical bases of cognitive aging, it is important to consider as many regional structure-function relationships as possible. A considerable proportion of variance among brain regional volumes, age, and cognitive indices is common, and although many brain regions are involved in cognition, a multivariate approach, in which mutual influences of multiple regions are controlled, should be emphasized. For example, in some studies the associations between volumes of certain brain regions and cognitive performance disappear when statistical controls are applied (Paul et al., 2007; Raz et al., 1998).

Although studies that explore neuroanatomical correlates of cognitive aging in animal models are rare, their results generally corroborate findings in humans. One such study has recently reported a negative correlation between the extent of the "aging" pattern that includes a substantial prefrontal component in the aging primate brain and performance on delayed response (DR), but not delayed non-matching-to-sample task (DNMS; Alexander et al., 2008). Note that DR is considered a standard measure of working memory and is sensitive to frontal lesions in monkeys.

There are, however, reports of negative correlations between prefrontal cortical volume and executive function proficiency (Duarte et al., 2006; Salat, Kaye, and Janowsky, 2002; Van Petten et al., 2004). It must be noted, however, that those studies were conducted not on samples spanning the full adult age range but on older (above 60 years of age) persons. In such samples that are composed of older adults with superior cognitive aptitude (Duarte et al., 2006; Van Petten et al., 2004), cognitive reserve (see Chapter 6 in this volume for a detailed discussion) may play a role in suppressing or even reversing the correlations between brain structure and cognition.

The most frequently examined structure-function association in the studies of brain aging is probably the link between hippocampal volume and memory performance. One may surmise that such focused attention is based on the fact that Alzheimer's disease (AD), which is associated with advanced age, is characterized by deterioration of the medial temporal lobe and accompanied by severe impairment of episodic memory. Although some earlier studies revealed positive correlations between memory performance and hippocampal volume in older adults (Golomb et al., 1994), recent meta-analysis of MRI studies indicated that the relationship between hippocampal volume and memory was nil (Van Petten, 2004). However, examination of the effect sizes across studies used in Van Petten's meta-analysis reveals that in the samples that contain a significant number of older participants, a small but positive effect of hippocampal volume on memory is observed. Thus it is possible that in the case of memory and the hippocampus, the structure-function relationship does not reveal itself until old age. Alternately, such association may reflect an admixture of preclinical cases with dementia (Sliwinski and Buschke, 1999). Indeed, research on samples combining healthy adults and persons at various stages of cognitive impairment show that once persons with significantly smaller hippocampi and significant memory deficits are added to the sample, the relationship between HC volume and memory becomes clear (de Leon et al., 2004; Petersen et al., 2000). In one study that found no association between hippocampal volume and memory in the adult life span sample, a strong trend was observed in a small subsample of older participants (Raz et al., 1998). In a recent study of an age-restricted sample of older adults (average age 81 years), larger hippocampi were associated with better performance on memory tests (Zimmerman et al., 2008). Notably, in the same sample, magnetic resonance spectroscopy (MRS) revealed relatively higher signals of neuronal viability marker, NAA, in persons with better mnemonic performance. That finding suggests that the better memory in older people with larger hippocampi was probably due to a better preservation of that region rather than to inborn or maturational advantages.

It is also possible that the relationship between the hippocampus and memory may be more subtle than the correlations between the whole hippocampal volume and simple memory measures can capture. For example, memory performance was positively associated with regional volumes of smaller subdivisions of the hippocampus (Hackert et al., 2002), and when memory was assessed at much longer delays than is customary in laboratory studies (Walhovd et al., 2004, 2006).

Acquisition of specific cognitive skills may be affected by aging, in addition to or because of age-related deficits in memory and executive functions. In several studies the associations between age differences in skill acquisition and procedural learning and neuroanatomy were examined. Specific associations between age differences in perceptual-motor skills and reduction in the striatal and/or cerebellar volumes were observed (Dimitrova et al., 2008; Kennedy and Raz, 2005; Raz et al., 2000; Woodruff-Pak et al., 2001). Age-related deficits in spatial navigation were shown to be mediated by hippocampal and prefrontal volume (Driscoll et al., 2003; Moffat et al., 2007). The latter emerges as a significant mediator of age-related differences in cognitive (Head et al., 2002) and perceptual (Kennedy et al., 2009) skills.

Speed of processing has been found to correlate with thalamic volume, above and beyond the total brain volume effect (Van der Werf et al., 2001), although no cortical regions were examined in that study. Speed and accuracy of mental image processing was associated with prefrontal volume in addition to the effect of age (Raz et al., 1999). Thus it is unclear whether the effect is specific to the thalamus or is associated with age-related differences in a broader network of structures. The observed associations between speed of processing and specific regional volumes, rather than global brain size, contradict the expectations of the "globalist" view of cognitive aging.

Because aging is linked to deterioration of the white-matter microstructure, indices of water diffusion that are sensitive to such changes may prove more useful than volumetry in providing clues to neural mechanisms of cognitive aging. To date, the associations between those indices of white matter integrity (mostly FA) and cognition were examined in several studies, which produced inconsistent results. In primates, higher FA in the frontal tracts is associated with better executive performance but unrelated to learning or memory (Makris et al., 2007). In healthy volunteers, working memory, various executive functions, and fluid intelligence have been shown to correlate with white matter integrity indices such as FA, ADC, or mean diffusivity (Charlton et al., 2006; Deary et al., 2006; Grieve et al., 2007; Kennedy and Raz, 2009; Madden et al., 2007; O'Sullivan et al., 2001; Shenkin et al., 2005; Sullivan et al., 2006).

As myelin is crucial for error-free fast conduction, it would be plausible to hypothesize that diffusion-based indices of white-matter integrity would be associated with differences in processing speed. However, somewhat counter-intuitively, in some samples speed of processing was associated with reduced FA and *higher* mean diffusivity across the brain (Charlton et al., 2006). No significant associations between the diffusion indices of the corpus callosum and inter-hemispheric transfer time were found in normal elderly (Schulte et al., 2005). Nonetheless, others reported associations between white-matter integrity and various measures of speed of processing (Bucur et al., 2008; Deary et al., 2006; Kennedy and Raz, 2009; Madden et al., 2004). Episodic memory performance has been associated with white matter integrity in some samples (Bucur et al., 2008; Kennedy and Raz, 2009;

Persson et al., 2006), but not in others (Deary et al., 2006; Grieve et al., 2007; Shenkin et al., 2005). Literature on white matter measures and specific cognitive skills is very meager, but there is at least one report of association between integrity of a specific tract (the inferior fronto-occipital fasciculus) and age-related decline in face recognition performance (Thomas et al., 2008).

Another index of white matter integrity, which is particularly sensitive to myelin content of the tissue, MTR, showed no reliable correlations with cognitive performance in three studies (Deary et al., 2006; Fazekas et al., 2005; van der Hiele et al., 2007). Notably, the magnitude of the correlations did not vary across the lobes, in spite of significant differences in the magnitude of age-related differences in MTR (Deary et al., 2006). Also of note is that correlations with several other cognitive indices, including highly plausible measures such as reaction time and speed of tapping, were nonsignificant, although the Fazekas et al. (2005) study found a marginal effect of frontal MTR on fine motor dexterity. In one study, MTR histogram was a better predictor of cognition than total brain volume or T2 lesion volume (Lee et al., 2004), but less sensitive than DTI (Schiavone et al., 2009). If, however, the variability across studies that used other neuroimaging methods is any indication, these few findings cannot be taken as definitive and more investigations of MT-based correlates of cognitive aging are needed, especially studies that take care to reliably measure specific regions of interest rather than using global indices of the brain.

Longitudinal follow-up design addresses some of the above-mentioned problems inherent to the cross-sectional studies of high-commonality variables. Individual differences that the participants bring to the study are controlled, and there is a lesser likelihood (although by no means an impossibility) that persons who remained healthy for the duration of the study harbor preclinical disease. Although longitudinal studies of the aging brain and cognition are still scarce, some significant findings have been reported.

Global changes in brain structure are associated with weakening of cognitive performance. Total WMH burden assessed at the age of 80 correlated with long-term declines in general intelligence scores while showing no association with concurrent cognition (Garde et al., 2000), and longitudinal rate of WMH progression predicted cognitive decline (Garde et al., 2005). A 5-year longitudinal study of middle-aged and older adults found that a link between declines in working memory and regional (fusiform gyrus) brain shrinkage was observed in persons with vascular risk but not in healthy participants (Raz et al., 2007). Although entorhinal cortical volume hardly declines with age, persons whose entorhinal cortex evidenced significant shrinkage had reduced (though not pathologically low) memory scores at follow-up (Rodrigue and Raz, 2004). Notably, they were more likely to experience entorhinal shrinkage if they had relatively low fluid intelligence at baseline (Raz et al., 2008). In a 3-year longitudinal study of older adults, declines in multiple measures of cognition were associated with smaller regional volumes in the prefrontal, parietal, and medial-temporal cortices at follow-up (Tisserand et al., 2004).

Because entorhinal and hippocampal shrinkage (De Toledo-Morell et al., 2004; Devanand et al., 2007) predict cognitive deterioration in older adults and transition to dementia, longitudinal changes in medial-temporal structures attracted the attention of investigators of normal aging. In one sample, the rate of hippocampal shrinkage correlated negatively with memory scores at follow-up, regardless of age and sex (Cohen et al., 2006a). In older (74 years old on average) adults, declines in episodic memory were associated with shrinkage of the hippocampus but not with generalized shrinkage of the cerebral cortex (Kramer et al., 2007). Longitudinal decline in delayed recall was greater in persons who had smaller hippocampi at baseline (Tupler et al., 2006). Unfortunately, in neither study were measures of entorhinal volume obtained, and in a study that compared the influence of entorhinal and hippocampal shrinkage adjusted for age, the effect of hippocampal shrinkage on memory was nil, whereas reduction in entorhinal volume occurred in persons with lower memory scores (Rodrigue and Raz, 2004). In sum, as with cross-sectional differences, longitudinal shrinkage of medial-temporal structures is more likely to emerge as a significant predictor of memory performance when older participants are involved.

In summary, the search for the structural basis of age-related declines in cognitive performance has so far yielded limited and somewhat contradictory results. Gross brain changes and individual differences bordering on pathology are indeed associated with lower cognitive performance. Age-related declines in specific cognitive functions may be related to focal declines in brain structure, but also depend on global or broadly defined regional alterations of brain anatomy. On the other hand, the findings of associations between *better* cognitive performance and *smaller* regional volumes remain to be explained. Such inconsistent and contradictory findings underscore two frustrating aspects of inquiry into neuroanatomical correlates of cognitive aging. First, calendar age, as a variable, exerts a very strong and at times overpowering influence on the other variables in the model (the commonality effect, see Lindenberger and Pötter [1998] for a concise discussion of the problem). Second, the associations between brain areas and cognitive tasks are hypothesized on the basis of studies on patients with lesions and degenerative disease that have relatively circumscribed initial focal damage. Those hypotheses may stand on shaky ground when applied to a gradual and less focal process of normal aging.

Because the associations between cognition and brain structural integrity seem stronger in samples with increased risk for pathology, it is important to detect and quantify such risks in samples recruited for studies of ostensibly healthy aging. One can only wonder how many of the observed declines are attributable to physiological aging and how many are due to the influence of the incipient age-related brain. In that context, it is important to examine the factors that can modify, positively or negatively, the expected trajectories of neural and cognitive aging.

Modifiers of Brain Aging

Multiple factors influence brain aging. Some accelerate it; others may slow it down and delay its negative consequences. As one suspects on the basis of the general law of entropy, preventing the former may be easier than promoting the latter. The following is a brief survey of the negative and positive modifiers of aging.

Cardiovascular, circulatory, and respiratory risk factors. The brain is the major consumer of blood supply and even a relatively brief interruption of blood flow, as well as the concomitant reduction in supply of oxygen and glucose, induces significant changes in brain structure. Those changes are evident on in vivo MRI images. For example 10 minutes of experimental ischemia results in significant expansion of the ventricles and reduction of the hippocampal volume in mice (McDaniel et al., 2001). It has been hypothesized more than half a century ago, that arterial hypertension, a highly prevalent chronic age-related condition (see Messerli, Williams, and Ritz [2007] for a review), may preferentially target executive functions and by inference, their neural substrates, especially the prefrontal cortex (Apter, Halstead, and Heimburger, 1951).

Studies in hypertensive rats and humans suggest that the prefrontal cortex may be more vulnerable to hypertension than other brain regions (Raz et al., 2003c; Sabbatini, Tomassoni, and Amenta, 2001). Surgically induced hypertension causes exaggerated executive function deficits in primates that are otherwise observed in the course of normal aging (Moore et al., 2002, 2006). In humans, essential hypertension enhances the effects of aging on prefrontal and medial temporal regions (Carmichael et al., 2007; DeLeew et al., 2001; den Heijer et al., 2005; Goldstein et al., 2002, 2005; Ikram et al., 2008; Raz et al., 2003c; Salerno et al., 1992; Schmidt et al., 1996; Strassburger et al., 1997). A meta-analysis of the relevant literature shows that WMH burden, a known correlate of vascular risk, is linked to moderate deficits in executive functions and memory (Gunning-Dixon and Raz, 2000). Longitudinal studies suggest that hypertension may accelerate age-related shrinkage of the hippocampus (Raz et al., 2005), which is further exacerbated by presence of lacunar infarcts (Du et al., 2006). When persons with identifiable strokes or diagnosed hypertension are eliminated from the sample, the association between WMH load and cognitive decline is significantly reduced (Head et al., 2002; Prins et al., 2005). Unfortunately, although controlling hypertension by medication alleviates cognitive declines, persons who are treated for high blood pressure may still show isolated neuroanatomical and cognitive deficits (den Heijer et al., 2005; Dufouil et al., 2001; Fukuda and Kitani, 1995; Head et al., 2002; Kennedy and Raz, submitted, 2007; Raz et al., 2005; Tzourio et al., 1999; but see van Swieten et al., 1991). Little is known about the effects of mild hypertension on the white matter microstructure. However, there is some evidence that in a lifespan sample of healthy adults, age differences in FA of some regions (temporal and occipital white matter) were substantially exacerbated by hypertension (Kennedy and Raz, 2007, submitted). Detremental effects of hypertension on the occipital white matter, a region frequently considered insensitive to aging, resemble its effects on the occipital WHM and the volume of pericalcarine cortex (Raz et al., 2007).

Multiple metabolic markers of cardiovascular impairment convey additional risk of structural brain differences that are usually associated with aging in general. An example of such a marker is homocysteine (Hcy), an amino acid synthesized from dietary methionine with vitamins B6 and B12 as co-factors and considered a marker for vascular disease (Wierzbicki, 2007). Excess of Hcy is associated with atrophy of the hippocampus (den Heijer et al., 2003; Williams et al., 2002), reduced total gray matter volume (Whalley et al., 2003), and ventriculomegaly (Sachdev et al., 2002). Increased plasma homocysteine predicts cognitive slowing and other neuropsychological deficits (Dufouil et al., 2003; Teunissen et al., 2003), although it is unclear how strong those differences are in healthy adults without other vascular risk factors. Further research is needed to establish whether vascular risk factors such as homocysteine have a differential effect on the brain structure.

The course of brain aging and cognitive performance in the later part of adulthood may be affected by multiple interrelated factors that determine brain oxygenation such as sleep apnea (Foley et al., 2004) and chronic obstructive pulmonary disease (COPD; Antonelli Incalzi et al., 2003; Ortapamuk and Naldoken, 2006). Reduction in direct indices of pulmonary function such as forced expiratory volume and forced vital capacity is linked to increased WMH burden and ventricular enlargement, but not to hippocampal volume in healthy elderly (Sachdev et al., 2006). Chronic

disorders of the respiratory system such as asthma and COPD are associated with significantly lower performance on age-sensitive tasks such as delayed recall and working memory (Liesker et al., 2004; Moss et al., 2005; Saunamäki and Jehkonen, 2007), even at preclinical levels of hypoxia (Liesker et al., 2004). Notably, the pattern of perfusion deficits in COPD appears to accentuate age effects in the anterior, mainly prefrontal, regions (Antonelli Incalzi et al., 2003).

Sleep disturbances, not necessarily complicated by apnea, are frequent among older adults: their prevalence increases with age (Ancoli-Israel, 2005; Zisapel, 2007), and their negative cognitive effects have been demonstrated (Ancoli-Israel, 2005; Bastien et al., 2003; Foley et al., 1999; Hornung, Danker-Hopfe, and Heuser, 2005, 2007; McEwen, 2006; Yaffe et al., 2007). The effects of sleep disruption may be expressed on the cellular level, i.e., in impaired neurogenesis (Guzman-Marin et al., 2007). Normative sleep is important for maintaining many cognitive operations in young adults. Sleep deprivation not only results in impairment of age-sensitive vital functions such as blood pressure regulation and glucose metabolism but also appears to affect age-sensitive structures such as the prefrontal cortex (Boonstra et al., 2007; Hennevin, Huetz, and Edeline, 2007; McEwen, 2006). Thus, it is plausible that age-related sleep disturbances may account for a significant share of variance in aging cognition. Yet, there are no comprehensive studies of the possible associations of sleep problems with age-related changes in brain structure and their influence on cognitive performance. In part, the dearth of relevant investigations may be explained by the extremely labor-intensive nature of sleep studies, that makes data collection on reasonably large samples rather difficult. Nonetheless, investigations of the modifying effects of sleep disturbances on the aging brain and cognition seem long overdue.

Stress. At the most basic level stress is defined as an external influence that disturbs systemic homeostasis (McEwen, 2007; Pardon, 2007). Stress response or *allostasis* is defined as an "adaptive process for actively maintaining stability through change (McEwen and Stellar, 1993; Sterling and Eyer, 1988). So defined, stress is a part of life, and eliminating it entirely seems neither feasible nor desirable. However, when allostatic load exceeds certain levels, when it turns into chronic assault on the vital systems, and when it is not alleviated by an adaptive response, the consequences for the organism may be dire. Because the adaptive stress response is based on the activity of the hypothalamic-pituitary-adrenal (HPA) axis, the system believed to be intimately involved in the physiology of aging, the link between allostasis and aging is highly plausible, and it may be expressed on the level of neuroanatomical changes (see McEwen, 2007; Pardon, 2007 for reviews).

Animal studies reveal significant changes in brain structure and function that can be linked to acute and chronic increase in allostatic load. The connections between stress, acute and chronic, and structural brain changes are complex and sometimes contradictory. Stress affects fundamental processes of cellular plasticity. It reduces the number of spine synapses and impairs generation of LTP in the CA1 and CA3 regions of the hippocampus and causes dendritic shortening in the medial prefrontal cortex (McEwen, 2007). Chronic stress induces excitotoxicity and alters calcium homeostasis in the dentate gyrus (Joëls et al., 2007). In contrast, in the amygdala and orbitofrontal cortex allostatic load actually enhances dendritic growth (Joëls et al., 2007; McEwen, 2007). All those changes are believed to be mediated by glucocorticoids and excitatory amino acids, as well as neuroplasticity promoters such as BDNF (McEwen, 2007). In a unique dissociation study that combined MRI imaging with histology, excessive levels of the stress hormone cortisol caused reduction in the volume of the anterior cingulate gyrus but not the whole brain or retrosplenial cortex of rodents (Cerqueira et al., 2005). In primates, the magnitude of stress response was shown to be negatively associated with hippocampal volume (Lyons et al., 2001, 2007). Notably, the effects of increased allostatic load appear stronger in the regions known for their elevated plasticity and neurogenesis, e.g., the dentate gyrus and CA3 sector of the hippocampus; and indeed, an increase in allostatic load has a detrimental effect on both neurogenesis and plasticity (Joëls et al., 2007). In addition to the outlined effects on cellular structure, chronic stress may also exert its negative influence on the brain by promoting inflammation and cytokine production (Sorrells and Sapolsky, 2007).

In contrast to the multiplicity of animal (mainly rodent) studies of neuroanatomical changes brought by stress, the human literature is quite limited, and studies on brain, stress, and aging are extremely scarce. In human studies, safe manipulations of acute stress are difficult, and chronic stress induction is patently unethical. Thus, although short term alterations in cognitive performance and its brain correlates can be measured with mild stress manipulations in the laboratory, the long term effects of chronic stress on the human brain can be gauged only through indirect evidence and the use of historical information. One of the phenomena that may inform us about the effects of stress on aging is mood disorders.

Depression, which is prevalent in older adults (Gareri, De Fazio, and De Sarro, 2002), is exacerbated and probably initiated by stressful life events and is linked to hyperactivity of the HPA (Swaab, Bao, and Lucassen, 2005). In patients with depression, the volume of the hippocampus and amygdala, as well as the prefrontal cortex, may be significantly reduced in comparison to healthy controls (Drevets et al., 1997; Sheline, Gado, and Kraemer, 2003; Sheline et al., 1999). Postmortem investigations suggest, however, that reduction of the hippocampal and prefrontal volume in depression may reflect a significant loss of glia, not only of neurons or dendritic processes (Rajkowska, 2003). Disruption of fronto-striatal connections by vascular changes in the prefrontal white matter may explain in part the excessive vulnerability of hypertensive older adults to depression (Hoptman et al., 2008).

Because stress response is associated with release of cortisol, assessing individual differences in its levels may provide insight into the effects of stress on the brain. Indeed, basal cortisol levels were found to correlate with both memory performance and hippocampal (but not temporal lobe or parahippocampal) volumes in older adults and young men (Lupien et al., 1998; Pruessner et al., 2007). In another sample the negative links between hippocampal volume, cortisol increase and memory were observed only in persons with a specific genetic variant of serotonin transporter gene (O'Hara et al., 2007). Thus, genetic predisposition may modify brain response to stress and, in some individuals, promote faster cognitive aging.

Another source of comparative information on stress and the brain is Cushing syndrome. In Cushing syndrome, which is characterized by chronic elevation of cortisol levels, a progressive reduction in the hippocampal volume has been observed (Bourdeau et al., 2005). On the other hand, chronic adminstation of medications that induce elevation of glucocorticoids is not associated with differences in hippocampal volume (Coluccia et al., 2008). Notably, treatment of Cushing syndrome results in reduction of cortisol levels, increase in hippocampal volume, and improvement of verbal learning (Starkman et al., 2003). Thus,

neuroanatomical effects of glucocorticoid excess, similar to those observed in chronic stress, may be malleable.

Lifestyle and life history associated with chronic stress or lack thereof may modify brain aging. Severe stress that is sufficient to cause post-traumatic stress syndrome (PTSD) is linked, in a dose-response manner, to reduced volume of the hippocampus and, to a lesser extent, amygdala as well as developmental deficits in the prefrontal cortex and white matter (Karl et al., 2006). Developmental predisposition to PTSD and other negative effects of stress is underscored by a finding that early life stress, operationalized through an inventory of adverse childhood events, is associated with reduced volumes of anterior cingulate cortex and caudate nucleus, though not the hippocampus or amygdala (Cohen et al., 2006b).

Although the consequences of living in pain or bliss are not easy to quantify, both present natural experiments that allow some appraisal of the effects of stress on human brain. Thus, an interesting insight into possible structural effects of stress was provided by a study of chronic pain patients, which demonstrated that prolonged suffering, regardless of the type of pain, was associated with a considerably reduced volume of the prefrontal cortex in a dose-response manner (Apkarian et al., 2004). Notably, no effects on the hippocampus were observed in that sample. To compare, in a small sample study of middle-age adults, persons who were habitually engaged in a relaxation practice (Zen meditation) for more than 3 years, showed no age-related differences in gray matter volume that were observed in healthy controls (Pagnoni and Cekic, 2007). It must be noted, however, that in interpreting the results of both studies, subject selection is a threat to validity. Negative or positive associations with a certain lifestyle or practices may reflect self-selection and predisposition that are impossible to control in a cross-sectional study, although dose-response effects (Apkarian et al., 2004) mitigate that problem to some extent.

One of the difficulties in translating the findings from animal literature to humans is that the former focuses mainly on the hippocampus (McEwen, 2007), whereas human studies have a broader focus. They consistently indicate the importance of cortical and striatal circuits in mediating allostatic effects on brain structure. Such a shift in emphasis, or at least a broadening of the search net, is consistent with the findings that indicate increased density of glucocorticoid receptors in the human cortex, especially in the association regions (Perlman et al., 2007).

In sum, the physiology of stress response is such that repeated and chronic stress may predispose the brain to premature aging. Yet, little is known about the actual modifying effect of stress on the trajectories of cerebral and cognitive aging in humans. Stress may play a complex role in modifying the course of aging; but to assess its effects, more studies with significantly greater statistical power and attention to more cerebral regions than just the hippocampus will be necessary. In addition, more comparative neuroimaging studies will certainly help to tease apart the connections between localized changes in structural plasticity and specific parameters of allostasis.

Aerobic fitness. Although the neurobiology of effects produced by vigorous aerobic activity is not yet well understood, the effects of exercise on circulatory and pulmonary systems are well known (Dishman et al., 2006). Aging is not kind to athletic prowess, as it is associated with a steady decline in peak oxygen utilization capacity, and the rate of decline accelerates from 3% in the 20s to more than 20% per decade in the 70s, especially in men (Fleg et al., 2005; Hollenberg et al., 2006). In that context, a growing body of research lends support to the notion that aerobic fitness has a positive effect on the brain and cognition of older adults (Cotman and Berchtold, 2002; Kramer and Erickson, 2007). Although the literature is still relatively limited, the general conclusion is that executive functions and the brain regions associated with them may enjoy some degree of protection in individuals who show higher levels of aerobic fitness (Colcombe and Kramer, 2003; Colcombe et al., 2003; Lesniak and Dubbert, 2001).

Notably, the regions that are most vulnerable (and probably most malleable) in normal aging (Raz, 2000, 2004c) appear to benefit the most from fitness-promoting interventions. Such a regional pattern provides additional support for speculation that late-life plasticity may be a viable phenomenon driving the positive effects of exercise (Greenwood, 2007; Kramer and Erickson, 2007). An intriguing finding lending further support to that idea has been reported recently in a sample of 59 older adults defined as "healthy but sedentary." In that study, the participants in a 6-month program of aerobic training evidenced a significant enlargement of measured brain tissue (via VBM). In contrast, no change was observed in persons who took part in a stretching exercise program or in young adults (Colcombe et al., 2006).

Thus, if age-related declines represent "the dark side of plasticity" (Raz, 2007), exercise, by enhancing the latter, may help to brighten the picture to some extent. More research is needed on possible interaction between beneficial interventions such as aerobic training and negative modifiers, such as hypertension with genetic predisposition (see Raz [2006] for a brief review). In addition, research on fitness manipulation in older adults needs to address several potential confounding factors, such as improved hydration in people who participate in the exercise program. After all, significant fluctuations in water intake have been shown to affect volumes of cerebral structures measured on MRI scans (Duning et al., 2005), although if hydration is important in tissue volume changes, one would expect the effects to be global rather than regional. Moreover, reduction in hydration is a significant problem at least in some elderly who have impaired thirst perception, decreased glomerular filtration rate and other impairments of the urinary system (Luckey and Parsa, 2003).

Hormone replacement therapy. The endocrine system undergoes profound age-related changes, which bear unfavorably on the brain and cognition (Janowsky, 2006; Moffat, 2005). When there is a belief that some of the declines are caused by a deficit in sex hormones, replenishing the latter appears a reasonable therapeutic strategy. The link between the levels of circulating hormones and neural as well as cognitive well-being is complicated and unclear. Higher levels of estrogen per se do not convey neural advantages on older women or men (den Heijer et al., 2003); and in older men, a link between blood levels of bioavailable testosterone and cerebral atrophy as well as elevated WMH burden has been reported (Irie et al., 2006). In one study of men in the seventh decade of their lives, higher blood testosterone levels predicted larger cerebral hemispheres, as well as frontal and parietal lobes, while correlating negatively with the occipital lobe volume and showing no relationship with WMH burden (Lessov-Schlager et al., 2005). Nonetheless, hormone replacement therapy (HRT) has been viewed as a promising neuroprotective strategy. Although some research has been conducted in men (Moffat, 2005), most of the HRT is synonymous with administration of female hormones to women.

Animal studies support the view of estrogen as a neuroprotector (McEwen, 2002; Van Amelsvoort, Compton, and Murphy, 2001). In human literature, especially in longitudinal studies, estrogen replacement seems to show promising effects, with evidence of reduction in WMH burden (Schmidt et al., 1996);

slower total brain shrinkage (Cook et al., 2002); larger hippocampal (Eberling et al., 2003) and cerebellar (Ghidoni et al., 2006) volumes; increased rCBF in medial temporal and association cortices (Maki and Resnick, 2000); and slower shrinkage of the age-sensitive cortical regions (dorsolateral prefrontal cortex and prefrontal white and fusiform gyrus; Raz et al., 2004b; Erickson et al., 2005). However, these encouraging results of multiple small studies have been offset by the results of large-scale clinical trials, in which HRT was associated with higher prevalence of cerebral infarcts (Luoto et al., 2000) and dementia (Shumaker et al., 2003). This apparent conflict between overwhelmingly optimistic predictions of experimental studies and alarming findings of the large-scale clinical trials needs to be resolved by greater attention to the demographics of the samples, selection of specific treatment approaches, and refinement of measurement instruments. One of the reasons for that discrepancy may be a time-sensitive nature of HRT, which, as was suggested by several researchers, may be effective only within a critical time window (Lord et al., 2008; also see Genazzani et al. [2007] for a review). Another possibility may be failure to counteract the negative pro-inflammatory action of estrogen (Straub, 2007) while capitalizing on its neuroprotective qualities. Finally, some women may be not able to benefit from at least some aspects of estrogen's neuroprotective action due to genetic predisposition. For example, in women who are homozygotic for T allele of C677T MTHFR, a gene controlling metabolism of homocysteine (Frosst et al., 1995), HRT does not reduce homocysteine levels (Brown et al., 1999).

Genetic Factors in Aging of the Brain and Cognition

Like any property of the organism, brain structure and function are determined to a large extent by the action of genes—alone, in their mutual interactions, or in interaction with the environment. Several studies used classic population genetics methods to examine the heritability of brain structural properties. Their results support the notion that across the life span the factors that regulate structural aspects of the brain are under significant genetic control. Only a handful of studies estimated heritability of brain structural properties, and they revealed significant differences among the examined structures. Heritability of the intracranial volume, total brain size, lateral ventricles, and cross-sectional area of the corpus callosum are rather high, ranging between 62% and 94% (Bartley and Jones, 1997; Pfefferbaum et al., 2000; Scamvougeras et al., 2003; Sullivan et al., 2001). By comparison, gyral-sulcal patterns show lower heritability, between 10% and 60% (Bartley and Jones, 1997; Carmelli et al., 1998; see Winterer and Goldman [2003] for a review). A study that examined local differences in brain structure in a sample of middle-aged twins revealed an interesting pattern of genetic dependency. It indicated that heritability was highest in the dorsolateral prefrontal cortex (areas 9 and 46) and lowest in the posterior occipito-parietal regions (Thompson et al., 2001). Thus the structures that are most vulnerable to aging may be under the greatest genetic control. Evidence to the contrary seems to come from a twin study of DTI-based white matter integrity in the corpus callosum. That study, while showing high heritability for callosal microstructure, revealed a substantially greater relative share of genetic variance in the posterior rather than anterior, putatively more age-sensitive, CC (Pfefferbaum et al., 2001).

Heritability of WMH load is also quite high (Atwood et al., 2004; Carmelli et al., 1998; Turner et al., 2004), although little is known about the influence of genes on the course of WMH expansion. By comparison, the volume of the hippocampus, a structure with demonstrated vulnerability to multiple environmental pathogens, is under significantly less genetic control, with heritability estimated at only 40% (Sullivan et al., 2001). Therefore, most of the variability in hippocampal volume is induced by environmental events, disease, or interactions of the two. Notably, a longitudinal assessment of heritability indicated that although the genetic component of the variance in corpus callosum area ventricular size remained stable across a 4-year follow-up, the contribution of the environmental component to ventricular size increased significantly (Pfefferbaum et al., 2004). Thus, some brain structures appear differentially more sensitive than others to environmental insults, for a variety of reasons. The increase of environmental influence on the hippocampus may reflect its vulnerability to multiple pathogens and insults such as hypoxia, ischemia, stress, and extreme mood and sleep disturbances; whereas the ventricular system's propensity to show increasing environmental variance may be due to its nature as a summary index of multiple CNS systems.

The genes are numerous, their functions are multiple, and the interactions are complex. So it is unlikely that we will be able to find a definitive answer to the question of genetic determination of the aging of the brain and cognition. Moreover, advances in computer and genomic technology have produced a powerful shotgun approach to genetic data mining known as whole-genome scans (Rao, 1998). As a result, millions of single nucleotide polymorphisms (SNPs) can be discovered and linked to a bewildering variety of traits and diseases. The dangers of such technology producing an unchecked avalanche of false positives propagated by loose replication criteria have been clearly demonstrated (Sullivan, 2007), although a reasonable balance of false positives against false negatives is well advised (Rao, 1998). Multiple factors, such as biased stratification between cases and controls, assortative mating, and other epigenetic phenomena, must be taken into account to prevent unqualified acceptance of chance findings. While a concerted effort to control for spurious findings, along with preserving the power of the method, is underway (e.g., Price et al., 2006; Zhao et al., 2007), several specific genes and SNPs have been linked to distinct neural and cognitive variation in healthy adults and to their developmental trajectories with a reasonable consistency and thus merit further examination. Below we review the findings pertaining to the selected genetic factors linked to neuroanatomical variation.

COMT. Many aspects of prefrontal cortical activity are controlled by dopamine, and dopaminergic transmission shows significant age-related declines (see Bäckman and Farde, 2004; Bäckman et al., 2006 and Chapter 5 for a review). One of the key determinants of the efficiency of dopaminergic function is catechol-O-methyl transferase, COMT, a catabolizing enzyme whose activity limits the dopamine flux, especially in the prefrontal circuits (Tunbridge et al., 2004). The levels of COMT are heritable (Weinshilboum and Raymond, 1977), and the degree to which COMT can limit availability of dopamine is controlled by a COMT gene (Tenhunen et al., 1994). A common Val158Met substitution in that gene locus affects the thermostability of the protein and leads to a significant decrease in the activity of the enzyme in the brain (Chen et al., 2004).

Several studies in young and middle-aged adults show that the COMT Val158Met polymorphism affects cognitive performance and that COMT Met carriers perform better than Val carriers on executive tasks (Barnett et al., 2007; Bruder et al., 2005; Caldú et al., 2007; Diaz-Asper et al., 2008; Tan et al., 2007) and, according to some studies, in an allele-dosage fashion (Egan et al., 2001). They

also show lower variability of reaction time on continuous performance tasks (MacDonald et al., 2007; Stefanis et al., 2005). Epistatic interactions between the COMT gene and the genes that control metabotropic glutamate receptor activity (GRM3) and dopamine transporter gene (DAT) expression have been observed. The combination of suboptimal variants of each gene produced greater and more wide-spread task-specific prefrontal activation and altered the normal pattern of prefrontal-parietal coupling during performance of a working memory task (Tan et al., 2007). Persons who carry two Val alleles of the COMT gene and 9-repeat alleles of DAT showed greater activation of the prefrontal cortex on a working memory task than those who did not have that combination of genes at the same levels of performance (Caldú et al., 2007).

There are very few studies of COMT Val158Met polymorphism and age-related differences in cognition. A longitudinal study of older adults suggests that the Met allele of the COMT gene may play a protective role (de Frias et al., 2005). In contrast, a study of healthy elderly revealed no effects of the COMT genotype on memory and speed of processing (O'Hara et al., 2006). Moreover, Val/Val men performed better than heterozygotes and Met/Met men on a test of delayed recall. The Met allele was associated with better performance on a combination of cognitive tests, including measures of memory and fluid intelligence in a group of older adults (Starr et al., 2007). In that study, a dose-response effect of the Met allele on cognition was observed. Other recent cross-sectional studies showed independent negative effects of advanced age and the Val/Val COMT genotype on fluid intelligence, memory, and speed of processing, but not on inhibition (Raz et al., 2009); and in a study of extreme age groups of Met and Val homozygotes, a significant COMT genotype $\times$ age interaction was observed, with Met homozygosity being associated with improved executive performance of older but not younger adults (Nagel et al., 2008).

The results of cognitive and functional MRI studies strongly suggest that the COMT gene may be involved in age-related vulnerability of the prefrontal regions. However, at the time of this writing, only a few studies have examined the effect of the COMT genotype on regional brain volumes in healthy adults. Zinkstok et al. (2006) found age-related differences in gray and white matter density, but only in women. In that sample, female Val carriers evidenced larger gray matter density in the temporal and parietal lobes and the cerebellum as well as increased frontal white matter density. Further, female Met homozygotes evidenced age-related decrease in gray matter density in the parietal lobe and decreased white matter density in the frontal lobes, the parahippocampal gyrus, and the corpus callosum (Zinkstok et al., 2006). These findings contradict the expectations based on cognitive findings that suggest that the Val allele is associated with poorer performance on tests of executive functions. The same group found a similar association between Val homozygocity and larger prefrontal cortices in adults with Velo-cardio-facial syndrome (VCFS), a chromosomal abnormality associated with deletions at chromosome 22q11I, cognitive impairment, and psychosis (Van Amelsvoort et al. 2007). However, another VBM study also reported greater prefrontal gray matter in val homozygotes and greater hippocampal gray matter in met carriers (Cerasa et al., 2008). Honea et al. (2009) used VBM to find decreased gray matter in the hippocampus and parahippocampal gyrus in val carriers and val homozygotes compared to met homozygotes, but also found decreased gray matter in the dorsolateral prefrontal cortex in the met carriers.

A volumetric study examined the regional volumes of several ROIs in healthy middle-aged adults and found that Val homozygotes had smaller temporal lobes and hippocampi than Met carriers, with no difference in the volumes of the caudate or cerebral hemispheres (Taylor et al., 2007b). The frontal regions were not examined in that study. These results are more in line with the expected detrimental effect of the val allele and/or neuroprotective effect of the met allele. More studies are needed before the stability of the association between COMT Val homozygocity and larger brain (especially prefrontal) volumes is established. If it is replicated, it may serve as a basis for a plausible explanation of the above-mentioned findings of negative correlations between prefrontal volumes and executive performance (Duarte et al., 2006; Van Petten et al., 2004; Salat, Kaye, and Janowsky, 2002). Alternatively, these descrepancies may be explained by a U-shaped relationship between regional brain volumes and COMT activity, where its effects vary from the very low to the very high activity haplotypes (Honea et al., 2009). In sum, COMT seems to be reliably associated with reduced executive functions regardless of age. Interaction between COMT genotypes and aging is unclear, and relatively little is known about the effect of Val158Met polymorphism on structural brain aging, although it seems to exert its influence on the age-sensitive aspects of neuroanatomy.

BDNF. Brain-derived neurotrophic factor (BDNF) is a promoter of neural plasticity and a potent modulator of LTP, a putative correlate of memory consolidation (see Lynch et al. [2007] for a review). Cognitive differences associated with BDNF Val/Met polymorphism were investigated in several studies. In two studies, Met allele carriers evidenced reduced recognition memory and decreased HC activation at encoding on fMRI experiments (Mattay and Goldberg, 2004), as well as poorer episodic memory in comparison to Val-homozygous individuals (Ho et al., 2006; Raz et al. 2008). However, a study of healthy older adults from the Scottish Mental Survey sample revealed no difference in memory and a significant effect on fluid reasoning tests that went in the opposite direction: Met homozygotes outperformed the heterozygotes and the latter did better than Val/Val homozygotes (Harris et al., 2006, 2007). The reason for that discrepancy is unknown. It is possible that the Met/Met carriers were a selected group of healthy survivors with a potentially detrimental genotype who by the selection criteria were cognitively intact in their late seventies and early eighties.

Several studies reported significant differences in the volume of the hippocampus and other medial temporal structures were associated with BDNF Val66Met polymorphism. Healthy volunteers, homozygous for Val BNDF allele, have larger volumes of the hippocampal formation compared to Val/Met heterozygotes (Bueller et al., 2006; Frodl et al., 2007; Szeszko et al., 2005). In a recent study, middle-aged adults who carried BDNF 66Met allele evidenced reduced volume of the amygdala in comparison to their younger counterparts, whereas no difference was observed in the BDNF Val66 homozygotes (Sublette et al., 2008). In a small sample study, healthy BDNF 66Met carriers had significantly smaller parahippocampal and left superior frontal gyri than the Val homozygotes (Takahashi et al., 2008).

One study of healthy adults revealed a significant age-related volume reduction in the dorsolateral prefrontal cortex (Nemoto et al., 2006). BDNF 66Val homozygotes also had larger anterior cingulate, temporal, and parietal cortices, and the negative correlation between bilateral prefrontal volumes and age was observed only in the Met carriers (Nemoto et al., 2006). Furthermore, in the same study, female Met carriers showed more widespread age-associated volume reduction in the prefrontal cortex than male Met carriers (Nemoto et al., 2006). In another sample, Met allele carriers had smaller temporal and occipital lobar gray matter volumes and significantly less density in prefrontal, fusiform, and secondary

visual cortices (Ho et al., 2006). A recent study showed that Met allele carriers may have smaller volume of the posterior superior cerebellar vermis (Agartz et al., 2006).

In sum, the studies of BDNF Val66Met polymorphism are scarce, and those that exist produced contradicting results, except maybe for relatively consistent evidence of the negative effect of the BDNF 66Met allele on hippocampal volume. Unfortunately, investigation of the effects of the Met BDNF allele on brain and cognition is hampered by the fact that that allele may be so dysfunctional that only very few persons would pass the health screening criteria to enter the study. The frequency of Met/Met BDNF carriers in selective healthy samples is about 2% (Raz et al., 2008). Those who survive with their cognitive abilities intact may represent a special group with other factors working to offset the negative effects of the Met allele.

ApoE. The role of the ApoE ε4 allele as a significant risk factor for early-onset Alzheimer's disease is well established (Corder, Saunders, and Strittmatter, 1993; Reiman, 2007; see more in Chapter 9). However, its effect in normal cognitive and brain aging are less clear. A recent meta-analysis found that although ApoE ε4 has a significant effect on cognition in normal elderly, the magnitude of the effect is very modest (Small et al., 2004). More recent longitudinal studies reveal stronger associations between the decline of episodic memory and the ε4 allele of the ApoE gene (Caselli et al., 2004; Tupler et al., 2006), especially in persons older than 60 years of age (Baxter et al., 2003). The negative effects of the ApoE ε4 allele on cognition may find stronger expression in functions that are necessary for proper function of memory encoding and retrieval systems but are not measured directly by standard memory tests. For example, declines in performance on a visual search task assessed over 1 year were significantly greater in carriers of ε4 than in other healthy middle-aged and older adults, and the effect on spatial attention and learning was dose-dependent (Greenwood et al., 2005a, 2005b; Negash et al., 2007). In contrast, the influence of ApoE ε4 on working memory may be confined to homozygotes (Greenwood et al., 2005a), with no effect on age-insensitive implicit learning (Negash et al., 2007).

Cross-sectional studies of samples with a wide age range have shown that ApoE ε4 carriers evidence a significantly thinner cortical mantle and reduced volume of cerebral cortex and cerebellum. The genotype effect was especially strong in the anterior prefrontal and temporal as well as inferior parietal cortices, and fusiform gyri (Espeseth et al., 2008; Wishart et al., 2006). No association between the ε4 allele of the ApoE gene and the area of the corpus callosum was found in a representative sample of older adults (Anstey et al., 2007). Other large-sample studies suggested that in the older adults, ApoE ε4 effects on cortical atrophy and cognitive performances may be limited to ε4 homozygous individuals, a relatively rare group in the general population and probably even more difficult to find in the selective healthy samples (Lemaître et al., 2005; Lind et al., 2006). Notably age-related variability in brain parameters may be reduced in that group (Lind et al., 2006). An interesting result was recently reported regarding age-related differences in an MRI parameter associated with iron content, R2 relaxation time. In a sample of healthy adults, age-related declines in R2 (and implied increases in iron deposits) were associated in a dose-response manner with the presence of the ε4 allele (Bartzokis et al., 2007). Moreover, carriers of a rare ε2 allele of the ApoE gene were less likely to show increased R2, implying a protective role for that allele.

Longitudinal studies of the ApoE ε4 effects on brain structure are mostly confined to assessment of hippocampal volume changes. The rate of hippocampal shrinkage is greater among ε4+ compared with ε4- individuals (Cohen et al., 2001; Jack et al., 2007; Jak et al.,

2007; Lind et al., 2006; Moffat et al., 2000; van de Pol et al., 2007; but see Cohen et al. [2006a] for a contradictory finding); and persons without the ε4 allele show slower overall brain shrinkage than ε4 carriers (Chen et al., 2007). No associations between hippocampal volume and ApoE ε4 presence were found in a study of healthy adults that revealed longitudinal decline in episodic memory (Tupler et al., 2006). Moreover, studies that revealed an association between HC shrinkage and ε4+ genotype showed no cross-sectional association between HC volume and that allele (Jak et al., 2007).

The effects of ApoE ε4 on brain structure may appear quite early in a person's life and express themselves in a reduction of glucose metabolism in the regions that are vulnerable to AD (Reiman et al., 2004). In a large sample of typical older adults, there was a higher subcortical (but not periventricular) WMH volume than in ApoE ε3/3 carriers irrespective of hypertension; whereas participants with both hypertension and at least one ApoE ε4 allele had the highest degree of WMH (De Leeuw et al., 2004). Other risk factors may interact with ApoE ε4 to produce synergistically enhanced risk. For example, the negative effects of prolonged stress on memory are stronger in ApoE ε4 carriers compared to their ε4-free peers (Peavy et al., 2007). Epistatic interactions with other genes may augment the effect of ApoE ε4. For example, having one copy of ε4 and being a homozygote for the T allele of a nicotinic receptor gene CHRNA4 is associated with reduced white matter volume, whereas no difference is observed for other ε4 carriers (Espeseth et al., 2006).

Other polymorphisms have been linked to variations in brain morphometry and volume. One recent example is of the PLXNB3 gene, which controls plexin B3, one of the proteins that serve as semaphorine receptors and are crucial for axonal growth. The relatively novel (human-specific) A haplotype was linked to increased volume of cerebral white matter as well as higher verbal ability (Rujescu et al., 2007). An association was also reported between the Tyrosine for Histidine substitution (His452Tyr) polymorphism of the serotonin receptor 2A gene (5-HT2A) and reduced volumes of temporal lobe cortical regions and white matter (Filippini et al., 2006).

In sum, the first years since the advent of the genomic revolution have already yielded some evidence to support the claims for significant genetic determination of some of the most fundamental aspects of cerebral and cognitive aging. This evidence, however, has been thus far assembled mostly from a few single SNP studies. Given the complexity of behaviors and the multifaceted nature of genetic control of the basic biochemical processes, it is safe to presume that the role of specific genes in brain aging and its consequences will be clarified through examination of epistatic interactions and the combined effects of single genes on specific aspects of brain and behavior. The first evidence of the fruitfulness of such an approach has been recently published (Espeseth et al., 2008; Reiman et al., 2007; Tan et al., 2007), and is expected to multiply.

Conclusions

This overview of the extant literature on the brain and cognitive aging and their modifiers suggests that the human brain shrinks with age, and brain shrinkage is selective and differential.

1. According to cross-sectional studies, the prefrontal cortices emerge as the most vulnerable region of the aging brain, whereas some but not all sensory cortices show virtually no aging-related differences.

2. Longitudinal studies are still too scarce and incomplete in the breadth and details of their assessment. Nonetheless, while converging with cross-sectional investigations in highlighting the prefrontal cortices as the regions of increased vulnerability, they implicate other tertiary association cortices (e.g., the inferior parietal), the neostriatum, the hippocampus, and the cerebellum to the same extent. It is hoped that the next decade will produce more longitudinal results that will further elucidate the nature of age-related change in brain structure.

3. The application of new neuroimaging methods depends on developing new methods of data reduction that distill the vast amounts of data to meaningful indicators of brain structural properties. Semi-automated methods such as VBM may aid in conducting studies of the aging brain on a larger scale, and they may become a standard first-pass approach to the analysis of large brain samples. However, because of their significant limitations, they need to be followed by manual measures of the target regions.

4. Unlike cortical tissue, the white matter exhibits a nonlinear relationship with age, as far as its gross volume, or pathological changes (e.g., WMH) are concerned. The regional specificity of age differences in microstructural integrity is unclear. Development of new methods of analysis that would allow investigation of connectivity changes in the aging white matter may reveal more subtle effects that thus far remain unnoticed. Longitudinal studies combining multiple structural techniques should shed light on the timing and order of precedence of white and gray matter changes in the context of normal and pathological aging.

5. The search for the neuroanatomical basis of cognitive aging has so far yielded limited and somewhat contradictory results. Whereas brain alterations that approach a pathological scale are indeed associated with lower cognitive performance, age-related declines in cognitive functions are not always observed in healthy older adults. Global brain shrinkage is associated with reduction in cognitive performance, and some age-sensitive cognitive processes are harmed by regional shrinkage as well. However, in some studies, *better* cognitive performance was linked to *smaller* regional volumes. Those findings remain unexplained. Although still too scarce, longitudinal studies combining neuroanatomical and cognitive measures appear more successful in revealing structure-function relationships than cross-sectional studies.

6. Multiple modifiers shape the trajectories of the brain and cognitive aging. Vascular risk factors such as hypertension increase age-related shrinkage in the prefrontal cortices, white matter, and the hippocampus, and they significantly increase white matter pathology load and rate of proliferation. Age-associated pulmonary and metabolic disorders may also exacerbate age-related brain shrinkage, but there are not enough data to confirm or deny this claim. Stress and mood disorders also may negatively influence the normal course of aging. These conditions may serve as negative modifiers of aging, even in the absence of full-blown clinical disease. However, although the research evidence for the negative impact of hypertension is consistent, other candidates for the role of negative

modifiers are supported by rather meager evidence and await larger, better designed studies.

7. Brain volumes (total as well as regional) are under significant genetic control, as is the propensity to acquire white matter pathology. However, some areas that exhibit significant age declines are also vulnerable to multiple environmental influences. The genomic revolution has propelled the study of genetic modifiers of aging beyond gross assessment of heritability into examination of the influence exerted by specific polymorphisms on specific functions. This evidence, however, is still being collected, and has been confined thus far to a few single SNPs. Thus what is needed is an examination of epistatic interactions and the combined effects of single genes, as well as interactions among genes and vascular risk factors on well-measured aspects of the brain and behavior.

8. Several positive modifiers of aging have been suggested. Evidence of a beneficial effect of aerobic exercise on the brain and cognitive aging is mounting, and is in dire need of replications. The role of sex hormones as positive modifiers of brain aging remains controversial. It needs to be examined in studies with manageable though not too small samples, detailed measures, and attention to the timing and nature of the therapeutic intervention. Further research into the genetic modifiers of aging may improve the success rate of therapeutic interventions designed to alleviate its negative effects.

9. Advancement in the knowledge of brain-behavior relationships in aging is hampered by the lack of clarity of understanding the biological meaning of the neuroimaging findings. There is significant need for systematic study of a sufficiently large number of animals (preferably primates) across a life span age range that would be followed for a long period, which would allow multiple assessments of groups of animals staggered in time via MRI and postmortem histology. All the methodological prerequisites for such a study are in place.

Acknowledgments

This work was supported in part by National Institutes of Health grant R37 AG-11230, and by the Max Planck Institute for Human Development in Berlin, where the first author was a Visiting Scientist during his work on this chapter.

References

Abe, O., Aoki, S., Hayashi, N., Yamada, H., Kunimatsu, A., Mori, H., et al. (2002). Normal aging in the central nervous system: Quantitative MR diffusion-tensor analysis. *Neurobiology of Aging*, 23: 433–441.

Aboitiz, F., Rodriguez, E., Olivares, R., and Zaidel, E. (1996). Age-related changes in fibre composition of the human corpus callosum: Sex differences. *Neuroreport*, 7: 1761–1764.

Agartz, I., Sedvall, G. C., Terenius, L., Kulle, B., Frigessi, A., Hall, H., and Jonsson, E. G. (2006). BDNF gene variants and brain morphology in schizophrenia. *American Journal of Medical Genetics B Neuropsychiatr Genetics.* 141: 513–523.

Aggleton, J. P. and Brown, M. W. (1999). Episodic memory, amnesia, and the hippocampal-anterior thalamic axis. *Behavioral and Brain Sciences*, 22: 425–444.

Alexander, G. E., Chen, K., Merkley, T. L., Reiman, E. M., Caselli, R. J., Aschenbrenner, M., et al. (2006). Regional network of magnetic resonance imaging gray matter volume in healthy aging. *Neuroreport*, 17: 951–956.

Alexander, G. E., Chen, K., Aschenbrenner, M., Merkley, T. L., Santerre-Lemmon, L. E., et al. (2008). Age-related regional network of magnetic resonance imaging gray matter in the rhesus macaque. *Journal of Neuroscience*, 28: 2710–2718.

Allen, J. S., Bruss, J., Brown, C. K., and Damasio, H. (2005). Methods for studying the aging brain: Volumetric analyses versus, VBM [Commentary]. *Neurobiology of Aging*, 26: 1275–1278.

Ancoli-Israel, S. (2005). Sleep and aging: Prevalence of disturbed sleep and treatment considerations in older adults. *Journal of Clinical Psychiatry*, 66, (Suppl 9): 24–30.

Anstey, K. J., Mack, H. A., Christensen, H., Li, S. C., Reglade-Meslin, C., Maller, J., et al. (2007). Corpus callosum size, reaction time speed and variability in mild cognitive disorders and in a normative sample. *Neuropsychologia*, 45: 1911–1920.

Antonelli Incalzi, R., Marra, C., Giordano, A., Calcagni, M. L., Cappa, A., Basso, S., et al. (2003). Cognitive impairment in chronic obstructive pulmonary disease—a neuropsychological and spect study. *Journal of Neurology*, 250: 325–332.

Apkarian, A. V., Sosa, Y., Sonty, S., Levy, R. M., Harden, R. N., Parrish, T. B., et al. (2004). Chronic back pain is associated with decreased prefrontal and thalamic gray matter density. *Journal of Neuroscience*, 24: 10410–10415.

Apter, N. S., Halstead, W. C., and Heimburger, R. F. (1951). Impaired cerebral functions in essential hypertension. *American Journal of Psychiatry*, 107: 808–813.

Ardekani, S., Kumar, A., Bartzokis, G., and Sinha, U. (2007). Exploratory voxel-based analysis of diffusion indices and hemispheric asymmetry in normal aging. *Magnetic Resonance Imaging*, 25, 154–167.

Artero, S., Tiemeier, H., Prins, N. D., Sabatier, R., Breteler, M. M., and Ritchie K. (2004). Neuroanatomical localisation and clinical correlates of white matter lesions in the elderly. *Journal of Neurology Neurosurgery and Psychiatry*, 75: 1304–1308.

Ashburner, J. A., and Friston, K. J. (2000). Voxel-based morphometry—the methods. *Neuroimage*, 11: 805–821.

Atwood, L. D., Wolf, P. A., Heard-Costa, N. L., Massaro, J. M., Beiser, A., D'Agostino, R. B., et al. (2004). Genetic variation in white matter hyperintensity volume in the Framingham Study. *Stroke*, 35: 1609–1613.

Au, R., Massaro, J. M., Wolf, P. A., Young, M. E., Beiser, A., Seshadri, S., et al. (2006). Association of white matter hyperintensity volume with decreased cognitive functioning: The Framingham Heart Study. *Archives of Neurology*, 63: 246–250.

Bäckman, L. and Farde, L. (2004). The role of dopamine systems in cognitive aging. In Cabeza, R., Nyberg, L., and Park, D. C. (eds), *Cognitive Neuroscience of Aging: Linking Cognitive and Cerebral Aging*, pp 58–84. New York: Oxford University Press.

Bäckman, L., Nyberg, L., Lindenberger, U., Li, S. C., and Farde L. (2006). The correlative triad among aging, dopamine, and cognition: Current status and future prospects. *Neuroscience and Biobehavioral Review*, 30: 791–807.

Barnett, J. H., Jones, P. B., Robbins, T. W., and Müller U. (2007). Effects of the catechol-O-methyltransferase Val158Met polymorphism on executive function: a meta-analysis of the Wisconsin Card Sort Test in schizophrenia and healthy controls. *Molecular Psychiatry*,12: 502–509.

Bartley, A. J. and Jones, D. W. (1997). Weinberger, D. R.Genetic variability of human brain size and cortical gyral patterns. *Brain*, 120: 257–269.

Bartzokis, G. (2004). Quadratic trajectories of brain myelin content: unifying construct for neuropsychiatric disorders. *Neurobiology of Aging*, 25: 49–62.

Bartzokis, G., Lu, P. H., Geschwind, D. H., Edwards, N., Mintz, J., and Cummings, J. L. (2006). Apolipoprotein E genotype and age-related myelin breakdown in healthy individuals: Implications for cognitive decline and dementia. *Archives of General Psychiatry*, 63: 63–72.

Bartzokis, G., Lu, P. H., Geschwind, D. H., Tingus, K., Huang, D., Mendez, M. F., et al. (2007). Apolipoprotein E affects both myelin breakdown and cognition: Implications for age-related trajectories of decline into Dementia. *Biological Psychiatry*, 62: 1380–1387.

Basser, P. J., Mattiello, J., and Le Bihan, D. (1994). Estimation of the effective self-diffusion tensor from the, NMR spin echo. *Journal of Magnetic Resonance*, 103: 247–254.

Bastien, C. H., Fortier-Brochu, E., Rioux, I., LeBlanc, M., Daley, M., and Morin, C. M. (2003). Cognitive performance and sleep quality in the elderly suffering from chronic insomnia. Relationship between objective and subjective measures. *Journal of Psychosomatic Research*, 54: 39–49.

Bastin, M. E., Clayden, J. D., Pattie, A., Gerrish, I. F., Wardlaw, J. M., and Deary, I. J. (2007). Diffusion tensor and magnetization transfer MRI measurements of periventricular white matter hyperintensities in old age. *Neurobiology of Aging*, Jul 10 [Epub ahead of print].

Baxter, L. C., Caselli, R. J., Johnson, S. C., Reiman, E., and Osborne D. (2003). Apolipoprotein E epsilon 4 affects new learning in cognitively normal individuals at risk for Alzheimer's disease. *Neurobiology of Aging*, 24: 947–952.

Benedetti, B., Charil, A., Rovaris, M., Judica, E., Valsasina, P., Sormani, M. P., et al. (2006). Influence of aging on brain gray and white matter changes assessed by conventional, MT, and DT MRI. *Neurology*, 66: 535–539.

Bhagat, Y. A. and Beaulieu, C. (2004). Diffusion anisotropy in subcortical white matter and cortical gray matter: Changes with aging and the role of CSF-suppression. *Journal of Magnetic Resonance Imaging*, 20: 216–227.

Bookstein, F. L., (2001). Voxel-based morphometry should not be used with imperfectly registered images. *Neuroimage*, 14: 1454–1462.

Boonstra, T. W., Stins, J. F., Daffertshofer, A., and Beek, P. J. (2007). Effects of sleep deprivation on neural functioning: an integrative review. *Cellular and Molecular Life Sciences*, 64: 934–946.

Bourdeau, I., Bard, C., Forget, H., Boulanger, Y., Cohen, H., and Lacroix A. (2005). Cognitive function and cerebral assessment in patients who have Cushing's syndrome. *Endocrinology Metabolism Clinics of North America*, 34: 357–369.

Brickman, A. M., Zimmerman, M. E., Paul, R. H., Grieve, S. M., Tate, D. F., Cohen, R. A., et al. (2006). Regional white matter and neuropsychological functioning across the adult lifespan. *Biological Psychiatry*, 60: 444–453.

Brown, C. A., McKinney, K. Q., Young, K. B., and Norton, H. J. (1999). The C677T methylenetetrahydrofolate reductase polymorphism influences the homocysteine-lowering effect of hormone replacement therapy. Molecular Genetics and Metabolism, 67: 43–48.

Bruder, G. E., Keilp, J. G., Xu, H., Shikhman, M., Schori, E., Gorman, J. M., et al. (2005). Catechol-O-methyltransferase (COMT) genotypes and working memory: associations with differing cognitive operations. *Biological Psychiatry*, 58: 901–907.

Brunk, U. T. and Terman, A. (2002). The mitochondrial-lysosomal axis theory of aging: accumulation of damaged mitochondria as a result of imperfect autophagocytosis. *European Journal of Biochemistry*, 269: 1996–2002.

Buckner, R. L. (2004). Memory and executive function in aging and AD: multiple factors that cause decline and reserve factors that compensate. *Neuron*, 44: 195–208.

Bucur, B., Madden, D. J., Spaniol, J., Provenzale, J. M., Cabeza, R., White, L. E., et al. (2008). Age-related slowing of memory retrieval: contributions of perceptual speed and cerebral white matter integrity. *Neurobiology of Aging*, 7: 1070–1079.

Bueller, J. A., Aftab, M., Sen, S., Gomez-Hassan, D., Burmeister, M., Zubieta, J. K. (2006). BDNF Val66Met allele is associated with reduced hippocampal volume in healthy subjects. *Biological Psychiatry*, 59: 812–815.

Bunce, D., Anstey, K. J., Christensen, H., Dear, K., Wen, W, and Sachdev, P. (2007). White matter hyperintensities and within-person variability in community-dwelling adults aged 60–64 years. *Neuropsychologia*, 45: 2009–2015.

Burke, S. N. and Barnes, C. A. (2006). Neural plasticity in the ageing brain. *Nature Review Neuroscience*, 7: 30–40.

Caldú, X., Vendrell, P., Bartrés-Faz, D., Clemente, I., Bargalló N, Jurado, M. A., et al. (2007). Impact of the COMT Val(108/158) Met and DAT genotypes on prefrontal function in healthy subjects. *Neuroimage*, Jul 4 [Epub ahead of print].

Cameron, H. A., and McKay, R. D. (1999). Restoring production of hippocampal neurons in old age. *Nature Neuroscience*, 2: 894–897.

Cardenas, V. A., Du, A. T., Hardin, D., Ezekiel, F., Weber, P., Jagust, W. J., et al. (2003). Comparison of methods for measuring longitudinal brain change in cognitive impairment and dementia. *Neurobiology of Aging*, 24: 537–544.

Carmelli, D., DeCarli, C., Swan, G. E., Jack, L. M., Reed, T., Wolf, P. A., et al. (1998). Evidence for genetic variance in white matter hyperintensity volume in normal elderly male twins. *Stroke*, 29: 1177–1181.

Carmichael, O. T., Kuller, L. H., Lopez, O. L., Thompson, P. M., Dutton, R. A., et al. (2007). Acceleration of cerebral ventricular expansion in the Cardiovascular Health Study. *Neurobiology of Aging*, 28: 1316–1321.

Caselli, R. J., Reiman, E. M., Osborne, D., Hentz, J. G., Baxter, L. C., Hernandez, J. L., et al. (2004). Longitudinal changes in cognition and behavior in asymptomatic carriers of the APOE e4 allele. *Neurology*, 62: 1990–1995.

Cerasa, A., Gioia, M. C., Labate, A., Liguori, M., Lanza, P., and Quattrone, A. (2008). Impact of catechol-O-methyltransferase Val108/158 Met genotype on hippocampal and prefrontal gray matter volume. *Neuroreport*, 19: 405–408.

Cerqueira, J. J., Catania, C., Sotiropoulos, I., Schubert, M., Kalisch, R., Almeida, O. F., et al. (2005). Corticosteroid status influences the volume of the rat cingulate cortex – a magnetic resonance imaging study. *Journal of Psychiatric Research*, 39: 451–460.

Charlton, R. A., Barrick, T. R., McIntyre, D. J., Shen, Y., O'Sullivan, M., Howe, F. A., et al. (2006). White matter damage on diffusion tensor imaging correlates with age-related cognitive decline. *Neurology*, 66: 217–222.

Chen, J., Lipska, B. K., Halim, N., Ma, Q. D., Matsumoto, M., Melhem, S. et al. (2004). Functional analysis of genetic variation in catechol-O-methyltransferase (COMT): Effects on mRNA, protein, and enzyme activity in postmortem human brain. *American Journal of Human Genetics*, 75: 807–821.

Chen, K., Reiman, E. M., Alexander, G. E., Caselli, R. J., Gerkin, R., Bandy, D., et al. (2007). Correlations between apolipoprotein E epsilon4 gene dose and whole brain atrophy rates. *American Journal of Psychiatry*, 164: 916–921.

Chen, X. J., Kovacevic, N., Lobaugh, N. J., Sled, J. G., Henkelman, R. M., and Henderson, J. T. (2005). Neuroanatomical differences between mouse strains as shown by high-resolution 3D MRI. *Neuroimage*, 29: 99–105.

Chepuri, N. B., Yen, Y. F., Burdette, J. H., Li, H., Moody, D. M., and Maldjian, J. A. (2002). Diffusion anisotropy in the corpus callosum. *American Journal of Neuroradiology*, 23: 803–808.

Chun, T., Filippi, C. G., Zimmerman, R. D., and Ulug, A. M. (2000). Diffusion changes in the aging human brain. *American Journal of Neuroradiology*, 21: 1078–1083.

Cohen, R. M., Small, C., Lalonde, F., Friz, J., and Sunderland, T. (2001). Effect of apolipoprotein E genotype on hippocampal volume loss in aging healthy women. *Neurology*, 57: 2223–2228.

Cohen, R. M., Szczepanik, J., McManus, M., Mirza, N., Putnam, K., Levy, J., et al. (2006a). Hippocampal atrophy in the healthy is initially linear and independent of age. *Neurobiology of Aging*, 27, 1385–1394.

Cohen, R. A., Grieve, S., Hoth, K. F., Paul, R. H., Sweet, L., Tate, D., et al. (2006b). Early life stress and morphometry of the adult anterior cingulate cortex and caudate nuclei. *Biological Psychiatry*, 59: 975–982.

Colcombe, S. J. and Kramer, A. F. (2003). Fitness effects on the cognitive function of older adults: a meta-analytic study. *Psychological Science*, 14: 125–130.

Colcombe, S. J., Erickson, K. I., Raz, N., Webb, A. G., Cohen, N. J., McAuley, E., et al. (2003). Aerobic fitness reduces brain tissue loss in aging humans. *Journal of Gerontology Series A: Biological Sciences and Medical Sciences*, 58A: 176–180.

Colcombe, S. J., Erickson, K. I., Scalf, P. E., Kim, J. S., Prakash, R., McAuley, E., et al. (2006). Aerobic exercise training increases brain volume in aging humans. *Journal of Gerontology Series A: Biological Sciences and Medical Sciences*, 61: 1166–1170.

Coluccia, D., Wolf, O. T., Kollias, S., Roozendaal, B., Forster, A., and de Quervain, D. J. F. (2008). Glucocorticoid therapy-induced memory deficits: Acute versus chronic effects. *Journal of Neuroscience*, 28: 3474–3478.

Cook, I. A., Morgan, M. L., Dunkin, J. J., David, S., Witte, E., Lufkin, R., et al. (2002). Estrogen replacement therapy is associated with less progression of subclinical structural brain disease in normal elderly women: A pilot study. *International Journal of Geriatric Psychiatry*, 17: 610–618.

Corder, E. H., Saunders, A. M., and Strittmatter, W. J. (1993). Gene dose of apolipoprotein E type 4 allele and the risk of Alzheimer's disease in late onset families. *Science*, 261: 921–923.

Cordonnier, C., Al-Shahi Salman, R., and Wardlaw, J. (2007). Spontaneous brain microbleeds: Systematic review, subgroup analyses and standards for study design and reporting. *Brain*, 130: 1988–2003.

Cotman, C. W. and Berchtold, N. C. (2002). Exercise: A behavioral intervention to enhance brain health and plasticity. *Trends Neuroscience*, 25: 295–301.

Crum, W. R., Griffin, L. D., Hill, D. L. G., and Hawkes, D. J. (2003). Zen and the art of medical image registration: correspondence, homology, and quality. *Neuroimage*, 20: 1425–1437.

Dauguet, J., Peled, S., Berezovskii, V., Delzescaux, T., Warfield, S. K., Born, R., and Westin, C. F. (2007). Comparison of fiber tracts derived from in-vivo DTI tractography with 3D histological neural tract tracer reconstruction on a macaque brain. *NeurIimage*, 37: 530–538.

Davatzikos, C. (2004). Why voxel-based morphometric analysis should be used with great caution when characterizing group differences. *Neuroimage*, 23: 17–20.

DeCarli, C., Massaro, J., Harvey, D., Hald, J., Tullberg, M., Au, R., et al. (2005). Measures of brain morphology and infarction in the framingham heart study: Establishing what is normal. *Neurobiology of Aging*, 26: 491–510.

de Frias, C. M., Annerbrink, K., Westberg, L., Eriksson, E., Adolfsson, R., abdNilsson, L. G. (2005). Catechol O-methyltransferase Val158Met polymorphism is associated with cognitive performance in nondemented adults. *Journal of Cognitive Neuroscience*, 17: 1018–1025.

De Leeuw, F. E., De Groot, J. C., and Breteler, M. M. B. (2001). White matter changes: Frequency and risk factors. In Pantoni, L., Inzitari, D., Wallin A. (eds), *The Matter of White Matter: Clinical and Pathophysiological Aspects of White Matter Disease Related to Cognitive Decline and Vascular Dementia* (pp. 19–33). Utrecht, The Netherlands: Academic Pharmaceutical Productions.

De Leeuw, F. E., Richard, F., de Groot, J. C., van Duijn, C. M., Hofman, A., Van Gijn, J., et al. (2004). Interaction between hypertension, apoE, and cerebral white matter lesions. *Stroke*, 35: 1057–1060.

de Leon, M. J., DeSanti, S., Zinkowski, R., Mehta, P. D., Pratico, D., Segal, S., et al. (2004). MRI and CSF studies in the early diagnosis of Alzheimer's disease. *Journal of Internal Medicine*, 256: 205–223.

De Toledo-Morrell, L., Stoub, T. R., Bulgakova, M., Wilson, R. S., Bennett, D. A., Leurgans, S., et al. (2004). MRI-derived entorhinal volume is a good predictor of conversion from MCI to AD. *Neurobiology of Aging*, 25: 1197–1203.

den Heijer, T., Geerlings, M. I., Hofman, A., de Jong, F. H., Launer, L. J., Pols, H. A., et al. (2003). Higher estrogen levels are not associated with larger hippocampi and better memory performance. *Archives of Neurology*, 60: 213–220.

den Heijer, T., Launer, L. J., Prins, N. D., van Dijk, E. J., Vermeer, S. E., Hofman, A., (2005). Association between blood pressure, white matter lesions, and atrophy of the medial temporal lobe. *Neurology*, 64: 263–267.

Deary, I. J., Bastin, M. E., Pattie, A., Clayden, J. D., Whalley, L. J., Starr, J. M., et al. (2006). White matter integrity and cognition in childhood and old age. *Neurology*, 66: 505–512.

Devanand, D. P., Pradhaban, G., Liu, X., Khandji, A., De Santi, S., Segal, S., et al. (2007). Hippocampal and entorhinal atrophy in mild cognitive impairment: Prediction of Alzheimer disease. *Neurology*, 68: 828–836.

Diaz-Asper, C. M., Goldberg, T. E., Kolachana, B. S., Straub, R. E., Egan, M. F., and Weinberger, D. R. (2008). Genetic variation in Catechol-O-Methyltransferase: Effects on working memory in schizophrenic patients, their siblings, and healthy controls. *Biological Psychiatry*, 63: 72–79.

Dickerson, B. C., Goncharova, I., Sullivan, M. P., Forchetti, C., Wilson, R. S., Bennett, D. A., et al. (2001). MRI-derived entorhinal and hippocampal atrophy in incipient and very mild Alzheimer's disease. *Neurobiology of Aging*, 22: 747–754.

Dickstein, D. L., Kabaso, D., Rocher, A. B., Luebke, J. I., Wearne, S. L., and Hof, P. R. (2007). Changes in the structural complexity of the aged brain. *Aging Cell*, 6: 275–284.

Dimitrova, A., Gerwig, M., Brol, B., Gizewski, E. R., Forsting, M., Beck, A., et al. (2008). Correlation of cerebellar volume with eyeblink conditioning in healthy subjects and in patients with cerebellar cortical degeneration. *Brain Research*, 1198: 73–84.

Dishman, R. K., Berthoud, H. R., Booth, F. W., Cotman, C. W., Edgerton, V. R., Fleshner, M. R., et al. (2006). Neurobiology of exercise. *Obesity* (Silver Spring), 14: 345–356.

Dorion, A. A., Salomon, O., Zanca, M., Duyme, M., and Capron, C. (2001). Magnetic resonance imaging and cerebral volumic evaluation: Comparison of four post-processing techniques. *Computers in Biology and Medicine*, 31: 215–227.

Douaud, G., Gaura, V., Ribeiro, M. J., Lethimonnier, F., Maroy, R., Verny, C., et al. (2006). Distribution of gray matter in Huntington's disease patients: A combined, ROI-based and voxel-based morphometric study. *Neuroimage*, 32: 1562–1575.

Drapeau, E., Mayo, W., Aurousseau, C., Le Moal, M., Piazza, P. V., and Abrous, D. N. (2003). Spatial memory performances of aged rats in the water maze predict levels of hippocampal neurogenesis. *Proceedings of the National Academy of Sciences of the USA*, 100: 14385–14390.

Drapeau, E., Montaron, M. F., Aguerre, S., and Abrous, D. N. (2007). Learning-induced survival of new neurons depends on the cognitive status of aged rats. *Neuroscience*, 27: 6037–6044.

Drevets, W. C., Price, J. L., Simpson, J. R Jr, Todd, R. D., Reich, T., Vannier, M., et al. (1997). Subgenual prefrontal cortex abnormalities in mood disorders. *Nature*, 386: 824–827.

Driscoll, I., Hamilton, D. A., Petropoulos, H., Yeo, R. A., Brooks, W. M., Baumgartner, R. N., et al. (2003). The aging hippocampus: Cognitive, biochemical and structural findings. *Cerebral Cortex*, 13: 1344–1351.

Driscoll, I., Howard, S. R., Stone, J. C., Monfils, M. H., Tomanek, B., Brooks, W. M., et al. (2006). The aging hippocampus: A Multi-level analysis in the rat. *Neuroscience*, 139: 1173–1185.

Du, A. T., Schuff, N., Chao, L. L., Kornak, J., Jagust, W. J., Kramer, J. H., et al. (2006). Age effects on atrophy rates of entorhinal cortex and hippocampus. *Neurobiology of Aging*, 27: 733–740.

Du, A. T., Schuff, N., Zhu, X. P., Jagust, W. J., Miller, B. L., Reed, B. R., et al. (2003). Atrophy rates of entorhinal cortex in AD and normal aging. *Neurology*, 60: 481–486.

Duarte, A., Hayasaka, S., Du, A., Schuff, N., Jahng, G. H., Kramer, J., et al. (2006). Volumetric correlates of memory and executive function in normal elderly, mild cognitive impairment and Alzheimer's disease. *Neuroscience Letters*, 406: 60–65.

Dufouil, C., Alperovitch, A., Ducros, V., and Tzourio, C. (2003). Homocysteine, white matter hyperintensities, and cognition in healthy elderly people. *Annals of Neurology*, 53: 214–221.

Dufouil, C., Chalmers, J., Coskun, O., Besancon, V., Bousser, M. G., Guillon, P., et al. (2005). PROGRESS, MRI Substudy Investigators. Effects of blood pressure lowering on cerebral white matter hyperintensities in patients with stroke: the, PROGRESS (Perindopril Protection Against Recurrent Stroke Study) Magnetic Resonance Imaging Substudy. *Circulation*, 112: 1644–1650.

Dufouil, C., de Kersaint-Gilly, A., Besancon, V., Levy, C., Auffray, E., Brunnereau, L., et al. (2001). Longitudinal study of blood pressure and white matter hyperintensities: The, EVA, MRI Cohort. *Neurology*, 56: 921–926.

Duning, T., Kloska, S., Steinsträter, O., Kugel, H., Heindel, W., and Knecht, S. (2005). Dehydration confounds the assessment of brain atrophy. *Neurology*, 64: 548–550.

Eberling, J. L., Wu, C., Haan, M. N., Mungas, D., Buonocore, M., and Jagust, W. J. (2003). Preliminary evidence that estrogen protects against age-related hippocampal atrophy. *Neurobiology of Aging*, 24: 725–732.

Egan, M. F., Goldberg, T. E., Kolachana, B. S., Callicott, J. H., Mazzanti, C. M., Straub, R. E., et al. (2001). Effect of, COMT Val108/158 Met genotype on frontal lobe function and risk for schizophrenia. *Proceedings of the National Academy of Sciences of the USA*, 98: 6917–6922.

Engelter, S. T., Provenzale, J. M., Petrella, J. R., DeLong, D. M., and MacFall, J. R. (2000). The effect of aging on the apparent diffusion coefficient of normal-appearing white matter. *American Journal of Roentgenology*, 175: 425–430.

Erickson, K. I., Colcombe, S. J., Raz, N., Korol, D. L., Scalf, P., Webb, A., et al. (2005). Selective sparing of brain tissue in postmenopausal women receiving hormone replacement therapy. *Neurobiology of Aging*, 26: 1205–1213.

Eriksson, P. S., Perfilieva, E., Björk-Eriksson, T., Alborn, A. M., Nordborg, C., Peterson, D. A., et al. (1998). Neurogenesis in the adult human hippocampus. *Nature Medicine*, 4: 1313–1317.

Espeseth, T., Greenwood, P. M., Reinvang, I., Fjell, A. M., Walhovd, K. B., Westlye, L. T., et al. (2006). Interactive effects of APOE and CHRNA4 on attention and white matter volume in healthy middle-aged and older adults. *Cognitive Affective and Behavioral Neuroscience*, 6: 31–43.

Espeseth, T., Westlye, L. T., Fjell, A. M., Walhovd, K. B., Rootwelt, H., and Reinvang, I. (2008). Accelerated age-related cortical thinning in healthy carriers of apolipoprotein E varepsilon4. *Neurobiology of Aging*, 29: 329–340.

Fazekas, F., Ropele, S., Enzinger, C., Gorani, F., Seewann, A., Petrovic, K., et al. (2005). MTI of white matter hyperintensities. *Brain*, 128(Pt 12): 2926–2932.

Fernando, M. S., Simpson, J. E., Matthews, F., Brayne, C., Lewis, C. E., Barber, R., et al. (2006). MRC cognitive function and ageing neuropathology study group. *Stroke*, 37: 1391–1398.

Filippini, N., Scassellati, C., Boccardi, M., Pievani, M., Testa, C., Bocchio-Chiavetto, L., et al. (2006). Influence of serotonin receptor 2A His452Tyr polymorphism on brain temporal structures: A volumetric, MR study. *European Journal of Human Genetics*, 14: 443–449.

Fjell, A. M., Walhovd, K. B., Reinvang, I., Lundervold, A., Salat, D., Quinn, B. T., et al. (2006). Selective increase of cortical thickness in high-performing elderly–structural indices of optimal cognitive aging. *Neuroimage*, 29: 984–994.

Flechsig, P. (1901). Developmental (myelogenetic) localisation of the cerebral cortex in the human subject. *Lancet*, October 19, 1027–1029.

Fleg, J. L., Morrell, C. H., Bos, A. G., Brant, L. J., Talbot, L. A., Wright, J. G., et al. (2005). Accelerated longitudinal decline of aerobic capacity in healthy older adults. *Circulation*, 112: 674–682.

Foley, D., Ancoli-Israel, S., Britz, P., and Walsh, J. (2004). Sleep disturbances and chronic disease in older adults: Results of the 2003 National Sleep Foundation Sleep in America Survey. *Journal of Psychosomatic Research*, 56: 497–502.

Foley, D. J., Monjan, A. A., Masaki, K. H., Enright, P. L., Quan, S. F., and White, L. R. (1999). Associations of symptoms of sleep apnea with cardiovascular disease, cognitive impairment, and mortality among older Japanese-American men. *Journal of American Geriatrics Society*, 47: 524–528.

Frodl, T., Schüle, C., Schmitt, G., Born, C., Baghai, T., Zill, P., et al. (2007). Association of the brain-derived neurotrophic factor Val66Met polymorphism with reduced hippocampal volumes in major depression. *Archives of General Psychiatry*, 64: 410–416.

Frosst, P., Blom, H. J., Milos, R., Goyette, P., Sheppard, C. A., Matthews, R. G., et al. (1995). A candidate genetic risk factor for vascular disease: A common mutation in methylenetetrahydrofolate reductase. *Nature Genetics*, 10: 111–113.

Fukuda, H. and Kitani, M. (1995). Differences between treated and untreated hypertensive subjects in the extent of periventricular hyperintensities observed on brain, MRI. *Stroke*, 26: 1593–1597.

Furutani, K., Harada, M., Minato, M., Morita, N., and Nishitani, H. (2005). Regional changes of fractional anisotropy with normal aging using statistical parametric mapping (SPM). *Journal of Medical Investigation*, 52: 186–190.

Garde, E., Mortensen, E. L., Krabbe, K., Rostrup, E., and Larsson, H. B. (2000). Relation between age-related decline in intelligence and cerebral white-matter hyperintensities in healthy octogenarians: a longitudinal study. *Lancet*, 356: 628–634.

Garde, E., Lykke Mortensen, E., Rostrup, E., and Paulson, O. B. (2005). Decline in intelligence is associated with progression in white matter hyperintensity volume. *Journal of Neurology Neurosurgery and Psychiatry*, 76: 1289–1291.

Gareau, P. J., Rutt, B. K., Karlik, S. J., and Mitchell, J. R. (2000). Magnetization transfer and multicomponent T2 relaxation measurements with histopathologic correlation in an experimental model of MS. *Journal of Magnetic Resonance Imaging*, 11: 586–595.

Gareri, P., De Fazio, P., and De Sarro G. (2002). Neuropharmacology of depression in aging and age-related diseases. *Ageing Research Review*, 1: 113–134.

Ge, Y., Grossman, R. I., Babb, J. S., Rabin, M. L., Mannon, L. J., and Kolson, D. L. (2002). Age-related total gray matter and white matter changes in normal adult brain. Part II: Quantitative magnetization transfer ratio histogram analysis. *American Journal of Neuroradiology*, 23: 1334–1341.

Genazzani, A. R., Pluchino, N., Luisi, S., and Luisi, M. (2007). Estrogen, cognition and female ageing. *Human Reproduction Update*, 13: 175–187.

Ghidoni, R., Boccardi, M. Benussi, L., Testa, C., Villa, A., Pievani, M., et al. (2006). Effects of estrogens on cognition and brain morphology: Involvement of the cerebellum. *Maturitas*, 54: 222–228.

Greenwood, P. (2007). Functional plasticity in cognitive aging: Review and hypothesis. *Neuropsychology*, 21: 657–673.

Greenwood, P. M., Lambert, C., Sunderland, T., and Parasuraman R. (2005a). Effects of apolipoprotein E genotype on spatial attention, working memory, and their interaction in healthy, middle-aged adults: Results from the National Institute of Mental Health's BIOCARD study. *Neuropsychology*, 19: 199–211.

Greenwood, P. M., Sunderland, T., Putnam K, Levy J, Parasuraman R. (2005b). Scaling of visuospatial attention undergoes differential longitudinal change as a function of APOE genotype prior to old age: Results from the NIMH BIOCARD study. *Neuropsychology*, 19: 830–840.

Grieve, S. M., Williams, L. M., Paul, R. H., Clark, C. R., and Gordon E. (2007). Cognitive aging, executive function, and fractional anisotropy: A diffusion tensor MR imaging study. *American Journal of Neuroradiology*, 28: 226–235.

Goldstein, I. B., Bartzokis, G., Guthrie, D., and Shapiro, D. (2002). Ambulatory blood pressure and brain atrophy in the healthy elderly. *Neurology*, 59: 713–719.

Goldstein, I. B., Bartzokis, G., Guthrie, D., and Shapiro, D. (2005). Ambulatory blood pressure and the brain: A 5-year follow-up. *Neurology*, 64: 1846–1852.

Golomb, J., Kluger, A., de Leon, M. J., Ferris, S. H., Convit, A., Mittelman, M. S., et al. (1994). Hippocampal formation size in normal human aging: A correlate of delayed secondary memory performance. *Learning and Memory*, 1: 45–54.

Gong, Q.-Y., Sluming, V., Mayes, A., Keller, S., Barrick, T., Cezayirli, E., et al.. (2005). Voxel-based morphometry and stereology provide convergent evidence of the importance of medial prefrontal cortex for fluid intelligence in healthy adults. *Neuroimage*, 25: 1175–1186.

Good, C. D., Johnsrude, I. S., Ashburner, J., Henson, R. N., Friston, K. J., and Frackowiak, R. S. (2001). A voxel-based morphometric study of ageing in 465 normal adult human brains. *Neuroimage*, 14: 21–36.

Good, C.D., Scahill, R. I., Fox., N.C., Ashburner, J., Friston, K. J., Chan., D., et al. (2002). Automatic differentiation of anatomical patterns in the human brain: Validation with studies of degenerative dementias. *Neuroimage*, 17: 29–46.

Gould, E. (2007). How widespread is adult neurogenesis in mammals? *Nature Review Neuroscience*, 8: 481–488.

Gunning-Dixon, F. M. and Raz, N. (2000). The cognitive correlates of white matter abnormalities in normal aging: A quantitative review. *Neuropsychology*, 14: 224–232.

Gunning-Dixon, F. M. and Raz, N. (2003). Neuroanatomical correlates of selected executive functions in middle-aged and older adults: A prospective MRI study. *Neuropsychologia*, 41: 1929–1941.

Guzman-Marin, R., Bashir, T., Suntsova, N., Szymusiak R., and McGinty, D. (2007). Hippocampal neurogenesis is reduced by sleep fragmentation in the adult rat. *Neuroscience*, 148: 325–333.

Hackert, V. H., den Heijer, T., Oudkerk, M., Koudstaal, P. J., Hofman, A., and Breteler, M. M. (2002). Hippocampal head size associated with verbal memory performance in nondemented elderly. *Neuroimage*, 17: 1365–1372.

Harris, S. E., Fox, H., Wright, A. F., Hayward, C., Starr, J. M., Whalley, L. J., and Deary, I. J. (2006). The brain-derived neurotrophic factor Val66Met polymorphism is associated with age-related change in reasoning skills. *Molecular Psychiatry*, 11: 505–513.

Harris, S. E., Fox, H., Wright, A. F., Hayward, C., Starr, J. M., Whalley, L. J., et al. (2007). A genetic association analysis of cognitive ability and cognitive ageing using 325 markers for 109 genes associated with oxidative stress or cognition. *BMC Genetics*, Jul 2, 8: 43.

Haug, H. (1985). Are neurons of the human cerebral cortex really lost during aging? A morphometric examination. In: Tarber, J., Gispen, W. H. (eds), *Senile Dementia of Alzheimer Type* (pp. 150–163). Berlin: Springer-Verlag.

Head, D., Buckner, R. L., Shimony, J. S., Williams, L. E., Akbudak, E., Conturo, T. E., et al. (2004). Differential vulnerability of anterior white matter in nondemented aging with minimal acceleration in dementia of the Alzheimer type: Evidence from diffusion tensor imaging. *Cerebral Cortex*, 14: 410–423.

Head, D., Raz, N., Gunning-Dixon, F., Williamson, A., and Acker, J. D. (2002). Age-related shrinkage of the prefrontal cortex is associated with executive, but not procedural aspects of cognitive performance. *Psychology and Aging*, 17: 72–84.

Head, D., Rodrigue, K. M., Kennedy, K. M., and Raz, N. (2008). Neuroanatomical and cognitive mediators of age-related differences in episodic memory. *Neuropsychology*, 22: 491–507.

Heiland, S., Sartor, K., Martin, E., Bardenheuer, H. J., and Plaschke, K. (2002). In vivo monitoring of age-related changes in rat brain using quantitative diffusion magnetic resonance imaging and magnetic resonance relaxometry. *Neuroscience Letters*, 334: 157–160.

Helenius, J., Soinne, L., Perkio, J., Salonen, O., Kangasmaki, A., Kaste, M., Carano, R. A., Aronen, H. J., and Tatlisumak, T. (2002). Diffusion-weighted MR imaging in normal human brains in various age groups. *AJNR American Journal of Neuroradiology, 23*, 194–199.

Hennevin, E., Huetz, C., and Edeline, J. M. (2007). Neural representations during sleep: from sensory processing to memory traces. *Neurobiology of Learning and Memory*, 87: 416–440.

Ho, B. C., Milev, P., O'Leary, D. S., Librant A, Andreasen, N. C., and Wassink, T. H. (2006). Cognitive and magnetic resonance imaging brain morphometric correlates of brain-derived neurotrophic factor Val66Met gene polymorphism in patients with schizophrenia and healthy volunteers. *Archives of General Psychiatry*, 63: 731–740.

Hofman, P. A., Kemerink, G. J., Jolles, J., and Wilmink, J. T. (1999). Quantitative analysis of magnetization transfer images of the brain: Effect of closed head injury, age and sex on white matter. *Magnetic Resonance in Medicine*, 42: 803–806.

Holland, C. M., Smith, E. E., Csapo, I., Gurol, M. E., Brylka, D. A., Killiany, R. J., et al. (2008). Spatial Distribution of White-Matter Hyperintensities in Alzheimer Disease, Cerebral Amyloid Angiopathy, and Healthy Aging. *Stroke*, 39: 1127–1133.

Hollenberg, M., Yang, J., Haight, T. J., and Tager, I. B. (2006). Longitudinal changes in aerobic capacity: Implications for concepts of aging. *Journals of Gerontology Series A Biological Sciences and Medical Sciences*, 61:851–858.

Honea, R., Verchinski, B. A., Pezawas, L., Kolachana, B. S., Callicott, J. H., Mattay, V. S., Weinberger, D. R., and Meyer-Lindenberg, A. (2009). Impact of interacting functional variants in COMT on regional gray matter volume in human brain. *Neuroimage*, 45:44–51.

Hoptman, M. J., Gunning-Dixon, F. M., Murphy, C. F., Ardekani, B. A., Hrabe, J., Lim, K. O., Etwaroo, G. R., Kanellopoulos, D., and Alexopoulos, G. S. (2008). Blood pressure and white matter integrity in geriatric depression. *Journal of Affective Disorders*. [Epub ahead of print].

Hornung, O. P., Danker-Hopfe, H., and Heuser, I. (2005). Age-related changes in sleep and memory: commonalities and interrelationships. *Expeimental Gerontology*, 40: 279–285.

Hornung, O. P., Regen, F., Danker-Hopfe, H., Schredl, M., and Heuser I. (2007). The relationship between REM sleep and memory consolidation in old age and effects of cholinergic medication. *Biological Psychiatry*, 61: 750–757.

Huang, L., Ling, X. Y., and Liu, S. R. (2006). Diffusion tensor imaging on white matter in normal adults and elderly patients with hypertension. *Chinese Medical Journal*, 119: 1304–1307.

Hugenschmidt, C. E., Peiffer, A. M., Kraft, R. A., Casanova, R., Deibler, A. R., Burdette, J. H., et al. (2008). Relating imaging indices of white matter integrity and volume in healthy older adults. *Cerebral Cortex*, 18: 433–442.

Ikram, M. A., Vrooman, H. A., Vernooij, M. W., van der Lijn, F., Hofman, A., van der Lugt, A., et al. (2008). Brain tissue volumes in the general elderly population: The Rotterdam scan study. *Neurobiology of Aging*, 29: 882–890.

Irie, F., Strozyk, D., Peila, R., Korf, E. S., Remaley, A. T., Masaki, K., et al. (2006). Brain lesions on MRI and endogenous sex hormones in elderly men. *Neurobiology of Aging*, 27: 1137–1144.

Jack, C. R. Jr, Petersen, R. C., Xu, Y., O'Brien, P. C., Smith, G. E., Ivnik, R. J., et al. (2000). Rates of hippocampal atrophy correlate with change in clinical status in aging and AD. *Neurology*, 55: 484–489.

Jack, C. R., Petersen, R. C., Grundman, M., Jin, S., Gamst, A., Ward, C. P., et al. (2007). Members of the Alzheimer's Disease Cooperative Study (ADCS). Longitudinal MRI findings from the vitamin E and donepezil treatment study for MCI. *Neurobiology of Aging*, Apr 21 [Epub ahead of print].

Jak, A. J., Houston, W. S., Nagel, B. J., Corey-Bloom, J., and Bondi, M. W. (2007). Differential cross-sectional and longitudinal impact of APOE genotype on hippocampal volumes in nondemented older adults. *Dementia and Geriatric Cognitive Disorders*, 23: 382–389.

Janowsky, J. S. (2006). The role of androgens in cognition and brain aging in men. *Neuroscience*, 138: 1015–1020.

Jernigan, T. L., Archibald, S. L., Fenema-Notestine, C., Gamst, A. C. Stout, J. C., Bonner, J., et al. (2001). Effects of age on tissues and regions of the cerebrum and cerebellum, *Neurobiology of Aging*, 22: 581–594.

Jernigan, T. L., Gamst, A. C., Fennema-Notestine, C., and Ostergaard, A. L. (2003). More "mapping" in brain mapping: statistical comparison of effects. *Human Brain Mapping*, 19: 90–95.

Joëls, M., Karst, H., Krugers, H. J., and Lucassen, P. J. (2007). Chronic stress: Implications for neuronal morphology, function and neurogenesis. *Frontiers in Neuroendocrinology*, 28: 72–96.

Kaes, T. (1907). *Die Grosshirnrinde des Menschen in ihren Massen und in ihrem Fasergehalt. Ein gehirnanatomischer Atlas mit erläuterndem Text und schematischer Zeichnung*, Jena, Germany: Fischer Verlag.

Karl, A., Schaefer, M., Malta, L. S., Dörfel, D., Rohleder, N., and Werner, A. (2006). A meta-analysis of structural brain abnormalities in PTSD. *Neuroscience and Biobehavioral Review*, 30: 1004–1031.

Kemper, T. (1994). Neuroanatomical and neuropathological changes during aging and dementia. In: Albert, M.L. and Knoefel, J. (eds), *Clinical Neurology of Aging* (pp. 3–67). New York: Oxford University Press.

Kempermann, G., Gast, D., and Gage, F. H. (2002). Neuroplasticity in old age: sustained fivefold induction of hippocampal neurogenesis by long-term environmental enrichment. *Annals of Neurology*, 52: 135–143.

Kempermann, G., Kuhn, H. G., and Gage, F. H. (1997). Genetic influence on neurogenesis in the dentate gyrus of adult mice. *Proceedings of the National Academy of Sciences of the USA*, 94: 10409–10414.

Kempermann, G., Kuhn, H. G., and Gage, F. H. (1998). Experience-induced neurogenesis in the senescent dentate gyrus. *Journal of Neuroscience*, 18: 3206–3212.

Kennedy, K. M. and Raz, N. (2005). Age, sex, and regional brain volumes predict perceptual-motor skill acquisition. *Cortex*, 41: 560–569.

Kennedy, K. M. and Raz, N. (2007). Regional white matter integrity and cognitive performance: The effects of age and vascular risk factors. A paper presented at the Annual Meeting of the Society for Neuroscience, San Diego, CA, November 4, 2007.

Kennedy, K. M. and Raz, N. (submitted). Hypertension is a Negative Modifier of Age-Related Regional Differences in White Matter Microstructure.

Kennedy, K. M. and Raz, N. (2009). Aging white matter and cognition: Differential effects of regional variations in diffusion properties on memory, executive functions, and speed. *Neuropsychologia*, 47: 916–927.

Kennedy, K. M., Erickson, K. I., Rodrigue, K. M., Voss, M. W., Colcombe, S. J, Kramer, A. F., et al. (2008a). Age-related differences in regional brain volumes: A Comparison of manual volumetry with optimized Voxel-Based Morphometry. *Neurobiology of Aging*, Feb 12 [Epub ahead of print] doi:10.1016/j.neurobiolaging.2007.12.020.

Kennedy, K. M., Partridge, T., and Raz, N. (2008b). Age-related differences in acquisition of perceptual-motor skills: Working memory as a mediator. *Aging, Neuropsychology and Cogition*, 15: 165–183.

Kennedy, K. M., Rodrigue, K. M., Head, D., Gunning-Dixon, F., and Raz, N. (2009). Neuroanatomical and cognitive mediators of age-related differences in perceptual priming and learning. *Neuropsychology*, in press.

Keuker, J. I., Luiten, P. G., and Fuchs E. (2003). Preservation of hippocampal neuron numbers in aged rhesus monkeys. *Neurobiology of Aging*, 24: 157–165.

Kimura, H., Meaney, D. F., McGowan, J. C., Grossman, R. I., Lenkinski, R. E., Ross, D. T., et al. (1996). Magnetization transfer imaging of diffuse axonal injury following experimental brain injury in the pig: Characterization by magnetization transfer ratio with histopathologic correlation. *Journal of Computer Assisted Tomography*, 20: 540–546.

Kochunov, P., Mangin, J. F., Coyle, T., Lancaster, J., Thompson, P., Riviere, D., et al. (2005). Age-related morphology trends of cortical sulci. *Human Brain Mapping*, 26: 210–220.

Kochunov, P., Thompson, P. M., Lancaster, J. L., Bartzokis, G., Smith, S., Coyle, T., et al. (2007). Relationship between white matter fractional anisotropy and other indices of cerebral health in normal aging: tract-based spatial statistics study of aging. *Neuroimage*, 35: 478–487.

Kraemer, H. C., Yesavage, J. A., Taylor, J. L., and Kupfer D. (2000). How can we learn about developmental processes from cross-sectional studies, or can we? *American Journal of Psychiatry*, 157: 163–171.

Kramer, A. F. and Erickson, K. I. (2007). Capitalizing on cortical plasticity: Influence of physical activity on cognition and brain function. *Trends in Cognitive Sciences*, 11: 342–348.

Kramer, J. H., Mungas, D., Reed, B. R., Wetzel, M. E., Burnett, M. M., Miller, B. L., et al. (2007). Longitudinal MRI and cognitive change in healthy elderly. *Neuropsychology*, 21: 412–418.

Kuhn, H. G., Dickinson-Anson, H., and Gage, F. H. (1996). Neurogenesis in the dentate gyrus of the adult rat: Age-related decrease of neuronal progenitor proliferation. *Journal of Neuroscience*, 16: 2027–2033.

Laule, C., Vavasour, I. M., Moore, G. R., Oger, J., Li, D. K., Paty, D. W., et al. (2004). Water content and myelin water fraction in multiple sclerosis. A T2 relaxation study. *Journal of Neurology*, 251: 284–293.

Leaper, S. A., Murray, A. D., Lemmon, H. A., Staff, R. T., Deary, I. J., Crawford, J. R., et al. (2001). Neuropsychologic correlates of brain white matter lesions depicted on MR images: *1921 Aberdeen Birth Cohort Radiology*, 221: 51–55.

Lee, K. Y., Kim, T. K., Park, M., Ko, S., Song, I. C., and Cho, I. H. (2004). Age-related changes in conventional and magnetization transfer MR imaging in elderly people: Comparison with neurocognitive performance. *Korean Journal of Radiology*, 5: 96–101.

Lehmbeck, J. T., Brassen, S., Weber-Fahr, W., and Braus, D. F. (2006). Combining voxel-based morphometry and diffusion tensor imaging to detect age-related brain changes. *Neuroreport*, 17: 467–470.

Lemaître, H., Crivello, F., Dufouil, C., Grassiot, B., Tzourio, C., Alperovitch, A., et al. (2005). No epsilon4 gene dose effect on hippocampal atrophy in a large MRI database of healthy elderly subjects. *Neuroimage*, 24: 1205–1213.

Lenaz, G., Bovina, C., D'Aurelio, M., Fato, R., Formiggini, G., Genova, M. L., et al. (2002). Role of mitochondria in oxidative stress and aging. *Annals of the New York Academy of Sciences*, 959: 199–213.

Lenroot, R. K. and Giedd, J. N. (2006). Brain development in children and adolescents: insights from anatomical magnetic resonance imaging. *Neuroscience and Biobehavioral Review*, 30: 718–729.

Lesniak, K. T. and Dubbert, P. M. (2001). Exercise and hypertension. *Current Opinion in Cardiology*, 16: 356–359.

Lessov-Schlaggar, C. N., Reed, T., Swan, G. E., Krasnow, R. E., DeCarli, C., Marcus, R., et al. (2005). Association of sex steroid hormones with brain morphology and cognition in healthy elderly men. *Neurology*, 65: 1591–1596.

Lexa, F. J., Grossman, R. I., and Rosenquist, A. C. (1994). Dyke Award paper. MR of wallerian degeneration in the feline visual system: characterization by magnetization transfer rate with histopathologic correlation. *American Journal of Neuroradiology*, 15: 201–212.

Liesker, J. J., Postma, D. S., Beukema, R. J., ten Hacken, N. H., van der Molen, T., Riemersma, R. A., et al. (2004). Cognitive performance in patients with COPD. *Respiratory Medicine*, 98: 351–356.

Lind, J., Larsson, A., Persson, J., Ingvar, M., Nilsson, L. G., Bäckman, L., et al. (2006). Reduced hippocampal volume in non-demented carriers of the apolipoprotein E epsilon4: Relation to chronological age and recognition memory. *Neuroscience Letters*, 396: 23–27.

Lindenberger, U. and Pötter, U. (1998). The complex nature of unique and shared effects in hierarchical linear regression: Implications for developmental psychology. *Psychological Methods*, 3: 218–230.

Liu, R. S. N, Lemieux, L., Bell, G. S., Sisodiya, S. M., Shovron, S. D., Sander, J. W. A. S, et al. (2003). Longitudinal study of brain morphometrics using quantitative magnetic resonance imaging and difference image analysis. *Neuroimage*, 20: 22–33.

Lord, C., Buss, C., Lupien, S. J., and Pruessner, J. C. (2008). Hippocampal volumes are larger in postmenopausal women using estrogen therapy compared to past users, never users and men: A possible window of opportunity effect. *Neurobiology of Aging*, 29: 95–101.

Luckey, A. E. and Parsa, C. J. (2003). Fluid and electrolytes in the aged. *Archives of Surgery*, 138: 1055–1060.

Luoto, R., Manolio, T., Meilahn, E., Bhadelia, R., Furberg, C., Cooper, L., et al. (2000). Estrogen replacement therapy and MRI-demonstrated cerebral infarcts, white matter changes, and brain atrophy in older women: The Cardiovascular Health Study. *Journal of American Geriatric Society*, 48: 467–472.

Lupien, S. J., de Leon, M., de Santi, S., Convit, A., Tarshish, C., Nair, N. P., et al. (1998). Cortisol levels during human aging predict hippocampal atrophy and memory deficits. *Natue Neuroscience*, 1: 69–73.

Lupien, S. J., Evans, A., Lord, C., Miles, J., Pruessner, M., Pike, B., et al. Hippocampal volume is as variable in young as in older adults: Implications for the notion of hippocampal atrophy in humans. *Neuroimage*, 34: 479–485.

Lynch, G., Rex, C. S., and Gall, C. M. (2007). LTP consolidation: Substrates, explanatory power, and functional significance. *Neuropharmacology*, 52: 12–23.

Lyons, D. M., Parker, K. J., Zeitzer, J. M., Buckmaster, C. L., and Schatzberg, A. F. (2007). Preliminary evidence that hippocampal volumes in monkeys predict stress levels of adrenocorticotropic hormone. *Biological Psychiatry*, 62: 1171–1174.

Lyons, D. M., Yang, C., Sawyer-Glover, A. M., Moseley, M. E., and Schatzberg, A. F. (2001). Early life stress and inherited variation in monkey hippocampal volumes. *Archives of General Psychiatry*, 58: 1145–1151.

MacDonald, A. W. 3rd, Carter, C. S., Flory, J. D., Ferrell, R. E., and Manuck, S. B. (2007). COMT val158Met and executive control: a test of the benefit of specific deficits to translational research. *Journal of Abnormal Psychology*, 116: 306–312.

Madden, D. J., Spaniol, J., Whiting, W. L., Bucur, B., Provenzale, J. M., Cabeza, R., et al. (2007). Adult age differences in the functional neuroanatomy of visual attention: a combined fMRI and DTI study. *Neurobiology of Aging*, 28: 459–476.

Madden, D. J., Whiting, W. L., Huettel, S. A., White, L. E., MacFall, J. R., and Provenzale, J. M. (2004). Diffusion tensor imaging of adult age differences in cerebral white matter: Relation to response time. *Neuroimage*, 21: 1174–1181.

Maki, P. M. and Resnick, S. M. (2000). Longitudinal effects of estrogen replacement therapy on PET cerebral blood flow and cognition. *Neurobiology of Aging*, 21: 373–383.

Makris, N., Papadimitriou, G. M., van der Kouwe, A., Kennedy, D. N., Hodge, S. M., Dale, A. M., et al. (2007). Frontal connections and cognitive changes in normal aging rhesus monkeys: A DTI study. *Neurobiology of Aging*, 28: 1556–1567.

Marner, L., Nyengaard, J. R., Tang, Y., Pakkenberg B. Marked loss of myelinated nerve fibers in the human brain with age. *Journal of Comparative Neurology*, 462: 144–152.

Mattay, V. S. and Goldberg, T. E. (2004). Imaging genetic influences in human brain function. *Current Opinion in Neurobiology*, 14: 239–247.

McArdle, J. J., Ferrer-Caja, E., Hamagami, F., and Woodcock, R. W. (2002). Comparative longitudinal structural analyses of the growth and decline of multiple intellectual abilities over the life span. *Developmetal Psychology*, 38: 115–142.

McEwen, B. (2002). Estrogen actions throughout the brain. *Recent Progress in Hormone Research*, 57: 357–384.

McEwen, B. S. (2006). Sleep deprivation as a neurobiologic and physiologic stressor: Allostasis and allostatic load. *Metabolism*, 55: S20–S23.

McEwen, B. S. (2007). Physiology and neurobiology of stress and adaptation: central role of the brain. *Physiological Reviews*, 87: 873–904.

McEwen, B. S. and Stellar, E. (1993). Stress and the individual. Mechanisms leading to disease. *Archives of Internal Medicine*, 153: 2093–2101.

McDaniel, B., Sheng, H., Warner, D. S., Hedlund, L. W., and Benveniste, H. (2001). Tracking brain volume changes in C57BL/6J and ApoE-deficient mice in a model of neurodegeneration: A 5-week longitudinal micro-MRI study. *Neuroimage*, 14: 1244–1255.

McLaughlin, N. C. R., Paul, R. H., Grieve, S. M., Williams, L. M., Laidlaw, D., DiCarlo, M., et al. (2007). Diffusion tensor imaging of the corpus callosum: A cross-sectional study across the lifespan. *International Journal of Developmental Neuroscience*, 25: 215–221.

Mehta, R. C., Pike, G. B., and Enzmann, D. R. (1995). Magnetization transfer MR of the normal adult brain. *American Journal of Neuroradiology*, 16: 2085–2091.

Mehta, R. C., Pike, G. B., and Enzmann, D. R. (1996). Magnetization transfer magnetic resonance imaging: a clinical review. *Top Magnetic Resonance Imaging*, 8: 214–230.

Merboldt, K. D., Hanicke, W., and Frahm, J. (1985). Self-diffusion NMR imaging using stimulated echoes. *Journal of Magnetic Resonance*, 64: 479–486.

Merrill, D. A., Karim, R., Darraq, M., Chiba, A. A., and Tuszynski, M. H. (2003). Hippocampal cell genesis does not correlate with spatial learning ability in aged rats. *Journal of Comparative Neurology*, 459: 201–207.

Merrill, D. A., Roberts, J. A., and Tuszynski, M. H. (2000). Conservation of neuron number and size in entorhinal cortex layers II, III, and V/VI of aged primates. *Journal of Comparative Neurology*, 422: 396–401.

Messerli, F. H., Williams, B., and Ritz, E. (2007). Essential hypertension. *Lancet*, 370: 591–603.

Mezzapesa, D. M., Rocca, M. A., Pagani, E., Comi, G., and Filippi, M. (2003). Evidence of subtle gray-matter pathologic changes in healthy elderly individuals with nonspecific white-matter hyperintensities. *Archives of Neurology*, 60: 1109–1112.

Miyahira, Y., Yu, J., Hiramatsu, K., Shimazaki, Y., and Takeda, Y. (2004). [Brain volumetric MRI study in healthy elderly persons using statistical parametric mapping]. *Seishin Shinkeigaku Zasshi*, 106: 138–151 [Article in Japanese; English abstract].

Moffat, S. D. (2005). Effects of testosterone on cognitive and brain aging in elderly men. *Annals of the New York Academy of Sciences*, 1055: 80–92.

Moffat, S. D., Szekely, C. A., Zonderman, A. B., Kabani, N. J., and Resnick, S. M. (2000). Longitudinal change in hippocampal volume as a function of apolipoprotein E genotype. *Neurology*, 55: 134–136.

Moffat, S. D., Kennedy, K. M., Rodrigue, K. M., and Raz, N. (2007). Extrahippocampal contributions to age differences in human spatial navigation. *Cerebral Cortex*, 17: 1274–1282.

Moss, M., Franks, M., Briggs, P., Kennedy, D., and Scholey, A. (2005). Compromised arterial oxygen saturation in elderly asthma sufferers results in selective cognitive impairment. *Journal of Clinical Experimental Neuropsychology*, 27: 139–150.

Mottershead, J. P., Schmierer, K., Clemence, M., Thornton, J. S., Scaravilli, F., Barker, G. J., et al. (2003). High field MRI correlates of myelin content and axonal density in multiple sclerosis – a post-mortem study of the spinal cord. *Journal of Neurology*, 250: 1293–1301.

Moore, T. L., Killiany, R. J., Rosene, D. L., Prusty, S., Hollander, W., and Moss, M. B. (2002). Impairment of executive function induced by hypertension in the rhesus monkey (Macaca mulatta). *Behavioral Neuroscience*, 116: 387–396.

Moore, T. L., Killiany, R. J., Herndon, J. G., Rosene, D. L., and Moss, M. B. (2006). Executive system dysfunction occurs as early as middle-age in the rhesus monkey. *Neurobiology of Aging*, 27: 1484–1493.

Moseley, M. (2002). Diffusion tensor imaging and aging – a review. *NMR Biomedicine*, 15: 553–560.

Naganawa, S., Sato, K., Katagiri, T., Mimura, T., and Ishigaki, T. (2003). Regional ADC values of the normal brain: differences due to age, gender, and laterality. *European Radiology*, 13: 6–11.

Nagel, I. E., Chicherio, C., Li, S.-C., von Oertzen, T., Sander, T., Villringer, A., et al. (2008). Human aging magnifies genetic effects on executive functioning and working memory. *Frontiers in Human Neuroscience*, 2:1. Epub 2008 May 3.

Negash, S., Petersen, L. E., Geda, Y. E., Knopman, D. S., Boeve, B. F., Smith, G. E., et al. (2007). Effects of ApoE genotype and mild cognitive impairment on implicit learning. *Neurobiology of Aging*, 28: 885–893.

Nemoto, K., Ohnishi, T., Mori, T., Moriguchi, Y., Hashimoto, R., Asada, T., et al. (2006). The Val66Met polymorphism of the brain-derived neurotrophic factor gene affects age-related brain morphology. *Neuroscience Letters*, 397: 25–29.

Nesvåg, R., Lawyer, G., Varnäs, K., Fjell, A. M., Walhovd, K. B., Frigessi, A., et al. (2008). Regional thinning of the cerebral cortex in schizophrenia: Effects of diagnosis, age and antipsychotic medication. *Schizophrenia Research*, 98: 16–28.

Nusbaum, A. O., Tang, C. Y., Buchsbaum, M. S., Wei, T. C., and Atlas, S. W. (2001). Regional and global changes in cerebral diffusion with normal aging. *American Journal of Neuroradiology*, 22: 136–142.

O'Hara, R., Miller, E., Liao, C. P., Way, N., Lin, X., and Hallmayer, J. (2006). COMT genotype, gender and cognition in community-dwelling, older adults. *Neuroscience Letters*, 409: 205–209.

O'Hara, R., Schröder, C. M., Mahadevan, R., Schatzberg, A. F., Lindley, S., Fox, S., et al. (2007). Serotonin transporter polymorphism, memory and hippocampal volume in the elderly: Association and interaction with cortisol. *Molecular Psychiatry*, 12: 544–555.

Ortapamuk, H. and Naldoken, S. (2006). Brain perfusion abnormalities in chronic obstructive pulmonary disease: Comparison with cognitive impairment. *Annals of Nuclear Medicine*, 20: 99–106.

O'Sullivan, M., Jones, D. K., Summers, P. E., Morris, R. G., Williams, S. C. R., and Markus, H. S. (2001). Evidence for cortical 'disconnection' as a mechanism of age-related cognitive decline. *Neurology*, 57: 632–638.

Ota, M., Obata, T., Akine, Y., Ito, H., Ikehira, H., Asada, T., et al. (2006). Age-related degeneration of corpus callosum measured with diffusion tensor imaging. *Neuroimage*, 31: 1445–1452.

Pagnoni, G. and Cekic, M. (2007). Age effects on gray matter volume and attentional performance in Zen meditation. *Neurobiology of Aging*, 28: 1623–1627.

Pardon, M. C. (2007). Stress and ageing interactions: A paradox in the context of shared etiological and physiopathological processes. *Brain Research Review*, 54: 251–73.

Paul, R., Grieve, S. M., Chaudary, B., Gordon, N., Lawrence, J., Cooper, N., et al. (2007). Relative contributions of the cerebellar vermis and prefrontal lobe volumes on cognitive function across the adult lifespan. *Neurobiology of Aging*, Sep 13 [Epub ahead of print].

Peavy, G. M., Lange, K. L., Salmon, D. P., Patterson, T. L., Goldman S, Gamst, A. C., et al. (2007). The effects of prolonged stress and APOE genotype on memory and cortisol in older adults. *Biological Psychiatry*, 62: 472–478.

Perlman, W. R., Webster, M. J., Herman, M. M., Kleinman, J. E., and Weickert, C. S. (2007). Age-related differences in glucocorticoid receptor mRNA levels in the human brain. *Neurobiology of Aging*, 28: 447–458.

Persson, J., Nyberg, L., Lind, J., Larsson, A., Nilsson, L.-G., Ingvar, M., et al. (2006). Structure-function correlates of cognitive decline in aging. *Cerebral Cortex*, 16: 907–915.

Peters, A. and Sethares, C. (2002). Aging and the myelinated fibers in prefrontal cortex and corpus callosum of the monkey. *Journal of Comparative Neurology*, 442: 277–291.

Petersen, R. C., Jack, C. R. Jr, Xu, Y. C., Waring, S. C., O'Brien, P. C., Smith, G. E., et al. (2000). Memory and MRI-based hippocampal volumes in aging and AD. *Neurology*, 54: 581–587.

Pfefferbaum, A., and Sullivan, E. V. (2003). Increased brain white matter diffusivity in normal adult aging: Relationship to anisotropy and partial voluming. *Magnetic Resonance in Medicine*, 49: 953–961.

Pfefferbaum, A., Adalsteinsson, E., and Sullivan, E. V. (2005). Frontal circuitry degradation marks healthy adult aging: Evidence from diffusion tensor imaging. *Neuroimage*, 26: 891–899.

Pfefferbaum, A., Sullivan, E. V., and Carmelli, D. (2001). Genetic regulation of regional microstructure of the corpus callosum in late life. *Neuroreport*, 12: 1677–1681.

Pfefferbaum, A., Sullivan, E. V., and Carmelli, D. (2004). Morphological changes in aging brain structures are differentially affected by time-linked environmental influences despite strong genetic stability. *Neurobiology of Aging*, 25: 175–183.

Pfefferbaum, A., Sullivan, E. V., Rosenbloom, M. J., Mathalon, D. H., and Lim, K. O. (1998). A controlled study of cortical gray matter and ventricular changes in alcoholic men over a 5-year interval. *Archives of General Psychiatry*, 55: 905–912.

Pfefferbaum, A., Sullivan, E. V., Swan, G. E., and Carmelli, D. (2000). Brain structure in men remains highly heritable in the seventh and eighth decades of life. *Neurobiology of Aging*, 21: 63–74.

Pierpaoli, C., Jezzard, P., Basser, P. J., Barnett, A., and DiChiro, G. (1996). Diffusion tensor MR imaging of the human brain. *Radiology*, 201: 637–648.

Price, A. L., Patterson, N. J., Plenge, R. M., Weinblatt, M. E., Shadick, N. A., and Reich, D. (2006). Principal components analysis corrects for stratification in genome-wide association studies. *Nature Genetics*, 38: 904–909.

Prins, N. D., van Dijk, E. J., den Heijer T, Vermeer, S. E., Jolles, J., Koudstaal, P. J., et al. (2005). Cerebral small-vessel disease and decline in information processing speed, executive function and memory. *Brain*, 128: 2034–2041.

Pruessner, M., Pruessner, J. C., Hellhammer, D. H., Bruce Pike, G., and Lupien, S. J. (2007). The associations among hippocampal volume, cortisol reactivity, and memory performance in healthy young men. *Psychiatry Research*, 155: 1–10.

Rabbitt, P., Ibrahim, S., Lunn, M., Scott, M., Thacker, N., Hutchinson, C., et al. (2008). Age-associated losses of brain volume predict longitudinal cognitive declines over 8 to 20 years. *Neuropsychology*, 22: 3–9.

Rajkowska, G. (2003). Depression: What we can learn from postmortem studies. *Neuroscientist*, 9: 273–284.

Rao, D. C. (1998). CAT scans, PET scans, and genomic scans. *Genetics of Epidemiology*, 15: 1–18.

Rau, P. R., Sellner, J., Heiland, S., Plaschke, K., Schellinger, P. D., Meyding-Lamadé, U. K., et al. (2006). Apparent diffusion coefficient in the aging mouse brain: a magnetic resonance imaging study. *Life Science*, 78: 1175–1180.

Raz, N. (2000). Aging of the brain and its impact on cognitive performance: Integration of structural and functional findings. In: Craik, F. I. M. and Salthouse, T. A. (eds), *Handbook of Aging and Cognition – II* (pp. 1–90). Mahwah, NJ: Erlbaum.

Raz, N. (2004). The aging brain observed in vivo: Differential changes and their modifiers. In: Cabeza, R., Nyberg, L., and Park, D. C. (eds), *Cognitive Neuroscience of Aging: Linking Cognitive and Cerebral Aging* (pp. 17–55). New York: Oxford University Press.

Raz, N. (2006). Societal factors in cognitive aging: One eye wide shut? In: Schaie, K. W. and Carstensen, L.L. (eds), *Social Structures, Aging, and Self-Regulation in the Elderly* (pp. 9–12). New York, NY: Springer.

Raz, N. (2007). Which side of plasticity? A comment on Greenwood. *Neuropsychology*, 21: 676–677.

Raz, N., Briggs, S. D., Marks, W., and Acker, J. D. (1999). Age-related deficits in generation and manipulation of mental images: II. The role of dorsolateral prefrontal cortex. *Psychology and Aging*, 14: 436–445.

Raz, N., Dixon, F. M., Head, D. P., Dupuis, J. H., and Acker, J. D. (1998). Neuroanatomical correlates of cognitive aging: Evidence from structural MRI. *Neuropsychology*, 12: 95–106.

Raz, N., Gunning, F. M., Head, D., Dupuis, J. H., McQuain, J. M., Briggs, S. D., et al. (1997). Selective aging of human cerebral cortex observed *in vivo*: Differential vulnerability of the prefrontal gray matter. *Cerebral Cortex*, 7: 268–282.

Raz, N., Gunning-Dixon, F., Head, D., Rodrigue, K., Williamson, A., Acker, J. D. (2004c). Aging, sexual dimorphism, and hemispheric asymmetry of the cerebral cortex: Replicability of regional differences in volume. *Neurobiology of Aging*, 25: 377–396.

Raz, N., Lindenberger, U., Rodrigue, K. M., Kennedy, K. M., Head, D. Williamson, A., et al. (2005). Regional brain changes in aging healthy adults: General trends, individual differences, and modifiers. *Cerebral Cortex*, 15: 1676–1689.

Raz, N., Lindenberger, U., Ghisletta, P., Rodrigue, K. M., Kennedy, K. M., and Acker, J. D. (2008). Neuroanatomical correlates of fluid intelligence in healthy adults and persons with vascular risk factors. *Cerebral Cortex*, 18: 718–726.

Raz, N. and Rodrigue, K. M. (2006). Differential aging of the brain: patterns, cognitive correlates and modifiers. *Neuroscience and Biobehavioral Review*, 30: 730–748.

Raz, N., Rodrigue, K. M., Kennedy, K. M., Head, D., Gunning-Dixon, F. M., Acker, J. D. (2003a). Differential aging of the human striatum: Longitudinal evidence. *American Journal of Neuroradiology*, 24: 1849–1856.

Raz, N., Rodrigue, K. M., Kennedy, K. M., Dahle C, Head D, Acker, J. D. (2003b). Differential age-related changes in the regional metencephalic volumes in humans: A five-year follow-up. *Neuroscience Letters*, 349: 163–166.

Raz, N., Rodrigue, K. M., and Acker, J. D. (2003c). Hypertension and the brain: Vulnerability of the prefrontal regions and executive functions. *Behavior Neuroscience*, 17: 1169–1180.

Raz, N., Rodrigue, K. M., Head, D., Kennedy, K. M., and Acker, J. D. (2004a). Differential aging of the medial temporal lobe: A study of a five-year change. *Neurology*, 62: 433–439.

Raz, N., Rodrigue, K. M., Kennedy, K. M., and Acker, J. D. (2004b). Hormone replacement therapy and age-related brain shrinkage: Regional effects. *NeuroReport*, 15: 2531–2534.

Raz, N., Torres, I. J., Briggs, S. D., Spencer, W. D., Thornton, A. E., Loken, W., et al. (1995). Selective neuroanatomical abnormalities in Down's syndrome and their cognitive correlates: Evidence from MRI morphometry. *Neurology*, 45: 356–366.

Raz, N., Rodrigue, K. M., Kennedy, K. M., and Acker, J. D. (2007). Vascular health and longitudinal changes in brain and cognition in middle-aged and older adults. *Neuropsychology*, 21: 149–157.

Raz, N., Rodrigue, K. M., Kennedy, K. M., and Land, S. (2009). Genetic and vascular modifiers of age-sensitive cognitive skills: Effects of, COMT, BDNF, ApoE and hypertension. *Neuropsychology*, 23: 105–116.

Raz, N., Williamson, A., Gunning-Dixon, F., Head, D., and Acker, J. D. (2000). Neuroanatomical and cognitive correlates of adult age differences in acquisition of a perceptual-motor skill. *Microscopy Research and Technique*, 51: 85–93.

Reed, B. R., Eberling, J. L., Mungas, D., Weiner, M., Kramer, J. H., Jagust, W. J. (2004). Effects of white matter lesions and lacunes on cortical function. *Archives of Neurology*, 61: 1545–1550.

Reiman, E. M. (2007). Linking brain imaging and genomics in the study of Alzheimer's disease and aging. *Annals of the New York Academy of the Sciences*, 1097: 94–113.

Reiman, E. M., Chen, K., Alexander, G. E., Caselli, R. J., Bandy, D., Osborne D, et al. (2004). Functional brain abnormalities in young adults at genetic risk for late-onset Alzheimer's dementia. *Proceedings of the National Academy of Sciences of the USA*, 101: 284–289.

Reiman, E. M., Webster, J. A., Myers, A. J., Hardy, J., Dunckley, T., Zismann, V. L., et al. (2007). GAB2 alleles modify Alzheimer's risk in APOE epsilon4 carriers. *Neuron*, 54: 713–720.

Resnick, S. M., Pham, D. L., Kraut, M. A., Zonderman, A. B., and Davatzikos, C. (2003). Longitudinal magnetic resonance imaging studies of older adults: A shrinking brain. *Journal of Neuroscience*, 23: 3295–3301.

Rodrigue, K. M. and Raz, N. (2004). Shrinkage of the entorhinal cortex over five years predicts memory performance in healthy adults. *Journal of Neuroscience*, 24: 956–963.

Rovaris, M., Iannucci, G., Cercignani, M., Sormani, M. P., De Stefano, N., Gerevini, S., et al. Age-related changes in conventional, magnetization transfer, and diffusion-tensor MR imaging findings: study with whole-brain tissue histogram analysis. *Radiology* 227: 731–738.

Rujescu, D., Meisenzahl, E. M., Krejcova, S., Giegling, I., Zetzsche, T., Reiser, M., et al. (2007). Plexin B3 is genetically associated with verbal performance and white matter volume in human brain. *Molecular Psychiatry*, 12: 190–194, 115.

Rusinek, H., De Santi, S., Frid, D., Tsui, W. H., Tarshish, C. Y., Convit, A., et al. Regional brain atrophy rate predicts future cognitive decline: 6-year longitudinal MR imaging study of normal aging. *Radiology*, 229: 691–696.

Sabbatini, M., Tomassoni, D., and Amenta, F. (2001). Hypertensive brain damage: comparative evaluation of protective effect of treatment with dihydropyridine derivatives in spontaneously hypertensive rats. *Mechanisms of Ageing and Development*, 122: 2085–2105.

Sachdev, P. S., Anstey, K. J., Parslow, R. A., Wen, W., Maller, J., Kumar, R., et al. (2006). Pulmonary function, cognitive impairment and brain atrophy in a middle-aged community sample. *Dementia and Geriatric Cognitive Disorders*, 21: 300–308.

Sachdev, P. S., Valenzuela, M., Wang, X. L., Looi, J. C., and Brodaty, H. (2002). Relationship between plasma homocysteine levels and brain atrophy in healthy elderly individuals. *Neurology*, 58: 1539–1541.

Salat, D. H., Buckner, R. L., Snyder, A. Z., Greve, D. N., Desikan, R. S., Busa, E., et al. (2004). Thinning of the cerebral cortex in aging. *Cerebral Cortex*, 14: 721–730.

Salat, D. H., Kaye, J. A., Janowsky, J. S. Greater orbital prefrontal volume selectively predicts worse working memory performance in older adults. *Cerebral Cortex*, 12: 494–505.

Salat, D. H., Tuch, D. S., Greve, D. N., van der Kouwe, A. J., Hevelone, N. D., Zaleta, A. K., et al. (2005). Age-related alterations in white matter microstructure measured by diffusion tensor imaging. *Neurobiology of Aging*, 26: 1215–1227.

Salerno, J. A., Murphy, D. G., Horwitz, B., DeCarli, C., Haxby, J. V., Rapoport, S. I., et al. (1992). Brain atrophy in hypertension. A volumetric magnetic resonance imaging study. *Hypertension*, 20: 340–348.

Saunamäki, T. and Jehkonen, M. (2007). A review of executive functions in obstructive sleep apnea syndrome. *Acta Neurologica Scandinavica*, 115: 1–11.

Scamvougeras, A., Kigar, D. L., Jones, D., Weinberger, D. R., and Witelson, S. F. (2003). Size of the human corpus callosum is genetically determined: An MRI study in mono and dizygotic twins. *Neuroscience Letters*, Feb 27 338(2): 91–94.

Schiavone, F., Charlton, R. A., Barrick, T. R., Morris, R. G., and Markus, H. S. (2009). Imaging age-related cognitive decline: A comparison of diffusion tensor and magnetization transfer MRI. *Journal of Magnetic Resonance Imaging*, 29: 23–30.

Schmahmann, J. D., Pandya, D. N., Wang, R., Dai, G., D'Arceuil, H. E., de Crespigny, A. J., et al. (2007). Association fibre pathways of the brain: parallel observations from diffusion spectrum imaging and autoradiography. *Brain*, 130(Pt 3): 630–653.

Schmidt, R., Fazekas, F., Reinhart, B., Kapeller, P., Fazekas, G., Offenbacher, H., et al. (1996). Estrogen replacement therapy in older women: A neuropsychological and brain MRI study. *Journal of American Geriatric Society*, 44: 1307–1313.

Schretlen, D., Pearlson, G. D., Anthony, J. C., Aylward, E. H., Augustine, A. M., Davis, A., et al. (2000). Elucidating the contributions of processing speed, executive ability, and frontal lobe volume to normal age-related differences in fluid intelligence. *Journal of the International Neuropsychological Society*, 6: 52–61.

Schulte, T., Sullivan, E. V., Muller-Oehring, E. M., Adalsteinsson, E., and Pfefferbaum, A. (2005). Corpus callosal microstructural integrity influences interhemispheric processing: a diffusion tensor imaging study. *Cerebral Cortex*, 15: 1384–1392.

Shamy, J. L., Buonocore, M. H., Makaron, L. M., Amaral, D. G., Barnes, C. A., and Rapp, P. R. (2006). Hippocampal volume is preserved and fails to predict recognition memory impairment in aged rhesus monkeys (Macaca mulatta). *Neurobiology of Aging*, 27: 1405–1415.

Sheline, Y. I., Gado, M. H., and Kraemer, H. C. (2003). Untreated depression and hippocampal volume loss. *American Journal of Psychiatry*, 160: 1516–1518.

Sheline, Y. I., Sanghavi M, Mintun, M. A., and Gado, M. H. (1999). Depression duration but not age predicts hippocampal volume loss in medically healthy women with recurrent major depression. *Journal of Neuroscience*, 19: 5034–5043.

Shenkin, S. D., Bastin, M. E., Macgillivray, T. J., Deary, I. J., Starr, J. M., Rivers, C. S., et al. (2005). Cognitive correlates of cerebral white matter lesions and water diffusion tensor parameters in community-dwelling older people. *Cerebrovascular Disease*, 20: 310–318.

Shumaker, S. A., Legault, C., Thal, L., Wallace, R. B., Ockene, J. K., Hendrix, S. L., et al. (2003). WHIMS Investigators. Estrogen plus progestin and the incidence of dementia and mild cognitive impairment in postmenopausal women: the Women's Health Initiative Memory Study: A randomized controlled trial. *Journal of American Medical Association*, 289: 2651–2662.

Silver, N. C., Barker, G. J., MacManus, D. G., Tofts, P. S., and Miller, D. H. (1997). Magnetisation transfer ratio of normal brain white matter: A normative database spanning four decades of life. *Journal of Neurology Neurosurgery and Psychiatry*, 62: 223–228.

Siwak-Tapp, C. T., Head, E., Muggenburg, B. A., Milgram, N. W., and Cotman, C. W. (2008). Region specific neuron loss in the aged canine hippocampus is reduced by enrichment. *Neurobiology of Aging*, 29: 39–50.

Sliwinski, M. and Buschke, H. (1999). Cross-sectional and longitudinal relationships among age, cognition, and processing speed. *Psychology of Aging*, 14: 18–33.

Small, B. J., Rosnick, C. B., Fratiglioni, L., and Backman, L. (2004). Apolipoprotein E and cognitive performance: a meta-analysis. *Psychology of Aging*, 19: 592–600.

Smith, D. E., Roberts, J., Gage, F. H., and Tuszynski, M. H. (1999). Age-associated neuronal atrophy occurs in the primate brain and is reversible by growth factor gene therapy. *Proceedings of the National Academy of Sciences of the USA*, 96: 10893–10898.

Söderlund, H., Nilsson, L. G., Berger, K., Breteler, M. M., Dufouil, C., Fuhrer, R., et al. (2006). Cerebral changes on MRI and cognitive function: the CASCADE study. *Neurobiology of Aging*, 27: 16–23.

Sorrells, S. F. and Sapolsky, R. M. (2007). An inflammatory review of glucocorticoid actions in the CNS. *Brain Behavior and Immunity*, 21: 259–272.

Spearman, C. (1904). General intelligence objectively determined and measured. *American Journal of Psychology*, 15: 201–293.

Spilt, A., Goekoop, R., Westendorp, R. G., Blauw, G. J., de Craen, A. J., and van Buchem, M. A. (2006). Not all age-related white matter hyperintensities are the same: a magnetization transfer imaging study. *American Journal of Neuroradiology*, 27: 1964–1968.

Stadlbauer, A., Salomonowitz, E., Strunk, G., Hammen, T., and Ganslandt, O. (2008a). Quantitative diffusion tensor fiber tracking of age-related changes in the limbic system. *European Radiology*, 18: 130–137.

Stadlbauer, A., Salomonowitz, E., Strunk, G., Hammen, T., and Ganslandt, O. (2008b). Age-related degradation in the Central Nervous System: Assessment with Diffusion-Tensor Imaging and quantitative fiber tracking. *Radiology*, 247: 179–188.

Staff, R. T., Murray, A. D., Deary, I. J., and Whalley, L. J. (2006). Generality and specificity in cognitive aging: A volumetric brain analysis. *Neuroimage*, 30: 1433–1440.

Stan, A. D., Ghose, S., Gao, X.-M., Roberts, R. C., Lewis-Amezcua, K. L., Hatanpaa, K. J., et al. (2006). Human postmortem tissue: What quality markers matter? *Brain Research*, 1123: 1–11.

Starkman, M. N., Giordani, B., Gebarski, S. S., and Schteingart, D. E. (2003). Improvement in learning associated with increase in hippocampal formation volume. *Biological Psychiatry*, 53: 233–238.

Starr, J. M., Fox, H., Harris, S. E., Deary, I. J., and Whalley, L. J. (2007). COMT genotype and cognitive ability: a longitudinal aging study. *Neuroscience Letters*, 421: 57–61.

Stefanis, N. C., van Os, J., Avramopoulos, D., Smyrnis, N., Evdokimidis, I., and Stefanis, C. N. (2005). Effect of COMT Val158Met polymorphism on the continuous performance test, identical pairs version: Tuning rather than improving performance. *American Journal of Psychiatry*, 162: 1752–1754.

Sterling, P. and Eyer, J. (1988). Allostasis: a new paradigm to explain arousal pathology. In: S. Fisher and J. Reason (eds), *Handbook of Life Stress, Cognition and Health* (pp. 629–649). New York: Wiley.

Strassburger, T. L., Lee, H. C., Daly, E. M., Szczepanik J, Krasuski, J. S., Mentis, M. J., et al. (1997). Interactive effects of age and hypertension on volumes of brain structures. *Stroke*, 28: 1410–1417.

Straub, R. H. (2007). The complex role of estrogens in inflammation. *Endocrine Reviews*, 28: 521–574.

Sublette, M. E., Baca-Garcia, E., Parsey, R. V., Oquendo, M. A., Rodrigues, S. M., Galfalvy, H., et al. (2008). Effect of BDNF Val66Met polymorphism on age-related amygdala volume changes in healthy subjects. *Progress in Neuropsychopharmacology and Biological Psychiatry*, 32:1652–1655.

Sullivan, E. V., Adalsteinsson, E., Sood, R., Mayer, D., Bell, R., McBride, W., et al. (2006a). Longitudinal brain magnetic resonance imaging study of the alcohol-preferring rat. Part I: adult brain growth. *Alcohol Clinical Experimental Research*, 30: 1234–1247.

Sullivan, E. V., Adalsteinsson, E., and Pfefferbaum, A. (2006b).elective age-related degradation of anterior callosal fiber bundles quantified in vivo with fiber tracking. *Cerebral Cortex*, 16: 1030–1039.

Sullivan, E. V. and Pfefferbaum, A. (2003). Diffusion tensor imaging in normal aging and neuropsychiatric disorders. *European Journal of Radiology*, 45: 244–255.

Sullivan, E. V. and Pfefferbaum, A. (2006c). Diffusion tensor imaging and aging. *Neuroscience and Biobehavioral Review*, 30: 749–761.

Sullivan, E. V., Pfefferbaum, A., Swan, G. E., and Carmelli, D. (2001). Heritability of hippocampal size in elderly twin men: equivalent influence from genes and environment. *Hippocampus*, 11: 754–762.

Sullivan, P. F. (2007). Spurious genetic associations. *Biological Psychiatry*, 61: 1121–1126.

Swaab, D. F., Bao, A. M., and Lucassen, P. J. (2005). The stress system in the human brain in depression and neurodegeneration. *Ageing Research Review*, 4: 141–194.

Szeszko, P. R., Lipsky, R., Mentschel, C., Robinson, D., Gunduz-Bruce, H., Sevy, S., et al. (2005). Brain-derived neurotrophic factor val66met polymorphism and volume of the hippocampal formation. *Molecular Psychiatry*, 10: 631–636.

Takahashi, T., Suzuki, M., Tsunoda, M., Kawamura, Y., Takahashi, N., and Tsuneki, H., et al. (2008). Association between the brain-derived neurotrophic factor Val66Met polymorphism and brain morphology in a Japanese sample of schizophrenia and healthy comparisons. *Neuroscience Letters*, 435: 34–39.

Tan, H. Y., Chen, Q., Sust, S., Buckholtz, J. W., Meyers, J. D., Egan, M. F., et al. (2007). Epistasis between catechol-O-methyltransferase and type II metabotropic glutamate receptor 3 genes on working memory brain function. *Proceedings of the National Academy of Sciences of the USA*, 104: 12536–12541.

Tapiola, T., Pennanen, C., Tapiola, M., Tervo, S., Kivipelto, M., Hänninen, T. et al. (2008). MRI of hippocampus and entorhinal cortex in mild cognitive impairment: A follow-up study. *Neurobiology of Aging*, 29: 31–38.

Taylor, W. D., Bae, J. N., MacFall, J. R., Payne, M. E., Provenzale, J. M., Steffens, D. C., et al. (2007a). Widespread effects of hyperintense lesions on cerebral white matter structure. *American Journal of Roentgenology*, 188: 1695–1704.

Taylor, W. D., Züchner, S., Payne, M. E., Messer, D. F., Doty, T. J., MacFall, J. R., et al. (2007b). The COMT Val158Met polymorphism and temporal lobe morphometry in healthy adults. *Psychiatry Research*, 155: 173–177.

Tenhunen, J., Salminen, M., Lundstrom, K., Kiviluoto, T., Savolainen, R., and Ulmanen, I. (1994). Genomic organization of the human catechol O-methyltransferase gene and its expression from two distinct promoters. *European Journal of Biochemistry*, 223: 1049–1059.

Teunissen, C. E., Blom, A. H., Van Boxtel, M. P., Bosma, H., de Bruijn, C., Jolles, J., et al. (2003). Homocysteine: a marker for cognitive performance? A longitudinal follow-up study. *Journal of Nutrion Health and Aging*, 7: 153–159.

Thomas, C., Moya, L., Avidan, G., Humphreys, K., Jung, K. J., Peterson, M. A., et al. (2008). Reduction in white matter connectivity, revealed by diffusion tensor imaging, may account for age-related changes in face perception. *Journal of Cognitive Neuroscience*, 20: 268–284.

Thompson, P. M., Cannon, T. D., Narr, K. L., van Erp, T., Poutanen, V. P., Huttunen, M., et al. (2001). Genetic influences on brain structure. *Nature Neuroscience*, 4: 1253–1258.

Tisserand, D. J., Pruessner, J. C., Arigita, E. J. S., van Boxtel, M. J., Evans, A. C., Jolles, J., et al. (2002). Regional frontal cortical volumes decrease differentially in aging: an MRI study to compare volumetric approaches and voxel-based morphometry. *Neuroimage*, 17: 657–669.

Tisserand, D. J., van Boxtel, M. P., Pruessner, J. C., Hofman, P., Evans, A. C., and Jolles, J. (2004). A voxel-based morphometric study to determine individual differences in gray matter density associated with age and cognitive change over time. *Cerebral Cortex*, 14: 966–973.

Tullberg, M., Fletcher, E., DeCarli, C., Mungas, D., Reed, B. R., Harvey, D. J., et al. (2004). White matter lesions impair frontal lobe function regardless of their location. *Neurology*, 63: 246–253.

Tunbridge, E. M., Bannerman, D. M., Sharp, T., and Harrison, P. J. (2004). Catechol-O-methyltransferase inhibition improves set-shifting performance and elevates stimulated dopamine release in the rat prefrontal cortex. *Journal of Neuroscience*, 24: 5331–5335.

Tupler, L. A., Krishnan, K. R., Greenberg, D. L., Marcovina, S. M., Payne, M. E., Macfall, J. R., et al. (2007). Predicting memory decline in normal elderly: Genetics, MRI, and cognitive reserve. *Neurobiology of Aging*, 28: 1644–1656.

Turner, S. T., Jack, C. R., Fornage, M., Mosley, T. H., Boerwinkle, E., and de Andrade, M. (2004). Heritability of leukoaraiosis in hypertensive sibships. *Hypertension* 43: 483–487.

Tzourio, C., Dufouil, C., Ducimetiere, P., and Alperovitch, A. (1999). Cognitive decline in individuals with high blood pressure: A longitudinal study in the elderly. EVA Study Group. Epidemiology of vascular aging. *Neurology*, 53: 1948–1952.

Van Amelsvoort, T., Compton, J., and Murphy, D. (2001). In vivo assessment of the effects of estrogen on the human brain. *Trends in Endocrinology and Metabolism*, 12: 273–276.

Van Amelsvoort, T., Zinkstok, J., Figee, M., Daly, E., Morris, R., Owen, M. J., et al. (2007). Effects of a functional, C. O.MT polymorphism on brain anatomy and cognitive function in adults with velo-cardio-facial syndrome. *Psychological Medicine*, 38: 89–100.

van der Flier, W. M., van den Heuvel, D. M., Weverling-Rijnsburger, A. W., Bollen, E. L., Westendorp, R. G., van Buchem, M. A., et al. (2002). Magnetization transfer imaging in normal aging, mild cognitive impairment, and Alzheimer's disease. *Annals of Neurology*, 52: 62–67.

van der Flier, W. M., van Straaten, E. C., Barkhof, F., Ferro, J. M., Pantoni, L., Basile, A. M., et al. (2005). LADIS study group. Medial temporal lobe atrophy and white matter hyperintensities are associated with mild cognitive deficits in non-disabled elderly people: the LADIS study. *Journal of Neurology Neurosurgery and Psychiatry*, 76: 1497–500.

van der Hiele, K., Vein, A. A., van der Welle, A., van der Grond, J., Westendorp, R. G., Bollen, E. L., van Buchem, M. A., van Dijk, J. G., and Middelkoop, H. A. (2007). EEG and MRI correlates of mild cognitive impairment and Alzheimer's disease. *Neurobiology of Aging*, 28: 1322–1329.

van der Kouwe, A. J., Benner, T., Salat, D. H., and Fischl, B. (2008). Brain morphometry with multiecho, MPRAGE. *Neuroimage*, 40: 559–569.

van de Pol, L. A., van der Flier, W. M., Korf, E. S., Fox, N. C., Barkhof, F., and Scheltens, P. (2007). Baseline predictors of rates of hippocampal atrophy in mild cognitive impairment. *Neurology*, 69: 1491–1497.

Van Der Werf, Y. D., Tisserand, D. J., Visser, P. J., Hofman, P. A., Vuurman E, Uylings, H. B., et al. (2001). Thalamic volume predicts performance on tests of cognitive speed and decreases in healthy aging. A magnetic resonance imaging-based volumetric analysis. *Brain Research, Cognitvie Brain Research*, 11: 377–385.

Van Petten, C. (2004). Relationship between hippocampal volume and memory ability in healthy individuals across the lifespan: review and meta-analysis. *Neuropsychologia*, 42: 1394–1413.

Van Petten, C., Plante, E., Davidson, P. S., Kuo, T. Y., Bajuscak L, and Glisky, E. L. (2004). Memory and executive function in older adults: Relationships with temporal and prefrontal gray matter volumes and white matter hyperintensities. *Neuropsychologia*, 42: 1313–1335.

van Swieten, J. C., Geyskes, G. G., Derix, M. M., Peeck, B. M., Ramos, L. M., van Latum, J. C., et al. (1991). Hypertension in the elderly is associated with white matter lesions and cognitive decline. *Annals of Neurology*, 30: 825–830.

Verhaeghen, P. and Salthouse, T. A. (1997). Meta-analyses of age-cognition relations in adulthood: Estimates of linear and nonlinear age effects and structural models. *Psychological Bulletin*, 122: 231–249.

Vermeer, S. E., Longstreth, W. T., and Koudstaal, P. J. (2007). Silent brain infarcts: a systematic review. *Lancet Neurology*, 6: 611–619.

Vernooij, M. W., van der Lugt, A., Ikram, M. A., Wielopolski, P. A., Niessen, W. J., Hofman, A., et al. (2008a). Prevalence and risk factors of cerebral microbleeds: the Rotterdam Scan Study. *Neurology*, 70: 1208–1214.

Vernooij, M. W., Ikram, M. A., Wielopolski, P. A., Krestin, G. P., Breteler, M. M., and van der Lugt, A. (2008b). Cerebral microbleeds: Accelerated 3D T2*-weighted GRE MR imaging versus conventional 2D T2*-weighted GRE MR imaging for detection. *Radiology*, 248: 272–277 [Epub 2008 May 9].

Walhovd, K. B. and Fjell, A. M. (2007). White matter volume predicts reaction time instability. *Neuropsychologia*, Jun 11 45(10): 2277–2284.

Walhovd, K. B., Fjell, A. M., Reinvang, I., Lundervold, A., Fischl, B., Quinn, B. T., et al. (2004). Size does matter in the long run: hippocampal and cortical volume predict recall across weeks. *Neurology*, 63: 1193–1197.

Walhovd, K. B., Fjell, A. M., Reinvang, I., Lundervold, A., Dale, A. M., Eilertsen, D. E., et al. (2005a). Effects of age on volumes of cortex, white matter and subcortical structures. *Neurobiology of Aging*, 26: 1261–1270.

Walhovd, K. B., Fjell, A. M., Reinvang, I., Lundervold, A., Fischl, B., Salat, D., et al. (2005b) Cortical volume and speed-of-processing are complementary in prediction of performance intelligence. *Neuropsychologia*, 43: 704–713.

Walhovd, K. B., Fjell, A. M., Dale, A. M., Fischl, B., Quinn, B. T., Makris, N., et al. (2006). Regional cortical thickness matters in recall after months more than minutes. *Neuroimage*, 31: 1343–1351.

Weinshilboum, R. M. and Raymond, F. A. (1977). Inheritance of low erythrocyte catechol-o-methyltransferase activity in man. *American Journal of Human Genetics*, Mar 29(2): 125–135.

Whalley, L. J., Staff, R. T., Murray, A. D., Duthie, S. J., Collins, A. R., Lemmon, H. A., et al. (2003). Plasma vitamin C, cholesterol and homocysteine are associated with grey matter volume determined by MRI in non-demented old people. *Neuroscience Letters*, 341: 173–176.

Wierzbicki, A. S. (2007). Homocysteine and cardiovascular disease: a review of the evidence. *Diabetes and Vascular Disease Research*, 4: 143–150.

Williams, J. H., Pereira, E. A., Budge, M. M., and Bradley, K. M. (2002). Minimal hippocampal width relates to plasma homocysteine in community-dwelling older people. *Age Ageing*, 31: 440–444.

Winterer, G. and Goldman, D. (2003). Genetics of human prefrontal function. *Brain Research. Brain Research Reviews*, 43: 134–163.

Wishart, H. A., Saykin, A. J., McAllister, T. W., Rabin, L. A., McDonald, B. C., Flashman, L. A., et al. (2006). Regional brain atrophy in cognitively intact adults with a single APOE epsilon4 allele. *Neurology*, 67: 1221–1224.

Woodruff-Pak, D. S., Vogel, R. W. III, Ewers, M., Coffey, J., Boyko, O. B., Lemieux, S. K. (2001). MRI-assessed volume of cerebellum correlates with associative learning. *Neurobiology of Learning and Memory*, 76: 342–357.

Wozniak, J. R. and Lim, K. O. (2006). Advances in white matter imaging: a review of in vivo magnetic resonance methodologies and their applicability to the study of development and aging. *Neuroscience and Biobehavioral Review*, 30: 762–774.

Xu, Y., Valentino, D. J., Scher, A. I., Dinov, I., White, L. R., et al. (2008). Age effects on hippocampal structural changes in old men: The HAAS. *Neuroimage*, 40: 1003–1015.

Yaffe, K., Blackwell, T., Barnes, D. E., Ancoli-Israel, S., and Stone, K. L. (2007). Study of osteoporotic fractures group: Preclinical cognitive decline and subsequent sleep disturbance in older women. *Neurology*, 69: 237–242.

Yoshita, M., Fletcher, E., Harvey, D., Ortega, M., Martinez, O., Mungas, D. M.,et al. (2006). Extent and distribution of white matter hyperintensities in normal aging, MCI, and AD. *Neurology*, 67: 2192–2198.

Zhang, L., Dean, D., Liu, J. Z., Sahgal, V., Wang, X., and Yue, G. H. (2007). Quantifying degeneration of white matter in normal aging using fractal dimension. *Neurobiology of Aging*, 28: 1543–1555.

Zhang, Y. T., Zhang, C. Y., Zhang, J., and Li, W. (2005). Age-related changes of normal adult brain structure: Analysed with diffusion tensor imaging. *Chinese Medical Journal*, 118: 1059–1065.

Zhao, K., Aranzana, M. J., Kim, S., Lister, C., Shindo, C., Tang, C., et al. (2007). An Arabidopsis example of association mapping in structured samples. *PLoS Genetics*, 3: e4.

Zimmerman, M. E., Brickman, A. M., Paul, R. H., Grieve, S. M., Tate, D. F., Gunstad, J., et al. (2006). The relationship between frontal gray matter volume and cognition varies across the healthy adult lifespan. *American Journal of Geriatr Psychiatry*, 14: 823–833.

Zimmerman, M. E., Pan, J. W., Hetherington, H. P., Katz, M. J., Verghese, J., Buschke, H., et al. (2008). Hippocampal neurochemistry, neuromorphometry, and verbal memory in nondemented older adults. *Neurology*, 70: 1594–1600.

Zinkstok, J., Schmitz, N., van Amelsvoort, T., de Win, M., van den Brink, W., Baas, F., et al. (2006). The COMT val(158)met polymorphism and brain morphometry in healthy young adults. *Neuroscience Letters*, 405: 34–39.

Zisapel, N. (2007). Sleep and sleep disturbances: Biological basis and clinical implications. *Cellular and Molecular Life Sciences*, 64: 1174–1186.

5

Dopaminergic Modulation of Cognition in Human Aging

Shu-Chen Li*, Ulman Lindenberger, Lars Nyberg, Hauke R. Heekeren, and Lars Bäckman*

Brain aging involves neurofunctional, neuroanatomical, and neurochemical changes, and the dynamic interactions between these levels (see Cabeza, Nyberg, and Park, 2005; Lindenberger, Li, and Bäckman, 2006 for recent reviews). There are about 100 billion nerve cells in the human brain and each of these neurons communicates with at least 1,000 other neurons via synaptic mechanisms. Over 99% of all synapses in the brain use neurochemical transmissions. This chapter addresses age-related neurochemical changes that affect neuronal signal transduction. We focus specifically on age-related impairments in dopamine (DA) systems and their relationships to cognitive deficits later in life. Other neurotransmitter systems—most notably acetylcholine, norepinephrine, serotonin, and glutamate—also undergo alterations during the adult life course (see Morgan and May, 1990; Segovia et al., 2001 for reviews). Thus far, however, the DA systems have attracted the most attention and there is mounting evidence that DA is a key neurotransmitter in the context of cognitive aging. Molecular imaging methods for assessing age-related decline in pre- and post-synaptic markers of the dopaminergic systems, as well as more recent genomic imaging, multimodal imaging, and computational neuroscience approaches to investigate how dopaminergic modulation affects cognitive aging will be particularly highlighted here.

It was only a half century ago that DA was discovered as an independent transmitter in the nervous system, as opposed to a precursor of other transmitters (see Björklund and Dunnett, 2007 for review). The dopaminergic systems have, however, already been widely studied in the context of aging research, owing mainly to (a) the number of well-characterized biomarkers for their pre- and post-synaptic components, (b) the marked age-related decrements observed, and (c) broad involvement of DA in a wide range of cognitive functions and Parkinson's disease. In the following section, we first describe the major DA systems in the human brain and methods for imaging these systems. Then we review evidence for DA's role in cognition and the relationship between age-related declines in DA systems and cognitive aging. In the last section, we highlight emerging themes and novel approaches that are amenable for investigating

dopaminergic modulation in the aging brain and its functional-consequences. Although this chapter focuses on DA systems, age-related changes in other transmitter systems are likely to also interact with dopaminergic systems to affect cognitive functions. Outstanding issues regarding other transmitter systems that are likely to interact with dopamine in affecting cognitive functions will be discussed as well.

DA Systems in the Human Brain

Originating in the mid-brain, DA neurons have wide innervations to various subcortical and cortical regions that make up the nigrostriatal, mesocortical, and mesolimbic (see Lewis and Sesack, 1997 for review), as well as the thalamic dopaminergic systems (Sánchez-González et al., 2005; see Figure 5.1 for a schematic diagram of the four pathways). The nigrostriatal and mesolimbic pathways form the two major subcortical DA systems. The cell bodies of the nigrostriatal DA system are located in the substantia nigra in the ventral mesencephalon. The neurons project to the striatum—a region with dense dopaminergic innervations. The mesolimbic DA system originates from a more diffuse collection of neurons in the ventral mesencephalon, medial to the substantia nigra. This region is called the ventral tegmentum. One portion of the neurons here projects to limbic regions such as the nucleus accumbens, the amygdala, the hippocampus, and the anterior cingulate cortex. A third pathway, referred to as the mesocortical DA system, also originates from the ventral tegmentum and projects throughout the neocortex. A fourth pathway that projects to the thalamus, and may be independent from the nigrostriatal and mesolimbic systems, has only recently been identified in the primate brain (Sánchez-González et al., 2005). In line with findings in primates, the thalamus in humans is also innervated by dopamine. For instance, relatively high dopamine D2-receptor binding in the thalamus has been identified in both receptor imaging (e.g., Ito et al., 2008) and in postmortem (Rieck et al., 2004) studies.

---

* Corresponding authors: Shu-Chen Li (shuchen@mpib-berlin.mpg.de) Lars Bäckman (Lars.Backman.1@ki.se)

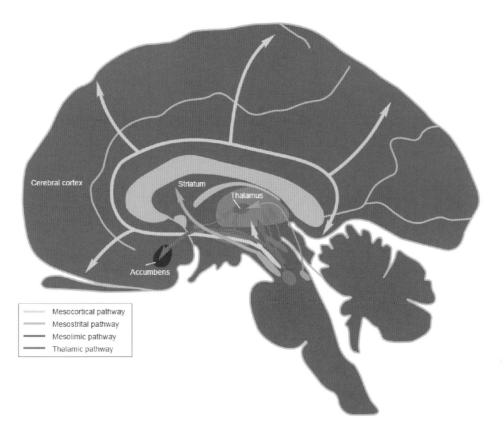

Figure 5–1 A schematic diagram of major dopaminergic pathways in the human brain. (Adapted from Bäckman and Farde, 2005 and Sánchez-González et al., 2005; special thanks to the lab of C. Cavada for providing an earlier draft of the figure.)

Post- and Pre-synaptic Components of DA Systems

The physiological effects of DA are mediated by binding to any of the five currently identified receptor subtypes (D1–D5). The DA receptor subtypes have distinct anatomical distributions in the brain (Meador-Woodruff, 1994) and can thus be viewed as markers for different clusters of DA-related functions. The five subtypes are grouped into two families on the basis of structural homology and biochemical characteristics. The family of D1-like receptors includes the D1 and D5 subtypes and the family of D2-like receptors including the D2, D3, and D4 subtypes. DA receptors exhibit tissue- and cell-specific expressions that are modulated during development, aging, and in conditions such as Parkinson's disease (Laurier, O'Dowd, and George, 1994; Schambra et al., 1994; Stoessl and de la Fuente-Fernandez, 2003). The molecular mechanisms regulating expressions of DA receptors are not well understood, and research in this area is just starting (e.g., Pasuit, Li, and Kuzhikandathil, 2004). The paucity of knowledge makes the task of developing distinct biomarkers for DA receptors difficult and complicates the interpretations of findings. In the following, the two receptor families are referred to as D1 and D2 receptors, as these are the most highly expressed DA receptor subtypes in the human brain. In addition, most of the ligands currently used for receptor imaging do not differentiate among the respective family members.

D1 receptors are more abundant than D2 receptors, reflecting high concentration not only in the striatum but also throughout the neocortex (Hall et al., 1994). D2 receptors are highly concentrated in the striatum. Lower concentrations are expressed in the brain stem and thalamus and concentrations are minute throughout the neocortex (Kessler et al., 1993). Cortically, the D2 receptors have a regional-specific laminar distribution, located in Lamina 2 of the lower temporal cortex and in Lamina 6 of the remaining neocortex (Kohler, Ericson, and Radesater, 1991).

Early work with rodents suggested an anterior-to-posterior gradient of dopaminergic projections to the neocortex, with a preferential DA innervation of the frontal cortex (Ungerstedt, 1971). This generally accepted assumption has, however, not been confirmed by more recent in vitro (Hall et al., 1994; Kessler et al., 1992) and in vivo (Farde et al., 1997) data. Specifically, studies in human subjects demonstrate a homogenous distribution of D1 receptors across the neocortex, and a preferential localization of D2 receptors in the ventral temporal cortex. The species differences in receptor distribution are consistent with findings that dopaminergic terminals are restricted to the frontal lobes in rodents, whereas they are more widely distributed, though with varying degrees of concentrations, across the entire cortex in monkeys and humans (Brown and Goldman, 1977; Gaspar et al., 1989).

Most DA receptors are located on postsynaptic neurons, although a small proportion is expressed on dopamine nerve terminals. The autoreceptors that are presynaptically located on nerve terminals (Carlsson, 1975) regulate dopamine synthesis and release and belong to the family of D2-like receptors (Roth, 1984). DA is synthesized at the presynaptic terminal—a process that is determined by the enzyme tyrosine hydroxylase (TH) that converts tyrosine to the DA precursor, dopa (see Figure 5.2). The DA transporter (DAT) is a membrane-bound protein that serves as a regulator of the synaptic concentration of DA at nerve terminals (Giros et al., 1992). The DAT provides a rapid and efficient

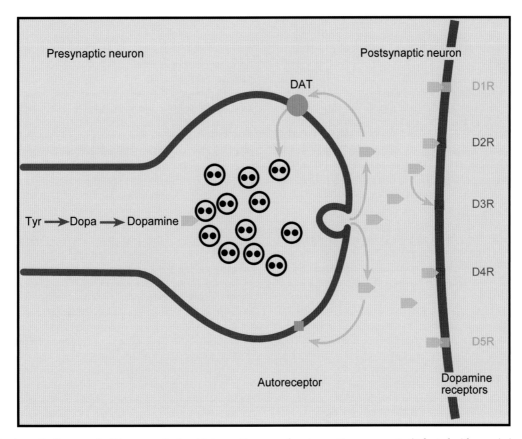

Figure 5–2   A schematic diagram of a DA synapse in the striatum with pre- and postsynaptic components. (Adapted with permission from Bäckman and Farde, 2005; copyright Oxford University Press.)

mechanism for reuptake of synaptic dopamine, and is essential for the regulation of dopamine neurotransmission (Giros et al., 1996). It has been suggested that the concentration of DAT may serve as a marker of the homeostatic tone of the DA system (Jaber et al., 1997; Jones et al., 1998). In addition, it should be noted that a small population of presynaptic D2 receptors also participate in the regulation of DA release (Roth, 1984). The highest concentration of the DAT is found in the striatum, with much lower concentration in the brain stem and the thalamus (Ito et al., 2008). Importantly, DAT is not expressed in the neocortex, where the noradrenaline transporter serves as a regulator of DA concentration. Other than the DAT, which is a DA specific transporter, the vesicular monoamine transporter (VMAT) is another presynaptic protein that transports monoamines, including DA, norepinephrine, and serotonin (Chen et al., 2008; Taylor et al., 2000). The VMAT— specifically the type-2 transporter VMAT2—transports intracellular monoamines into the synaptic vesicles and is expressed in all monoaminergic neurons. In the striatum, 95% of the VMAT2 binding takes place in dopaminergic neurons (Taylor et al., 2000). A schematic illustration of the different components of the striatal DA synapse is shown in Figure 5.2.

Imaging Dopaminergic Systems

The concentration of most receptor proteins in the brain is in the nanomolar range. Such low concentrations cannot be detected using magnetic resonance (MR)-based techniques. The nuclear medicine imaging techniques, positron emission tomography

(PET) and single photon emission tomography (SPECT), are ideal for this purpose, as they have a clear sensitivity advantage over MR-based techniques (Bäckman and Farde, 2005). The PET and SPECT techniques employ radioactive tracers to generate images reflecting the distribution of ligands (i.e., signal triggering molecules that bind to specific target receptors of transmitters) for specific molecules in the brain, and they can be used to study the synthesis and release of neurotransmitters and the availability of receptors (see McGuire et al., 2008 for review). PET detects rather short-lived radionuclides that decay via release of a positron, whereas SPECT detects more long-lived radionuclides that decay by release of a gamma ray.

Various ligands for imaging the different pre- and postsynaptic markers of the dopaminergic systems in the human brain have been developed (see Cropley et al., 2006; Halldin et al., 2001, for overviews). PET studies on biochemical markers for specific neurotransmission systems depend on the availability of suitable ligands that can be rapidly labeled with short-lived radionuclides such as carbon-11, which has a half-life of 20.3 minutes. An advantage of radio-labeling with carbon-11, by substitution of the naturally occurring carbon-12, is that the structure and properties of the molecule remain unchanged. When conducting a PET study, a trace amount of about 1 μg of the radioligand is injected intravenously and brain radioactivity is measured continuously for about one hour while the subject lies on a scanner table with the head fixated. The relatively long acquisition time is one reason for the excellent test-retest reproducibility, which is usually within 5% of discrepancy (Nordström et al., 1992). The binding potential (BP) is a commonly used parameter in PET research on neuroreceptor binding. This parameter represents the ratio Bmax/ Kd, where Bmax is the concentration of a protein in a brain region and Kd is the apparent in vivo affinity of the radioligand for the receptor.

The benzazepine [11C]SCH23390 was the first radioligand developed for PET visualization of the D1 receptor (Farde et al., 1987) and has since been a reference ligand for this purpose. [11C]NNC112 is a more recently developed ligand that provides a higher signal-to-noise ratio for cortical D1 receptors (Halldin et al., 1998). The most commonly used radioligand for PET examination of D2 receptors is [11C]raclopride (Farde et al., 1986). This ligand is suitable for quantification in regions with a high density of D2 receptors (i.e., the striatum). Another radioligand, [11C]FLB457, has a very high affinity for D2 receptors and is one example of ligands suitable for visualization of low-density D2 populations in the limbic system and the neocortex (Farde et al., 1997). More recently, the BP of [11C]FLB457 in the hippocampus has been found to be positively correlated with measures of episodic memory and executive control in young adults (Takahashi et al., 2006).

The L-[18F]DOPA was the first radiotracer developed for imaging of the presynaptic DA neuron (Garnett et al., 1983). PET studies with L-[18F]DOPA provide the rate constant k_3, which is assumed to serve as an index of DA synthesis. The tracer 6-[18F]fluoro-L-m-tyrosine (FMT) is another marker for quantifying presynaptic DA synthesis (Cools et al., 2008; Eberling et al., 2004; Nahmias et al., 1995). Further, different cocaine analogues have been developed for quantifying DAT BP. Of these, [123I] ß-CIT is the most widely used ligand for SPECT imaging of the DAT (Neumeyer et al., 1991). This ligand, however, also has an affinity for serotonin and noradrenaline transporters. Analogues such as [11C]ß-CIT-FE (Farde et al., 2000) and [11C] PE2I (Halldin et al., 2003) provide a more selective signal and are currently used in PET studies. In particular, [11C]PE2I is also promising for detailed examination of extrastriatal DAT populations, such as those in the midbrain. Regarding PET imaging of striatal VMAT, [11C]dihydrotetrabenazine (DTBZ) is a commonly used ligand (Frey et al., 1995).

In summary, various ligands have been developed for imaging different components of the dopaminergic systems using PET or SPECT techniques. It is currently possible to use a range of molecular imaging methods to assess striatal or extrastriatal dopamine D1 and D2 receptor binding, DAT binding, and endogenous DA synthesis rate, with some ligands being appropriate for the striatal ([11C]raclopride) and others for the extrastriatal (e.g., [11C]FLB457) components of the DA systems (see Frankle, 2007 for review). Efforts at establishing a normative molecular imaging database of DA systems in healthy individuals are emerging (Ito et al., 2008). With these methodological developments, receptor imaging technologies provide new avenues for understanding the age-related decline in pre- and postsynaptic mechanisms of DA systems and their implications for cognitive deficits in late life.

DA and Cognition

Data from animal work, clinical and pharmacological research, candidate gene association studies, and computational neuroscience all converge to demonstrate a major influence of dopaminergic modulation on a wide range of cognitive functions. Ample evidence from animal studies shows that lesions on the

DA systems at multiple sites (e.g., prefrontal cortex, nucleus accumbens, subthalamic nucleus) cause impairment in higher-order cognitive functions such as attention, memory, and inhibition (see Bäckman et al., 2006, for review). Clinical studies on patient groups with severe alterations of the DA systems (e.g., Parkinson's disease and Huntington's disease) reveal deficits in several cognitive functions such as executive functioning, episodic memory, and cognitive speed (Brown and Marsden, 1990; Brandt and Butters, 1986). Moreover, PET studies show strong relations between DA biomarkers and cognitive performance assessed outside the scanner in both Parkinson's (Bruck et al., 2005) and Huntington's (Bäckman et al., 1997) patients.

A range of association studies with candidate genes implicating dopaminergic neurotransmission provided further support for the DA-cognition link. For example, the COMT enzyme degrades DA in the prefrontal cortex (Weinshilboum et al., 1999). A common val/met polymorphism accounts for much of the enzymatic activity (val > met), resulting in less DA availability in frontal D1 receptors among val carriers (Egan et al., 2001). In executively demanding tasks (e.g., working memory, Wisconsin Card Sorting) an advantage of met carriers has been found (see Goldberg and Weinberger, 2004 for review). Relatedly, variations in the DAT gene (i.e., number of tandem repeats) are associated with DAT availability in the striatum (more repeats > fewer repeats), translating into less synaptic dopamine for persons with more repeats (Maher et al., 2002). Alleles with 9 or 10 repeats are most common (Mitchell et al., 2000). Behavioral evidence shows lower performance among 10-repeat carriers in tasks assessing speed and attention (Loo et al., 2003) as well as response inhibition (Cornish et al., 2005).

Whereas gene-association studies on the DA-cognition link build on individual differences in genetic predispositions for dopaminergic modulation, pharmacological studies intervene directly with activity in the dopaminergic systems. Pharmacological manipulations of the DA systems (i.e., increased activity through agonists or decreased activity through antagonists) have been shown to affect cognition in humans and animals alike. In general, agonist studies indicate performance benefits in cognitive tasks (e.g., working memory, speed, attention, and reinforcement learning), whereas antagonist studies show decrements in the same task domains (Halliday et al., 1994; Luciana and Collins, 1997; Pizzagalli et al., 2008; Ramaekers et al., 1999; Sawaguchi and Goldman-Rakic, 1991; Servan-Schreiber et al., 1998). However, the effects of these compounds are not entirely consistent. In particular, they tend to vary with dosage and baseline cognitive capacity (Kimberg and D'Esposito, 2003; Kimberg, D'Esposito, and Farah, 1997). These findings have been interpreted in terms of an inverted U-shaped function relating DA levels to cognitive performance (Cai and Arnsten, 1997; Cools et al., 2001; Goldman-Rakic, Muly, and Williams, 2000; Knutson and Gibbs, 2007; Li and Sikström, 2002). Evidence in favor of this account was obtained in a study that combined molecular genetics with pharmacology and brain imaging (Mattay et al., 2003). In this study, val carriers of the COMT gene (less frontal DA signaling) had to recruit more frontal tissue than met carriers to achieve the same performance level in a working-memory task, a pattern suggesting lower neural efficiency among val carriers. Under the influence of a DA agonist, however, the pattern was reversed, with the val carriers showing a more efficient frontal response and the met carriers a less efficient response. Obviously, this pattern of data provides direct support for the viability of the inverted U-shape account of DA and cognition.

In addition to these lines of empirical evidence, various computational approaches have been introduced to understand the mechanisms whereby dopaminergic modulation affects cognition (see Rolls et al., 2008 for review). These attempts range from realistic biophysical firing rate models of how D1 and D2 receptors affect the stability of working memory representations (Durstewitz, Seamans, and Sejnowksi, 2000; see also Seamans and Yang, 2004, for review) to more abstract models of dopaminergic effects on the dynamic connectivity between prefrontal cortex and basal ganglia (O'Reilly and Frank, 2006). Other models focus on DA's general computational role in affecting the signal-to-noise ratio of neuronal signal transduction (Cohen and Servan-Schreiber, 1992; Li, Lindenberger, and Sikström, 2001) or outcome-based valuation in reinforcement learning (see Montague, Hyman, and Cohen, 2004 for review).

Although the different computational approaches differ in their level of analysis and biophysical specificity, one basic assumption shared by most theories is that dopaminergic modulation influences the properties of neuronal representations of cognitive and perceptual events. For instance, a two-stage model of dopaminergic modulation of working memory aims at capturing the dynamic interactions between DA and NMDA receptors in affecting the neuronal representations of memory items in the prefrontal cortex (Durstewitz, Seamans, and Sejnowksi, 2000). Specifically, when D2 receptor modulation predominates during the first stage, the prefrontal cortex (PFC)network is supposed to be in an exploratory state with multiple weak representations. However, in a second stage, when D1 receptor modulation predominates, heightened inhibitory mechanisms weed out weaker representations, and enhance the representation of the stronger inputs (Seamans and Yang, 2004; see Figure 5.3a). This effect is nicely paralleled by results from other models that aim at explicating the computational effect of dopaminergic modulation on the signal-to-noise ratio of information processing at a more molar level (Cohen and Servan-Schreiber, 1992; Li, Lindenberger, and Sikström, 2001). As the gain parameter of a neural network's activation function is attenuated or increased to mimic deficient or excessive dopaminergic modulation, respectively, the

Figure 5–3 (**a**) A two-stage model of dopaminergic modulation of memory representations in the prefrontal cortex. Plotted are simulations of activation in PFC. Peaks denote activated states, corresponding to the sustained recurrent activity required to hold items in working memory. The left panel shows the exploration state, where D2 modulation predominates, with a net reduction in inhibition resulting in multiple weak representations. The right panel shows the representation sharpening state, where D1 modulation predominates, with a net increase in inhibition resulting strong focused representation. (Adapted with permission from Seamans and Yang, 2004, copyright Elsevier.) Dopamine modulates the signal-to-noise ratio of neural information processing and affects the (**b**) distinctiveness of memory representations (**c**) and memory span. Simulating deficient or excessive dopaminergic modulation, by respectively attenuating or increasing the gain parameter (G) of the activation function of a neural network, results in less distinctive internal representations. Less distinctive representations, in turn, result in limited memory spans. (Adapted with permission from Li and Sikström, 2002; copyright Elsevier.)

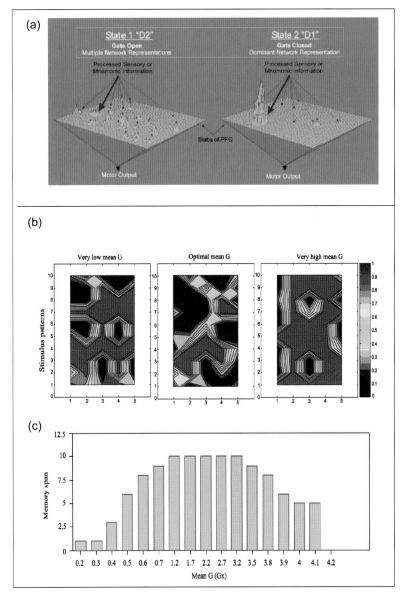

distinctiveness of stored memory items' internal presentations is reduced. Less distinctive representations result in more limited memory span, and account for the aforementioned inverted-U function relating DA signaling to working memory performance (Li and Sikström, 2002; see Figure 5.3b and 5.3c).

Changes in DA Systems during Aging

During the course of normal aging, dopaminergic systems undergo substantial decline (see Figure 5.4 and Table 5.1 for overview). Much of the work on the relationship between aging and DA neurotransmission has focused on the caudate and the putamen—two major nuclei in the striatal complex with dense dopaminergic innervation from the substantia nigra. Thus, the conditions for reliable analyses of DA biomarkers are particularly favorable in the striatum. There is strong evidence for age-related losses of pre- and postsynaptic biochemical markers of the nigrostriatal DA system. Regarding presynaptic mechanisms, both PET and SPECT studies (Erixon-Lindroth et al., 2005; Mozley et al., 2001) indicate marked age-related losses of the DAT in the striatum (see Figure 5.4a), the average decline estimated to be 5–10% per decade from early to late adulthood. For postsynaptic mechanisms, molecular imaging work reveals age-related losses of both striatal D1 (Suhara et al., 1991; Wang et al., 1998) and D2 (Antonini et al., 1993; Nordström et al., 1992) receptor densities of comparable magnitude as found for the DAT (see Figure 5.4a and 5.4b). Age-related decline in receptor density might contribute to dendritic spine loss (Lacor, 2007). An issue for future research to determine is

Table 5–1   Cross-sectional estimates of percentage of decade-by-decade decline in dopamine D2 receptor binding mechanisms in various extrastriatal regions reported in two studies.

Brain Regions	Kaassinen et al. 2000 %	Inoue et al. (2001) %
Frontal	11	14
Temporal	10	12
Parietal	–	13
Occipital		12
Hippocampus	10	12
Amygdala	7	–
Thalamus	5	5

the temporal ordering between age-related changes in DA markers and corresponding anatomical alterations, such as changes in dendritic morphology and grey-matter and white-matter integrity.

A similar downward age trajectory is seen for the mesocortical and mesolimbic dopaminergic pathways. Thus, marked age-related losses in D2 receptor binding have been observed throughout the neocortex as well as in the hippocampus, amygdala, and thalamus. Table 5.1 summarizes cross-sectional estimates of percent reduction per decade in D2 binding efficacy in various extrastriatal regions from two independent studies with Asian and Caucasian samples (Inoue et al., 2001; Kaasinen et al., 2000). Figure 5.4 (c, d)

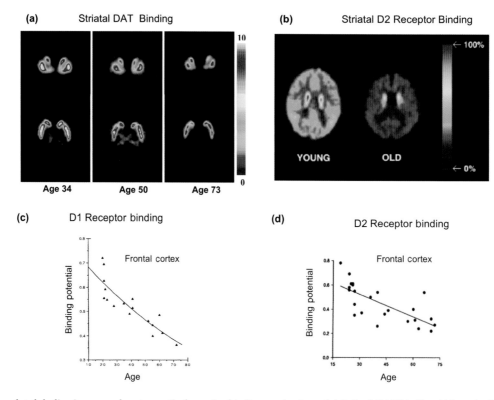

Figure 5–4   Age-related decline in pre- and postsynaptic dopamine binding mechanisms: (**a**) Striatal DAT binding (Adapted with permission from Erixon-Lindroth et al., 2005; copyright Elsevier.); (**b**) Striatal D2 receptor binding (Adapted with permission from Kaasinen and Rinne, 2002; copyright Elsevier.); (**c**) D1 receptor binding in frontal cortex (Adapted with permission from Suhara et al., 1991; copyright Springer-Verlag.); (**d**) D2 receptor binding in frontal cortex. (Adapted with permission from Kaasinen and Rinne 2002; copyright Elsevier.)

portrays a decline in D1 and D2 receptor binding in the frontal cortex across the adult lifespan.

The general age-related decline of DA systems may have multiple sources, including neuronal loss in the substantia nigra, loss of synapses, and a decrease of biomarker proteins per neuron with advancing age (see Bäckman et al., 2006 for review). There is an age-related reduction of DA cell bodies in substantia nigra, with an average loss of around 3% per decade (Fearnley and Lees, 1991). In a unique study, post-mortem cell counts in the substantia nigra were highly related to an ante-mortem imaging marker for DA synthesis capacity (Snow et al., 1993). This suggests that neuronal number influences the total synthesis rate of DA. There is also a reduction of synapses that progresses from childhood through adulthood to old age, which may reflect both adaptive, plastic processes during development and predominantly nonadaptive loss in late life (Gopnic, Meltzoff, and Kuhl, 1999). Finally, there is evidence suggesting an age-related decrease in the number of biomarker proteins per cell. Specifically, work with rodents has demonstrated substantial age-related losses in steady-state levels and synthesis of D2 receptor messenger ribonucleic acid (mRNA; Mesco et al., 1993). Relatedly, human work shows that the age-related decrease in DAT mRNA may exceed the extent of neuronal loss (De Keyser et al., 1990; Seeman et al., 1987; Severson et al., 1982). Thus, the bottom line is that age-related alterations in neuronal number, synapses, and protein concentrations may all contribute to the general decline of DA systems with advancing adult age.

The fact that similar age patterns are seen for DATs and postsynaptic markers suggests that the expression of transporters and receptors may reflect adaptation of major dopaminergic pathway components. One possibility derived from work on knockout mice is that the loss of DATs initially results in increased DA concentrations; increased DA levels may subsequently lead to down regulation of neurotransmission in postsynaptic neurons (Shinkai et al., 1997; Zhang et al., 1995).

The Correlative Triad: Dopamine, Cognition, and Aging

So far, we have reviewed evidence indicating (a) a marked negative relationship between adult age and multiple DA markers, and (b) that DA is implicated in a range of cognitive functions. There is also strong evidence of a negative relationship between adult age

and performance in tasks assessing various cognitive abilities, including executive functioning, episodic memory, and speed (see Craik and Salthouse, 2007 for reviews). The fact that performance in the very same task domains is influenced by DA functions suggests that there might be a correlative triad among adult age, DA, and cognition. In examining this triad, the key issue is whether alterations in dopaminergic neuromodulation over the lifespan can be empirically linked to age-related cognitive changes. Although relatively few studies have addressed this issue, the data pattern is strikingly consistent.

Wang et al. (1998) reported strong relationships among age, striatal D1 receptor binding, and performance in a psychomotor test. Similar results were obtained in a study examining the association between age, striatal D2 receptor binding, and finger-tapping performance (Yang et al., 2003). Although these studies reported bivariate correlations only, the results are important in that they document the correlative triad within the same groups of participants.

In a seminal study, Volkow et al. (1998) assessed striatal D2 binding in conjunction with the testing of executive and motor functioning, as well as perceptual speed across the adult life span. In line with earlier studies (Antonini et al., 1993, Nordström et al., 1992), D2 receptor binding decreased with advancing age and there were negative relationships between age and performance in cognitive tests. Of critical importance, partial correlations revealed moderate-to-strong relationships between D2 binding and cognitive and motor performance, also after controlling for chronological age. These results suggest that age-related decreases in DA function are related to deficits in both cognitive and motor functioning, and that DA activity may influence performance irrespective of age.

These findings were corroborated in a related study (Bäckman et al., 2000) that examined striatal D2 binding and cognitive performance (episodic memory and perceptual speed) in an adult life-span sample. The key finding was that statistical control of D2 binding effectively eliminated the influence of age on cognitive performance, whereas D2 binding contributed to performance over and above that of age (see Table 5.2). The results provide further evidence for the view that DA is implicated in age-related cognitive deficits as well as in cognitive functioning in general.

Other research has extended these findings to presynaptic DA markers such as DATs. Mozley et al. (2001) reported age-related reductions of DATs in the striatum along with age-related deficits in verbal episodic memory. Importantly, striatal DAT binding was

Table 5–2 Hierarchical regression analyses showing the relative influences of age and dopamine D2 receptor binding on key measures of cognitive aging. (Adapted with permission from Bäckman et al., 2000; copyright American Psychiatric Publishing.)

Regression Variable	Tests of Perceptual Speed		Tests of Episodic Memory	
	Dots	Trial Making A	Word Recognition	Face Recognition
Age First				
Age	0.52	0.34	0.13	0.27
D2 binding	0.11	0.22	0.27	0.24
Both Age and D2	0.63	0.56	0.40	0.51
D2 Binding first				
D2 binding	0.61	0.55	0.38	0.48
Age	0.02	0.01	0.02	0.03
Both D2 and Age	0.63	0.56	0.40	0.51

Table 5–3   Hierarchical regression analyses showing the relative influences of age and dopamine transport (DAT) binding on key measures of cognitive aging (presented are R2). (Adapted with permission from Erixon-Lindroth et al., 2005; copyright Elsevier.)

Regression Variable	Tests of Episodic Memory		Tests of Executive Function	
	Word Recognition	Face Recognition	Working Memory	Letter Fluency
Age First				
Age	0.31	0.28	0.40	0.15
DAT binding	0.24	0.13	0.13	0.16
Both Age and DAT	0.55	0.41	0.53	0.31
DAT Binding first				
DAT binding	0.46	0.40	0.49	0.30
Age	0.09	0.01	0.04	0.01
Both DAT and Age	0.55	0.41	0.53	0.31

strongly associated with memory performance in both younger and older adults. An age-related decrease of DAT density in the caudate and putamen was also documented by Erixon-Lindroth et al. (2005). This study revealed age-related deficits in tests of episodic memory, working memory, and word fluency, but not in a test of general knowledge. As in the Bäckman et al. (2000) study on D2 receptors, the age-related cognitive deficits were completely mediated by DAT density, although DAT density contributed to the performance variation in memory and fluency independent of age. The latter finding was substantiated by the result that DAT density also was related to performance in the age-insensitive knowledge test (Table 5.3).

Taken together, the available evidence shows that pre- and postsynaptic markers of the nigrostriatal dopamine system are strong general correlates of cognitive performance, as well as powerful mediators of the cognitive changes that occur across adulthood and old age. In light of DA's critical role in age-related cognitive deficits, a range of new research themes and paradigms has recently been proposed for furthering our understanding of the mechanisms through which the DA systems change and affect cognition during aging. In the remainder of this chapter we will highlight some of these new approaches and emerging themes, as well as delineate some outstanding issues for future research on the aging-DA-cognition link.

Emerging Themes and Novel Approaches

In terms of new themes in cognitive aging research, the issues of (a) whether the relationhip between DA and cognitive deficits is domain-general or function-specific, (b) reduction in adaptive flexibility (or plasticity) when confronted with cognitive challenges or intervention, (c) age-related increases of noise (or fluctuation) in neural and cognitive processes, and (d) changes in decision-making processes, could all be linked to age-related declines in dopaminergic modulation. With regard to new research paradigms, genomic imaging and pharmacological intervention approaches are extended to investigate the functioning of the various DA systems. Similarly, multimodal imaging approaches that combine receptor imaging and functional imaging are particularly important for understanding the dynamics of dopaminergic modulation. Below we present these new approaches in turn.

General or Specific Dopaminergic Effects on Cognitive Aging

Extant evidence seems to suggest that, during the process of aging different aspects of DA systems are similarly affected (Bäckman et al., 2006). In this regard, there is a discrepancy between human and animal research concerning the specificity of the DA-cognition relationship. Studies on aging (Bäckman et al., 2000; Erixon-Lindroth et al., 2005; Volkow et al., 1998), as well as corresponding research on patients with basal ganglia disorders (Bäckman et al., 1997; Lawrence et al., 1998), show that markers of D1, D2, and DAT binding in both the caudate and the putamen show strong-relationships to each other, as well as to cognitive performance. By contrast, dissociative patterns have been found in monkeys both with regard to receptor subtypes as well as regions in the fronto-striatal network. For example, Williams and Goldman-Rakic (1995) showed that a D1 agonist modulated working-memory fields, whereas a D2 agonist caused changes in the integration of motor and motivational capacities. Wang et al. (2004) found that D2 receptors modulated memory-guided saccades in a working-memory task, whereas D1 receptors modulated persistent memory-related activity.

To be sure, most of the studies involving primates are based on acute pharmacological challenges, whereas the human studies address interindividual variability over several decades. The possibility for adaptive regulatory mechanisms (Shinkai et al., 1997; Zhang et al., 1995) reducing the chance of finding selective effects is obviously greater in the latter case. Also, in contrast to single-cell recordings, one might question whether the measurement devices in human research (e.g., PET) are sensitive enough to detect potential differences between different DA markers regarding their role in cognitive functions. In particular, it is still difficult to apply PET imaging in a dynamic, event-related sense, which is central for deciphering functional specificities. At the same time, relatively few molecular-imaging studies have addressed the DA-cognition relationship, and the research is characterized by small sample sizes. Thus, the general failure to obtain differential relationships among brain regions as well as different biochemical markers may reflect the limited nature of the database along with low statistical power in individual studies.

Using a sample of middle-aged adults, Cervenka et al. (2008) recently examined whether D2 receptor binding in different regions within the striatal complex are selectively implicated in

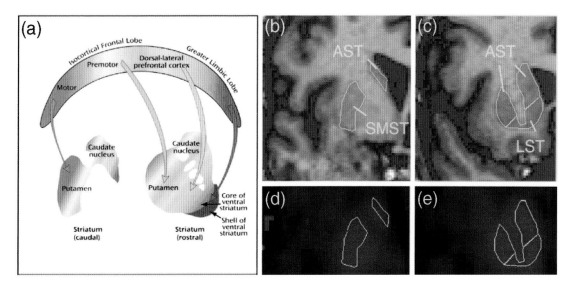

Figure 5–5 (**a**) A schematic figure of the anatomical connectivity in striatum. (**b, c**) Coronal MRI sections depicting manually drawn ROIs for striatum in one subject—posterior and anterior to the anterior commissure, respectively. Right hemisphere is showed, left side of the image is lateral. (**d, e**) Corresponding PET sections showing [11C]raclopride binding in the same subject, with ROIs superimposed. LST = limbic striatum; AST = associative striatum; and SMST = sensorimotor striatum. (Adapted with permission from Cervenka et al., 2008; copyright Elsevier.)

episodic memory, knowledge, and word fluency. They subdivided the striatum into ventral (nucleus accumbens, ventral caudate, and putamen), associative (mostly caudate, dorsal putamen), and sensorimotor (mostly putamen, dorsolateral caudate) compartments (see Figure 5.5; Alexander, DeLong, and Strick, 1986; Martinez et al., 2003; Parent and Hazrati, 1995). Of chief interest was whether D2 binding in the ventral striatum would be especially critical to episodic memory. Supportive evidence for this hypothesis comes from fMRI research showing that coactivation of ventral tegmentum, nucleus accumbens, and hippocampus strongly predicts episodic recall of reward-related items (Adcock et al., 2006; Wittmann et al., 2005). Relatedly, the BOLD signal in ventral tegmentum has been found to reflect reward probability (D'Ardenne et al., 2008). Furthermore, initial evidence from pharmacological fMRI work in humans and in rodents suggests that BOLD responses increase with drug-induced DA releases in ventral striatum and nucleus accumbens (see Knutson and Gibbs, 2007 for review).

In general, the data from Cervenka et al. (2008) were in agreement with the hypothesis: First, the relationship between ventral striatal D2 binding and episodic memory was stronger than for the other striatal compartments. Conversely, D2 binding in associative and sensorimotor striatum was more strongly related to performance in the knowledge and fluency tasks compared to ventral striatum (see Table 5.4). Thus, these findings extend the fMRI observations (Adcock et al., 2006; Wittman et al., 2005) to the

level of neuromodulation and suggest that the striatum, at least in part, may be functionally compartmentalized regarding higher-order cognition. This approach could be extended to brain regions outside the striatum in addressing several important issues. For example, could it be that age-related dopamine losses in a particular brain area (e.g., putamen) are more critical than DA losses in other areas (e.g., frontal cortex, hippocampus) for certain domains of cognitive functioning (e.g., psychomotor speed), whereas the opposite pattern holds true for other cognitive domains (e.g., working memory)? Of interest is also whether potential regional selectivity regarding the DA-cognition link remains the same or is attenuated in aging. The latter outcome would suggest dedifferentiation of the dopamine system in advanced age—a pattern that has often been found for various cognitive abilities (Chen, Myerson, and Hale, 2002; de Frias et al., 2007; Grady, 2002; Li et al., 2004; Lindenberger and Baltes, 1994).

DA Release during Cognitive Activity

Until recently, cognitive performance in molecular imaging studies linking DA functions to cognition was assessed outside the scanner; thus the biomarker (e.g., receptor densities) was related to the off-line cognitive markers (see Cropley et al., 2006 for review). There is, however, emerging evidence for the actual release of dopamine during cognitive activity. A paradigm used to address

Table 5–4 Relationship between D2 binding potential in striatal subregions and cognitive performance (presented are correlation coefficients). (Adapted with permission from Cervenka et al., 2008; copyright Elsevier.)

	Paired Associate Learning	Word Recognition	Delayed Pattern Recognition	Information	Category Fluency
Limbic	0.67	0.56	0.47	0.33	0.42
Associative	0.66	0.44	0.39	0.59	0.69
Sensorimotor	0.50	0.29	0.24	0.48	0.72

this issue involves contrasting DA binding in two conditions varying in cognitive load. DA release is inferred if the BP is lower under the high-load condition compared with the low-load condition. This is so because the binding of the ligand to receptors is supposed to compete more fiercely with endogenous DA when conditions are more cognitively challenging. For instance, an early study showed that the [11C]raclopride-labeled D2 receptor binding in the striatum is reduced when individuals played a video game that required goal-directed motor activities in comparison to the baseline condition (Koepp et al., 1998). More recently, a range of studies using similar paradigms also found reduced DA receptor binding during cognitive activities. Specifically, in young adults there is evidence for DA release in frontal cortex and hippocampus during working-memory performance (Aalto et al., 2005; see Figure 5.6), and evidence for striatal DA release during both card-sorting (Monchi, Ko, and Strafella, 2006) and sequential learning (Badgaiyan, Fischman, and Alpert, 2007).

A recent PET D2 receptor imaging study also showed that caudate BP was sensitive to the demands of cognitive control, suggesting increased endogenous DA release due to increased executive requirements (Sawamoto et al., 2008). However, this task-induced alteration of D2 binding was not observed in Parkinson patients, likely reflecting deficient striatal DA modulation in this disease.

The fact that it is possible to demonstrate DA release in young adults during cognitive activity (Aalto et al., 2005; Badgaiyan, Fischman, and Alpert, 2007; Monchi, Ko, and Strafella, 2006; Sawamoto et al., 2008) opens up the opportunity for interesting age-comparative work on this topic. We know that age-related cognitive deficits are especially pronounced in tasks that require active (executive) stimulus-processing (Craik and Salthouse, 2007). We also know that DA markers are strongly related to performance in executively demanding tasks (Bäckman et al., 2000; Erixon-Lindroth et al., 2005; Volkow et al., 1998). Given these observations, we might hypothesize that age differences observed in executively demanding tasks

partly reflect the fact that such tasks require excessive DA release to be successfully performed (Mattay et al., 2003). As a result, age-related DA losses should be particularly detrimental relative to less demanding tasks.

Karlsson et al. (2008) examined this hypothesis by measuring D1 receptor binding in young and old adults while they performed the Multi-Source Interference Task (Bush et al., 2003) compared to that while they were at rest. This task measures the ability to inhibit prepotent responses. Although age-group differences were relatively small, the young outperformed the old with regard to both accuracy and latency. In line with corresponding work on D2 receptors (Aalto et al., 2005; Monchi, Ko, and Strafella, 2006), the young adults showed less binding of the ligand to striatal D1 receptors during the interference task compared with baseline. This may reflect displacement because of competition with endogenous DA as a function of the cognitive challenge (Laruelle, 2000). The apparent increased release of DA in the young was seen in the ventral, associative, and sensorimotor compartments of the striatum. Most intriguingly, the pattern of data was very different for the old sample, which showed no differences whatsoever in D1 receptor binding between the two conditions. This null effect suggests unaltered DA release during executive performance in old adults—a less responsive neurotransmitter system in face of a cognitive challenge.

Another paradigm for examining activity-dependent DA release is cognitive intervention or training research. Animal studies show that habitual exercise increases plasticity of the dopaminergic systems. Specifically, wheel-running training in rats increased tyrosine hydroxylase mRNA expressions and reduced D2 autoreceptor mRNA in the substantia nigra, as well as increased postsynaptic D2 receptor mRNA in caudate and putamen (Foley and Fleshner, 2008). These results suggest that habitually physically active animals may have an enhanced ability to increase DA synthesis and reduce D2 autoreceptor-mediated inhibition of DA neurons in the nigra, as compared to sedentary animals. Thus far, there is no direct evidence for age-related changes in training or activity-induced DA release in humans. Combining molecular imaging with cognitive intervention, future research should examine whether these findings on activity-dependent plasticity in DA synaptic mechanisms may generalize to humans, and whether the extent of this type of plasticity is affected by aging. To this end, a recent fMRI study on the effects of cognitive training showed that an age-related deficit in task-relevant striatal activation might constrain the transfer of learning in older adults (Dahlin et al., 2008).

Several outstanding issues remain to be investigated in research on DA and cognitive activity. These include the relationship between DA release and BOLD activation in fMRI studies (Knutson and Gibbs, 2007), and how this relationship might change with advancing age. Further, behavioral studies demonstrate that, although young adults typically benefit more than old adults from cognitive training, there is still a sizable cognitive reserve capacity in aging (Hill, Bäckman, and Stigsdotter-Neely, 2000; Nyberg et al., 2003). Thus, it would be of interest to examine whether the negative findings for D_1 binding in older adults reported by Karlsson et al. (2008) are modifiable through systematic training. Relatedly, investigating training-related changes in transient neurocognitive processes that could be linked to D_2 receptors (Bilder et al., 2004), such as updating (O'Reilly, 2006), constitutes an interesting avenue for future research. How the dynamic relationship between transient (D2-related) and sustained (D1-related) DA systems (Grace et al., 2007) might change with age

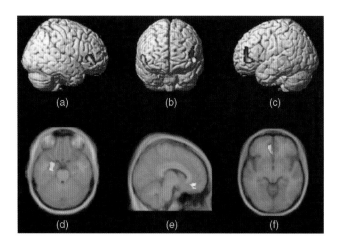

Figure 5–6 Molecular imaging findings of DA release during cognitive activity. Compared with a vigilance task, DA D2 receptor binding (with [11C]FLB 457 as the tracer) decreased during a working memory task bilaterally in the ventrolateral frontal cortex (**a–c**) and in the left medial temporal lobe (**d**). Compared with resting state baseline, both the vigilance task (**e**) and the working memory task (**f**) induced a decrease in D2 receptor binding in left ventral anterior cingulated. (Adapted with permission from Aalto et al., 2005; copyright Society of Neuroscience 2005.)

and is modulated by genetic background (e.g., COMT status; de Frias et al., 2008) will also be a key issue in cognitive DA research in the years to come.

Deficient Dopaminergic Modulation and Decreased Processing Robustness

Recent empirical evidence and theoretical models suggest that increased within-person performance fluctuations flag suboptimal neuronal information processing (see MacDonald, Nyberg, and Bäckman, 2006 for review). Empirically, higher levels of within-person behavioral variability on sensorimotor, perceptual, and cognitive tasks are often accompanied by lower mean levels of performance, and are indicative of processing alterations associated with aging or pathology (e.g., ADHD, traumatic brain injury, schizophrenia, Parkinson's disease, and dementia; see MacDonald, Nyberg, and Bäckman, 2006 for review). Within-person performance fluctuations (e.g., from trial to trial or session to session in reaction time or memory tasks) increase with advancing age for a variety of cognitive functions (Li et al., 2004), indicating decreases in processing robustness in late life. Conversely, during child development, performance fluctuations decrease as brain and cognitive functions mature (see Figure 5.7a).

It is critical to note that age-related differences in within-person fluctuations are not simply an artifact of mean-level differences, for these are routinely partialed out in the analysis of within-person variability. On a cognitive level, performance fluctuations are thought to reflect momentary lapses of attention—a failure to exert executive control (West et al., 2002). Consequently, it has been argued that the frontal lobes may be particularly crucial for maintaining stability, hence minimizing performance fluctuations (Stuss et al., 2003). The fact that patients with frontotemporal dementia show higher performance fluctuation than Alzheimer patients at the same severity level (Murtha et al., 2002) supports this contention. Furthermore, longitudinal data demonstrate that older adults who exhibit higher within-person fluctuations declined more in executive functioning over several years than their more stable counterparts (see Figure 5.7b; Lövdén, Li, Shing, and Lindenberger, 2007).

Of specific interest here is the link between dopaminergic modulation and processing fluctuation observed at the behavioral and neuronal levels. Animal studies have shown that DA receptor reductions, as observed during aging, not only slow down performance but also increase performance variability (MacRae, Spirduso, and Wilcox, 1988; Schultz et al., 1989). Prefrontal broadband noise derived from electroencephalogram (EEG) is increased in patients with schizophrenia, a condition marked by

Figure 5–7 (**a**) Lifespan age differences in processing robustness as measured by the inverse of fluctuations in cognitive reaction times. Older adults and children show less robust processing. (Adapted from Li et al., 2004 with permission; copyright Blackwell 2004.) (**b**) Individual differences in processing robustness predict 13-year longitudinal decline in executive functioning measured by the category fluency test. (Adapted from Lövdén et al., 2007 with permission; Copyright Elsevier Science 2007.)

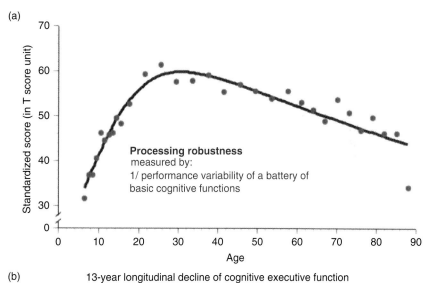

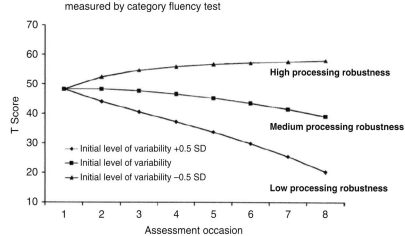

dysfunctional dopaminergic neuromodulation. A review of more recent findings concludes that those groups of individuals who exhibit high performance fluctuations are often characterized by alterations in DA functions (MacDonald, Nyberg, and Bäckman, 2006). Indeed, neurocomputational work on DA, aging, and cognition suggests that reduced DA activity increases neuronal noise and results in less distinctive internal representations of percepts of memory items, which, in turn, leads to increased performance fluctuations (Li, Lindenberger, and Sikström, 2001) and altered dynamics of interactions between extrinsic neuronal noise and perceptual noise (Li, von Oertzen, and Lindenberger, 2006).

In the first attempt to directly link DA to processing fluctuations, MacDonald et al. (in press) measured extrastriatal D2 binding in the anterior cingulate, frontal cortex, and hippocampus in a middle-aged group. Processing fluctuation was assessed in terms of within-person variability in reaction time during episodic memory retrieval and concept formation. Because the sample was relatively age-homogeneous, between-person differences in D2 binding and processing fluctuation were relatively small. Nevertheless, there were systematic negative correlations between D2 binding and processing fluctuation across all three brain regions examined (rs ranging from −.30 to −.45). Thus, these data indicate that, even within normal ranges, reduced availability of DA may result in more fluctuating behavior.

In a related vein, polymorphisms of the gene coding for catechol O-methyltransferase (COMT), which catabolizes DA in the frontal cortex, are systematically related to performance variability. As noted, relative to monozygotic carriers of the met allele of COMT, the degradation rate of DA in the synaptic cleft is about three to four times faster in monozygotic carriers of the val allele (Lotta et al., 1995), who also show higher noise levels in EEGs (Winterer et al., 2004) and fMRI (Winterer et al., 2006) brain signals during perceptual and cognitive tasks. In line with these findings, recent genomic studies with young adults show that reaction times while performing simple cognitive tasks fluctuated more in COMT val homozygotes than in met homozygotes (Stefanis et al., 2005). These studies suggest that future research could benefit from combining individual differences in genetic predispositions for DA signaling with behavioral and imaging studies to more directly examining the relationship between deficient dopaminergic modulation and reduced processing robustness in old age. In this context, the computational approach of stochastically reducing the slope of the sigmoidal activation to simulate aging-related decline in dopaminergic modulation (Li, Lindenberger, and Sikström, 2001) suggests that increased processing fluctuation may contribute to age-related decline in perceptual decision making. More specifically, as aging or individual differences in genetic polymorphisms affecting neuromodulation may lead to suboptimal gain modulation of neuronal signal-to-noise ratio (Figure Figure 5.8a), the extent of random processing fluctuation increases (Figure 5.8b). This results in less distinctive perceptual representations (Figure 5.8c). Future studies

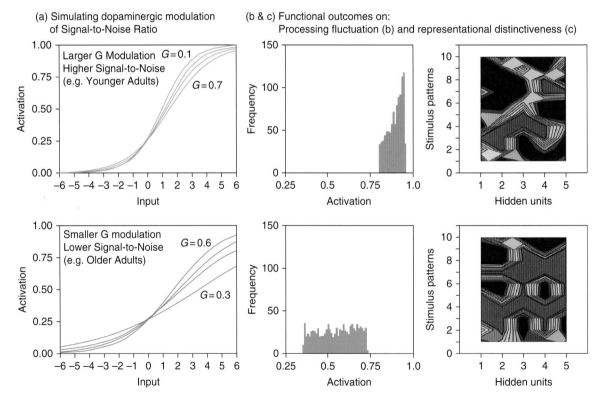

Figure 5–8 Schematic diagram relating functional effects of dopaminergic modulation of neuronal noise to processing characteristics of evidence accumulation. (**a**) The role of DA in affecting neuronal signal-to-noise ratio is modeled by the gain parameter (G) of the sigmoidal activation function (Li, Lindenberger, and Sikström, 2001; Servan-Schreiber et al., 1990). The neuronal input-response mapping functions of individuals with optimal dopaminergic modulation because of advantageous DA genotype are captured by steeper activation functions with higher G and signal-to-noise ratio. (**b**) G modulation of signal-to-noise ratio results in less random activation variability in networks simulating optimal DA modulation and greater variability in networks simulating suboptimal DA modulation. (**c**) The internal stimulus representations are more distinctive (with fewer units overlapping in representing different stimuli) in networks with optimal DA modulation than in networks with suboptimal DA modulation. (Adapted with permission from Li et al., 2001; copyright Elsevier.)

should directly examine the interactions between individual differences in DA-relevant genotypes and aging-related deficits in dopaminergic modulation on processing fluctuation and the distinctiveness of neural representations underlying perception and memory.

Dopamine, Aging, and Decision Making

During the past decade, evidence from research at neurophysiological, neuroimaging, and behavioral levels has converged on the view that perception and cognition are gradual processes of evidence accumulation amidst noisy sensory information and signal processing. According to this view, perceptual decisions (e.g., deciding whether a human face or a physical object, such as a house, was seen) are made by accumulating sensory information until a threshold is reached, at which point the decision process concludes and a motor response is elicited (Heekeren, Marrett, and Ungerleider, 2008 for review; see Figure 5.9). Moment-to-moment fluctuations in the sampling of evidence for choice options reflect noise in the sensory input as well as in the decision process. Formal sequential sampling models of sensory evidence accumulation account for memory and decision performance, and related biophysical models link ramping neuronal firing rates with rates of sensory information integration. Single-cell recording studies in monkeys, as well as human EEG and fMRI research, provide support for these models (Heekeren, Marrett, and Ungerleider, 2008).

Sequential sampling models of perceptual decision-making postulate that signal processing is inherently noisy (see Bogacz, 2007 for review). However, noise is typically treated as a primitive in these models, and the neurobiological mechanisms affecting its properties and functional consequences for cortical dynamics are left unspecified. As indicated by empirical and computational findings reviewed above (Li et al., 2001; Serven-Schreiber et al., 1990; Winterer & Weinberger, 2004), DA's noise-tuning function may affect the quality of perceptual representations, which underlie perceptual decisions.

Hence, three strands of evidence for (a) pervasive decline in dopaminergic modulation during aging, (b) DA's noise-tuning effect on perceptual decision-making, and (c) DA's influences on reward-based decision-making (see Schultz, 2006 for review) suggest a possible triadic relationship between aging, neuromodulation, and reward-based decision-making (Li et al., 2007). Currently, there is limited evidence on neurofunctional correlates of reward-based decision-making in the context of aging. Using a probabilistic object reversal task, Mell et al. (2005) found deficits in instrumental learning in older adults. Compared to younger adults, older adults collected fewer reward points throughout the task and needed more trials to learn the stimulus-response associations. In a subsequent fMRI study, the poor behavioral performance in older adults was linked to reduced brain activation in ventral striatum (Marschner et al., 2005; Mell et al., 2005). Relatedly, Larkin et al. (2007) found that younger and older adults differed in both self-reported and neural responsiveness to anticipated monetary gains

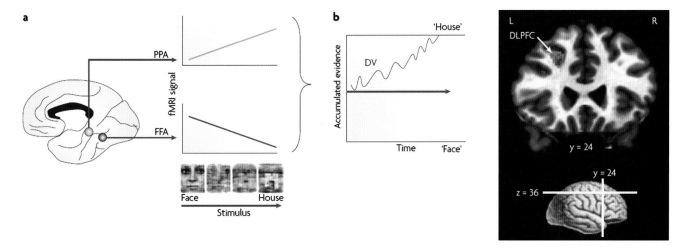

Figure 5–9 Representation of sensory evidence in low-level sensory regions and perceptual decision-making in the posterior dorsal lateral prefrontal cortex. (**a**) Schematic diagram of the representation of sensory evidence in category-selective brain regions. When participants had to decide whether an image was a face or a house, there was a greater response in face-selective regions (the fusiform face area (FFA)—red line) to clear images of faces than to degraded images of faces. In addition, house-selective brain regions (the parahippocampal place area (PPA)) showed a greater response to clear images of houses than to degraded images of houses (blue line). (**b**) The comparison of sensory evidence in higher-level brain regions. Neurophysiological data, as well as modeling studies, suggest that a decision variable is computed by comparing the output of pools of selectively tuned lower-level sensory neurons. In this example, the output of category-specific brain regions (the FFA and the PPA) is integrated over time. The decision variable (DV) drifts between the two boundaries and once one of them has crossed, the corresponding decision is made (here, 'house'). (Adapted from Heekeren, Marrett, and Ungerleider, 2008, with permission; copyright Nature Publishing Group 2008.)

and losses. Specifically, older adults exhibited intact striatal and insular activation during gain anticipation, but reduced activation during loss anticipation. Although these studies did not directly examine the impact of aging-related decline in dopaminergic modulation in affecting reward-based decision-making, DA's involvement can be inferred given the rich dopaminergic innervation in the striatum and related regions relevant to reward processing.

DA-relevant Genes and Cognition: Magnified Effects in Old Age

Genetic polymorphisms relevant for DA synthesis, catabolism, presynaptic and postsynaptic effects have been identified and their functional consequences are currently under intense investigation (see Green, Munafo, and DeYoung, 2008; Mattay et al., 2008; Meyer-Lindenberg and Weinberger, 2006 for reviews). As noted in previous sections, allelic variations in COMT genotype have been linked to cognitive performance, with met carriers (higher dopamine availability in PFC) outperforming val carriers (lower DA availability in PFC; see Goldberg and Weinberger, 2004 for review). In studies with younger adults, however, effect sizes are small and findings are inconsistent (see Barnett et al., 2007 for meta-analytic evidence). Relatively few studies have assessed the effects of the COMT genotype on cognition in aging. The available evidence, however, suggests a more robust advantage of met carriers in late adulthood (de Frias et al., 2004, 2005; Harris et al., 2005; O'Hara et al., 2006; Starr et al., 2007). A magnification of gene- related COMT effects on cognitive performance should, in fact, be expected on the basis of the inverted U-shaped function relating DA levels to cognition (Cai and Arnsten, 1997; Li, Lindenberger, and Sikström, 2001; Li and Sikström, 2002). Specifically, as aging results in marked DA losses, the inverted U-shaped curve implies that the cognitive difference between older met and val carriers of the COMT gene is greater than that between younger met and val carriers (Lindenberger et al., 2008; Figure 5.10).

Nagel et al. (2008) tested this hypothesis directly in a recent large-scale study. Using two measures that draw heavily on frontal

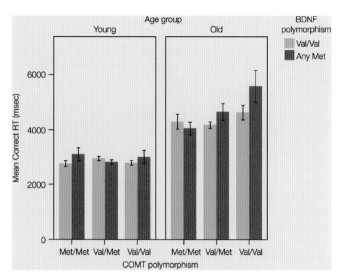

Figure 5–11 Mean reaction for correct WCST responses as a function of age, COMT, and BDNF genotype. The age x COMT interaction accounted for 4.1%, and the age x COMT x BDNF interaction for 3.1 % of the variance (Adapted with permission from Nagel et al., 2008; copyright Frontiers of Human Neurosciences.)

integrity, the Wisconsin Card Sorting Test (WCST), and a test of spatial working memory, Nagel et al. (2008) demonstrated COMT genotype x age interactions in the expected direction: Whereas differences between met and val carriers were small or nonexistent in the young sample, a met advantage was observed in the old sample. Furthermore, the effect of COMT genotype not only interacted with age but also with the gene coding for brain-derived neurotrophic factor (BDNF). Older adults carrying two COMT Val alleles and at least one BDNF Met allele took particularly long time to respond, resulting in an age x gene x gene interaction (see Figure 5.11). Thus, although genetic status does not change across adulthood, the functional effects of genotype variation may change because of age-related constraints on brain resources, such as deficits in various aspects of DA modulation (Lindenberger et al., 2008).

In addition to the COMT gene, effects of genes affecting the DAT, as well as different receptors (e.g., DRD1, DRD2, and DARPP-32) on cognitive aging at the brain and behavioral levels, are interesting avenues for further investigation of the mechanisms through which deficits in different components of the DA systems affect cognitive aging (Deary et al., 2004; Mattay et al., 2008).

Pharmacological Intervention

In young adults, DA agonists typically enhance performance (Luciana and Collins, 1997), whereas DA antagonists impair performance (Ramaekers et al., 1999) across a variety of cognitive tasks. Furthermore, consistent with the inverted U-shaped function, the effects of DA on cognition and brain activity seem to be modified by COMT genotype, such that val carriers (lower baseline DA levels) show a more efficient frontal response, whereas met carriers (higher baseline DA levels) show a less efficient frontal response following administration of a DA agonist (Mattay et al., 2003). These patterns of data open up for a series of interesting research questions regarding the role of DA

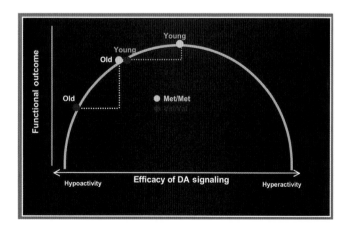

Figure 5–10 An inverted U-shaped function linking the strength of frontal DA signaling in early vs. late adulthood to performance. The shape of the curve implies that the difference in performance between older met and val carriers is greater than the difference between younger met and val carriers of the COMT gene. (Adapted with permission from Nagel et al., 2008; copyright Frontiers of Human Neurosciences.)

in cognitive aging. Preliminary answers are emerging for some of these questions.

First, we may ask whether dopamine antagonists, in addition to lowering performance, might lead to a pattern of brain activation during cognitive performance (e.g., working memory) in young adults that resembles that which is typically exhibited by older adults under placebo conditions (e.g., more diffuse activation). In an fMRI study, Fischer et al. (2008) addressed this issue by examining whether brain activation patterns in young adults under the influence of a dopaminergic antagonist during a spatial working memory task would resemble those of older adults under normal conditions. Three groups were studied: young-placebo (YP), young-antagonist (YA), and old-placebo (OP). Two initial findings from this study provide support for this assumption. First, the YP group showed greater activity in task-relevant frontal and parietal regions than the YA and OP groups. Second, the two latter groups showed more widespread activity in regions associated with expenditure of effort to cope with the task demands (e.g., anterior cingulate cortex, cerebellum). These preliminary findings may reflect the fact that depletion of DA (whether ontogenetically or pharmacologically) decreases the signal-to-noise ratio in relevant networks, resulting in lowered neural efficiency.

We may also ask whether a dopamine agonist would alter the brain activation patterns of older people in the opposite direction (i.e., more specific and associated with better performance). This research issue may profit from considering COMT gene-related differences in DA signaling. On the basis of the inverted U-shaped relationship between DA levels and cognitive/brain function, older val carriers may be expected to exhibit the largest cognitive improvement and the most pronounced increase in neural efficiency from a DA agonist. Young val carriers and older met carriers may also show some improvement, whereas young met carriers may deteriorate, because their initially high dopamine levels lead to suboptimally high dopamine levels in conjunction with a dopamine agonist (cf. Mattay et al., 2003). Evidence that speaks to these issues is on its way.

Methodological Fusion: Multimodal Imaging

Research on neuromodulation of cognition and how this link is affected by aging has produced many exciting findings, with new possibilities for methodological fusion. Molecular imaging techniques are suitable means for investigating pre- and postsynaptic DA system mechanisms, whereas functional neuroimaging techniques provide evidence on neural circuitries engaged during cognitive processing. Further, more than half of the genes in the human genome are expressed in the brain (Hariri and

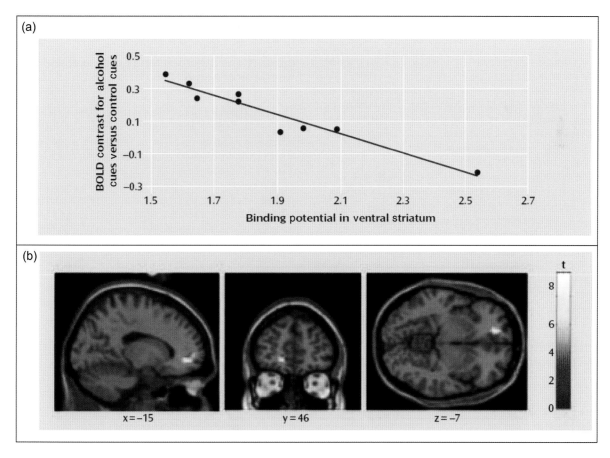

Figure 5–12   Findings from a multimodal imaging study of the dopaminergic modulation of addiction. Panels (**a**) and (**b**) show a scatterplot and the localization, respectively, of the correlation between D2 receptor binding potential in ventral striatum and functional brain activation elicited by alcohol-associated stimuli, beyond the activation produced by abstract and neutral control stimuli in the left medial prefrontal cortex of the alcoholics. (Adapted with permission from Heinz et al., 2004; copyright American Psychiatric Publishing.)

Weinberger, 2003; Meyer-Lindenberg and Weinberger, 2006). Thus, multimodal imaging approaches combining molecular imaging and functional imaging can be further augmented with candidate gene association research to study age-related differences in dopaminergic modulation of cognition. By collecting PET-based data on pre- or postsynaptic mechanisms of the DA systems and functional imaging data during cognitive activity on the same individuals, age-related differences in the relationship between neurotransmission and functional brain activation can be more directly investigated.

Multimodal imaging approaches have been applied in the context of psychiatric research. For instance, by combining PET imaging of D2 receptors (with the benzamide radioligand [^{18}F]DMFP) and fMRI of alcohol cue-related brain activity, Heinz et al. (2004) showed that D2 BP in the nucleus accumbens and ventral striatum is correlated both with the behavioral measures of alcohol craving and functional brain activation elicited by alcohol cues in the medial prefrontal cortex (see Figure 5.12). More recently, Meyer-Lindenberg et al. (2007) combined individual differences in genetic polymorphism (DARPP-32) affecting D1 receptors in striatum with structural MR and fMRI, and showed that the DARPP-32 gene affects striatal volume and functional activation, as well as connectivity to the prefrontal cortex in schizophrenic patients.

Outside the context of clinical research, Schott et al. (in press) used PET imaging of D2 receptors (with [11C]raclopride) and fMRI to examine the relationship between DA release in ventral striatum and reward-related functional brain activity in the same brain region. Consistent with the view that DA agonism affects the BOLD signal (Knutson and Gibbs, 2007), Schott et al. (in press) observed a strong relationship between striatal DA release and the magnitude of the BOLD response.

In another recent study in a group of middle-aged and older adults, Landau et al. (2008) found that a PET marker of DA synthesis capacity was related to load-dependent PFC activation during a working-memory task, corroborating the point that dopaminergic neurotransmission is related to PFC-related functions. Extending the DA-BOLD relationship to the domain of episodic memory, Nyberg et al. (2008) showed a positive association between striatal D2 binding and BOLD activation in the lateral prefrontal cortex during a long-term memory updating task in a sample of healthy older adults (Nyberg et al., 2008). How the relationship between PET-derived indicators of DA activity and functional brain activation might change over the life course, and the extent to which these changes are modulated by other age-associated neurochemical changes and genetic background, constitute key questions for future research.

Interactions Between DA and Other Transmitters and Epistasis Between DA-related Genes

In addition to the dopaminergic systems, future theoretical and empirical work should consider other transmitter systems, such as the glutamatergic system. NMDA receptors interact with DA in regulating PFC-related cognitive functions (see Castner and Williams, 2007 for review) and there is also recent evidence that the COMT polymorphism and the glutamate receptor 3 gene (GRM3) interact in affecting working memory functions in the PFC (Tan et al., 2007). Delineating the interactions between different

transmitter systems would require investigations that encompass multiple genes linked to multiple transmitter systems. The degree to which these interactions change across adulthood is a major issue in future research in the cognitive neuroscience of aging.

Computational theories may be helpful in exploring the complex interactions between multiple systems. For instance, some aspects of the interactions between NMDA and DA receptors have been modeled in a two-state model dopaminergic modulation of neuronal representations in the PFC (Durstewitz, Seamans and Sejnowksi, 2000), where D1 receptor modulation results in long-lasting NMDA currents and increased inhibition that sharpens memory representations. On this basis, predictions of the interactions between DA and NMDA in affecting age differences in working memory functions can be mapped onto individual differences in genotype profiles with respect to, for example, D1, D2, and NMDA receptors. Specifically, individuals with similar D2 and NMDA receptor genotypes who differ in D1 receptor type may express different brain functional and behavioral patterns with respect to the exploration and filtering states of working memory processing, and these differences may increase with advancing age.

In addition to DA's interactions with other transmitters, the different components of DA modulation (e.g., synthesis, presynaptic and postsynaptic mechanisms) also influence each other in affecting cognitive functioning. Recent findings indicate that the COMT and DAT genes interact with each other in affecting hippocampal memory functions (Bertolino et al., 2008) and reward processing (Yacubian et al., 2007); the extent to which these interactions change during the aging process remains unknown.

Interactions Between Neurochemical and Anatomical Aging

The general decline of DA systems with advancing adult age, which commences in early adulthood and comprises declines in receptors may affect dendritic loss (Lacor, 2007) and trigger or accentuate other physiological changes in the aging brain, such as grey matter loss, by compromising the functional integrity of subcortical-cortical connections. Consistent with this hypothesized trajectory of age-related brain changes, evidence suggests that alterations in various DA biomarkers may have an earlier onset and progress more rapidly across the lifespan compared to changes in gray or white matter (Bäckman et al., 2000; Raz et al., 2000). The temporal relation between changes in transmitter systems and anatomical alterations of the aging process could be directly addressed by longitudinal studies combining MR-based measures of regional volumes and structural connectivity with PET-based measures of transmitter availability.

Concluding Remarks

Fifty years after the discovery of DA as a neurotransmitter, much is now known about its critical involvement in a wide range of cognitive functions. Theoretical and recent empirical evidence converge to suggest that DA's influence on various cognitive functions (e.g., working memory, reward processing, and processing robustness) may be traced back to its basic role in affecting neural signal transduction (Girault and Greengard, 2004), such as by modulating the signal-to-noise ratio of neural gain function (Cohen and Servan-Schreiber, 1992; Li, Lindenberger, and

Sikström, 2001). Furthermore, much is also known about how the different DA components decline during usual and pathological aging. With recent methodological advances in molecular imaging, various components of the DA systems can now also be scrutinized in great detail.

Capitalizing on these developments, research on dopaminergic modulation of human cognitive aging is currently in an unprecedented exciting phase, empowered with genomic, molecular, and functional brain-imaging technologies. Age-comparative studies combining genomic approaches with multimodal imaging will be able to investigate the effects of aging on the DA-cognition association at multiple levels, by cross-linking genetic influences on the various components of the DA systems with measures of receptor binding efficacy and functional brain activity. In addition, given that the DA systems are not acting in isolation in affecting brain and cognitive processes, future research should also systematically investigate the interactions between DA and other transmitters, for instance, serotonin, glutamate, and gamma-aminobutyric acid (GABA), that are relevant to aging and cognition. In addition to working memory, the most commonly investigated DA modulated cognitive function, there is emerging interest in the influences of DA modulation on: (a) the robustness of the aging cognitive system, (b) aging-related limits in cognitive plasticity (e.g., altered transient response to cognitive challenges or reduced long-term enhancement from cognitive intervention), and (c) aging-related differences in reward-based decision-making subserving goal-directed behavior. In conclusion, by combining new methodologies that allow the integration of DA modulation of aging and cognition at various levels with the broadening of investigated phenomena, the perspectives for future research on DA modulation of cognitive aging will be both deepened and widened.

References

Aalto, S., Brück, A., Laine, M., Någren, K., and Rinne, J. O. (2005). Frontal and temporal dopamine release during working memory and attention tasks in healthy humans: A PET study using the high-affinity dopamine D_2 receptor ligand [11C] FLB 457. *Journal of Neuroscience*, 25: 2471–2477.

Adcock, R. A., Thangavel, A., Whitfield-Gabrieli, S., Knutson, B., and Gabrieli, J. D. E. (2006). Reward-motivated learning: Mesolimbic activation precedes memory formation. *Neuron*, 50: 507–517.

Alexander, G. E., DeLong, M. R., and Strick, P. L. (1986). Parallel organization of functionally segregated circuits linking basal ganglia and cortex. *Annual Review of Neuroscience*, 9: 357–381.

Antonini, A., Leenders, K. L., Reist, H., Thomann, R., Beer, H.-F., and Locher, J. (1993). Effect of age on D2 dopamine receptors in normal human brain measured by positron emission tomography and [11C] raclopride. *Archives of Neurology*, 50: 474–480.

Bäckman, L. and Farde, L. (2005). The role of dopamine functions in cognitive aging. In R. Cabeza, L. Nyberg, and D. C. Park (eds), *Cognitive Neuroscience of Aging: Linking Cognitive and Cerebral Aging* (pp. 58–84). New York: Oxford University Press.

Bäckman, L., Ginovart, N., Dixon, R. A., Robins Wahlin, T. B., Wahlin, Å., Halldin, C., and Farde, L. (2000). Age-related cognitive deficits mediated by changes in the striatal dopamine system. *American Journal of Psychiatry*, 157: 635–637.

Bäckman, L., Nyberg, L., Lindenberger, U., Li, S.-C., and Farde, L. (2006). The correlative triad among aging, dopamine, and cognition: Current status and future prospects. *Neuroscience and Biobehavioral Reviews*, 30: 791–807.

Bäckman, L., Robins-Wahlin, T.-B., Lundin, A., Ginovart, N., and Farde, L. (1997). Cognitive deficits in Huntington's disease are predicted by dopaminergic PET markers and brain volumes. *Brain*, 120: 2207–2217.

Badgaiyan, R. D., Fischman, A. J., and Alpert, N. M. (2007). Striatal dopamine release in sequential learning. *NeuroImage*, 38: 549–556.

Barnett, J. H., Jones, P. B., Robbins, T. W., and Müller, U. (2007). Effects of the catechol-O-methyltransferase Val/158Met polymorphism on executive function: A meta-analysis of the Wisconsin Card Sorting in schizophrenia and healthy controls. *Molecular Psychiatry*, 12: 502–509.

Bertolino, A., Giorgio, D. A., Blasi, G., Sambataro, F., Caforio, G., Sinibaldi, L. et al. (2008). Epistasis between dopamine regulating genes identifies a nonlinear response of the human hippocampus during memory tasks. *Biological Psychiatry*, 64: 226–234.

Bilder, R. M., Volavka, J., Lachman, H. M., and Grace, A. A. (2004). The catechol-O-methyltransferase polymorphism: Relations to the tonic-phasic dopamine hypothesis and neuropsychiatric disorders. *Neuropsychopharmacology*, 29: 1943–1961.

Björklund, A. and Dunnett, S. B. (2007). Dopamine neuron systems in the brain: An update. *Trends in Neuroscience*, 30: 194–202.

Bogacz, R. (2007) Optimal decision-making theories: Linking neurobiology with behaviour. *Trends Cognitive Science*, 11: 118–125.

Brandt, J. and Butters, N. (1986). The neuropsychology of Huntington's disease. *Trends in Neuroscience*, 9: 118–120.

Brown, R. G. and Marsden, C. D. (1990). Cognitive function in Parkinson's disease: From description to theory. *Trends in Neuroscience*, 13: 21–29.

Brown, R. M. and Goldman, P. S. (1977). Catecholamines in neocortex of Rhesus monkey: Regional distribution and ontogenetic development. *Brain Research*, 124, 576–580.

Bruck, A., Aalto, S., Nurmi, E., Bergman, H. Rinne, J. O. (2005). Cortical 6-%F18&fluoro-L-dopa uptake and frontal cognitive functions in early Parkinson's disease. *Neurobiology of Aging*, 26: 891–898.

Bush, G., Shin, L. M., Holmes, J., Rosen, B. R., and Vogt, B. A. (2003). The Multi-Source Interference Task: Validation study with fMRI in individual subjects. *Molecular Psychiatry*, 8: 60–70.

Cabeza, R., Nyberg, L., and Park, D. (2005). *Cognitive Neuroscience of Aging.* New York: Oxford University Press.

Cai, J. X. and Arnsten, A. F. (1997). Dose-dependent effects of the dopamine receptor agonists A77636 and SKF81297 on spatial working memory in aged monkeys. *Journal of Pharmacology and Experimental Therapeutics*, 283: 183–189.

Carlsson, A. (1975). Drugs acting through dopamine release. *Pharmacological Therapy*, 1; 401–405.

Castner, S. A. and Williams, G. (2007). Tuning the engine of cognition: A focus on NMDA/D1 receptor interactions in prefrontal cortex. *Brain and Cognition*, 63: 94–122.

Cervenka, S., Bäckman, L., Cselényi, Z., Halldin, C., and Farde, L. (2008). Associations between dopamine D2-recptor binding and cognitive performance indicate functional compartmentalization of the human striatum. *NeuroImage*, 40: 1287–1295.

Chen, J., Myerson, J., and Hale, S. (2002). Age-related dedifferentiation of visuospatial abilities. *Neuropsychologia*, 40: 2050–2056.

Chen, M. K., Kuwabara, H., Zhou, Y., Adams, R. J., Brasic, J. R., McGlothan, J. L. et al. (2008). VMAT2 and dopamine neuron loss in a primate model of Parkinson's disease. *Journal of Neurochemistry*, 105: 78–90.

Cohen, J. D. and Servan-Schreiber, D. (1992). Context, cortex, and dopamine: A connectionist approach to behavior and biology in schizophrenia. *Psychological Review*, 99: 45–77.

Cools, R., Braker, R. A., Sahakian, B. J., and Robbins, T. W. (2001). Enhanced or impaired cognitive function in Parkinson's disease as a function of dopaminergic medication and task demands. *Cerebral Cortex*, 11: 1136–1143.

Cools, R., Gibbs, S. E., Miyakawa, A., Jagust, W., and D'Esposito, M. (2008). Working memory capacity predicts dopamine synthesis capacity in the human striatum. *Journal of Neuroscience*, 28: 1208–1212.

Cornish, K. M., Manly, T., Savage, R., Swanson, J., Morisano, D., Butler, N., Grant, C., Cross, G., Bentley, L., and Hollis, C. P. (2005). Association of the dopamine transporter (DAT1) 10/10-repeat genotype with ADHD symptoms and response inhibition in a general population sample. *Molecular Psychiatry*, 10: 686–698.

Craik, F. I. M. and Salthouse, T. (2007). *The Handbook of Aging and Cognition.* New York : Psychological Press.

Cropley, V. L., Fujita, M., Innis, R. B., and Nathan, P. J. (2006). Molecular imaging of the dopaminergic system and its association with human cognitive function. *Biological Psychiatry* 59: 898–907.

Dahlin, E., Neely Stigsdotter, A., Larsson, A., Bäckman, L., and Nyberg, L. (2008). Transfer of learning after updating training mediated by the striatum. *Science*, 320: 1510–1512.

D'Ardenne, K., McClure, S. M., Nystrom, L. E., and Cohen, J. D. (2008). Bold responses reflecting dopaminergic signals in the human ventral tegmental area. *Science*, 318: 1264–1267.

Deary, I. J., Wright, A. F., Harris, S. E. Whalley, L. J., and Starr, J. M. (2004). Searching for genetic influences on normal cognitive aging. *Trends in Cognitive Sciences*, 8: 178–184.

de Frias, C. M., Annerbrink, K., Westberg, L., Eriksson, E., Adolfsson, R., and Nilsson L.-G. (2004). COMT gene polymorphism is associated with declarative memory in adulthood and old age. *Behavior Genetics*, 34: 533–539.

de Frias, C. M., Annerbrink, K., Westberg, L., Eriksson, E., Adolfsson, R., Nilsson, L.-G. (2005). Catechol O-methyltransferase Val^{158}Met polymorphism is associated with cognitive performance in nondemented adults. *Journal of Cognitive Neuroscience*, 17: 1018–1025.

de Frias, C. M., Lövdén, M., Lindenberger, U., and Nilsson, L.-G. (2007). Revisiting the dedifefrentiation hypothesis with longitudinal multi-cohort data. *Intelligence*, 35: 381–392.

de Frias, C. M., Marklund, P., Eriksson, E., Larsson, A., Öman, L., Annerbrink, L. et al. (2008). *Influence of COMT Gene Polymorphism on fMRI-Assessed Sustained and Transient Activity during a Working Memory Task*. Manuscript submitted for publication.

De Keyser, J., De Backer, J. P., Vauquelin, G., and Ebinger, G. (1990). The effect of aging on the D1 dopamine receptors in human frontal cortex. *Brain Research*, 528, 308–310.

Durstewitz, D., Seamans, J. K., and Sejnowksi, T. J. (2000). Dopamine-mediated stablization of delay-period activity in network model of prefrontal cortex. *Journal of Neurophysiology*, 93: 1733–1750.

Eberling, J. L., Pivirotto, P., Bringas, J., and Bankiewicz, K. S. (2004). Comparison of two methods for the analysis of [18F]-6-fluoro-L-*m*-tyrosine PET dopamineta. *NeuroImage*, 23: 358–363.

Egan, M. F., Goldberg, T. E., Kolachana, B. S., Callicott, J. H., Mazzanti, C. M., Straub, R. E. et al. (2001). Effect of COMT Val108/158Met genotype on frontal lobe function and risk for schizophrenia. *Proceedings of the National Academy of Sciences of the USA*, 98: 6917–6922.

Erixon-Lindroth, N., Farde, L., Robins Wahlin, T. B., Sovago, J., Halldin, C., and Bäckman, L. (2005). The role of the striatal dopamine transporter in cognitive aging. *Psychiatry Research: Neuroimaging*, 138: 1–12.

Farde, L., Ginovart, N., Halldin, C., Chou, Y., Olsson, H., and Swahn, C. (2000). A PET-study of [11C]b-CIT-FE binding to the dopamine transporter in the monkey and human brain. *International Journal of Clinical Neuropsychopharmacology*, 3: 203–214.

Farde, L., Hall, H., Ehrin, E., and Sedvall, G. (1986). Quantitative analysis of D2 dopamine receptor binding in the living human brain by PET. *Science*, 231: 258–261.

Farde, L., Halldin, C., Stone-Elander, S., and Sedvall, G. (1987). PET analysis of human dopamine receptor subtypes using 11C-SCH 23390 and 11C-raclopride. *Psychopharmacology*, 92: 278–284.

Farde, L., Suhara, T., Nyberg, S., Karlsson, P., Nakashima, Y., Hietala, J. et al. (1997). A PET-study of [11C]FLB 457 binding to extrastriatal D2-dopamine receptors in healthy subjects and antipsychotic drug treated patients. *Psychopharmacology*, 133: 396–404.

Fearnley, J. M. and Lees, A. J. (1991). Aging and Parkinsońs disease: Substantia nigra regional selectivity. *Brain*, 114: 2283–2301.

Fischer, H., Nyberg, L., Karlsson, P., Farde, L., Karlsson, S., MacDonald, S. W. S. et al. (2008). *Simulating Cognitive Aging: Effects of a Dopaminergic Antagonist on Brain Activation Patterns in Young Adults*. Manuscript submitted.

Foley, T. E. and Fleshner, M. (2008). Neuroplasticity of dopamine circuits after exercise: Implications for central fatigue. *Neuromolecular Medicine*, 10: 67–80.

Frankle, W. G. (2007). Neuroreceptor imaging studies in schizophrenia. *Harvard Review of Psychiatry*, 15: 213–232.

Frey, K. A., Vander Borght, T. M., Killbourn, J. N., DaSilva, J. E., Carey, J. E., and Kuhl, D. E. (1995). In vivo imaging of the brain vesicular monoamine transporter. *Journal Nuclear Medicine*, 36: 2252–2260.

Garnett, E. S., Firnau, G., and Nahmias, C. (1983). Dopamine visualized in the basal ganglia of living man. *Nature*, 305: 137–138.

Gaspar, P., Berger, B., Febvret, A., Vigny, A., and Henry, J. P. (1989). Catecholamine innervation of the human cerebral cortex as revealed by comparative immunohistochemistry of tyroxine-hydroxylase and dopamine-beta-hydroxylase. *Journal of Comparative Neurology*, 279: 249–271.

Girault. J. A. and Greengard, P. (2004). The neurobiology of dopamine signaling. *Archives of Neurology*, 61: 641–644.

Giros, B., El Mestikawy, S., Godinot, N., Zheng, K. Q., Han, H., Yangfeng, T. et al. (1992). Cloning, pharmacological characterization, and chromosome assignment of the human dopamine transporter. *Molecular Pharmacology*, 3: 383–390.

Giros, B., Jaber, M., Jones, S. R., Wightman, R. M., and Caron, M. G. (1996). Hyperlocomotion and indifference to cocaine and amphetamine in mice lacking the dopamine transporter. *Nature*, 379: 606–612.

Goldberg, T. E. and Weinberger, D. R. (2004). Genes and the parsing of cognitive processes. *Trends in Cognitive Sciences*, 8: 325–335.

Goldman-Rakic, P. S., Muly, E. C., and Williams, G. V. (2000). D1 receptors in prefrontal cells and circuits. *Brain Research Review*, 31: 295–301.

Gopnic, A., Meltzoff, A., and Kuhl, P. (1999). *The Scientist in the Crib: What Early Learning Tells Us About the Mind*. New York: HarperCollins.

Grace, A. A., Floresco, S. B., Goto, Y., and Lodge, D. J. (2007). Regulation of firing of dopaminergic neurons and control of gioal-directed behaviors. *Trends in Neurosciences*, 30: 220–227.

Grady, C. L. (2002). Age-related differences in face processing: A meta-analysis of three functional neuroimaging experiments. *Canadian Journal of Experimental Psychology*, 56: 208–220.

Green, A. E., Munafo, M. R., DeYoung, C. G. (2008). Using genetic data in cognitive neuroscience: from growing pains to genuine insights. *Nature Reviews Neuroscience*, 9: 710–720.

Hall, H., Sedvall, G., Magnusson, O., Kopp, J., Halldin, C., and Farde, L. (1994). Distribution of D1- and D2-dopamine receptors and dopamine and its metabolites in the human brain. *Neuropsychopharmacology*, 11: 245–256.

Halldin, C., Erixon-Lindroth, N., Pauli, S., Chou, Y. H., Okubo, Y. Karlsson, P. et al. (2003). [11C]PE2I: A highly selective radioligand for PET examination of the dopamine transporter in monkey and human brain. *European Journal of Nuclear Medicine*, 30: 1220–1230.

Halldin, C., Foged, C., Karlsson, P., Swahn, C.-G., Sedvall, G., and Farde, L. (1998). [11C]NNC 112: A radioligand for PET examination of striatal and extrastriatal D1-dopamine receptors. *Journal of Nuclear Medicine*, 39: 2061–2068.

Halldin, C., Gulyas, B., Langer, O., and Farde, L. (2001). Brain radioligands – State of the art and new trends. *Quarterly Journal of Nuclear Medicine*, 45: 139–152.

Halliday, R., Naylor, H., Brandeis, D., Callaway, E., Yano, L., and Herzig, K. (1994). The effect of d-amphetamine, clonidine, and yohimbine on human information processing. *Psychophysiology*, 31: 331–337.

Hariri, A. R. and Weinberger, D. R. (2003). Imaging genomics. *British Medical Bulletin*, 65: 259–270.

Harris, S. E., Wright, A. F., Hayward, C., Starr, J. M., Whalley, L. J., and Deary, I. J. (2005). The functional COMT polymorphism, Val158Met, is associated with logical memory and the personality trait intellect/imagination in a cohort of healthy 79 year olds. *Neuroscience Letters*, 385: 1–6.

Heekeren, H. R., Marrett, S., and Ungerleider, L. G. (2008) The neural systems that mediate human perceptual decision making. *Nature Reviews Neuroscience*, 9: 467–479.

Heinz, A., Siessmeier, T., Wrase, J., Hermann, D., Grusser, S. M. Flor, H. et al. (2004). Correlation between dopamine D-2 receptors in the ventral striatum and central processing of alcohol cues and craving. *American Journal of Psychiatry*, 161: 1783–1789.

Hill, R. D., Bäckman, L., and Stigsdotter-Neely, A. (eds). (2000). *Cognitive Rehabilitation in Old Age*. New York: Oxford University Press.

Inoue, M., Suhara, T., Sudo, Y., Okubo, Y., Yasuno, F. , Kishimoto, T. et al. (2001). Age-related reduction of extrastriatal dopamine D2 receptor measured by PET. *Life Sciences*, 69: 1079–1084.

Ito, H., Takahashi, H., Arakawa, R., Takano, H., and Suhara, T. (2008). Normal database of dopaminergic neurotransmission system in human brain measured by positron emission tomography. *NeuroImage*, 39: 555–565.

Jaber, M., Jones, S., Giros, B., and Caron, M. G. (1997). The dopamine transporter: A crucial component regulating dopamine transmission. *Movement Disorders*, 12, 629–633.

Jones, S. R., Gainetdinov, R. R., Jaber, M., Giros, B., Wightman, R. M., and Caron, M. G. (1998). Profound neural plasticity in response to inactivation of the dopamine transporter. *Proceedings of the National Academy of Sciences of the USA*, 95: 4029–4034.

Kaasinen, V. and Rinne, J. O. (2002). Functional imaging studies of dopamine system and cognition in normal aging and Parkinson's disease. *Neuroscience and Biobehavioral Reviews*, 26: 785–793.

Kaasinen, V., Vilkman, H., Hietala, J., Nagren, K., Helenius, H. Olsson, H. et al. (2000). Age-related D2/D3 receptor loss in extrastriatal regions of the human brain. *Neurobiology of Aging*, 21: 683–688.

Karlsson, S., Nyberg, L., Karlsson, P., Farde, L., Fischer, H., MacDonald, S. W. S. et al. (2008). *Age-related differences in reduction of dopamine D₁ receptor binding measured with [11 C] SCH 23390 during cognitive activity compared to resting state*. Manuscript submitted.

Kessler, R. M., Whetsell, W. O., Ansari, M. S. et al. (1993). Identification of extrastriatal dopamine D2 receptors in post mortem human brain with [125I]epipride. *Brain Research*, 609: 237–243.

Kimberg, D. Y. and D'Esposito, M. (2003). Cognitive effects of the dopamine receptor agonist pergolide. *Neuropsychologia*, 41: 1020–1027.

Kimberg, D. Y., D'Esposito, M., and Farah, M. J. (1997). Effects of bromocriptine on human subjects depend on working memory capacity. *NeuroReport*, 8: 3581–3585.

Koepp, M. J., Gunn, R. N., Lawrence, A. D., Cunningham, V. J., Dagher, A., Jones, T. et al. (1998). Evidence for striatal dopamine release during a video game. *Nature*, 393: 266–268.

Kohler, C., Ericson, H. and Radesater, A. C. (1991). Different laminar distributions of dopamine D1 and D2 receptors in the rat hippocampal region. *Neuroscience Letters*, 126: 107–109.

Knutson, B. and Gibbs, S. E. B. (2007). Linking nucleus accumbens dopamine and blood oxygenation. *Psychopharmacology*, 191: 813–822.

Lacor, P. N. (2007). Advances on the understanding of synaptic pathology in AD. *Current Genomics*, 8: 486–508.

Larkin, G. R. S., Gibs, S. E. B., Khanna, K., Nielsen, L., Castensen, L., and Knuston, B. (2007). Anticipation of mentary gain but not loss in healthy older adults. *Nature Neuroscience*, 10: 787–791.

Laruelle, M. (2000). Imaging synaptic neurotransmission with in vivo binding competition techniques: A critical review. *Journal of Cerebral Blood Flow and Metabolism*, 20: 423–451.

Laurier, L. G., O'Dowd, B. F., and George, S. R. (1994). Heterogeneous tissue-specific transcription of dopamine receptor subtype messenger RNA in rat brain. *Brain Research and Molecular Brain Research*, 25: 344–350.

Lawrence, A. D., Weeks, R. A., Brooks, D. J., Andrews, T. C., Watkins, L. H. A., Harding, A. E. et al. (1998). The relationship between dopamine receptor binding and cognitive performance in Huntington's disease. *Brain*, 121: 1343–1355.

Lewis, D. A. and Sesack, S. R. (1997). Dopamine systems in the primate brain. In E. F. Bloom, A. Björklund, and T. Hökfelt (eds), *The Primate Nervous System Part 1* (pp. 263–375). Amsterdopaminem: Elsevier.

Li, S.-C., Biele, G., Mohr, P. N. C, and Heekeren, H. (2007). Aging and neuroeconomics: Insights from research on neuromodulation of reward-based decision making. *Analyse and Kritik*, 29: 97–111.

Li, S.-C., Lindenberger, U., and Sikström, S. (2001). Aging cognition: From neuromodulation to representation to cognition. *Trends in Cognitive Sciences*, 5: 479–486.

Li, S.-C., Lindenberger, U., Hommel, B., Aschersleben, G., Prinz, W., and Baltes, P. B. (2004). Transformations in the couplings among intellectual abilities and constituent cognitive processes across the lifespan. *Psychological Science*, 15: 155–163.

Li, S.-C. and Sikström, S. (2002). Integrative neurocomputational perspectives on cognitive aging, neuromodulation, and representation. *Neuroscience and Biobehavioral Reviews*, 26: 795–808.

Li, S.-C., von Oertzen, T., and Lindenberger, U. (2006). A neurocomputational model of stochastic resonance and aging. *Neurocomputing*, 69: 1553–1560.

Lindenberger, U. and Baltes, P. B. (1994). Sensory functioning and intelligence in old age: A strong relation. *Psychology and Aging*, 9: 339–355.

Lindenberger, U., Li, S.-C., and Bäckman, L. (2006). (eds). Special issue: Brain-behavior dynamics across the lifespan. *Neurosience and Biobehavioral Reviews*, 30: 713–885.

Lindenberger, U., Nagel, I. E., Chicherio, C., Li, S.-C., Heekeren, H., and Bäckman, L. (2008). Age-related decline in brain resources modulates genetic effects on cognitive functioning. *Frontier in Neuroscience*, 2, 234–244.

Loo, S. K., Specter, E., Smolen, A., Hopper, C., Teale, P. D., and Reite, M. L. (2003). Functional effects of the DAT1 polymorphism on EEG measures in ADHD. *Journal of the American Academy of Child and Adolescent Psychiatry*, 42: 986–993.

Lotta, T., Vidgren, J., Tilgmann, C., Ulmanen, I., Julkunen, I., and Taskinen, J. (1995). Kinetics of human soluble and membrane-bound catechol-O-methyltransferase: A revised mechanism and description of the termolabile variant of the enzyme. *Biochemistry*, 34: 4202–4210.

Lövdèn, M., Li, S.-C., Shing, Y. L., and Lindenbeger, U. (2007). Within-person trial-to-trial variability precedes and predicts cognitive decline in old and very old age: Longitudinal data from the Berlin Aging Study. *Neuropsychologia*, 45: 2827–2838.

Luciana, M. and Collins, P. F. (1997). Dopamine modulates working memory for spatial but not object cues in normal humans. *Journal of Cognitive Neuroscience*, 9: 330–347.

MacDonald, S. W. S., Cervenka, S., Farde, L., Nyberg, L., and Bäckman, L. (in press). Extrastriatal Dopamine D2 receptor binding modulates intraindividual variability in episodic memory and executive functioning. *Neuropsychologia*.

MacDonald, S. W. S., Nyberg, L., and Bäckman, L. (2006). Intra-individual variability in behavior: Links to brain structure, neurotransmission, and neuronal activity. *Trends in Neurosciences*, 29: 474–480.

MacRae, P. G., Spirduso, W. W., and Wilcox, R. E. (1988). Reaction time and nigrostriatal dopamine function: The effects of age and practice. *Brain Research*, 451: 139–146.

Maher, B. S., Marazita, M. L., Ferrell, R. E., and Vanyukov, M. M. (2002). Dopamine system genes and attention deficit hyperactivity disorder: A meta-analysis. *Psychiatric Genetics*, 12: 207–215.

McGuire, P., Howes, O. D., Stone, J., and Fusar-Poli, P. (2008). Functional neuroimaging in schizophrenia: Diagnosis and drug discovery. *Trends in Pharmacological Sciences*, 29: 91–98.

Marschner, A., Mell, T., Wartenburger, I., Villringer, A., Reischies, F. M., and Heekeren, H. R. (2005). Reward-based decision making and aging. *Brain Research Bulletin*, 67: 382–390.

Mattay, V. S., Goldberg, T. E., Fera, F., Hariri, A. R., Tessitore, A., and Egan, M. F. (2003). Catechol-O-methyltransferase val(258)-met genotype and individual variation in he brain responses to amphetamine. *Proceedings of the National Academy of Sciences of the USA*, 100: 6186–6191.

Mattay, V. S., Goldberg, T. E., Sambataro, F., and Weinberger, D. R. (2008). Neurobiology of cognitive aging: Insights from imaging genetics. *Biological Psychology*, 79: 9–22.

Meador-Woodruff, J. H. (1994). Update on dopamine receptors. *Annals of Clinical Psychiatry*, 6: 79–90.

Mell, T., Heekeren, H. R., Marschner, A., Wartenburgerm, I., Villringer, A., and Reischies, F. M. (2005). Effect of aging on stimulus-related association learning. *Neuropsychologia*, 43: 554–563.

Mesco, E. R., Carlsson, S. G., Joseph, J. A., and Roth, G. S. (1993). Decreased striatal D2 dopamine receptor mRNA synthesis during aging. *Molecular Brain Research*, 17: 160–162.

Meyer-Lindenberg, A. and Weinberger, D. R. (2006). Intermediate phenotypes and genetic mechanisms of psychiatric disorders. *Nature Reviews Neuroscience*, 7: 818–827.

Meyer-Lindenberg, A., Straub, R. E., Lipska, B. K., Verchinski, B. A., Goldberg, T., and Callicott, J. H. et al. (2007). Genetic evidence implicating DARPP-32 in human frontostriatal structure, function, and cognition. *Journal of Clinical Investigations*, 117: 672–682.

Martinez, D., Silfstein, M., Broft, A., Mawlawi, O., Hwang, D.-R., Huang, Y. et al. (2003). Imaging human mesolimbic dopamine transmission with positron emission tomography. Part II: Amphetamine-induced dopamine release in the functional subdivisions of the striatum. *Journal of Cerebral Blood Flow and Metabolism*, 23: 285–300.

Mitchell, R. J., Howlett, S., Earl, L., McComb, J., Schanfield, M. S., Briceno, I. et al. (2000). Distribution of the´VNTR polymorphism in the human dopamine transporter gene in world populations. *Human Biology*, 72: 295–304.

Monchi, O., Ko, J. H., and Strafella, A. P. (2006). Striatal dopamine release during performance of executive functions: A [11C] raclopride PET study. *Neuroimage*, 33: 907–912.

Montague, P. R., Hyman, S. E., and Cohen, J. D. (2004). Computational roles for dopamine in behavioural control. *Nature*, 431: 760–767.

Morgan, D. G. and May, P. C. (1990). Age-related changes in synaptic neurochemistry. In Schneider and Row (eds), *Handbook of the Biology of Aging* (pp. 219–250). New York: Academic Press.

Mozley, L. H., Gur, R. C., Mozley, P. D., and Gur, R. E. (2001). Striatal dopamine transporters and cognitive functioning in healthy men and women. *American Journal of Psychiatry*, 158: 1492–1499.

Murtha, S., Cismaru, R., Waechter, R., and Chertkow, H. (2002). Increased variability accompanies frontal lobe damage in dementia. *Journal of the International Neuropsychological Society*, 8: 360–372.

Nagel, I. E., Chicherio, C., Li, S.-C., von Oertzen, T., Sander, T., Villringer, A. et al. (2008). Human aging magnifies genetic effects on executive functioning and working memory. *Frontiers in Human Neuroscience*, 2: 1–8.

Nahmias, C., Wahl, L. et al. (1995). A probe for intracerebral aromatic amino-acid decarboxylase activity: distribution and kinetics of [18F]6-fluoro-L-*m*-tyrosine in the human brain. *Movement Disorder*, 10: 298–304.

Neumeyer, J. L., Wang, S., Milius, R. A., Baldwin, R. M., Zeaponce, Y., Hoffer, P. B. et al. (1991). [^{123}I]-2-b -carbomethoxy-3b-(4-iodophenyl)-tropane: High-affinity SPECT radiotracer of monoamine reuptake sites in brain. *Journal of Medicinal Chemistry*, 34: 3144–3146.

Nordström, A. L., Farde, L., Pauli, S., Litton, J. E., and Halldin, C. (1992). PET analysis of [11C] raclopride binding in healthy young adults and schizpenrenic patients: Reliability and age effects. *Human Psychopharmacology*, 7: 157–165.

Nyberg, L., Sandblom, J., Jones, S., Stigsdotter-Neely, A., Petersson, K. M., Ingvar, M., and Bäckman, L. (2003). Neural correlates of training-related memory improvement in adulthood and aging. *Proceedings of the National Academy of Sciences of the USA*, 100: 13728–13733.

Nyberg, L., Andersson, M., Forsgren, L., Jakobsson-Mo, S., Larsson, A., Marklund, P. et al. (2008). Striatal dopamine D2 binding is related to frontal BOLD response during updating of long-term memory representations. Manuscript submitted.

O'Hara, R., Miller, E., Liao, C. P., Way, N., Lin, X. Y., and Hallmayer, J. (2006). COMT genotype, gender, and cognition in community dwelling, older adults. *Neuroscience Letters*, 409: 205–209.

O'Reilly, R. C. (2006). Biological based computational models of high-level cognition. *Science*, 314: 91–94.

O'Reilly, R. C. and Frank, M. J. (2006). Making working memory work: a computational model of learning in the frontal cortex and basal ganglia. *Neural Computation*, 18: 283–328.

Parent, A. and Hazrati, L. N. (1995). Functional anatomy of the basal ganglia. I. The cortico-basal ganglia-thalamo-cortical loop. *Brain Research Review*, 20: 91–127.

Pasuit, J. B., Li, Z., and Kuzhikandathil, V. (2004). *Journal of Neurochemistry*, 89: 1508–1519.

Pizzagalli, D. A., Evins, A. E., Schetter, E. C., Frank, M. J., Pajtas, P. E., Santesso, D. L., and Culhane, M. (2008). Single dose of a dopamine agonist impairs reinforcement learning in humans: Behavioral evidence from a laboratory-based measure of reward responsiveness. *Psychopharmacology*, 196: 221–232.

Ramaekers, J. G., Louwerens, J. W., Muntjewerff, N. D., Milius, H., de Bie, A., Rosenzweig, P. et al. (1999). Psychomotor, cognitive, extrapyramidopaminel and affective functions of healthy volunteers during treatment with an atypical (amisulpiride) and a classic (haloperidol) antipsychotic. *Journal of Clinical Psychopharmacology*, 19: 209–221.

Raz, N., Williamson, A., Gunning-Dixon, F., Head, D., and Acker, J. D. (2000). Neuroanatomical and cognitive correlates of adult age differences in acquisition of a perceptual-motor skill. *Microscopy Research and Technique, a Special Issue on Neuroimaging and Memory*, 51: 85–93.

Rieck, R. W., Ansari, M. S., Whetsell, Jr., W. O., Deutch, A. Y., Kessler, R. M. (2004). Distribution of dopamine D2-like receptors in the human thalamus: autoradiographic and PET studies. *Neuropsychopharmacology*, 29: 362–372.

Rolls, E. T., Loh, M., Deco, G., and Winterer, G. (2008). Computational models of schizophrenia and dopamine modulation in the prefrontal cortex. *Nature Reviews Neuroscience*, 9: 696–709.

Roth, R. H. (1984). CNS dopamine autoreceptors: Distribution, pharmacology, and function. *Annals of the New York Academy of Sciences*, 430: 27–53.

Sánchez-González, M. A., García-Cabezas, M. A., Rico, B., and Cavada, C. (2005). The primate thalamus is a key target for brain dopamine. *Journal of Neuroscience*, 25: 6076–6083.

Sawaguchi, T. and Goldman-Rakic, P. S. (1991). D$_1$ dopamine receptors in prefrontal cortex: Involvement in working memory. *Science*, 251: 947–950.

Sawamoto, N., Piccini, P., Hotton, G., Pavese, N., Thielemans, K., and Brooks, D. J. (2008). Cognitive deficits and striato-frontal dopamine release in Parkinson's disease. *Brain*, 131: 1294–1302.

Schambra, U. B., Duncan, G. E., Breese, G. R., Fornaretto, M. G., Caron, M. G., and Fremeau, J. R. (1994). Ontogeny of D1a and D2 dopamine receptor subtypes in rat brain using *in situ* hybridization and receptor binding. *Neuroscience*, 62: 65–85.

Schott, B. H., Minuzzi, L., Krebs, R. M., Elmenhorst, D., Lang, M., Winz, O. H. et al. (2008). Mesolimbic fMRI activations during reward anticipation correlate with reward-related ventral striatal dopamine release. *Journal of Neuroscience*, 28: 14311–14319.

Schultz, W., Studer, A., Romo, R., Sundstrom, E., Jonsson, G., and Scarnati, E. (1989). Deficits in reaction-times and movement times as correlates of hypokinesia in monkeys with MPTP-induced striatal dopamine depletion. *Journal of Neurophysiology*, 61, 651–668.

Schultz, W. (2006). Behavioral theories and the neurophysiology of reward. *Annual Review of Psychology*, 57: 87–115.

Seamans, J. K. and Yang, C. R. (2004). The principal features and mechanisms of dopamine modulation in the prefrontal cortex. *Progress in Neurobiology*, 74: 1–57.

Seeman, P., Bzowej, N. H., Guan, H. C., Bergeron, C., Becker, L. E., Reynolds, G. P. et al. (1987). Human brain dopamine receptors in children and aging adults. *Synapse*, 1: 399–404.

Segovia, G., Porras, A., Arco, A. D., and Mora, F. (2001). Glutamatergic neurotransmission in aging: A critical perspective. *Mechanisms of Ageing and Development*, 122: 1–29.

Servan-Schreiber, D., Printz, H., and Cohen, J. D. (1990). A network model of catecholamine effects: Gain, signal-to-noise ratio, and behavior. *Science*, 249: 892–895.

Servan-Schreiber, D., Carter, C. S., Bruno, R. M., and Cohen, J. D. (1998). Dopamine and the mechanisms of cognition: Part II. D-amphetamine effects in human subjects performing a selective attention task. *Biological Psychiatry*, 43: 723–729.

Severson, J. A., Marcusson, J., Winblad, B., and Finch, C. E. (1982). Age-correlated loss of dopaminergic binding sites in human basal ganglia. *Journal of Neurochemistry*, 39: 1623–1631.

Shinkai, T., Zhang, L., Mathias, S. A., and Roth, G. S. (1997). Dopamine induces apoptosis in cultured rat striatal neurons: Possible mechanism of D2-dopamine receptor neuron loss during aging. *Journal of Neuroscience Research*, 47: 393–399.

Snow, B. J., Tooyama, I., McGeer, E. G., Yamada, T., Calne, D. B., Takahashi, H. et al. (1993). Human positron emission tomographic [18F]fluorodopa studies correlate with dopamine cell counts and levels. *Annals of Neurology*, 34: 324–330.

Starr, J. M., Fox, H., Harris, S. E., Deary, I. J., and Whalley, L. J. (2007). COMT genotype and cognitive ability: A longitudinal aging study. *Neuroscience Letters*, 421: 57–61.

Stefanis, N. C., van Os, J., Avramopoulos, D., Smyrnis, N., Evdokimidis, I., and Stefanis, C. N. (2005). Effect of COMT Val(158)Met polymorphism on the continuous performance test, identical pairs version: Tuning rather improving performance. *American Journal of Psychiatry*, 162: 1753–1754.

Stoessl, A. J. and de la Fuente-Fernandez, R. (2003). Dopamine receptors in Parkinson's disease: imaging studies. *Advanced Neurology*, 91: 65–71.

Stuss, D. T., Murphy, K. J., Binns, M. A., and Alexander, M. P. (2003), Staying on the job: The frontal lobes control individual performance variability. *Brain*, 126: 2363–2380.

Suhara, T., Fukudopamine, H., Inoue, O., Itoh, T., Suzuki, K., Yamasaki, T., Tateno, Y. (1991). Age-related changes in human D1 dopamine receptors measured by positron emission tomography. *Psychopharmacology*, 103: 41–45.

Takahashi, H., Kato, M., Hayashi, M., Okubo, Y., Takano, A., Ito, H. et al. (2006). Memory and frontal lobe functions: Possible relations with dopamine D2 receptors in the hippocampus. *NeuroImage*, 34: 1643–1649.

Tan, H. Y., Chen, Q, Sust, S., Buckholtz, W., Meyers, J. D., Egan, M. F. et al. (2007). Epistasis between catechol-O-Methyltransferase and type II metabotropic glutamate receptor 3 genes on working brain function. *Proceedings of the National Academy of Sciences of the USA*, 104: 12536–12541.

Taylor, S. F., Koeppe, R. A., Tandon, R., Zubieta, J. K., and Frey, K. A. (2000). In vivo measurement of the vesicular monoamine transporter in schizophrenia. *Neuropsychopharmacology*, 6: 667–675.

Ungerstedt, U. (1971). *On the Anatomy, Pharmacology, and Function of the Nigrostriatal Dopamine System*. Stockholm: Norstedts.

Volkow, N. D., Gur, R. C., Wang, G. J., Fowler, J. S., Moberg, P. J., Ding, Y. S. et al. (1998). Association between decline in brain dopamine activity with age and cognitive and motor impairment in healthy individuals. *American Journal of Psychiatry*, 157: 344–349.

Wang, M., Vijayraghavan, S., and Goldman-Rakic, P. S. (2004). Selective D2 receptor actions on the functional circuit of working memory. *Science*, 303: 853–856.

Wang, Y., Chan, G. L. Y., Holden, J. E., Dobko, T., Schulzer, M. E., Huser, J. M. et al. (1998). Age-dependent decline of dopamine D1 receptors in human brain: A PET study. *Synapse*, 30: 56–61.

Weinshilboum, R. M., Otterness, D. M., and Szumlanski, C. L. (1999). Methylation pharmacogenetics: Catechol-O-methyltransferase, thiopurine methyltransferase, and histamine N-methyltransferase. *Annual Review of Pharmacology and Toxicology*, 39: 19–52.

West, R., Murphy, K. J., Armilio, M. L., Craik, F. I. M., and Stuss, D. T. (2002). Lapses of intention and performance variability reveal age-related increases in fluctuations of executive control. *Brain and Cognition*, 49: 402–419.

Winterer, G., Coppola, R., Goldberg, T. E., Egan, M. F., Jones, D. W., Sanchez, C. E., and Weinberger, D. R. (2004). Prefrontal broadband noise, working memory, and genetic risk for schizophrenia. *America Journal of Psychiatry*, 161: 490–500.

Winterer, G. and Weinberger D. R. (2004) Genes, dopamine and cortical signal-to-noise ratio in schizophrenia. *Trends in Neuroscience*, 27: 683–690.

Winterer, G., Musso, F., Vucurevic, G., Stoeter, P., Konrad, A., Seker, B. et al. (2006). COMT genotype predicts BOLD signal and noise characteristics in prefrontal circuits. *Neuroimage*, 32: 1722–1732.

Williams, G. V. and Goldman-Rakic, P. S. (1995). Modulation of memory fields by dopamine D1 receptors in prefrontal cortex. *Nature*, 376: 572–575.

Wittmann, B. C., Schott, B. H., Guderian, S., Frey, J. U., Heinze, H. J., Duzel, E. (2005). Reward-related FMRI activation of dopaminergic midbrain is associated with enhanced hippocampus-dependent long-term memory formation. *Neuron*, 5: 459–467.

Yacubian, J., Sommer, T., Schroeder, K., Gläscher, J., Kalisch, R., Leuenberger, B. et al. (2007). Gene-gene interaction associated with neural reward sensitivity. *Proceedings of the National Academy of Sciences of the USA*, 104: 8125–8130.

Yang, Y. K., Chiu, N. T., Chen, C. C., Chen, M., Yeh, T. L., and Lee, I. H. (2003). Correlation between fine motor activity and striatal dopamine D2 receptor density in patients with schizophrenia and healthy controls. *Psychiatry Research: Neuroimaging*, 123: 191–197.

Zhang, L., Ravipati, A., Joseph, J., and Roth, G. S. (1995). Aging-related changes in rat striatal D2 dopamine receptor mRNA-containing neurons: A quantitative nonradioactive in situ hybridization study. *Journal of Neuroscience*, 15: 1735–1740.

6

Cognitive Reserve and Aging

Yaakov Stern

The idea of reserve against brain damage stems from the repeated observation that there is not a direct relationship between the degree of brain pathology or brain damage and the clinical manifestation of that damage. For example, Katzman et al. (1989) described 10 cases of cognitively normal elderly women who were discovered to have advanced Alzheimer's disease (AD) pathology in their brains at death. They speculated that these women did not express the clinical features of AD because their brains were larger than average, providing them with "brain reserve." In more recent cohort studies it has been estimated that approximately 25% of individuals who have neuropathologic evidence of AD post-mortem are not demented during their lives (Ince, 2001).

Brain reserve (Katzman, 1993) is an example of what might be called passive models of reserve, where reserve derives from brain size or neuronal count. The models are passive because reserve is defined in terms of the amount of brain damage that can be sustained before reaching a threshold for clinical expression. The threshold model (Satz, 1993), one of the best articulated passive models, revolves around the construct of brain reserve capacity (BRC). While BRC is a hypothetical construct, concrete examples of BRC might include brain size or synapse count. The model recognizes that there are individual differences in BRC. It also presupposes that there is a critical threshold of BRC. Once BRC is depleted past this threshold, specific clinical or functional deficits emerge.

In contrast, the cognitive reserve (CR) model suggests that the brain actively attempts to cope with brain damage by using pre-existing cognitive processing approaches, or by enlisting compensatory approaches (Stern, 2002). Individuals with more CR would be more successful at coping with the same amount of brain damage. Thus, the same amount of brain damage or pathology will have different effects on different people, even if BRC (e.g., brain size) is held constant. The concept of CR provides a ready explanation for why many studies have demonstrated that higher levels of intelligence, and of educational and occupational attainment, are good predictors of which individuals can sustain greater brain damage before demonstrating functional deficit. Rather than positing that these individuals' brains are grossly anatomically different than those with less reserve (e.g., they have more synapses), the cognitive reserve hypothesis posits that they process tasks in a manner that allows them to cope better with brain damage. Brain reserve and cognitive reserve concepts are not mutually exclusive, and it likely that both are involved in providing reserve against brain damage.

Measures of Reserve

For advocates of the idea of brain reserve, anatomic measures such as brain volume, head circumference, synaptic count, or dendritic branching are effective measures of reserve. Mounting evidence suggests that many of these measures are malleable over the lifetime, and influenced by life experience. Therefore, brain reserve may represent a summation of many aspects of life experience that are also thought to summate into CR.

Variables descriptive of lifetime experience are the most commonly used proxies for CR. These include measures of socioeconomic status, such as income or occupational attainment. Educational attainment has also been a widely used proxy for reserve, probably because it is relatively easy to ascertain. Degree of literacy might be a better marker for CR than number of years of formal education because it is a more direct measure of educational attainment (Manly et al., 2003, 2005). Finally, specific measured attributes have been used as indices of reserve, including IQ, and measures of various cognitive functions.

Education might also be a marker for innate intelligence, which may, in turn, be genetically based or a function of exposures. Some studies suggest that an estimate of IQ, or premorbid IQ might actually be a more powerful measure of reserve in some cases (Albert and Teresi, 1999; Alexander et al., 1997). Still, education or other life experiences probably impart reserve over and above that obtained from innate intelligence. Studies have demonstrated separate or synergistic effects for higher educational and occupational attainment and leisure activities, suggesting that each of these life experiences contributes independently to reserve (Evans et al., 1993; Mortel et al., 1995; Rocca et al., 1990; Stern et al., 1994, 1995). A prospective study showed that an estimated IQ at age 53 was separately influenced by childhood cognition, educational attainment, and adult occupation (Richards and Sacker, 2003). These observations stress that CR is not fixed; at any point in one's lifetime it results from a combination of exposures.

The simplest explanation for how CR forestalls the clinical effects of AD pathology does not posit that experiences associated with more CR directly affect brain reserve or the development of AD pathology. Rather, CR allows some people to better cope with the pathology and remain clinically more intact for longer periods of time. This has been the working assumption underlying the design and interpretation of many of my studies. However, as mentioned above, many of the factors associated with CR may also have direct impact on the brain itself. There is a demonstrated relationship between IQ and brain volume (Willerman et al., 1991). Thus, child development literature suggests that intracranial brain volume and aspects of lifetime exposure are predictive of differential susceptibility to the effects of traumatic brain injury (Kesler et al., 2003). Also, it is now clear that stimulating environments and exercise promote neurogenesis in the dentate of animals (Brown et al., 2003; van Praag et al., 2005). In addition, there is evidence to suggest that environmental enrichment might act directly to prevent or slow the accumulation of AD pathology (Lazarov et al., 2005). Thus, a more complete accounting of CR would have to integrate these complex interactions between genetics, the environmental influences on brain reserve and pathology, and the ability to actively compensate for the effects of pathology.

Epidemiologic Evidence for CR

The concept of reserve is relevant to any situation where the brain sustains injury. In addition, it will be argued that the concept of reserve should be extended to encompass variations in healthy individuals' performance, particularly when they must perform at their maximum capacity. Nevertheless, many of the studies discussed in this chapter will be framed around aging and AD, with the implicit assumption that the discussion has implications for brain damage in general. Both aging and AD have some unique advantages for examining disease-induced changes in brain function. Both are more likely than conditions such as stroke to affect similar anatomic sites across subjects, allowing for better generalization. Both are also slowly progressive, providing a more sensitive indicator of the severity of brain insult required before cognitive networks change. On the other hand, the potential for adaptation of recovery might vary between slowly progressive and acute pathologies, so studies of aging and AD may not always have direct implications for studies of other conditions.

Many studies have examined the relation of CR proxy variables to incident dementia. A meta-analysis examined cohort studies of the effects of education, occupation, premorbid IQ and mental activities on dementia risk (Valenzuela and Sachdev, 2005). A summary analysis was based on an integrated total of 29,279 individuals from 22 studies. The median follow-up was 7.1 years. The summary overall risk of incident dementia for individuals with high brain reserve compared to low was 0.54 (95%CI 0.49–0.59, $p < 0.0001$)—a decreased risk of 46%. Eight out of 33 datasets showed no significant effect, while 25 out of 33 demonstrated a significant protective effect. The authors found a significant negative association between incident dementia risk (based on differential education) and the overall dementia rate for each cohort ($r = -0.57$, $p = 0.04$), indicating that in negative studies there was a lower overall risk of incident dementia in the cohort.

There is also evidence for the role of education in age-related cognitive decline, with several studies of normal aging reporting slower cognitive and functional decline in individuals with higher educational attainment (Albert et al., 1995; Butler, Ashford, and Snowdon, 1996; Chodosh et al., 2002; Christensen et al., 1997; Colsher and Wallace, 1991; Farmer et al., 1995; Lyketsos, Chen, and Anthony, 1999; Snowdon, Ostwald, and Kane, 1989). These studies suggest that the same education-related factors that delay the onset of dementia also allow individuals to cope more effectively with brain changes encountered in normal aging. In an ethnically diverse cohort of nondemented elders in New York City, increased literacy was also associated with a slower decline in memory, executive function, and language skills (Manly et al., 2005).

In contrast to the studies above, in which greater reserve was associated with better outcomes, a series of studies of patients with AD have suggested that those with higher reserve have poorer outcomes. In a prospective study of AD patients matched for clinical severity at baseline (Stern et al., 1995), patients with greater education or occupational attainment died sooner than those with less attainment. Although at first these findings appear contra-intuitive, they are consistent with the CR hypothesis. The hypothesis predicts that at any level of assessed clinical severity, the underlying pathology of AD is more advanced in patients with CR than in those with CR. This would result in the clinical disease emerging when pathology is more advanced, as suggested by the incidence studies reviewed above. This disparity in degree of pathology would be present at more advanced clinical stages of the disease as well. At some point, the greater degree of pathology in the high reserve patients would result in more rapid death. Although one study did not replicate this finding (Geerlings, et al., 1997), a follow-up study by the same group, using patients with more advanced dementia, did (Geerlings et al., 1999). Higher measured CR has also been associated with more rapid cognitive decline in patients with AD (Stern et al., 1999; Scarmeas et al., 2006). Explanation of this finding is along similar lines. At some point AD pathology must become too severe to support the processes that mediate CR. This point should arrive at an earlier stage of clinical severity in patients with higher CR because the underlying AD pathology is more severe.

Imaging Studies of CR

Several imaging studies of CR in AD used resting cerebral blood flow (CBF) as a surrogate for AD pathology (DeCarli et al., 1992; Friedland, Brun, and Bundinger, 1985; McGeer et al., 1990). Our original functional imaging study found that, in patients matched for overall severity of dementia, the parietotemporal flow deficit was greater in those with more years of education (Stern et al., 1992). This observation was confirmed in a later PET study (Alexander et al., 1997). After controlling for clinical dementia severity, higher education was correlated with reduced cerebral metabolism in prefrontal, premotor, and left superior parietal association areas. The negative correlations are consistent with the CR hypothesis' prediction that at any given level of clinical disease severity, a subject with a higher level of CR should have greater AD pathology (i.e., lower CBF). These studies support the idea that although pathology was more advanced in patients with higher education, the clinical manifestations of the disease were comparable to those in patients with lower education and less pathology. Presumably the patients with more education had more cognitive reserve. We made a similar observation for occupational attainment (Stern et al., 1995) and later for leisure activities (Scarmeas et al., 2003a). These findings were confirmed in a prospective study with subsequent neuropathological analysis. Education was found to modify the association between AD pathology and levels of cognitive function: for the same degree of brain pathology there was better cognitive function with each year of education (Bennett et al., 2003).

Neural Mechanisms Underlying CR

The neural implementation of CR might take two forms: neural reserve and neural compensation (Stern et al., 2005; Stern, 2006). The idea behind neural reserve is that there is natural interindividual variability in the brain networks or cognitive processes that underlie the performance of any task. This variability could be in the form of differing efficiency or capacity of these networks, or in greater flexibility in the networks that can be invoked to perform a task. While healthy individuals may invoke these networks when coping with increased task demands, the networks could also help an individual cope with brain pathology. An individual whose networks are more efficient, have greater capacity, or are more flexible, might be more capable of coping with the challenges imposed by brain pathology.

Neural compensation refers to the process by which individuals suffering from brain pathology use brain structures or networks (and thus cognitive strategies) not normally used by individuals with intact brains to compensate for brain damage. "Neural compensation" is reserved for a situation where it can be demonstrated that the more impaired group is using a different network than the unimpaired group.

Distinguishing between these two possible neural implementations of CR becomes particularly important when attempting to formulate and interpret functional imaging studies that investigate CR. Consideration of these possible neural mechanisms can guide the design and classification of research that intends to study the neural implementation of CR. The following set of research questions provides a framework for investigating the neural underpinnings of CR. This will help clarify the underlying rationale behind some of the studies that have been conducted. To simplify the discussion, these questions will be framed in terms of the effects of age-related brain changes on cognition and how these may be mediated by CR. Work from our group will be used to explore the implications of each of these questions.

1. Do old and young subjects use the same or different networks to mediate task performance?

This is the basic question that underlies the differentiation between neural reserve and neural compensation. If elders use the same network as younger individuals, but to a greater or lesser degree, this differential activation cannot be considered compensatory according to the definition put forward above. Of course, most imaging studies in aging essentially are asking this question, even if they are not studying CR.

Addressing the question of whether task-related activation in two groups is the same or different is complicated by several issues. Figure 6.1 illustrates some hypothetical data that may help to clarify these concepts. Increasing task demand is on the x-axis. This refers to a hypothetical within-subject manipulation where the difficulty of the task is increased in a parametric manner. The y-axis represents task-related activation either at one particular brain location or throughout some brain network. The figure demonstrates hypothesized curves relating task demand to task-related activation in young and old individuals. Note that at any fixed level of task difficulty, a task might be relatively more difficult or demanding for one group than for another. For example, if a young group and an old group are given a seven-word memory test, this task might be trivial for the young subjects, but demanding for the older subjects. This divergence in relative difficulty for the two groups might lead to differences in task-related activation in any particular brain area or network.

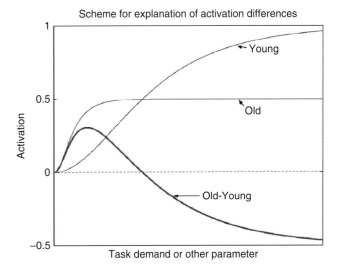

Figure 6–1 Hypothetical relationship between task demand and activation in old and young.

Note in the Figure that at relatively low task demand, greater activation might be seen in old people than in young people. Conversely, at greater task demand, greater activation might be seen in the young subjects than in the old. Therefore, differential activation in and of itself is very difficult to interpret. Using the same task at different levels of difficulty, one might find greater or less activation in any brain area in young subjects. However, these differences do not necessarily indicate that the two groups are using different brain networks to mediate task performance. To begin making inferences from differential activation across groups, the investigator must have an understanding of or good control over the relative difficulty of the task in the groups. One may do this by carefully matching task performance across the groups. For example, several investigators have taken great pains to ensure that, as a group, old and young subjects' behavioral performance on their activation task was matched. An alternate approach, which was implemented in some of the studies described below, is to titrate task difficulty in each individual subject to ensure that each subject is performing the task at a comparable level. More recently, my group has moved to attempting to understand the nature of task-related activation over a range of task difficulty, and the way in which this may differ with young and old subjects.

Another difficulty in determining whether two groups are using the same or different networks derives from the approaches used to analyze imaging data. Thus, in Figure 6.2, we have situations where the same task, at different levels of task demand, may yield greater and lesser activation in the two groups. This could be because the underlying neural network differs in the two groups, or that the network is actually the same but is operating at different efficiencies and capacities. Voxel-based analyses of imaging data as traditionally applied are not sufficient to make this discrimination. The existence of voxel-wise differences in the case illustrated in Figure 6.2 does not imply distinct spatial patterns. To illustrate this concept, note that groups A and B in Figure 6.2 express identical brain networks, but to different degrees. This is a reasonable expectation if, for example, an older group expressed the same brain network as a younger group, but with less efficiency. When comparing thresholded maps between groups, one might

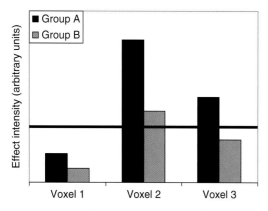

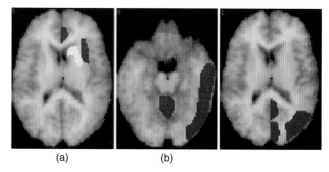

Figure 6–2 Example of two groups expressing the same pattern of activation, but to different degrees. If comparing thresholded maps between groups, one might incorrectly conclude the activation of voxel 3 uniquely in group A.

Figure 6–3 Covariance patterns (topographies) expressed by healthy elderly and AD subjects. Weights for each region's participation in the topography are overlaid on standard, Tailarach-transformed axial MRI sections, with positive weights indicated in red and negative weights indicated in yellow. (**a**) The healthy elders' topography: higher SLS was associated with increased activation and left anterior cingulate and interior insula, and decreased activation of left basal ganglia. (**b**) AD topography: higher SLS was associated with increased activation of left posterior temporal cortex, calcarine cortex, posterior cingulate, and the vermis.

incorrectly conclude that activation of voxel 3 is unique in group A. One solution to this problem is to use analytic approaches that investigate spatial covariance patterns, as opposed to comparing groups on a voxel-by-voxel basis. Another approach, demonstrated in the section for Question 3 below, is to examine how task-related activation relates to some other variable, like performance or CR. If the relationship differs in young and old individuals, then one can reasonably conclude that there is some difference in how these areas mediate performance in the two groups.

In our first imaging study (Stern et al., 2000), we tried to determine whether or not the pathology of AD alters the brain networks subserving performance on a memory task, while carefully controlling for task difficulty. This study used a serial recognition task—one of the two tasks that has been used in all of the imaging studies described here. We used a continuous nonverbal recognition task in a series of studies that address this issue. The basic task consists of the serial presentation of a set of words or shapes, followed by a series of the same number of recognition probes. For each probe, the subject uses a button press to indicate whether or not they just saw the item. There are two task conditions. In the low-demand condition, each study item is followed by a recognition probe. In the titrated-demand condition, subjects study a longer list of items, and then respond to an equally long set of recognition probes. Prior to scanning, the study list size (SLS) of the titrated-demand condition is adjusted for each subject such that recognition accuracy is 75%. This procedure is intended to match task difficulty (as operationalized by level of performance) across subjects. This, in turn, allows us to interpret activation differences without the concern that they are simply related to differential difficulty of the task across subjects or groups. In the present study, $H_2{}^{15}O$ PET was used to measure regional cerebral blood flow in AD patients and healthy elders during the performance of a verbal version of the serial recognition task. In healthy elders, a network of brain areas involving left anterior cingulate, anterior insula, and left basal ganglia, was activated during the titrated-demand (vs. low) condition. Higher study list size in the titrated-demand condition was associated with increased recruitment of this network, indicating that subjects who could recruit the network to a greater degree could perform the task better. Only three AD patients expressed this network in a manner similar to controls. The remaining 11 AD patients recruited a different

network during task performance, consisting of left posterior temporal cortex, calcarine cortex, posterior cingulate, and the vermis. In these patients (but not in controls), higher study list size in the titrated-demand condition was associated with increased activation of this network (Figures 6.3 and 6.4). We hypothesized that this alternate network may be used by the AD patients to compensate for the effects of AD pathology.

We also explored this issue during the performance of a version of a Sternberg letter task, based on one published originally by Rypma et al. (Rypma et al., 1999). This is the second task used in the studies reported here. In the letter version of this task, subjects study one, three, or six letters for three seconds, and then follow with a seven-second retention period. They are then presented with a single probe letter, and must indicate whether that letter is a member of the previously studied set. One straightforward behavioral measure from this task is the increase in reaction time associated with making this decision as the set size increases. This slope of the reaction time over set size (RT slope) is considered to be a measure of processing speed.

We compared fMRI data of 40 young subjects and 18 old subjects during the performance of this task (Zarahn et al., 2007). We used multivariate linear modeling, which is a covariance approach to analyzing the data. This analytic approach can directly assess whether the same or different spatial patterns of brain areas are responsive to increasing task difficulty during performance of each phase of the task, in young and old subjects. We found that the two groups used the same brain network during the encoding phase. Similarly, we found that the two groups used the same network during the recognition (or probe) phase of the task. However, we found that during the retention phase of the task there were two spatial patterns, one expressed by both young and old subjects, and the second only by the older subjects. This analysis demonstrates that the neural networks underlying the performance of this aspect of the task differ in young and old individuals. By definition, the network used by the old subjects alone can be considered neural compensation. The issue of whether and how this additional network benefits performance is addressed in the next question.

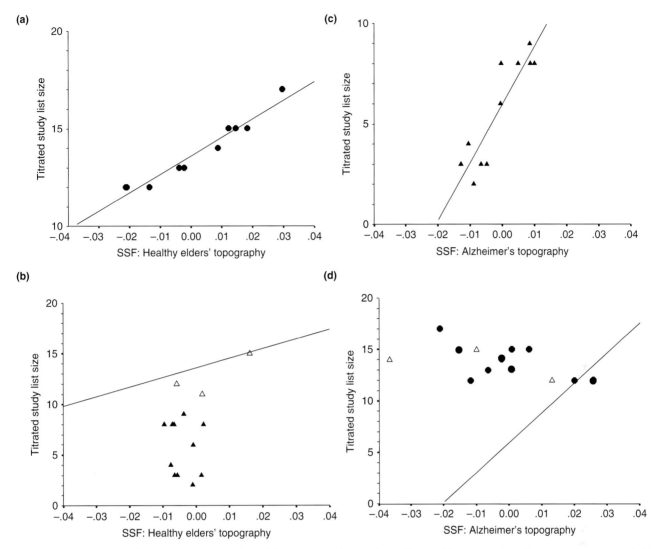

Figure 6–4   Scatter plots of the SLS attained in the titrated-demand condition and its predictor, subjects expression of a topography as quantified by the subject scaling factor. Healthy elderly individuals are represented with closed circles, AD patients with low SLS with closed triangles, and patients with high SLS with open triangles. (**a**) Correlation between healthy elders' SLS with an expression of their topography. (**b**) Scatter plot of the relation between SLS in high-and low-SLS AD patients and expression of healthy elders' topography. The regression line of Figure 6.4a. is reproduced for a reference. Notice that the data for the high SLS AD patients fall along the regression line, suggesting that these individuals are expressing this network in the same way as healthy controls. (**c**) Correlation between SLS in low-SLS AD patients and expression of their topography. (**d**) Scatter plot of high-SLS AD patients and healthy elders' SLS and expression of the AD patient topography. The regression line of Figure 6.4c is reproduced for reference. Notice that the data for the healthy elders and the high-SLS AD patients do not fall along the regression line, suggesting that their expression of this network is not related to test performance.

2. If young and old subjects use the same network, a) are there individual differences in efficiency and capacity of this network as a function of proxy measures of CR, and b) does age affect the network's efficiency or capacity?

If young and old subjects use the same underlying neural network for performing a task, then CR might be mediated through differential efficiency and capacity of this network. Figure 6.1 illustrates some hypothetical data that may help clarify these concepts. The figure demonstrates hypothesized curves relating task demand to task-related activation in young and old individuals. Note two features of these curves. First, the rate of rise in the curve might

be an index of the efficiency of the system. Thus, in this hypothetical example, the rate of rise is much slower in the young subjects than in the old subjects. This might indicate that the brain network is more efficient in the younger subjects. Simplistically, at any particular level of difficulty, the task can be mediated by less activation in the young people than in the old. A second feature of these curves is that they reach an asymptote, potentially indicative of the capacity of the system. In these hypothetical curves, the brain network has a greater capacity in the younger subjects than in the older subjects, suggesting that it might continue to respond effectively in the face of increased task demand. Intuitively, these concepts of efficiency and capacity of brain networks might be important components underlying cognitive reserve, such that networks with greater efficiency and capacity might be more able to withstand disruption and still operate effectively. One might predict that individuals with higher reserve would show greater efficiency and/or greater capacity. It is worth noting that differential efficiency and capacity can occur within young or older people, as opposed to just between them. To the extent that efficiency and capacity correlate with proxy measures of CR, we might conclude that this these features may be neural mechanisms underlying reserve.

In one study (Habeck et al., 2003), we analyzed the data from 17 young subjects who underwent fMRI while performing a spatial version of the serial recognition task. In this task, the items to be remembered were complex shapes that were constructed to be difficult to name. As in the verbal version of the task, there were two conditions: low demand, where only one shape was studied and recognized at a time; and titrated demand, where the study set size was adjusted such that each subject's recognition accuracy was 75%. Imaging data were analyzed using a covariance approach—ordinal trend canonical variates analysis (OrTCVA) (Habeck et al., 2005). This analysis attempted to identify a covariance pattern (or "brain network") whose expression increases from the low- to titrated-demand condition for as many subjects as possible. Once such a brain network was identified, we examined the relationship between individual subjects' change in network expression across the two conditions and their National Adult Reading Test (NART) scores.

Ordinal trend analysis was first performed on imaging data from the study phase of the task. There, we identified a covariance pattern whose change in expression from the low- to the titrated-demand condition increased for 15 of the 17 subjects. This brain network reflects activity in all areas of the brain, however some areas are more involved in this network than others. Further, the identification of a covariance pattern implies that change in activation in one area is related to change in another area. This relationship can be positive or negative. Thus, as the brain network expression increases, some brain areas show increased activation and some areas show decreased activation. Areas that were associated with increases in activation from the low- to titrated-demand condition for the majority of subjects were found in cerebellar locations. Areas associated with decreased activity from low- to titrated-demand conditions were attained in the precuneus, anterior singular gyrus, bilateral thalamus, right insular, right middle temporal gyrus, and bilateral inferior frontal gyrus. The key finding for our purposes was that the larger the increase in network expression from low- to titrated-demand condition was in a subject, the lower their NART IQ was (Figure 6.5). That is, subjects with lower CR showed the greatest changes in expression of this brain network across the two difficulty conditions.

Thus, this analysis identified a brain network that showed increased expression as the load associated with the task increased. Further, this change in activation across tasks was associated with CR: individuals with lower CR showed greater levels change in network expression. This brain network, therefore, appears to be differentially expressed as a function of CR. We consider this network a good example of the concept of neural reserve. Further, the fact that higher CR was associated with less activation of this network suggests that CR is associated with greater efficiency in the neural activation underlying task performance.

Another analysis focused on fMRI data from 40 young subjects performing the Sternberg letter task (Habeck et al., 2005). Using ordinal trend analysis, we identified a covariance pattern whose expression during the retention phase increased systematically with set size in almost all subjects. The degree to which this pattern's

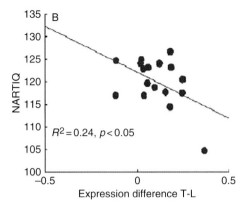

Figure 6–5 Correlation of NARTIQ with increase in expression of the covariance pattern found during study from low- to titrated-demand conditions.

expression increased correlated significantly with RT slope such that individuals with larger increases in pattern expression had larger RT slope. This correlation suggests a link between processing efficiency, as measured by RT slope and network expression, where individuals with greater efficiency, as indicated by lower RT slope, require a smaller increase in network expression as set size increases. Further, change in network expression across set sizes also correlated with NART scores. Thus, individuals with higher IQ demonstrated greater efficiency in network expression. In our theoretical framework, this would be an estimate of neural reserve.

In a subsequent analysis, the data from young subjects performing the Sternberg letter task (described above) was compared to that from healthy elderly subjects using a different analytic approach (Zarahn et al., 2007). Here, we used multivariate linear modeling (MLM). This technique begins with a contrast of interest derived from the general linear model approach (such as that used in SPM). In this case, we considered load-related changes in activation during the different phases of the task in both young and old subjects. MLM uses a singular value decomposition (SVD) followed by sequential latent root testing to systematically assess how many significant latent spatial patterns are present. Because the analyses considered two contrasts at a time (one for young and one for old), it can be used to determine whether the pattern of task-related activation was similar or different in the two groups. If only one significant pattern is found, this indicates that both young and old are using the same pattern. If two patterns are found, the second pattern consists of aspects of task-related activation that differ between the two groups. The analysis determined that for the stimulus and probe phases of the task, load-related activation in each task phase could be summarized with a single spatial network used by both young and old groups. Expression of the common network noted during the probe phase was more inefficient in the elder subjects. That is, elders expressed it to a greater degree despite their poorer performance. This is a demonstration of how age-related neural changes can limit the efficiency of a network, while the network itself remains unchanged. The findings from the retention phase are discussed below, because significant patterns were found and this finding is suggestive of neural compensation

We conducted a similar analysis of another version of the Sternberg task that used one, two, or three nonverbal stimuli as the items to be remembered (unpublished data). While this task has the same structure as the Sternberg letter task, the nature of the stimuli makes it much more demanding. Analysis of the Sternberg shape task also showed that load-related activation during the stimulus and probe phases could each be described in both the young and old subjects by a single spatial pattern. Again, this indicates young and old individuals use similar brain networks during the performance of these task phases. In this case, we found that activation of the network noted during the probe phase was greater in the young subjects than in the old. Thus, in this case, the better performance by the younger subjects was accompanied by increased expression of the underlying brain network. This suggests a capacity difference in this case, with younger subjects able to activate this network to a greater degree.

In summary, in the task that used a stimulus set that is well practiced and easier to encode, we noted a difference in efficiency, with the elder subjects more inefficient than the younger subjects. However, with more challenging stimuli that are more difficult to encode we were able to demonstrate a capacity difference, with increased capacity of the younger subjects' brain network accompanied by superior performance. We are still investigating the implications of differential expression of these networks within each group. For example, what are the implications of one younger subject being able to recruit the network noted during shape encoding to a greater degree than another subject? One possibility is that this increased capacity may put this subject in a better position to confront age-related changes in the brain and maintain function.

3. If young and old subjects use a different network, what is the nature of the compensatory activation? Are individual differences in eliciting the compensatory activation associated with CR?

This question gets to the implementation of neural compensation. This different network can take several forms. One possibility is that the impaired group uses a completely different set of brain areas (or network) than the unimpaired group. Another possibility is that the impaired group continues to use the same brain areas, but that the relationship between activation in these areas is reorganized. Note that the term "neural compensation" does not imply that the alternate mode of processing is associated with improved task performance. While this is an important question to be asked in regard to a compensatory network, demonstrating a relationship between differential expression of a compensatory network and superior performance is not required. That is because it is possible that a compensatory network could serve to maintain performance when the network that usually mediates performance is damaged. In this case, network expression might not be associated with superior performance, but simply with the maintenance of the ability to perform.

Of course, this does not eliminate the possibility that a compensatory network can be associated with superior performance. In the "compensatory reallocation" model, those who make use of a compensatory network perform better than those who do not. An example of this is the hemispheric asymmetry reduction in older adults or HAROLD hypothesis (Cabeza, 2002). In summary, this hypothesis posits that better-functioning older adults will evidence additional compensatory activation in homologous areas contralateral to those typically activated by younger adults. In contrast, poorer functioning elders will not evidence this compensatory activation.

One PET study (Stern et al., 2005) examined the nonverbal serial recognition task described above in 17 young adults and 19 healthy elderly adults. The cognitive reserve variable that we used in this study was a factor score that summarized years of education and scores on two IQ indices—the NART and WAIS-R vocabulary scores. Subjects were scanned while performing the low- and titrated-demand tasks. We use covariance analysis to identify a set of functionally connected regions that changed in expression across the two task conditions and were differentially expressed by the young and elderly subjects. That is, this analysis specifically sought out a covariance pattern that was differentially expressed by the two groups, and therefore represents altered task-related activation in the older subjects. The regions most active in this brain network consisted of right hippocampus, posterior insula, thalamus, and right and left operculum; and concomitant deactivation in right lingual gyrus, inferior parietal lobe, association cortex, left posterior cingulate, and right and left calcarine cortex.

Since young subjects operate without the burden of any age-related physiologic changes, we began by evaluating expression of this network in the young group. The mean expression of this network in the young subjects was lower than that in the old subjects, but the correlation between network expression and reserve was positive. Thus, in the transition from low- to titrated-demand conditions, the higher their level of CR, the more young subjects increased their activation in regions with positive loadings, with concomitantly decreased activation in regions with negative loadings. The differential utilization of this topography by young subjects as a function of CR is consistent with our prediction of the behavior of a neural reserve network.

In the elder subjects, the correlation between the CR index and their expression of the age-related topography was negative. That is, the higher their level of CR, the more old subjects increased their activation in regions with negative loadings and decreased their activation in regions with positive loadings in the transition from low- to titrated-demand conditions. Thus, as in the young subjects, individual differences in elder subjects' network expression in response to increased task demand correlated with a measure of CR. However, the direction of this relationship was the opposite of that seen in the young subjects.

Since the young subjects have no age-related neural changes, we can speculate that the different relationship between CR and topographic expression in the two groups is due to some age-related physiological change in the older subjects. As a response to these changes, and perhaps as a function of longer-term brain adaptation, the older subjects make use of an altered network, causing the activation of the regions captured in the covariance pattern to switch signs. This results in higher CR being associated with increased utilization of some brain areas, with more positive network expression in one group, and more negative expression in the other. The age-related changes in network expression are thus most consistent with our definition of neural compensation.

We also noted evidence of neural compensation in the analyses of the Sternberg letter task described above, where 40 young subjects and 18 old subjects' activation data were evaluated (Zarahn et al., 2007). As mentioned above, we noted in those analyses that load-related activation during the stimulus and probe phases could be characterized by one spatial pattern, while activation during the retention phase of the task could be best characterized by two spatial patterns. The first pattern was used by both young and old subjects, and consisted of areas often associated with working memory (Figure 6.6a). Regions that increased with memory load included the mid-line cerebellum,

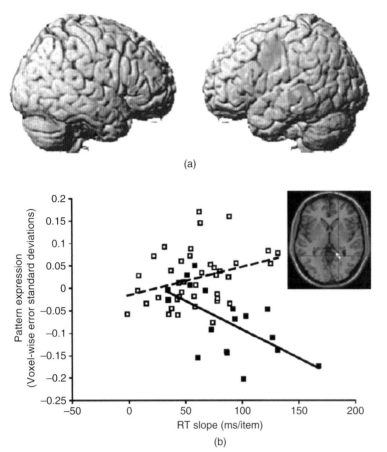

Figure 6–6 (**a**) Scaled first latent spatial pattern (red: positive voxel weights; green: negative voxel weights) for slope of fMRI response amplitude vs. set size associated with memory set retention delay. (**b**) Observed expressions of latent spatial pattern 2 of load-dependent processing (i.e., fMRI slope) during the retention delay are plotted vs. RT slope; elder (filled square), young (open square). An axial slice of the suprathreshold negative spatial weights of latent spatial pattern 2 is shown as an inset.

left insula/inferior frontal gyrus, left hippocampus, right middle/superior frontal gyri, left inferior/middle frontal gyri into the precentral gyrus, left inferior/superior parietal lobule, right cingulate gyrus into medial/superior frontal gyri, and left medial/superior gyri. Regions in the mid-line cingulate, left medial/superior temporal gyri, right medial frontal gyrus, and left cingulate gyrus signal decreased with increased working memory load. In contrast, the second pattern was used only by the older subjects (Figure 6.6b). The primary brain area in this pattern that increased expression with memory load was the right parahippocampal gyrus (and left parahippocampal gyrus at a slightly less stringent alpha level), although in the case of any spatial pattern, all areas of the brain are weighted to different degrees as being part of that pattern. Interestingly, the more older subjects used this additional network, the poorer their performance was on the task (Figure 6.6b). In the original article describing these results, we considered two alternate explanations for this observation. The first was that this additional activation in the elders represents dedifferentiation. The concept of dedifferentiation suggests that regional processing specification decreases with aging due to increased levels of noise or decreased levels of functional integration (Li, Lindenberger, and Sikstrom, 2001) (Rajah and D'Esposito, 2005). One might argue that since the more older subjects use this second network the poorer they perform, use of this network cannot be considered compensatory, and is consistent with dedifferentiation. An alternate view is that use of the second network is compensatory. According to this view, this network is needed to maintain function because age-related neural changes impair the efficacy of the first network. Those individuals who need to use the second network more are doing so because the

first network is more impaired. Thus, compensation in this case would be associated with maintenance of function as opposed to improved function. Testing this idea requires some measure of age-related neural change. The prediction would be that individuals who express the second network are more likely to have age-related neural change that impairs the performance of the primary network.

In recent analyses (Steffener et al., 2009), we used voxel-based morphometry to measure gray matter density in subjects who participated in the study. The idea was to consider brain atrophy a proxy for age-related neural changes. These analyses demonstrated that increased expression of the second network is correlated with focal atrophy (i.e., reduced rate matter density) in the left precentral gyrus of the primary network. Thus, greater activation of the second network was seen in elders whose expression of the first common network was most impaired. This observation lends support to the idea of a compensatory network that is not necessarily associated with improved performance.

4. Is there some unique, CR-related activation that is independent of the specific demands of the task at hand?

To this point I have discussed how variability in task-related activation might give clues to the nature of CR. That is, we are positing that CR is mediated by differential expression of the networks typically used to mediate task performance, or by differential recruitment of new compensatory networks in the face of brain damage. Since this approach centers around the networks that directly underlie task performance, it does not address an alternate concept of how CR is neurally mediated. Since CR allows someone to cope for a longer time with aging or AD pathology, it is unlikely that the brain networks subserving cognitive reserve are equivalent to those that are required to perform any particular task. Rather, it is more likely that a more general "cognitive reserve network" would be elicited by many tasks. By subserving some general (as opposed to task-specific) function, CR might allow someone to cope with pathology and maintain effective functioning for a longer period of time. Since the nature and underlying cognitive operations of such a network are not clear, the task at hand might be described as studying the relationship between task-related brain activation and proxies for CR, as opposed to performance of the task itself.

We have addressed this question by using CR proxies as covariates in our imaging analyses. This allows us to study the aspects of task-related activation that vary as a function of CR, whether or not this activation is directly associated with measures of performance on the activation task. Furthermore, in one study we sought to determine whether such CR-related activation could be noted across two tasks with different processing demands. That is, could we derive a generic CR network that might be operating across multiple tasks?

Two analyses of data from our continuous nonverbal recognition task investigated activation during the performance of that task that correlated with the measurement of CR. We explored how individual differences in CR are related to changes in neural activity as the subjects move from the low- to the titrated-demand task. Our prediction was that certain aspects of task-related activation would be related to CR. The first study (Stern et al., 2003) used 19 healthy young adults between the ages of 18 and 30. We used the NART raw score as a proxy measure for CR. The data analysis approach in this study was to do a voxel-wise comparison to find brain areas in which the change in event-related fMRI response amplitude from low- to titrated-demand conditions (T-L) correlated with an individual subject's NART scores. During the study phase of the task (i.e., when subjects were viewing the shapes to remember them later), positive correlations between T-L and NART were seen in the left middle frontal gyrus, and negative correlations were seen in the right superior frontal gyrus, middle frontal gyrus, precentral gyrus, medial frontal gyrus, and insular. We also found brain areas that showed correlations between task-related activation and NART scores during the recognition phase of the task. Thus, the primary finding of this study was that, both during study and during subsequent retrieval, brain areas were noted where there was a systematic relationship between CR and brain activation. These correlations point to aspects of processing that differ as a function of CR in healthy young adults. Note that the aspects of task-related activation that correlated with CR are not necessarily those that would be seen in an analysis that simply focused on areas whose activation changed from the simple to the titrated-demand condition. Therefore, this analytic approach might yield more direct information about the neural implementation of CR.

The second analysis (Scarmeas et al., 2003b) used the same nonverbal activation task. In this study, we used PET to study 17 young and 19 elderly healthy subjects and again, we use NART and WAIS-R scores as a cognitive reserved variable. This study used a similar analytic approach to that described above. We searched for voxels in which there was a correlation between the CR measure and the change in activation from the low- to the titrated-demand condition. As in our initial study, areas where such a correlation is found would be likely candidates for mediating CR. Indeed, we found such areas both in the young and old subjects. The more crucial analysis (from a theoretical point of view) was to search for areas in which the relationship between task-related activation and CR differed in young and old subjects. For example, the relationship between task-related activation and CR in the cingulate gyrus was positive in the young subjects, and negative in the old. If we assume that people with more CR are doing a task in a more optimal manner, then the positive relationship in the young would suggest that it is more adaptive to show increased activation at this brain location as a task gets more difficult. However, the older subjects with more reserve are doing exactly the opposite. This finding suggests that there has been some reorganization of the brain areas underlying CR in the old subjects vs. the young subjects. We hypothesized that the source of this change in brain utilization is the age-related neural changes in the older group. Thus, this study points to a set of brain areas associated with CR that differ between the old and young.

In the two analyses described to this point, we explored the neural implementation of CR by examining the relationships between task-related activation and putative proxies for CR, including IQ measures. However, these relationships were explored only within single tasks. In another study (Stern et al., 2008), we sought to determine whether there is a network subserving CR that was active across tests of verbal and object working memory, each of which has differing cognitive-processing demands. Young and elder subjects were scanned with fMRI while performing one of two versions of the Sternberg task; one version used letters as the stimuli to be encoded and recognized, while the other used shapes that were difficult to name. Load-dependent fMRI signal corresponding to each trial component (i.e., stimulus presentation, retention delay, and probe) and task (letter or shape) were regressed onto putative CR variables. We then used multivariate linear modeling, separately for each trial component, to summarize the imaging data – CR relationships. We wished to determine if there were patterns of CR-related brain activity whose latent predictors had similar and sizeable contributions from both the letter and shape tasks. Such a pattern, expressed across two tasks with divergent processing demands, would be a likely candidate for a generic neural substrate underlying CR.

In each phase, a CR-related pattern was identified that was expressed only during performance of the letter task. Of more interest to the intent of this current analysis, in the young group, a second spatial pattern was identified in the stimulus presentation phase that manifested similar relationships between CR and load-related activation across both the letter and shape working memory (WM) tasks (Figure 6.7). In the elder group, expression of this pattern as a function of CR differed in directionality across the two tasks, indicating that it was not expressed consistently across the two tasks as a function of CR.

These analyses focused on identifying spatial patterns of activation that systematically differ as a function of CR. The derived spatial patterns therefore have no relationship with the neural networks associated with the specific demands of the stimulus presentation, retention delay, or probe phases of these two types of Sternberg tasks. Separate analyses demonstrated that the stimulus presentation phase activated different brain areas in the letter and shape tasks. This would be expected given the divergent demands associated with processing verbal and nonverbal stimuli.

Similarly, the analysis did not concern itself with whether differential expression of a CR-related spatial pattern is associated

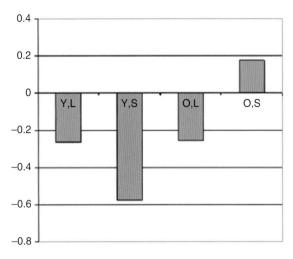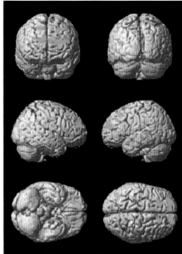

Figure 6–7   The spatial pattern identified during the encoding phase that was expressed as both a verbal and spatial task as a function of CR. A plot of the latent predictor weights for each of the independent variables in the model is presented. Codes for the variables are Y = young; E = Elder; L = letter; S = shape. The surface rendering of the positively (red) and negatively (green) weighted aspects of the spatial pattern is also presented. In young subjects, pattern expression was negatively related to the CR scores in both the letter and shape tasks. This indicates that brain areas with negative weights showed increased expression with increasing levels of CR in both tasks. Similar directionality of pattern expression was noted for the elders during performance of the letter but not the shape task, and the degree of pattern expression did not reach significance in the elders.

with better or worse performance. In fact, we explicitly eliminated the possibility of such a relationship in the analytic design. This reduces the chance that CR-related network expression is influenced by differences in performance across individuals. We relied on the processing effort in these tasks (by looking at load-related activation) to elicit CR-related networks independent of performance. This means that a high-CR young person, although badly performing in a high-demand task, will still show a pure instantiation of the CR-network. The inference that we wish to draw is that these networks might represent the neural instantiation of CR, or alternately that the ability to invoke these networks might underlie the benefits that CR imparts. Because this pattern reflects a CR-related network that is used by healthy individuals, it meets our previously proposed criteria for neural reserve (Stern et al., 2005).

Older subjects' expression of this pattern did not reach significance. This may be due to more limited power in detecting a relationship between CR and pattern expression in this smaller group (N = 18 for elders vs. 40 for the young subjects). Still, it is of interest to note that with the elders, pattern expression was not consistent across the two tasks. Notably, the direction of pattern expression was similar to that in the young subjects for the letter task, but not the shape task. Follow-up studies are needed to test the idea that the CR-related pattern can be used by elders in the simpler letter task, but not in the more challenging shape task.

Many of the areas included in the common CR pattern here have been noted in studies of control processes, such as task-switching (Braver, Reynolds, and Donaldson, 2003; Wager, Jonides, and Reading, 2003), as well as in some studies of working memory (Wager and Smith, 2006). In the fMRI study described above, using a continuous recognition task for nonverbal stimuli (Stern et al., 2003), we found several of the same areas noted here were differentially activated as a function of CR during both the encoding and retrieval phases of the task. As in the current study, increased expression of these areas was associated with higher measured CR. These consistent findings across studies and tasks

provide a preliminary suggestion that control processes may be an important component of some aspects of CR.

In summary, in young (but not old) subjects, a spatial pattern or brain network was noted whose expression as task load increases correlates with measures of CR during performance of a verbal and a object-working memory task. This network, therefore, appears to represent a nontask-specific neural instantiation of CR—more specifically, of neural reserve.

This study raises two important sets of questions that must be addressed in future studies. First, it will be of interest to see if expression of this CR-related network by younger subjects can be detected during the performance of tasks not used in the current study. If the network is expressed across multiple tasks, it would support the idea that it mediates a general feature of CR.

Perhaps more important is determining whether differential expression of this pattern actually imparts reserve against the neural effects of aging. One way to address this question would be to measure the expression of this network in a set of younger subjects, and then follow them over time, with the prediction that higher expression will predict slower progression of age-related cognitive changes. An alternate approach is to develop measures of age-related pathology. Higher expression should then able to counteract the effects of age-related pathology.

Conclusions

In summary, there is strong epidemiologic evidence for the idea that CR mediates between brain changes or pathology, and the clinical manifestation of that pathology. The concept of CR strongly relies on the idea that there can be individual differences in how tasks are processed that can allow some people to cope better than others with brain changes in general, and aging in particular. This chapter presents a systematic approach for exploring the neural implementation of CR. The approach recognizes that reserve may be mediated in many different ways. Neural reserve recognizes that old and young individuals may use the same networks to mediate task performance, albeit with different levels of efficiency and capacity. This inter-individual variability is present even within these two groups, and differences in neural reserve may be one mechanism underlying cognitive reserve. On the other hand, there are clearly situations where older individuals adopt new, compensatory networks, pre-sumably in response to age-related changes in the brain. This neural compensation again can vary across individuals in its expression and success. Evaluating neural compensation in imaging studies is often hampered by the difficulty in measuring the underlying results in compensation. Simply relating the degree of expression of compen-satory activation to performance is not sufficient. As demonstrated above, compensatory activation can be accompanied by both better and poorer performance. In either case, CR might also be mediated in part via neural compensation.

Another key consideration is whether reserve is mediated via variability in the expression of the specific brain networks associated with the task at hand, or whether there may be one or more general reserve-related networks whose expression is associated with CR across many different tasks. This translates into the question of whether CR is task-specific, or represents some generalized cognitive function that is associated with the performance of multiple tasks. The epidemiologic evidence suggests that a set of lifetime exposures translates into a cognitive reserve that mediates the brain changes associated with aging or AD. This makes it attractive to speculate that a general reserve-related network may be identified.

This issue is also is important for considering whether it will be possible to intervene to impart increased CR and thereby slow the effects of advancing age or AD pathology. Research-to-date suggests that cognitive training only benefits the task used in training itself and does not generalize to other tasks or behaviors. For example, in the Advanced Cognitive Training for Independent and Vital Elderly (ACTIVE) study, a national sample of 2,802 older adults were randomly assigned to receive memory training, proces-sing speed training, reasoning training, or no training (i.e., non-contact control group) over ten 60- to 75-minute training sessions. While domain-specific improvements in cognitive function were noted, the improvements did not transfer to other domains (e.g., receiving training in processing speed did not also convey improvements on reasoning scores) and also did not improve the participants' ability to perform everyday tasks such as food preparation, driving, or handling medications (Ball et al., 2002).

Better understanding of the neural mediation of CR may provide suggestions for targets and approaches for increasing CR and improving performance across a range of tasks. The possibility of using an imaging approach to measure CR would also have other practical implications. Imaging could then be used as a meaningful outcome in cognitive interventions. It would also be important for understanding an individual's true clinical status at any age, which would be some combination of underlying age-related brain changes and that individual's CR in the face of those changes. Two individuals who appear the same clinically could differ widely on those underlying measures, and this could have strong implications for prognosis and treatment. These considerations underline the importance of continued investigation of the neural representation of cognitive reserve.

Acknowledgements

This work was supported by a grant from the National Institutes on Aging (RO1 AG26158).

References

Albert, M. S., Jones, K., Savage, C. R., Berkman, L., Seeman, T., Blazer, D. et al. (1995). Predictors of cognitive change in older persons: MacArthur studies of successful aging. *Psychology and Aging*, 10: 578–589.

Albert, S. M. and Teresi, J. A. (1999). Reading ability, education, and cognitive status assessment among older adults in Harlem, New York City. *American Journal of Public Health*, 89: 95–97.

Alexander, G. E., Furey, M. L., Grady, C. L., Pietrini, P., Mentis, M. J., and Schapiro, M. B. (1997). Association of premorbid function with cerebral metabolism in Alzheimer's disease: Implications for the reserve hypoth-esis. *American Journal of Psychiatry*, 154: 165–172.

Ball, K., Berch, D. B., Helmers, K. F., Jobe, J. B., Leveck, M. D., Marsiske, M. et al. (2002). Effects of cognitive training interventions with older adults: a randomized controlled trial. *Journal of the American Medical Association*, 288: 2271–2281.

Bennett, D. A., Wilson, R. S., Schneider, J. A., Evans, D. A., Mendes De Leon, C. F., Arnold, S. E. et al. (2003). Education modifies the relation of AD pathology to level of cognitive function in older persons. *Neurology*, 60(12): 1909–1915.

Braver, T. S., Reynolds, J. R., and Donaldson, D. I. (2003). Neural mechanisms of transients and sustained cognitive control during task switching. *Neuron*, 39: 713–726.

Brown, J., Cooper-Kuhn, C. M., Kemperman, G., van Praag, H., Winkler, J., and Gage, F. H. (2003). Enriched environment and physical activity stimulate hippocampal but not olfactory bulb neurogenesis. *European Journal of Neuroscience*, 17: 2042–2046.

Butler, S. M., Ashford, J. W., and Snowdon, D. A. (1996). Age, education, and changes in the Mini-Mental State Exam scores of older women: findings from the Nun Study. *Journal of the American Geriatrics Society*, 44: 675–681.

Cabeza, R. (2002). Hemispheric asymmetry reduction in older adults: The HAROLD model. *Psychology & Aging*, 17: 85–100.

Chodosh, J., Reuben, D. B., Albert, M. S., and Seeman, T. E. (2002). Predicting cognitive impairment in high-functioning community-dwelling older persons: MacArthur Studies of Successful Aging. *Journal of the American Geriatrics Society*, 50: 1051–1060.

Christensen, H., Korten, A. E., Jorm, A. F., Henderson, A. S., Jacomb, P. A., Rodgers, B. et al. (1997). Education and decline in cognitive performance: Compensatory but not protective. *International Journal of Geriatric Psychiatry*, 12: 323–330.

Colsher, P. L. and Wallace, R. B. (1991). Longitudinal application of cognitive function measures in a defined population of community-dwelling elders. *Annals of Epidemiology*, 1: 215–230.

DeCarli, C., Atack, J. R., Ball, M. J., Kay, J. A., Grady, C. L., Fewster, P. et al. (1992). Post-mortem regional neurofibrillary tangle densities but not senile plaque densities are related to regional cerebral metabolic rates for glucose during life in Alzheimer's disease patients. *Neurodegeneration*, 1: 113–121.

Evans, D. A., Beckett, L. A., Albert, M. S., Hebert, L. E., Scherr, P. A., Funkenstein, H. H. et al. (1993). Level of education and change in cognitive function in a community population of older persons. *Annals of Epidemiology*, 3: 71–77.

Farmer, M. E., Kittner, S. J., Rae, D. S., Bartko, J. J., and Regier, D. A. (1995). Education and change in cognitive function: The epidemiologic catch-ment area study. *Annals of Epidemiology*, 5: 1–7.

Friedland, R. P., Brun, A., and Bundinger, T. F. (1985). Pathological and positron emission tomographic correlations in Alzheimer's disease. *Lancet*, 1–228.

Geerlings, M. I., Deeg, D. J. H., Penninx, B. W., Schmand, B., Jonker, C., Bouter, L. M. et al. (1999). Cognitive reserve and mortality in dementia: The role of cognition, functional ability and depression. *Psychological Medicine*, 29: 1219–1226.

Geerlings, M. I., Deeg, D. J. H., Schmand, B., Lindeboom, J., and Jonker, C. (1997). Increased risk of mortality in Alzheimer's disease patients with higher education? A replication study. *Neurology*, 49: 798–802.

Habeck, C., Hilton, H. J., Zarahn, E., Flynn, J., Moeller, J. R., and Stern, Y. (2003). Relation of cognitive reserve and task performance to expression of regional covariance networks in an event-related fMRI study of non-verbal memory. *Neuroimage*, 20: 1723–1733.

Habeck, C., Krakauer, J. W., Ghez, C., Sackeim, H. A., Eidelberg, D., Stern, Y. et al. (2005). A new approach to spatial covariance modeling of functional brain imaging data: Ordinal trend analysis. *Neural Computation*, 17: 1602–1645.

Habeck, C., Rakitin, B. C., Moeller, J., Scarmeas, N., Zarahn, E., Brown, T. et al. (2005). An event-related fMRI study of the neural networks underlying the encoding, maintenance, and retrieval phase in a delayed-match-to-sample task. *Brain Research Cognitive Brain Research*, 23: 207–220.

Ince, P. G. (2001). Pathological correlates of late-onset dementia in a multicenter community-based population in England and Wales. *Lancet*, 357: 169–175.

Katzman, R. (1993). Education and the prevalence of dementia and Alzheimer's disease. *Neurology*, 43: 13–20.

Katzman, R., Aronson, M., Fuld, P., Kawas, C., Brown, T., Morgenstern, H. et al. (1989). Development of dementing illnesses in an 80-year-old volunteer cohort. *Annals of Neurology*, 25: 317–324.

Kesler, S. R., Adams, H. F., Blasey, C. M., and Bigler.E. D. (2003). Premorbid intellectual functioning, education, and brain size in traumatic brain injury: An investigation of the cognitive reserve hypothesis. *Applied Neuropsychology*, 10: 153–162.

Lazarov, O., Robinson, J., Tang, Y. P., Hairston, I. S., Korade-Mirnics, Z., Lee, V. M. et al. (2005). Environmental enrichment reduces Abeta levels and amyloid deposition in transgenic mice. *Cell*, 120: 701–713.

Li, S. C., Lindenberger, U., and Sikstrom, S. (2001). Aging cognition: from neuromodulation to representation. *Trends Cognitive Science*, 5: 479–486.

Lyketsos, C. G., Chen, L.-S., and Anthony, J. C. (1999). Cognitive decline in adulthood: An 11.5-year follow-up of the Baltimore epidemiologic catchment area study. *American Journal of Psychiatry*, 156: 58–65.

Manly, J. J., Schupf, N., Tang, M. X., and Stern, Y. (2005). Cognitive decline and literacy among ethnically diverse elders. *Journal of Geriatic Psychiatry and Neurology*, 18: 213–217.

Manly, J. J., Touradji, P., Tang, M.-X., and Stern, Y. (2003). Literacy and memory decline among ethnically diverse elders. *Journal of Clinical and Experimental Neuropsychology*, 5: 680–690.

McGeer, E. G., McGeer, P. L., Harrop, R., Akiyama, H., and Kamo, H. (1990). Correlations of regional postmortem enzyme activities with premortem local glucose metabolic rates in Alzheimer's disease. *Journal of Neuroscience Research*, 27: 612–619.

Mortel, K. F., Meyer, J. S., Herod, B., and Thornby, J. (1995). Education and occupation as risk factors for dementia of the Alzheimer and ischemic vascular types. *Dementia*, 6: 55–62.

Rajah, M. N. and D'Esposito, M. (2005). Region-specific changes in prefrontal function with age: A review of PET and fMRI studies on working and episodic memory. *Brain*, 128: 1964–1983.

Richards, M. and Sacker, A. (2003). Lifetime antecedents of cognitive reserve. *Journal of Clinical and Experimental Neuropsychology*, 25: 614–624.

Rocca, W. A., Bonaiuto, S., Lippi, A., Luciani, P., Turtu, F., Cavarzeran, F. et al. (1990). Prevalence of clinically diagnosed Alzheimer's disease and other dementing disorders: A door-to-door survey in Appignano, Macerata Province, Italy. *Neurology*, 40: 626–631.

Rypma, B., Prabhakaran, V., Desmond, J. E., Glover, G. H., and Gabrieli, J. D. (1999). Load-dependent roles of frontal brain regions in the maintenance of working memory. *Neuroimage*, 9: 216–226.

Satz, P. (1993). Brain reserve capacity on symptom onset after brain injury: A formulation and review of evidence for threshold theory. *Neuropsychology*, 7: 273–295.

Scarmeas, N., Albert, S. M., Manly, J., Stern, Y. (2006). Education and rates of cognitive decline in incident Alzheimer's disease. *Journal of Neurology, Neurosurgery, and Psychiatry*, 77: 308–316.

Scarmeas, N., Zarahn, E., Anderson, K. E., Habeck, C. G., Hilton, J., Flynn, J. et al. (2003a). Association of life activities with cerebral blood flow in Alzheimer disease – Implications for the cognitive reserve hypothesis. *Archives of Neurology*, 60: 359–365.

Scarmeas, N., Zarahn, E., Anderson, K. E., Hilton, H. J., Flynn, J., Van Heertum, R. L. et al. (2003b). Cognitive reserve modulates functional brain responses during memory tasks: A PET study in healthy young and elderly subjects. *Neuroimage*, 19: 1215–1227.

Snowdon, D. A., Ostwald, S. K., and Kane, R. L. (1989). Education, survival and independence in elderly Catholic sisters, 1936-1988. *American Journal of Epidemiology*, 130: 999–1012.

Steffener, J., Brickman, A. M., Rakitin, B. C., Gazes, Y., and Stern, Y. (2009). The impact of structure on age-related changes in working memory functional activity. *Brain Imaging and Behavior*, doi:10.1007/s11682-008-9056-x.

Stern, Y. (2002). What is cognitive reserve? Theory and research application of the reserve concept. *Journal of the International Neuropsychological Society*, 8: 448–460.

Stern, Y. (2006). Cognitive reserve and Alzheimer disease. *Alzheimer Disorder Association Disorder*, 20: 112–117.

Stern, Y., Albert, S., Tang, M. X., and Tsai, W. Y. (1999). Rate of memory decline in AD is related to education and occupation: Cognitive reserve? *Neurology*, 53: 1942–1957.

Stern, Y., Alexander, G. E., Prohovnik, I., and Mayeux, R. (1992). Inverse relationship between education and parietotemporal perfusion deficit in Alzheimer's disease. *Annals of Neurology*, 32: 371–375.

Stern, Y., Alexander, G. E., Prohovnik, I., Stricks, L., Link, B., Lennon, M. C. et al. (1995). Relationship between lifetime occupation and parietal flow: Implications for a reserve against Alzheimer's disease pathology. *Neurology*, 45: 55–60.

Stern, Y., Gurland, B., Tatemichi, T. K., Tang, M. X., Wilder, D., and Mayeux, R. (1994). Influence of education and occupation on the incidence of Alzheimer's disease. *Journal of the American Medical Association*, 271: 1004–1010.

Stern, Y., Habeck, C., Moeller, J., Scarmeas, N., Anderson, K. E., Hilton, H. J. et al. (2005). Brain networks associated with cognitive reserve in healthy young and old adults. *Cereb.Cortex*, 15: 394–402.

Stern, Y., Moeller, J. R., Anderson, K. E., Luber, B., Zubin, N., Dimauro, A. et al. (2000). Different brain networks mediate task performance in normal aging and AD: Defining compensation. *Neurology*, 55: 1291–1297.

Stern, Y., Tang, M. X., Denaro, J., and Mayeux, R. (1995). Increased risk of mortality in Alzheimer's disease patients with more advanced educational and occupational attainment. *Annals of Neurology*, 37: 590–595.

Stern, Y., Zarahn, E., Habeck, C., Holtzer, R., Rakitin, B. C., Kumar, A. et al. (2008). A common neural network for cognitive reserve in verbal and object working memory in young but not old. *Cerebral Cortex*, 18: 959–967.

Stern, Y., Zarahn, E., Hilton, H. J., Delapaz, R., Flynn, J., and Rakitin, B. (2003). Exploring the neural basis of cognitive reserve. *Journal of Clinical and Experimental Neuropsychology*, 5: 691–701.

Valenzuela, M. J. and Sachdev, P. (2005). Brain reserve and dementia: a systematic review. *Psychological Medicine*, 35: 1–14.

van Praag, H., Shubert, T., Zhao, C., and Gage, F. H. (2005). Exercise enhances learning and hippocampal neurogenesis in aged mice. *Journal of Neuroscience*, 25: 8680–8685.

Wager, T. D., Jonides, J., and Reading, S. (2003). Neuroimaging of shifting attention: A meta-analysis. *Neuroimage*, 22: 1679–1693.

Wager, T. D. and Smith, E. E. (2006). Neuroimaging studies of working memory: A meta-analysis. *Cognitive, Affective, and Behavioral Neuroscience*, 3: 255–274.

Willerman, L., Schultz, R., Rutledge, J. N., and Bigler. E. D. (1991). In vivo brain size and intelligence. *Intelligence*, 15: 223–228.

Zarahn, E., Rakitin, B., Abela, D., Flynn, J., and Stern, Y. (2007). Age-related changes in brain activation during a delayed item recognition task. *Neurobiological Aging*, 28: 784–798.

7

Compensatory Reorganization of Brain Networks in Older Adults

Cheryl L. Grady

Introduction

Age differences in cognitive function have been studied for many years, with much of this work focusing on memory. This rich literature has shown that older adults have particular difficulty with episodic memory, defined as the conscious recollection of events that have occurred in a person's experience (Tulving, 1983). In the laboratory, these age differences in episodic memory are seen in a reduced ability to learn and retrieve both verbal and nonverbal material, such as a list of words (for a review see Craik and Bosman, 1992). Reductions in recall of real-life, autobiographical memories have also been reported (Levine et al., 2002; Piolino et al., 2002). Age-related difficulties in episodic memory may be related to deficits in encoding new material (Craik and Byrd, 1982), as well as reductions in how well information can be retrieved (Burke and Light, 1981). Substantial age-related declines also are seen in working memory tasks (for reviews see Balota, Dolan, and Duchek, 2000; Zacks, Hasher, and Li, 2000), but semantic memory, or the accumulation of knowledge about the world, is maintained in older adults (Craik and Jennings, 1992).

In recent years, functional neuroimaging has been used to study how these differences in memory between young and old adults are expressed in terms of brain activity. When brain activity in young and older adults is compared on a task, there are at least three possible outcomes in any given brain area: (1) young and old groups could have equivalent brain activity, (2) older adults could show less activity, or (3) older adults could show greater activity. Reduced activity in the elderly can reasonably be assumed to reflect a reduced level of functioning, particularly when accompanied by poorer performance on the task. Equivalent activity is generally considered evidence for spared function in the elderly, although if performance is lower in the older group this may indicate reduced neural efficiency (Zarahn et al., 2007). The major challenge facing researchers in this field is how to interpret increased recruitment of brain regions in older subjects as compared to younger participants. From the earliest experiments in this field (e.g., Grady et al., 1994), it was clear that age differences in brain activity patterns could take the form of both decreases and increases of activity in older adults compared to their younger counterparts, with increases found frequently in the prefrontal cortex. This led to the suggestion that increased frontal activity can compensate for reduced activity elsewhere in the brain (Cabeza et al., 1997; Grady et al., 1994). Much of the subsequent work has continued to explore this idea; indeed many, if not most, of the published

neuroimaging papers on cognitive aging have interpreted at least some aspect of their results in the context of compensatory mechanisms, either as evidence for or against the idea. The best evidence for compensation would be to find a direct link between task performance and activity in a region that is over-recruited by older adults. A number of experiments have taken this approach, whereas others claim compensation when performance in young and old adults is equivalent but the older adults still activate some brain area more than the younger adults. At the current time, it seems safe to state that at least some age-related differences in brain activity are likely to be compensatory, but certainly one cannot make this claim for all such differences. In this review, the evidence supporting the notion of compensatory brain activity in older adults will be assessed, as well as evidence that speaks against this interpretation.

Evidence for Compensation in Aging

From the first PET experiment comparing younger and older adults, in this case using a series of perceptual tasks (Grady et al., 1992, 1994), there was evidence that older adults exhibited increased prefrontal activity to a greater degree than younger adults in response to cognitive tasks. Since that time, there has been ample support for this finding, particularly during memory tasks, from both PET and fMRI experiments (e.g., Cabeza et al., 2004; Grady, McIntosh, and Craik, 2005; Gutchess et al., 2005; Madden et al., 1999; Morcom et al., 2003; Reuter-Lorenz et al., 2000). However, simply finding increased activity in older adults as compared to younger adults is not necessarily evidence for a compensatory mechanism. To search for evidence in favor of a compensation hypothesis, one approach that has been taken is to determine the relationship between prefrontal activity and task performance in older adults. If the older adults who perform better on memory tasks recruit the prefrontal cortex to a greater degree than those performing less well, this would suggest that increased frontal activity can compensate for some of the structural and functional changes that occur in the brains of older people. Such findings have been reported in a number of studies, including those in which the older sample is divided into high and low performing groups (Cabeza et al., 2002), and those that use an individual differences approach to correlating performance measures and prefrontal activity (Grady et al., 2003, 2005).

Another approach is to match the performance in young and old groups so that any age-related increases in brain activity cannot be attributed to differences in ability to perform the task per se, and thus are more likely to be compensatory. Several recent studies of this type have lent support to the compensation hypothesis, and have done so in a variety of cognitive domains. In the realm of attentional processes, Madden et al. (2007) utilized a visual search task and found more reliance on a top-down frontoparietal attention network in older adults, whereas young adults utilized the occipital cortex to a greater extent. They suggested that this may reflect compensation for a decline in the efficiency of bottom-up processes mediated by visual cortical regions, allowing older adults to maintain performance at the level of younger adults. Recent evidence in the memory domain comes from Daselaar et al. (2006), who used a verbal recognition task to assess recollection and familiarity, and matched performance on a subject-by-subject basis in the two age groups. They found a disassociation within the medial temporal lobes between recollection-related activity in hippocampus, which was reduced in older adults, and familiarity-related activity in the rhinal cortex, which was increased in older adults relative to the younger group. Older adults also showed reduced functional connectivity within a hippocampal-parietotemporal network, but increased connectivity within a rhinal-frontal network. The authors interpreted these findings as evidence that older adults compensate for hippocampal deficits by relying more on rhinal cortex, possibly through a top-down frontal modulation. Nielson et al. (2006) looked at a task tapping semantic memory for famous people, in which there were no group differences in accuracy of performance, and both young and old adults scored at better than 90% accuracy levels. Both groups engaged a number of regions during the task, including posterior cingulate, right hippocampus, temporal lobe, and left prefrontal regions. Older adults had more extensive and greater magnitude of activation in the left prefrontal cortex. The results of these three studies support the idea that older adults use additional functional recruitment to support task performance, particularly in frontal regions, even when the task is a relatively easy one. In addition, this support is boosted by the fact that there were no confounding performance differences related to age.

In some studies, investigators have been able to compare brain activity between young and old adults on memory tasks where performance is the same, as well as tasks where the older group performs more poorly. In this case, if older adults have an over-recruitment of the prefrontal cortex in both kinds of tasks, then this activity is less likely to be due solely to reduced performance per se, and more likely to be a true age difference that may be compensatory. In one such study, Fernandes et al. (2006) compared young and old adults on verbal recognition memory tasks under both full and divided attention. Older adults were less accurate in the full-attention condition, but showed the same amount of memory interference as young adults during the divided-attention condition. The older adults had more prefrontal activation than young adults during both conditions, although the location of this over-recruitment was in dorsolateral prefrontal cortex during the full-attention condition, and in ventral prefrontal cortex during the divided-attention condition (Figure 7.1a). Fernandes et al. concluded that the increased frontal activity in older adults during retrieval under full attention could be influenced by task difficulty, as the older adults performed more poorly than the younger group. However, increased prefrontal activity in older adults during the divided attention condition is unlikely to reflect task difficulty or simple performance differences, because the interference effects were the same in both younger and older groups. A second study used a 1-back task to assess working memory for spatial (sound

location) and nonspatial (sound category) auditory information in young and older adults (Grady, Yu, and Alain, 2008). Older adults were less accurate on the category task, but there was no age difference on the location task. In both groups, there was increased activity for category memory in the left anterior temporal and ventral prefrontal cortex, and increased activity for location working memory in the right inferior parietal cortex and dorsal prefrontal cortex. There were no reliable age differences in this pattern of activity, however older adults had more activity than younger adults in the left ventrolateral frontal cortex during both tasks (Figure 7.1b). In both of these studies, over-recruitment of the prefrontal regions may reflect a compensatory function that is better adapted to maintain performance for some tasks than for others. These studies also suggest that the dorsal and ventral regions of the prefrontal cortex influence performance differently in older adults (this issue will be discussed in greater detail in the next section).

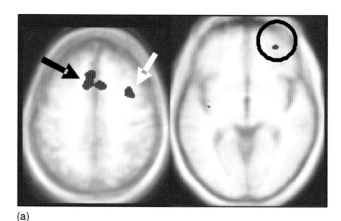

(a)

(b)

Figure 7–1   Brain areas where activity was greater in older adults compared to younger adults during two auditory tasks—(**a**) word recognition (adapted from Fernandes et al., 2006), and (**b**) working memory (adapted from Grady, Yu, and Alain, 2008)—are shown on average structural MRIs. Dorsal regions of lateral prefrontal cortex (white arrows) and medial prefrontal cortex (black arrows) were more active in older adults during performance of a task where accuracy was reduced relative to young adults (word recognition under full attention in (**a**) and category working memory in (**b**)). Regions of ventral prefrontal cortex were more active in older adults during tasks where performance measures were not different from those seen in young adults: memory interference under divided attention (black circle in (**a**)); location working memory as well as category working memory (yellow region in black circle in (**b**)).

A third approach to assessing compensatory brain activity in the context of task performance in young and old adults is to use the so-called "subsequent memory effect." This involves examining brain activity during encoding for items that are subsequently remembered or forgotten when memory is tested later in the experimental session. In this way, one can examine memory in older and younger adults with the assurance that encoding processes, while not necessarily equal between groups, are nevertheless adequate to support successful recognition. Using this approach, Morcom et al. (2003) measured brain activity in young and old adults while they made animacy decisions about words. Activity was then examined for those words that were later successfully recognized. Activity during the animacy task in the left ventral prefrontal cortex and the left hippocampus was greater for subsequently recognized words in both age groups. However, older adults also showed the same association between more activity and subsequent recognition in anterior regions of the bilateral prefrontal cortex. Gutchess et al. (2005) used a similar approach to study scene encoding in young and older adults. Compared to activity for forgotten items, activity during encoding of scenes that were subsequently remembered was greater in the ventral frontal and lateral occipital regions for both younger and older adults. Older adults showed less activation than young adults in the parahippocampus bilaterally, and more activation than young adults in the left dorsolateral frontal cortex. A similar approach was used by Nielson et al. to study inhibitory control in healthy young and older adults (Nielson, Langenecker, and Garavan, 2002). In this study, similar to examining trials associated with successful encoding, the investigators looked at trials where participants successfully inhibited a prepotent response. Activation during successful inhibition occurred predominantly in right prefrontal and parietal regions, regardless of age, but was more extensive (bilaterally and prefrontally) in the older group. These results using the approach of examining only successful trials, both for memory and inhibitory function, are consistent with a compensatory interpretation—that older adults engage frontal areas to a greater degree when processing is sufficient to support performances at levels equivalent to those seen in younger adults.

This apparent compensatory activity is not limited to over-recruitment of the prefrontal cortex, but also extends to distributed cognitive networks. For example, a study of the functional connectivity of the hippocampus during encoding found different patterns in young and old adults, as well as differences in the way in which this connectivity was related to recognition performance (Grady et al., 2003). In this experiment, young and older adults carried out animacy tasks on pictures of common objects. Both groups showed increased activity in the medial temporal regions during object encoding (Grady et al., 1999). When the functional connectivity of the hippocampus to activity in the rest of the brain was assessed, and the relation of activity in this identified network *as a whole* to subsequent recognition was determined, an interesting age difference was found. When young adults were encoding objects, hippocampal activity was correlated with activity in the ventral prefrontal and extrastriate regions, and increased activity in all these regions was associated with better recognition. In contrast, older adults showed correlations between hippocampal activity and more dorsal prefrontal and parietal regions, and positive correlations between activity in these regions and better memory performance (see Figure 7.2b). This ventral/dorsal distinction seen with age suggests a shift in the cognitive resources utilized from more perceptually based processes (mediated by the extrastriate cortex and its connections to the ventral prefrontal cortex) to processes involved in executive functions and cognitive control (mediated by more dorsal prefrontal and parietal regions). This result also can be seen as evidence for compensation, as older adults showed an encoding network that differed from that seen in young adults, and those individuals best able to recruit this network showed better memory. Similar evidence for recruitment of age-specific networks for face encoding (Grady et al., 2002), delayed visual discrimination (Della-Maggiore et al., 2000; McIntosh et al., 1999), and recognition tasks (Grady McIntosh, and Craik, 2005; Stern et al., 2005) has also been reported. All of these studies suggest that aging results in the modification of large-scale network operations, which, in turn, has an impact on various forms of memory.

Although the studies reviewed so far have shown fairly consistent age differences in how prefrontal activity is related to memory performance, few experiments have directly addressed the generality of this finding across multiple cognitive domains. In one of these, a meta-analysis of brain activity in young and old adults was carried out using data across three face-processing

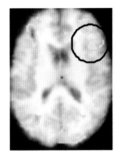 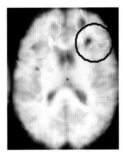 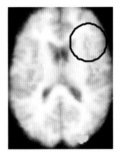

(a) Over-recruitment during face processing   **(b) Encoding activity related to better memory**   **(c) Recognition activity related to better memory**

Figure 7–2 Brain areas with age differences in activity are shown on average structural MRIs. In (**a**), the regions shown in yellow and red were active in older adults compared to a baseline task across three types of face-processing tasks (young adults showed activation only for memory tasks) (Grady, 2002). Yellow/red areas shown in (**b**) were those where activity during the encoding of objects was functionally correlated to activity in the hippocampus and was associated with better subsequent recognition performance in older adults (Grady, McIntosh, and Craik, 2003). Yellow/red areas shown in (**c**) were those where activity during recognition of words and objects was associated with better recognition performance in older adults (Grady, McIntosh, and Craik, 2005). A similar region of the ventral prefrontal cortex appearing in all three images is outlined with black circles.

experiments: episodic memory, working memory, and degraded face perception (Grady, 2002). Each experiment contained an easy face-matching condition and a more difficult processing condition. Young adults showed greater activity in the bilateral prefrontal cortex during the memory tasks, compared to face-matching, but no difference in prefrontal activity between degraded and nondegraded perception. Older adults, on the other hand, had greater prefrontal activity in both memory and degraded perceptual tasks as compared to matching (Figure 7.2a). This suggests that increased prefrontal activity is task-specific in young adults, but is a more general response to increased cognitive effort or need for resources in old adults. Another study by Cabeza et al. (2004) scanned younger and older adults while they performed three different tasks: working memory, visual attention, and episodic retrieval. In all three tasks, older adults showed less occipital and hippocampal activity, and more prefrontal and parietal activity compared to younger adults (Figure 7.3). The age reductions across the three tasks were interesting in light of suggestions that there is a "common cause" for cognitive aging (Salthouse, Atkinson, and Berish, 2003; Salthouse and Ferrer-Caja, 2003), and indicate that both sensory and memory processing could be influenced by such a common cause. The prefrontal increase was interpreted as further evidence for functional compensation in the elderly participants. Taken together with the meta-analysis, these results indicate that some of the age differences in brain activity that have been reported—particularly alterations of prefrontal activity—generalize across task conditions and may play a compensatory role in multiple cognitive domains.

It is worth considering whether the evidence to date has pointed to any specific prefrontal region or regions as being a major player in compensatory mechanisms. A recent review of episodic and working memory experiments (Rajah and D'Esposito, 2005) concluded that aging results in the dedifferentiation of function—or loss of task-selectivity (Grady, 2002)—in

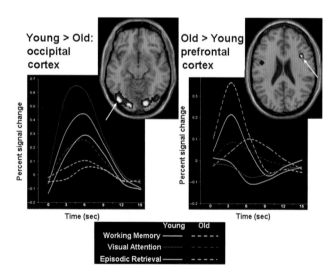

Figure 7–3   Data are shown from a study of age differences in brain activity across three types of task: working memory, visual attention and episodic retrieval (Cabeza et al., 2004). This figure shows task-independent age effects—i.e., those that were seen across all tasks. Compared to younger adults, older adults showed weaker activity in the occipital cortex but greater activity in frontal regions. The hemodynamic time-course plots are from the regions indicated with white arrows. (Adapted from Roberto Cabeza et al; 2004 with permission; Copyright Oxford University Press 2004.)

bilateral ventral prefrontal regions and functional deficits in the right dorsal prefrontal cortex. The authors further suggested that even when older adults recruit the right dorsal frontal area, this does not help them perform the task, but that activity in the left dorsal and anterior prefrontal cortex may be compensatory. The more recent studies reviewed here are broadly consistent with these conclusions. For example, both Gutchess et al. (2005) and Nielson et al. (2006) found greater activation of the left prefrontal cortex in older adults as compared to younger adults, in the left dorsolateral and ventrolateral areas, respectively. Also consistent with the suggestion of Rajah and D'Esposito are the data shown in Figure 7.1, which show that older adults recruit the right dorsolateral prefrontal cortex, but do so in the context of poorer performance than that seen in younger adults. This figure, as well as Figure 7.2, shows regions of ventrolateral prefrontal cortex that are recruited nonselectively in older adults—i.e., is over-recruited across multiple types of tasks. However, it can be seen (Figure 7.2b and 7.2c) that right (as well as left) ventral frontal cortex activity also can be compensatory in the sense that it is engaged in those older adults who perform better on the task. Therefore, it would seem that dedifferentiation (or nonselectivity) and compensation are not mutually exclusive characteristics of brain activation in older adults. In addition, there is continuing evidence that ventral and dorsal regions of the prefrontal cortex may play different roles in the aging process, and that laterality of over-recruitment in the elderly may also influence performance measures.

Another aspect of the compensation hypothesis that has been addressed in only a few studies is the idea that increased prefrontal activity in older adults occurs because there is decreased activity elsewhere in the brain. It was originally suggested that over-recruitment of prefrontal regions occurred in response to decreased activity in early visual processing regions in older adults (Grady et al., 1994). The study by Gutchess et al. (2005) recently found significant negative correlations between the ventral frontal and parahippocampal activity only in old adults, which would be consistent with the idea that frontal activity was related to reduced task-related activity in the medial temporal cortex. Payer et al. (2006) examined brain activity during working memory tasks for faces and houses to examine the relationship between altered activity in the visual cortex and prefrontal activity. These tasks were used because young adults typically have selective activation for faces and houses in different parts of ventral visual cortex (e.g., Haxby et al., 2001; Maurer et al., 2007). Although both groups showed selective activity for faces and houses, this selectivity was reduced with age, which was interpreted as a type of dedifferentiation. In addition, older adults showed bilateral activation in the prefrontal region, whereas younger adults had right hemisphere activity, although no direct group comparisons were reported. The finding that apparently greater prefrontal activations for the old were concurrent with reduced visual selectivity led the authors to suggest that prefrontal activity may compensate for dedifferentiated object recognition mechanisms in the visual cortex. Thus, there is some direct evidence that the prefrontal cortex is over-recruited in older adults in response to decreased activity, or a reduction in task-selective activity, elsewhere in the brain.

One of the major outstanding issues in this field is how compensation in the elderly actually works, and which cognitive processes are engaged. A recent model of how compensation might evolve during memory retrieval was proposed by Velanova et al. (2007). According to this model, executive and cognitive control resources are required both early in the retrieval process, as well as late (Figure 7.4). Young adults are able to engage early resources to

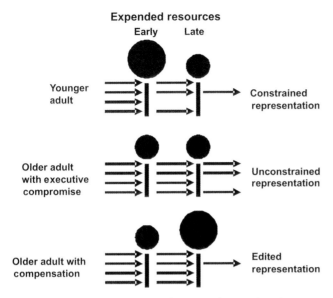

Expended resources

Early   Late

Younger adult — Constrained representation

Older adult with executive compromise — Unconstrained representation

Older adult with compensation — Edited representation

Figure 7–4 The load-shift model of executive function in aging proposed by Velanova et al. (2007). Memory retrieval is considered to be a set of processes automatically elicited by a cue that are constrained by early-selection processes and edited by late-selection processes. Resources, represented by circles, can be expended at early- and late-selection stages to aid effective memory retrieval. In (**a**), young adults are hypothesized to rely on a combination of early- and late-selection processes, with more resources used to constrain processing through top-down mechanisms at early-selection stages. In (**b**), due to compromise in executive function, older adults fail to constrain processing at the early-selection stage. As a result, representations are poorly constrained. To compensate, older adults expend greater resources to edit the retrieval event at late-selection stages in (c). (Adapted from Katerina Velanova et al., 2007 with permission; Copyright Oxford University Press 2007.)

constrain the amount of information necessary to determine if a stimulus is old or new, and hence there is less demand on later processes. However, with aging there is a reduction in these early resources so that more reliance on later resources—so-called "back-end" processing—is needed to compensate. Support for this model was found in two experiments of word recognition, in which an age-related increase was found in both the ventral and dorsal prefrontal cortex that appeared to occur after parietal activity that indicated a successful retrieval decision had been reached. This is an interesting hypothesis that would account for some of the results reviewed here, although clearly it will need further testing. For example, the proposed age deficit in early top-down processing will need to be distinguished from any age differences in early bottom-up attentional changes.

Finally, there is recent evidence of the limits of compensation. A study by Mattay et al. (2006) revealed a similar distribution of cortical activity between younger and older subjects during a series of n-back working memory tasks with increasing load levels. However, there was a significant group difference in the dorsolateral prefrontal cortex bilaterally. In the 1-back task, when the older group performed as well as the younger group, they showed greater prefrontal activity. At higher working-memory loads, however, when they performed worse than the younger adults, this relative increase was absent. These results suggest that compensatory mechanisms, such as additional prefrontal activity, can be called upon to maintain proficiency in task performance. As cognitive demand increases, however, compensation cannot be maintained and performance declines.

Evidence Against Compensation

In this section, we will consider situations in which over-recruitment of brain regions in the elderly appears not to be compensatory, or at least is not directly related to task performance. One such example comes from a study by Springer et al. (2005) that examined the relations among years of education, brain activity during memory tasks, and task performance in young and older adults. Elderly individuals showed a positive correlation between years of education and prefrontal recruitment, but young adults did not show such a relationship. However, increased frontal activity in the older group was not associated with better memory performance, leading to the suggestion that prefrontal activity might have a general function that, when engaged, can facilitate a variety of cognitive processes but may or may not affect task accuracy directly. Although not inconsistent with the idea of compensation, per se, this result indicates that the impact of increased frontal activity in the elderly may not always be seen on a particular task. Similarly, Zarahn et al. (2007) have proposed a type of compensation that could have a beneficial effect on performance relative to what performance would have been without the engagement of an age-specific pattern, even if this pattern is not associated with better task performance in a cross-sectional sense. This conclusion was based on a study using a Sternberg-type recognition task with varying set sizes. In this experiment, a pattern of activity distinguishing older from younger adults was expressed more strongly in those older adults who performed the slowest on the task. Because the better-performing elderly had brain activation more similar to that seen in young adults, these data would not be consistent with the notion of compensation as it typically is considered, but would be consistent with the idea that the lower-performing individuals might have performed even worse had they not engaged the age-specific pattern of activity. It should be noted, however, that this particular relationship between age differences in brain activity and performance was found for reaction time, whereas most other studies looked at compensation in terms of accuracy.

Another important thing to keep in mind is that even if activity in the prefrontal cortex is related to better performance in older adults, other regions may not show this effect. Wierenga et al. (2006) studied naming ability with age, using a task that typically activates the left frontal region in young adults. Although there was no difference in overall naming accuracy between the groups, or in the left prefrontal activation, activity in the right inferior frontal gyrus was increased in older adults, compared to the young, and was positively correlated with greater naming accuracy. This is consistent with the idea that over-recruitment of right-hemisphere homologues in the left prefrontal regions benefits performance in the elderly (Cabeza, 2002). However, activity in other right-hemisphere regions was not related to better naming, indicating that additional activity is not always compensatory in older adults. It is also important to consider the task demands in relation to compensatory activity, because less-complex sensory or motor tasks might not show the same relation between over-recruitment of brain activity and performance that is found using more complex cognitive tasks. Indeed, such a finding was reported recently (Riecker et al., 2006) in an experiment using a finger-tapping task that increased in rate of tapping. Although older adults had more ipsilateral motor-related activity (including activity in frontal regions) than young adults, this overactivation did not increase with an increased rate of tapping. The authors concluded that, because the frontal recruitment was not related to functional demand, the age increase did not necessarily reflect reorganization to compensate for the neurobiological changes of aging. Nevertheless, this finding is consistent with the idea of nonspecific compensation proposed by Springer et al. and Zarahn et al.

Finally, a critical question in this field is whether age differences in brain activity thought to be compensatory can be elicited through training of specific cognitive processes in older adults. That is, if over-recruitment of the prefrontal cortex is compensating for some age decline in brain structure or function, then prefrontal activity should increase accordingly in older adults who are trained on a particular task (and thereby improve their performance). This would have the effect of increasing the age differences in prefrontal activity, particularly if young adults showed lateralized activity in one hemisphere or the other during the task in question, and the training-induced increase in older adults occurred in the opposite hemisphere. This has not been studied yet to any great degree, but one recent study examined this issue in the context of training on a dual-task paradigm. In this study, participants carried out two visual tasks (color detection and letter detection), either singly or simultaneously (Erickson et al., 2007). A subset of young and older adults then received five hours of training on the tasks over a several-week period. Both young and old trained groups showed improved performance on the tasks, both in accuracy and reaction times. In terms of pretraining brain activity, young adults had more activity in the left ventral prefrontal cortex, and older adults had more activity in the dorsal prefrontal cortex bilaterally. After training, older adults showed an increase in left ventral prefrontal cortex activity and a decrease in dorsal prefrontal cortex activity, such that age differences in these regions were no longer apparent in the trained groups. In addition, these changes in prefrontal activity were correlated with improved reaction time on the dual task in older adults. No differences over time were seen in the untrained groups. This result clearly does not support the idea that behavioral improvement after training reflects compensatory increases of frontal activity to levels above that seen in younger adults. If anything, activity in the older adults after training was more similar to that seen in the young group. One explanation for these findings is that older adults prior to training needed additional cognitive control to perform the dual tasks, indicated by more dorsal prefrontal activity, and that the training allowed them to reduce their dependence on these control processes. Again, it should be noted that the relationships seen here between brain activity and performance were also found for reaction times, so it is not known if a similar relationship would hold for accuracy as well. Clearly more studies will need to be done to address this issue using other kinds of tasks, as it may well be that dual task performance and memory retrieval, for example, draw on different processes and will respond differently to training.

Unresolved Issues

It is clear from the evidence to date that healthy aging is associated with alterations of the brain networks that underlie cognition. Further, these alterations are frequently, although not invariably, associated with better task performance, and hence provide evidence in favor of the compensation hypothesis. This evidence has fueled considerable interest in the neuroscience of cognitive aging, and in the process has uncovered more questions about how such compensation might work and how it might arise. The remaining section of this chapter will review these questions and how we might go about answering them.

One question is whether changes in brain activity with age indicate that young and old adults use different cognitive processes to carry out the same task, even if they presumably follow the same set of instructions, or whether different brain areas come to be used for the same cognitive process over time. That is, does a given cognitive process become represented differently in the brain as we age? Another way of expressing this question is to ask if these differences that we see in brain activity with age are changes in how cognition is carried out by the brain, or changes in strategy use by older adults. This is a difficult issue, and it is not clear how one can separate brain activity and behavioral strategy. A more tractable question to ask may be which comes first: the change in brain function necessitating a change in behavior, or a change in behavior that is reflected in brain activity. Although it may be very difficult to distinguish between these two alternatives except by longitudinal studies, one recent study attempted to address this question cross-sectionally in a group of adults between the ages of 20 and 87 years of age (Grady, Springer, Hongwanishkul, McIntosh, and Winocur, 2006). Both encoding and recognition tasks were examined and contrasted with a fixation baseline. Across all encoding and recognition tasks, linear increases of activity with age were found in areas that normally decreased during task performance (e.g., medial frontal and parietal regions), whereas activity in regions with task-related activation (e.g., dorsolateral prefrontal cortex) decreased with age (Figure 7.5). Interestingly, the age differences in memory performance were *not* linear; that is, the middle-aged adults performed as well as the younger adults, but the oldest participants showed typical reductions in memory. These results suggest that there is a gradual, age-related reduction in the ability to suspend non-task-related (so-called "default-mode" activity, Raichle et al., 2001) and engage areas for carrying out memory tasks, and that the brain changes may occur before behavioral changes are seen. This suggests that a change in brain function necessitates a change in behavioral strategy, but clearly more work needs to be done in this area.

There also are issues regarding functional connectivity that have yet to be resolved. For example, results to date indicate that older adults engage different brain networks even when their performance on the task in question is equivalent to that seen in young adults. This raises the question of whether old and young groups will *always* be different in terms of their cognitive networks, or whether there are some task conditions in which these would be the same. It is possible (and perhaps likely) that for simple perceptual or sensorimotor tasks, such as pressing a button to a specified stimulus, the recruited network would not differ with age. This, however, has not been tested directly. Clearly, there must be constraints on the degree to which networks can be altered, as well as aspects that remain invariant with age, but these limits have not been determined. In addition, almost all tasks involve more than one cognitive process, as well as motor components, so that multiple networks are probably active simultaneously. Little is known about how these processes and networks interact with one another in young adults, much less in older adults.

Another interesting question is the extent to which the network alterations seen in older adults are due to changes in the function of the brain regions themselves, or to structural changes in these areas or in the white matter tracts that connect the regions. Recent evidence (see review by Buckner, 2004) indicates that age differences in white matter are more prominent in frontal than posterior brain areas. Others have also reported that frontal gray matter regions have more atrophic changes in older adults than other brain areas (Raz, 2000). Communication between cortical

Figure 7–5   (a) Brain regions where activity during encoding and recognition tasks is correlated with age are shown on average structural MRIs (data are from Grady et al., 2006). Activity in the yellow/orange regions (default mode regions) increased with age, and those shown **in blue** (task-related regions) decreased with age during the tasks. The graphs in (**b**) and (**c**) show plots of brain scores that result from a multivariate analysis that assessed the age/activity correlation across the tasks. As the brain score becomes more positive, activity in the orange regions increases, whereas more negative brain scores are associated with more activity in the blue regions. The graphs show linear changes with age in these activity patterns across all memory tasks.

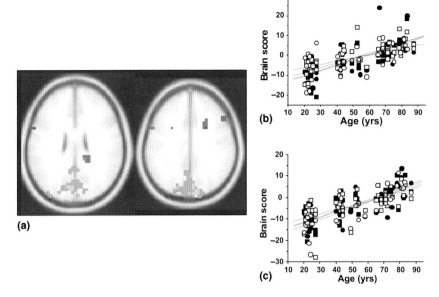

regions, therefore, could be reduced or altered because the neurons in the regions themselves have altered function or because the fibers that connect them are damaged or less efficient. The impact on cognition of changes with age in white matter have been documented (e.g., DeCarli et al., 1995; Garde et al., 2000; Gunning-Dixon and Raz, 2000; Pfefferbaum et al., 2000) and a few studies have now looked at the impact of these structural changes on functional activation. Unfortunately, the results of these studies have not been consistent. Nordahl et al. (2006) used structural MRI to quantify the extent of white matter hyperintensities (WMH) in a group of cognitively normal elderly individuals, and tested whether these measures were predictive of the magnitude of prefrontal activity observed during the performance of an episodic retrieval task and a verbal working-memory task. Results showed that increases in both global and regional dorsal prefrontal WMH volume were associated with decreases in frontal task-related activity. In addition, frontal WMH volume was associated with decreased activity in medial temporal and anterior cingulate regions during episodic retrieval, and decreased activity in the posterior parietal and anterior cingulate cortex during working memory performance. These results suggest that disruption of white matter tracts, especially within the prefrontal cortex, may be a mechanism for age-related reductions in both memory functioning and brain activation. On the other hand, Persson et al. (2006) scanned older adults during an episodic encoding task, and found that reductions in white matter integrity of the corpus callosum (measured with diffusion tensor imaging, or DTI) were associated with *increased* activation in the right prefrontal cortex. The authors suggested that increased activation is either caused by structural disruption or is a compensatory response to such disruption. Madden et al. (2007) also examined brain activity and white matter integrity with DTI and found that there was an age-related reduction in white matter integrity that was more pronounced for anterior brain regions than for posterior regions (as others have noted). However, white matter integrity did not specifically mediate the age-related increase in activation of the frontoparietal attentional network. Thus, it is still far from clear how changes in white matter integrity influence neural communication and activation levels in the elderly. It may be that changes

in the myelin that are detected via DTI result in subtle alterations in neural function that can be compensated for by increased activity, whereas disruptions caused by more severe damage underlying specific cortical areas (i.e., WMH in the frontal lobes) may lead to alterations of function that are more difficult to adapt to. It is also possible that damage to white matter in the corpus callosum has a different impact on brain activity than damage to white matter *underlying* the cortex.

The way in which one can reconcile the structural and functional imaging results in older adults also has been something of a puzzle. That is, structural scanning shows that frontal regions are more vulnerable to age-related atrophy than other areas, yet these are precisely the areas that are often more active in older adults as compared to younger adults. This would seem to present a paradox; however, there has been a recent attempt to explain these two sets of data by Greenwood (2007). According to her theory, regional changes such as thinning of the cortex and dendritic shrinking in specific brain areas leads to plasticity surrounding these areas in an attempt to lessen their impact. For example, there could be cellular changes, as well as changes in neural connectivity. This would be reflected in increased activation on functional neuroimages in older adults compared to younger adults, which is, of course, what has been observed. Of course, this hypothesis needs to be tested, but it does provide a starting point for reconciling two apparently disparate sets of data. Clearly we have much to learn about the complex interplay between brain structure and function, and how this interaction is affected by age.

Conclusion

Functional neuroimaging has provided some intriguing insights into the field of cognitive aging, but provided us with some new challenges as well. Evidence to date would suggest that increased recruitment of the prefrontal cortex, and functional interactions between prefrontal and other brain regions, including the medial temporal lobes, are associated with better memory performance in older adults. These alterations in memory networks may be compensatory, at least for some types of tasks. The use of network approaches to image analysis has considerable potential to inform us about how brain areas work together to mediate memory function, and how these networks change with age. The challenge facing future research will be to understand the task conditions that promote compensation in older adults, the role of the various brain areas in aiding cognitive function, and how these compensatory mechanisms can be elicited to enhance quality of life.

References

Balota, D. A., Dolan, P. O., and Duchek, J. M. (2000). Memory changes in healthy older adults. In E. Tulving and F. Craik (eds), *The Oxford Handbook of Memory* (pp. 395–410). New York: Oxford University Press.

Buckner, R. L. (2004). Memory and executive function in aging and AD: multiple factors that cause decline and reserve factors that compensate. *Neuron*, 44: 195–208.

Burke, D. M. and Light, L. L. (1981). Memory and aging: the role of retrieval processes. *Psychological Bulletin*, 90: 513–546.

Cabeza, R. (2002). Hemispheric asymmetry reduction in older adults: The HAROLD model. *Psychology and Aging*, 17: 85–100.

Cabeza, R., Anderson, N. D., Locantore, J. K., and McIntosh, A. R. (2002). Aging gracefully: compensatory brain activity in high-performing older adults. *NeuroImage*, 17: 1394–1402.

Cabeza, R., Daselaar, S. M., Dolcos, F., Prince, S. E., Budde, M., and Nyberg, L. (2004). Task-independent and task-specific age effects on brain activity during working memory, visual attention and episodic retrieval. *Cerebral Cortex*, 14: 364–375.

Cabeza, R., Grady, C. L., Nyberg, L., McIntosh, A. R., Tulving, E., Kapur, S., et al. (1997). Age-related differences in neural activity during memory encoding and retrieval: A positron emission tomography study. *Journal of Neuroscience*, 17: 391–400.

Craik, F. I. M. and Bosman, E. A. (1992). Age-related changes in memory and learning. In H. Bouma and J. Graafmans (eds), *Gerontechnology: Proceedings of the First International Conference on Technology and Aging* (pp. 79–92). Eindhoven: IOS Press.

Craik, F. I. M. and Byrd, M. (1982). Aging and cognitive deficits: The role of attentional resources. In F. I. M. Craik and S. Trehub (eds), *Aging and Cognitive Processes* (pp. 191–211). New York: Plenum Press.

Craik, F. I. M., and Jennings, J. M. (1992). Human memory. In F. I. M. Craik and T. A. Salthouse (eds), *The Handbook of Aging and Cognition* (pp. 51–110). Hillsdale, NJ: Lawrence Erlbaum.

Daselaar, S. M., Fleck, M. S., Dobbins, I. G., Madden, D. J., and Cabeza, R. (2006). Effects of healthy aging on hippocampal and rhinal memory functions: an event-related fMRI study. *Cerebral Cortex*, 16: 1771–1782.

DeCarli, C., Murphy, D. G., Tranh, M., Grady, C. L., Haxby, J. V., Gillette, J. A., et al. (1995). The effect of white matter hyperintensity volume on brain structure, cognitive performance, and cerebral metabolism of glucose in 51 healthy adults. *Neurology*, 45: 2077–2084.

Della-Maggiore, V., Sekuler, A. B., Grady, C. L., Bennett, P. J., Sekuler, R., and McIntosh, A. R. (2000). Corticolimbic interactions associated with performance on a short-term memory task are modified by age. *Journal of Neuroscience*, 20: 8410–8416.

Erickson, K. I., Colcombe, S. J., Wadhwa, R., Bherer, L., Peterson, M. S., Scalf, P. E., et al. (2007). Training-induced plasticity in older adults: effects of training on hemispheric asymmetry. *Neurobiology of Aging*, 28: 272–283.

Fernandes, M. A., Pacurar, A., Moscovitch, M., and Grady, C. L. (2006). Neural correlates of auditory recognition under full and divided attention in young and old adults. *Neuropsychologia*, 44: 2452–2464.

Garde, E., Mortensen, E. L., Krabbe, K., Rostrup, E., and Larsson, H. B. (2000). Relation between age-related decline in intelligence and cerebral white- matter hyperintensities in healthy octogenarians: A longitudinal study. *Lancet*, 356: 628–634.

Grady, C. L. (2002). Age-related differences in face processing: A meta-analysis of three functional neuroimaging experiments. *Canadian Journal of Experimental Psychology*, 56: 208–220.

Grady, C. L., Bernstein, L., Siegenthaler, A., and Beig, S. (2002). The effects of encoding task on age-related differences in the functional neuroanatomy of face memory. *Psychology and Aging*, 17: 7–23.

Grady, C. L., Haxby, J. V., Horwitz, B., Ungerleider, L. G., Schapiro, M. B., Carson, R. E., et al. (1992). Dissociation of object and spatial vision in human extrastriate cortex: Age-related changes in activation of regional cerebral blood flow measured with [^{15}O]water and positron emission tomography. *Journal of Cognitive Neuroscience*, 4: 23–34.

Grady, C. L., Maisog, J. M., Horwitz, B., Ungerleider, L. G., Mentis, M. J., Salerno, J. A., et al. (1994). Age-related changes in cortical blood flow activation during visual processing of faces and location. *Journal of Neuroscience*, 14: 1450–1462.

Grady, C. L., McIntosh, A. R., and Craik, F. I. (2003). Age-Related differences in the functional connectivity of the hippocampus during memory encoding. *Hippocampus*, 13: 572–586.

Grady, C. L., McIntosh, A. R., and Craik, F. (2005). Task-related activity in prefrontal cortex and its relation to recognition memory performance in young and old adults. *Neuropsychologia*, 43: 1466–1481.

Grady, C. L., McIntosh, A. R., Rajah, M. N., Beig, S., and Craik, F. I. M. (1999). The effects of age on the neural correlates of episodic encoding. *Cerebral Cortex*, 9: 805–814.

Grady, C. L., Springer, M. V., Hongwanishkul, D., McIntosh, A. R., and Winocur, G. (2006). Age-related changes in brain activity across the adult lifespan. *Journal of Cognitive Neuroscience*, 18: 227–241.

Grady, C. L., Yu, H., and Alain, C. (2008). Age-related differences in brain activity underlying working memory for spatial and nonspatial auditory information. *Cerebral Cortex*, 18: 189–199.

Greenwood, P. M. (2007). Functional plasticity in cognitive aging: Review and hypothesis. *Neuropsychology*, 21: 657–673.

Gunning-Dixon, F. M., and Raz, N. (2000). The cognitive correlates of white matter abnormalities in normal aging: A quantitative review. *Neuropsychology*, 14: 224–232.

Gutchess, A. H., Welsh, R. C., Hedden, T., Bangert, A., Minear, M., Liu, L. L., et al. (2005). Aging and the neural correlates of successful picture encoding: Frontal activations compensate for decreased medial temporal activity. *Journal of Cognitive Neuroscience*, 17: 84–96.

Haxby, J. V., Gobbini, M. I., Furey, M. L., Ishai, A., Schouten, J. L., and Pietrini, P. (2001). Distributed and overlapping representations of faces and objects in ventral temporal cortex. *Science*, 293: 2425–2430.

Levine, B., Svoboda, E., Hay, J., Winocur, G., and Moscovitch, M. (2002). Aging and autobiographical memory: dissociating episodic from semantic retrieval. *Psychology and Aging*, 17: 677–689.

Madden, D. J., Spaniol, J., Whiting, W. L., Bucur, B., Provenzale, J. M., Cabeza, R., et al. (2007). Adult age differences in the functional neuroanatomy of visual attention: a combined fMRI and DTI study. *Neurobiology of Aging*, 28: 459–476.

Madden, D. J., Turkington, T. G., Provenzale, J. M., Denny, L. L., Hawk, T. C., Gottlob, L. R., et al. (1999). Adult age differences in the functional neuroanatomy of verbal recognition memory. *Human Brain Mapping*, 7: 115–135.

Mattay, V. S., Fera, F., Tessitore, A., Hariri, A. R., Berman, K. F., Das, S., Meyer-Lindenberg, A., et al. (2006). Neurophysiological correlates of age-related changes in working memory capacity. *Neuroscience Letters*, 392: 32–37.

Maurer, D., O'Craven, K. M., Le Grand, R., Mondloch, C. J., Springer, M. V., Lewis, T. L., et al. (2007). Neural correlates of processing facial identity based on features versus their spacing. *Neuropsychologia*, 45: 1438–1451.

McIntosh, A. R., Sekuler, A. B., Penpeci, C., Rajah, M. N., Grady, C. L., Sekuler, R., et al. (1999). Recruitment of unique neural systems to support visual memory in normal aging. *Current Biology*, 9: 1275–1278.

Morcom, A. M., Good, C. D., Frackowiak, R. S., and Rugg, M. D. (2003). Age effects on the neural correlates of successful memory encoding. *Brain*, 126: 213–229.

Nielson, K. A., Douville, K. L., Seidenberg, M., Woodard, J. L., Miller, S. K., Franczak, M., et al. (2006). Age-related functional recruitment for famous name recognition: An event-related fMRI study. *Neurobiology of Aging*, 27: 1494–1504.

Nielson, K. A., Langenecker, S. A., and Garavan, H. (2002). Differences in the functional neuroanatomy of inhibitory control across the adult life span. *Psychology and Aging*, 17: 56–71.

Nordahl, C. W., Ranganath, C., Yonelinas, A. P., Decarli, C., Fletcher, E., and Jagust, W. J. (2006). White matter changes compromise prefrontal cortex function in healthy elderly individuals. *Journal of Cognitive Neuroscience*, 18: 418–429.

Payer, D., Marshuetz, C., Sutton, B., Hebrank, A., Welsh, R. C., and Park, D. C. (2006). Decreased neural specialization in old adults on a working memory task. *Neuroreport*, 17: 487–491.

Persson, J., Nyberg, L., Lind, J., Larsson, A., Nilsson, L. G., Ingvar, M., et al. (2006). Structure-function correlates of cognitive decline in aging. *Cerebral Cortex*, 16: 907–915.

Pfefferbaum, A., Sullivan, E. V., Hedehus, M., Lim, K. O., Adalsteinsson, E., and Moseley, M. (2000). Age-related decline in brain white matter anisotropy measured with spatially corrected echo-planar diffusion tensor imaging. *Magnetic Resonance in Medicine*, 44: 259–268.

Piolino, P., Desgranges, B., Benali, K., and Eustache, F. (2002). Episodic and semantic remote autobiographical memory in ageing. *Memory*, 10: 239–257.

Raichle, M. E., MacLeod, A. M., Snyder, A. Z., Powers, W. J., Gusnard, D. A., and Shulman, G. L. (2001). A default mode of brain function. *Proceedings of the National Academy of Sciences of the USA*, 98: 676–682.

Rajah, M. N. and D'Esposito, M. (2005). Region-specific changes in prefrontal function with age: a review of PET and fMRI studies on working and episodic memory. *Brain*, 128: 1964–1983.

Raz, N. (2000). Aging of the brain and its impact on cognitive performance: Integration of structural and functional findings. In F. I. M. Craik and T. A. Salthouse (eds), *Handbook of Aging and Cognition – II* (pp. 1–90). Mahwah, NJ: Lawrence Erlbaum.

Reuter-Lorenz, P. A., Jonides, J., Smith, E. E., Hartley, A., Miller, A., Marshuetz, C., et al. (2000). Age differences in the frontal lateralization of verbal and spatial working memory revealed by PET. *Journal of Cognitive Neuroscience*, 12: 174–187.

Riecker, A., Groschel, K., Ackermann, H., Steinbrink, C., Witte, O., and Kastrup, A. (2006). Functional significance of age-related differences in motor activation patterns. *Neuroimage*, 32: 1345–1354.

Salthouse, T. A., Atkinson, T. M., and Berish, D. E. (2003). Executive functioning as a potential mediator of age-related cognitive decline in normal adults. *Journal of Experimental Psychology: General*, 132: 566–594.

Salthouse, T. A. and Ferrer-Caja, E. (2003). What needs to be explained to account for age-related effects on multiple cognitive variables? *Psychology and Aging*, 18: 91–110.

Springer, M. V., McIntosh, A. R., Winocur, G., and Grady, C. L. (2005). The relation between brain activity during memory tasks and years of education in young and old adults. *Neuropsychology*, 19: 181–192.

Stern, Y., Habeck, C., Moeller, J., Scarmeas, N., Anderson, K. E., Hilton, H. J., et al. (2005). Brain networks associated with cognitive reserve in healthy young and old adults. *Cerebral Cortex*, 15: 394–402.

Tulving, E. (1983). *Elements of Episodic Memory*. New York: Oxford University Press.

Velanova, K., Lustig, C., Jacoby, L. L., and Buckner, R. L. (2007). Evidence for frontally mediated controlled processing differences in older adults. *Cerebral Cortex*, 17: 1033–1046.

Wierenga, C. E., Benjamin, M., Gopinath, K., Perlstein, W. M., Leonard, C. M., Rothi, L. J., et al. (2008). Age-related changes in word retrieval: Role of bilateral frontal and subcortical networks. *Neurobiology of Aging*, 29: 436–451.

Zacks, R. T., Hasher, L., and Li, K. Z. H. (2000). Human memory. In F. I. M. Craik and T. A. Salthouse (eds), *The Handbook of Aging and Cognition* (2nd ed., pp. 200–230). Mahwah, NJ: Erlbaum.

Zarahn, E., Rakitin, B., Abela, D., Flynn, J., and Stern, Y. (2007). Age-related changes in brain activation during a delayed item recognition task. *Neurobiology of Aging*, 28: 784–798.

8

Cross-Species Imaging Applied to the Aging Brain: Dissociating Alzheimer's Disease from Normal Aging

Sidonie T. Jones and Scott A. Small

Age-related Hippocampal Dysfunction: Framing the Debate

As commonly experienced, and as neuropsychologically documented, our cognitive abilities decline with advancing years (Zelinski and Burnight, 1997). Fortunately, age-related cognitive decline is not diffuse, but rather aging targets select cognitive domains. The ability to consciously memorize new and complex experiences—for example, learning the name of a new acquaintance—is one cognitive domain particularly sensitive to the aging process (Small et al., 1999). This cognitive ability requires the hippocampal formation (Amaral and Witter, 1989)—a brain structure nestled deep in the temporal lobes (Figure 8.1).

One contributing cause to age-related hippocampal dysfunction is undoubtedly Alzheimer's disease (AD), a gradually progressive disorder that typically manifests in later life. Anatomically, AD targets the hippocampal formation early on (Amaral and Witter, 1989), presenting as mild forgetfulness, but ultimately AD sweeps through the neocortical mantle, devastating most cognitive abilities and leaving dementia in its wake (Jacobs et al., 1995; Masur et al., 1994). Within each affected area, AD progresses through different pathophysiological stages. Early on, AD causes neurons to malfunction (Selkoe, 2002), manifesting as metabolic and synaptic failure, before causing neurons to die. Accordingly, a distinction is sometimes made between the early "cell sickness" stage vs. the later "cell death" stage of AD (Small, 2005).

Not every aging individual with age-related hippocampal dysfunction progresses to AD dementia, raising the possibility that the aging process itself might affect hippocampal function. A wide range of nonhuman studies support this possibility (Barnes, 1994; Erickson and Barnes, 2003; Gallagher and Rapp, 1997). All aging nonhuman mammals manifest hippocampal dysfunction, yet no species besides our own develop AD. Thus, all species develop nonAD age-related memory decline, and it would seem unlikely that humans would be spared this species-wide process. Nevertheless, the possibility still exists that in humans, age-related hippocampal dysfunction uniformly reflects the early stages of AD, and that if humans live long enough, all will develop full-fledged AD.

Thus, despite over a century of research, there is still residual debate about whether age-related hippocampal dysfunction is etiologically homogenous reflecting the earliest stages of AD, or is age-related hippocampal dysfunction etiologically heterogenous, reflecting both early AD and the normal wear and tear of the normal aging process.

The Functional Organization of the Hippocampal Formation Can Inform this Debate

In principle, the microanatomy of the hippocampal formation may help in resolving this debate. The hippocampal formation is a complex structure made up of separate but interconnected subregions (Amaral and Witter, 1989): the entorhinal cortex, the dentate gyrus, the CA1 and CA3 subfields, and the subiculum (Figure 8.1). Because the subregions are connected in a unidirectional manner, the hippocampal formation functions as a circuit. Thus, a lesion in any individual hippocampal subregion will equivalently interrupt the circuit, leading to overlapping memory deficits.

Importantly, each hippocampal subregion houses a distinct population of neurons, unique in their molecular expression profiles (Zhao et al., 2001). It is this molecular uniqueness that accounts for why each hippocampal subregion is differentially vulnerable to mechanisms of dysfunction (Small, 2001). So, for example, transient hypoxemia causes memory deficits by targeting the CA1 subfield because of high expression of glutamate receptors in CA1 neurons; while, in contrast, an adrenalectomy causes overlapping memory deficits by targeting the dentate gyrus because neurons in this subregion express relatively high concentrations of corticosteroid receptors.

Based on this anatomical and molecular organization, the following hypothesis can be made: if AD and normal aging are

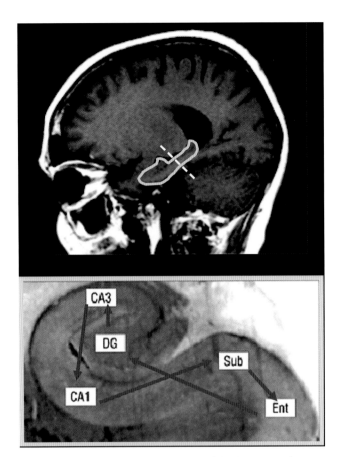

Figure 8–1   The functional organization of the hippocampal formation. The hippocampal formation is a cylindrical structure that spans the anterior to longitudinal extent of the medial temporal lobes (**demarcated in blue** in the upper panel). The microanatomy of the hippocampal formation (bottom panel) is best appreciated by viewing a transverse slice through the body of the hippocampal formation (stippled line in the upper panel). The hippocampal formation is made up of the anatomically and molecularly distinct subregions—the entorhinal cortex (EC), the dentate gyrus (DG) and the CA1 and CA3 subfields (bottom panel). The hippocampal subregions are interconnected, giving rise to the hippocampal circuit. The circuit organization of the hippocampal formation accounts for why dysfunction in any individual hippocampal subregion will equivalently interrupt the circuit, causing overlapping memory deficits. The molecular organization of the hippocampal formation accounts for why each hippocampal subregion is differentially vulnerable to mechanisms of dysfunction.

indeed pathologically separate processes, then the odds are high that they will target different hippocampal subregions (Small, 2001). Establishing whether this anatomical dissociation exists, therefore, is an effective approach for addressing the debate about whether age-related hippocampal dysfunction is etiologically heterogeneous.

Optimizing Cross-Species Imaging to Address the Debate

To test this hypothesis, an imaging technique is needed that fulfills three basic requirements (Figure 8.2). First, a technique needs to be sensitive to neuronal function, not just structure. As already mentioned, the early stages of AD are characterized by cell sickness, not cell death. Animal studies have established that insofar that aging

causes memory decline, it does so by interrupting neuronal physiology—again, a form of cell sickness—with a notable absence of cell loss (Rapp and Gallagher, 1996). Second, the technique needs to have sufficient spatial resolution to interrogate the hippocampus as a circuit. Because of its circuit organization, lesions in one hippocampal subregion will secondarily affect the function of other subregions, and will affect the circuit as a whole. Thus, in order to pinpoint the primary subregion targeted by a particular mechanism of dysfunction, a technique needs to assess each hippocampal subregion individually, but also simultaneously account for circuit-wide effects.

Third, the technique needs to have cross-species capabilities, so that the same "imaging readout" can be generated in humans and animal models. As discussed below, a technique that fulfills this cross-species requirement can be exploited to confirm any findings in humans using animal models. The ability to apply this technique to mice, in particular, would provide a bridge between molecular biology and functional imaging by exploiting transgenic engineering.

Since the early studies by Kety and Schmidt (Small, 2004), functional brain imaging has come to imply a method that detects changes in regional energy metabolism. Energy metabolism is best defined as the rate with which cells produce ATP, which requires the consumption of oxygen and glucose from the blood stream in neurons. Visualizing ATP directly is challenging, but imaging techniques have been developed that can visualize correlates of oxygen and glucose consumption. With the use of radiolabeled glucose, PET can quantify the regional rates of glucose uptake. In contrast, MRI-based techniques have typically relied on the second ingredient of ATP production—oxygen consumption—to visualize correlates of energy metabolism. Because of hemodynamic coupling, oxygen consumption is correlated with cerebral blood flow (CBF), cerebral blood volume (CBV), and deoxyhemoglobin content, and all these correlates can be estimated with MRI.

All forms of functional imaging engage in "stimulus mapping." Namely, metabolism is by definition a dynamic process—is never "at rest"—and is always responding to internal and external cues or stimuli. It is important to clearly define the stimulus of interest, since this will dictate how to optimize a functional imaging study. For example, a common utility of functional imaging is sensory representation—mapping areas of the brain that transiently show shifts in metabolism coupled to an external and brief stimulus (for example, as in our previous studies, asking which areas of the hippocampus respond to "faces" or "names") (Figure 8.3). Temporal resolution is, therefore, key for sensory representations to map an acute metabolic event. In clinical neuroscience, however, it is the disease itself that is the stimulus (albeit an internal one), and by and large most diseases of the brain affect the brain chronically, reflected by changes in basal metabolism. Thus, although in our early experiments we performed acute-on-chronic experiments, more recently we have focused on imaging the basal, disease-related state. Compared to acute imaging, basal metabolic imaging provides the following important advantages: (1) basal metabolic measures are more tightly coupled to the stimulus under investigation (disease states); (2) basal metabolic measures are easier to quantify, and quantification is extremely important when comparing diseased and control brains; and (3) for technical reasons, basal metabolism allows us to increase our spatial resolution, visualizing the hippocampal subregions.

Measuring glucose uptake with PET has earned the right to be considered the gold standard approach for mapping basal metabolic brain changes. Unfortunately, PET technologies simply

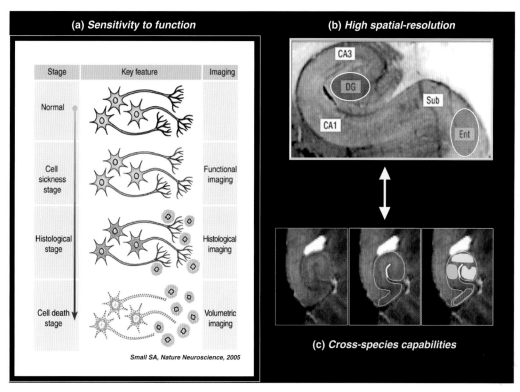

Figure 8–2 An imaging technique that fulfills the following three requirements is well-suited for dissociating Alzheimer's disease from normal aging. (a). *Sensitivity to function.* A technique that is sensitive to "cell-sickness" can capture the earliest stages of AD. **(b) *High spatial resolution.*** A technique that has very high spatial resolution can evaluate the functional integrity of multiple hippocampal subregions, individually and simultaneously. **(c) *Cross-species capabilities.*** A technique that generates the same imaging "readout" across species can confirm human findings in animal models—in particular, genetically-modified mice.

Figure 8–3 Alzheimer's diseases and normal aging affect basal brain metabolism. Functional imaging maps changes in brain metabolism that are always shifting in response to internal or external stimuli. Mapping transient internal (e.g., seizures) or external (e.g., flashing faces) stimuli is achieved with high temporal resolution. However, mapping slow internal (e.g., Alzheimer's disease or aging) or external (e.g., memorizing a face) stimuli is achieved with slower temporal resolution. Changes in basal metabolism are also easier to quantify and allow enhanced spatial resolution.

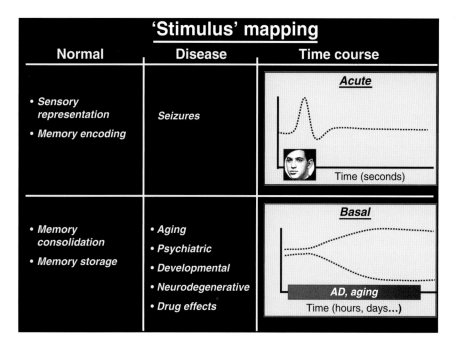

cannot achieve the spatial resolution required to visualize hippocampal subregions. Because of this, we have turned our attention instead to MRI technologies and their promise of high spatial resolution, specifically exploring the three remaining "functional imaging" variables—CBF, deoxyhemoglobin, and CBV. Our

exploratory studies showed that we would not achieve sufficiently high enough spatial resolution with typical CBF techniques such as ASL. Deoxyhemoblogin turned out to have sufficient spatial resolution, and as is discussed below, yielded some interesting results, but it is limited by the inability to quantify the signal. Fortunately,

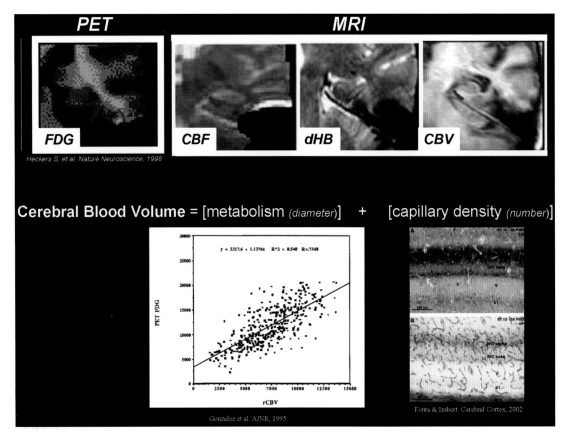

Figure 8–4   Basal metabolism can be mapped with PET or MRI. Mapping glucose uptake (a correlate of glucose metabolism) with PET is the gold standard technique for mapping basal metabolism. However, PET cannot achieve the required high spatial resolution. Mapping CBF, deoxyhemoglobin content (dHB), or CBV—all correlates of oxygen metabolism—can be achieved with MRI. Among these, CBV turns out to be the best imaging variable.

our last variable (CBV) fulfilled all of our starting requirements, and is currently the technique that we use most extensively in cross-species studies (Figure 8.4).

Cross-species Imaging Applied to Humans, Non-human Primates, and Transgenically-engineered Mice

By quantifying cell loss in the post-mortem tissue of AD patients, studies have suggested that either the entorhinal cortex or the CA1 subfield are the hippocampal subregions most vulnerable to AD (Braak and Braak, 1996; Fukutani et al., 2000; Giannakopoulos et al., 2003; Price et al., 2001; Schonheit, Zarski, and Ohm, 2004; Shoghi-Jadid et al., 2002). In many of these studies, the entorhinal cortex and the CA1 subfield were not assessed simultaneously, accounting in part for the reported inconsistencies. More generally, however, isolating the hippocampal subregion most vulnerable to AD is difficult when relying on post-mortem studies alone. Not only are post-mortem studies biased against the earliest and most discriminatory stages of disease, but these studies cannot assess the cell-sickness stage of AD (Selkoe, 2002).

As discussed above, variants of fMRI that are sensitive to basal correlates of neuronal function are well-suited to aiding in resolving this debate. In one of our first studies, an MRI measure sensitive to basal levels of deoxyhemoglobin was used to assess the hippocampal subregions in patients with AD dementia compared to age-matched controls (Small et al., 2000). This MRI measure has proven capable of detecting cell sickness in individual hippocampal subregions. Univariate analysis revealed that normalized signal intensity was reduced in all hippocampal subregions in patients compared to controls. Nevertheless, when the hippocampus was analyzed as a circuit—namely, using a multivariate model to analyze signals from all hippocampal subregions simultaneously—the entorhinal cortex was found to be the primary site of dysfunction in AD (Small et al., 2000).

This study suggests that the entorhinal cortex, not the CA1 subfield, is the hippocampal subregion most vulnerable to AD—agreeing with some, though not all, post-mortem studies. Nevertheless, the patients assessed in this study already had severe dementia, indicating that that they had already progressed from the cell-sickness to the cell-death stage of AD. Furthermore, this study does not inform us about the hippocampal subregions most vulnerable to normal aging.

Both of these issues were addressed in a second study, in which 70 subjects across the age span (from 20–88 years of age) were imaged with the same MRI measure (Small et al., 2002). Importantly, all subjects were healthy. The older age groups in particular were carefully screened against any evidence of dementia. The starting assumption made in this study was that some of the older subjects were in the earliest stage of AD and some subjects were aging normally. The question was how to make this distinction since there is no independent indicator to determine who had early AD and who did not. This is true even if the hippocampal formation of all subjects could be examined post-mortem, because, as mentioned, the earliest stages of AD may be microscopically invisible. Instead, formal parametric criteria were used to distinguish a "pathological" pattern of decline (i.e., related to Alzheimer's disease) vs. a "normal" pattern of decline. Specifically, since the effect of normal aging on the brain is, by definition, a stochastic process, the variance of signal intensity among an older age group should be equal to the variance among a younger age group, although a shift in the mean is expected. In contrast, since it is a disease, AD should affect a subgroup within an older age group, which should significantly broaden the variance of signal intensity compared to a younger age group.

Applying this and other criteria, the results of this study showed that age-related changes in the entorhinal cortex fulfilled the criteria for pathological decline; in contrast, age-related changes in the dentate gyrus, and to a lesser extent in the subiculum, fulfilled the criteria for normal aging (Small et al., 2002). These findings not only confirm, but also extend, the results of the previous study. First, the entorhinal cortex indeed appears to be the hippocampal subregion most vulnerable to AD, even during the early cell-sickness stage. Second, these findings provided the first evidence that the dentate gyrus might be the hippocampal subregion that is most vulnerable to normal aging.

This study had a number of limitations. First, despite the strict criteria, independent verification of which older subjects did or did not have early AD was not possible. Second, although the MRI measure used is sensitive to basal deoxyhemoglobin levels, these images are also sensitive to other, nonmetabolic tissue constituents that are potential confounds (Small et al., 2000; Small, 2003).

These potential limitations were addressed in a third study. First, a cohort of aging individuals was needed that indisputably were free of AD. Because this cohort is difficult, or even impossible, to identify in human subjects, we turned to aging nonhuman primates instead. Like all mammals, monkeys develop age-related hippocampal dysfunction, yet they do not develop the known molecular or histological hallmarks of AD. Second, because of the stated limitations of imaging techniques sensitive to deoxyhemoglobin content, we relied on MRI to generate regional measures of CBV. Previous studies have established that CBV is a hemodynamic variable tightly correlated with brain metabolism, capable of detecting brain dysfunction in the hippocampus and other brain regions (Bozzao et al., 2001; Gonzalez et al., 1995; Harris et al., 1998; Wu et al., 1999).

In the third study, the hippocampal subregions of 14 rhesus monkeys were imaged across the age span, from 7–31 years of age (Small et al., 2004). In a remarkable parallel to the previous human study, age-related decline in CBV was observed only in the dentate gyrus, and to a lesser extent the subiculum. Notably, CBV measured from the entorhinal cortex, and the CA1 subregion remained stable across the lifespan. Indeed, when all subregions were analyzed simultaneously—in accordance with the circuit organization of the hippocampus—the dentate gyrus was the primary subregion that declined with age. Furthermore, since all monkeys were assessed cognitively, we found that a decline in dentate gyrus CBV was the only subregion that correlated with a decline in memory performance (Small et al., 2004).

Despite the reliance on CBV to investigate aging monkeys, this third study also had a number of limitations. The first limitation applies to all functional imaging. As derived from Fick's principle (Small, 2004), all hemodynamic variables—deoxyhemoglobin, CBV, or CBF—are correlates of oxygen metabolism. Nevertheless, they are only *indirect* correlates. The possibility always exists that these measures are confounded by changes in vascular physiology, and not

underlying neuronal physiology. Thus, we cannot exclude the possibility that there is something unique to the vascular system within the dentate gyrus that caused a shrinkage of CBV, independent of dentate gyrus physiologic dysfunction. The second limitation of the monkey MRI study has to do with the cellular complexity of any brain subregion, including the dentate gyrus. Although the granule cells are the primary neurons of the dentate gyrus, the dentate gyrus contains other types of neurons, as well as glial cells. Even if the CBV measure does reflect underlying cellular function, MRI cannot be relied on to isolate the cells that govern this observed effect.

A fourth study was designed to address these concerns. Here, in vitro imaging was used, directly visualizing correlates of neuronal physiology. Aging rats were investigated who, like humans and monkeys, develop age-related hippocampal dysfunction. Immunocytochemisty was used to visualize the behaviorally-induced expression of *Arc* in the hippocampal subregions of aging rats. *Arc* is an immediate early gene whose expression has been shown to correlate with spike activity and with long-term plasticity in hippocampal neurons (Guzowski et al., 1999, 2000, 2001). Rats of different ages were allowed to explore a novel place and then were sacrificed and processed for *Arc* staining. *Arc* expression was quantified in the granule cells of the dentate gyrus and in the pyramidal neurons of the CA1 and CA3 subregions. The dentate gyrus was the only hippocampal subregion whose neurons were found to have a significant age-related decline in *Arc* expression (Small et al., 2004). Thus, this study confirms and extends the prior studies, showing that it is in fact neuronal, not vascular, physiology that underlies the aging effect. Moreover, this study established that aging primarily targets the granule cells of the dentate gyrus.

The previous studies relied on different species to suggest that AD and aging target different hippocampal subregions. Recently, a number of transgenically engineered mouse models of AD have been developed that result in mice developing AD-like pathology relatively early in life. Thus, we reasoned that generating CBV maps of the mouse hippocampal formation would allow us to more formally disambiguate AD from normal aging in the same species. Although the logic is obvious, generating CBV maps in the minuscule mouse hippocampus is not trivial. To achieve this goal, we needed to construct a mouse MRI laboratory *de novo*, housing a very high field-dedicated mouse scanner and various small animal devices to monitor various physiological parameters that can affect functional imaging variables. Furthermore, we needed to develop a unique approach for generating CBV maps safely and longitudinally over time (Moreno et al., 2006).

We have recently applied this imaging approach to image a mouse model of AD expressing a disease-causing mutation in the amyloid precursor protein (APP) that develops AD-like hippocampal changes early in life. By imaging nearly 60 mice—mutants and their wildtype littermates over the mouse lifespan—a clear dissociation was established between AD and normal aging. Specifically, entorhinal dysfunction was observed early on in the mutant mice and it progressed over time to affect all hippocampal subregions. In contrast, aging itself was found to differentially target the dentate gyrus (Moreno et al., 2007) (examples of cross-species CBV mapping can be seen in Figure 8.5.).

Implications of Resolving the Debate

By interrogating the functional integrity of the hippocampal circuit in humans and animals, a double anatomical dissociation has emerged that distinguishes early AD from normal aging. During

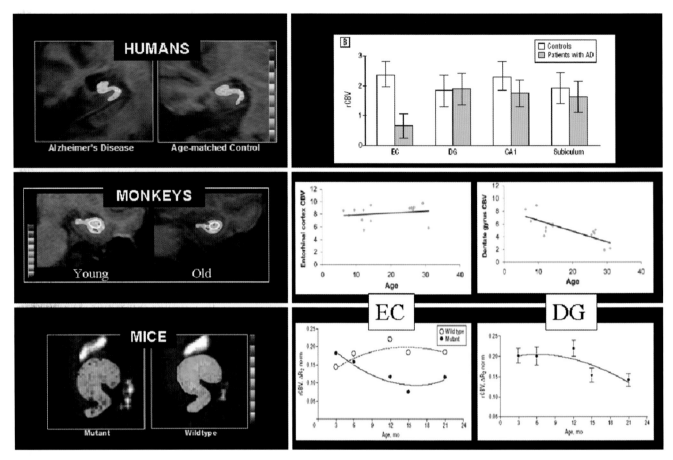

Figure 8–5   Examples of cross-species CBV mapping in Alzheimer's disease and aging. Comparing hippocampal CBV maps between patients with Alzheimer's disease vs. age-matched controls suggests that the disease differentially targets the EC while differentially sparing the DG (upper panels). Hippocampal CBV maps in rhesus monkeys across their lifespan suggest that aging differentially targets the DG while differentially sparing the EC. Hippocampal CBV maps in a transgenic mouse model of Alzheimer's disease that develops Alzheimer-like changes at a relatively young age suggest that the disease differentially targets the EC, while aging differentially targets the DG.

its earliest stages, AD targets the entorhinal cortex and spares the dentate gyrus; while in contrast, normal aging spares the entorhinal cortex but targets the dentate gyrus (Figure 8.6).

This anatomical profiling has three important implications. First, the anatomical dissociation establishes that AD and normal aging are two pathogenically separate processes, forevermore putting an end to the possibility that age-related memory decline might solely represent AD. Second, the anatomical dissociation, and the ability to visualize this dissociation in living subjects, can be exploited as a diagnostic tool. Although we currently do not have effective treatments for AD, arresting or even reversing the cell-sickness stage of AD on theoretical grounds is more likely than treating the cell-death stage of AD. Currently, relying on cognitive measures alone, we cannot accurately diagnose AD during its early cell-sickness stage because it cognitively overlaps with normal aging. Imaging techniques that can assess the functional integrity of the hippocampal subregions—in particular, the entorhinal cortex and the dentate gyrus—are well-suited to achieve this diagnostic goal. Testing the diagnostic capabilities of any technique requires large-scale, epidemiologically rigorous, prospective studies. One such study is currently underway, testing whether the imaging approaches discussed in this chapter can be used to diagnose AD during its earliest stages.

Finally, pinpointing the hippocampal neurons most vulnerable to AD and to aging is a required first step for uncovering the

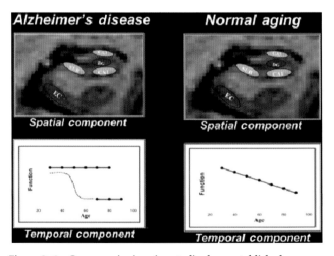

Figure 8–6   Cross-species imaging studies have established spatiotemporal patterns of hippocampal dysfunction that dissociate Alzheimer's disease from normal aging. Spatially, Alzheimer's disease is characterized by differential dysfunction in the EC with relative sparing of the DG, while the reverse pattern is observed in normal aging. Temporally, Alzheimer's disease is characterized by stable dysfunction over time and across age groups, while a linear decline in function is observed in normal aging.

molecular causes of each process. By isolating the molecular defects that underlie the rare autosomal-dominant form of AD, and by expressing these molecules in cell culture and in transgenic mice, tremendous strides have been made to uncover the molecular biology of AD. Nevertheless, the primary molecules whose defects underlie autosomal-dominant AD are normal in sporadic AD—the common form that accounts for over 95% of all cases. Thus, the primary molecular defects of the vast majority of AD remain unknown. Pinpointing the entorhinal cortex as the site of greatest vulnerability provides an anatomical handle with which to tackle this problem. Specifically, comparing the molecular profiles of the entorhinal cortex of affected and unaffected brains at the mRNA or protein level holds great promise for uncovering heretofore unidentified pathogenic molecules underlying sporadic AD. In a similar fashion, mapping age-related changes in the molecular profiles of the dentate gyrus in healthy brains may lead to insights into the molecular causes of memory decline associated with normal aging.

Age-related hippocampal dysfunction has emerged as a serious societal problem. As life expectancy is expanding, most of us do not simply want to live longer, but rather we would like to age with cognitive grace, remaining intellectually engaged in our information-rich environments. As discussed in this chapter, and in accordance with fundamental principles of clinical neuroscience, pinpointing the population of neurons differentially vulnerable to aging and to AD is an important first step towards developing effective diagnostics and, one day, even ameliorating the age-related slide into forgetfulness.

References

Amaral, D. G. and M. P. Witter (1989). The three-dimensional organization of the hippocampal formation: A review of anatomical data. *Neuroscience*, 31(3): 571–591.

Barnes, C. A. (1994). Normal aging: Regionally specific changes in hippocampal synaptic transmission. *Trends Neuroscience*, 17(1): 13–18.

Bozzao, A., Floris, R. Baviera, M. E., Apruzzese, A., and Simonetti, G. (2001). Diffusion and perfusion MR imaging in cases of Alzheimer's disease: Correlations with cortical atrophy and lesion load. *American Journal of Neuroradiology*, 22(6): 1030–1036.

Braak, H. and E. Braak (1996). Evolution of the neuropathology of Alzheimer's disease. *Acta Neurolgica Scandinavica*, Suppl 165: 3–12.

Erickson, C. A. and C. A. Barnes (2003). The neurobiology of memory changes in normal aging. *Experimenatl Gerontology*, 38(1–2): 61–69.

Fukutani, Y., Cairns, N. J., Shiozawa, M., Sasaki, K., Sudo, S., Isaki, K. et al. (2000). Neuronal loss and neurofibrillary degeneration in the hippocampal cortex in late-onset sporadic Alzheimer's disease. *Psychiatry and Clinical Neuroscience*, 54(5): 523–529.

Gallagher, M. and P. R. Rapp (1997). The use of animal models to study the effects of aging on cognition. *Annual Review of Psychology*, 48: 339–370.

Giannakopoulos, P., Herrmann, F. R., Bussière, T., Bouras, C., Kövari, E., Perl, D. P. et al. (2003). Tangle and neuron numbers, but not amyloid load, predict cognitive status in Alzheimer's disease. *Neurology*, 60(9): 1495–1500.

Gonzalez, R. G., Fischman, A. J., Guimaraes, A. R., Carr, C. A., Stern, C. E., Halpern, E. F. et al. (1995). Functional MR in the evaluation of dementia: correlation of abnormal dynamic cerebral blood volume measurements with changes in cerebral metabolism on positron emission tomography with fludeoxyglucose F 18. *American Journal of Neuroradiology*, 16(9): 1763–1770.

Guzowski, J. F., Lyford, G. L., Stevenson, G. D., Houston, F. P., McGaugh, J. L., Worley, P. F. et al. (2000). Inhibition of activity-dependent arc protein expression in the rat hippocampus impairs the maintenance of long-term potentiation and the consolidation of long-term memory. *Journal of Neuroscience*, 20(11): 3993–4001.

Guzowski, J. F., McNaughton, B. L., Barnes, C. A., and Worley, P. F. (1999). Environment-specific expression of the immediate-early gene Arc in hippocampal neuronal ensembles. *Nature Neuroscience* 2(12): 1120–1124.

Guzowski, J. F., Setlow, B., Wagner, E. K., and McGaugh, J. L. (2001). Experience-dependent gene expression in the rat hippocampus after spatial learning: A comparison of the immediate-early genes Arc, c-fos, and zif268. *Journal of Neuroscience*, 21(14): 5089–5098.

Harris, G. J., Lewis, R. F., Satlin, A., English, C. D., Scott, T. M., Yurgelun-Todd, D. A. et al. (1998). Dynamic susceptibility contrast MR imaging of regional cerebral blood volume in Alzheimer disease: A promising alternative to nuclear medicine. *American Journal of Neuroradiology*, 19(9): 1727–1732.

Jacobs, D. M., Sano, M., Dooneief, G., Marder, K., Bell, K. L., Stern, Y. (1995). Neuropsychological detection and characterization of preclinical Alzheimer's disease [comment] [see comments]. *Neurology*, 45(5): 957–962.

Masur, D. M., Sliwinski, M., Lipton, R. B., Blau, A. D., and Crystal, H. A. (1994). Neuropsychological prediction of dementia and the absence of dementia in healthy elderly persons [see comments]. *Neurology*, 44(8): 1427–1432.

Moreno, H., Wu, W. E., Brown, T., and Small, S. (2006). Longitudinal mapping of mouse cerebral blood volume with MRI. *NMR in Biomedicine*, 19(5): 535–543.

Moreno, H., Wu, W. E., Lee, T., Brickman, A., Mayeux, R., Brown, T. R. et al. (2007). Imaging the abeta-related neurotoxicity of Alzheimer disease. *Archives of Neurology*, 64(10): 1467–1477.

Price, J. L., Ko, A. I., Wade, M. J., Tsou, S. K., McKeel, D. W., and Morris, J. C. (2001). Neuron number in the entorhinal cortex and CA1 in preclinical Alzheimer disease. *Archives of Neurology*, 58(9): 1395–1402.

Rapp, P. R. and M. Gallagher (1996). Preserved neuron number in the hippocampus of aged rats with spatial learning deficits. *Proceedings of the National Academy of Sciences of the USA* 93(18): 9926–9930.

Schonheit, B., Zarski, R., and Ohm, T. G. (2004). Spatial and temporal relationships between plaques and tangles in Alzheimer-pathology. *Neurobiology of Aging*, 25(6): 697–711.

Selkoe, D. J. (2002). Alzheimer's disease is a synaptic failure. *Science*, 298(5594): 789–791.

Shoghi-Jadid, K., Small, G. W., Agdeppa, E. D., Kepe, V., Ercoli, L. M., Siddarth, P. et al. (2002). Localization of neurofibrillary tangles and beta-amyloid plaques in the brains of living patients with Alzheimer disease. *American Journal of Geriatric Psychiatry*, 10(1): 24–35.

Small, S. A. (2001). Age-related memory decline; current concepts and future directions. *Archives of Neurology*, 58: 360–364.

Small, S. A. (2003). Measuring correlates of brain metabolism with high-resolution MRI: A promising approach for diagnosing Alzheimer disease and mapping its course. *Alzheimer Disease Association Disorder*, 17(3): 154–161.

Small, S. A. (2004). Quantifying cerebral blood flow: Regional regulation with global implications. *Journal of Clinical Investment*, 114(8): 1046–1048.

Small, S. A. (2005). Alzheimer disease, in living color. *Nature Neuroscience*, 8(4): 404–405.

Small, S. A., Chawla, M. K., Buonocore, M., Rapp, P. R., and Barnes, C. A. (2004). From the cover: Imaging correlates of brain function in monkeys and rats isolates a hippocampal subregion differentially vulnerable to aging. *Proceedings of the National Academy of Sciences of the USA*, 101(18): 7181–7186.

Small, S. A., Nava, A. S., Perera, G. M., Delapaz, R., and Stern, Y. (2000). Evaluating the function of hippocampal subregions with high-resolution MRI in Alzheimer's disease and aging [In Process Citation]. *Microscopy Research and Technique*, 51(1): 101–108.

Small, S. A., Stern, Y., Tang, M., and Mayeux, R. (1999). Selective decline in memory function among healthy elderly. *Neurology*, 52(7): 1392–1396.

Small, S. A., Tsai, W. Y., DeLaPaz, R, Mayeux, R., and Stern, Y. (2002). Imaging hippocampal function across the human life span: is memory decline normal or not? *Annals of Neurology*, 51(3): 290–295.

Small, S., Wu, E. X., Bartsch, D., Perera, G. M., Lacefield, C. O., DeLaPaz, R. et al. (2000). Imaging physiologic dysfunction of individual hippocampal subregions in humans and genetically modified mice. *Neuron*, (28): 653–664.

Wu, R. H., Bruening, R., Noachtar, S., Arnold, S., Berchtenbreiter, C., Bartenstein, P. et al. (1999). MR measurement of regional relative cerebral blood volume in epilepsy. *Journal of Magnetic Resonance Imaging*, 9(3): 435–440.

Zelinski, E. M. and K. P. Burnight (1997). Sixteen-year longitudinal and time lag changes in memory and cognition in older adults. *Psychological Aging*, 12(3): 503–513.

Zhao, X., Lein, E. S., He, A., Smith, S. C., Aston, C., and Gage, F. H. (2001). Transcriptional profiling reveals strict boundaries between hippocampal subregions. *Journal of Comparative Neurology*, 441(3): 187–196.

9

Genetics and Imaging in Alzheimer's Disease

Susan Y. Bookheimer

Because interventions are more likely to delay or slow disease progression rather than reverse it, a major goal in Alzheimer's disease (AD) research is to identify individuals likely to develop AD in the earliest possible stages. Neuroimaging has proven critical in identifying brain changes associated with AD in vivo, providing more definitive diagnosis during life, and drawing associations between preclinical stages found in MCI and more advanced AD. To identify the at-risk, clinically normal population, imaging alone is not practical, as it is expensive, the analysis is time-consuming, and it is still too nonspecific to serve this purpose alone. The additional information provided by genetic risk has the potential to greatly improve the identification of individuals more likely to develop AD. Genetic status as an independent biomarker for AD, however, is equally insufficient, as all genetic risk factors are clearly not known, and genetic risk alone in most cases is not sufficiently predictive of AD for clinical utility. This chapter will present recent data combining genetic information with imaging to address the question of whether this combination may serve as a valid biomarker for AD, whether there is evidence for added value, and whether the combined information has proven useful in understanding the pathogenesis of AD or is a valid predictor of future AD. The focus will be on whether the combined data has added predictive value over either imaging or genetic data individually.

There are several potential benefits of combined genetic risk and imaging in AD research. One is in increasing diagnostic accuracy in living patients, which improves our ability to study AD pathophysiology in living subjects with more reliability. Many cases of dementia, including frontotemporal lobar degeneration (FTLD), Lewy body dementia, vascular disease, and dementias of unknown pathology, may appear similar to AD in clinical presentation. A characteristic imaging profile, in combination with a known AD risk gene, would increase the likelihood of an AD diagnosis. This would be a potential benefit to AD research in that one would expect less variability in the sample and thus increased power. Another important goal in AD research is to identify individuals at risk for developing the disorder. While genotype alone is not a good predictor of AD—except in the rare familial Alzheimer's Dementias (FAD)—genetics, in combination with imaging, may potentially become a reliable metric of incipient AD in the preclinical or presymptomatic stage. Understanding the pathogenesis of AD from the asymptomatic stage through to disease may be enhanced by accurate identification of those at greatest risk; such research is effectively impractical without a strong likelihood that a

large proportion of the subjects will evidence decline. Finally, identifying at-risk individuals may allow an earlier and potentially more efficacious evaluation of interventions. In this chapter, we will discuss the state of the science for combining imaging and genetics in both early-and late-onset genetic risk individuals, identifying which of the imaging measures have proven most valuable in the diagnosis of AD, and predicting risk and outcome in the preclinical stages.

Genetic Risk for AD: Autosomal Dominant Genetic Variants

There are two broad categories of genetic contributors to AD to consider: rare genes that are fully penetrant, autosomal dominant, and predict AD with certainty; and more common polymorphisms that confer an increased risk for AD. Of the former, the principal actors are mutations of the presenilin genes PS-1 and PS-2, and variants in the amyloid precursor protein or APP 717 valine to glycine mutation (see Serretti et al., 2007; Ertekin-Taner, 2007 for recent reviews). The three familial AD risk genes share a common mechanism involving beta-amyloid deposition. Carriers of these genetic variants develop the same neuropathological hallmarks of AD, and typically confer an earlier age of onset. Extended families with these genetic variants provide important information that is highly beneficial to AD imaging research. Because carriers will certainly get the disease, investigators can identify early brain changes in a truly healthy or preclinical state. Since these individuals tend to have an early age of onset, other brain changes characteristic of aging generally, rather than AD specifically, should be less apparent, making it possible to differentiate those imaging markers specific to the disease process. A potential weakness in studying these genes is whether the pathological hallmarks observed in these rare cases are equivalent to those in the typical late-onset AD presentation, although most studies to date appear to show similar patterns of brain changes. Because these cases may be identified many years before the disease is evident and followed throughout the onset, they are ideally suited to understanding the progression of brain changes, and thus contribute to our understanding of the pathogenesis of AD in relation to imaging findings. Several imaging studies have examined brain changes in patients with these variants in the preclinical state, and longitudinally, using a range of imaging methods. The primary disadvantage of using FAD in AD research is that they account for a very small percentage of AD cases, and as a practical matter are difficult to study: PS-1, PS-2, and APP together account for about 5% of AD cases overall (Signorini et al., 2004). Of these, the PS-1 mutations are the most common and have generated the most imaging studies, typically producing results similar to those in AD using a variety of techniques.

PS-1 and Imaging: Mutations in the PS-1 gene on chromosome 14 are frequently associated with dementia, usually (but not always) of the Alzheimer's type. The PS-1 gene is affected by multiple mutations: over 130 have been reported (Signorini et al., 2004) and the presentation of dementia appears to vary with the precise mutation. For instance, the PS-1 mutation at codon 183 reported by Dermaut et al. (2004) is associated with a Picks presentation without apparent amyloid plaques; other mutations have resulted in less common presentations, including FTD (Tang-Wai et al., 2002; Zekanowski et al., 2006) and language impairment (Godbolt et al., 2004). Numerous mutations in PS-1 have been associated with AD, and generally involve abnormal cleavage of the amyloid precursor protein to produce insoluble A-beta 42 or 43, as opposed to A-beta 40, which is soluble and not associated with AD. There may be presentations of several different dementias within families with PS-1 mutations (Snider et al., 2005).

FDG PET and PS-1: Mosconi et al. (2006) examined the relative abnormalities in glucose metabolism vs. MRI volumes in PS-1 mutation carriers. Interestingly they found that glucose metabolism was reduced in all of the mutation carriers across a range of brain regions, including the hippocampus and entorhinal cortex (EC), but also neocortical regions—particularly the intraparietal regions. Importantly, this pattern was similar to that found in sporadic AD, which tends to support the generalizability of studying these rare cases to understand the pathogenesis of AD.

Amyloid PET: Amyloid imaging using Pittsburgh Compound B (PIB) offers a novel approach to understanding the pathophysiology in preclinical AD (discussed in more detail in Chapter 15). A study by Klunk et al. (2007) measured amyloid using PIB PET in five PS-1 presymptomatic and five symptomatic PS-1 carriers in relation to 12 with sporadic AD and 18 controls. Interestingly, the PS-1 mutation carriers displayed increased amyloid in the striatum, while showing some cortical amyloid signal, though substantially less than in sporadic AD. Indeed, the PS-1 mutation carriers with AD did not demonstrate the regional pattern of PIB signal found consistently in AD. PIB is a relatively new compound, and the relationship of PIB signal with AD pathology is still under debate. These data would tend to suggest that either the amyloid pathology in these PS-1 mutation carriers is fundamentally different than in sporadic AD, limiting the utility of studying FAD patients as a surrogate for the more common sporadic AD, or the data may reflect a limitation of the PIB probe in identifying true AD pathology. In contrast with the PIB findings, FDG PET showed a classic AD pattern of hypometabolism in PS-1 mutation carriers, arguing against a fundamental difference in pathology between PS-1 and sporadic AD (Mosconi et al., 2006). However the cohorts studied had different mutations of PS-1, and it is possible that the pathology in PS-1 is mutation-specific, even among those associated with AD.

MRI: Although PS-1 is the more common of the FAD mutations, few studies have systematically analyzed MRI images in PS-1 carriers. An early report in a PS-1 family described white matter MRI abnormalities in parietal cortex consistent with pathology in sporadic AD, though the measurements were qualitative (Aoki et al., 1997). Mosconi and colleagues (Mosconi et al., 2006) compared MRI volumetry to FDG-PET in differentiating PS-1 carriers from controls in a small cohort. The PS-1 carriers showed

significant reductions in volume in the left intraparietal area alone, and while other regions such as the hippocampus were smaller, they were not significantly so for this group of seven subjects. In contrast, glucose metabolism in the same regions differed significantly in most measured regions, and showed larger effect sizes in predicting genetic status in all regions compared to MRI volumetry. No studies to date have studied MRI volumes longitudinally in PS-1 carriers.

Diffusion Tensor Imaging (DTI): White matter changes in AD are increasingly recognized as important in the pathophysiology of AD, and DTI is an optimal tool for examining WM integrity. Only one study to date has examined DTI in FAD. Ringman et al. (2007) measured fractional anisotropy in a relatively large cohort of preclinical and nonsymptomatic PS-1 carriers in comparison to noncarriers and two carriers with dementia. Preclinical carriers (nondemented but with areas of mild decline) showed reduced FA in whole brain and in frontohippocampal pathways relative to noncarriers, specifically finding that an area of the fornix was the strongest predictor of mutation status, with reduced FA found even in presymptomatic carriers who had normal cognition.

FMRI in PS-1: To date, only one study has used functional MRI during memory activation in presymptomatic PS-1 mutation carriers. This study examined five members of a PS-1 family—two with the mutation, one young and one old—with fMRI (Mondadori et al., 2006). In an episodic memory task, the young mutation carrier showed relatively increased fMRI activation compared to the noncarriers, while the older (near age of onset) carrier showed a decrease in activation. This result is similar to most other fMRI studies, indicating decreased fMRI activation during memory tasks in AD and memory-impaired subjects, but increased activation (in most studies) of APOE-4 carriers with normal cognition (Bondi et al., 2005; Bookheimer et al., 2000; Smith et al., 2002).

Amyloid Precursor Protein (APP): Several recent studies have examined serial MRI in amyloid precursor protein (APP) 717 valine-glycine mutation carriers. An earlier report by Fox et al. (1996) measured the volume of the hippocampus in addition to clinical measures in seven carriers of the mutation, with three evidencing cognitive decline over the course of the 3-year follow-up period. Those who declined showed a significant loss in hippocampal (HC) volume. Notably, the variability in HC volume at baseline was such that those later declining could not have been identified on the basis of volume alone, although on average the normalized volume was less than controls and nondecliners. This study suggests that rate of HC volume decline may herald an impending decline in cognition associated with AD. A more recent study that also mapped control subjects longitudinally (Ridha et al., 2006) similarly found that the rate of HC atrophy predicted future cognitive decline in APP carriers, suggesting that rate-of-change metrics identified AD risk 2–3 years earlier than static measures.

Summary of FAD-imaging Studies: The autosomal dominant genetic forms of early Alzheimer's are an attractive target for AD-risk research because of their potential to identify early imaging markers of AD. Because the patients develop the disease early, there is far less concern with the general effects of normal aging on imaging measures that plague AD-risk research, and the certainty that mutation carriers will develop the disease allows for minimal data loss and quick results. Both the PS-1 and APP carrier studies have generally supported a similarity in pathology to sporadic AD, particularly for FDG-PET and HC volumetry on MRI, and the lone studies using fMRI and DTI show similar promise. However, the only study of amyloid deposition using the PIB compound revealed disparate results for PS-1 and sporadic AD, which casts doubt on the similarity of the rare genetic variants of common forms. This result may prove to be a specific problem with either the PIB compound or with the specific PS-1 mutations in the published sample (Klunk et al., 2007), and clearly requires further investigation, perhaps with other amyloid-PET compounds. Research on imaging in FAD will necessarily have limited applicability for larger scale studies, such as those testing interventions where large N's would be necessary. The rare nature of these genetic variants limits the utility of their study to smaller-scale investigations of AD pathology rather than interventions, and thus will have limited clinical utility. The benefits of studying FAD will therefore likely be limited to investigations that can tolerate small sample sizes or are of a more exploratory nature, unless multiple laboratories collaborate.

AD Risk Genes: Common Polymorphisms

The other major genetic approach examines common polymorphisms that confer a risk for AD. These include the APOE-4 allele, ubiquilin-1, systatin-C, and several other candidate genes. However, with the exception of the APOE-4 allele on chromosome 19, most of these other AD risk genes have failed to replicate in some linkage studies or have weak associations to AD (Bertram and Tanzi, 2004b).

As an example, the ubiquilin-1 gene has been identified in two major genetic linkage studies. Bertram et al. (2005), focusing on linkage peaks in 9q22, examined single nucleotide polymorphisms on genes in this region in over 400 multiplex families. Positive results were cross-validated with a smaller independent sample, and identified the UBQLN1 polymorphism in both, specifically on intron eight. However, Brouwers et al. (2006) analyzed the same polymorphism and failed to replicate in two independent samples. Smemo et al. (2006) obtained a similar result in over 1,500 cases without detecting an association. However, a separate study of 978 cases found modest effect sizes for at least two haplotypes in the UBQLN1 gene (Kamboh et al., 2006). But seven polymorphisms in this region tested by Slifer et al. (2006) in two data sets—a family-based set and a second, independent case-control cohort— failed to show a consistent association.

In contrast, the apolipoprotein epsilon-4 (APOE-4) allele on chromosome 19 has demonstrated an association with AD consistently. The frequency of the APOE-4 allele is approximately .16 in the population generally but .4 in AD, while the more common APOE-3 allele has a frequency of about .78 (Strittmatter and Roses, 1995). The odds ratio of developing AD with the E4 allele is approximately three times that of those with APOE-3, and in homozygous carriers, about 15 times (Bertram and Tanzi, 2004a). Presence of the APOE-4 allele lowers the age of onset of AD, and has a dose-related effect on incidence (Corder et al., 1993) that may account for nearly 50% of the genetic variance in AD, and while it is certain that at least several additional genes must contribute to AD (estimated 4–11: Bertram and Tanzi, 2004b), it is unlikely that any other gene will be found to account for more cases of AD than APOE-4. This strong genetic association has made APOE-4 a compelling target for AD research, and imaging studies of APOE-4 have examined individuals from childhood through AD diagnosis.

By recruiting subjects with a positive family history of AD, especially in first degree relatives, it is possible to significantly enrich a sample from an estimated base rate of 20% probability

of APOE-4 to nearly 50% (Small et al., 2000). Ideally, then, if one could follow older APOE-4 subjects into the age range wherein most subjects develop AD, a large minority of subjects should develop cognitive decline and ultimately AD. This approach defines the genetic risk studies that constitute most imaging genetics research into AD. Therefore, the remainder of this chapter will focus on imaging studies in APOE-4 carriers.

PET and APOE Status: FDG PET shows a consistent and well-validated characteristic profile of hypometabolism in AD; it is increasingly used in differential clinical diagnoses in AD, as well as in research (Foster et al., 2007; Jagust et al., 2007), and can identify healthy controls at risk for cognitive decline (Mosconi et al., 2007a). Indeed, Jagust et al. (2007) found PET to be more accurate than both an initial and final complete clinical evaluation for dementia.

In patients with AD, the presence of the APOE-4 allele produces more extensive regional hypometabolism even when dementia severity is similar (Mielke et al., 1998). One study (Mosconi et al., 2004) found that in APOE-4 patients with AD (compared to those without APOE), the regional hypometabolism extended beyond, and was adjacent to, the regions typically associated with AD—particularly, intraparietal cortex and frontal and inferior temporal cortex. A separate study in a larger cohort (Drzezga et al., 2005) found that APOE-4 subjects with AD showed significantly reduced glucose metabolism throughout the cortex but particularly in regions most associated with AD, including bilateral temporal, parietal, posterior cingulated, and prefrontal cortical areas.

More recently, studies from several independent labs have demonstrated reductions in cerebral glucose metabolism in APOE-4 carriers with MCI, age-associated memory impairment, older healthy controls, and even younger healthy controls. Among the first studies to use PET in nondemented subjects were those by Reiman et al. (1996) and Small et al. (1995). Reiman studied older, normal adults (age 50–65) who were APOE 4/4 homozygotes, in comparison to APOE-4 noncarriers—all with a family history of AD. Regions in which APOE-4 subjects had FDG hypometabolism compared to noncarriers were essentially overlapping, though of less severity, as compared with prior studies of AD patients from the same laboratory. Similarly, Small et al. (1995) showed reduced metabolism in E-4-carrying relatives of AD patients compared to relatives without the risk allele—again, in the same spatial distribution as is characteristic of AD (Figure 9.1). More recently, similar reports of reduced metabolism in APOE-4 carriers have been reported in younger adults. Reiman et al. (2005) examined PET in normal volunteers in their 20's and 30's with the APOE-4 allele. As in their studies of older adults, the young carriers showed a similar pattern of hypometabolism prominently in the posterior cingulated parietal and temporal lobes, and also in the frontal cortex.

The severity of abnormal glucose metabolic patterns in APOE-4 carriers is also modulated by subjective memory complaints in older subjects without dementia; Mosconi et al. (2007b) found an interaction between APOE-4 and subjective memory complaints in nondemented subjects aged 45–70. Hypometabolism associated with this interaction was greatest in parahippocampal and inferior frontal and temporal cortex; Small et al. (1999) found similar results in an earlier study.

Prediction of Decline with PET: The usefulness of combining PET and genetic risk is greatest if the combined metrics predict cognitive decline and conversion to AD. Several recent reports have followed subjects longitudinally to track changes in diagnosis, cognitive tests, or imaging parameters.

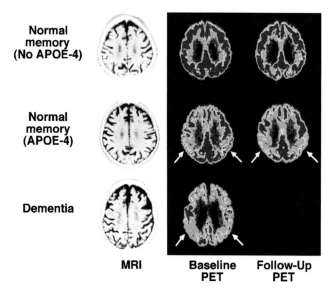

Figure 9–1   PET scans showing glucose metabolic patterns in normal elderly without the APOE-4 allele (top), with the allele (center) and with AD (bottom), showing a similar spatial pattern of metabolic decline in the genetically at-risk, but normally functioning subject. (Adapted from Small et al., 2000.)

Drzezga et al. (2005) combined genetic risk status and PET in predicting conversion from MCI to AD in a longitudinal study. In an average follow-up of 16-months, 40% converted to AD. Notably, less than half of the MCI patients had FDG PET scans clearly indicative of AD pathology. However, PET was highly predictive of a conversion to AD—significantly more so than genotype alone. They also calculated sensitivity and specificity of combining both metrics. Using various weightings, they were able to either predict AD with relatively lower sensitivity and higher specificity (67% and 100%, respectively) or higher sensitivity and lower specificity (100% vs. 44%, respectively). In fact, PET alone was a better overall predictor of decline (92% sensitivity, 92% specificity). However, the sample size was relatively small and there was no cross-validation. Mosconi et al. (2004) performed a similar study examining the added value of genotype and FDG PET on prediction of conversion in a small cohort of subjects (eight converters, 29 nonconverters). While PET alone was an excellent predictor of conversion (84% diagnostic accuracy), FDG plus APOE-4 was superior, with 100% sensitivity and 90% specificity (94% accuracy overall).

Amyloid Imaging in Genetic Risk: Two major amyloid imaging PET ligands have been reported in AD and AD risk—Pittsburgh Compound B and DDNP. One study has examined amyloid in APOE-4 subjects: Rowe et al. (2007) studied PIB PET in patients with AD, Lewy Body dementia, or frontotemporal dementia, as compared to controls; a post-hoc analysis of APOE-4 showed increased PIB binding in demented subjects with the risk allele, but no relation to dementia severity. Similarly, Kemppainen et al. (2007) examined PIB binding in MCI patients with and without APOE-4. They found a trend for MCI patients with APOE-4 to show greater PIB binding than those without APOE-4. Pike et al. (2007) studied PIB binding in AD, MCI, and control subjects. In examining the frequency of APOE-4 in the MCI sample, they found that while 83% of MCI patients with a high PIB signal had APOE-4, 23% of those without significant PIB binding had APOE-4, suggesting that genetic risk plays a critical

role in differentiating MCI patients with AD-like pathology from those without. Using FDDNP, a different amyloid binding agent that appears to have a different mechanism and characteristic distribution than PIB (Small et al., 2006), Small et al. (2009) found increased DDNP binding in older normal controls (mean age 66) with the APOE-4 allele in the medial temporal region. No other studies to date have examined amyloid imaging markers in normal subjects with APOE-4, and none have studied subjects longitudinally with amyloid PET in combination with genetics.

Summary of PET-APOE-4 Research: In general, PET (particularly FDG) is highly predictive of AD and conversion to AD, and correlates well with APOE-4 status. Is the predictive value of PET and APOE status better than genetic risk alone? Virtually all of the studies of PET in genetic risk for AD combine imaging data across subjects in their predictions. While useful from a research perspective, these existing results do not speak to the pressing clinical question of identifying which individuals are at greatest risk for declining or developing AD. Likewise, as a group, APOE-4 carriers are more likely to develop AD, but the gene alone is not a sufficient predictor—indeed, the majority of heterozygotes will not develop AD. The combined genetics and imaging data in PET are unanimous in showing greater imaging changes in carriers compared to controls, and an increasing likelihood of declining cognitively or developing AD. However, few studies to date have used combinatory models to predict which individuals are likely to decline among those with genetic risk. None have explicitly examined what specific PET values and metrics are most reliable, nor have they used sensitivity and specificity figures of combined measures in a cross-validation study. Given the number of studies performed to date, it is not unlikely that data exist to build these models; however, as of yet, there are no published studies of this nature. Therefore, while the present data are very promising, further work is needed to optimize and validate combined imaging and genetic data.

MRI

Numerous studies have reported on structural MRI metrics such as ventricular enlargement and global and regional volume loss in AD. Here, we will focus on more current and sensitive MRI measures in APOE-4 carriers, both static and in longitudinal analysis. These include voxel-based techniques, measurements of grey matter thickness, hippocampal volume, and entorhinal cortex volume.

MRI in AD and MCI

Entorhinal cortex (EC) volume is significantly reduced in Alzheimer's disease and may be the earliest and most significantly affected structure in AD. Nonetheless, the presence of the APOE-4 allele in AD appears to intensify structural MRI abnormalities. In one study, AD patients with the APOE-4 allele showed a 45% loss in ERC volume vs. 27% in APOE-3 AD patients, relative to controls (Juottonen et al., 1998), a highly significant effect of genotype. Decreased hippocampal volumes have also been found in APOE-4 carriers with mild cognitive impairment (Farlow et al., 2004; Jack et al., 1999) as well as APOE-4 subjects without AD (Reiman et al., 1998).

Longitudinal Change Metrics: A difficulty with MRI volumetric measures is that there is tremendous variability across individuals in terms of brain size, and even accounting for whole

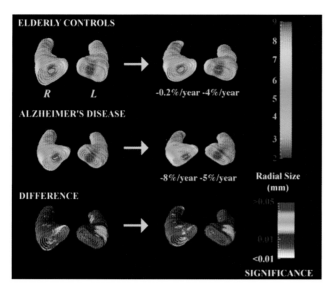

Figure 9–2 Based on maps of radial atrophy in the hippocampus, this figure demonstrates the annualized percent change in hippocampal size on each point on the surface in distance from the center. While older controls lose volume at a rate of between .2% and 4% per year, AD patients lose 5%–8% of HC volume annually. The bottom panel shows the spatial distribution of statistically significant differences between normal aging and AD, indicating a preferential loss of tissue in the anterior ventral hippocampal region—i.e., nearest the entorhinal cortex. (Adapted from Thompson et al., 2004.)

brain volume, smaller structures like the hippocampus vary substantially. Using a surface model of the hippocampus, Thompson et al. (2004) mapped the rate of change in hippocampal atrophy by plotting the amount of shrinkage from the center of the hippocampus using a surface model. The rate of change of the right hippocampus was 8.25 in AD compared to .2% in controls (no left hippocampal changes were found) (Figure 9.2).These rate-of-change measures were more sensitive than static volume measures of the hippocampus; similar approaches have been used in MRI reports of subjects with MCI to predict conversion. Van de Pol et al. (2007) followed a large cohort (over 300) of patients with MCI with serial MRI—measuring HC and whole brain volumes—and divided subjects into groups based on the rate of atrophy in 2 years. APOE-4 significantly correlated with atrophy rate, as did age and general cognition. Although this study did not follow subjects to determine conversion to AD, they demonstrated that combining risk factors predicted atrophy rates in the hippocampus.

In normal elderly, longitudinal mapping of HC and ERC volume shows similarly accelerated atrophy rates in genetically at-risk subjects without cognitive impairment. For instance, Chen et al. (2007) studied normal, older volunteers with the APOE-4 allele; they reported that, despite maintained cognitive performance, atrophy rates were significantly higher in APOE-4 subjects. A separate 6-year follow-up study (Rusinek et al., 2003) examined cognitive decline in normal elderly subjects using 2-year longitudinal change analysis on MRI, finding atrophy rate predictive of cognitive decline, but did not include genetic data. A recent report (Jak et al., 2007) compared cross-sectional and longitudinal HV volumetric data in a cohort of elderly subjects over an average of 17 months. They found that the rate of HC atrophy in APOE-4 subjects was over 9%, compared to 3% without APOE-4, and longitudinal data were superior to cross-sectional data in revealing relationships with APOE-4.

Does genetic risk data add to the predictive value of structural MRI? Tupler et al. (2007) conducted a 5-year longitudinal study of a large cohort of normal elderly using neuropsychological measures, MRI volumes, and APOE-4 status as predictors of change in memory performance. They found that baseline memory, APOE status, and left (but not right) hippocampal volume predicted memory decline in a stepwise regression, although MRI added only marginally to the prediction value. However, they used a static MRI measure and noted significant variability in HC volume at baseline.

MRI and Genetic Status in Younger, Healthy Controls

It is generally presumed that reduced EC volume in APOE-4 subjects represents a preclinical state in which the EC has atrophied as a result of the underlying pathology without reaching a critical decline to produce memory impairment.

This notion is challenged, however, by several studies reporting grey matter changes in healthy subjects with APOE-4 across a wide age range. Wishart et al. (2006a) found reduced volume in medial temporal and frontal regions predominantly using a voxel-based morphometric approach in a large mixed-age (19–80) cohort (Figure 9.3). Lind et al. (2006) found similar results using hippocampal volume, and further reported a correlation between volume loss and memory performance. More convincing is a recent study of EC thickness in children. Shaw et al. (2007) measured entorhinal cortex thickness in 239 healthy children and adolescents with serial MRI using a voxel-based analysis approach. Those with APOE-4 allele had a thinner EC than APOE-3 carriers who, in turn, had thinner EC than those with the neuroprotective APOE-2 allele (Figure 9.4). Notably, they found no evidence for age-progressive or longitudinal tissue loss in the EC. These data would tend to suggest that reduced ERC thickness or volume represents a lifelong risk factor for AD, rather than indicating progressive atrophy associated with Alzheimer pathology.

White Matter-based MRI Techniques: There is increasing interest in generally identifying WM abnormalities in AD, and in genetic risk for AD. In one recent DTI study (Persson et al., 2006), normal elderly with the APOE-4 allele had reduced fractional anisotropy in the posterior callosum and medial temporal white matter, consistent with the early regional localization of AD pathology. Bartzokis et al. (2006, 2007) have used different MR techniques to examine myelin integrity in AD and APOE-4. Using a dual spin echo sequence MRI, they calculated transverse relaxation time (T2) in late vs. earlier myelinating regions of the brain. APOE-4 subjects showed a steeper decline in T2 relaxation, which is related to reduced myelin integrity, prominent in later myelinating regions of the white matter—specifically, frontal white matter and the genu of the corpus callosum (Bartzokis et al., 2006). This line of research suggests a very different basis for the pathology in AD associated with APOE-4, arguing in favor of a myelin breakdown mechanism leading to the cognitive deficits associated with AD. Bartzokis et al. (2007) has demonstrated a relationship between cognition and transverse relaxation rate in APOE-4 subjects, which supports this model. The relationship between the T2 relaxation rate and more traditional methods of reduced volume in structures like the HC and EC remains unknown; nor do we understand how T2 relaxation might relate to either of the amyloid imaging probes, which may potentially be sensitive to the presence of myelin breakdown products.

Left   Right

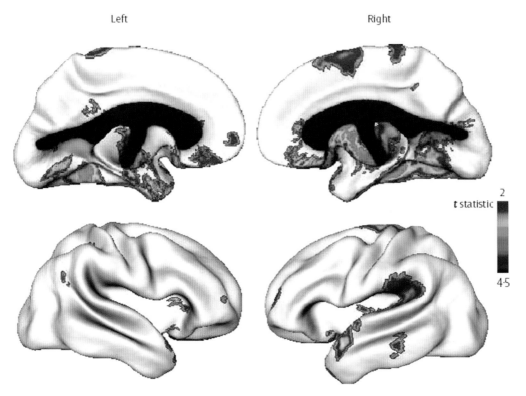

Figure 9–3   Regions of reduced grey matter density in APOE-3/4 vs. APOE 3/3 control subjects. (Adapted from Wishart et al., 2006a.)

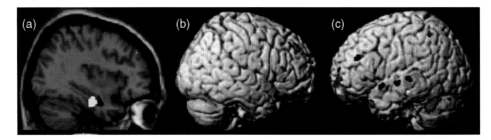

Figure 9–4   Statistical map of cortical thickness in children, showing significantly thinner cortex among children with the APOE-4 allele compared to those without APOE-4. Note the prominent decrease in cortical thickness around the entorhinal region. (Adapted from Shaw et al., 2007.)

FMRI and Genetic Risk

Cognitive activation studies in patients with Alzheimer's disease—using PET or fMRI—typically show a reduction in cerebral blood flow during performance on a range of cognitive tasks (Grady et al., 1993; Sperling, 2007). Activation studies of this nature, however, are confounded with the poorer performance among AD patients on the cognitive tasks used during imaging, which has a strong influence on activation magnitude (Just et al., 1996). Using fMRI during a challenging memory paired-associates learning task, Bookheimer et al. (2000) found a significant increase in cerebral activation among APOE-4 compared to APOE-3 normal elderly subjects who were matched for performance on the task (see Figure 9.5). This result suggested that prior to the onset of cognitive symptoms, at-risk subjects may compensate for declining function by drawing on more cognitive resources, resulting in increased activation in broad cortical and medial temporal brain regions (see also Chapters 6 and 7). These results were specific to memory challenge. In a separate study using the same subjects,

genetic groups performing a very challenging task that did not include an episodic memory component showed no differences in fMRI activation (Burggren and Bookheimer, 2002).

Since these initial reports, several other laboratories have replicated this general finding. Bondi et al. (2005) used a picture novelty task with normal elderly subjects and demonstrated increased fMRI activation in APOE-4 subjects who were matched for neuropsychological performance. Using a verbal paired associated memory task, Han et al. (2007) found that the compensatory response was prominent in the right hemisphere as well as the hippocampus. Similarly, Smith et al. (2002) demonstrated a pattern of increased brain activation on a fluency task while maintaining performance in subjects at risk for AD. A separate study (Dickerson et al., 2005) found increases in activation in the EC region among MCI patients with the APOE-4 allele compared to MCI patients without genetic risk. In contrast, a few studies have found disparate results. Bassett et al. (2006) recruited a large cohort of subjects with a dense family history of AD (two relatives). In this sample, a compensatory response was found for subjects with a

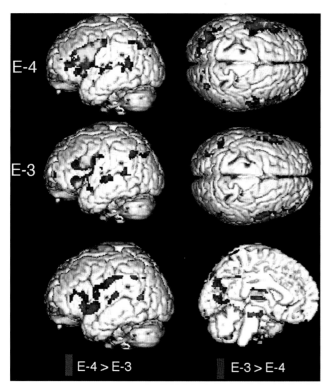

Figure 9–5 Brain regions showing increased fMRI activation for APOE-4 compared to APOE-3 subjects during associative encoding. (Adapted from Bookheimer et al., 2000.)

strong family history of AD, but no main effect for APOE-4. A separate report (Johnson et al., 2006) similarly found that a family history of AD modulated the effects of APOE-4 on brain activation during encoding of novelty pictures. However, Fleisher et al. (2005) combined both family history (FH) and APOE status to establish groups with either a high risk for AD (positive for both APOE and FH) or a low risk (positive for neither); they found increased fMRI activity during a novel word-pair encoding test among high-risk subjects.

In general, fMRI activation studies in healthy subjects using memory tasks have supported a compensatory model in which genetically at-risk subjects show increased activity relative to those without the genetic risk. Studies in which APOE-4 subjects did not show increased activation have typically involved recruiting subjects with a dense family history of AD in the APOE-3 groups. Those that use verbal or paired associate stimuli have generally proven more robust than nonmemory tasks like digit span (Burggren and Bookheimer, 2002) or word classification (Lind et al., 2006), although one study of working memory also found evidence for a compensatory response for APOE-4 subjects (Wishart et al., 2006b). Mixed results have been found with the picture encoding paradigm, which makes minimal demands on hippocampal encoding systems, as demonstrated by high-resolution fMRI (Zeineh et al., 2000).

FMRI studies are particular difficult to compare, as subtle differences in task choice, task difficulty, and subject performance can have profound effects on activation patterns. Because cognition in the at-risk population can vary markedly depending upon their age and proximity to likely disease onset, it will be difficult to use fMRI as a predictive measure of AD risk until the relationship between declining task performance and blood flow is well

characterized in longitudinal exams. It is interesting to note that the sole MEG study of memory activation in normal APOE-4 subjects showed a similar compensation pattern to the majority of fMRI studies (Filbey et al., 2006).

Several studies have related fMRI activation to clinical outcome in AD risk. In MCI, Dickerson et al. (2004) related functional MRI activation to cognition after a 2.5-year follow-up. Separating subjects into decliners and maintainers, they found that MCI patients who later declined had increased fMRI activation at baseline, consistent with a compensatory hypothesis. However, they found no difference in the percentage of subjects declining with the APOE-4 vs. APOE-3 genotype, and no independent effect of genotype on fMRI activation. One study used fMRI during memory performance to predict outcome in healthy, at-risk subjects. Bookheimer et al. (2000) performed a 2-year cognitive follow-up in genotyped normal elderly subjects, finding that the magnitude of fMRI increase at baseline correlated with memory decline, measured as individual memory change scores.

Comparison of Imaging Markers in Genetic Risk: Of the imaging methods reviewed here, FDG PET and MRI assessment of EC volume have received the most study, and perhaps predictably have demonstrated promise in predicting outcome when combined with genetic status. A few reports have attempted a side-by-side comparison of FDG and MRI in prediction value. For instance, Mosconi et al. (2006) reported significantly greater predictive value of PET compared to MRI volumetry of the HC, finding PET to be a superior predictor; however they did not evaluate the relative benefit of combining imaging and APOE status. We know of no studies that have attempted to combine more than one imaging technique with APOE to predict AD diagnosis, conversion to AD, or cognitive decline. To the extent that different imaging tools are independent in the pathology they are measuring, there may be advantages to using several techniques, even if they differ in their predictive power. For instance, the most sensitive locus of pathology in FDG PET for AD prediction is in the intraparietal and posterior cingulate cortex, while in MRI it is in the EC of hippocampus; PIB signal appears strongest in precuneus, frontal cortex, and caudate in AD patients. These data would suggest that the measures may have independent predictive value and, if so, this would suggest a need for combining measures and developing regression formulas for prediction.

Combined Genetic Risk and Imaging for Evaluating Treatment in AD

Assessing the efficacy of interventions for AD typically involves either demonstrating a direct effect on AD—i.e., improvement in cognitive status—or a longer-term benefit of slowing or preventing cognitive decline or conversion to AD in at-risk, MCI, or early AD subjects. Studies using rate of AD conversion to evaluate interventions are difficult to conduct because of the need to recruit large N's; estimates of the conversion rate in MCI over a few years ranges from 10%–50% (Modrego, 2006), and potential treatment effects may be difficult to evaluate when a majority of subjects are not expected to decline in an interval reasonable for conducting such studies. The optimal long-term goal would be to intervene even prior to clinical MCI in subjects that are at-risk for AD, and evaluating intervention efficacy in this population would be far more difficult. Genetic risk alone is not sufficient to determine AD risk, since most APOE-4 carriers are heterozygotes, and the lifetime risk by age 90 is still less than 50% (Martinez et al., 1998).

Identifying likely decliners by combining imaging with genetic risk to evaluate interventions would potentially facilitate the evaluation of new interventions, particular those of a neuroprotective nature. To date, however, very little work has examined the relative benefit of combining imaging measures and APOE status to measure treatment efficacy.

One open-label study examined the response to rivastigmine in patients with AD (no placebo control), using MRI measures of medial temporal lobe atrophy as a dependent measure and APOE genotype as a modulating variable (Visser et al., 2005). They found no relationship between medial temporal lobe atrophy and genotype on outcome, although there was a trend for patients with greater atrophy to show cognitive decline across the treatment interval.

A study by Hashimoto et al. (2005) examined the effect of Donepezil treatment on hippocampal atrophy in a placebo-controlled trial of mild AD. In this study, they found that treatment slowed the rate of HC atrophy. APOE status also related to the degree of HC atrophy, but there was no interaction between drug and genotype on imaging outcome. Upon examining the rate of atrophy on the genetic risk groups, a greater rate of atrophy was found in all subjects with APOE-4, and the effects of treatment on atrophy were more reliable than the effects of treatment on the AD assessment scale (ADAS). While this study did not expressly look at the added value of genetics, it did demonstrate the utility of imaging measure as a surrogate marker for drug efficacy.

A new multicenter study of Aricept in MCI (Jack et al., 2008), however, did not show an overall beneficial effect of Aricept on HC atrophy, although there was a trend in that direction for the APOE-4 subjects. Because atrophy rates were significantly greater in subjects who ultimately converted to AD, the study supports the notion of using imaging as a dependent measure for drug efficacy, and is suggestive that APOE-status may enhance that effect. However, if it is assumed that a treatment response would only be observed in subjects who are undergoing decline associated with preclinical AD, it seems possible that a study such as this is adversely affected by including many MCI subjects who are ultimately found to be "maintainers."

The few studies to date that have examined treatment efficacy and APOE have not suggested a differential treatment response depending upon genotype, which is encouraging because it suggests that preselecting subjects on the basis of genotype will not mediate any potential treatment effects. However, to truly use imaging and genetics in combination (rather than separately evaluating genetic contributions to the atrophy rate dependent measure), an approach might identify the APOE-4 carriers who also had abnormal HC volumes at baseline, and determine the effects of intervention on those subjects. Such an approach might be beneficial in preclinical studies, where treatment effects may be diluted by adding subjects who are unlikely to experience cognitive decline and thus unlikely to show treatment benefits. As of this writing, no studies to date have used such an approach.

Summary

Using a vast array of modalities, studies of Alzheimer's and AD risk combining genetics and imaging have identified imaging "hallmarks" of AD in preclinical populations. Increasingly, these studies have pinpointed the earliest pathological changes in at-risk subjects; it is likely that some of these measures, particularly those focusing on rate of change in HC or EC volume, white matter breakdown, parietal hypometabolism on PET, and (potentially)

abnormally increased cerebral activation on fMRI, begin to change many years before disease onset, and will ultimately prove to be reliable predictors of change. In several ways, these metrics are serving as reliable surrogate markers in AD. Imaging as a surrogate marker for diagnosis, particularly PET measures but also HC volume, are highly valued markers of disease, countermanding earlier insistence on reserving a confident diagnosis to post-mortem analysis. While post-mortem analysis is indeed the gold standard for quality research, the best imaging measures make this considerably less important than in prior years. With an imaging and genetic risk marker, a correct diagnosis is highly likely. Confidence in these metrics for surrogate markers should move research on intervention and drug discovery in AD forward.

As surrogate markers for disease prediction—i.e., a diagnosis of a preclinical state—combined imaging and genetics offers the best combination the science has to offer. Of the imaging methods reported, FDG PET continues to be the most sensitive and reliable. As noted above, a few studies have reported sensitivity and specificity figures with FDG PET for differential diagnosis of AD, and for predicting conversion, with excellent results. Similar data are not yet available for MRI measures, though it is apparent that several—particularly EC and HC—volumetric rates of change, are sensitive even in preclinical and presymptomatic, healthy controls with a risk gene. Analysis of PET data is less complicated and time-consuming as the most sensitive MRI measures, EC and HC volume, though new approaches in automated MR analysis may soon make these studies more practical and thus clinically relevant. While amyloid imaging is a very promising new tool, limited work to date has combined this method with genetics, and some reports (Klunk et al., 2007) are inconsistent with the known pathology in AD.

Across all imaging modalities, it is likely that metrics of change over time, rather than static measures, are the most promising in predicting disease risk and conversions.

Despite the plethora of data supporting the combination of genetic risk and imaging, there remains a serious deficiency in the research—the existing studies focus on differences in imaging parameters at the group level, whereas ultimately the goal will be to predict individuals who are most likely to decline. While it is likely that the data exist today to derive appropriate predictive models, the sensitivity and specificity of combined metrics have never been established, nor are there any published validation studies using predictive models. Such models will be essential to identifying which of the many imaging modalities—and metrics within those modalities—add unique predictive value over clinical information, genetic status, or clinical evaluation of imaging studies in isolation. Because all of the imaging methods discussed here are expensive—both in acquisition and data processing time and expertise—analysis of the costs relative to the benefits will be important in the future. Above all, the value of any of these tools as a reliable predictor of risk in individuals continues to depend upon the promise of viable interventions, without which limits the utility of imaging genetics in AD research.

References

Aoki, M., Abe, K. Ikeda, M., Tsuda, T., Kanai, M., Shoji, M. et al. (1997). A presenilin-1 mutation in a Japanese family with Alzheimer's disease and distinctive abnormalities on cranial MRI. *Neurology*, 48(4): 1118–1120.

Bartzokis, G., Lu, P. H., Geschwind, D. H., Edwards, N., Mintz, J., and Cummings, J. L. (2006). Apolipoprotein E genotype and age-related myelin breakdown in healthy individuals: Implications for cognitive decline and dementia. *Archives of General Psychiatry*, 63(1): 63–72.

Bartzokis, G., Lu, P. H., Geschwind, D. H., Tingus, K., Huang, D., Mendez, M. F. et al. (2007). Apolipoprotein E affects both myelin breakdown and cognition: Implications for age-related trajectories of decline into dementia. *Biological Psychiatry*, 62(12): 1380–1387.

Bassett, S. S., Yousem, D. M., Cristinzio, C., Kusevic, I., Yassa, M. A., Caffo, B. S. et al. (2006). Familial risk for Alzheimer's disease alters fMRI activation patterns. *Brain*, 129(Pt. 5): 1229–1239.

Bertram, L., Hiltunen, M., Parkinson, M., Ingelsson, M., Lange, C, Ramasamy, K. et al. (2005). Family-based association between Alzheimer's disease and variants in UBQLN1. *New England Journal of Medicine*, 352(9): 884–894.

Bertram, L. and Tanzi, R. E. (2004a). The current status of Alzheimer's disease genetics: What do we tell the patients? *Pharmacological Research*, 50(4): 385–396.

Bertram, L. and Tanzi, R. E. (2004b). Alzheimer's disease: One disorder, too many genes? *Human Molecular Genetics*, 13 Spec No 1: R135–R141.

Bondi, M. W., Houston, W. S., Eyler, L. T., and Brown, G. G. (2005). fMRI evidence of compensatory mechanisms in older adults at genetic risk for Alzheimer disease. *Neurology*, 64(3): 501–508.

Bookheimer, S. Y., Strojwas, M. H., Cohen, M. S., Saunders, A. M., Pericak-Vance, M. A., Mazziotta, J. C. et al. (2000). Patterns of brain activation in people at risk for Alzheimer's disease. *New England Journal of Medicine*, 343(7): 450–456.

Brouwers, N., Sleegers, K., Engelborghs, S., Bogaerts, V., van Duijn, C. M., De Deyn, P. P. et al. (2006). The UBQLN1 polymorphism, UBQ-8i, at 9q22 is not associated with Alzheimer's disease with onset before 70 years. *Neuroscience Letters*, 392(1–2): 72–74.

Burggren, A. C. and Bookheimer, S. Y. (2002). Structural and functional neuroimaging in Alzheimer's disease: An update. *Current Topics in Medicinal Chemistry*, 2(4): 385–393.

Chen, K., Reiman, E. M., Alexander, G. E., Caselli, R. J., Gerkin, R., Bandy, D. et al. (2007). Correlations between apolipoprotein E epsilon4 gene dose and whole brain atrophy rates. *American Journal of Psychiatry*, 164(6): 916–921.

Corder, E. H., Saunders, A. M., Strittmatter, W. J., Schmechel, D. E., Gaskell, P. C., Small, G. W. et al. (1993). Gene dose of apolipoprotein E type 4 allele and the risk of Alzheimer's disease in late onset families. *Science*, 261(5123): 921–923.

Dermaut, B., Kumar-Singh, S., Engelborghs, S., Theuns, J., Rademakers, R., Saerens, J. et al. (2004). A novel presenilin 1 mutation associated with Pick's disease but not beta-amyloid plaques. *Annals of Neurology*, 55(5): 617–626.

Dickerson, B. C., Salat, D. H., Bates, J. F., Atiya M., Killiany R. J., and Greve D. N. et al. (2004). Medial temporal lobe function and structure is mild cognitive impairment. *Annals of Neurology*, 56: 27–35.

Dickerson, B. C., Salat, D. H., Greve, D. N., Chua, E. F., Rand-Giovannetti, E., Rentz, D. M. et al. (2005). Increased hippocampal activation in mild cognitive impairment compared to normal aging and AD. *Neurology*, 65(3): 404–411.

Drzezga, A., Riemenschneider, M., Strassner, B., Grimmer, T., Peller, M., Knoll, A. et al. (2005). Cerebral glucose metabolism in patients with AD and different APOE genotypes. *Neurology*, 64(1): 102–107.

Ertekin-Taner, N. (2007). Genetics of Alzheimer's disease: A centennial review. *Neurology Clinics*, 25(3): 611–667.

Farlow, M. R., He, Y., Tekin, S., Xu, J., Lane, R., and Charles, H. C. (2004). Impact of APOE in mild cognitive impairment. *Neurology*, 63(10): 1898–1901.

Filbey, F. M., Slack, K. J., Sunderland, T. P., and Cohen, R. M. (2006). Functional magnetic resonance imaging and magnetoencephalography differences associated with APOEepsilon4 in young healthy adults. *Neuroreport*, 17(15): 1585–1590.

Fleisher, A. S., W. S. Houston, Eyler, L. T., Frye, S., Jenkins, C., Thal, L. J., Bondi, M. W. (2005). Identification of Alzheimer disease risk by functional magnetic resonance imaging. *Archives of Neurology*, 62(12): 1881–1888.

Foster, N. L., Heidebrink, J. L., Clark, C. M., Jagust, W. J., Arnold, S. E., Barbas, N. R. et al. (2007). FDG-PET improves accuracy in distinguishing frontotemporal dementia and Alzheimer's disease. *Brain*, 130(Pt. 10): 2616–2635.

Fox, N. C., Warrington, E. K., Stevens, J. M., and Rossor, M. N. (1996). Atrophy of the hippocampal formation in early familial Alzheimer's disease. A longitudinal MRI study of at-risk members of a family with an amyloid precursor protein 717Val-Gly mutation. *Annals of the New York Academy of Sciences*, 777: 226–232.

Godbolt, A. K., Beck, J. A., Collinge J., Garrard, P., Warren, J. D., Fox, N. C. et al. (2004). A presenilin 1 R278I mutation presenting with language impairment. *Neurology*, 63(9): 1702–1704.

Grady, C. L., Haxby, J. V., Horwitz, B., Gillette, J., Salerno, J. A., Gonzalez-Aviles, A. et al. (1993). Activation of cerebral blood flow during a visuo-perceptual task in patients with Alzheimer-type dementia. *Neurobiological Aging*, 14(1): 35–44.

Han, S. D., Houston, W. S., Jak, A. J., Eyler, L. T., Nagel, B. J., Fleisher, A. S. et al. (2007). Verbal paired-associate learning by APOE genotype in non-demented older adults: fMRI evidence of a right hemispheric compensatory response. *Neurobiology of Aging*, 28(2): 238–247.

Hashimoto, M., Kazui, H., Matsumoto, K., Nakano, Y., Yasuda, M., and Mori, E. (2005). Does donepezil treatment slow the progression of hippocampal atrophy in patients with Alzheimer's disease? *American Journal of Psychiatry*, 162(4): 676–682.

Jack, C. R., Jr., Petersen, R. C., Xu, Y. C., O'Brien, P. C., Smith, G. E., Ivnik, R. J. et al. (1999). Prediction of AD with MRI-based hippocampal volume in mild cognitive impairment. *Neurology*, 52(7): 1397–13403.

Jack, C. R., Jr., Petersen, R. C., Grundman, M., Jin, S., Gamst, A., Ward, C. P. et al. (2008). Longitudinal MRI findings from the vitamin E and donepezil treatment study for MCI. *Neurobiology of Aging*, 29(9): 1285–1295.

Jagust, W., Reed, B., Mungas, D., Ellis, W., and Decarli, C. (2007). What does fluorodeoxyglucose PET imaging add to a clinical diagnosis of dementia? *Neurology*, 69(9): 871–877.

Jak, A. J., Houston, W. S., Nagel, B. J., Corey-Bloom, J., and Bondi, M. W. (2007). Differential cross-sectional and longitudinal impact of APOE genotype on hippocampal volumes in nondemented older adults. *Dementia Geriatrics and Cognitive Disorders*, 23(6): 382–389.

Johnson, S. C., Schmitz, T. W., Trivedi, M. A., Ries, M. L., Torgerson, B. M., Carlsson, C. M. et al. (2006). The influence of Alzheimer disease family history and apolipoprotein E epsilon4 on mesial temporal lobe activation. *Journal of Neuroscience*, 26(22): 6069–6076.

Juottonen, K., Lehtovirta, M., Helisalmi, S., Riekkinen, P. J., Sr, and Soininen, H. (1998). Major decrease in the volume of the entorhinal cortex in patients with Alzheimer's disease carrying the apolipoprotein E epsilon4 allele. *Journal of Neurology, Neurosurgery and Psychiatry*, 65(3): 322–327.

Just, M. A., Carpenter, P. A. et al. (1996). Brain activation modulated by sentence comprehension. *Science*, 274: 114–116.

Kamboh, M. I., Minster, R. L., Feingold, E., DeKosky, S. T. (2006). Genetic association of ubiquilin with Alzheimer's disease and related quantitative measures. *Molecular Psychiatry*, 11(3): 273–279.

Kemppainen, N. M., Aalto, S., Wilson, I. A., Någren, K., Helin, S., Brück, A. et al. (2007). PET amyloid ligand [11C]PIB uptake is increased in mild cognitive impairment. *Neurology*, 68(19): 1603–1606.

Klunk, W. E., Price, J. C., Mathis, C. A., Tsopelas, N. D., Lopresti, B. J., Ziolko, S. K., Bi, W. et al. (2007). Amyloid deposition begins in the striatum of presenilin-1 mutation carriers from two unrelated pedigrees. *Journal of Neuroscience*, 27(23): 6174–6184.

Lind, J., Larsson, A., Persson, J., Ingvar, M., Nilsson, L. G., Bäckman, L. et al. (2006). Reduced hippocampal volume in non-demented carriers of the apolipoprotein E epsilon4: Relation to chronological age and recognition memory. *Neuroscience Letters*, 396(1): 23–27.

Lind, J., Persson, J., Ingvar, M., Larsson, A., Cruts, M., Van Broeckhoven, C. et al. (2006). Reduced functional brain activity response in cognitively intact apolipoprotein E epsilon4 carriers. *Brain*, 129(Pt 5): 1240–1248.

Martinez, M., Campion, D., Brice, A., Hannequin, D., Dubois, B., Didierjean, O. et al. (1998). Apolipoprotein E epsilon4 allele and familial aggregation of Alzheimer disease. *Archives of Neurology*, 55(6): 810–816.

Mielke, R., Zerres, K., Uhlhaas, S., Kessler, J., and Heiss, W. D. (1998). Apolipoprotein E polymorphism influences the cerebral metabolic pattern in Alzheimer's disease. *Neuroscience Letters*, 254(1): 49–52.

Modrego, P. J. (2006). Predictors of conversion to dementia of probable Alzheimer type in patients with mild cognitive impairment. *Current Alzheimer Research*, 3(2): 161–170.

Mondadori, C. R., Buchmann, A., Mustovic, H., Schmidt, C. F., Boesiger, P., Nitsch, R. M. et al. (2006). Enhanced brain activity may precede the diagnosis of Alzheimer's disease by 30 years. *Brain*, 129(Pt 11): 2908–2922.

Mosconi, L., Brys, M., Glodzik-Sobanska, L., De Santi, S., Rusinek, H., and de Leon, M. J. (2007a). Early detection of Alzheimer's disease using neuroimaging. *Experimental Gerontology*, 42(1–2): 129–138.

Mosconi, L., Brys, M., Switalski, R., Mistur, R., Glodzik, L., Pirraglia, E. et al. (2007b). Maternal family history of Alzheimer's disease predisposes to reduced brain glucose metabolism. *Proceedings of the National Academy of Sciences of the USA*, 104(48): 19067–19072.

Mosconi, L., Nacmias, B., Sorbi, S., De Cristofaro, M. T., Fayazz, M., Tedde, A. et al. (2004). Brain metabolic decreases related to the dose of the ApoE e4 allele in Alzheimer's disease. *Journal of Neurology, Neurosurgery and Psychiatry*, 75(3): 370–376.

Mosconi, L., Perani, D., Sorbi, S., Herholz, K., Nacmias, B., Holthoff, V. et al. (2004). MCI conversion to dementia and the APOE genotype: A prediction study with FDG-PET. *Neurology*, 63(12): 2332–2340.

Mosconi, L., Sorbi, S., de Leon, M. J., Li, Y., Nacmias, B., Myoung, P. S. et al. (2006). Hypometabolism exceeds atrophy in presymptomatic early-onset familial Alzheimer's disease. *Journal of Nuclear Medicine*, 47(11): 1778–1786.

Persson, J., Lind, J., Larsson, A., Ingvar, M., Cruts, M., Van Broeckhoven, C. et al. (2006). Altered brain white matter integrity in healthy carriers of the APOE epsilon4 allele: A risk for AD? *Neurology*, 66(7): 1029–1033.

Pike, K. E., Savage, G., Villemagne, V. L., Ng, S., Moss, S. A., Maruff, P. et al. (2007). Beta-amyloid imaging and memory in non-demented individuals: Evidence for preclinical Alzheimer's disease. *Brain*, 130(Pt 11): 2837–2844.

Reiman, E. M., Caselli, R. J., Yun, L. S., Chen, K., Bandy, D., Minoshima, S. et al. (1996). Preclinical evidence of Alzheimer's disease in persons homozygous for the epsilon 4 allele for apolipoprotein E. *New England Journal of Medicine*, 334(12): 752–758.

Reiman, E. M., Chen, K., Alexander, G. E., Caselli, R. J., Bandy, D., Osborne, D. et al. (2005). Correlations between apolipoprotein E epsilon4 gene dose and brain-imaging measurements of regional hypometabolism. *Proceedings of the National Academy of Sciences of the USA*, 102(23): 8299–8302.

Reiman, E. M., Uecker, A., Caselli, R. J., Lewis, S., Bandy, D., de Leon, M. J. et al. (1998). Hippocampal volumes in cognitively normal persons at genetic risk for Alzheimer's disease. *Annals of Neurology*, 44(2): 288–291.

Ridha, B. H., Barnes, J., Bartlett, J. W., Godbolt, A., Pepple, T., Rossor, M. N. et al. (2006). Tracking atrophy progression in familial Alzheimer's disease: a serial MRI study. *Lancet Neurology*, 5(10): 828–834.

Ringman, J. M., O'Neill, J., Geschwind, D., Medina, L., Apostolova, L. G., Rodriguez, Y. et al. (2007). Diffusion tensor imaging in preclinical and presymptomatic carriers of familial Alzheimer's disease mutations. *Brain*, 130(Pt 7): 1767–1776.

Rowe, C. C., Ng, S., Ackermann, U., Gong, S. J., Pike, K., Savage, G. et al. (2007). Imaging beta-amyloid burden in aging and dementia. *Neurology*, 68(20): 1718–1725.

Rusinek, H., De Santi, S., Frid, D., Tsui, W. H., Tarshish, C. Y., Convit, A. et al. (2003). Regional brain atrophy rate predicts future cognitive decline: 6-year longitudinal MR imaging study of normal aging. *Radiology*, 229(3): 691–696.

Serretti, A., Olgiati, P., and De Ronchi, D. (2007). Genetics of Alzheimer's disease. A rapidly evolving field. *Journal of Alzheimers Disease*, 12(1): 73–92.

Shaw, P., Lerch, J. P., Pruessner, J. C., Taylor, K. N., Rose, A. B., Greenstein, D. et al. (2007). Cortical morphology in children and adolescents with different apolipoprotein E gene polymorphisms: An observational study. *Lancet Neurology*, 6(6): 494–500.

Signorini, S., Ghidoni, R, Barbiero, L., Benussi, L., and Binetti, G. (2004). Prevalence of pathogenic mutations in an Italian clinical series of patients with familial dementia. *Current Alzheimer Research*, 1(3): 215–218.

Slifer, M. A., Martin, E. R., Bronson, P. G., Browning-Large, C., Doraiswamy, P. M., Welsh-Bohmer, K. A. et al. (2006). Lack of association between UBQLN1 and Alzheimer disease. *American Journal of Medical Genetics B Neuropsychiatric Genetics*, 141(3): 208–213.

Small, G. W., Chen, S. T., Komo, S., Ercoli, L., Bookheimer, S., Miller, K. et al. (1999). Memory self-appraisal in middle-aged and older adults with the apolipoprotein E-4 allele. *American Journal of Psychiatry*, 156(7): 1035–1038.

Small, G. W., Ercoli, L. M., Silverman, D. H., Huang, S. C., Komo, S., Bookheimer, S. Y. et al. (2000). Cerebral metabolic and cognitive decline in persons at genetic risk for Alzheimer's disease. *Proceedings of the National Academy of Sciences of the USA*, 97(11): 6037–6042.

Small, G. W., Kepe, V., Ercoli, L. M., Siddarth, P., Bookheimer, S. Y., Miller, K. J. et al. (2006). PET of brain amyloid and tau in mild cognitive impairment. *New England Journal of Medicine*, 355(25): 2652–2663.

Small, G. W., Mazziotta, J. C., Collins, M. T., Baxter, L. R., Phelps, M. E., Mandelkern, M. A. et al. (1995). Apolipoprotein E type 4 allele and cerebral glucose metabolism in relatives at risk for familial Alzheimer disease. *Journal of American Medical Association*, 273(12): 942–947.

Small, G. W., Siddarth, P., Burggren, A. C., Kepe, V., Ercoli, L. M., Miller, K. J. et al. (2009). Influence of cognitive status, age, and APOE-4 genetic risk on brain FDDNP positron-emission tomography imaging in persons without dementia. *Archives of General Psychiatry*, 66(1): 81–87.

Smemo, S., Nowotny, P., Hinrichs, A. L., Kauwe, J. S., Cherny, S., Erickson, K. et al. (2006). Ubiquilin 1 polymorphisms are not associated with late-onset Alzheimer's disease. *Annals of Neurology*, 59(1): 21–26.

Smith, C. D., Andersen, A. H., Kryscio, R. J., Schmitt, F. A., Kindy, M. S., Blonder, L. X. et al. (2002). Women at risk for AD show increased parietal activation during a fluency task. *Neurology*, 58(8): 1197–1202.

Snider, B. J., Norton, J., Coats, M. A., Chakraverty, S., Hou, C. E., Jervis, R. et al. (2005). Novel presenilin 1 mutation (S170F) causing Alzheimer disease with Lewy bodies in the third decade of life. *Archives of Neurology*, 62(12): 1821–1830.

Sperling, R. (2007). Functional MRI studies of associative encoding in normal aging, mild cognitive impairment, and Alzheimer's disease. *Annals of the New York Academy of Sciences*, 1097: 146–155.

Strittmatter, W. J. and Roses, A. D. (1995). Apolipoprotein E and Alzheimer disease. *Proceedings of the National Academy of Sciences of the USA*, 92(11): 4725–4727.

Tang-Wai, D., Lewis, P., Boeve, B., Hutton, M., Golde. T, Baker, M. et al. (2002). Familial frontotemporal dementia associated with a novel presenilin-1 mutation. *Dementia Geriatrics and Cognitive Disorders*, 14(1): 13–21.

Thompson, P. M., Hayashi, K. M., De Zubicaray, G. I., Janke, A. L., Rose, S. E., Semple, J. et al (2004). Mapping hippocampal and ventricular change in Alzheimer disease. *Neuroimage*, 22(4): 1754–1766.

Tupler, L. A., Krishnan, K. R., Greenberg, D. L., Marcovina, S. M., Payne, M. E., MacFall, J. R. et al. (2007). Predicting memory decline in normal elderly: Genetics, MRI, and cognitive reserve. *Neurobioloy of Aging*, 28(11): 1644–1656. Epub 2006 Aug 17.

van de Pol, L. A., van der Flier, W. M., Korf, E. S., Fox, N. C., Barkhof, F., and Scheltens, P. (2007). Baseline predictors of rates of hippocampal atrophy in mild cognitive impairment. *Neurology*, 69(15): 1491–1497.

Visser, P. J., Scheltens, P., Pelgrim, E., Verhey, F. R., and Dutch ENA-NL-01 Study Group. (2005). Medial temporal lobe atrophy and APOE genotype do not predict cognitive improvement upon treatment with rivastigmine in Alzheimer's disease patients. *Dementia Geriatrics and Cognitive Disorders*, 19(2–3): 126–133.

Wishart, H. A., Saykin, A. J., McAllister, T. W., Rabin, L. A., McDonald, B. C., Flashman, L. A. et al. (2006a) Regional brain atrophy in cognitively intact adults with a single APOE epsilon4 allele. *Neurology*, 67(7): 1221–1224.

Wishart, H. A., Saykin, A. J., Rabin, L. A., Santulli, R. B., Flashman, L. A., Guerin, S. J. et al. (2006b) Increased brain activation during working memory in cognitively intact adults with the APOE {epsilon}4 allele. *American Journal of Psychiatry*, 163(9): 1603–1610.

Zeineh, M. M., Engel, S. A., and Bookheimer, S. Y., (2000). Application of cortical unfolding techniques to functional MRI of the human hippocampal region. *Neuroimage*, 11(6 Pt 1): 668–683.

Zekanowski, C., Golan, M. P., Krzyśko, K. A., Lipczyńska-Łojkowska, W., Filipek, S., Kowalska, A. et al. (2006). Two novel presenilin 1 gene mutations connected with frontotemporal dementia-like clinical phenotype: Genetic and bioinformatic assessment. *Experimental Neurology*, 200(1): 82–88.

Part II

Clinical Applications

Imaging Cognitive Decline in Aging: Predicting Decline with Structural Imaging

Jeffrey Kaye

The focus of this chapter is predicting cognitive decline or dementia in normal older people using structural imaging. Key questions to be addressed include: What are the major methods, both clinical and imaging, that may help us to predict decline? What pathologies do structural changes preceding decline suggest are developing in the brain? What is the evidence from structural studies that anatomical changes are present before behavioral ones or precede the diagnosis of mild cognitive impairment or dementia? Does imaging provide information about the pace of future decline? What are the limitations of these studies? What are the implications of structural imaging outcomes for application to the conduct of treatment studies or future research?

The utility of structural imaging in the detection or prediction of cognitive decline or dementia may be encapsulated by answering a key question. How can a static image, a brief biopsy of time, indicate that a person has or will have dementia in the future? This question like any in medicine is tied to the degree to which the captured image can be most tightly linked to the known pathologies of the disease and the resultant clinical changes of interest. Thus in this context, the images are proxies for the pathology of disease. In a cross-sectional or first-time study of a brain, one is performing a process that is not much different from the classic correlation of the phenotype of the disease with the brain at autopsy. The obvious advantage of imaging is that one has the flexibility of performing many "autopsies" as symptoms unfold or even when the individual is asymptomatic. The obvious disadvantage is that the imaging measure during life is always indirect and brief. Nevertheless, fundamentally, this inferred state of the brain at the time of the snapshot forms the basis for all subsequent clinical conclusions to be made about the individual.

The most common concept and frequently studied variable in structural images is brain atrophy, presumptively reflecting a general loss of brain parenchyma. This process will be the emphasis of this chapter. Other aspects of structural imaging relating either to unique properties of the brain that can be assessed with specialized imaging techniques such as white matter integrity (discussed in Chapter 17), or deposits of amyloid (discussed in Chapter 14) will be reviewed as appropriate. There is great overlap between the structural and functional domains. For example, imaging of lesions of biochemical measures of aging or dementia pathology such as amyloid deposition using positron emission tomography (PET) is commonly referred to as functional or molecular imaging. However, the snapshot of amyloid provided by these PET images is a static picture of a structural or biochemical change, i.e., largely the amount of a particular chemical species found at a brief time-point occupying a particular compartment of brain. These images by themselves do not define when the amyloid accumulation began, whether it will continue to progress or, most importantly, what the functional clinical consequence of this change is likely to be in the future. This general concept of understanding what one is observing at various time-scales is an important overarching concept that will be a major theme of this chapter.

What Underlies Brain Volume loss Detected with Structural Imaging and What this Ulltimately Predicts

Since the premise of neuroimaging in aging and Alzheimer's disease is that the image reflects salient pathologies, it is useful to keep in mind what those pathologies are in terms of how they may be anticipated to affect structural imaging change, an issue covered in greater detail in Chapter 3. The identification of relevant pathologies underlying imaging appearances essentially began with Alzheimer himself at the end of the 19th Century when he became interested in "atherosclerotic brain atrophy" finally describing the signal clinical-pathological correlation for his 57-year-old patient, Auguste D., that to this day we ascribe to most cases of dementia (Maurer and Maurer, 2003). Thus the gold standard for the pathological diagnosis of the most common cause of adult onset dementia, Alzheimer's disease, is widely conceived of as the result of the deposition of amyloid in plaques and intraneuronal neurofibrillary tangles. These pathologies are associated microscopically with neuron loss and presumptively result in the macroscopic loss of brain parenchyma labeled "atrophy." Importantly, Alzheimer as a student of brain atrophy was impressed that he had found a new entity that could lead to atrophy that was distinct from the general paresis of syphilis, as well as major atherosclerotic change assumed at the time to be the primary cause of atrophy in old age. This view obviously fell out of favor at the end of the past century when the similarities between pre- and senile dementia were emphasized (Katzman, 1976). Ironically,

Alzheimer may have been more prescient than we have imagined since, in practice, we have come to realize that the picture is clearly more complex than a simple formula of plaques and tangles leading to eventual atrophy.

Recent community-based brain autopsy series report that it is in fact uncommon to find these lesions in a pure culture among the aging, i.e., there are likely to be multiple coincident pathologies accumulating with aging (Bennett et al., 2006; Hulette et al., 1998; Katzman et al., 1988; Schmitt et al., 2000). These include, non-specific gliosis and hippocampal sclerosis, changes in the white matter, changes in cerebrospinal fluid dynamics, Lewy bodies and a host of vascular changes. These studies suggest an as yet to be understood aggregate or enabling role for these other pathologies. The potential importance of these or other pathologies has been further emphasized by the discovery in these studies that notable subgroups of elderly die with large numbers of amyloid plaques and neurofibrillary tangles, but clearly remain cognitively intact prior to death, seemingly unaffected by the classic "Alzheimer" pathologies thought to lead unequivocally to brain damage, atrophy and cognitive impairment. Thus, the quantitative accrual of several pathologies can lead to the phenotype of cognitive impairment often referred to as "mild cognitive impairment" (or other related syndromes) in its less severe form or to frankly manifest dementias. Where the lesions lie, the rate of their accumulation and the relationship of one to the other are all factors underlying the ultimate macroscopic view that most imaging modalities provide at this time. High-field imaging and other evolving methods may provide a higher resolution view of brain regions in the near future and help to disentangle the various potential pathologies. This may add further complexity to our concept of what is occurring structurally in the aging and dementia-susceptible brain, but hopefully will also provide an improved understanding of these relationships.

Given this background, what evidence is there that the underlying pathologies that have been commonly regarded as tied to the atrophy of aging or dementia can be connected to changes observed with structural imaging? Although there was considerable imaging evidence, beginning with x-ray computed tomography (CT) and then later magnetic resonance imaging (MRI), that one could distinguish various control or normative groups from those with clinical dementia, it was only in the early 1990s that imaging pathological correlations directed at understanding the relationship of the presumptive causes of the atrophy being imaged (and the basis for the clinical classification in all these studies) were reported. These tended to be small studies with only a few cases dying dementia-free, a situation that holds to this day. This is not surprising given the fact that one needs to follow large numbers of subjects with annual scans until death to end up with sufficient sample sizes for comparison. Since it is rare that an individual dies suddenly without the effects of some disease, it is thus difficult to ultimately know what the atrophy of "normal" aging is. Nevertheless, the studies that have been reported are key to our fundamental understanding of what we are inferring when we compare various measures of atrophy to clinical states.

One of the first studies to examine the relationship of structural imaging to post-mortem neuropathologic change was the result of following 44 patients with Alzheimer's disease to autopsy (and thus histopathologically verified) who had had a CT scan within a year of their death (Jobst et al., 1992). Using a surrogate measure of medial temporal lobe atrophy, the minimum thickness of the medial temporal lobe measured linearly on axial CT scans, the histopathologically confirmed Alzheimer's disease cases were shown to have dramatically narrowed MTL widths, compared to age-matched cognitively normal CT-imaged control cases (none of whom came to autopsy at the time). Follow-up of this cohort and approach extended this observation longitudinally to show a clear progression of atrophy in this region which was noted to be quite rapid, on the order of 15% per year in these later stage Alzheimer's disease patients compared to control cases. In the three control cases without Alzheimer's neuropathology who also came to autopsy there was very little atrophy observed (1.5% per year) by comparison. Although these cases were based on pathological criteria that were amyloid-weighted (Khachaturian, 1985), and the measurements of atrophy as well as regional pathology were both indirect, they nevertheless suggested an important relationship between the general presence of classic Alzheimer's disease pathology in the brain with atrophy in the medial temporal lobes.

Other series with more direct imaging-pathological correlative approaches have investigated specific lesion types. In a study of 13 Alzheimer's disease patients and nine age-matched control subjects, *postmortem* coronal slices assessed with 7-tesla MR microscopy were compared to corresponding histopathologic sections focusing on the hippocampal formations (Huesgen et al., 1993). Neuritic plaques and neurofibrillary tangles (NFT) were quantified. The mean cross-sectional area of the hippocampus in the Alzheimer's disease brain was decreased by 31% compared to the control group. The width of the gray matter in the CA1 region of the hippocampus correlated with the total hippocampal area. The atrophy was significantly correlated with hippocampal NFT counts, but not with neuritic plaque counts. A later postmortem MRI study of hippocampal volume including a much larger number of subjects (24) dying cognitively intact within a year of their death also found a significant association of hippocampal volume with NFT rated by Braak stage (a semiquantitative rating) (Gosche et al., 2002). Hippocampal volume was a better indicator of NFT pathology than a delayed recall memory test administered within the year before death.

Another postmortem MRI study examined other important aspects of the relationship of hippocampal imaged volume to histopathologic change (Bobinski et al., 2000). In this study of 11 postmortem Alzheimer's disease cases and four normal elderly control subjects subregional (hippocampus, hippocampus/subiculum and hippocampus/parahippocampal gyrus), postmortem volumes were directly measured and correlated with 1.5 Tesla MR images of these same regions. Importantly, stereologically determined neuron counts were also made and these were correlated with the MR obtained volumes as well. For all regions of the hippocampus the MRI- and histology-based measurements were strongly correlated (r^2 ranging from .89–.97). Strong correlations between the MRI subvolumes and neuronal counts were found for the hippocampus (r^2 0.90) and the hippocampus/subiculum subvolume (r^2 0.84) as well. These postmortem studies directly link neuron loss of the hippocampus to volumes obtained with MRI. To the extent that NFT pathology reflects neuronal loss these results are concordant with prior postmortem MR-histological studies.

These studies focusing on hippocampal histology in relation to *postmortem* MR imaging do not address the relationship of *antemortem* MR atrophy to postmortem histopathology (which most closely bridges clinical application). There are few studies that have addressed this issue. One study of ante-mortem MR imaging—postmortem histopathology in the hippocampus—provides further support that NFT are correlated with observed hippocampal atrophy on MRI (Jack et al., 2002). In this study, 25 "typical aging" (based on neuropathological criteria; some were likely cognitively impaired) subjects were compared to a group of 23 elderly with

AD (based on Reagan neuropathological criteria) as well as nine with other dementias. Significant correlations (.39 for all cases; .69 AD, cases only) were found between normalized hippocampal volume scores and Braak NFT stage. Because the Braak stage is a measure of degree of dispersion of NFT outside the hippocampus, this study (and others using Braak staging as a NFT measure) did not directly verify the relation of NFT within the hippocampus itself to atrophy of this brain region. The relationship of amyloid plaques was also not investigated. Importantly, this study included non-AD cases and found that hippocampal atrophy related to Braak NFT staging was not specific for AD.

Another study further examined the specific association of ante-mortem MRI hippocampal volume and postmortem hippocampal pathology by assessing neuron number and size in a series of 20 brains imaged a mean of 2.6 years prior to death (Zarow et al., 2005). In this series containing not only AD cases, but also ischemic vascular dementia cases and noncognitively impaired controls, the same phenomenon of correlating neuron number (in the CA1 region, but *not* CA2 of hippocampus in this study) with ante-mortem MRI observed in the postmortem studies was found even though the MR images were obtained over 2 years prior to death. There were high correlations with neuron number ($r = .72$) and postmortem volume ($r = 0.54$). Although Braak scores were available for these cases, they were not examined with regard to MRI-determined ante-mortem volumes or other histopathology such as neuritic plaque or amyloid angiopathy. The important principle that this study confirmed was that overall volume loss measured by hippocampal MRI is a reflection of neuron loss in this region. However, although this volume (and indirectly neuronal loss) is strongly associated with AD-specific pathology (i.e., NFT densities), any pathology that damages or reduces the number of neurons in this critical region will also reduce the MRI measured hippocampal volume.

There have been few ante-mortem MRI studies correlating postmortem AD histopathology outside of the hippocampus ((Jagust, 2008; Silbert et al., 2003). In a study of 29 seniors (15 cognitively intact and 24 cognitively impaired) imaged serially with their last scan a mean of 2.3 years before death, NFT were quantified using a 4-level rating scale and neuritic plaques were counted. The histopathology assessment was conducted in the hippocampus as well as across six neocortical regions. As in the prior studies there was a significant relationship found between postmortem NFT score and ante-mortem hippocampal volume. The cortical region volume was not significantly correlated with *either* NFT scores or plaque counts. However, ventricular volume was significantly correlated with *both* NFT scores and plaque counts. The observation in this study that the ante-mortem *rate* of volume loss in the hippocampus did not correlate to NFT scores found postmortem (only the last hippocampal volume) is important for later consideration of the role of rates of change in predicting cognitive loss. This suggests that the pace of volume loss in the hippocampus over time is slow, driven by other or additional pathologies than NFT or that there already is significant volume loss by the time NFT have appeared. On the other hand, the rate of ventricular volume increase with time was significantly correlated with both cortical NFT and plaque counts. The rate of volume change may be considered an integrated measure of accumulating pathology over time and, given the difficulty of obtaining MRI in subjects close to the time of their death when they may be frail or very impaired, may provide a more accurate index of change.

A larger autopsy series has further examined the ante-mortem MRI volume, postmortem AD histopathology correlation (Jagust, 2008). In this study of 93 cases carrying the ante-mortem diagnoses of AD, vascular dementia, mixed dementia, cognitive impairment without dementia and normal, MRIs were obtained a mean of 2.7 years before death. This study constructed pathological subcategories based on classic AD pathology (Braak and CERAD staging) and vascular pathologies to create categories of AD, cerebrovascular disease, normal, and other (cognitively impaired without significant pathology). Ante-mortem MRI derived volumes (cortical gray matter, hippocampal, white matter hyperintensities and lacunes) were then examined with regard to the pathological categories using multivariate associations of MR volumes with pathologic groups (AD, cerebrovascular disease or hippocampal sclerosis). Significant associations were found for the cortical gray matter volume and AD, subcortical vascular, and arteriosclerosis pathology groups. Ante-mortem hippocampal volume was associated with AD pathology and hippocampal sclerosis. The fact that AD and vascular pathologies contributed to only 25% of the variance in cortical gray matter volume highlights the potential difficulty in equating a particular volume change to a specific pathology.

In summary, the best evidence to date suggests that hippocampal volume loss measured with MRI is an index of neuron loss and NFT accumulation at the time of scan. Few studies have reported the relationship of ante-mortem volume to postmortem pathologies outside of the hippocampus addressing the relationship of amyloid as well. These studies suggest a more complicated picture. Ventricular volume change appears best indexed by NFT and amyloid-associated pathologies, but cortical volume change is not as specifically tied to these pathologies. The impact of vascular pathologies which are challenging to comprehensively quantify not only ante-mortem, but postmortem as well, are likely significant contributors to cortical volumes measured with MRI. More study of the basic causes of cerebral atrophy, the major outcome measure of volumetric imaging, is needed. This is especially important in light of the use of volumetric imaging as a biomarker for treatment studies or for diagnostic predictions (a topic discussed in more detail in Chapter 19). If, for example, cortical atrophy is poorly related to amyloid deposition itself, especially over the time interval of a treatment study, then an anti-amyloid therapy should not be assessed with cortical volume changes except to the extent that brain volume sparing by itself is accepted as an independent surrogate marker of clinical efficacy. In this specific case one might suggest ventricular volume change based on our current limited knowledge.

Structural Changes Identify Those Destined for Cognitive Impairment: The CT Era

Regardless of uncertainties in the underlying pathophysiology leading to brain volume loss identified with structural imaging techniques, the clear direction of the field has been to consistently observe that *any* imaging technique that can reliably measure brain loss consistently finds group differences, but with notable overlap in these measures when comparing groups of normal older people to appropriately matched elders with cognitive impairment (Figure 10.1 demonstrates this point using MR images). This was clearly the case beginning with CT studies in the 1970s and 1980s where measurement of CSF spaces were generally taken as a proxy for brain loss presumptively reflecting aging and neurodegenerative disease processes. It was apparent in these early studies (as it is to this day) that there was a continuing challenge to differentiate between what has come to be a commonly posed dichotomy of "aging" vs. "disease" or "dementia-related" change. Thus, whether various linear measures (Earnest et al., 1979; Gomori et al., 1984; Gyldensted, 1977; Hahn and Rim, 1976; Haug 1977; Meese et al.,

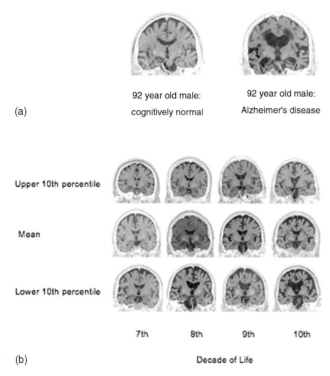

(a)

92 year old male: cognitively normal

92 year old male: Alzheimer's disease

Upper 10th percentile

Mean

Lower 10th percentile

7th   8th   9th   10th

(b)   Decade of Life

Figure 10–1 Images depicting the range and overlap of brain atrophy between cognitively intact and impaired individuals, as well as across age. Panel (a) portrays the clear cross-sectional contrast typically seen between age and sex-matched "normals" and "dementia patients". Panel (b) compares representative coronal images selected from an archive of over 2,500 MRI brain scans from cognitively intact adults. Each brain is identified by decade of life and by the relative degree of atrophy, compared to the brains of other cognitively healthy volunteers of similar age. Total brain volumes, corrected for head size, were measured using a standard volumetric analysis method (Mueller, 1998) to calculate the distribution of brain atrophy by decade. Atrophy identified as falling within the mean volume for a particular decade falls within the 45th to 55th percentiles of the statistical norms for that decade's subgroup. Note the similarity of the brain in the Alzheimer's Disease case in Panel (a) to the representative scan for a cognitively intact 90-year-old falling in the lower 10th percentile for brain atrophy shown in Panel (b). (All images from the NIA-Layton Aging and Alzheimer's Disease Center at Oregon Health & Science University.)

1980), planimetric (cross-sectional areas of regions of interest) (Barron, Jacobs, and Kinkel, 1976; Stafford et al., 1988; Zatz and Jernigan, 1983), or volumetric measures (Ito et al., 1981; Kaye et al., 1992; Pfefferbaum, Zatz, and Jernigan, 1986; Takeda and Matsuzawa, 1984, Takeda, 1985; Yamaura et al., 1980; Zatz, Jernigan, and Ahumada, 1982) of CSF spaces were used, one consistently identified by-decade enlargement of CSF spaces (ventricles and sulcal spaces) among normative aging samples.

Regardless of technique, in general, two important conclusions from these studies were that the expansion of these spaces was *not linear* with aging and, further, that the *variance in measurements increased with increasing age*. Other studies assessed the functional impact of this CT-measured atrophy, first examining correlations of this CT-demonstrated atrophy with cognitive measures and, second, how this atrophy compared between healthy cognitively intact groups and people with dementia (usually designated "dementia of the Alzheimer's type" in these older studies). In these studies the additional observation of importance was that *the medial temporal*

lobe (measured by linear indices) was smaller (or more narrow) in those who were demented (Jobst et al., 1992).

It is remarkable that despite large age-associated increases in CSF spaces or other related measures, it was never clearly demonstrated with these CT studies that there was a strong relationship to various measures of cognitive function, either with general cognitive measures (using composite summary scores) or with specific cognitive domains (Ito et al., 1981; Yeo et al., 1987). Simply stated, when age was statistically controlled in most analyses, even including dementia patients (Bigler et al., 1985; George et al., 1983; Naugle et al., 1985), it seemingly obscured any robust relationship of atrophy to cognition. This has always seemed counterintuitive in that the studies comparing age-matched (and thus presumably "controlled" for age) normal subjects to dementia patients consistently have shown group mean differences between the nondemented and demented subjects (Gado et al., 1982; George et al., 1983; Ichimiya et al., 1986; Jobst et al., 1992; Massman et al., 1986). However, there was always overlap among individual subject groups. Explanations for these seemingly disparate results have generally focused on two fronts: the measurements or the subjects. In terms of the CT measures these were only broad or indirect indices of brain atrophy (such as temporal width, ventricular or total CSF volume). More specific measures (not possible with CT), such as hippocampal or gyral volumes, might be considered to correlate more specifically with the cognitive actions most frequently trafficking through those regions. With regard to subject effects on discerning the relationship between atrophy and cognition, it is often noted that subjects in aging studies are by definition "normal elderly" and, thus, there is a relatively narrow range or variability possible in terms of cognitive function, especially when most studies focus on a restricted age range across the lifespan. This testing effect, often referred to as a ceiling or plateau effect of the test instruments in their normal range, may be intrinsic to the boundaries set on the range of performance characteristic for being considered functionally intact. As will be noted later, these issues continue to be important today.

One of the important observations of the earlier structural imaging studies was that if indeed some of the difficulties in discerning the relationship between cognitive change or dementia to atrophy were the result of noise or measurement insensitivity (both imaging based as well as clinically based), then methodologically, longitudinal studies may offer a means to disentangle these effects. Repeated measures over time tend to dampen measurement error or variance itself ("measure twice, cut once"). Further, the repeated measures of a longitudinal study allow an individual to be a control for themselves, thus decreasing, in theory, some of the interindividual variability of measurement. In addition, if change is not linear over time, then repeated measures will afford the ability to model a trajectory or curve of change which can only be very imprecisely inferred by cross-sectional analysis of subjects captured at a single age or a particular stage of disease. Of course, longitudinal imaging studies themselves have practical limitations, such as the need for long observation periods (and attendant subject drop-out or potential measurement noise due to scanner changes) to go beyond simple two-point rate estimates as opposed to true curve modeling.

Despite the challenges of longitudinal studies, several CT-based longitudinal studies of brain atrophy suggested the power of these study designs early on. These studies, beginning with linear measures of atrophy taken at two time-points (usually a baseline and follow-up (Brinkman and Largen, 1984; Gado et al., 1983; Jobst et al., 1994), or with volumetric CSF space measurements (de Leon et al., 1989; Luxenberg et al., 1987; Shear et al., 1995) surveyed over time (e.g., several years of follow-up) were consistent in detecting progressive atrophy. Using the widely adopted metric of annual change (often percent loss/year), these studies showed remarkable and rather rapid rates of brain loss of up to 10% per year in individuals with dementia of the Alzheimer's type. Limited sample sizes did not provide the ability to adequately evaluate the relationship between rate of cognitive decline and rate of brain loss in these studies. Further, these studies did not follow many unaffected individuals who later became demented, the strongest test of the relevance of structural changes to cognitive loss. These limitations were addressed as MR imaging eclipsed CT for research study of structural changes associated with aging and dementia.

Structural Changes Identify those Destined for Cognitive Impairment: The MRI Era

Concepts Key to MR-based Predictions of Dementia

The review of these older CT studies is of more than simple historical interest. Despite neuroimaging being a field intensely driven by rapid technological evolution where technique feasibility ultimately drives the questions that can be asked, the lessons and conclusions from these early studies have stood the test of time and have been recapitulated with improved imaging capabilities. Thus, improved resolution afforded by 3D MR imaging has improved discrimination that has significantly reduced the variance characteristic of older CT studies, but has not changed the basic insights obtained from studies of brain aging and dementia of the past. What has changed dramatically with the advent of MR imaging has been the ability to analyze important regional changes, especially in

the hippocampus and related areas that was not feasible with CT. This became immediately apparent beginning with the first MR study of hippocampal volume comparing control subjects to Alzheimer's disease cases (Seab et al., 1988). Further, although MR imaging in the context of this discussion is utilized largely as a tool to appraise regional structural change and, thus, may be thought of as a rather static view of the brain, MR in fact, in its classic application to brain anatomy is an inherently functional methodology applying a time series transformation of the state of water (or other) molecules making up different tissue types under controlled conditions. Accordingly, MR imaging of not only tissue volumes of regional or functionally important structures can be surveyed, but the structural integrity of specific pathways or the presence of lesions may also be readily assessed by varying the MR pulse sequence or experiment protocol. Other major advances in the field have not been in the MR hardware or technique itself, but in the software and study designs. Thus, several important techniques for analyzing the data in different ways, as well as transformations in conceptualizing the transition to cognitive impairment, have provided additional important new insights.

It is the latter area that is worth some discussion in considering the available data that speaks to structural changes leading to or associated with cognitive transitions in aging. There are many models now proposed to conceptualize the view that change is gradually reaching some *threshold* where brain volume or structure no longer supports normal cognition. As this threshold is crossed, the trajectory increasingly points to an increased risk for frank dementia. A key to detecting this threshold or projecting forward in predictive models when structural change will lead to clinically significant cognitive impairment is defining the cognitive threshold for meaningful change. In short, all knowledge in this area refers back to defining the clinical prodrome of cognitive change. This concept is graphically illustrated in Figure 10.2.

Figure 10–2 Working model of how different brain aging rates as indexed by brain atrophy or any related phenotype links to the emergence of the dementia phenotype. Subject A has a similar rate of brain aging of quantitative phenotype as Subject B, but begins with greater brain volume or reserve. This results in a longer period for Subject A before entering a zone where cognitive impairment begins to be detected clinically or psychometrically. Note that because of changing characteristics of aging trajectories (transitioning from slow more linear change to more curvilinear change) individual differences at a single cross-section in time at later ages may appear to be magnified, although the rates of change have remained relatively constant. Although Subject C also has a similar early rate of brain atrophy as Subject A and B, and starts at a similar starting point as Subject B, intrinsic events and/or extrinsic brain insults later in life precipitously change this trajectory resulting in an earlier onset of prodromal dementia symptoms and eventual dementia. The difference in the starting points or at any point in time along the Y axis is considered a relative reserve capacity difference between subjects and takes into account not only how fast one changes, but how far one has traveled. In practice contemporary longitudinal studies are able to describe with real data only relatively brief continuous time-frames extracted and analyzed during the later decades of life.

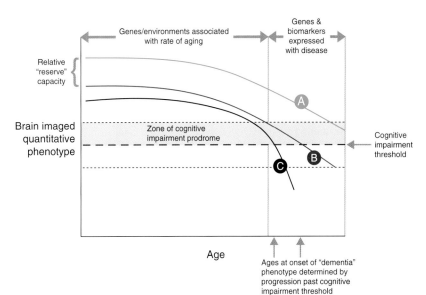

Many clinical prodromes leading to or increasing the risk of dementia have been defined over the past five decades of cognitive aging research (Ebly, Hogan, and Parhad, 1995; Kral, 1962; Petersen, 1999; Ritchie, Artero, and Touchon, 2001; Wolf et al., 1998). Thus, the notion of subtle changes in cognition that precede dementia is not new. Currently the cognitive aging prodrome most frequently referred to in research is the syndrome termed "mild cognitive impairment" or "MCI." It is a construct in evolution. Several symposia and debates continue to better define this prodromal concept and its implications. At this time, although the general definition of MCI is clear, there is no specific definition that has been adopted for standard application of this evolving concept (Jack Jr et al., 2005; Luis et al., 2003; Petersen, 2004) .

For evaluation of research results in this chapter on structural brain imaging changes most tied to the cognitive decline of aging that predict dementia, the particular variants of MCI where memory impairment is prominent—often referred to as amnestic MCI—is most relevant as available data suggests that this form frequently leads to dementia and, more specifically, Alzheimer's disease. In general, people with amnestic forms of MCI have a memory complaint, which is associated with objective test evidence of a delayed recall deficit 1–1.5 SD lower than typical for their age group, while other tested cognitive domains remain relatively spared. Importantly, they have minimal functional decline. As should be apparent from this general definition, the devil is in the details in defining meaningful cognitive change. Inconsistencies in who is labeled with MCI derive from several sources including differences in subject populations studied, in assessments and rating scales employed, and in the use of various reference standards (Busse, 2003; Petersen 2004). Thus, for example, simple differences such as the form of the delayed recall task chosen to define memory loss (such as a 10-word, 12-word or 15-word list learning or paragraph recall task), or the definition of functional impairment among the aging may create important differences in who is defined as having MCI. Accordingly, this creates overlap in who is identified with MCI when varying MCI criteria are applied to the same individuals.

The precision of MCI definition may be particularly important to interpret the relationship of brain aging to cognition in the "MCI range." First, the incidence of MCI in younger elderly increases 2–4 times in those aging past age 85 (Busse, 2003), emphasizing the importance of MCI in the oldest old and challenging the definition of normal aging. Second, MCI diagnoses obtained by using subjective input from the older person and an informant may be problematic as memory complaints increase with advanced age (Jonker, 2000). This is particularly challenging for the oldest old where 50% or more of nondemented seniors see themselves as having degraded memory or cognitive function. Third, a lower level of "normal for age" at advanced age makes the concept of certifying a 90-year-old scoring within 1.0–1.5 standard deviations from the mean of their peer age group as having no MCI problematic. For example, a "low normal" (1 SD below the mean) score for an 87-year-old would be considered defective performance for a 60-year-old on delayed story recall (Wechsler, 1997). Thus, psychometric cutpoints, although critical for objective classification, are based on preconceived, arbitrary notions of age normality. Finally, the challenge of comorbid effects on detecting MCI may be particularly important as individuals age. Medications, intermittent or chronic medical illnesses, and motor and sensory impairments may all affect cognitive function either as reported or tested. These comorbid conditions impact the completeness of assessment and drop-out from study. They also have great potential to influence the imaging characteristics of the brain itself.

I have spent considerable space on the importance of understanding the challenges of defining when and how cognitive decline is identified in order to set the stage for review of the contemporary MR imaging data supporting when and where structural change can be detected that presages cognitive decline. I have also emphasized that because the dynamics of cognitive decline with aging and dementia occur over decades, the most accurate predictions of future cognitive decline are derived from longitudinal observations. Single time-point predictions are snapshots of a particular point on the transition curve and, thus, where in time one takes this assay of brain structure determines the predictive power of these cross-sectional measurements. Accordingly, these cross-sectional studies may be best thought of as measures of how far across the arc of brain loss a person has traveled, but without knowing with how much brain they began their aging journey. Thus, predictions in cross-sectional structural MRI studies of future cognitive decline may be thought of as basing how much brain volume (or "reserve") a subject has left at the time of measurement being predictive of when a later cognitive decline threshold will be crossed.

In this discussion we have focused on brain volume present during the period of run-up to the emergence of clinically manifested early cognitive decline. Implicit in this discussion has been the notion of reserve that translates in structural imaging terms as more brain is better. This has been referred to as the "bigger is better" hypothesis (Van Petten, 2004). Within the hippocampus this may be true, but highly dependent on age, since among younger adults, smaller may in fact be better. Thus, significant negative correlations are seen between hippocampal volume and memory performance during adolescence and younger adulthood (Chantome et al., 1999; Foster et al., 1999). Later in life the relationship is characterized by overall great variability in structure size relative to cognitive performance, a variance that may in part be born by developmental and genetic programs playing out decades earlier that is enhanced by accumulating environmental events. The relevance here is that determining when the most important structural signature of change foretelling future dementia occurs may be marked by the intrinsic and extrinsic influences taking place many decades earlier.

It is not likely that the many early environmental events driving brain atrophy found in later life will be easily uncovered and specified. To some degree it is anticipated that the genetic components may be at least partially identified as the relationship of genetic polymorphisms to brain size, morphology and atrophy may become increasingly amenable to study. However, this seemingly fixed, heritable component to the brain atrophy equation may also be difficult to specify. For example, imaging studies of cognitively intact monozygotic twins in their seventh decade of life have shown that their hippocampal volumes are no more similar than those of unrelated individuals with up to 20% differences in volume found between "identical" twin pairs (Plassman et al., 1997). This should not be surprising since, regardless of zygosity, second-born twins have a smaller intracranial volume than first-born or singleton siblings, suggesting that *overall* brain growth is influenced most or is dominated more by nongenetic factors during early development (Hulshoff Pol et al., 2004). Nevertheless, although information for the hippocampus is limited, it has been shown that temporal lobe gray matter volume already shows a decreasing proportion of its variance attributable to heritable mechanisms by the teen years (Gregory et al., 2006). This decrease in heritability of brain volume with age extends to other gray matter regions and the ventricles, but not the cerebellum or white matter structures (Wallace et al., 2006). The relationship of genetic influences on hippocampal volume or atrophy is complex. Exemplifying this complexity, for example, are observations that have been made on the best established specific genetic risk factor for AD, apolipoprotein E (APOE) relative to hippocampal volume. Thus, specifically with regard to the twin data just noted, despite a discordance of hippocampal volume in twin pairs, a smaller hippocampus is observed in those twins carrying an APOE, epsilon 4 allele (Plassman et al., 1997). The data linking APOE mediated effects to hippocampal volume changes in adult life is highly variable with some studies finding no association, some finding an association with volume and some finding an association not with volume per se, but with hippocampal asymmetry (Cherbuin, 2007). It is likely that these mixed results reflect the known variability of effect of APOE alleles especially relative to age as well as other demographic factors such as gender, ethnicity and health status that play important roles in the clinical outcomes associated with this polymorphism (Cherbuin, 2007; Farrer et al., 1997).

These studies highlight the intricate mixture of genetic and nongenetic determinants of brain atrophy unfolding over a lifetime. Thus, the arrow of time always results in atrophy, but with considerable variability even among cognitively intact individuals in the later decades of life. The fact that these individuals have normal cognitive function at an advanced age when atrophy of most structures is universal suggests that it is the relative amount of tissue lost from whatever state of the brain had previously been capable of supporting normal function that is important. This speaks to the importance of also considering a more dynamic model where not only structure of a single region is important, but the structure and function within and among regions is considered.

Timing is Everything: MR Volumetrics Suggest Regional and Time-sensitive Predictors of Cognitive Decline

The relationship of MRI measures to clinically manifest syndromes of cognitive impairment (MCI, Alzheimer's disease and other dementias) is addressed in Chapters 12 and 16. As noted in the review of earlier CT studies and then with the advent of MRI as we will emphasize, several tenets of brain atrophy have emerged. Without question there is more atrophy in medial temporal lobe structures (Bobinski et al., 1999; Callen et al., 2001; Convit, De Leon, and Tarshish, 1997; Csernansky et al., 2000; De Santi et al., 2001; De Toledo-Morrell et al., 2000; Den Heijer et al., 2006; Du, Schuff, and Amend, 2001; Foundas et al., 1997; Geroldi et al., 2000; Jack et al., 2000; Jack Jr., 1992; 1997, Jack Jr., 1998, Jack Jr., 1992; Juottonen, 1998, Juottonen, 1999; Karas et al., 2004; Kaye, 1997, 2005; Kesslak, Nalcioglu, and Cotman, 1991; Kidron et al., 1997; Korf et al., 2004; Krasuski et al., 1998; Laakso et al., 1998; Ohnishi et al., 2001; Pennanen et al., 2004; Seab, 1988; Xu et al., 2000), extra-temporal regions (Cuenod, 1993; Du, Schuff, and Amend, 2001; Foundas, 1997; Kaye et al., 2005; Kesslak, Nalcioglu, and Cotman, 1991; Kidron et al., 1997; Lehericy et al., 1994; Lehtovirta et al., 1995; Murphy et al., 1993; Salat, Kaye, and Janowsky, 2001; Scahill et al., 2002; Stoub et al., 2005; Tanabe et al., 1997; Teipel et al., 2002; Thompson et al., 2004), and whole brain (Du, Schuff, and Amend, 2001; Fox et al., 2000, Kaye et al., 2005; Ohnishi et al., 2001; Seab et al., 1988; Tanabe et al., 1997), as well as enlargement of CSF spaces (Carmichael et al., 2007; Convit

et al., 1993; Convit, De Leon, and Tarshish, 1997; Cuenod, 1993; Du, Schuff, and Amend, 2001; Kaye et al., 2005; Lehericy et al., 1994; Murphy et al., 1993; Seab et al., 1988; Tanabe et al., 1997; Thompson et al., 2004) when MCI or early AD patients are compared to age-appropriate controls. Consistent overlap is found in mean volumes between comparison groups.

Since presumably the patients in these cross-sectional studies all began somewhere in life with volumes closer to, if not the same as those who populate the normal groups, not surprisingly in longitudinal studies one also generally finds increased rates of change in all these regions in the impaired groups, but again as in cross-sectional comparisons, with overlapping mean rates of volume change between groups (Carmichael et al., 2007; Convit et al., 1993; Convit, De Leon, and Tarshish, 1997; De Santi et al., 2001; De Toledo-Morrell et al., 2000; Du, Schuff, and Amend, 2001; Erten-Lyons et al., 2006; Fotenos et al., 2005; Fox, 1996; Fox et al., 1996, 2000; Jack et al., 2000; Jack, 2004; Jack Jr., et al., 1998; Kaye, 1997; Kaye et al., 1997, 2005; Laasko et al., 2000; Rusinek et al., 2003; Schott et al., 2003; Teipel et al., 2002; Xu et al., 2000). The key issue that these studies present with regard to prediction is when do these volume changes begin relative to when cognitive decline is observed? To most unambiguously answer this question, we focus on those MRI studies that have observed groups of individuals who were carefully examined and found to be cognitively intact and then followed clinically until a defined change or conversion to a cognitively (Werring et al., 2004) impaired state was recognized (Table 10.1). For this kind of assessment MR images must be obtained at least at one time-point prior to becoming cognitively impaired.

Several approaches have been taken to prospectively identifying volumetric change relevant to future cognitive decline. Practically speaking, because the magnitude of both the volume changes as well as the frequency of intact older persons transitioning to mild cognitive decline in any given year is small (about 0.8%–2.6% per year (Palmer and Fratigloini, 2006) an important method for study has been to focus on populations at highest risk (or at greatest risk) for dementia. Among these approaches some have focused on early-onset, autosomal dominant or familial forms of Alzheimer's disease, in which known mutations such as in the amyloid precursor protein (APP) or presenilin 1 (PS1) genes, essentially guarantee that those carrying these mutations will develop dementia with associated MRI-detected brain volume loss. This principle has been demonstrated in a series of reports beginning with a group of cognitively intact family members carrying an APP mutation who were followed over a 3-year period (Fox et al., 1996). Three of the seven family members carrying the mutation subsequently became affected and were shown to not only have smaller hippocampal volumes at the onset of the observation period, but on serial MRI, also showed a greater rate of hippocampal atrophy. The fact that the hippocampus was already smaller while unaffected is of particular interest, suggesting that structural change is already present at least a couple of years prior to onset. A similar study of five subjects carrying either an APP ($n = 2$) or PS1 ($n = 3$) mutation who began with "presymptomatic" Alzheimer's disease (it is not clear if they had MCI initially) and then subsequently, over a 2–3 year period, progressed to Alzheimer's dementia were assessed for baseline volumes of medial temporal lobe structures (hippocampus, entorhinal cortex), temporal lobe and whole brain volumes, as well as the rate of change in these volumes from baseline to dementia (Schott et al., 2003). Similar to the earlier familial Alzheimer's disease study, the baseline hippocampal and entorhinal volumes were

Table 10–1 Summary of prospective MRI volume studies of cognitively normal subjects who progress to MCI or dementia

	Age of Cohort (mean yrs (SD))*	N (MCI converters/total normal at baseline)	Base-Line Predictor of MCI or Dementia	Rate Predictor of MCI or Dementia	Comments
Fox et al. (1996)	45 (5)	3/7	Hippocampus	NA	FAD cases with APP mutation
Schott et al. (2003)	42.9 (4.5)	5/NA	Hippocampus, Entorhinal Cortex	Total brain, temporal lobe, hippocampus, and entorhinal cortex	FAD cases with APP ($n=2$) and Presenilin 1 ($n=3$) mutations
Kaye et al. (1997)	88.6 (3.6)	12/30	Hippocampus	Temporal lobe volume	
Marquis et al. (2001)	83.2 (7.9)	45/108	Hippocampus	NA	Hippocampal prediction independent of delayed recall or motor function at baseline
Rusinek et al. (2003)	69.8 (5.4)	13/45	(% of CSF in brain, not significant)**	Med Temp Lobe	Interval for determining rate spanned period past conversion; medial temporal lobe was not independent of age and sex
Jack Jr et al. (2005)	81.9 (7.5)***	13/91	NA	Ventricular volume	Interval from last scan to conversion, >3 years
Jagust et al. (2008)	69.5 (5.8)	6/60	Hippocampus, Entorhinal Cortex	NA	EC predicted rate of memory decline when converters were removed from analysis (analysis not based on those developing MCI itself)
den Heijer et al. (2006)	73.4 (8.0)	35/511	Hippocampus, Amygdala	NA	Endpoint was dementia; results did not change if those with MCI ($n=16$) at baseline were excluded
Erten-Lyons (2006)	85.3 (5.6)	37/55	Hippocampus	Total brain, Ventricular, Temporal horn volume	Predictor volumes are for 23 subjects converting to progressing MCI; Stable MCI subjects followed for mean of 5.4 yrs without conversion to dementia
Carmichael et al. (2007)	72.7 (3.6)	59/255	(Ventricular volume not significant)	NA	Long conversion surveillance interval (up to 5 years) from baseline scan may have diminished effect
Carmichael et al. (2007)	83.9 (3.9)	29/104	NA	(Ventricular volume, not significant)	Long inter-scan interval (5 years) relative to possible conversion may have diminished effect
Carlson et al. (2008)	83.5±7.4	37/72	NA	Ventricular Volume	Ventricular volume expansion accelerated 2 years prior to conversion to MCI

Abbreviations: FAD = Familial Alzheimer's Disease; NA = Not analyzed or Not applicable

* Age is mean of normal groups at baseline or first scan used for rate calculations.

** Baseline whole-brain atrophy (% of CSF in brain) was different between stable and converters, but did not predict conversion in a multiple regression model including rate of medial temporal lobe atrophy.

*** Mean age of healthy group at second scan (baseline ages, not given) smaller than age-matched control subjects. Atrophy rates for total brain, temporal lobe, hippocampus, and entorhinal cortex were significantly increased in patients compared with control subjects.

Given the 3-year window of follow-up, one can only speculate as to how far back in time this structural change may have begun. Linear extrapolation backward of this familial Alzheimer's disease-based data suggested medial temporal lobe atrophy commenced 3.5 years from onset of dementia symptoms . The fact that this form of familial Alzheimer's disease has onset typically before the sixth decade of life suggests that these observations are less confounded by aging affects on the brain. On the other hand, the genetic nature of the disorder raises the possibility that individuals may developmentally begin life with less brain reserve. However, those not demonstrating any cognitive symptoms and carrying an APP mutation were noted to have volumes similar to age-matched controls (Fox et al., 1996) suggesting that the genetically driven pathology leading to dementia in these cases does not macroscopically affect structural brain reserve until the decade of risk.

Another approach to enhancing the opportunity of observing a cognitively intact individual's transition to cognitive impairment is to follow those at increased risk for cognitive decline based on advanced age. This approach takes advantage of the fact that the incidence of dementia doubles with each successive 5-year interval after age 65, resulting in up to half of all people over age 85 (commonly referred to as the oldest old) with MCI or dementia. This means that by increasing the age of the unimpaired cohort there is a greater likelihood of observing decline within a reasonable number of interval scans. This design was used in a study of 30 oldest old who were observed for up to 4 years with annual MRI scans in which 12 subjects became impaired over a mean 4-year follow-up period (Kaye et al., 1997). In this latter group initial hippocampal volumes were smaller in those who eventually became cognitively impaired. Neither the parahippocampus nor the rest of the temporal lobe was significantly smaller at initial scan in this study. When rates of change were evaluated in the three regions there were clear time-dependent changes in rates of volume loss regardless of whether one became cognitively impaired or not. However, only the rate of temporal lobe volume loss, and not the hippocampal rate of atrophy, was significantly greater in those destined to develop MCI.

An expanded sample from the same cohort was followed for a longer period of time and examined with regard to the ability of a baseline or earlier hippocampal volume to predict future cognitive decline. In this cohort of 108 elderly (mean age, 83), 48 developed cognitive impairment over a period of up to 6 years. Hippocampal volume assessed at the baseline visit significantly predicted, independent of memory and other neurological function, cognitive decline at a mean of 4 years later (Marquis, 2002). The hippocampus at baseline of those that would develop persistent cognitive impairment was 10% smaller than age-appropriate control subjects.

A large population-based study has similarly examined whether the hippocampus and amygdala predict incident dementia (Den Heijer, 2006). In this study of 511 cognitively intact seniors followed for an average of 6 years, 35 developed dementia. Of interest, the hazard ratio of the prediction of dementia was similar (about 3 for hippocampus, 2 for amygdala) regardless of whether the survival analysis was performed comparing the dementia cases to those individuals who had MCI ($n = 16$) or other levels of memory impairment or complaint at baseline. Precise timing of these atrophy measures relative to the degree of mild cognitive decline was limited by the design of this study where the endpoint

was dementia and clinical assessments were done in three successive 2-year waves over the 6-year follow-up period. However, an estimate of how long before clinical onset of dementia atrophy became apparent was made by grouping those who developed dementia into three equally sized cohorts based on the time between baseline and clinical onset of dementia. This resulted in median times since baseline scan of 2.0, 4.9, and 6.3 years. These three time-to-dementia groups were then plotted according to the average volume difference in these groups. In this analysis, there was significant atrophy in hippocampus and amygdala compared to the age-appropriate control subjects 6 years prior to the onset of dementia. The amount of atrophy depended on the time from diagnosis to dementia ranging from 5% (at 6 years from diagnosis) to 17% 2 years away from diagnosis. This timing of hippocampal brain loss forms a consistent picture relative to the earlier prediction studies (Figure 10.3).

Another important population-based study has looked at a Latino population. This prospective study of 60 cognitively intact older Latinos followed for a mean of 3.8 years did not specifically examine the predictive power of volumes determined while cognitively intact, but did relate these initial volumes to rates of change in delayed recall in the six who converted to MCI or dementia compared to those who did not (Jagust, 2006). It was concluded that the entorhinal cortex volume was importantly related to memory decline in the converters because although both hippocampal and entorhinal cortex volumes were significantly related to rates of memory decline in the entire group, when the six MCI converters were removed from the analysis only the entorhinal cortex predicted rate of decline.

Other prospective studies have examined medial temporal lobe volumes in cognitively healthy subjects and their relationship to future cognitive decline in different, but complementary ways to these studies. In a study of 45 younger elderly, mean age 69 years, brain atrophy was assessed at a baseline; follow-up MR assessments were conducted up to 40 months later (Rusinek, 2003). A standard medial temporal lobe (MTL) region containing hippocampus, entorhinal cortex and other temporal lobe gray and white matter, as well as the total amount of brain CSF (ventricular and extraventricular) were measured. By the end of the observation period, 13 subjects had developed mild cognitive impairment. The rate of

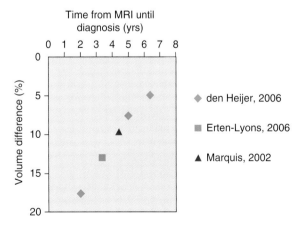

Figure 10–3 A plot of the baseline volume differences in hippocampal volume of cohorts of cognitively intact subjects compared to those that later developed MCI or dementia relative to the time from baseline MRI to diagnosis. Despite different data sources, a linear trend is noted. (Adapted from Den Heijer, 2006; Erten-Lyons, 2006; Marquis, 2002.)

brain atrophy between the baseline and first follow-up examination was assessed by using an automated procedure that included spatial co-registration of the two images and regional brain boundary shift analysis. At baseline, the measures of whole brain and MTL atrophy (percent CSF) were significantly different between those that developed MCI and those that did not. In a logistic regression analysis of the baseline measures including age, sex, whole brain and MTL atrophy and whole brain and MTL atrophy rates (percentages per year), only the MTL atrophy *rate* predicted who would develop MCI. Since the MTL rate calculation included the second time-point when subjects had already developed MCI, it was not possible to determine whether this increased rate was driven by an acceleration of atrophy seen closer to the time of MCI onset.

A later study addressed this timing issue by calculating the rate of volume change *before* the onset of MCI (Jack Jr., 2005). However, in this study the rates of change in hippocampus, entorhinal cortex, whole brain and ventricular volumes were each calculated using an approximate 1-year change score where the second volume used to calculate the rate was obtained within a median of 3.4 years before the clinical detection of MCI. Importantly, despite the rather remote time period when the rate of change was calculated relative to the time when the subjects were noted to be impaired, a significantly greater rate of ventricular enlargement and whole brain atrophy was seen in 13 of 72 initially cognitively intact seniors who developed MCI. Hippocampal rate of atrophy contrary to the earlier study (Kaye, 1997) was not predictive of developing MCI. Because the rates were determined a few years prior to the diagnosis of MCI, it is possible that an accelerating rate of hippocampal volume loss would have been predictive closer to the time of the emergence of MCI symptoms. The predictive power of the baseline volumes obtained approximately 4 years prior to conversion to MCI was not analyzed in this study.

The importance of the interval from baseline clinical assessment and scan to the period that elapses for follow-up clinical assessment and MRI is emphasized by a recent study of a subgroup from the U.S. Cardiovascular Health Study (Carmichael et al., 2007). In this study at baseline there were 255 subjects scanned while cognitively intact. The ventricular brain ratio (the volume of the ventricles relative to the brain) at baseline did not predict the future conversion of the 59 subjects who were observed to have MCI up to 6 years later. The rate of ventricular volume change also did not differ in a subset of 104 seniors (29 developing MCI) with follow-up scans when compared to the MCI converters within that time interval as well (Carmichael et al., 2007). Because beginning volumes and rates of change of volume may not coincide with the progression of cognitive decline and subsequent incidence rates of MCI, this may have obscured the relation of the volumes to predict MCI. An important additional consideration is that this population was derived from a population-based sample that may have had important subject characteristics that differed from other studies. Less than half of the originally normal subjects were available for follow-up scans, 18% of the baseline normal cohort was African-American while 40% of the MCI converters were African-American, only two of the 29 subjects converting to MCI had amnestic MCI and the group in general may have had more comorbidities or other factors that might modulate effects or present different results.

As the field has progressed several important points have emerged. First, whether a single volume obtained prior to the onset of MCI may predict future clinical decline depends on how distant the initial scan is from the determination of the onset of MCI. Second, in order to pinpoint the timing of atrophic change

relative to the onset of MCI symptoms, it is important to attempt to capture the rate of change with scans that have been obtained close to the first clinical designation of MCI. Third, all MCI may not be the same. In general, most prospective studies to date (except as noted [Carmichael et al., 2007; Jagust et al., 2006]) have primarily involved selected cohort studies of well-educated people of European ancestry. Differences in subject characteristics may be important because such factors as medical comorbidities, education and socioeconomic status may be associated with differing rates of clinical progression. Finally, refining the timing and understanding of the trajectory of brain volume changes relative to clinical symptoms needs to take into account that all MCI may not be the same. This goes beyond the already discussed challenges of specifying what cognitive domains are involved in MCI. There are so-called "back-converters" (people who appear to have only transient cognitive change, but revert to normal), as well as people with apparently stable MCI who do not progress to dementia or Alzheimer's disease for many years. Further, the rates of change among reported populations have been modeled linearly. This has primarily been a function of necessity driven by the limited number of time-points and follow-up evaluations available for analysis. However, these considerations are important since one of the major gains to be made through understanding presymptomatic atrophy is to be able to apply preventative treatments at the most effective time-points. Presumably the most desirable periods for intervention is when there is less atrophy and the rate of brain loss is at a minimum.

Some of these points have begun to be addressed. In a study of 55 cognitively intact seniors (ages 75–95; mean 85) followed until conversion to MCI (or not), the rate of change in brain atrophy was calculated with the last time-point used in the rate calculation acquired in the year *before* the onset of MCI (Erten-Lyons, 2006). This study further analyzed the data with respect to the stability of MCI by considering the 14 subjects who developed and then remained stable with MCI for a mean of 5.4 years at the time of study separately from the other 23 MCI "progressors," all but one of whom (who developed vascular dementia) were documented to go on to develop Alzheimer's disease. In the baseline comparison of total brain, ventricular, temporal horn, hippocampal, and total intracranial volume, only the hippocampal volume was different among the three groups (smaller in the progressing MCI patients). The hippocampus was 13% smaller at baseline in those who developed progressive MCI a mean of 3.4 years later. On the other hand, the rate of change of the whole brain, ventricular and temporal horn volumes were all significantly greater in those that would develop progressing MCI (Figure 10.4).

This study, as well as the prior studies, modeled brain loss using simple linear models. These studies suggest that the hippocampus and related structures are atrophic at some point prior to MCI symptoms, but that the rate of change of these specific limbic system structures is either not rapidly changing or changing little during this prodromal period. However, clear change over time can be detected during this prodrome in larger extra-limbic regions indexed by rates of volume change in whole brain or ventricular volumes. Given the long prodromal process, and the large rates of gross change detected in these large regions going back to CT-scan studies, there must be a point where this more rapid acceleration begins. This has been addressed in a longitudinal study of individuals cognitively intact at entry who were followed up to 15 consecutive years with annual MRI scans and assessment for cognitive decline consistent with MCI (Carlson, 2008). During the study period, 37 of 79 subjects developed MCI. A mixed effects model

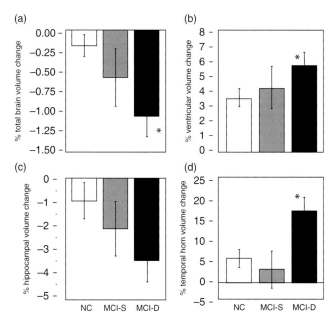

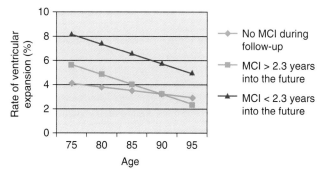

Figure 10–5 The graph shows the age at which a particular rate of ventricular expansion would be expected if a person belonged to one of three groups: Those not developing MCI, those developing MCI, but at least 2.3 years from the clinically detectable time of conversion and those for which MCI will develop within 2.3 years. For example, if a person is diagnosed with MCI at an age greater than 78.3 years then the rate of ventricular volume expansion from 75 to 76 years of age is 5.6%, or if the person is diagnosed with MCI prior to age 87.3 then the rate of ventricular volume expansion from 85 to 86 years of age is 6.5%. (Adapted from Carlson, 2008.)

Figure 10–4 Bar graphs showing annualized percentage change in brain volumes by whether subjects remained cognitively normal (NC) or developed stable (MCI-S) or progressing to dementia (MCI-D) MCI. Panels show: (a) total brain volume change, (b) ventricular volume change, (c) hippocampal volume change, (d) temporal horn volume change. Asterisk (*) indicates that accounting for age, sex, and interval between scans there was a significant difference from the NC and MCI-S groups. (Adapted from Erten-Lyons, 2006. Reproduced with permission from *American Academy of Neurology.*)

with a change point modeled the pattern of brain volume loss (assessed as ventricular expansion) in healthy aging compared to subjects diagnosed with MCI. The brain loss trajectory of subjects developing MCI during follow-up differed from those aging without cognitive impairment. First, the expansion of ventricular volume in cognitively intact subjects did not change appreciably over the 20-year age span covered (75–95 years) in terms rates of change (decelerating from 4.1 to 3% over the two decades) (Figure 10.5). However, the annual rates of expansion were greater in those who developed cognitive impairment during follow-up compared to those who did not. Further, subjects who developed MCI had an acceleration of ventricular volume expansion approximately 2.3 years prior to clinical diagnosis of MCI.

Summary and Conclusions

The convergence of existing data suggests that the medial temporal lobe and, in particular, the hippocampus, whether in young adults with familial Alzheimer's disease, population-based studies, selected cohort studies or an ethnic minority study is clearly more atrophic and predicts dementia at least within the decade before clinical symptom onset. The hippocampus and entorhinal cortex atrophy slowly since at least linear *rates* of atrophy in these regions across studies in normal elderly are consistently modest in magnitude (from 1% to 5% per year) and do not appear to markedly increase with transitions to early states of cognitive impairment. Thus, the rates of hippocampal change in normal (ranging from 0.8% to 2.3%) (Du et al., 2004; Erten-Lyons et al., 2006; Jack et al., 2004; Jack Jr, et al., 2005; Kaye et al., 2005; Mueller, Moore, and

Kerr, 1998; Wang et al., 2003), MCI (1.8% to 4.3% per year) (Erten-Lyons et al., 2006; Jack Jr. et al., 2005) or mild Alzheimer's disease (2.9%–5.1% per year) (Jack, 2004; Jack Jr., 2005; Kaye et al., 2005; Wang et al., 2003) subjects are not very different and demonstrate considerable overlap. These rather small and constant rates of atrophy are not strongly predictive of future cognitive decline during the prodromal period.

The dynamics of hippocampal change lead one to ponder the apparent paradox of hippocampal volumes measured cross-sectionally, clearly distinguishing impaired vs. nonimpaired populations while the rate of hippocampal change is a poor predictor of future clinical state. This may be due to our failure to think in terms of several phenomena which may all play some role. First, there may be a threshold effect. Although the rate of volume loss is small and fairly constant the long-term clinical effect may not be equivalent for each successive year. A 1% rate of change per year may not sound like much, but after 10 years one has lost 10% of volume simply adding the losses. However, this accounting does not assume what may be a functional compound interest effect, i.e., as more volume is lost compensation may not be proportionally as effective. Second, the measurements of hippocampal volume relative to clinical change may not be best described as simply linear (as is the common modeling practice) and thus the measurements may be relatively too coarse and infrequent to capture the true trajectory of change beyond this assumption. Thus, a rapid curvilinear acceleration of hippocampal atrophy above the slower base rate may be needed to result in clinically manifest impairment; this needs to be captured to be measured. Third, hippocampal volume measured on MRI is not solely a reflection of neuron loss. Physiologic or other functional measures can also play an important role in compensation. These are not obviously measured when focusing solely on morphometrics. Related to this is the relative atrophy and effective continuing function of regions that are connected to the hippocampus. Studies often treat the hippocampus in isolation. It is likely that because of the critical role played by this region, there are circuits and activity that we fail to account for that would better characterize the relationship of the rate loss of the hippocampus to future clinical outcome. Clearly, much work is still needed with regard to more precisely specifying the trajectory of change in the important medial temporal lobe region and its clinical consequences.

On the other hand, indices of more widespread or cortical atrophy and, in particular, the ventricular system do appear to show presymptomatic rates of atrophy that are a good predictor of future cognitive decline. The magnitude of the rates of change in general (ranging from 2% to 10% per year overall) are increasingly greater as one compares groups that remain cognitively intact (ventricular volumes ranging from 1.7% to 5.5%/yr) (Carmichael et al., 2007; Jack et al., 2004; Jack Jr. et al., 2005; Kaye et al., 2005; Mueller, Moore, and Kerr, 1998) with those that go on to develop progressing MCI (ventricular volumes ranging from 3.4% to 7.4%/yr) (Carmichael et al., 2007; Jack et al., 2004; Kaye et al., 2005) or mild Alzheimer's disease (4.3%–9.9%) (Carmichael et al., 2007; Jack et al., 2004; Kaye et al., 2005). The trajectory of this change appears to modestly decelerate overall with age until a more abrupt acceleration of change heralds the onset of MCI or dementia symptoms within a couple of years of this increased rate of ventricular enlargement (Figure 10.6). This 2–3 year window prior to symptom onset would seem to be the minimum critical time zone to apply treatments preventing dementia. Ultimately, the preclinical cognitive trajectories of change also need to be considered when designing prevention studies as well since meaningful cognitive decline is the primary functional outcome or endpoint. Fortunately, the periods of most divergent (from rates of cognitively intact subjects) preclinical cognitive change appear to also be within a similar 3–4 year window (Howieson et al., 2008). With this in mind, the period of observation for a prevention study where MRI volumetrics as an outcome measure would likely need to begin is prior to the 2–3 year period of more rapid preclinical atrophy. The role of more frequent imaging and identifying other

regions of interest and methods of assessment (as further noted below) in the measurement mix is a high research priority. At this time, the clearly divergent preclinical trajectories of atrophy (as well as of cognitive measures) several years before clinically manifested MCI suggest that indices of total brain atrophy or ventricular system expansion may be particularly useful for tracking and predicting those at greatest risk for cognitive decline.

These conclusions raise additional important future directions. The focus of this chapter has been on the key areas for which the best structural imaging evidence exists for predicting cognitive decline. Important developments continue in the field. First, there is evidence from comparing rates of volume change obtained at different clinical time-periods across multiple regions, that there are differential rates of atrophy not only related to cognitive state of decline, but by region of the brain (Kaye et al., 2005). More study of these subregional changes and the relationship of one area to another as cognitive impairment emerges and progresses is needed. The use of hypothesis-free exploration of regions most sensitive to change has been afforded by several mapping techniques (Chetelat et al., 2002; Scahill et al., 2002; Whitwell et al., 2007). These studies suggest additional areas of exploration for the future such as the precuneus and posterior cingulate, posterior temporal and parietal cortices among other regions. Second, we have focused on structural imaging in terms of atrophy. Other important structural changes in the brain are amenable to MRI assessment such as cortical thickness (Singhl et al., 2006), integrity of white matter tracts with diffusion tensor imaging (DTI) (Rosea et al., 2000), whole brain magnetization transfer imaging of axonal damage (Van Der Flier et al., 2002) or the presence of microhemorrhages with T2*-weighted gradient-echo imaging (Werring et al., 2004). Third, since multiple pathologies may lead to different structural signatures of damage over

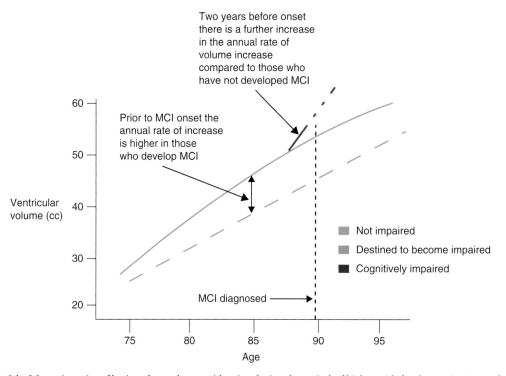

Figure 10–6 Model of the trajectories of brain volume change with aging during the period of highest risk for dementia. A two-phase trajectory is proposed with a slower increase in rate of volume loss in those who retain cognitive function, while those destined to develop dementia differ in rates over a decade before dementia symptoms appear and then have a more rapid acceleration of atrophy within a couple of years of diagnosed MCI. Ventricular volume is given as an example, but total brain volume would be expected to mirror this picture. (Adapted from Carlson, 2008.)

time, further imaging-pathological correlation is needed. This is particularly important for applying these neuroimaging markers toward monitoring treatment effects in clinical trials. The choice of imaging method should ideally reflect the mechanism of action of the drug to be tested with regard to how the drug's targeted pathology may affect brain morphology (or function). For example, the affect of an anti-amyloid drug may not be best assessed by methods that track hippocampal atrophy since the size of the hippocampus has not been shown to be strongly related to amyloid pathology. Fourth, the structure of the brain does not exist in isolation. For purposes of review it makes sense to isolate approaches, but functional studies employing many functional MRI (fMRI) and positron emission tomography (PET) methods (see next chapter), although providing different information, are nevertheless highly complementary to structural imaging. In addition, other data can be profitably integrated into the prediction models including information from other biomarkers such as those found in blood or CSF, as well as markers of genetic risk, as these all become increasingly more available. In parallel, more precise and objective specification when clinically meaningful change occurs will also improve the clinical-imaging correlation. This will be facilitated with the advent of more frequent home-based automated assessments of function using such methods as ubiquitous or embedded computing and automated speech recognition-based cognitive testing (Kaye, 2008).

Finally, as our knowledge about the underlying pathophysiology of cognitive decline leading to dementia grows, we need to continually incorporate this information into imaging research. There are, likely, many factors that may modulate aging of the brain and resultant atrophy over time. These include genetic traits, health habits, environments, or drugs. These are often unknown or have not been well controlled in most imaging studies. They are particularly important in understanding longitudinal outcomes in aging as well as in treatment studies. These new data will guide the optimal use of structural imaging in the understanding of how to optimize brain health for a lifetime.

References

Barron, S., Jacobs, L., and Kinkel, W. (1976). Changes in size of normal lateral ventricles during aging determined by computerized tomography. *Neurology*, 26: 1011–1043.

Bennett, D., Schneider, J., Arvanitakis, Z., Kelly, J., Aggarwal, N., Shah, R. et al. (2006). Neuropathology of older persons without cognitive impairment from two community-based studies. *Neurology*, 66: 1837–1844.

Bigler, E. D., Hubler, D. W., Cullum, C. M., and Turkheimer, E. (1985). Intellectual and memory impairment in dementia. Computerized axial tomography volume correlations. *Journal of Nervous Mental Disorders*, 173: 347–352.

Bobinski, M., de Leon, M., Convit, A., De Santi, S., Wegiel, J., Tarshish, C., Saint Louis, L., and Wisniewski, H. (1999). MRI of entorhinal cortex in mild Alzheimer's disease. *Lancet*, 353: 38–40.

Bobinski, M., Leon, M., Weigel, J., Desanti, S., Convit, A., Saint Louis, L. et al. (2000). The histological validation of post mortem MRI—determined hippocampal volume in Alzheimer's disease. *Neuroscience*, 95: 721–725.

Brinkman, S. and Largen, J. (1984). Changes in brain ventricular size with repeated CAT scans in suspected Alzheimer's disease. *American Journal of Psychiatry*, 141: 81–83.

Busse, A., Bischkopf, J., and Riedel-Heller, S. (2003). Mild cognitive impairment: Prevalence and incidence according to different diagnostic criteria. Results of the Leipzig Longitudinal Study of the Aged (LEILA75+). *British Journal of Psychiatry*, 182: 449–454.

Callen, D., Black, S., Gao, F., Caldwell, C., and Szalai, J. (2001). Beyond the hippocampus: MRI volumetry confirms widespread limbic atrophy in AD. *Neurology*, 57: 1669–1674.

Carlson, N., Moore, M., Dame, A., Howieson, D., Silbert, L., Quinn, J. et al. (2008). Trajectories of brain loss in aging and the development of cognitive impairment. *Neurology*, 70: 828–833.

Carmichael, O., Kuller, L., Lopez, O., Thompson, P., Dutton, R., Lu, A. et al. (2007). Cerebral ventricular changes associated with transitions between normal cognitive function, mild cognitive impairment, and dementia. *Alzheimer's Disease and Associated Disorders*, 21: 14–24.

Carmichael, O., Kuller, L., Lopez, O., Thompson, P., Dutton, R., Lu, A. et al. (2007). Ventricular volume and dementia progression in the Cardiovascular Health Study. *Neurobiology of Aging*, 28: 3389–3397.

Chantome, M., Perruchet, P., Hasboun, D., Dormont, D., Sahel, M., Sourour, N. et al. (1999). Is there a negative correlation between explicit memory and hippocampal volume? *Neuroimage*, 10: 589–595.

Cherbuin, N., Leach, L., Christensen, H., and Anstey, K. (2007). Neuroimaging and APOE genotype: A systematic qualitative review. *Dementia and Geriatric Cognitive Disorders*, 24: 348–362.

Chetelat, G., Desgranges, B., de La Sayette, V., Eustache, V., and Baron, J. (2002). Mapping gray matter loss with voxel-based morphometry in mild cognitive impairment. *NeuroReport*, 13: 1939–1943.

Convit, A., De Leon, M., and Tarshish, C. (1997). Specific hippocampal volume reductions in individuals at risk for Alzheimer's disease. *Neurobiology of Aging*, 18: 131–138.

Convit, A., De Leon, M., Golomb, J., George, A., Tarshish, C., Bobinski, M. et al. (1993). Hippocampal atrophy in Alzheimer's disease: Anatomic specificity and validation. *The Psychiatric Quarterly*, 64: 371–387.

Csernansky, J., Wang, L., Joshi, S., Miller, J., Gado, M., Kido, D. et al. (2000). Early DAT is distinguished from aging by high-dimensional mapping of the hippocampus. Dementia of the Alzheimer type. *Neurology*, 55: 1636–1643.

Cuenod, C., Denys, A., Michot, J., Jehenson, P., Forette, F., Kaplan, D. et al. (1993). Amygdala atrophy in Alzheimer's disease. *Archives of Neurology*, 50: 941–945.

de Leon, M., George, A., Reisberg, B., Ferris, S., Kluger, A., Stylopoulos, L. et al. (1989). Alzheimer's disease: Longitudinal CT studies of ventricular change. *American Journal of Roentgenology*, 152: 1257–1262.

De Santi, S., De Leon, M., Rusinek, H., Convit, A., Tarshish, C., Roche, A. et al. (2001). Hippocampal formation glucose metabolism and volume losses in MCI and AD. *Neurobiology of Aging*, 22: 529–539.

De Toledo-Morrell, L., Goncharova, I., Dickerson, B., Wilson, R., and Bennett, D. (2000). From healthy aging to early Alzheimer's disease: In vivo detection of entorhinal cortex atrophy. *Annals of the New York Academy of Sciences*, 911: 240–253.

Den Heijer, T., Geerlings, M., Hoebeek, F., Hofman, A., Koudstaal, P., and Breteler, M. (2006). Use of hippocampal and amygdalar volumes on magnetic resonance imaging to predict dementia in cognitively intact elderly people. *Archives of General Psychiatry*, 63: 57–62.

Du, A., Schuff, N., and Amend, D. (2001). Magnetic resonance imaging of the entorhinal cortex and hippocampus in the mild cognitive impairment and Alzheimer's disease. *Journal of Neurology, Neurosurgery and Psychiatry*, 71: 441–447.

Du, A., Schuff, N., Kramer, J., Ganzer, S., Zhu, X., Jagust, W. et al. (2004). Higher atrophy rate of entorhinal cortex than hippocampus in AD. *Neurology*, 62: 422–427.

Earnest, M., Heaton, R., Wilkinson, W., and Manke, W. (1979). Cortical atrophy, ventricular enlargement and intellectual impairment in the aged. *Neurology*, 29: 1138–1143.

Ebly, E., Hogan, D., and Parhad, I. (1995). Cognitive impairment in the non-demented elderly: Results from the Canadian study of health and aging. *Archives of Neurology*, 52: 612–619.

Erten-Lyons, D., Howieson, D., Moore, M. M., Quinn, J., Sexton, G., Silbert, L. et al. (2006). Brain volume loss in MCI predicts dementia. *Neurology*, 66: 233–235.

Farrer, L., Cupples, L., Haines, J., Hyman, B., Kukull, W., Mayeux, R. et al. (1997). Effects of age, sex, and ethnicity on the association between apolipoprotein E genotype and Alzheimer disease. A meta-analysis. APOE and Alzheimer Disease Meta Analysis Consortium. *Journal of American Medical Association*, 278: 1349–1356.

Foster, J., Meikle, A., Goodson, G., Mayes, A., Howard, M., Sunram, S. et al. (1999). The hippocampus and delayed recall, bigger is not necessarily better? *Memory*, 7: 715–732.

Fotenos, A., Snyder, A., Girton, L., Morris, J., and Buckner, R. (2005). Normative estimates of cross-sectional and longitudinal brain volume decline in aging and AD. *Neurology*, 6: 1032–1039.

Foundas, A., Leonard, C., Mahoney, S., Agee, O., and Heilman, K. (1997). Atrophy of the hippocampus, parietal cortex and insula in Alzheimer's disease: A volumetric magnetic resonance imaging study. *Neuropsychiatry, Neuropsychology and Behavioral Neurology*, 10: 81–89.

Fox, N., Cousens, S., Scahill, R., Harvey, R., and Rossor, M. (2000). Using serial registered brain MRI to measure disease progression in Alzheimer's disease. *Archives of Neurology*, 57: 339–344.

Fox, N., Warrington, E., Freeborough, P., Hartikainen, P., Kennedy, A., Stevens, J. et al. (1996). Presymptomatic hippocampal atrophy in Alzheimer's diease. A longitudinal MRI study. *Brain*, 119: 2001–2007.

Gado, M., Hughes, C., Danziger, W., and Chi, D. (1983). Aging, dementia, and brain atrophy: A longitudinal computed tomographic study. *American Journal of Neuroradiology*, 4: 699–702.

Gado, M., Hughes, C. P., Danziger, W., Chi, D., Jost, G., and Berg, L. (1982). Volumetric measurements of the cerebrospinal fluid spaces in demented subjects and controls. *Radiology*, 144: 535–538.

George, A. E., de Leon, M. J., Rosenbloom, S., Ferris, S. H., Gentes, C., Emmerich, M. et al. (1983). Ventricular volume and cognitive deficit: A computed tomographic study. *Radiology*, 149: 493–498.

Geroldi, C., Laakso, M., DeCarli, C., Beltramello, A., Bianchetti, A., Soininen, H. et al. (2000). Geneotype and hippocampal asymmetry in Alzheimer's disease: A volumetric MRI study. *Journal of Neurology, Neurosurgery and Psychiatry*, 68: 93–96.

Gomori, J., Steiner, I., Melamed, E., and Cooper, G. (1984). The assessment of changes in brain volume using combined linear measurements: A CT scan study. *Neuroradiology*, 26: 21–24.

Gosche, K., Morimer, J., Smith, C., Markesbery, W., and Snowdon, D. (2002). Hippocampal volume as an index of Alzheimer's neuropathology. Findings from the Nun study. *Neurology*, 58: 1476–1482.

Gregory, L., Wallace, J., Schmitt, E., Lenroot, R., Viding, E., Ordaz, S. et al. (2006). A pediatric twin study of brain morphometry. *Journal of Child Psychology and Psychiatry*, 47: 987–993.

Gyldensted, C. (1977). Measurements of the normal ventricular system and hemispheric sulci of 100 adults with computed tomography. *Neuroradiology*, 14: 183–192.

Hahn, F. and Rim, K. (1976). Frontal ventricular dimensions on normal computed tomography. *American Journal of Roentgenology*, 126: 593–596.

Haug G. (1977). Age and sex dependence of the size of normal ventricles on computed tomography. *Neuroradiology*, 14: 201–204.

Howieson, D., Carlson, N., Moore, M., Wasserman, D., Abendroth, C., Payne-Murphy, J. et al. (2008). Trajectory of mild cognitive impairment onset. *Journal of the International Neuropsychological Society*, 14: 192–198.

Huesgen, C., Burger, P., Crain, B., and Johnson, G. (1993). In vitro MR microscopy of the hippocampus in Alzheimer's disease. *Neurology*, 43: 145–152.

Hulette, C., Welsh-Bohmer, K., Murray, M., Saunders, A., Mash, D., and McIntyre, L. (1998). Neuropathological and neuropsychological changes in "normal" aging: Evidence for preclinical Alzheimer disease in cognitively normal individuals. *Journal of Neuropathology and Experimental Neurology*, 57: 1168–1174.

Hulshoff Pol, H., Brans, R., van Haren, N., Schnack, H., Langen, M., Baare, W. et al. (2004). Gray and white matter volume abnormalities in monozygotic and same-gender dizygotic twins discordant for schizophrenia. *Biological Psychiatry*, 55: 126–130.

Ichimiya, Y., Kobayashi, K., Arai, H., Ikeda, K., and Kosaka, K. (1986). A computed tomography study of Alzheimer's disease by regional volumetric and parenchymal density measurements. *Journal of Neurology*, 233: 164–167.

Ito, M., Hatazawa, J., Yamaura, H., and Matsuzawa, T. (1981). Age-related brain atrophy and mental deterioration–a study with computed tomography. *British Journal of Radiology*, 54: 384–390.

Jack, C., Dickson, D., Parisi, J., Xu, Y., Cha, R., O'Brien, P. et al. (2002). Antemortem MRI findings correlate with hippocampal neuropathology in typical aging and dementia. *Neurology*, 58: 750–757.

Jack, C., Petersen, R., Xu, Y., O'Brien, P., Smith, G., Ivnik, R. et al. (2000). Rates of hippocampal atrophy correlate with change in clinical status in aging and AD. *Neurology*, 55: 484–489.

Jack, C., Shiung, M., Gunter, J., O'Brien, P., Weigand, S., Knopman, D. et al. (2004). Comparison of different MRI brain atrophy rate measures with clinical disease progression in AD. *Neurology*, 62: 591–600.

Jack, Jr. C., Petersen, R., Xu, Y., Waring, S., O'Brien, P., Tangalos, E. et al. (1997). Medial temporal atrophy on MRI in normal aging and very mild Alzheimer's disease. *Neurology*, 49: 786–794.

Jack, Jr. C., Peterson, R., Xu, Y., O'Brien, P., Waring, S. et al. (1998). Hippocampal atrophy and apolipoprotein E genotype are independently associated with Alzheimer's disease. *Annals of Neurology*, 43: 303–310.

Jack, Jr. C., Shiung, M., Weigand, S., O'Brien, P., Gunter, J., Boeve, B. et al. (2005). Brain atrophy rates predict subsequent clinical conversion in normal elderly and amnestic MCI. *Neurology*, 65: 1227–1231.

Jack, Jr. C., Petersen, R., O'Brien, P., and Tangalos, E. (1992). MR-based hippocampal volumetry in the diagnosis of Alzheimer's disease. *Neurology*, 42: 183–188.

Jagust, W., Gitcho, A., Sun, F., Kuczynski, B., Mungas, D., and Haan, M. (2006). Brain imaging evidence of preclinical Alzheimer's disease in normal aging. *Annals of Neurology*, 59: 673–681.

Jagust, J., Zheng, L., Harvey, D., Mack, W., Vinters, H., Weiner, M. et al. (2008). Neuropathological basis of magnetic resonance images in aging and dementia. *Annals of Neurology*, 63: 72–80.

Jobst, K., Smith, A., Szatmari, M., Molyneux, A., Esiri, M., King, E. et al. (1992). Detection in life of confirmed Alzheimer's disease using a simple measurement of medial temporal lobe atrophy by computed tomography. *Lancet*, 340: 1179–1183.

Jobst, K., Smith, D., Szatmari, M., Esiri, M., Jaskowski, A., Hindley, N. et al. (1994). Rapidly progressing atrophy of medial temporal lobe in Alzheimer's disease. *Lancet*, 343: 829–830.

Jonker, C., Geerlings, M., and Schmand, B. (2000) Are memory complaints predictive for dementia? A review of clinical and population-based studies. *International Journal of Geriatric Psychiatry*, 15: 983–991.

Juottonen, K., Laakso, M., Insausti, R., Lehtovirta, M., Pitkanen, A., Partanene, K. et al. (1998). Volumes of the entorhinal and perirhinal cortices in Alzheimer's disease. *Neurobiology of Aging*, 19: 15–22.

Juottonen, K., Laasko, M., Partanen, K., and Soininen, H. (1999). Comparative MR analysis of the entorhinal cortex and hippocampus in diagnosing Alzheimer disease. *American Journal of Neuroradiology*, 20: 139–144.

Karas, G., Scheltens, P., Rombouts, S., Visser, P., van Schijndel, R., Fox, N. et al. (2004). Global and local gray matter loss in mild cognitive impairment and Alzheimer's disease. *Neuroimage*, 23: 703–716.

Katzman, R. (1976). A pediatric twin study of brain morphometry. *Archives of Neurology*, 33: 217–218.

Katzman, R., Terry, R., DeTeresa, R., Brown, T., Davies, P., Fuld, P. et al. (1988). Clinical, pathological, and neurochemical changes in dementia: A subgroup with preserved mental status and numerous neocortical plaques. *Annals of Neurology*, 23: 138–144.

Kaye, J. (2008). Home-based technologies: a new paradigm for conducting dementia prevention trials. *Alzheimer's & Dementia*, 4: S60–S66.

Kaye, J., DeCarli, C., Luxenberg, J., and Rapoport, S. (1992). The significance of age-related enlargement of the cerebral ventricles in healthy men and women measured by quantitative computed x-ray tomography. *Journal of the American Geriatrics Society*, 40: 225–231.

Kaye, J., Moore, M., Dame, A., Quinn, J., Camicioli, R., Howieson, D. et al. (2005). Asynchronous regional brain volume losses in presymptomatic to moderate AD. *Journal of Alzheimer's Disease*, 8: 51–56.

Kaye, J., Swihart, T., Howieson, D., Dame, A., Moore, M., Karnos, T. et al. (1997). Volume loss of the hippocampus and temporal lobe in healthy elderly persons destined to develop dementia. *Neurology*, 48: 1297–1304.

Kesslak, J., Nalcioglu, O., and Cotman, C. (1991). Quantification of magnetic resonance scans for hippocampal and parahippocampal atrophy in Alzheimer's disease. *Neurology*, 41: 51–54.

Khachaturian, Z. (1985). Diagnosis of Alzheimer's disease. *Archives of Neurology*, 42: 1097–1105.

Kidron, D., Black, S., Stanchev, P., Buck, B., Szalai, J., Parker, J. et al. (1997). Quantitative MR volumetry in Alzheimer's disease. Topographic markers and the effects of sex and education. *Neurology*, 49: 1504–1512.

Korf, E., Wahlunch, L., Visser, P., and Scheltens, P. (2004). Medial Temporal lobe atrophy on MRI predicts dementia in patients with mild cognitive impairment. *Neurology*, 63: 94–100.

Kral, V. (1962). Senescent forgetfulness: Benign and malignant. *Canadian Medical Association Journal*, 86: 257–260.

Krasuski, J., Alexander, G., Horwitz, B., Daly, E., Murphy, D., Rapoport, S. et al. (1998). Volumes of medial temporal lobe structures in patients with Alzheimer's disease. *Biological Psychiatry*, 43: 60–68.

Laasko, M., Lehtovirta, M., Partanen, K., Reikkinen, P., and Soininen, H. (2000). Hippocampus in Alzheimer's disease: A 3-year follow-up MRI study. *Biological Psychiatry*, 47: 557–561.

Laakso, M., Soininen, H., Partanen, K., Lehtovirta, M., Hallikainen, M., Hanninen, T. et al. (1998). MRI of the hippocampus in Alzheimer's disease: Sensitivity, specificity, and analysis of the incorrectly classified subjects. *Neurobiology of Aging*, 19: 23–31.

Lehericy, S., Baulac, M., Chiras, J., Pierot, L., Martin, N., Pillon, B. et al. (1994). Amygdalohippocampal MR volume measurements in the early states of Alzheimer disease. *American Journal of Neuroradiology*, 15: 927–937.

Lehtovirta, M., Laakso, M., Soininen, H., Helisalmi, S., Mannermaa, A., Helkala, E. et al. (1995). Volumes of hippocampus, amygdala and frontal lobe in Alzheimer patients with different apolipoprotein E genotypes. *Neuroscience*, 67: 65–72.

Luis, C., Loewenstein, D., Acevedo, A., Barker, W., and Duara, R. (2003). Mild Cognitive Impairment: Directions for future research. *Neurology*, 61: 438–444.

Luxenberg, J., Haxby, J., and Creasey, H. et al. (1987). Rate of ventricular enlargement in dementia of the Alzheimer type correlates with rate of neuropsychological deterioration. *Neurology*, 37: 1135–1140.

Marquis, S., Moore, M., Howieson, D., Sexton, G., Payami, H., Kaye, J. et al. (2002). Independent predictors of cognitive decline in healthy elderly persons. *Archives of Neurology*, 59: 601–606.

Massman, P. J., Bigler, E. D., Cullum, C. M., and Naugle, R. I. (1986). The relationship between cortical atrophy and ventricular volume. *International Journal of Neuroscience*, 30: 87–99.

Maurer, K. and Maurer, I. (2003). *Alzheimer: The Life of a Physician and the Career of a Disease*. New York: Columbia University Press, p. 270.

Meese, W., Kluge, W., Grumme, T., and Hopfenmuller, W. (1980). CT evaluation of the CSF spaces of healthy persons. *Neuroradiology*, 19: 131–136.

Mueller, E., Moore, M., and Kerr, D. (1998). Brain volume preserved in healthy elderly through the eleventh decade. *Neurology*, 51: 1555–1562.

Murphy, D., DeCarli, D., Daly, E., Gillette, J., McIntosh, A., Haxby, J. et al. (1993). Volumetric magnetic resonance imaging in men with dementia of the Alzheimer type: Correlations with disease severity. *Biological Psychiatry*, 1: 612–621.

Naugle, R. I., Cullum, C. M., Bigler, E. D., and Massman, P. J. (1985). Neuropsychological and computerized axial tomography volume characteristics of empirically derived dementia subgroups. *Journal of Nervous and Mental Disease*, 173: 596–604.

Ohnishi, T., Matsuda, H., Tabira, T., Asada, T., and Uno, M. (2001). Changes in brain morphology in Alzheimer disease and normal aging: Is Alzheimer disease an exaggerated aging process? *American Journal of Neuroradiology*, 22: 1680–1685.

Palmer, K. and Fratigloini, L. (2006) Is mild cognitive impairment a distinct clinical entity? *Aging Health*, 2: 763–769.

Pennanen, C., Kivipelto, M., Tuomainen, S., Hartikainen, P., Hanninen, T., Laakso, M. et al. (2004). Hippocampus and entorhinal cortex in mild cognitive impairment and early AD. *Neurobiology of Aging*, 25: 303–310.

Petersen, R. (2004). Mild cognitive impairment as a diagnostic entity. *Journal of Internal Medicine*, 256: 183–194, 2004.

Petersen, R., Smith, G., Waring, S., Ivnik, R., Tangalos, E., and Kokmen, E. (1999). Mild cognitive impairment: Clinical characterization and outcome. *Archives of Neurology*, 56: 303–308.

Pfefferbaum, A., Zatz, L., and Jernigan, T. (1986). Computer interactive methods for quantifying cerebrospinal fluid and tissue in brain CT scans: Effects of aging. *Journal of Computer Assisted Tomography*, 10: 571–578.

Plassman, B., Welsh-Bohmer, K., Bigler, E., Johnson, S., Anderson, C., Helms, M. et al. (1997). Apolipoprotein E epsilon 4 allele and hippocampal volume in twins with normal cognition. *Neurology*, 48: 985–989.

Ritchie, K., Artero, S., and Touchon, J. (2001). Classification criteria for mild cognitive impairment. *Neurology*, 56: 37–42.

Rosea, S., Chena, F., Chalkb, J., Zelayad, F., Strugnellc, W., Bensonc, M. et al. (2000). Loss of connectivity in Alzheimer's disease: An evaluation of white matter tract integrity with colour coded MR diffusion tensor imaging. *Journal of Neurology, Neurosurgery and Psychiatry*, 5269: 528–530.

Rusinek, H., Santi, S., Frid, D., Wai-Hon, T., Tarshish, C., Convit, A. (2003). Regional brain atrophy rate predicts future cognitive decline: 6 year longitudinal MR Imaging study of normal aging. *Radiology*, 229: 691–696.

Salat, D., Kaye, J., and Janowsky, J. (2001). Selective preservation and degeneration within the prefrontal cortex in aging and Alzheimer disease. *Archives of Neurology*, 58: 1403–1408.

Scahill, R., Schott, J., Stevens, J., Rossor, M., and Fox, N. (2002). Mapping the evolution of regional atrophy in Alzheimer's disease: Unbiased analysis of fluid-registered serial MRI. *Proceedings of the National Academy of Sciences of the USA*, 99: 4703–4707.

Schmitt, F., Davis, D., Wekstein, D., Smith, C., Ashford, J., and Markesbery W. (2000). "Preclinical" AD revisited: Neuropathology of cognitively normal older adults. *Neurology*, 55: 370–376.

Schott, J., Fox, N., Frost, C., Scahill, R., Janssen, J., Chan, D. et al. (2003). Assessing the onset of structural change in familial Alzheimer's disease. *Annals of Neurology*, 53: 181–188.

Seab, J., Jagust, W., Wong, S., Roose, M., Reed, B., Budinger, T. (1988). Quantitative NMR measurements of hippocampal atrophy in Alzheimer's disease. *Magnetic Resonance Imaging*, 8: 200–208.

Shear, P., Sullivan, E., Mathalon, D., Lim, K., Davis, L., Yesavage, J. et al. (1995). Longitudinal volumetric computed tomographic analysis of regional brain changes in normal aging and Alzheimer's disease. *Archives of Neurology*, 52: 392–402.

Silbert, L., Quinn, J., Moore, M., Corbridge, E., Ball, M., Murdock, G. et al. (2003). Changes in premorbid brain volume predict AD pathology. *Neurology*, 61: 487–492.

Singhl, V., Chertkow, H., Lerch, J., Evans, A., Dorr, A., Kabani, N. (2006). Spatial patterns of cortical thinning in mild cogntive impairment and Alzheimer's disease. *Brain*, 129: 2885–2893.

Stafford, J., Albert, M., Naeser, M. et al. (1988). Age-related differences in computed tomographic scan measurements. *Archives of Neurology*, 45: 409–415.

Stoub, T., Bulgakova, M., Leurgans, S., Bennett, D., Fleischman, D., Turner, D. et al. (2005). MRI predictors of risk of incident Alzheimer disease: A longitudinal study. *Neurology*, 64: 1520–1524.

Takeda, S. and Matsuzawa, T. (1984). Measurement of brain atrophy of aging using X-ray computed tomography: Sex difference in 1045 normal cases. *Tohoku Journal of Expert Medicine*, 144: 351–359.

Takeda, S. and Matsuzawa, T. (1985). Age-related change in volumes of the ventricles, cisternae, and sulci: A quantitative study using computer tomography. *Journal of the American Geriatric Society*, 33: 264–268.

Tanabe, J., Amend, D., Schuff, N., DiSclafani, V., Ezekiel, F., Norman, D. et al. (1997). Tissue segmentation of the brain in Alzheimer disease. *American Journal of Neuroradiology*, 18: 115–123.

Teipel, S., Bayer, W., Alexander, G., Zebuhr, Y., Teichberg, D., Kulic, L. et al. (2002). Progression of corpus callosum atrophy in Alzheimer's disease. *Archives of Neurology*, 59: 243–348.

Thompson, P., Hayasahi, K., De Zubicaray, G., Janke, A., Rose, S., Semple, J. et al. (2004). Mapping hippocampal and ventricular change in Alzheimer's disease. *Neuroimage*, 22: 1754–1766.

Van Der Flier, W., Van Den Heuvel, D., Weverling-Rijnsburger, A., Bollen, E., Westendorp R, Van Buchem, M. et al. (2002). Magnetization transfer imaging in normal aging, mild cognitive impairment, and Alzheimer's disease. *Annals of Neurology*, 52: 62–67.

Van Petten, C. (2004). Relationship between hippocampal volume and memory ability in healthy individuals across the lifespan: Review and meta-analysis. *Neuropsychologia*, 42: 1394–1413.

Wallace, G., Schmitt, J., Lenroot, R., Viding, E., Ordaz, S., Rosenthal, M. et al. (2006). A pediatric twin study of brain morphometry. *Journal of Child Psychology and Psychiatry*, 47: 987–993, 2006.

Wang, L., Wank, J., Glick, I., Gado, M., Miller, M., Morris, J. et al. (2003). Changes in hippocampal volume and shape across time distinguish dementia of the Alzheimer's type from healthy aging. *Neuroimage*, 20: 667–682.

Wechsler, D. (1997). *Wechsler Memory Scale (WMS-III)*. San Antonio: The Psychological Corporation.

Werring, D., Frazer, D., Coward, L., Losseff, N., Watt, H., Cipolotti, L. (2004). Cognitive dysfunction in patients with cerebral microbleeds on T2-weighted gradient-echo MRI. *Brain*, 127: 2265–2275.

Whitwell, J., Petersen, R., Negash, S., Weigand, S., Kantarci, K., Ivnik, R. et al. (2007). Patterns of atrophy differ among specific subtypes of mild cognitive impairment. *Archives of Neurology*, 64: 1130–1138.

Wolf, H., Grunwald, M., Ecke, G., Zedlick, D., Bettin, S., Dannenberg, C. et al. (1998). The prognosis of mild cognitive impairment in the elderly. *Journal of Neural Transmission*, 54: 31–50.

Xu, Y., Jack, Jr C., O'Brien, P., Kokmen, E., Smith, G., Ivnik, R. et al. (2000). Usefulness of MRI measures of entorhinal cortex versus hippocampus in AD. *Neurology*, 54: 1760–1767.

Yamaura, H., Ito, M., Kubota, H., and Matsuzawa, T. (1980). Brain atrophy during aging: A quantitative sutdy with computed tomography. *Journal of Gerontology*, 35: 492–498.

Yeo, R., Turkheimer, E., Raz, N., and Bigler, E. (1987). Volumetric asymmetries of the human brain: Intellectual correlates. *Brain and Cognition*, 6: 15–23.

Zarow, C., Vinters, H., Ellis, W., Weiner, M., Mungas, D., White, L. et al. (2005). Correlates of hippocampal neuron number in Alzheimer's disease and ischemic vascular dementia. *Annals of Neurology*, 57: 896–903.

Zatz, L. and Jernigan, T. (1983). Th ventricular-braini ratio on computed tomography scans: Validity and proper use. *Psychiatry Research*, 8: 207–214.

Zatz, L., Jernigan, T., and Ahumada, A. (1982). Changes on computed cranial tomography with aging: Intercranial fluid volume. *American Journal of Neuroradiology*, 3: 1–11.

11

The Early Detection of Alzheimer's Disease with Positron Emission Tomography

Rachel Mistur, Lisa Mosconi, Remigiusz Switalski, Susan De Santi, Yi Li, Lidia Glodzik, Miroslaw Brys, Wai Tsui, Henry Rusinek, and Mony J. de Leon

Introduction

Alzheimer's disease (AD) is the leading cause of dementia in the elderly, accounting for up to 70% of dementia cases, and is the fourth leading cause of death in developed nations after heart disease, cancer, and stroke. AD is a progressive neurodegenerative disorder with insidious onset. AD is characterized by a precipitous decline in episodic memory and impairment in activities of daily living. Instrumental signs include aphasia, apraxia, and agnosia, together with general cognitive symptoms, such as impaired judgment, decision-making, and orientation (McKhann et al., 1984). Currently, a diagnostic test for AD is not available and the clinical diagnosis of AD remains a behavioral diagnosis after excluding other causes. This greatly limits the potential for early intervention and prevention research. Furthermore, it is estimated that between 50% and 90% of dementia cases are left undiagnosed by standard clinical examinations (Hebert et al., 2003).

The definitive diagnosis of AD is based on the postmortem observation of specific pathological lesions: intracellular neurofibrillary tangles (NFT), amyloid beta (Aß) deposition in the form of extracellular senile plaques and blood vessel deposits, associated with neuronal and synaptic loss, and atrophy in specific areas of the brain (Mirra et al., 1991; Price and Morris, 1999). Neurodegeneration in AD is estimated to begin as many as 20–30 years before the clinical manifestations become evident (Braak and Braak, 1991, 1996; Delacourte et al., 1999; Morris et al., 1996). During this preclinical phase, plaque and tangle load increase, and the first symptoms appear after specific brain circuits are structurally disrupted through synapse loss and neuronal death (see Morrison and Hof 1997 and Chapter 3 for review). It is widely recognized that the brain regions most vulnerable early in AD are in the medial temporal lobes (MTL, i.e., hippocampus, and transentorhinal, entorhinal cortex, and subiculum) (Braak and Braak, 1991, 1996; Delacourte et al., 1999). The pyramidal cells anatomically connected to the entorhinal cortex (EC) and the CA1 and subiculum regions of the hippocampus are particularly prone to NFT formation and degeneration, whereas primary sensory-motor and occipital areas and the cerebellum exhibit minimal neuronal loss (Braak and Braak 1991, 1996; Delacourte et al., 1999).

Disruption of the pyramidal neurons in the perforant path is thought to disconnect the hippocampus from the rest of the cortex, strongly contributing to the decline in memory observed in early AD (Hyman et al., 1984). There is an association between NFT staging and the severity of clinical status in AD. NFTs originate in the MTL, which plays a critical role in the neural control of memory functions, then begin to cluster in the adjacent inferior temporal and posterior cingulate cortex in mild AD, further disrupting episodic and autobiographic memory, and eventually disrupting the parieto-temporal and prefrontal association cortices, which are involved in the neural control of perception, attention, and language, in moderate and then severe dementia (Braak and Braak, 1996; Delacourte et al., 1999). Despite an initial predilection for the neocortex, Aß depositions are also found in the MTL at later stages of disease (Arriagada, Marzloff, and Hyman, 1992; Giannakopoulos et al., 1994; Ulrich, 1985). For many years, the aggregation of large Aβ fibrils was considered the key event in AD pathogenesis and the main determinant of neuronal degeneration (Selkoe, 1997). A recent reformulation of the amyloid cascade hypothesis states that Aβ oligomers (Aβ-derived diffusible ligand, ADDL), not fibrillar Aβ, confer greater neurotoxicity to neurons by disrupting nerve signaling pathways and subsequently causing neuronal cell death (Lambert et al., 1998).

While the causes of neurodegeneration in AD are under investigation, the early appearance of pathological lesions and the progressive nature of cognitive deterioration in AD indicate a great need for developing biological markers of disease that are sensitive to the brain changes that are expected to occur decades prior to the onset of clinical symptoms. Ideally, a biological measure would be predictive of AD in presymptomatic individuals. Criteria for a model biomarker of the disease have been proposed by the Consensus Group on Molecular and Biochemical Markers of Alzheimer's disease (Consensus Working Group, 1998). In short, an ideal biomarker for the disease should detect a fundamental

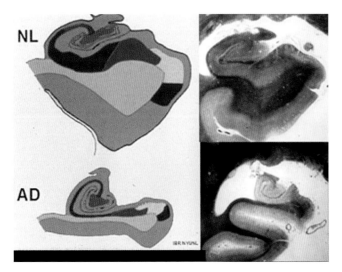

Figure 11–1 Postmortem evidence for atrophy in the hippocampal subfields and subiculum in AD. Schematic defines regions in color. (Adapted from Bobinski et al., 1995.)

characteristic of the neuropathology and be validated in neuropathologically confirmed cases, with sensitivity and specificity of no less than 80% (Consensus Working Group, 1998).

Several modalities show promise for developing early diagnostic tools for AD. These include: magnetic resonance imaging (MRI) structural measurements and positron emission tomography (PET) imaging of glucose metabolism of the MTL, PET imaging of Aβ deposits, and cerebrospinal fluid (CSF) biomarkers for tauopathy and Aβ. At present, none of these are recommended in any consensus guidelines for the diagnosis of AD, as they are not yet validated by large prospective studies.

Structural imaging, such as with MRI, plays an important part in the diagnosis of AD by identifying other causes of dementia, such as tumor, subdural hematoma, and cerebrovascular diseases marked by infarcts and white matter lesions (McKhann et al., 1984). Cerebral atrophy, visualized as enlarged ventricles and cortical sulci, can also be identified by CT and MRI, but there is significant overlap with normal aging and other dementias (Nestor et al., 2004). Nonetheless, several CT and MRI studies have shown that MTL atrophy is an early sign of AD (see Figures 11.1 and 11.2) and has value in predicting future dementia in non-demented subjects (see, among others, den Heijer et al., 2006; de Leon et al., 1988, 1989; Jack et al., 2000; Rusinek et al., 2003). For a detailed review of MRI studies in preclinical AD, see Chapters 10 and 12 in this book.

Ultimately, AD pathology has the effect of impairing neuronal function, which then leads to the clinical symptoms of dementia. Functional neuroimaging offers the unique capability to both

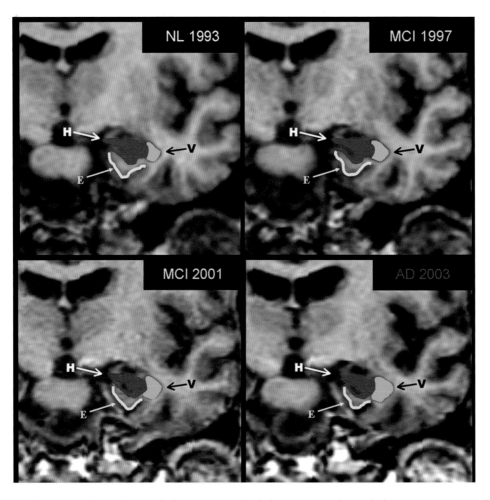

Figure 11–2 MRI scans of a normal elderly subject studied over 10 years who declines to MCI and AD. The hippocampus is painted red, the entorhinal cortex yellow, and the temporal horn of the lateral ventricle green. (Adapted from Blennow et al., 2006.)

visualize the direct effects of neuronal activity and quantitate the rates of specific biological processes at the tissue level in vivo. PET imaging with 2-[^{18}F]fluoro-2-Deoxy-D-glucose (FDG) has long been used to track AD-related brain changes by providing qualitative and quantitative estimates of the cerebral metabolic rate of glucose (CMRglc).

Glucose is the predominant source of energy for the brain. Early studies showed that glucose utilization could be measured and serve as an index of neuronal function (Sokoloff, 1977). Brain energy metabolism is mainly associated with brain glutamate signaling (Magistretti et al., 1999) as more than 80% of brain's neurons are excitatory and 90% of synapses are glutamatergic. Thus, glucose metabolism can be interpreted as an index of synaptic functioning and density (Attwell and Iadecola, 2002; Malonek and Grinvald, 1999; Rocher et al., 2004; Sokoloff, 1977). A recent FDG-PET study showed a significant correlation between CMRglc in vivo and levels of synaptophysin, a marker of synaptic density, assessed at *postmortem* (Rocher et al., 2004). Astrocytes also have metabolic demands and contribute to the FDG-PET signal (Magistretti and Pellerin, 1996; Pellerin and Magistretti, 1994). Other recent studies have shown that coupling between energy metabolism and neuronal activity may also be achieved through astrocyte uptake of glucose and lactate shuttling to neurons (Pellerin and Magistretti, 1994).

The present review will provide an overview of the experiences with FDG-PET in the study of AD and in the evaluation of the presymptomatic and preclinical stages of AD.

Alterations of Brain Glucose Metabolism in Alzheimer's Disease

One of the striking features of AD is the drastic reduction of CMRglc in specific brain areas. FDG-PET studies in AD demonstrate consistent and progressive CMRglc reductions, whose extent and topography correlate with symptom severity (see Mosconi, 2005 for review). Virtually all FDG-PET studies report that, compared to age-matched healthy normal controls, AD patients show both widespread global metabolic impairment (Ferris et al., 1980) and regional metabolic reductions involving the parietotemporal (Frackowiak et al., 1981; Friedland et al., 1981, 1983) (see Figure 11.3) and posterior cingulate cortices (Minoshima et al., 1997) (see Figure 11.4), and in advanced disease involvement of the frontal lobe (Foster et al., 1984). This pattern is seen in contrast to relative preservation of the primary motor and visual areas. Moreover, the cerebellum, thalamus and basal ganglia nuclei are relatively spared (Mazziotta and Phelps, 1986). In comparison to AD, normal aging is characterized by subtle and diffuse CMRglc reductions in the frontal cortex and anterior cingulate cortex (ACC), accompanied by small reductions in global CMRglc (Herholz et al., 2002).

These findings initially reported in the early 1980s, have been often replicated and this pattern of hypometabolism is largely accepted as a reliable in vivo hallmark of AD. Temporo-parietal abnormalities have high sensitivity in distinguishing AD from normal aging and, to some extent, from other neurodegenerative diseases such as frontotemporal and lewy body dementia (Silverman et al., 2001).

Interestingly, despite innumerable pathology reports and both in vivo CT and MRI studies identifying significant hippocampal formation damage in AD, for many years FDG-PET studies failed to report MTL abnormalities. This led to the paradoxical

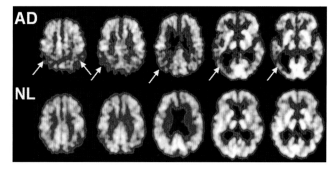

Figure 11–3   FDG-PET scans of a 70 year-old mild AD patient (top) and a cognitively normal subject (bottom). Arrows point to areas of hypometabolism in the AD patient, involving the parietal and temporal neocortex. (Adapted from Mosconi et al., 2008)

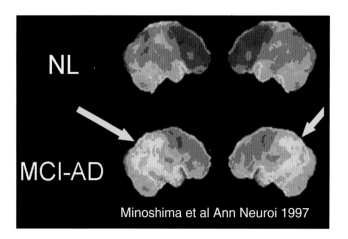

Figure 11–4   Parietotemporal lobe and posterior cingulate cortex hypometabolism in MCI and AD individuals, as compared to NL individuals. (Adapted from Minoshima et al., 1997.)

conclusion that the MTL was either not hypometabolic or maintained its metabolic rate as a compensatory mechanism against advancing disease (see Mosconi, 2005 for discussion). Only recently, owing to technical achievements leading to higher spatial resolution, improving resolution from nearly 2 cm to under 5 mm, enhanced detector sensitivity of PET instrumentation, and the use of anatomically precise brain sampling with MRI guidance, has there also appeared an increasing number of reports of MTL CMRglc abnormalities in AD that accompany the characteristic cortical hypometabolism (Figure 11.5) (de Leon et al., 1997b, 2001; De Santi et al., 2001; Mosconi et al., 2005b, 2006a, 2007e, 2008; Nestor et al., 2003; Ouchi et al., 1998). Characteristic patterns of MTL hypometabolism can be quantified on an individual basis using a FDG-PET visual rating scale developed by Mosconi et al. This FDG-PET scale arose from an earlier MRI scale of hippocampal atrophy (Figure 11.6) (de Leon et al., 1997a).

Despite these characteristic alterations, PET currently has limited clinical approval in the United States for the examination of cases that are difficult to distinguish between AD and FTD. The principal evidence that PET is of use for AD vs. FTD lies in a few reports that consistently identify frontal lobe changes in FTD with preservation of the parietotemporal association areas (Diehl-Schmid et al., 2007; Foster et al., 2007; Franceschi et al., 2005; Ishii et al., 1998b; Jeong et al., 2005; Mosconi et al., 2008). Frontal lobe damage is relatively absent in AD until the later stages

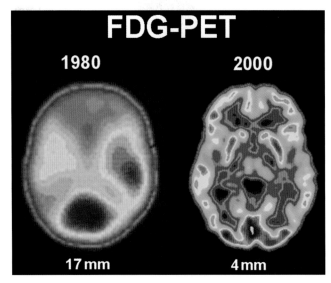

Figure 11–5 Higher spatial resolution and increased detector sensitivity of PET instrumentation has enabled more precise imaging of brain regions displaying CMRglc reductions. Comparison shows the PET III and the PET CTI 931. (Adapted from de Leon et al., 2008)

of disease, whereas parietotemporal association area defects are consistently identified (Foster et al., 1984). The use of PET in the differential diagnosis of dementia often involves comparison with Dementia with Lewy Bodies (DLB) (Albin et al., 1996; Minoshima et al., 2001; Mosconi et al., 2008), and vascular dementia (Barber et al., 2000; Szelies et al., 1994) as well as a host of other conditions reviewed in greater detail in Chapter 15.

The Early Diagnosis of AD

Importantly, MTL CMRglc reductions have been observed with FDG-PET before the onset of full AD symptoms and a growing list of observations has highlighted the importance of PET as a tool for detecting early disease and for estimating an increased risk for future dementia. This list of observations includes:

- Presymptomatic individuals carrying autosomal dominant mutations responsible for early-onset familial AD;
- Patients with Mild Cognitive Impairment, which is in many cases a prodrome to AD;
- Cognitively normal elderly who declined to MCI and AD several years after PET;
- Cognitively normal individual carriers of the Apolipoprotein E (ApoE) E4 allele, a susceptibility factor for late-onset AD;
- Cognitively normal subjects with subjective memory complaints;
- Cognitively normal subjects with a maternal family history of AD.

The main FDG-PET findings from these studies are reviewed below.

Conversion Studies

Presymptomatic Early-Onset Familial AD

Autosomal dominant mutations have been identified in three genes, i.e. amyloid precursor protein (APP, on chromosome 21), Presenilin 1 (PS1, on chromosome 14), and Presenilin 2 (PS2, on

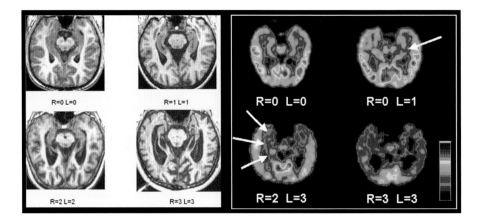

Figure 11–6 MRI hippocampal atrophy scale (left). Four MR scans depicting the rating scale evaluations for hippocampal formation atrophy. The rating from 0 to 3 is displayed, where 0 = no atrophy, 1 = questionable atrophy, 2 = mild atrophy, and 3 = moderate atrophy. All images were displayed using the neurological convention (left is left) (Adapted from de Leon et al., 1997a). FDG-PET MTL hypometabolism scale (right). Negative-angle axial PET views depicting examples of MTL ratings. The rating from 0 to 3 is displayed, where 0 = normal metabolism, 1 = questionable hypometabolism, 2 = mild hypometabolism, and 3 = moderate to severe hypometabolism. All images were displayed using the neurological convention (left is left). All PET scans were displayed using a 20-level color-coded scale (5% increments). The overall intensities for each scan were scaled so that the reference regions (i.e., sensorimotor strip, thalamus, and occipital cortex) were all viewed in the top 20% of the scale. Consequently, the MTL areas appear more in the middle range of the scale as compared with the occipital cortex, which appears at this plane. To achieve a scale point of 0, no areas of hypointensity should be seen in the MTL over any of three contiguous slices (3 mm thick). A scale point of 1 was assigned to questionable evidence for hypometabolism, defined as focal low activity typically in the junction between the head and the body of the hippocampus (single arrow). A scale point of 2 was assigned to mild but definite (i.e., localized) hypometabolism, which is typically diffuse (multiple arrows) with areas of preservation. A scale point of 3 was assigned to moderate to severe hypometabolism. To be considered indicative of regional MTL or cortical hypometabolism (scores 2 or 3), the observed regional abnormality had to be observed in at least two contiguous slices. (Adapted from Mosconi et al., 2006a.)

chromosome 1), which are associated with early-onset familial AD (FAD). FAD accounts for <5% of AD cases in the general population and is characterized by autosomal dominant inheritance with 100% penetrance and a predictable early age of symptom-onset for a given pedigree (see Tanzi and Bertram, 2001 for review). Therefore, the study of presymptomatic mutation carriers close to the expected age of dementia-onset provides unique information about preclinical AD-related brain changes in individuals who are destined to develop the disease.

Several FDG-PET studies have examined presymptomatic FAD, and showed parietotemporal, posterior cingulate, and frontal cortex hypometabolism in most FAD cases as compared to age-matched controls (Kennedy et al., 1995a, 1995b). A study by Kennedy et al. (1995a) (Kennedy et al., 1995a) showed that pre-symptomatic FAD individuals have whole brain CMRglc levels intermediate between controls and symptomatic FAD patients, which suggests a progression of global CMRglc impairment along the course of disease. However, these early studies only examined the neocortex. They did not examine the MTL, nor did they perform partial volume correction of the FDG-PET values. Since these patients also showed significant volume losses (atrophy) on MRI, it remained to be established whether the CMRglc reductions were an effect of an increasing CSF pool or reflected damage to the remaining tissue. The presence of brain atrophy and consequent partial volume effects of CSF in a particular region serve to lower the estimated CMRglc values on FDG-PET (see also Chapter 2).

We recently addressed this issue in an FDG-PET and MRI study of presymptomatic PS-1 carriers from families with early-onset FAD, examined an average of 13 years prior to the estimated age of disease-onset (Mosconi et al., 2006b). Our data show MTL and cortical hypometabolism in presymptomatic FAD. Furthermore, the CMRglc reductions in these individuals exceed tissue loss. Specifically, we compared CMRglc and volumes in several brain regions, including the hippocampus, entorhinal cortex (EC), posterior cingulate cortex (PCC), parietal and temporal cortices, and the whole brain, between FAD and age-matched non-carriers from the same families. Significant volume reductions in FAD, as compared to controls, were restricted to the parietal cortex. Conversely, CMRglc reductions on FDG-PET were observed in all regions examined, and remained significant after partial volume correction from MRI. After partial volume correction, the CMRglc reductions ranged from 13% (whole brain) to 21% (PCC), reflecting true reductions of brain glucose utilization per unit brain volume. After partial volume correction the MTL CMRglc were reduced 12% in the hippocampus and 20% in the EC. Overall, in the relative absence of structural brain atrophy, presymptomatic FAD patients showed widespread CMRglc reductions in the brain regions typically hypometabolic in clinically diagnosed dementia patients (Mosconi et al., 2006b). These results provide definitive evidence that CMRglc reductions precede clinical symptoms as well as gross structural brain changes. Similar observations have been made in the preclinical stages of late-onset AD.

Mild Cognitive Impairment

A successful strategy to examine the preclinical stages of sporadic AD has been the investigation of MCI patients. MCI is recognized by many as a transitional state between healthy aging and dementia, during which individuals are able to perform the usual activities of daily living, but suffer mild memory impairments and/or other cognitive difficulties exceeding those expected with normal aging. These symptoms reduce the quality of life for the patient and put

them at higher risk for developing AD (Gauthier et al., 2006; Petersen et al., 2001). Specifically, patients with salient memory deficits, e.g., amnestic MCI, decline to AD with an estimated conversion rate of 10%–30% per year in research settings (Gauthier et al., 2006; Petersen et al., 2001).

While parietotemporal and PCC hypometabolism is consensually recognized as the metabolic signature of AD, there is currently no specific pattern of hypometabolism considered to be a hallmark for MCI as related to AD (see Mosconi, 2005; Nestor, Scheltens, and Hodges, 2004 for recent reviews, and also Chapter 13). In keeping with the concept of MCI as an intermediate stage along the hypothesized continuum from normal aging to AD, MCI patients generally present with mild global and regional hypometabolism within the same brain regions typically affected in clinical AD, as compared to controls (Anchisi et al., 2005; Arnaiz et al., 2001; Chetelat et al., 2003; de Leon et al., 2001; De Santi et al., 2001; Drzezga et al., 2003, 2005; Herholz et al., 1999; Minoshima et al., 1997; Mosconi et al., 2005b, 2006a; Nestor et al., 2003), including an increasing numbers of reports of MTL CMRglc reductions.

The regional patterns of CMRglc reduction in MCI are milder and somewhat more variable than those found in AD; nevertheless, the patterns of reduction correspond to variations in the patterns of cognitive and behavioral abnormalities in individual patients (Anchisi et al., 2005l; Haxby et al., 1990). Importantly, FDG-PET studies in MCI showed that hippocampal hypometabolism is a consistent feature of MCI patients regardless of the neuropsychological profile (de Leon et al., 2001; De Santi et al., 2001; Mosconi et al., 2006a, 2008). Studies have shown a more diversified metabolic profile in non-amnestic MCI (i.e., patients with selective deficits in attention and language (Petersen et al., 2001)) who show either an absence of cortical hypometabolism or hypometabolism in brain regions including, but not restricted to, the anterior cingulate and parietotemporal cortices (Berent et al., 1999; de Leon et al., 2001; De Santi et al., 2001; Mosconi et al., 2006a; Reed et al., 1989). In contrast, amnestic MCI patients more consistently show pronounced abnormalities in the PCC and parietotemporal cortices (Chetelat et al., 2003; Drzezga et al., 2003; Minoshima et al., 1997; Mosconi et al., 2004; Nestor et al., 2003). Given the higher rate of decline to AD in amnestic than in non-amnestic MCI (Gauthier et al., 2006), these data suggest that the more severe and spatially extended CMRglc reductions in AD-specific regions may predispose these patients to develop AD in the near future.

In addition to cross-sectional examination of FDG-PET in the differentiation of MCI from normal aging, a growing body of longitudinal FDG-PET examinations has examined the predictive value of these measures in the decline from MCI to AD. Most studies focused on amnestic MCI patients and the data show that baseline CMRglc reductions are more pronounced in those MCI that later develop the symptoms of AD as compared to those who remained stable. The reported prediction accuracies range from 75% to 100% (Anchisi et al., 2005; Arnaiz et al., 2001; Chetelat et al., 2003; Drzezga et al., 2005; Herholz et al., 1999; Minoshima et al., 1997). Moreover, there is evidence showing that the metabolic changes in the declining MCI patients are progressive, and that longitudinal CMRglc measures both predict and correlate with decline to AD (Drzezga et al., 2003).

Decline from Normal Cognition to MCI and to AD

Very little work has been done with FDG-PET to monitor the progression from normal aging to sporadic AD. Such studies are limited because of the intrinsic difficulty of observing clinical change for a group with a low incidence of decline (1%–3%/year) and a slow progression of cognitive change (Petersen et al., 1999). To follow cognitively normal persons over time until they develop dementia requires large subject samples, long follow-up intervals, and great expense.

Only a few FDG-PET studies that monitored decline from normal to MCI (de Leon et al., 2001) or from normal to MCI and dementia (Jagust et al., 2006; Mosconi et al., 2008) have been published. In the first study, de Leon et al. (2001) studied 67 normal elderly of whom 48 completed a 3-year follow-up. It was observed that 11 declined to MCI and one to AD. They showed that reduced baseline CMRglc in the entorhinal cortex predicted the MCI diagnosis 3 years later with 83% sensitivity and 85% specificity (see Figure 11.7) (de Leon et al., 2001). Moreover, longitudinal CMRglc reductions were found in the EC, hippocampus, and lateral temporal cortex during the progression to MCI (see Figure 11.9). Importantly, these effects remained significant after correcting the CMRglc values for partial volume effects from MRI, suggesting that these early CMRglc reductions in MCI are independent of tissue loss and represent a real reduction of glucose consumption per gram brain tissue. However, considering that many MCI patients remain stable, it was not established whether the observed CMRglc reductions in MCI were in fact due to AD.

In 2006, Jagust and colleagues also looked at early metabolic changes with FDG-PET in cognitively normal individuals studied longitudinally (Jagust et al., 2006). Sixty subjects were followed for a mean of 4 years and received baseline FDG-PET scans and annual evaluations of global cognition, assessed by the Modified Mini-Mental State Examination (3MSE). Within this cohort, six subjects developed incident dementia or cognitive impairment after the initial visit. The results showed that baseline CMRglc reductions in the angular gyri, left mid-temporal gyrus, and left middle frontal gyrus predicted rate of change on the 3MSE, and was associated with faster cognitive decline (Jagust et al., 2006).

We recently published the first longitudinal FDG-PET study monitoring the conversion from normal cognition to AD. Mosconi et al. (2008) examined 77 normal elderly that were followed over 6–14 years with multiple FDG-PET examinations. Over this interval, 11 baseline normal subjects developed dementia, six of whom were diagnosed with AD, and 19 declined to MCI. Decline for both outcome groups occurred, on average, 8 years after the baseline exam. CMRglc in the hippocampus and cortical regions

were examined as predictors and correlates of change in clinical status. The baseline hippocampal CMRglc was the only regional predictor of future cognitive decline, and predicted decline from normal to AD with 81% accuracy, including two postmortem confirmed AD cases. The baseline hippocampal CMRglc also predicted decline from normal to MCI with 71% accuracy and from normal to another dementia with 77% accuracy. Hippocampal hypometabolism was also a significant predictor of the time to decline. On survival analysis, for individuals with hippocampal CMRglc ≤24 μmol/100 g/min, the predicted time to decline to AD was 7 years. For hippocampal CMRglc of 25–29 μmol/100 g/min, the predicted time to decline was 9.5 years, and for CMRglc ≥30 μmol/100 g/min, greater than 14 years (Figure 11.8). In AD, for every unit decrease in baseline hippocampal CMRglc, time to decline decreased by 8.7% (95% CI: 3.0%–14.1%) (χ2 (1) = 8.6, p = .003), which corresponds to a time ratio (TR) of 1.1 (95% CI: 1.0–1.4) years; the time to decline to other dementias is decreased by 4.7% (95% CI: .3%–8.9%) (χ2 (1) = 4.6, p < .05), for a TR of 1.0 (95% CI: 0.8–1.2) years; the time to decline in MCI is decreased by 7.2% (95% CI: 2.8%–11.5%) (χ2 (1) = 9.93, p < .01), for a TR of 1.08 (95% CI: 1.03–1.11) years. Furthermore, greater rates of hippocampal, PCC and temporal cortex CMRglc reductions were found in the declining as compared to the non-declining normal subjects (Mosconi et al., 2008).

In addition, these FDG-PET data provided direct evidence for a topographical progression of CMRglc abnormalities, which appear to originate in the MTL during the normal stages of cognition, extend to the PCC at the MCI stage of AD, and finally spread to the parietotemporal cortices in full-blown dementia (Mosconi et al., 2008). This finding is consistent with the progression of NFT pathology delineated by Braak and Braak (Braak and Braak, 1991). Overall, our results showed an association between reduced

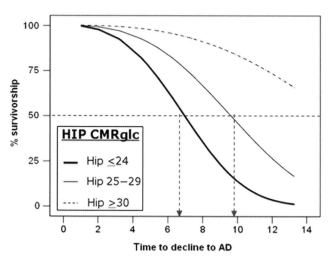

Figure 11–8 Hippocampal glucose metabolism and the risk for Alzheimer's disease (AD). Weibull survival regression curves of normal subjects whose hippocampal (Hip) metabolism (MRglc, μmol/(g min)) at baseline was ≤24 (bold line), 25–29 (plain line), and ≥30 (dashed line). The prediction model shows that for baseline Hip MRglc ≤24 μmol/(g min) the median predicted time to decline to AD is 7 years, for baseline Hip MRglc 25–29 μmol/(g min) the median predicted time to decline to AD is 9.5 years, and for baseline Hip MRglc ≥30 μmol/(g min) the median predicted time to decline to AD is greater than 14 years. The median estimated time to decline to AD for each tertile of Hip MRglc is indicated with dashed arrows. (Adapted from Mosconi et al., 2008.)

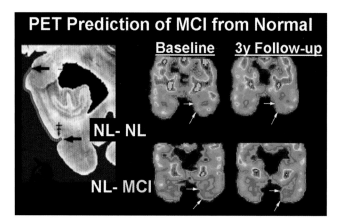

Figure 11–7 NL subjects who later declined to MCI show baseline CMRglc reductions in the EC. Figure shows the baseline and the follow-up scans for a patient who declined. Note the widespread and progressive changes over the three-year period. (Adapted from de Leon et al., 2001.)

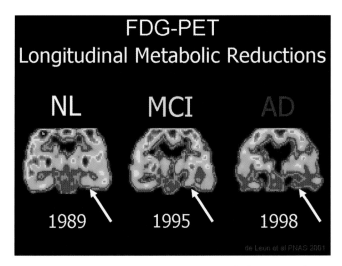

Figure 11–9 Progressive CMRglc reductions in the hippocampal formation (entorhinal cortex) of a patient who declined from NL to MCI and later AD over a 9-year period. (Adapted from de Leon et al., 2001.)

hippocampal CMRglc during normal aging, shorter times until onset of dementia, and increased risk for cognitive decline years in advance of clinical diagnosis.

Risk Factors for AD

Apolipoprotein E E4 Genotype

The epsilon 4 allele of the Apolipoprotein E (ApoE) gene on chromosome 19 is a widely recognized genetic risk factor for late-onset AD (Corder et al., 1993; Farrer et al., 1997). The ApoE gene codes for the production of lipoproteins, which mediate the transport of lipids throughout bodily fluids such as blood and cerebrospinal fluid. ApoE is specifically thought to maintain neuronal homeostasis by transporting lipids such as cholesterol and phospholipids, which are responsible for neuronal plasticity, throughout the central nervous system (Laws et al., 2003). ApoE also provides lipids needed to repair damaged nerve cell membranes. There are three common isoforms of the ApoE allele, including ApoE-2, ApoE-3, and ApoE-4. The ApoE-4 genotype is described as a risk factor since 40% of AD patients have at least one ApoE-4 allele, and there is a negative association between the dose of ApoE-4 allele and the mean age of onset of AD (Farrer et al., 1997).

The mechanism by which the ApoE-4 allele confers increased risk of future AD is under study, although it is believed that ApoE-4 may confer decreased plasticity of neuronal synapses and an inability to repair damaged neurons, as compared to the other allelic variants (Laws et al., 2003).

FDG-PET studies examining the effects of the ApoE-4 allele on CMRglc in non-demented individuals reported that, compared to non-carriers, cognitively normal individual ApoE-4 carriers have mild but definite CMRglc reductions in the same regions as clinically affected AD patients (Mosconi et al., 2008; Reiman et al., 1996, 1998, 2001, 2004; Small et al., 1995, 2000). This finding raises questions about the diagnostic interpretation of the PET scan of ApoE-4 carriers (Figure 11.10). There is evidence in middle-age ApoE-4 carriers that the metabolic reductions are progressive and correlate with reductions in cognitive performance (Reiman et al., 2001; Small et al., 1995). A study of cognitively

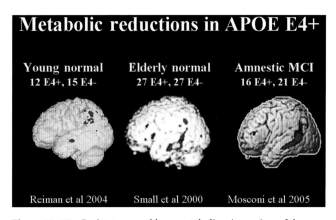

Figure 11–10 Parietotemporal hypometabolism in carriers of the ApoE-4 allele in young NL, elderly NL, and amnestic MCI, as compared to non-carriers in each group classification. (Adapted from Small et al., 2000; Reiman et al., 2004; Mosconi et al., 2005a.)

normal persons aged 50–63 having two ApoE-4 alleles showed a 25% decline in CMRglc over an interval of 2 years (Reiman et al., 2001). Moreover, the same pattern of hypometabolism was observed in 20 to 40-year-old carriers. These CMRglc reductions are considered the earliest brain abnormalities yet found in living persons at risk for AD (Reiman et al., 2004).

Nonetheless, these studies are limited by the relatively short follow-up intervals and it remains to be established whether the CMRglc reductions in the ApoE-4 carriers are predictive of decline to AD.

Subjective Memory Complaints

Subjective memory complaints (SMC) are widespread in the elderly community with a prevalence of 25%–50%, and for many represent a preclinical sign of incipient dementia (Geerlings et al., 1999). We recently published an FDG-PET study examining CMRglc in cognitively normal individuals with and without SMC (Mosconi et al., 2008). The results showed that normal individuals with SMC have significant CMRglc reductions in several brain regions, including the parahippocampal gyri (PHG), parietotemporal and inferior frontal cortex, fusiform gyrus and thalamus, as compared to demographically matched individuals with no such complaints (Figure 11.11). Hypometabolism in the PHG region, which anteriorly includes the entorhinal cortex (Bobinski et al., 1999), was the most significant predictor of SMC status, and distinguished subjects with and without SMC with 75% accuracy, with an odds ratio of 2.4 (95% Confidence Interval = 1.3–4.8, $p < .001$). In other words, normal individuals with SMC are more than twice as likely to have PHG deficits, compared to those with no complaints (Mosconi et al., 2008). Moreover, we also explored the effects of the ApoE genotype on CMRglc and showed a significant interaction between SMC and APOE status. Among subjects with SMC, carriers of the ApoE-4 genotype had the lowest CMRglc measures in the PHG, temporal and frontal cortices, and thalamus as compared to the three other subgroups. Again, the CMRglc reductions were most prominent in the PHG (18%).

Maternal Family History of AD

After advanced age, the most prominent demographic risk factor for developing AD is a first-degree family history of late-onset AD (Farrer et al., 1997). Normal individuals with a first-degree relative

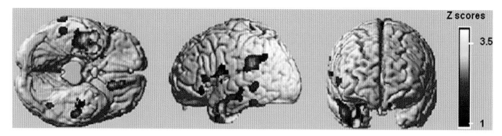

Figure 11–11 Statistical parametric maps showing CMRglc reductions in subjects with subjective memory complaints vs. control. Hypometabolic regions include middle temporal gyrus, inferior parietal lobe, parahippocampal gyrus, and inferior temporal and frontal gyri. Areas of hypometabolism are represented on a red-to-yellow color-coded scale, reflecting progressively higher Z scores, and displayed (from left to right). Figure shows the inferior, left lateral, and anterior views of a volume-rendered MRI. (Adapted from Mosconi et al., 2008.)

affected with AD, particularly those with an affected parent, have a 4- to 10-fold increased risk for developing AD, as compared to individuals with no family history (Cupples et al., 2004; Green et al., 2002; Silverman et al., 2005). We recently performed the first imaging study to compare individuals with a parental history of AD to those without, and to examine whether having a maternal or paternal history of AD affected CMRglc in normal individuals (Mosconi et al., 2007b). We examined the FDG-PET scans of 49 cognitively normal elderly grouped according to their family history of AD, and compared those with a maternal, paternal, or no family history of AD. The results revealed that individuals with a maternal history of AD show CMRglc reductions in the PCC/precuneus, parietotemporal and frontal cortices, and medial temporal lobes, as compared to individuals with no family history and those with an AD-affected father (Figure 11.12) (Mosconi et al., 2007b). Intriguingly, these are the brain regions typically affected in clinical AD patients. The results remained significant after accounting for other potential risk factors for AD, such as age, female gender, ApoE genotype, and presence of subjective memory complaints. The ApoE-4 genotype was represented in 22% of our maternal AD subjects and the same effects were found in the group

of ApoE-4 non-carriers. These data indicate that factors other than ApoE-4 genotype contributed to the CMRglc abnormalities.

The biological and genetic mechanisms that underlie the CMRglc reductions in individuals with maternal AD are not known. With all that is known about the molecular processes involved in glucose metabolism, hypometabolism may be due to, amongst other factors, a combination of defective mitochondrial function and possible mitochondrial DNA (mtDNA) mutations (Lin and Beal, 2006). The fact that mtDNA is entirely maternally inherited in humans, and diseases associated with mtDNA mutations often present as sporadic disorders (Lin and Beal, 2006), lends support to this hypothesis. Although other genetic mechanisms (i.e., epigenetic imprinting, chromosome X transmission, and mutations in nuclear DNA affecting mitochondrial function) could potentially account for these results, our findings suggest maternal transmission of hypometabolism in normal subjects at risk for AD.

As with the ApoE-4 genotype, it is necessary to longitudinally follow subjects in all family history categories to determine whether the observed CMRglc alterations predict the onset of AD and if they correlate with clinical decline over time. Our preliminary data suggest this possibility (data not published).

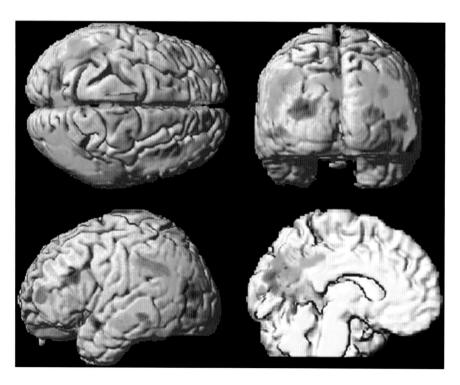

Figure 11–12 Brain regions showing reduced brain glucose metabolism in normal individuals with a maternal history of AD as compared to those with a paternal history of AD (in red), and to those with no family history of AD (in green). These same brain regions are typically hypometabolic in clinical AD patients (Adapted from Mosconi et al., 2007b.)

Increasing Diagnostic Specificity

While hypometabolism can reflect synapse dysfunction, remote changes in circuitry, and neuronal damage, CMRglc measures do not provide information on the specific pathology of AD. Recent evidence shows that CMRglc reductions correlate moderately well with regional densities of neurofibrillary pathology (NFT), but are not well correlated with amyloid plaque distribution (DeCarli et al., 1992). A ^{99m}Tc-HMPAO SPECT study showed that reduced cerebral perfusion correlated with Braak's stages of NFT distribution in AD, with both features originating in the MTL (Bradley et al., 2002). Further indirect evidence for a relationship between CMRglc reductions and AD pathology comes from studies that show agreement between postmortem diagnosis of AD and the parietotemporal hypometabolism detected *in vivo* with PET. In the largest series of cases available to date, the presence of cortical CMRglc abnormalities on ante-mortem FDG-PET correctly predicted postmortem AD diagnosis with 88% accuracy (Silverman et al., 2001). However, the major limitation to the use of FDG-PET in the diagnosis of AD is the lack of disease specificity. Recent evidence shows that FDG-PET pattern recognition, especially when facilitated by the use of automated voxel-based analysis techniques, discriminates AD, FTD, and DLB from controls and from each other with accuracies >90% (Mosconi et al., 2008). However, there is significant overlap in hypometabolic regions across neurodegenerative disorders.

Amyloid PET Imaging

An effective strategy to increase the diagnostic accuracy in AD would be to combine the sensitivity of FDG-PET with another modality that provides a disease-specific measure of pathology. Recently, several PET tracers for Aβ plaques have been developed. The best known tracer, N-methyl-[^{11}C] 2-(4′-methylaminophenyl)-6-hydroxybenzothiazole, also known as Pittsburgh Compound-B (PIB), binds to Aβ plaques in the brain (Klunk et al., 2004). For a detailed review of amyloid–PET imaging, please see Chapter 14. Several PIB-PET studies demonstrated significant PIB retention in AD patients as compared to controls, mostly evident in the middle- and prefrontal cortex, parietotemporal regions, PCC/precuneus, occipital lobes, thalamus and striatum (Kemppainen et al., 2006; Klunk et al., 2004; Mintun et al., 2006; Pike et al., 2007; Rowe et al., 2007). These regions are consistent with the known pattern of Aβ plaque deposition observed at postmortem, and correlate with reductions in CSF Aβ1-42 (Fagan et al., 2005). PIB-PET studies have shown significant PIB retention in the AD range in as many as 61% of MCI (Kemppainen et al., 2006; Mintun et al., 2006; Pike et al., 2007), and 22% of normal elderly (Mintun et al., 2006). These subjects may be at increased risk for developing AD. One follow-up PIB-PET publication indicates a lack of longitudinal progression (Engler et al., 2006), suggesting that amyloid deposition may plateau at the AD stage. At this early phase of development, PIB-PET has been shown to facilitate an improved differential diagnosis of the dementias (Drzezga et al., 2008; Mintun et al., 2006), although a recent study demonstrated that PIB may not be specific for dense, classical plaques (Mathis, Wang, and Klunk, 2004), as it rather seems to bind to a family of amyloid substrates ranging from diffuse plaques to plaques in the vascular system (i.e., cerebral amyloid angiopathy), and, to a lesser extent, also to NFT (Lockhart et al., 2007).

These data, together with the observation that many normal elderly have brain amyloid deposits, suggest that PIB-PET imaging may be more suitable to rule out AD, as a patient with negative PIB uptake is unlikely to have AD.

The 20-minute radioactive decay half-life of ^{11}C limits the use of PIB to centers with an on-site cyclotron, which hinders use of the tracer for routine clinical use. To overcome these limitations, tracers for imaging Aβ that are labeled with fluorine-18 (^{18}F, 110 minute half-life) have been developed. The first fluorinated Aβ PET tracer to become available is 2-(1-96-(2-^{18}F-fluoroethyl)(methyl)amino)-2-naphthyl)ethyldene)malono nitrile (^{18}F-FDDNP), which binds with high specificity to both Aβ fibrils and NFTs (Agdeppa et al., 2001; Small et al., 2006). ^{18}F-FDDNP binding was elevated in AD and MCI patients as compared with healthy elderly, and showed uptake in the MTL, yielding 100% diagnostic separation between AD and controls, and 95% between MCI and controls (Small et al., 2006). Moreover, tracer uptake showed good correlation with scores on memory and global cognition tests, as well as longitudinal progression for a subgroup of non-demented subjects that deteriorated over 2 years (Small et al., 2006). One potential early diagnostic advantage of ^{18}F-FDDNP over PIB is its capacity to bind NFT in addition to Aβ (de Leon et al., 2007b). It is known that neurofibrillary tangle pathology, unlike Aβ depositions, appears in the early stages of disease in the hippocampal formation (Braak and Braak, 1991) and increased NFT load in this region is associated with impairment of cognition (Powell et al., 2006). One issue raised is the narrow range of tracer binding across subjects and subsequently low percent change in binding across groups, ranging from 5%–8% increase in patients with MCI and AD relative to controls (de Leon, Mosconi, and Logan, 2007b). Further studies are needed to assess the extent to which ^{18}F-FDDNP increases both early diagnosis and diagnostic specificity.

At the present time, amyloid imaging studies have not yet reported on early diagnosis, or on predictions of longitudinal change. Additional validation studies are needed before Aβ imaging can enter into clinical practice.

CSF Biomarkers

Cerebrospinal fluid (CSF) is in direct contact with the brain and the molecular composition of CSF reflects biochemical changes in the central nervous system. Consequently, many studies have examined the CSF as a possible source for biomarkers of AD pathology. Several candidate diagnostic biomarkers have emerged. The most widely studied CSF analytes include markers for tau (i.e., total [T-tau] and hyperphosphorylated tau [P-tau] proteins) and Aβ pathology (i.e., peptide fragments of Aβ$_{40}$ and Aβ$_{42}$ amino-acid residues) and isoprostane (IsoP, a marker of lipid peroxidation and inflammation).

CSF tau studies. Two types of CSF measures for tau pathology have been used in AD: T-tau and markers for isoforms (X) of hyperphosphorylated (P) tau (P-TauX). T-tau, the first biomarker to be available, is the most widely used. Overall, CSF T-tau reflects both the normal metabolism of tau and the non-specific release of tau following neuronal damage, whereas P-tau231 reflects abnormal tau metabolism that is both sensitive and specific for AD (Mitchell and Brindle, 2003). The evidence consistently demonstrates elevated CSF concentrations of T-tau in AD and in MCI compared to NL controls (Brys et al., 2006). CSF T-tau is increased to around 300% in AD as compared to controls, probably as a result of neuronal and axonal degeneration, with a mean sensitivity of 84% and 91% specificity (Blennow and Hampel, 2003). Moreover, 11 studies show that CSF T-tau (and P-tauX in several studies) alone or in combination with Aβ42 predicts the conversion from MCI to AD (Blennow, de Leon, and Zetterberg, 2006). Equivalent prediction accuracies for CSF T-tau and P-tau231-235 were reported by Arai (Arai et al., 2000), by Hansson using P-tau181 (Hansson et al., 2006), and by our group (Brys et al., 2000) with P-tau231 (see Figure 11.14). However, reports about CSF X-tau levels in normal aging are limited and contradictory; some show age-related elevations in T-tau (Buerger nee et al., 1999) and others do not (Andreasen et al., 2001; Hulstaert et al., 1999). Our adult lifespan data shows age-related increases after age 60 for both P-tau231 and T-tau, and both demonstrate additive ε4 related effects (Glodzik-Sobanska et al., 2009) (see Figure 11.13). The T-tau level is not specific for AD, as CSF T-tau levels are also elevated in other neurodegenerative diseases (Arai et al., 1997; Mollenhauer et al., 2005). In acute stroke, the T-tau, but not the P-tau181 levels, were increased and later returned to normal (Hesse et al., 2001). However, P-tau231 offers reasonable diagnostic specificity for AD. Hampel and his co-investigators found that the levels of P-tau231, but not T-tau, were consistently elevated in AD as compared with frontotemporal dementia (FTD), Lewy body dementia (LBD), vascular dementia, and NL elderly controls (Buerger et al., 2002). More recent work extended the specificity of P-tau231 for AD to major depression (Buerger et al., 2003) and CJD (Buerger et al., 2006). Similarly, others demonstrated the advantage of P-tau181 over T-tau in comparisons between AD with FTD (Sjogren et al., 2001; Vanmechelen et al., 2000) and with non-AD dementias (Ishiguro et al., 1999; Parnetti et al., 2001). A recent longitudinal biomarker study using MRI showed that changes in the levels of

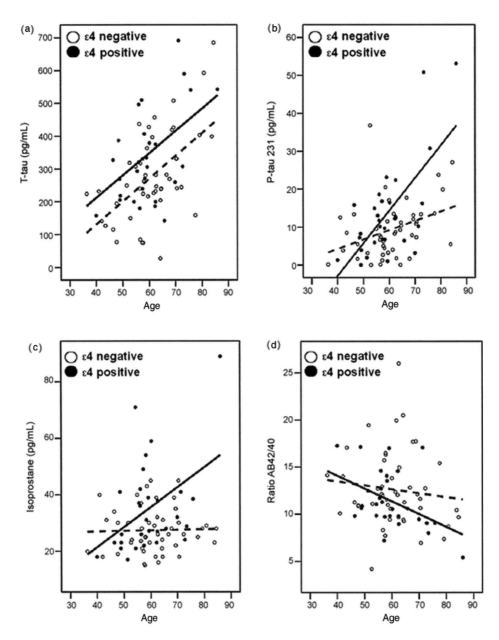

Figure 11–13   T-tau (a), P-tau231 (b), IP (c) concentrations and Aβ42/Aβ40 (d) in CSF as a function of age and ApoE genotype. Solid line: four positive group; dashed line: four negative group. (Adapted from Glodzik-Sobanska et al., 2009.)

P-tau231 were longitudinally associated with the change in the hippocampal volume in MCI patients (de Leon et al., 2006). However, there is very limited evidence for CSF tau levels to increase with clinical progression (de Leon et al., 2002, 2006), thus making the CSF measurement a potentially ancillary measurement to be used with modalities that do confer longitudinal information, such as FDG-PET or MRI. At present there are no reports of the combined use of tau biomarkers with FDG-PET in longitudinal designs.

CSF Aβ studies. CSF-Aβ$_{42}$ is reduced in AD to around 50% of control concentrations, which may be due to the deposition of the peptide in brain plaques or to reduced neuronal production. Cross-sectional CSF Aβ studies consistently show reduced Aβ42 levels in both late onset AD (Blennow, de Leon, and Zetterberg 2006; Brys et al., 2006) and MCI (Andreasen and Blennow 2005; Hansson et al., 2006), but there is a dearth of longitudinal data. The available longitudinal data show Aβ42 levels decrease in AD, but the magnitude of change has limited diagnostic value (Mollenhauer et al., 2005; Tapiola et al., 2000). The background effects of aging on CSF turnover and Aβ production and clearance are poorly understood (Bading et al., 2002; Silverberg et al., 2001, 2002). Peskind et al., recently showed that CSF Aβ42 reductions were increasingly found with old age and detected at younger ages in ε4 carriers (Peskind et al., 2006), and our data confirm that observation (Glodzik-Sobanska et al., 2009).

Fagan recently reported that CSF Aβ42 reductions are associated with PIB evidence for deposition, but that the relationship is bimodal rather than linear (Fagan et al., 2005). CSF Aβ42 reductions predict decline from MCI to dementia (Blennow, de Leon, and Zetterberg 2006) and from CDR = 0 to CDR > 0 when combined with T-tau or P-tau181 (Fagan et al., 2007). To date, only one study importantly showed that high CSF T-tau/Aβ42 or P-tau181/Aβ42 ratios, but not X-tau or Aβx measures alone, predicted decline from CDR = 0 (normal) to CDR > 0 (impaired) (Fagan et al., 2007).

The diagnostic utility of CSF Aβ40, a predominant feature of vascular amyloid, as an AD biomarker is less well understood than Aβ42. A limited number of reports have shown elevated CSF Aβ40 levels with increasing age (Fukuyama et al., 2000; Shoji et al., 2001). However, several cross-sectional studies failed to observe differences between AD and NL (Kanai et al., 1998; Mehta et al., 2000) and for this reason the Aβ42/40 ratio, controlling for overall Aβ production and clearance, is often used as a diagnostic marker.

CSF IsoP studies. Oxidative stress is a recognized feature of AD and other neurodegenerative diseases (Markesbery, 1997). Postmortem studies by both the Pratico and Montine groups show elevated brain (Montine et al., 1999b) and CSF IsoP levels (Montine et al., 1998) in AD. IsoP are isomers of enzymatically derived prostaglandins, which are produced by O_2 radical-catalyzed peroxidation of polyunsaturated fatty acids (Pratico, 1999). Most AD work has focused on IsoP's derived from prostaglandin $F_{2\alpha}$, which is a reliable marker of in vivo oxidative stress (Pratico et al., 2001a). These studies also demonstrate

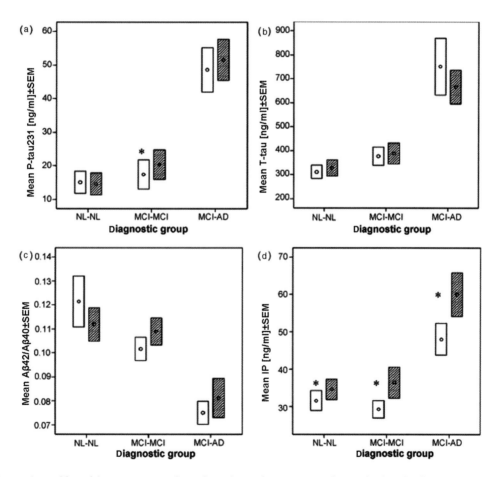

Figure 11–14 Comparison of five of the most commonly used CSF biomarkers in a 2-year longitudinal study of NL, stable MCI, and MCI patients declining to AD. (Adapted from Brys et al., 2000.)

correlations between neuronal oxidation (Montine et al., 1999b) and Braak staging (Montine et al., 1998). There is a growing awareness that IsoP changes are early features of AD that may even precede the development of fibrillar amyloid plaques (Markesbery et al., 2005; Nunomura et al., 2001; Pratico et al., 2001b). At postmortem CSF IsoP is elevated in MCI (Markesbery et al., 2005), and there is consensus that the levels are elevated in both AD (Montine et al., 1999a; Pratico et al., 2000) and MCI *in vivo* (de Leon et al., 2006; Pratico et al., 2002). In collaboration with Pratico, our CSF IsoP data show longitudinal elevations in MCI (de Leon et al., 2006) that accurately predict the decline from MCI to AD (Brys et al., 2000) (see Figure 11.14). Specifically, IsoP levels do change with clinical progression (Brys et al., 2000) and with progressive brain damage (de Leon et al., 2007a). While there is no mechanistic basis to expect that elevated IsoP levels are AD-specific, several studies show that CSF IsoP levels are higher in AD than FTD (Yao et al., 2003; Grossman et al., 2005) and other dementias (Montine et al., 2001).

Combining PET with CSF Biomarkers

Unfortunately, there is not much literature examining CSF biomarkers and PET. We recently published the first study to examine the relationship in normal subjects with subjective memory complaints (SMC) between hypometabolism on FDG-PET and CSF markers of AD pathology (Mosconi et al., 2008). Across all subjects, CMRglc in the MTL, parietotemporal and frontal cortices were significantly correlated with CSF levels of T-Tau, P-Tau$_{231}$ and IsoP, while no significant relationships with PET were found between CSF Aß$_{40}$ and Aß$_{42}$. ApoE-4 carriers with SMC showed the highest CSF T-Tau, P-Tau$_{231}$ and IsoP levels, and the lowest MTL CMRglc on PET, compared to all other subgroups. These data indicate a relationship between MTL CMRglc reductions, tau pathology and lipid membrane peroxidation in normal individuals at risk for late-onset AD, and suggest that the relationship between these biomarkers becomes tighter when subjects start to show memory deficits. Longitudinal follow-up examinations of these subjects are needed to determine whether the observed CSF and CMRglc abnormalities foreshadow clinical decline.

Conclusions

In recent years, several FDG-PET studies have shown that brain glucose hypometabolism in the hippocampal formation, combined with cortical abnormalities, is useful in accurately distinguishing AD from normal aging and, to some extent, from other dementias. These MTL changes can be found in both sporadic AD and early-onset FAD individuals, even at the stages where the patients are cognitively normal. For sporadic AD, this pattern of hypometabolism has also been reported among those at increased risk for developing AD, such as those with subjective memory complaints, carriers of the ApoE-4 genotype, and those with a maternal history of AD. Consequently, FDG-PET neuroimaging is a candidate modality for detecting brain changes in early AD.

There is considerable evidence that CMRglc is sensitive to progression effects (Mosconi et al., 2007a) and can be used as an outcome measure in long-term treatment studies of AD (Alexander et al., 2002; Reiman et al., 2001). A major advantage of PET over other clinically based assessments, such as cognitive performance, is the potential for reducing the sample sizes and study duration. It was estimated that, in order to detect a 33% treatment response with 80% power in a typical 1-year, double-blind, placebo-controlled treatment study, using the Mini Mental State Examination as an endpoint would require 224 AD patients per group, whereas as few as 36 patients per group would be needed for an FDG-PET study (Alexander et al., 2002).

Further longitudinal studies are necessary to examine whether the risk for developing different forms of dementia can be predicted based on the detection of individual FDG-PET patterns of CMRglc abnormalities among cognitively normal subjects or even subjects in the MCI stages of impairment.

There remains a great need to increase the preclinical diagnostic specificity, and to test whether combining the disease-sensitive CMRglc measures with pathology-specific biomarkers, such as with CSF measures of Aß or tauopathy proteins or amyloid PET imaging, would improve the differential diagnosis of AD and other dementing disorders prior to the onset of dementia.

Accurate characterization of the extent and nature of brain damage in individual patients, based on converging evidence from different biomarkers, could play an important role in the prediction of subjects' clinical course, in the selection of individualized treatment plans, and in screening patients with more uniform underlying pathology for targeted research and drug trials. Overall, CMRglc FDG-PET measures predict cognitive decline from normal aging with sensitivity and specificity greater than 80%, and correlate with clinical progression in AD. CMRglc is, therefore, a promising candidate biomarker for AD (Consensus Working Group, 1998).

Acknowledgements

We would like to thank the following laboratory directors for their respective CSF determinations: Drs. Pratico (Temple U) for the IsoP, Dr Pankaj Mehta (Institute for Basic Research) for the Aß$_{40}$ and Aß$_{42}$, Dr. Kaj Blennow (Salgrenska U) for T-tau and Dr. Ray Zinkowski (Applied Neurosolutions, Chicago) for the P-tau$_{231}$. This study was supported by National Institutes of Health/National Institute on Aging Grants AG13616, AG12101, AG08051, and AG022374; by the National Alzheimer's Disease Coordinating Center; by National Institutes of Health/National Center for Research Resources Grant M01-RR0096, and by the Alzheimer's Association.

References

Agdeppa, E. D., Kepe, V., Liu, J., Flores-Torres, S., Satyamurthy, N., Petric, A. et al. (2001). Binding characteristics of radiofluorinated 6-dialkylamino-2-naphthylethylidene derivatives as positron emission tomography imaging probes for beta-amyloid plaques in Alzheimer's disease. *Journal of Neuroscience*, 21: 1–5.

Albin, R. L., Minoshima, S., D'Amato, C. J., Frey, K. A., Kuhl, D. E., Sima, A. A. F. (1996). Fluoro-deoxyglucose positron emission tomography in diffuse lewy body disease. *Neurology*, 47: 462–466.

Alexander, G. E., Chen, K., Pietrini, P., Rapoport, S. I., Reiman, E. M. (2002). Longitudinal PET evaluation of cerebral metabolic decline in dementia: a potential outcome measure in Alzheimer's disease treatment studies. *American Journal of Psychiatry*, 159: 738–745.

Anchisi, D., Borroni, B., Franceschi, M., Kerrouche, N., Kalbe, E., Beuthien-Beumann, B. et al. (2005). Heterogeneity of brain glucose metabolism in mild cognitive impairment and clinical progression to Alzheimer disease. *Archives of Neurology*, 62: 1728–1733.

Andreasen, N. and Blennow K. (2005). CSF biomarkers for mild cognitive impairment and early Alzheimer's disease. *Clinical Neurology and Neurosurgery*, 107: 165–173.

Andreasen, N., Minthon, L., Davidsson, P., Vanmechelen, E., Vanderstichele, H., Winblad, B. et al. (2001). Evaluation of CSF-tau and CSF-Abeta42 as diagnostic markers for Alzheimer's disease in clinical practice. *Archives of Neurology* , 58: 373–379.

Arai, H., Ishiguro, K., Ohna, H., Moriyama, M., Itoh, N., Okamura, N. et al. (2000). CSF phosphorylated tau protein and mild cognitive impairment: A prospective study. *Experimental Neurology*, 166: 201–203.

Arai, H., Morikawa, Y., Higuchi, M., Matsui, T., Clark, C. M., Miura, M. et al. (1997). Cerebrospinal fluid tau levels in neurodegenerative diseases with distinct tau-related pathology. *Biochemical & Biophysical. Research Communications*, 236: 262–264.

Arnaiz, E., Jelic, V., Almkvist, O., Wahlund, L. O., Winblad, B., Valind, S. et al. (2001). Impaired cerebral glucose metabolism and cognitive functioning predict deterioration in mild cognitive impairment. *NeuroReport*, 12: 851–855.

Arriagada, P. V., Marzloff, K., and Hyman, B. T. (1992). Distribution of Alzheimer-type pathologic changes in nondemented elderly individuals matches the pattern in Alzheimer's disease. *Neurology*, 42: 1681–1688.

Attwell, D. and Iadecola, C. (2002). The neural basis of functional brain imaging signals. *Trends Neuroscience*, 25: 621–625.

Bading, J. R., Yamada, S., Mackic, J. B., Kirkman, L., Miller, C., Calero, M. et al. (2002). Brain clearance of Alzheimer's amyloid-beta40 in the squirrel monkey: A SPECT study in a primate model of cerebral amyloid angiopathy. *Journal of Drug Targeting*, 10: 359–368.

Barber, R., Ballard, C., McKeith, I. G., Gholkar, A., and O'Brien, J. T. (2000). MRI volumetric study of dementia with Lewy bodies: A comparison with AD and vascular dementia. *Neurology*, 54: 1304–1309.

Barber, R., Snowden, J. S., and Craufurd, D. (1995). Frontotemporal dementia and Alzheimer's disease: Retrospective differentiation using information from informants. *Journal of Neurology, Neurosurgery and Psychiatry*, 59: 61–70.

Berent, S., Giordani, B., Foster, N., Minoshima, S., Lajiness-O'Neill, R., Koeppe, R. et al. (1999). Neuropsychological function and cerebral glucose utilization in isolated memory impairment and Alzheimer's disease. *Journal of Psychiatric Research*, 33: 7–16.

Blennow, K. and de Leon, M. J., (2006). Zetterberg H. Alzheimer's disease. *Lancet Neurology*, 368: 387–403.

Blennow, K. and Hampel H. (2003). CSF markers for incipient Alzheimer's disease. *Lancet Neurology*, 2: 605–613.

Bobinski, M., de Leon, M. J., Convit, A., De Santi, S., Wegiel, J., Tarshish, C. Y. et al. (1999). MRI of entorhinal cortex in mild cognitive impairment. *Lancet*, 353: 38–40.

Bobinski, M., Wegiel, J., Wisniewski, H. M., Tarnawski, M., Reisberg, B., Mlodzik, B. et al. (1995). Atrophy of hippocampal formation subdivisions correlates with stage and duration of Alzheimer's disease. *Dementia*, 6: 205–210.

Braak, H. and Braak E. (1991). Neuropathological stageing of Alzheimer-related changes. *Acta Neuropathologica*, 82: 239–259.

Braak, H. and Braak E. (1996). Development of Alzheimer-related neurofibrillary changes in the neocortex inversely recapitulates cortical myelogenesis. *Acta Neuropathologica*, 92: 197–201.

Bradley, K. M., Bydder, G. M., Budge, M. M., Hajnal, J. V., White, S. J., Ripley, B. D. et al. (2002). Serial brain MRI at 3-6 month intervals as a surrogate marker for Alzheimer's disease. *The British Journal of Radiology*, 75: 506–513.

Brys, M., Mosconi, L., De Santi, S., Rich, K. E., and de Leon, M. J. (2006). CSF biomarkers for mild cognitive impairment. *Aging Health*, 2: 111–121.

Brys, M., Pirraglia, E., Rich, K., Rolstad, S., Mosconi, L., Switalski, R. et al. (2000). Prediction and longitudinal study of CSF biomarkers in mild cognitive impairment. *Neurobiology of Aging*, 30(5): 682–690.

Buerger nee, B. K., Padberg, F., Nolde, T., Teipel, S. J., Stubner, S., Haslinger, A. et al. (1999). Cerebrospinal fluid tau protein shows a better discrimination in young old (<70 years) than in old old patients with Alzheimer's disease compared with controls. *Neuroscience Letters*, 277: 21–24.

Buerger, K., Otto, M., Teipel, S. J., Zinkowski, R., Blennow, K., DeBernardis, J. et al. (2006). Dissociation between CSF total tau and tau protein phosphorylated at threonine 231 in Creutzfeldt-Jakob disease. *Neurobiology of Aging*, 27: 10–15.

Buerger, K., Zinkowski, R., Teipel, S. J., Tapiola, T., Arai, H., Blennow, K. et al. (2002). Differential diagnosis of Alzheimer disease with cerebrospinal fluid levels of tau protein phosphorylated at Threonine 231. *Archives of Neurology*, 59: 1267–1272.

Buerger, K., Zinkowski, R., Teipel, S. J., Arai, H., DeBernardis, J., Kerkman, D. et al. (2003). Differentiation of Geriatric Major Depression from Alzheimer's disease with CSF tau protein phosphorylated at Threonine 231. *American Journal of Psychiatry*, 160: 376–379.

Chetelat, G., Desgranges, B., De La Sayette, V., Viader, F., Eustache, F., Baron, J. C. (2003). Mild cognitive impairment: Can FDG-PET predict who is to rapidly convert to Alzheimer's disease? *Neurology*, 60: 1374–1377.

Consensus Working Group. (1998). Consensus report of the Working Group on: "Molecular and Biochemical Markers of Alzheimer's Disease". The Ronald and Nancy Reagan Research Institute of the Alzheimer's Association and the National Institute on Aging. *Neurobiology of Aging*, 19: 109–116.

Corder, E. H., Saunders, A. M., Strittmatter, W. J., Schmechel, D. E., Gaskell, P. C., Small, G. W. et al. (1993). Gene dose of apolipoprotein E type 4 Allele and the risk of Alzheimer's disease in late onset families. *Science*, 261: 921–923.

Cupples, L. A., Farrer, L. A., Sadovnik, A. D., Relkin, N., Whitehouse, P., Green, P. (2004). Estimating risk curves for first-degree relatives of patients with Alzheimer's disease: The REVEAL study. *Genetics in Medicine*, 6: 192–196.

de Leon, M. J., Convit, A., Wolf, O. T., Tarshish, C. Y., De Santi, S., Rusinek, H. et al. (2001). Fowler J. Prediction of cognitive decline in normal elderly subjects with 2-[18F]fluoro-2-deoxy-D-glucose/positron emission tomography (FDG/PET). *Proceedings of the National Academy of Sciences of the USA*, 98: 10966–10971.

de Leon, M. J., Desanti, S., Zinkowski, R., Mehta, P. D., Pratico, D., Segal, S. et al. (2006). Longitudinal CSF and MRI biomarkers improve the diagnosis of mild cognitive impairment. *Neurobiology of Aging*, 27: 394–401.

de Leon, M. J., George, A. E., Stylopoulos, L. A., Smith, G., Miller, D. C. (1989). Early marker for Alzheimer's disease: The atrophic hippocampus. *Lancet*, 2: 672–673.

de Leon, M. J., George, A. E., Golomb, J., Tarshish, C., Convit, A., Kluger, A. et al. (1997a). Frequency of hippocampal formation atrophy in normal aging and Alzheimer's disease. *Neurobiology of Aging*, 18: 1–11.

de Leon, M. J., McRae, T., Rusinek, H.,Convit, A., De Santi, S., Tarshish, C. et al. (1997b). Cortisol reduces hippocampal glucose metabolism in normal elderly but not in Alzheimer's disease. *Journal of Clinical Endocrinology and Metabolism*, 82: 3251–3259.

de Leon, M. J., McRae, T., Tsai, J. R., George, A. E., Marcus, D. L., Freedman, M. et al. (1988). Abnormal cortisol response in Alzheimer's disease linked to hippocampal atrophy. *Lancet*, 2: 391–392.

de Leon, M. J., Mosconi, L., Li, Y., De Santi, S., Yao, Y., Tsui, W. H. et al. (2007a). Longitudinal CSF isoprostane and MRI atrophy in the progression to AD. *Journal of Neurology*, 254: 1666–1675.

de Leon, M. J., Mosconi, L., and Logan J. (2007b). Seeing what Alzheimer saw. *Nature Medicine*; 13: 129–131.

de Leon, M. J., Segal, C. Y., Tarshish, C. Y., De Santi, S., Zinkowski, R., Mehta, P. D. et al. (2002). Longitudinal CSF tau load increases in mild cognitive impairment. *Neuroscience Letters*, 333: 183–186.

De Santi, S., de Leon, M. J., Rusinek, H., Convit, A., Tarshish, C. Y., Boppana, M. et al. (2001). Hippocampal formation glucose metabolism and volume losses in MCI and AD. *Neurobiology of Aging*, 22: 529–539.

DeCarli, C., Atack, J. R., Ball, M. J., Kay, J. F., Grady, C. L., Fewster, P. et al. (1992). Post-mortem regional neurofibrillary tangle densities but not senile plaque densities are related to regional cerebral metabolic rates for glucose life in Alzheimer's Disease patients. *Neurodegeneration*, 1: 113–121.

Delacourte, A., David, J. P., Sergeant, N., Buee, L., Wattez, A., Vermersch, P. et al. (1999). The biochemical pathway of neurofibrillary degeneration in aging and Alzheimer's disease. *Neurology*, 52: 1158–1165.

den Heijer, T., Geerlings, M. I., Hoebeek, F. E., Hofman, A., Koudstaal, P. J., Breteler, M. (2006). Use of hippocampal and amygdalar volumes on magnetic resonance imaging to predict dementia in cognitively intact elderly people. *Archives of General Psychiatry*, 63: 57–62.

Diehl-Schmid, J., Grimmer, T., Drzezga, A., Bornschein, S., Riemenschneider, M., Forstl, H. et al. (2007). Decline of cerebral glucose metabolism in frontotemporal dementia: a longitudinal 18F-FDG-PET-study. *Neurobiology of Aging* In Press, 28(1): 42–50.

Drzezga, A., Grimmer, T., Riemenschneider, M., Lautenschlager, N., Siebner, H., Alexopoulus, P. et al. (2005). Prediction of individual outcome in MCI by means of genetic assessment and 18F-FDG PET. *Journal of Nuclear Medicine*, 46: 1625–1632.

Drzezga, A., Grimmer, T., Henriksen, G., Stangier, I., Perneczky, R., Diehl-Schmid, J. et al. (2008). Imaging of amyloid plaques and cerebral glucose metabolism in semantic dementia and Alzheimer's disease. *Neuroimage*, 39: 619–633.

Drzezga, A., Lautenschlager, N., Siebner, H., Riemensneider, M., Willoch, F., Minoshima, S. et al. (2003). Cerebral metabolic changes accompanying conversion of mild cognitive impairment into Alzheimer's disease: A PET follow-up study. *European Journal of Nuclear Medicine and Molecular Imaging*, 30: 1104–1113.

Engler, H., Forsberg, A., Almkvist, O., Blomquist, G., Larsson, E., Savitcheva, I. et al. T(2006). Two-year follow-up of amyloid deposition in patients with Alzheimer's disease. *Brain*, 129: 2856–2866.

Fagan, A. M., Mintun, M. A., Mach, R. H., Lee, S., Dence, C. S., Shah, A. R. et al. (2005). Inverse relation between in vivo amyloid imaging load and cerebrospinal fluid. *Annals of Neurology*, 59: 512–519.

Fagan, A. M., Roe, C. M., Xiong, C., Mintun, M., Morris, J. C., Holtzman, D. M. (2007). Cerebrospinal fluid tau/beta-Amyloid42 ratio as a prediction of cognitive decline in nondemented older Adults. *Archives of Neurology*, doi:10.1001/archneur.64.3.noc60123.

Farrer, L. A., Cupples, L. A., Haines, J. L., Hyman, B., Kukull, W. A., Mayeux, R. et al. (1997). Effects of age, sex, and ethnicity on the association between apolipoprotein E genotype and Alzheimer disease. *Journal of American Medical Association*, 278: 1349–1356.

Ferris, S. H., de Leon, M. J., Wolf, A. P., Farkas, T., Christman, D. R., Reisberg, B. et al. (1980). Positron emission tomography in the study of aging and senile dementia. *Neurobiology of Aging*, 1: 127–131.

Foster, N. L., Chase, T. N., Mansi, L., Brooks, R., Fedio, P., Patronas, N. J. et al. (1984). Cortical abnormalities in Alzheimer's disease. *Annals of Neurology*, 16: 649–654.

Foster, N. L., Heidebrink, J. L., Clark, C. M., Jagust, W. J., Arnold, S. E., Barbas, N. R. et al. (2007). FDG-PET improves accuracy in distinguishing frontotemporal dementia and Alzheimer's disease. *Brain*, 130: 2616–2635.

Frackowiak, R. S. J., Pozzilli, C., Legg, N. J., DuBoulay, G. H., Marshall, J., Lenzi, G. L. et al. (1981). A prospective study of regional cerebral blood flow and oxygen utilization in dementia using positron emission tomography and oxygen-15. *Journal of Cerebral Blood Flow and Metabolism*, 1: S453–S454.

Franceschi, M., Anchisi, D., Pelati, O., Zuffi, M., Matarrese, M., Moresco, R. M. et al. (2005). Glucose metabolism and serotonin receptors in the frontotemporal lobe degeneration. *Annals of Neurology*, 57: 216–225.

Friedland, R. P., Budinger, T. F., Ganz, E., Yano, Y., Mathis, C. A., Koss, B. et al. (1983). Regional cerebral metabolic alterations in dementia of the Alzheimer type: Positron emission tomography with [18F] fluorodeoxyglucose. *Journal of Computer Assisted Tomography*, 7: 590–598.

Fukuyama, R., Mizuno, T., Mori, S., Nakajima, K., Fushiki, S., and Yanagisawa K. (2000). Age-dependent change in the levels of Abeta40 and Abeta42 in cerebrospinal fluid from control subjects, and a decrease in the ratio of Abeta42 to Abeta40 level in cerebrospinal fluid from Alzheimer's disease patients. *European Neurology*, 43: 155–160.

Gauthier, S., Reisberg, B., Zaudig, M., Petersen, R. C., Ritchie, K., Broich, K. et al. (2006). Mild cognitive impairment. *Lancet*, 367: 1262–1270.

Geerlings, M. I., Jonker, C., Bouter, L. M., Ader, H. J., and Schmand, B. (1999). Association between memory complaints and incident Alzheimer's disease in elderly people with normal baseline cognition. *American Journal of Psychiatry*, 156: 531–537.

Giannakopoulos, P., Hof, P. R., Mottier, S., Michel, J. P., and Bouras, C. (1994). Neuropathological changes in the cerebral cortex of 1258 cases from a geriatric hospital: retrospective clinicopathological evaluation of a 10-year autopsy population. *Acta Neuropathologica*, 87: 456–468.

Gilman, S., Koeppe, R., Little, R., An, H., Junck, L., Giordani, B. et al. (2005). Differentiation of Alzheimer's disease from dementia with Lewy bodies utilizing positron emission tomography with [18F]fluorodeoxyglucose and neuropsychological testing. *Experimental Neurology*, 191: S95–S103.

Glodzik-Sobanska, L., Pirraglia, E., Brys, M., De Santi, S., Mosconi, L., Rich, K. E. et al. (2009). The effects of normal aging and ApoE genotype on the levels of CSF biomarkers for Alzheimer's disease. *Neurobiology Aging*, 30(5): 672–681.

Green, R. C., Cupples, L. A., Go, R., Benke, K. S., Edeki, T., Griffith, P. A. et al. and the MIRAGE Study Group. (2002). Risk of dementia among white and African American relatives of patients with Alzheimer disease. *Journal of American Medical Association*, 287: 329–336.

Grossman, M., Farmer, J., Leight, S., Work, M., Moore, P., Van Deerlin, V. et al. (2005). Cerebrospinal fluid profile in frontotemporal dementia and Alzheimer's disease. *Annals of Neurology*, 57: 721–729.

Hansson, O., Zetterberg, H., Buchhave, P., Londos, E., Blennow, K., and Minthon L. (2006). Association between CSF biomarkers and incipient Alzheimer's disease in patients with mild cognitive impairment: A follow-up study. *Lancet Neurology*, 5: 228–234.

Haxby, J. V., Grady, C. L., Koss, E., Horwitz, B., Heston, L., Schapiro, M. et al. (1990). Longitudinal study of cerebral metabolic asymmetries and associated neuropsychological patterns in early dementia of the Alzheimer type. *Archives of Neurology*, 47: 753–760.

Hebert, L. E., Scherr, P. A., Bienias, J. L., Bennett, D. A., and Evans, D. A. (2003). Alzheimer disease in the US population: prevalence estimates using the 2000 census. *Archives of Neurology*, 60(8): 1119–1122.

Herholz, K., Nordberg, A., Salmon, E., Perani, D., Kessler, J., Mielke, R. et al. (1999). Impairment of neocortical metabolism predicts progression in Alzheimer's disease. *Dementia and Geriatric Cognitive Disorders*, 10: 494–504.

Herholz, K., Salmon, E., Perani, D., Baron, J. C., Holthoff, V., Frolich, L. et al. (2002). Discrimination between Alzheimer dementia and controls by automated analysis of multicenter FDG PET. *Neuroimage*, 17: 302–316.

Hesse, C., Rosengren, L., Andreasen, N., Davidsson, P., Vanderstichele, H., Vanmechelen, E. et al. (2001). Transient increase in total tau but not phospho-tau in human cerebrospinal fluid after acute stroke. *Neuroscience Letters*, 297: 187–190.

Higuchi, M., Tashiro, M., Arai, H., Okamura, N., Hara, S., Higuchi, S. et al. (2000). Glucose hypometabolism and neuropathological correlates in brains of dementia with Lewy bodies. *Experimental Neurology*, 162: 247–256.

Hulstaert, F., Blennow, K., Ivanoiu, A., Schoonderwaldt, H. C., Riemenschneider, M., De Deyn, P. P. et al. (1999). Improved discrimination of AD patients using β-amyloid (1-42) and tau levels in CSF. *Neurology*, 52: 1555–1562.

Hyman, B. T., Van Hoesen, G. W., Damasio, A. R., and Barnes, C. L. (1984). Alzheimer's disease: Cell-specific pathology isolates the hippocampal formation. *Science*, 225: 1168–1170.

Ishiguro, K., Ohno, H., Arai, H., Yamaguchi, H., Urakami, K., Park, J. M. et al. (1999). Phosphorylated tau in human cerebrospinal fluid is a diagnostic marker for Alzheimer's disease. *Neuroscience Letters*, 270: 91–94.

Ishii, K., Imamura, T., Sasaki, M., Yamaji, S., Sakamoto, S., Kitagaki, H. et al. (1998a). Regional cerebral glucose metabolism in dementia with Lewy bodies and Alzheimer's disease. *Neurology*, 51: 125–130.

Ishii, K., Sakamoto, S., Sasaki, M., Kitagaki, H., Yamaji, S., Hashimoto, M. et al. (1998b). Cerebral glucose metabolism in patients with frontotemporal dementia. *Journal of Nuclear Medicine*, 39: 1875–1878.

Jack, C. R., Petersen, R. C., Xu, Y., O'Brien, P. C., Smith, G. E., Ivnik, R. J. (2000). Rates of hippocampal atrophy correlate with change in clinical status in aging and AD. *Neurology*, 55: 484–489.

Jagust, W. J., Gitcho, A., Sun, F., Kuczynski, B., Mungas, D., Haan, M. (2006). Brain imaging evidence of preclinical Alzheimer's disease in normal aging. *Annals of Neurology*, 59: 673–681.

Jeong, Y., Cho, S. S., Park, J. M., Kang, S. J., Lee, J. S., Kang, E. et al. (2005). 18F-FDG PET findings in frontotemporal dementia: an SPM analysis of 29 patients. *Journal of Nuclear Medicine*, 46: 233–239.

Kanai, M., Matsubara, E., Isoe, K., Urakami, K., Nakashima, K., Arai, H. et al. (1998). Longitudinal study of cerebrospinal fluid levels of tau, A beta1-40, and A beta1-42(43) in Alzheimer's disease: a study in Japan. *Annals of Neurology*, 44: 17–26.

Kemppainen, N., Aalto, S., Wilson, I., Nagren, K., Helin, S., Bruck, A. et al. (2006). Voxel-based analysis of PET amyloid ligand [11C]PIB uptake in Alzheimer disease. *Neurology*, 67: 1575–1580.

Kennedy, A. M., Frackowiak, R. S. J., Newman, S. K., Bloomfield, P. M., Seaward, J., Roques, P. et al. (1995a). Deficits in cerebral glucose metabolism demonstrated by positron emission tomography in individuals at risk of familial Alzheimer's disease. *Neuroscience Letters*, 186: 17–20.

Kennedy, A. M., Newman, S. K., Frackowiak, R. S., Cunningham, V. J., Roques, P., Stevens, J. et al. (1995b). Chromosome 14 linked familial Alzheimer's disease: A clinico-pathological study of a single pedigree. *Brain*, 118: 185–205.

Klunk, W. E., Engler, H., Nordberg, A., Yanming, W., Blomqvist, G., Holt, D. P. et al. (2004). Imaging brain amyloid in Alzheimer's disease with Pittsburgh Compound-B. *Annals of Neurology*, 55: 306–319.

Lambert, M. P., Barlow, A. K., Chromy, B. A., Edwards, C., Freed, R., Liosatos, M. et al. (1998). Diffusible, nonfibrillar ligands derived from Abeta1-42 are potent central nervous system neurotoxins. *Proceedings of the National Academy of Sciences of the USA*, 11: 6448–6453.

Laws, S. M., Hone, E., Gandy, S., and Martins, R. N. (2003). Expanding the association between the APOE gene and the risk of Alzheimer's disease: possible roles for APOE promoter polymorphisms and alterations in APOE transcription. *Journal of Neurochemistry*, 84: 1215–1236.

Lin, M. T. and Beal, M. F. (2006). Mitochondrial dysfunction and oxidative stress in neurodegenerative diseases. *Nature*, 443: 787–795.

Lockhart, A., Lamb, J. R., Osredkar, T. et al. (2007). PIB is a non-specific imaging marker of amyloid-beta (A{beta}) peptide-related cerebral amyloidosis. *Brain*, 130: 2607–2615.

Magistretti, P. J. and Pellerin, L. (1996). The contribution of astrocytes to the 18F-2-deoxyglucose signal in PET activation studies. *Molecular. Psychiatry*, 1: 445–452.

Magistretti, P. J., Pellerin, L., Rothman, D. L., and Shulman, R. G. (1999). Energy on demand. *Science*, 283: 496–497.

Malonek, D. and Grinvald, A. (1999). Interactions between electrical activity and cortical microcirculation revealed by imaging spectroscopy: Implications for functional brain mapping. *Science*, 272: 551–554.

Markesbery, W. R. (1997). Oxidative stress hypothesis in Alzheimer's disease. *Free Radical Biology & Medicine*, 23: 134–147.

Markesbery, W. R., Kryscio, R. J., Lovell, M. A., and Morrow, J. D. (2005). Lipid peroxidation is an early event in the brain in amnestic mild cognitive impairment. *Annals of Neurology*, 58: 730–735.

Mathis, C. A., Wang, Y., and Klunk, W. (2004). Imaging [beta]-amyloid plaques and neurofibrillary tangles in the aging human brain. *Current Pharmaceutical Design*, 10: 1469–1492.

Mazziotta, J. C. and Phelps, M. E. (1986). Positron Emission Tomography studies of the brain. In: Phelps, M. E., Mazziotta, J. C., and Schelbert, H. (eds), *Positron Emission Tomography & Autoradiography: Principles & Applications for the Brain & Heart* (pp. 493–579). New York: Raven Press.

McKeith, I. G., Galasko, D., Kosaka, K., Perry, E. K., Dickson, D. W., Hansen, L. A. et al. (1996). Consensus guidelines for the clinical and pathologic diagnosis of dementia with Lewy bodies (DLB): Report of the consortium on DLB international workshop. *Neurology*, 47: 1113–1124.

McKhann, G., Drachman, D., Folstein, M., Katzman, R., Price, D., and Stadlan, E. M. (1984). Clinical diagnosis of Alzheimer's disease: Report of the NINCDS-ADRDA Work group under the auspices of department of health and human services task force on Alzheimer's disease. *Neurology*, 34: 939–944.

Mehta, P. D., Pirttila, T., Mehta, S. P., Sersen, E. A., Aisen, P. S., and Wisniewski, H. M. (2000). Plasma and cerebrospinal fluid levels of amyloid beta proteins 1-40 and 1-42 in Alzheimer disease. *Archives of Neurology*, 57: 100–105.

Minoshima, S., Foster, N. L., Sima, A. A., Frey, K. A., Albin, R. L., and Kuhl, D. E. (2001). Alzheimer's disease versus dementia with Lewy bodies: Cerebral metabolic distinction with autopsy confirmation. *Annals of Neurology*, 50: 358–365.

Minoshima, S., Giordani, B., Berent, S., Frey, K. A., Foster, N. L., and Kuhl, D. E. (1997). Metabolic reduction in the posterior cingulate cortex in very early Alzheimer's disease. *Annals of Neurology*, 42: 85–94.

Mintun, M. A. M., LaRossa, G. N., Sheline, Y. I. M., Dence, C. S. M, Lee, S. Y. P., Mach, R. H. P. et al. (2006). [11C]PIB in a nondemented population: Potential antecedent marker of Alzheimer disease. *Neurology*, 67: 446–452.

Mirra, S. S., Heyman, A., McKeel, D., Sumi, S. M., Crain, B. J., Brownlee, L. M. et al. (1991). The consortium to establish a registry for Alzheimer's disease (CERAD). Part II. Standardization of the neuropathologic assessment of Alzheimer's disease. *Neurology*, 41: 479–486.

Mitchell, A. and Brindle, N. (2003). CSF phosphorylated tau–does it constitute an accurate biological test for Alzheimer's disease? *International Journal of Geriatric Psychiatry*, 18: 407–411.

Mollenhauer, B., Bibl, M., Trenkwalder, C., Stiens, G., Cepek, L., Steinacker, P. et al. (2005). Follow-up investigations in cerebrospinal fluid of patients with dementia with Lewy bodies and Alzheimer's disease. *Journal of Neural Transmission*, 112: 933–948.

Montine, T. J., Beal, M. F., Cudkowicz, M. E., O'Donnell, H., Margolin, R. A., McFarland, L. et al. (1999a). Increased CSF F2-isoprostane concentration in probable AD. *Neurology*, 52: 562–565.

Montine, T. J., Kaye, J. A., Montine, K. S., McFarland, L., Morrow, J. D., and Quinn, J. F. (2001). Cerebrospinal fluid abeta42, tau, and f2-isoprostane concentrations in patients with Alzheimer disease, other dementias, and in age-matched controls. *Archives of Pathology & Laboratory Medicine*, 125: 510–512.

Montine, T. J., Markesbery, W. R., Morrow, J. D., and Roberts, L. J. (1998). Cerebrospinal fluid F2-isoprostane levels are increased in Alzheimer's disease. *Annals of Neurology*, 44: 410–413.

Montine, T. J., Markesbery, W. R., Zackert, W., Sanchez, S. C., Roberts, L. J., and Morrow, J. D. (1999b). The magnitude of brain lipid peroxidation correlates with the extent of degeneration but not with density of neuritic plaques or neurofibrillary tangles or with APOE genotype in Alzheimer's disease patients. *American Journal of Pathology*, 155: 863–868.

Morris, J. C., Storandt, M., McKeel, D. W., Rubin, E. H., Price, J. L., Grant, E. A. et al. (1996). Cerebral amyloid deposition and diffuse plaques in "normal" aging: Evidence for presymptomatic and very mild Alzheimer's disease. *Neurology*, 46: 707–719.

Morrison, J. H. and Hof, P. R. (1997). Life and death of neurons in the aging brain. *Science*, 278: 412–419.

Mosconi, L. (2005). Brain glucose metabolism in the early and specific diagnosis of Alzheimer's disease. *European Journal of Nuclear Medicine*, 32: 486–510.

Mosconi, L., Brys, M., Glodzik-Sobanska, L., De Santi, S., Rusinek, H., de Leon, M. J. (2007a). Early detection of Alzheimer's disease using neuroimaging. *Experimental Gerontology*, 42: 129–138.

Mosconi, L., Brys, M., Switalski, R., Mistur, R., Glodzik-Sobanska, L., Pirraglia, E. et al. (2007b). Maternal family history of Alzheimer's disease predisposes to reduced brain glucose metabolism. *Proceedings of the National Academy of Sciences of the USA*, 104: 19067–19072.

Mosconi, L., De Santi, S., Li, Y., Li, J., Zhan, J., Tsui, W. H. et al. (2006a). Visual rating of medial temporal lobe metabolism in mild cognitive impairment and Alzheimer's disease using FDG-PET. *European Journal of Nuclear Medicine*, 33: 210–221.

Mosconi, L., De Santi, S., Brys, M., Tsui, W. H., Pirraglia, E., Glodzik-Sobanska, L. et al. (2008). Hypometabolism and altered CSF markers in normal ApoE E4 carriers with subjective memory complaints. *Biological Psychiatry*, 63(6): 609–618.

Mosconi, L., De Santi, S., Li, J., Tsui, W. H., Li, Y., Boppana, M. et al. (2008). Hippocampal hypometabolism predicts cognitive decline from normal aging. *Neurobiology of Aging*, 29(5): 676–692.

Mosconi, L., Herholz, K., Prohovnik, I., Sorbi, S., Nacmias, B., De Cristofaro, M. T. R. et al. (2005a). Metabolic interaction between APOE genotype and onset age in Alzheimer disease. Implications for brain reserve. *Journal of Neurology, Neurosurgery and Psychiatry*, 76: 15–23.

Mosconi, L., Perani, D., Sorbi, S., Herholz, K., Nacmias, B., Holthoff, V. et al. (2004). MCI conversion to dementia and the APOE genotype: A prediction study with FDG-PET. *Neurology*, 63: 2332–2340.

Mosconi, L., Sorbi, S., de Leon, M. J., Li, Y., Nacmias, B., Bessi, V. et al. (2006b). Hypometabolism exceeds atrophy in presymptomatic early-onset familial Alzheimer's disease. *Journal of Nuclear Medicine*, 47: 1778–1786.

Mosconi, L., Tsui, W. H., De Santi, S., Rusinek, H., Li, J., Convit, A. et al. (2005b). Reduced hippocampal metabolism in mild cognitive impairment and Alzheimer's disease: Automated FDG-PET image analysis. *Neurology*, 64: 1860–1867.

Mosconi, L., Tsui, W. H., Rusinek, H., De Santi, S., Li, Y., Wang, G. J. et al. (2007e). Quantitation, regional vulnerability and kinetic modeling of brain glucose metabolism in mild Alzheimer's disease. *European Journal of Nuclear Medicine and Molecular Imaging*, 34: 1467–1479.

Mosconi, L., Tsui, W. H., Herholz, K., Pupi, A., Drzezga, A., Lucignani, G. et al. (2008). Multi-center standardized FDG-PET diagnosis of Mild Cognitive Impairment, Alzheimer's disease and other dementias. *Journal of Nuclear Medicine*, 49(3): 390–398.

Nestor, P. J., Fryer, T. D., Smielewski, P., and Hodges, J. R. (2003). Limbic hypometabolism in Alzheimer's disease and mild cognitive impairment. *Annals of Neurology*, 54: 343–351.

Nestor, P. J., Scheltens, P., and Hodges, J. R. (2004). Advances in the early detection of Alzheimer's disease. *Nature Medicine*, 10: S34–S41.

Nunomura, A., Perry, G., Aliev, G., Hirai, K., Takeda, A., Balraj, E. K. M. et al. (2001). Oxidative damage is the earliest event in Alzheimer's disease. *Journal of Neuropathology & Experimental Neurology*, 60: 759–767.

Ouchi, Y., Nobezawa, S., Okada, H., Yoshikawa, E., Futatsubashi, M., and Kaneko M. (1998). Altered glucose metabolism in the hippocampal head in memory impairment. *Neurology*, 51: 136–142.

Parnetti, L., Lanari, A., Amici, S., Gallai, V., Vanmechelen, E., Hulstaert, F., and Phospho-Tau International Study Group. (2001). CSF phosphorylated tau is a possible marker for discriminating Alzheimer's disease from dementia with Lewy bodies. Phospho-Tau International Study Group. Neurological Sciences: *Official Journal of the Italian Neurological Society and of the Italian Society of Clinical Neurophysiology*, 22: 77–78.

Pellerin, L. and Magistretti, P. J. (1994). Glutamate uptake into astrocytes stimulates aerobic glycolysis: A mechanism coupling neuronal activity to glucose utilization. *Proceedings of the National Academy of Sciences of the USA*, 91: 10625–10629.

Peskind, E. R., Li, G., Shofer, J., Quinn, J. F., Kaye, J. A., Clark, C. M. et al. (2006). Age and apolipoprotein E*4 allele effects on cerebrospinal fluid beta-amyloid 42 in adults with normal cognition. *Archives of Neurology*, 63: 936–939.

Petersen, R. C., Smith, G. E., Waring, S. C., Ivnik, R. J., Tangalos, E. G., Kokmen E. (1999). Mild cognitive impairment: Clinical characterization and outcome. *Archives of Neurology*, 56: 303–308.

Petersen, R. C., Stevens, J. C., Ganguli, M., Tangalos, E. G., Cummings, J. L., DeKosky, S. T. (2001). Practice parameter: Early detection of dementia: Mild cognitive impairment (an evidence-based review). Report of the quality standards subcommittee of the American Academy of Neurology. *Neurology*, 56: 1133–1142.

Pike, K. E., Savage, G., Villemagne, V. L., Ng, S., Moss, S. A., Maruff, P. et al. (2007). Beta-amyloid imaging and memory in non-demented individuals: evidence for preclinical Alzheimer's disease. *Brain*, 130: 2837–2844.

Powell, M. R., Smith, G. E., Knopman, D. S., Parisi, J. E., Boeve, B. F., Petersen, R. C. et al. (2006). Cognitive measures predict pathologic Alzheimer disease. *Archives of Neurology*, 63: 865–868.

Pratico, D. (1999). F2-isoprostanes: sensitive and specific non-invasive indices of lipid peroxidation in vivo. *Atherosclerosis*, 147: 1–10.

Pratico, D., Clark, C. M., Lee, V. M., Trojanowski, J. Q., Rokach, J., and Fitzgerald, G. A. (2000). Increased 8,12-iso-iPF2alpha-VI in Alzheimer's disease: correlation of a noninvasive index of lipid peroxidation with disease severity. *Annals of Neurology*, 48: 809–812.

Pratico, D., Clark, C. M., Liun, F., Lee, V. Y., and Trojanowski, J. Q. (2002). Increase of brain oxidative stress in mild cognitive impairment: a possible predictor of Alzheimer disease. *Archives of Neurology*, 59: 972–976.

Pratico, D., Lawson, J. A., Rokach, J., and Fitzgerald, G. A. (2001a). The isoprostanes in biology and medicine. *Trends in Endocrinology and Metabolism*, 12: 243–247.

Pratico, D., Uryu, K., Leight, S., Trojanowski, J. Q., and Lee, V. M. Y. (2001b). Increased lipid peroxidation precedes amyloid plaque formation in an animal model of Alzheimer amyloidosis. *Journal of Neuroscience*, 21: 4183–4187.

Price, J. L. and Morris, J. C. (1999). Tangles and plaques in nondemented aging and "preclinical" Alzheimer's disease. *Annals of Neurology*, 45: 358–368.

Reed, B. R., Jagust, W. J., Seab, J. P., and Ober, B. A. (1989). Memory and regional cerebral blood flow in mildly symptomatic Alzheimer's disease. *Neurology*, 39: 1537–1539.

Reiman, E. M., Caselli, R. J., Yun, L. S., Chen, K., Bandy, D., Minoshima, S. et al. (1996). Preclinical evidence of Alzheimer's disease in persons homozygous for the E4 allele for apolipoprotein E. *New England Journal of Medicine*, 334: 752–758.

Reiman, E. M., Caselli, R. J., Chen, K., Alexander, G. E., Bandy, D., and Frost J. (2001). Declining brain activity in cognitively normal apolipoprotein E epsilon 4 heterozygotes: A foundation for using positron emission tomography to efficiently test treatments to prevent Alzheimer's disease. *Proceedings of the National Academy of Sciences of the USA*, 98: 3334–3339.

Reiman, E. M., Chen, K., Alexander, G. E., Caselli, R. J., Bandy, D., Osborne, D. et al. (2004). Functional brain abnormalities in young adults at genetic risk for late-onset Alzheimer's dementia. *Proceedings of the National Academy of Sciences of the USA*, 101: 284–289.

Reiman, E. M., Uecker, A., Caselli, R. J., Lewis, S., Bandy, D., de Leon, M. J. et al. Hippocampal volumes in cognitively normal persons at genetic risk for Alzheimer's disease. *Annals of Neurology*, 44: 288–291.

Rocher, A. B., Chapon, F., Blaizot, X., Baron, J.-C., and Chavoix, C. (2004). Resting-state brain glucose utilization as measured by PET is directly related to regional synaptophysin levels: A study in baboons. *Neuroimage*, 20: 1894–1898.

Rowe, C. C., Ackermann, U., Browne, W., Mulligan, R., Pike, K. L., O'Keefe, G. et al. (2008). Imaging of amyloid beta in Alzheimer's disease with (18)F-BAY94-9172, a novel PET tracer: Proof of mechanism. *Lancet Neurology*, 7: 129–135.

Rowe, C. C., Ng, S., Ackermann, U., Gong, S.J., Pike, K., Savage, G. et al. (2007). Imaging {beta}-amyloid burden in aging and dementia. *Neurology*, 68: 1718–1725.

Rusinek, H., De Santi, S., Frid, D., Tsui, W., Tarshish, C., Convit, A. et al. (2003). Regional brain atrophy rate predicts future cognitive decline: 6-year longitudinal MR imaging study of normal aging. *Radiology*, 229: 691–696.

Santens, P., De Bleecker, J., Goethals, P., Strijckmans, K., Lemahieu, I., Slegers, G. et al. (2001). Differential regional cerebral uptake of (18)F-fluoro-2-deoxy-D-glucose in Alzheimer's disease and frontotemporal dementia at initial diagnosis. *European Neurology*, 45: 19–27.

Selkoe, D. J. (1997). Alzheimer's disease: genotypes, phenotype, and treatments. *Science*, 275: 630–631.

Shoji, M., Kanai, M., Matsubara, E., Tomidokoro, Y., Shizuka, M., Ikeda, Y. et al. (2001). The levels of cerebrospinal fluid Abeta40 and Abeta42(43) are regulated age-dependently. *Neurobiology of Aging*, 22(2): 209–215.

Silverberg, G. D. (2001). The cerebrospinal fluid production rate is reduced in dementia of the Alzheimer's type. *Neurology*, 57: 1763–1766.

Silverberg, G. D., Levinthal, E., Sullivan, E. V., Bloch, D. A., Chang, S. D., Leverenz, J. et al. (2002). Assessment of low-flow CSF drainage as a treatment for AD: Results of a randomized pilot study. *Neurology*, 59: 1139–1145.

Silverman, D. H. S., Small, G. W., Chang, C. Y., Lu, C. S., Kung de Aburto, M. A., Chen, W. et al. (2001). Positron emission tomography in evaluation of dementia: Regional brain metabolism and long-term outcome. *Journal of American Medical Association*, 286: 2120–2127.

Silverman, J. M., Ciresi, G., Smith, C. J., Marin, D. B., Schnaider-Beeri, M. (2005). Variability of familial risk of Alzheimer disease across the late life span. *Archives of General Psychiatry*, 62: 565–573.

Sjogren, M., Davidsson, P., Tullberg, M., Minthon, L., Wallin, A., Wikkelso, C. et al. (2001). Both total and phosphorylated tau are increased in Alzheimer's disease. *Journal of Neurology, Neurosurgery and Psychiatry*, 70: 624–630.

Small, G. W., Ercoli, L. M., Silverman, D. H. S., Huang, S. C., Komo, S., Bookheimer, S. et al. (2000). Cerebral metabolic and cognitive decline in persons at genetic risk for Alzheimer's disease. *Proceedings of the National Academy of Sciences of the USA*, 97: 6037–6042.

Small, G. W., Kepe, V., Ercoli, L. M., Siddarth, P., Bookheimer, S. Y., Miller, K. J. et al. (2006). PET of brain amyloid and tau in mild cognitive impairment. *New England Journal of Medicine*, 355: 2652–2663.

Small, G. W., Mazziotta, J. C., Collins, M. T., Baxter, L. R., Phelps, M. E., Mandelkern, M. A. et al. (1995). Apolipoprotein E type 4 allele and cerebral glucose metabolism in relatives at risk for familial Alzheimer disease. *Journal of American Medical Association*, 273: 942–947.

Sokoloff, L. (1977). Relation between physiological functions and energy metabolism in the central nervous system. *Journal of Neurochemistry*, 29: 13–26.

Szelies, B., Mielke, R., Herholz, K., and Heiss, W.-D. (1994). Quantitative topographical EEG compared to FDG PET for classification of vascular and degenerative dementia. *Electroencephalography and Clinical Neurophysiology*, 91: 131–139.

Tanzi, R. E. and Bertram, L. (2001). New frontiers in Alzheimer's disease genetics. *Neuron*, 32: 181–184.

Tapiola, T., Pirttila, T., Mikkonen, M., Mehta, P. D., Alafuzoff, I., Koivisto, K. et al. (2000). Three-year follow-up of cerebrospinal fluid tau, B-amyloid 42 and 40 concentrations in Alzheimer's disease. *Neuroscience Letters*, 280: 119–122.

Ulrich, J. (1985). Alzheimer changes in nondemented patients younger than sixty-five: Possible early stages of Alzheimer's disease and senile dementia of Alzheimer type. *Annals of Neurology*, 17: 273–277.

Vanmechelen, E., Vanderstichele, H., Davidsson, P., Van Kerschaver, E., Van Der Perre, B., Sjögren, M. et al. (2000). Quantification of tau phosphorylated at threonine 181 in human cerebrospinal fluid: a sandwich ELISA with a synthetic phosphopeptide for standardization. *Neuroscience Letters*, 285: 49–52.

Yao, Y., Zhukareva, V., Sung S., Clark, C. M., Rokach, J., Lee, V. M. et al. (2003). Enhanced brain levels of 8,12-iso-iPF2{alpha}-VI differentiate AD from frontotemporal dementia. *Neurology* 2003; 61: 475–478.

12

Structural Imaging of Mild Cognitive Impairment

Clifford R. Jack, Jr.

Clinical Aspects of Mild Cognitive Impairment

The construct of mild cognitive impairment (MCI) was described in the 1990s by Ronald Petersen and colleagues at the Mayo Clinic as the clinical transitional state between cognitive changes of normal aging and those of dementia (Petersen et al., 1995, 1999). The original criteria for mild cognitive impairment described the syndrome of amnestic MCI (aMCI). These criteria are listed in Table 12.1 and emphasize memory impairment with relatively preserved non-memory cognitive domains and preserved activities of daily living (Petersen, 2007). This clinical entity generally, but not always, was seen in subjects who later developed clinical Alzheimer's disease (AD). As will be described subsequently, subjects with aMCI on average occupy an intermediate position, both on imaging and also pathologically, between cognitively normal (CN) elderly subjects and those with AD. However, there is overlap among individual subjects clinically classified as CN, aMCI, and AD on psychometric, imaging, and pathologic indices. While overlap of individual subjects exists, it is important to remember that MCI is considered to represent a clinical state which usually represents the prodromal stages of a dementing condition and, thus, is different from normal aging.

Autopsy studies of subjects who died while clinically classified as aMCI reveal that the most typical autopsy findings are features that are intermediate between changes of normal aging and AD (Jicha et al., 2006; Markesbery et al., 2006; Petersen et al., 2006; Sabbagh et al., 2006). Typically, aMCI subjects have medial temporal lobe neurofibrillary pathology, on average Braak III–IV, which likely accounted for the clinically observed memory deficit. There is individual variation with some aMCI subjects falling into low (I–II) and some into high (V–VI) Braak stages. While most aMCI subjects have AD-like pathology, many have mixed pathologies, and some have non-AD pathology (Bennett et al., 2005; Jicha et al., 2006). In those with non-AD substrates, medial temporal lobe pathology such as hippocampal sclerosis is usually found which can account for the memory deficit. Most aMCI subjects have a low probability of having AD pathologically when staged using National Institute on Aging-Reagan criteria (Petersen et al., 2006).

Incidence and prevalence figures for MCI vary among published studies, largely due to differences in methodological implementation of the definition of the syndrome. However, a summary of the published literature would indicate that the overall prevalence of MCI is in the 12%–15% range among individuals age

65 years and older, and the incidence rates are in the 1% per year range, similar to those of AD (Lopez et al., 2003; Petersen, 2007). Rates at which aMCI subjects progress to dementia again vary among studies largely due to methodological differences. However, annual rates of progression of 12%–15% per year from aMCI to AD are representative of the literature (Petersen, 2007).

As noted above, the construct of MCI was originally formulated as amnestic MCI which was conceived as a transition stage between normal aging and AD. However, as investigation of this syndrome expanded several modifying concepts emerged. (1) It became apparent that not all subjects who met clinical criteria for aMCI evolved to AD. Some aMCI subjects progress to non-AD dementias while some do not decline clinically. (2) Neurodegenerative dementias other than AD also ought to have characteristic prodromal clinical phenotypes. (3) Since cerebrovascular disease is an often contributing factor to dementia alone or in combination with other pathologies, then it must contribute to clinical transitional states (i.e., MCI) as well. Indeed, preliminary results from a new epidemiological study of the prevalence and incidence of MCI in Rochester MN indicate that cerebrovascular disease is significantly more prevalent in both amnestic and non-amnestic MCI than in cognitively intact elderly subjects. Therefore, the concept of MCI has more recently been expanded. This expanded definition of MCI was the subject of an international conference in Stockholm in 2003 (Winblad et al., 2004). This conference resulted in the current diagnostic algorithm describing MCI that has been adopted by Alzheimer's Disease Centers and the Alzheimer's Disease Neuroimaging Initiative which are sponsored by the National Institute on Aging (Petersen et al., 2005).

Figure 12.1 illustrates a flow chart which operationalizes the definition of the expanded criteria for MCI (Petersen, 2007). The algorithm originates with a cognitive concern on the part of the patient or an informant. At the next step, the clinician must determine whether the patient's cognitive function is normal, compatible with dementia, or abnormal but not compatible with dementia. If the clinician believes that the patient is neither normal nor demented and there appears to have been a decline in cognitive function with regard to daily living activities, then the patient can be designated as having MCI. The next branch point involves determining the nature of the impairment. If the impairment is predominantly memory then the patient is designated as having aMCI. If the impairment or impairments are predominantly non-memory then the patient is designated as having non-amnestic MCI (naMCI). Further classification is usually based on neuropsychological testing. The clinician

Table 12–1　Original mild cognitive impairment criteria – amnestic MCI.

- memory complaint, preferably qualified by an informant
- memory impairment for age and education
- preserved general cognitive function
- intact activities of daily living
- not demented

determines whether the subject has impairment in isolation or whether more than one cognitive domain is impaired. For example, a subject with an isolated memory impairment is labeled single domain amnestic MCI. A subject with a memory impairment, but who also has impairments in one or more other cognitive domains such as language, executive or visual spatial ability, would be labeled multi-domain amnestic MCI. Similarly, if the patient does not have a significant memory impairment, but does have an isolated impairment in a single non-memory domain, the patient is labeled single domain non-amnestic MCI. Or, if the patient has impairments in more than one non-memory domain with preserved memory then the patient is labeled multi-domain non-amnestic MCI. A second layer of classification relates to the suspected etiology. Obviously, without autopsy the precise etiology or etiologies of the impairment cannot be known with certainty. However, a proposed etiologic classification can be made based on clinical or imaging findings. The full classification scheme is illustrated in Figure 12.2, with the clinical classification denoted horizontally and the proposed etiologic classification vertically (Petersen, 2007).

The utility of the construct of MCI has been questioned in some circles. The fact that some subjects who qualify for a diagnosis of aMCI do not have early AD has been interpreted negatively, i.e., to question the clinical utility of the MCI construct. The opposite point of view, however, is that all subjects who develop dementia (perhaps with the exception of sudden post-stroke dementia) must pass through a transitional phase from normal aging to dementia. From a clinical perspective, it is critical to accurately identify these subjects and classify them appropriately. The fact that some subjects who present clinically with aMCI will turn out to not have early AD does not invalidate the concept of MCI. MCI

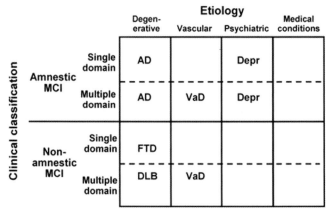

Figure 12–2　Clinical plus suspected etiological classification Scheme. (With permission from Petersen, 2007.)

subjects are clearly abnormal and the construct of MCI provides a framework by which these patients can be appropriately identified and categorized.

The remainder of this chapter will focus on imaging of MCI. Because the original definition, i.e., amnestic MCI, has been in clinical use for a much longer period of time than the more recently expanded definition, most imaging studies published to date have addressed only aMCI.

Relationship Between MRI and AD Pathology

Imaging can be viewed as an in vivo surrogate of tissue or organ pathology. The abnormal protein deposits, neurofibrillary tangles and amyloid plaques, which are stained and examined in order to render a pathologic diagnosis of AD are well known. However, a host of other histological abnormalities also occur in AD. These include, but are not limited to, neuron loss, neuron shrinkage,

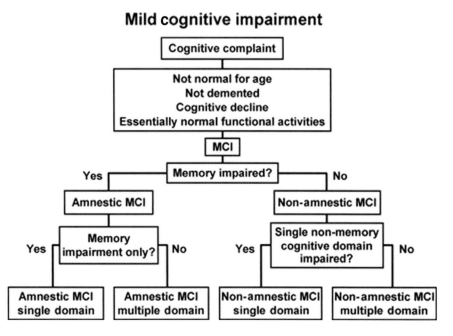

Figure 12–1　Expanded criteria for MCI operationalized. (With permission from Petersen, 2007.)

dendritic de-arborization, synapse loss, and glial activation. MRI is sensitive to these neuronal pathologies which characterize AD. In the first section of this chapter, the case was made that aMCI, usually but not always, represents a transitional phase between normal aging and AD, both clinically and pathologically. Therefore, it stands to reason that if imaging appropriately captures relevant pathologic changes in AD, then MR imaging studies that compare measurements in CN, aMCI, and AD subjects should demonstrate that aMCI subjects on average lie at an intermediate position between CN and AD subjects. Also, given that aMCI patients overlap both clinically and pathologically with subjects who are classified as CN and AD, one would expect analogous overlap on imaging. In the next few paragraphs, this chapter will review cross-sectional imaging studies in which subjects with aMCI have been compared to CN and AD subjects to demonstrate that these expectations are met.

While the bulk of MRI research in dementia has focused on structural imaging, MRI is a rich modality which is able to probe a number of different properties of tissue. Therefore, in addition to structural MRI, two other MRI techniques will be briefly reviewed, MRI spectroscopy and diffusion imaging, in order to demonstrate the generalizability of the relationship between MR imaging and clinical presentation along the spectrum of healthy aging to aMCI to AD.

Structural MRI

The properties of tissue that are assessed by structural MRI are volume (or volume loss, atrophy), thickness, or density of particular tissue compartments (e.g., gray matter). Imaging autopsy correlation studies have clearly documented the association between these imaging findings on MRI and neuronal pathology in AD—both neurofibrillary pathology and also pathological indices of neuron shrinkage and neuron loss. Hippocampal volumes measured from ante-mortem MRI scans correlate with Braak neurofibrillary tangle pathologic staging in both demented and non-demented subjects (Gosche et al., 2002; Jack et al., 2002). Ante-mortem hippocampal volume from MRI correlates with hippocampal neurofibrillary tangle density (Csernansky et al., 2004; Silbert et al., 2003) at autopsy and ante-mortem brain volume on MRI correlates with hippocampal plaque density (Csernansky et al., 2004). Ante-mortem rates of brain atrophy correlate with neurofibrillary tangle density and rates of ventricular expansion correlate with both plaque and tangle density at autopsy (Silbert et al., 2003). Excellent correlation is found between hippocampal volume measures obtained on either ante-mortem MRI (Zarow et al., 2005) or postmortem MRI (Bobinski et al., 2000) and hippocampal neuron cell counts in autopsy specimens. On the basis of these imaging-to-pathologic correlation studies, quantitative measures from structural MRI, such as hippocampal volume, are inferred to represent an approximate surrogate of the neuronal pathology – neuron loss, neuron shrinkage, and synapse loss—that occurs in AD. The stage or severity of neuronal pathology can be approximately inferred from quantitative structural MRI measures such as hippocampal volume.

The images in Figure 12.3 illustrate this principle visually; greater atrophy correlates with poorer cognitive performance. In general, however, for research studies, one would like to quantify the imaging data. There are two general approaches to image quantification. One is the region-of-interest (ROI)-based approach. The effect of measuring the volume of specific anatomic

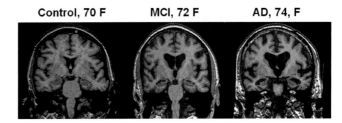

Figure 12–3   Structural MRI: atrophy and AD stage.

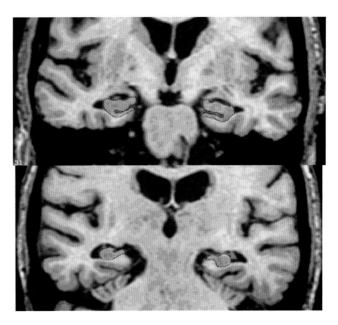

Figure 12–4   Hippocampal boarders delineated on MRI.

structures within user defined ROIs is to convert gray scale images into numbers. The most frequently targeted anatomic structure in ROI-based studies of AD and aMCI has been the hippocampus (Figure 12.4). Reasons for this are clear. The hippocampus is among the earliest and most severely affected structures in AD. And of equal importance, the anatomic properties of the hippocampus are such that its borders can be clearly delineated throughout its entire 3D extent on anatomic MRI. A relevant companion, medial temporal lobe structure, is the entorhinal cortex. While the entorhinal cortex boundaries are not as well defined as the hippocampus on MRI throughout its entire extent, this structure is biologically relevant because neurofibrillary pathology appears in the entorhinal cortex before the hippocampus.

A number of cross-sectional papers have assessed hippocampal or entorhinal cortex volume or thickness measurements from structural MRI in individuals with a mild impairment (Convit et al., 1995; De Santi et al., 2001; Dickerson et al., 2001, 2004; Du et al., 2001; Grundman et al., 2002; Killiany et al., 1993, 2002; Krasuski et al., 1998; Laakso et al., 1998; Parnetti et al., 1996; Pennanen et al., 2004; Xu et al., 2000). Some of these studies have employed the formal definition of amnestic MCI proposed by Petersen et al. (Petersen et al., 1999), while others have employed other criteria to define mild impairment, such as the clinical dementia rating scale (CDR) score of 0.5. Nonetheless, the conclusions drawn from these cross-sectional studies have been quite

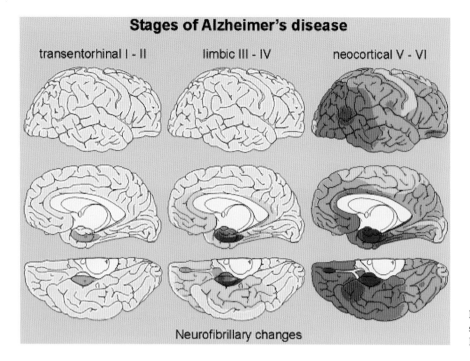

Figure 12–5 Braak neurofibrillary tangle staging. (With permission from Braak and Braak, 1991.)

uniform despite differences in methods and patient populations. In general, hippocampal or entorhinal cortex volume measurements in aMCI (or mildly impaired subjects) fall between those of CN and AD subjects. These studies validate the concept that structural MRI measures appropriately capture the underlying anatomic changes due to the pathologic progression of AD. And when evaluated from the opposite perspective (i.e., taking imaging as the gold standard), these studies support the notion that aMCI is, on average, an intermediate stage between CN and AD.

The second general approach taken to quantify structural imaging data has been labeled voxel-based analysis. Here statistical analyses are done at the level of the individual voxel rather than using user defined ROIs. For example, two different groups of subjects may be compared statistically on a per voxel basis throughout the brain. One of the most commonly used software programs for this is voxel-based morphometry (VBM) from the statistical parametric mapping (SPM) suite (Ashburner and Friston, 2000; Good et al., 2001). VBM pair-wise comparisons of AD subjects to CN reveal gray matter loss (i.e., atrophy) that corresponds to stage V–VI in the Braak (Braak and Braak, 1991) neurofibrillary tangle staging scheme, i.e., most severe in the medial temporal lobe, next most severe in the basal temporal neocortex, next most severe in lateral temporal-parietal association cortex and precuneus—posterior cingulate cortex, next in frontal association cortex, with relative sparing of the primary sensorimotor and visual areas (Figure 12.5) (Baron et al., 2001; Frisoni et al., 2002; Good et al., 2002; Karas et al., 2003; Rombouts et al., 2000; Senjem et al., 2005). In contrast, comparison of aMCI subjects to healthy controls reveals a much more limited topographic pattern of gray matter loss which is confined to and most extensive in the medial temporal lobe areas with extension into the basal and lateral temporal parietal neocortical areas and posterior cingulate/precuneus (Bell-McGinty et al., 2005; Chetelat et al., 2002; Ishii et al., 2005; Karas et al., 2004; Pennanen et al., 2005; Shiino et al., 2006; Trivedi et al., 2006; Whitwell et al., 2007a) (Figure 12.6). Hippocampal shape changes also differentiate mildly impaired subjects from CN and AD (Csernansky et al., 2000; Wang et al., 2003).

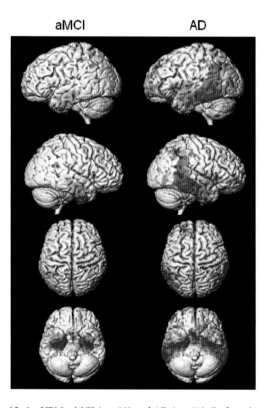

Figure 12–6 VBM: aMCI ($n = 88$) and AD ($n = 51$). Both patient groups were compared to a common group of age- and gender-matched CN subjects.

MRI Spectroscopy

The most common atomic nucleus studied in human MR spectroscopy is hydrogen. The metabolites which can be reliably measured in vivo with hydrogen spectroscopy (^{1}H MRS) at clinical field strengths are N-acetyl-aspartate (NAA), myo-inositol (mI), choline, creatinine, and lactate. The metabolites that are most relevant to AD are NAA, which is felt to be a measure of neuron and synapse density and neuron health, and mI, which is felt to be a measure of glial activation (Adalsteinsson et al., 2000; Meyerhoff et al., 1994; Miller et al., 1993; Schuff et al., 1997, 1998; Shonk and Ross, 1995; Shonk et al., 1995; Tedeschi et al., 1996). Many ^{1}H MRS studies report data as a ratio of either NAA or mI to creatinine, where creatinine is felt to be a non-changing reference metabolite. Another commonly reported metric is the NAA/mI ratio. Spectroscopic imaging can take one of two forms, chemical shift imaging or single voxel spectroscopy. Chemical shift imaging provides spatially resolved spectra, but is more artifact prone. Single voxel ^{1}H MRS provides data from only a single pre-selected region, or voxel-of-interest, but is less artifact prone than chemical shift imaging.

The number of spectroscopy ^{1}H MRS studies performed in MCI is significantly less than the number of structural MRI studies (Kantarci et al., 2002; Parnetti et al., 1997). Nonetheless, the reports that have been published indicate that both NAA and mI measures in aMCI subjects on average occupy an intermediate position when compared to CN and AD subjects, supporting the notion that this MRI modality, like structural MRI, is appropriately capturing the expected pathobiology of AD along the entire cognitive continuum.

Diffusion Imaging

Diffusion imaging is an MRI method by which the random motion of water protons and tissue may be quantified (Le Bihan et al., 1986; Stejskal and Tanner, 1965). Although proton diffusion can be quantified a number of ways by MR, the two most commonly used metrics are the apparent diffusion coefficient (ADC) and fractional anisotropy (FA). ADC is a scalar, nondirectional measure of the magnitude or ease with which water protons randomly diffuse through tissue. FA, on the other hand, is a measure of the directionality of this diffusion process. Tissue microstructure limits diffusion and imposes preferential directionality. AD is characterized by a loss of tissue microstructural complexity which results in increased ADC values. Likewise, loss of microstructural integrity in white matter tracts, where proton diffusion preferentially occurs parallel to the dominate direction of the tract, is characterized by a decrease in FA. Diffusion imaging can be categorized as diffusion-weighted imaging (DWI) in which diffusion encoding occurs only along the three cardinal axes of the magnet; or, as diffusion tensor imaging (DTI) in which diffusion encoding occurs along six or more directions which permits mathematical computation of a tensor. Most diffusion imaging studies in AD to date have been performed by computing ADC or FA values within user defined ROIs.

Diffusion MRI studies to date indicate that ADC values are increased, and FA are decreased, in AD subjects when compared to CN (Hanyu et al., 1997, 1998; Sandson et al., 1999). When both of these groups are compared with aMCI subjects, the ADC and FA values in aMCI subjects on average occupy an intermediate position between CN and AD subjects (Kantarci et al., 2001; Zhang et al., 2007). This supports the notion that this MRI modality is appropriately capturing the pathobiology of AD along the spectrum from healthy aging from aMCI to AD.

Prediction

As discussed above, MCI usually represents a transitional phase between normal aging and dementia. To date, imaging studies evaluating the relationship between imaging and prediction of dementia have largely focused on the transition from aMCI to AD, or from mild impairment defined as CDR 0.5 to AD. Once a diagnosis of MCI (here specifically aMCI) is made, then it would be highly desirable to be able to predict if and when these subjects will progress to dementia. There are subtle differences between "if" and "when" which merit discussion. Research studies on prediction have not followed every subject enrolled in the study to death. Therefore, these studies by definition are not designed to answer the question, "What information will predict if subjects will ever progress to dementia in their lifetime?". Instead, research studies enroll subjects and follow these subjects for variable lengths of time. These studies, therefore, are designed to answer the question, "What variables provide information about the hazard, or risk rate of progression to AD—i.e., when?". The appropriate study design and analytic method to address questions about risk rate are time dependent.

An example of such a study is illustrated in Figure 12.7. Here 80 aMCI subjects were identified at the point in time when they were enrolled in a longitudinal patient registry (Jack et al., 1999). Hippocampal volumes were measured at the time subjects were enrolled. Subjects were then followed longitudinally for an average of approximately 3 years; however, the follow-up times were variable among subjects. The event of interest was progression from aMCI to a clinical diagnosis of AD. Subjects were stratified into three groups on the basis of baseline hippocampal volumes which had been converted to hippocampal W scores. Hippocampal W scores can be thought of as age, gender, and total intracranial volume adjusted hippocampal Z scores with zero mean and standard deviation one among healthy elderly subjects. Negative W scores, therefore, indicate adjusted hippocampal volumes below the expected mean for cognitively normal elderly. W scores of −1.65 and 1.65 correspond to the 5th and 95th percentiles of the normal elderly distribution. The data indicate that in subjects with highly atrophic hippocampi (i.e., hippocampi at or less than the first percentile of normals) the risk of progression to AD was greatest. Subjects with non-atrophic hippocampi (i.e., hippocampal W scores at or larger than the 50th percentile of normals) had the lowest risk of progression to AD. Subjects with

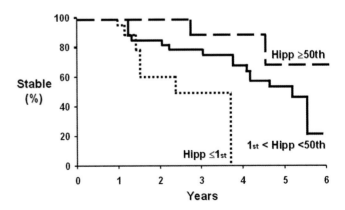

Figure 12–7 Baseline adjusted hippocampal volume: relationship to progression from MCI to AD. (With permission from Jack et al., 1999.)

intermediate hippocampal volumes had an intermediate risk of progression. These data are displayed in the appropriate survival curve format in Figure 12.7. Life table analysis estimates of the risk of progression from aMCI to AD within 3 years based on baseline hippocampal volume measures were: 9% for those aMCI subjects whose hippocampal W scores were at or greater than the 50th percentile of normals; 50% for subjects whose hippocampal volumes at baseline were at or less than the first percentile for normal controls, and 26% for those whose baseline hippocampal volumes were between the 1st and 50th percentile of normal controls. This result has been replicated by a number of independent groups in different samples of aMCI subjects (DeCarli et al., 2007; deToledo-Morrell et al., 2004; Geroldi et al., 2006; Korf et al., 2004; Laakso et al., 2000; Visser et al., 1999).

A study performed in a manner analogous to the aforementioned study showed that rates of atrophy are related to the risk of subsequent conversion from aMCI to AD (Jack et al., 2005). Here, rates of change of the whole brain and ventricle were computed from serial MRI studies prior to the starting point of the clinical observation period. And, subjects with greater rates of ventricular expansion and brain shrinkage were shown to have a higher risk of progression from aMCI to AD than subjects with lower rates of atrophy (Figure 12.8). Amnestic MCI subjects with higher (i.e., more abnormal) hippocampal ADC values from diffusion-weighted images have a greater risk of progression to AD than do subjects with lower (i.e., more normal) hippocampal diffusion measures (Kantarci et al., 2005) (Figure 12.9).

Other ROI-based studies have produced similar results when different definitions of "mild impairment" are used (Kaye et al., 1997; Marquis et al., 2002). For example, hippocampal and entorhinal cortex volumes of CDR 0.5 subjects who later progress to AD were more atrophic than were volume measures in CDR 0.5 subjects who did not progress to AD over the same observation period (Dickerson et al., 2001; Killiany et al., 2000, 2002). Hippocampal shape differences also predict onset of AD (Apostolova et al., 2006; Csernansky et al., 2005). Rates of atrophy measured in either asymptomatic or mildly affected subjects with familial AD predict subsequent dementia (Fox et al., 1996).

A recent VBM analysis of progression in MCI revealed an AD-like pattern of gray matter loss when aMCI subjects who do progress to AD within three years of the MRI scan were compared

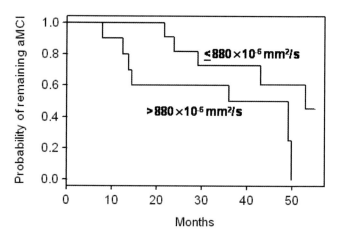

Figure 12–9   Hippocampal diffusion and progression from aMCI to AD. (With permission from Kantarci et al., 2005.)

to a group of cognitively normal elderly subjects (Whitwell et al., 2007c) (Figure 12.10). That is, the topographic distribution of gray matter loss in these MCI–progressor subjects was similar to that seen in subjects who have already progressed to AD. Conversely, when aMCI subjects who remained stable for three or more years after the MRI were compared to the same group of normal control subjects, no difference between stable aMCI subjects and controls in the topographic distribution of gray matter density was seen. These results imply that the overall topographic distribution of gray matter density is a predictor of time to progression from aMCI to AD. The positive predictive results in

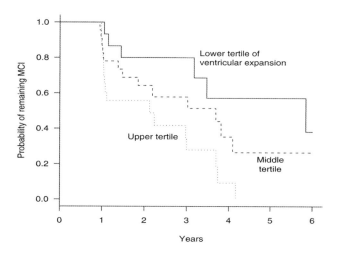

Figure 12–8   Rates of Atrophy and Progression from MCI to AD. (With permission from Jack et al., 2005.)

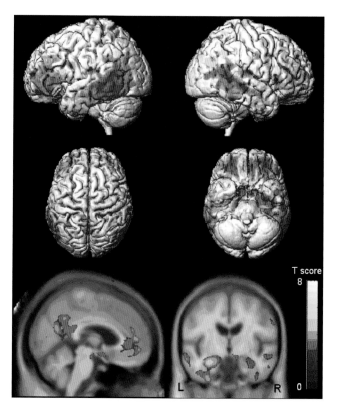

Figure 12–10   MCI-progressor vs. MCI-stable. VBM comparison (With permission from Whitwell et al., 2007c.)

this study need to be replicated, because some VBM studies that have compared aMCI progressors to stables have found negligible gray matter differences between the groups (Bozzali et al., 2006; Chetelat et al., 2005).

Both the VBM and ROI-based studies of prediction in aMCI are based on the underlying assumption that structural MRI is able to detect more severe AD pathology in subjects who are destined to progress than in subjects who are not destined to progress within a given period of time. The implication, therefore, is that the structural MRI is detecting disease stage in vivo.

Longitudinal Imaging Studies in aMCI

Because of the greater difficulty in obtaining longitudinal or serial imaging studies in well characterized subjects, fewer studies have been published on serial imaging than on cross-sectional imaging findings of aMCI subjects. The interest in longitudinal imaging measures in aMCI and, more generally, in dementia is more than academic. The current method of assessing disease progression in aMCI or AD is via serial clinical and neuropsychometric tests. Imaging can supplement these clinical/neuropyschometric indices with independent measures of disease progression. Imaging is also attractive because serial imaging measures potentially have less variability in measurement of disease progression than clinical and neuropsychometric assessments (Fox et al., 1999; Jack et al., 2003).

Studies of rates of change on serial MRI imply a different type of study design from the prediction studies mentioned above. In prediction studies, a measurement(s) from an MRI study is obtained at baseline. Subjects are then followed longitudinally to ascertain the relationship between risk of the event of interest (progression to AD) and the baseline exposure (MRI measurement). In contrast, longitudinal studies of rates of change on imaging imply that a series of imaging measurements are made concurrently with a series of clinical observations. Longitudinal MRI studies published in MCI and AD have provided estimates

of the rates of morphometric change over time and consistently demonstrate increased rates among AD and MCI relative to similarly aged CN subjects (Du et al., 2003, 2004; Fox and Freeborough, 1997; Freeborough and Fox, 1997; Jack et al., 1998, 2007a; Kaye et al., 1997; Teipel et al., 2002).

Given that AD is a progressive disease and that serial imaging can capture change over time, a logical question to ask in this context is "What is the correlation between change on serial imaging measures and change on concurrent clinical assessments?". Clinical assessments can take the form of clinical categorization (i.e., CN, aMCI or AD), or change on continuous measures of cognitive performance. An important feature of longitudinal imaging-clinical correlation studies is that the pathology underlying AD is progressive, not static. If serial imaging captures this essential element of the disease, then one expects good correlation between clinical and imaging indices of disease progression over concurrent periods of observation (Figure 12.11). One such study of aMCI evaluated rates of change of hippocampus in aMCI subjects who underwent two serial MRI studies from which annualized rates of hippocampal volume change were measured. In this study, aMCI subjects could either remain stable (i.e., remain MCI) or could progress to AD. The result that would be expected based on the biology of the disease is that rates of atrophy would be greater in those aMCI subjects who progressed to AD than in those aMCI subjects who remained clinically stable. And, this was the observed result (Jack et al., 2000). A follow-up study evaluated rates of atrophy of several different brain structures from two serial MRI studies and again found the biologically expected result. That is, rates of hippocampal, entorhinal cortex, whole brain and ventricular atrophy were uniformly greater in aMCI subjects who progressed to AD when compared to aMCI subjects who remained stable (Jack et al., 2004). An important feature of these studies is that the average observation period over which the serial MRI and serial clinical assessments were made was the same for aMCI subjects who remained stable vs. those who progressed to AD. Had the average observation interval not been the same, then the

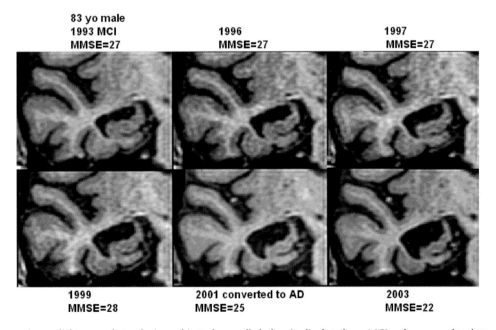

Figure 12–11 Progressive medial temporal atrophy in a subject who enrolled a longitudinal study as aMCI and progressed to dementia. Six serial MRI studies obtained over 10 years were spatially registered to illustrate progressive volume loss in the medial temporal lobe.

conclusions would have been invalid. Studies in which subjects with familial AD were evaluated serially have produced similar results – i.e., that change on images corresponds to concurrent longitudinal clinical assessments of change (Fox et al., 1999; Fox, Warrington, and Rossor, 1999; Scahill et al., 2003; Schott et al., 2003, 2005).

Several features of rates of atrophy on serial MRI deserve mention. One of these is the relationship with APOE. It is well established that APOE ε4 increases lifetime risk of AD and lowers mean age of onset. In the context of imaging, one can ask "Does APOE genotype influence rates of brain atrophy?" In a recent therapeutic study for aMCI, the relationship between rates of atrophy and APOE status was evaluated in the placebo arm (Jack et al., 2007a). Rates were greater in both APOE ε4 homozygotes and heterozygotes relative to APOE ε4 non-carriers. But rates were not different between APOE ε4 homozygotes and heterozygotes. These findings are relevant to planning future therapeutic and observational studies in aMCI that employ structural MRI as an outcome

measure. For example, studies should be powered based on an anticipated APOE ε4 effect on atrophy rates; therapeutic studies using MRI as an outcome measure could be designed to balance APOE ε4 status across treatment groups.

Longitudinal MRI studies published in aMCI and AD typically employ two scans acquired at different time-points from which a rate of change is calculated. However, by sampling two time-points per subject, characterization of longitudinal morphometric trajectory on a per subject basis is linear by default. In order to directly assess a change in rate with time in individual subjects—i.e., acceleration or deceleration—three or more time-points must be sampled in each subject. In the context of aMCI, one logical question to ask is, "Do rates of brain atrophy accelerate as subjects progress, or are rates constant over time?" The diagnosis of AD is a meaningful clinical event shared by all aMCI subjects who do progress. Analyzing brain and ventricular volumes relative to this index point is a logical way to anchor the series of serial MRI studies in aMCI-progressor subjects to a common clinically definable point in the natural history of the disease. In a recently published analysis of change in rate over time in aMCI subjects, rates of whole brain shrinkage and ventricular expansion were found to accelerate as subjects progressed from aMCI to AD (Figure 12.12) (Jack et al., 2007b). These results are illustrated in Figure 12.12 where each subject's series of MRI scans is aligned in time to the point at which a diagnosis of AD was made (time 0 in the figure). The change in rate (i.e., acceleration) of ventricular expansion as subjects converted from aMCI to AD was 1.7 cm³/yr. The analogous acceleration in brain shrinkage was 5.3 cm³/yr. These data match those obtained in younger individuals with mutations leading to early-onset AD where both hippocampal and brain atrophy rates accelerated relative to index points defined using either a fixed MMSE score or a diagnosis of dementia (Chan et al., 2003; Ridha et al., 2006). These data indicate that while the deviation from linearity is relatively minor, rates of both brain shrinkage and ventricular expansion do accelerate as subjects progress to AD. Using a linear estimate for a non-linear function will tend to be invalid when comparing rates of change across subjects who have significantly different inter-scan intervals, different intrinsic rates of change, or both. While such errors should be

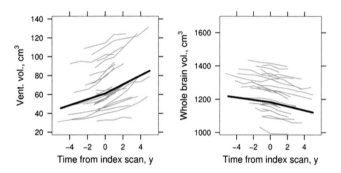

Figure 12–12 Rate Acceleration as aMCI progress to AD. Ventricular and whole brain atrophy before and after AD diagnosis in aMCI – progressors. The diagnosis of AD (i.e., the index scan) in each subject is indicated as time 0. Thin gray lines represent a random sample of 23 individual subject volumes over time, thick black line indicates average volume. Average volumes are shown assuming a woman with a total intracranial volume of 1.4 L whose index scan is at age 79. (With permission from Jack et al., 2007b.)

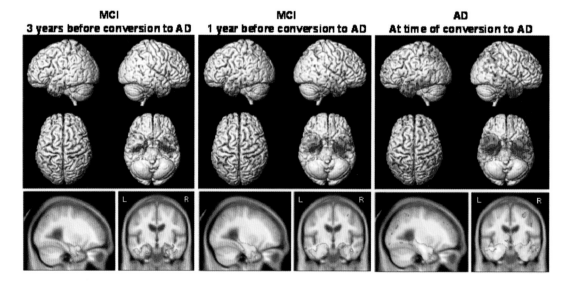

Figure 12–13 Voxel-wise methods capture time dependent Progression from aMCI to AD (*n* = 33). VBM maps from multiple MRI illustrate changing atrophy patterns as subjects progress from MCI to AD. (With permission from Whitwell et al., 2007b.)

fairly minor in studies of elderly aMCI subjects when the inter-scan interval is limited to a year or so, in future studies it might be useful to incorporate non-linearity in models of longitudinal morphometric change, especially when modeling change over periods exceeding 1–2 years.

Longitudinal voxel-wise studies have also been performed in aMCI. Two general approaches have been taken. One approach is to follow a group of subjects over time and generate 3D voxel-wise maps of gray matter loss at specific points in time of disease progression. An example of such a study is illustrated in Figure 12.13 (Whitwell et al., 2007b). Here a group of 33 aMCI subjects who all progressed to a diagnosis of AD were identified and all had MRI studies performed at specific points in time prior to the diagnosis of AD. In these 33 subjects, VBM maps were generated in the 33 aMCI compared to a group of CN subjects 3 years prior to conversion to AD, 1 year prior to conversion to AD, and at the time of conversion to AD. These group-wise VBM maps illustrate the topographic progression of gray matter loss at each of these three discrete points in time (Figure 12.13). Three years prior to conversion to AD, aMCI subjects had gray matter loss that was largely confined to the medial and basal temporal lobe and, to a lesser extent, lateral temporal neocortex—i.e., a pattern reminiscent of Braak stage III–IV. One year prior to conversion to AD, gray matter loss more heavily involved medial temporal lobe and lateral temporal neocortex and now extended to involve areas of parietal and frontal neocortex—i.e., a pattern reminiscent of Braak IV–V. At the time of conversion to AD, the pattern of gray matter loss now extended to more extensively involve temporal parietal and frontal association areas—i.e., a pattern reminiscent of Braak stage V.

A second way in which serial MRI studies have been evaluated in a voxel-wise manner is to perform a true 4D analysis at the voxel level. Several different groups have performed studies using elegant computational methods which illustrate changes in the hippocampal surface over time on serial imaging studies and also illustrate changes over the entire cerebral cortex over time (Chetelat et al., 2005; Fox et al., 2001; Freeborough and Fox, 1998; Scahill et al., 2002; Thompson et al., 2003).

Comparison of PIB and Structural MRI Measures in aMCI

While detailed information about amyloid imaging with positron emission tomography (PET) can be found in Chapter 14, it is important to relate these biochemical measures to changes in brain structure. Data from a study comparing structural MRI and amyloid imaging with Pittsburgh Compound B (PIB) in aMCI

provides interesting insight into the clinical construct of aMCI. In this study, 20 CN, 17 aMCI, and eight AD subjects were imaged with both MRI and PIB (Jack et al., 2007c). PIB retention was quantified as the ratio of uptake in cortical regions-of-interest to the uptake in the cerebellar ROI in images acquired 40–60 minutes post-injection. A global cortical PIB retention summary measure was derived from six cortical ROIs which demonstrated high PIB uptake in AD. Hippocampal volumes were measured in these subjects using standard methods and were converted to W scores using established methods which control for inter-subject variability in age, gender, and head size (Jack et al., 1997).

On average, AD subjects had high global cortical PIB retention and low hippocampal volume; CN subjects had low PIB uptake and high hippocampal volume, and group averages for aMCI subjects were intermediate on both PIB and hippocampal volume (Figure 12.14). Among all subjects in the study who demonstrated PIB retention, PIB tended to be located in the medial and lateral prefrontal, anterior and posterior cingulate/precuneus and lateral temporal and parietal cortical areas. The topographic distribution of PIB in PIB positive subjects was the same regardless of clinical category: CN, aMCI, or AD. A target-to-cerebellar ratio 1.5 was used to designate subjects as high PIB vs. low PIB cortical retention. All AD subjects fell above this ratio as did six out of 20 CN subjects and nine of 17 aMCI subjects.

One way to explain individual subjects in which a dissociation between current cognitive status and PIB retention is observed is to propose that amyloid deposition is an early event in the disease process ultimately leading to clinical AD. A hypothetical time line relating amyloid deposition, neuronal injury, and clinical symptoms is illustrated in Figure 12.15. In this hypothetical time line, amyloid deposition is established in the clinically presymptomatic phase of AD. Neuronal injury is a later event that precedes and parallels clinical decline. Amyloid deposition can be detected by PIB imaging and neuronal injury can be detected in vivo by MRI and fluorodeoxyglucose (FDG) PET (covered in greater detail in Chapter 13). The hypothetical time course outlined in Figure 12.15 presents several testable hypotheses which can be used to validate the theory. Among these are the following. One would expect to see individuals who are cognitively normal, with high PIB deposition and with little or no evidence of neuronal injury (atrophy on MRI). One would expect to find similar topographic patterns of PIB deposition in subjects whose cognitive status spans the range from CN to aMCI to AD. In contrast MRI measures of neuronal injury should be much more closely coupled with current cognitive status. Finally, one would expect to see good correlation between rates of change on serial MRI and cognitive change, and not so with rates of change on serial PIB studies. Data is emerging to support

Figure 12–14 Group-wise separation for global cortical PiB and hippocampal W score.

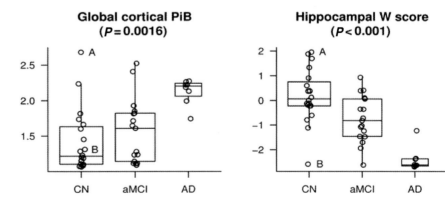

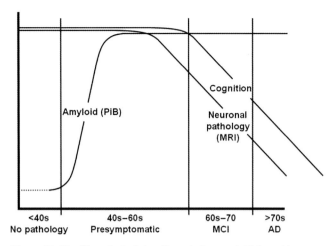

Figure 12–15 Hypothetical time line relating amyloid deposition, neuronal injury, and clinical symptoms.

each of the above testable hypotheses; however, at this point this scheme is just that—a hypothesis.

About half of the aMCI subjects in this study fell into the high PIB uptake range (global cortical-to-cerebellar retention ratio >1.5), and half fell into the low PIB retention range. While the proportion of PIB negative aMCI subjects in this study may be higher than seen in other studies, observing PIB negative aMCI subjects is consistent with results from several studies (Lopresti et al., 2005; Pike et al., 2007; Price et al., 2005; Rowe et al., 2007). Interestingly, no consistent differences in cognitive performance, including learning and memory, were seen between high vs. low PIB aMCI subjects. The upper left and lower right quadrants in Figure 12.16 represent concordant PIB and MRI findings (i.e., high PIB and low hippocampal W score, or vice versa), while the lower left and upper right panels represent subjects with discordant PIB and MRI findings. Of the 17 aMCI subjects in the study, PIB and

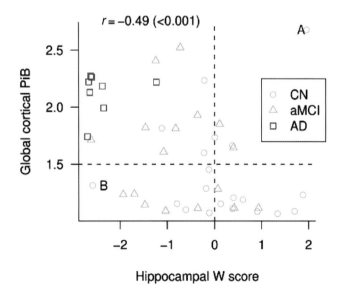

Figure 12–16 Scatter plot showing relationship between global cortical PiB retention and hippocampal W score.

MRI were discordant in seven. Five of these had low PIB retention and hippocampal W scores less than 0 (i.e., hippocampal atrophy). A hypothesis is that low PIB retention aMCI subjects who also have atrophic hippocampi have prodromal dementias other than AD, and at autopsy will be found to have pathologic substrates for their cognitive impairment other than AD. Conversely, aMCI subjects who lie in the high PIB retention range have prodromal AD which will be confirmed at autopsy. However, this is purely a hypothesis and longitudinal studies to autopsy are required to confirm or refute this.

MRI of MCI Subtypes

Because the expanded definition of MCI to include both amnestic and non-amnestic categories is relatively recent, little literature exists at this point on MCI subtypes (Bell-McGinty et al., 2005). In a recent study which examined single domain MCI subjects that were broken out by the specific cognitive domain involved, interesting correlations were observed (Whitwell et al., 2007a). Subjects who were labeled single domain non-amnestic MCI in whom the predominant domain of impairment was language displayed a selective left temporal pattern of gray matter loss (Figure 12.17). One could hypothesize that these subjects with single domain, predominantly language impairment, represent prodromal language-variant frontal temporal lobar degeneration subjects. It is also possible that the underlying pathology in such subjects is AD, but with an atypical anatomic distribution. Nonetheless, the anatomic-functional correlation in this group of naMCI subjects was quite good, with isolated language impairment predominantly loading onto the left temporal lobe. In the same study, MCI subjects who were labeled single domain non-amnestic, and in whom the predominant abnormality was in the attention/executive domain, illustrated a pattern of gray matter loss that was confined to the substantia innominata, hypothalamus, and the dorsal pontomesencephalic regions (Figure 12.18). This pattern has been identified in VBM studies of subjects with clinically defined dementia with Lewy bodies (Whitwell et al., 2007d). One can hypothesize, therefore, that single domain non-amnestic MCI, in whom the predominant domain is attention executive, are displaying a pattern that represents the form fruste of DLB. However, this is purely speculative at this point and longitudinal studies are required. Another interesting feature of this study was that when all non-amnestic subjects were grouped together and VBM analysis was performed no coherent pattern emerged. More specifically, there was no evidence of an AD-like pattern of gray matter loss in non-amnestic MCI subjects. This is in sharp contrast to the pattern that emerged in aMCI subjects who demonstrated a less advanced, but nonetheless AD-like pattern of gray matter loss (Figure 12.6).

Unpublished preliminary data from the Mayo Clinic indicate that while hippocampal ADC values on average are moderately increased in aMCI and more severely so in AD, these values do not differ between naMCI and CN subjects. While hippocampal volumes on average are moderately decreased in aMCI, and more severely so in AD, these values do not differ between naMCI and CN subjects. In ^{1}H MRS spectra obtained from the posterior cingulate gyrus, mI is elevated and NAA is depressed in aMCI and AD; however, these values are normal in naMCI subjects. Finally, Pike et al. (Pike et al., 2007) recently demonstrated that most (but not all) aMCI subjects are PIB positive, while all naMCI subjects studied ($n = 6$) were PIB negative.

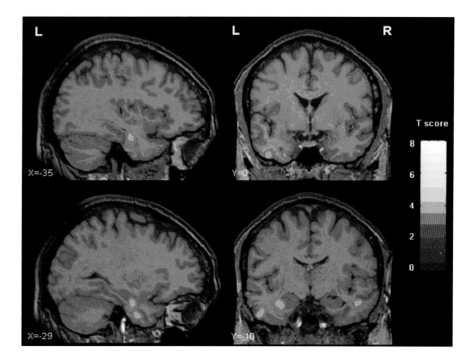

Figure 12–17   Non-amnestic MCI: language domain (*n* = 10). Patterns of gray matter atrophy identified in the non-amnestic single-domain MCI subjects with a language impairment compared to controls (*p* < 0.001, uncorrected). (With permission from Whitwell et al., 2007a.)

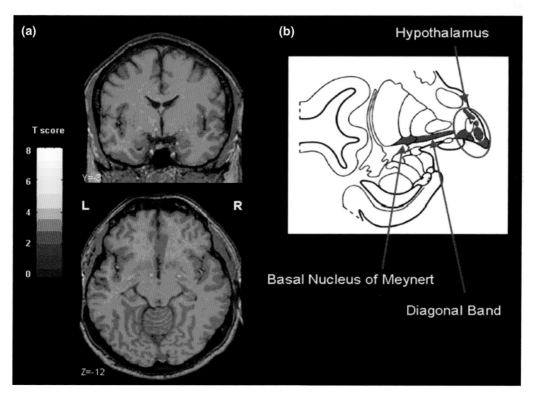

Figure 12–18   Non-amnestic MCI: attention/executive domain (*n* = 9). Patterns 1of gray matter atrophy identified in the non-amnestic single-domain MCI subjects with an attention/executive impairment compared to controls (*p* < 0.001, uncorrected). Panel (b) suggests that the pattern of atrophy identified in panel (a) involves the basal nucleus of Meynert, the diagonal band of the basal forebrain and the hypothalamus. (With permission from Whitwell et al., 2007a.)

What Has Imaging Taught Us About MCI?

MCI was originally conceived to describe a transitional clinical state between normal aging and AD—i.e. amnestic MCI. Multiple imaging studies indicate that when examined cross-sectionally, aMCI subjects on average lie at an intermediate position between CN and AD—precisely what one would expect if aMCI were a transition state. However, aMCI subjects are not all identical clinically, pathologically, or on imaging. Rather, aMCI encompasses a range of disease severity which is grouped under a common construct. Amnestic MCI subjects destined to progress to AD more rapidly have quantitative ROI and voxel-based MRI findings that are more "AD-like" than MCI subjects who are destined to progress to AD more slowly or not at all. Similarly, aMCI subjects who concurrently progress to AD have more "AD-like" rates of atrophy on serial MRI than MCI subjects who do not progress.

Further study has revealed that while most subjects who meet clinical criteria for aMCI progress to AD, not all do. A minority of aMCI subjects progress to non-AD dementias, and some do not seem to progress clinically on long-term follow-up. Amyloid imaging studies reveal that a proportion of subjects who meet clinical criteria for aMCI do not have evidence of amyloid binding (Jack et al., 2007c; Pike et al., 2007; Rowe et al., 2007). Therefore, aMCI may best be conceived as a risk factor for dementia, but not a diagnosis of early AD. This is completely consistent with the original formulation of the construct of aMCI (Petersen et al., 1995). In those aMCI subjects who do go onto AD, aMCI represented prodromal AD. Conversely, in aMCI subjects who do not go on to AD, aMCI represented the prodrome of non-AD dementia, or it represented static nonprogressive lifelong memory impairment.

Available data indicates that naMCI subjects typically have MRI imaging findings that are distinct from aMCI and AD. The fact that most naMCI subjects studied with PIB to date (although the number is small) have been negative is telling. One might think, therefore, that naMCI typically represents the prodromal presentation of non-AD dementia(s). This may well be true; however, the syndrome of naMCI has not been studied fully enough to make this determination.

References

Adalsteinsson, E., Sullivan, E. V., Kleinhans, N., Spielman, D. M., and Pfefferbaum, A. (2000). Longitudinal decline of the neuronal marker N-acetyl aspartate in Alzheimer's disease. *Lancet*, 355: 1696–1697.

Apostolova, L. G., Dutton, R. A., Dinov, I. D., Hayashi, K. M., Toga, A. W., Cummings, J. L., et al. (2006). Conversion of mild cognitive impairment to Alzheimer's disease predicted by hippocampal atrophy maps. *Archives of Neurology*, 63: 693–699.

Ashburner, J. and Friston, K. J. (2000). Voxel-based morphometry—the methods. *Neuroimage*, 11: 805–821.

Baron, J. C., Chetelat, G., Desgranges, B., Perchey, G., Landeau, B., de la Sayette, V., et al. (2001). In vivo mapping of gray matter loss with voxel-based morphometry in mild Alzheimer's disease. *Neuroimage*, 14: 298–309.

Bell-McGinty, S., Lopez, O. L., Meltzer, C. C., Scanlon, J. M., Whyte, E. M., Dekosky, S. T., et al. (2005). Differential cortical atrophy in subgroups of mild cognitive impairment. *Archives of Neurology*, 62: 1393–1397.

Bennett, D. A., Schneider, J. A., Bienias, J. L., Evans, D. A., and Wilson, R. S. (2005). Mild cognitive impairment is related to Alzheimer disease pathology and cerebral infarctions. *Neurology*, 64: 834–841.

Bobinski, M., de Leon, M. J., Wegiel, J., Desanti, S., Convit, A., Saint Louis, L. A., et al. (2000). The histological validation of post mortem magnetic resonance imaging-determined hippocampal volume in Alzheimer's disease. *Neuroscience*, 95: 721–725.

Bozzali, M., Filippi, M., Magnani, G., Cercignani, M., Franceschi, M., Schiatti, E., et al. (2006). The contribution of voxel-based morphometry in staging patients with mild cognitive impairment. *Neurology*, 67: 453–460.

Braak, H. and Braak E. (1991). Neuropathological staging of Alzheimer-related changes. *Acta Neuropathologica*, 82: 239–259.

Chan, D., Janssen, J. C., Whitwell, J. L., Watt, H. C., Jenkins, R., Frost, C., et al. (2003). Change in rates of cerebral atrophy over time in early-onset Alzheimer's disease: longitudinal MRI study. *Lancet*, 362: 1121–1122.

Chetelat, G., Desgranges, B., De La Sayette, V., Viader, F., Eustache, F., and Baron JC. (2002). Mapping gray matter loss with voxel-based morphometry in mild cognitive impairment. *Neuroreport*, 13: 1939–1943.

Chetelat, G., Landeau, B., Eustache, F., Mezenge, F., Viader, F., de la Sayette, V., et al. (2005). Using voxel-based morphometry to map the structural

changes associated with rapid conversion in MCI: A longitudinal MRI study. *Neuroimage*, 27: 934–946.

Convit, A., de Leon, M. J., Tarshish, C., De Santi, S., Kluger, A., Rusinek, H., et al. (1995). Hippocampal volume losses in minimally impaired elderly. *Lancet*, 345: 266.

Csernansky, J. G., Hamstra, J., Wang, L., McKeel, D., Price, J. L., Gado, M., et al. (2004). Correlations between antemortem hippocampal volume and postmortem neuropathology in AD subjects. *Alzheimer Disease Association Disorder*, 18: 190–195.

Csernansky, J. G., Wang, L., Joshi, S., Miller, J. P., Gado, M., Kido, D., et al. (2000). Early DAT is distinguished from aging by high-dimensional mapping of the hippocampus. Dementia of the Alzheimer type. *Neurology*, 55: 1636–1643.

Csernansky, J. G., Wang, L., Swank, J., Miller, J. P., Gado, M., McKeel, D., et al. (2005). Preclinical detection of Alzheimer's disease: Hippocampal shape and volume predict dementia onset in the elderly. *Neuroimage*, 25: 783–792.

DeCarli, C., Frisoni, G. B., Clark, C. M., Harvey, D., Grundman, M., Petersen, R. C., et al. (2007). Qualitative estimates of medial temporal atrophy as a predictor of progression from mild cognitive impairment to dementia. *Archives of Neurology*, 64: 108–115.

De Santi, S., de Leon, M. J., Rusinek, H., Convit, A., Tarshish, C. Y., Roche, A., et al. (2001). Hippocampal formation glucose metabolism and volume losses in MCI and AD. *Neurobiology of Aging*, 22: 529–539.

deToledo-Morrell, L., Stoub, T. R., Bulgakova, M., Wilson, R. S., Bennett, D. A., Leurgans, S., et al. (2004). MRI-derived entorhinal volume is a good predictor of conversion from MCI to AD. *Neurobiology of Aging*, 25: 1197–1203.

Dickerson, B. C., Goncharova, I., Sullivan, M. P., Forchetti, C., Wilson, R. S., Bennett, D. A., et al. (2001). MRI-derived entorhinal and hippocampal atrophy in incipient and very mild Alzheimer's disease. *Neurobiology of Aging*, 22: 747–754.

Dickerson, B. C., Salat, D. H., Bates, J. F., Atiya, M., Killiany, R. J., Greve, D. N., et al. (2004). Medial temporal lobe function and structure in mild cognitive impairment. *Annals of Neurology*, 56: 27–35.

Du, A. T., Schuff, N., Amend, D., Laakso, M. P., Hsu, Y. Y., Jagust, W. J., et al. (2001). Magnetic resonance imaging of the entorhinal cortex and hippocampus in mild cognitive impairment and Alzheimer's disease. *Journal of Neurology, Neurosurgery & Psychiatry*, 71: 431–432.

Du, A. T., Schuff, N., Zhu, X. P., Jagust, W. J., Miller, B. L., Reed, B. R., et al. (2003). Atrophy rates of entorhinal cortex in AD and normal aging. *Neurology*, 60: 481–486.

Du, A. T., Schuff, N., Kramer, J. H., Ganzer, S., Zhu, X. P., Jagust, W. J., et al. (2004). Higher atrophy rate of entorhinal cortex than hippocampus in AD. *Neurology*, 62: 422–427.

Fox, N. C. and Freeborough, P. A. (1997). Brain atrophy progression measured from registered serial MRI: Validation and application to Alzheimer's disease. *Journal of Magnetic Resonance Imaging*, 7: 1069–1075.

Fox, N. C., Crum, W. R., Scahill, R. I., Stevens, J. M., Janssen, J. C., Rossor, M. N. (2001). Imaging of onset and progression of Alzheimer's disease with voxel-compression mapping of serial magnetic resonance images. *Lancet*, 358: 201–205.

Fox, N. C., Scahill, R. I., Crum, W. R., and Rossor, M. N. (1999). Correlation between rates of brain atrophy and cognitive decline in AD. *Neurology*, 52: 1687–1689.

Fox, N. C., Warrington, E. K., and Rossor, M. N. (1999). Serial magnetic resonance imaging of cerebral atrophy in preclinical Alzheimer's disease. *Lancet*, 353: 2125.

Fox, N. C., Warrington, E. K., Freeborough, P. A., Hartikainen, P., Kennedy, A. M., Stevens, J. M., et al. (1996). Presymptomatic hippocampal atrophy in Alzheimer's disease. A longitudinal MRI study. *Brain*, 119 (Pt 6): 2001–2007.

Freeborough, P. A. and Fox, N. C. (1997). The boundary shift integral: an accurate and robust measure of cerebral volume changes from registered repeat MRI. *IEEE Trans Medical Imaging*, 16: 623–639.

Freeborough, P. A. and Fox, N. C. (1998). Modeling brain deformations in Alzheimer disease by fluid registration of serial 3D MR images. *Journal of Computer Assisted Tomography*, 22: 838–843.

Frisoni, G. B., Testa, C., Zorzan, A., Sabattoli, F., Beltramello, A., Soininen, H., et al. (2002). Detection of grey matter loss in mild Alzheimer's disease with voxel based morphometry. *Journal of Neurology, Neurosurgery and Psychiatry*, 73: 657–664.

Geroldi, C., Rossi, R., Calvagna, C., Testa, C., Bresciani, L., Binetti, G., et al. (2006). Medial temporal atrophy but not memory deficit predicts progression to dementia in patients with mild cognitive impairment. *Journal of Neurology, Neurosurgery and Psychiatry*, 77: 1219–1222.

Good, C. D., Johnsrude, I. S., Ashburner, J., Henson, R. N., Friston, K. J., and Frackowiak, R. S. (2001). A voxel-based morphometric study of ageing in 465 normal adult human brains. *Neuroimage*, 14: 21–36.

Good, C. D., Scahill, R. I., Fox, N. C., Ashburner, J., Friston, K. J., Chan, D., et al. (2002). Automatic differentiation of anatomical patterns in the human brain: Validation with studies of degenerative dementias. *Neuroimage*, 17: 29–46.

Gosche, K. M., Mortimer, J. A., Smith, C. D., Markesbery, W. R., and Snowdon, D. A. (2002). Hippocampal volume as an index of Alzheimer neuropathology: findings from the Nun Study. *Neurology*, 58: 1476–1482.

Grundman, M., Sencakova, D., Jack, C. R., Jr., Petersen, R. C., Kim, H. T., Schultz, A., et al. (2002). Brain MRI hippocampal volume and prediction of clinical status in a mild cognitive impairment trial. *Journal of Molecular Neuroscience*, 19: 23–27.

Hanyu, H., Sakurai, H., Iwamoto, T., Takasaki, M., Shindo, H., and Abe, K. (1998). Diffusion-weighted MR imaging of the hippocampus and temporal white matter in Alzheimer's disease. *Journal of Neurological Sciences*, 156: 195–200.

Hanyu, H., Shindo, H., Kakizaki, D., Abe, K., Iwamoto, T., and Takasaki, M. (1997). Increased water diffusion in cerebral white matter in Alzheimer's disease. *Gerontology*, 43: 343–351.

Ishii, K., Kawachi, T., Sasaki, H., Kono, A. K., Fukuda, T., Kojima, Y., et al. (2005). Voxel-based morphometric comparison between early- and late-onset mild Alzheimer's disease and assessment of diagnostic performance of z score images. *American Journal of Neuroradiology*, 26: 333–340.

Jack, C. R., Jr., Dickson, D. W., Parisi, J. E., Xu, Y. C., Cha, R. H., O'Brien, P. C., et al. (2002). Antemortem MRI findings correlate with hippocampal neuropathology in typical aging and dementia. *Neurology*, 58: 750–757.

Jack, C. R., Jr., Petersen, R. C., Grundman, M., Jin, S., Gamst, A., Ward, C. P., et al. (2007a). Longitudinal MRI findings from the vitamin E and donepezil treatment study for MCI. *Neurobiology of Aging.*, 29(9): 1285095

Jack, C. R., Jr., Petersen, R. C., Xu, Y. C., Waring, S. C., O'Brien, P. C., Tangalos, E. G., et al. (1997). Medial temporal atrophy on MRI in normal aging and very mild Alzheimer's disease. *Neurology*, 49: 786–794.

Jack, C. R., Jr., Petersen, R. C., Xu, Y., O'Brien, P. C., Smith, G. E., Ivnik, R. J., et al. (1998). Rate of medial temporal lobe atrophy in typical aging and Alzheimer's disease. *Neurology*, 51: 993–999.

Jack, C. R., Jr., Petersen, R. C., Xu, Y. C., O'Brien, P. C., Smith, G. E., Ivnik, R. J., et al. (1999). Prediction of AD with MRI-based hippocampal volume in mild cognitive impairment. *Neurology*, 52: 1397–1403.

Jack, C. R., Jr., Petersen, R. C., Xu, Y., O'Brien, P. C., Smith, G. E., Ivnik, R. J., et al. (2000). Rates of hippocampal atrophy correlate with change in clinical status in aging and AD. *Neurology*, 55: 484–489.

Jack, C. R., Jr., Shiung, M. M., Gunter, J. L., O'Brien, P. C., Weigand, S. D., Knopman, D. S., et al. (2004). Comparison of different MRI brain atrophy rate measures with clinical disease progression in AD. *Neurology*, 62: 591–600.

Jack, C. R., Jr., Shiung, M. M., Weigand, S. D., O'Brien, P. C., Gunter, J. L., Boeve, B. F., et al. (2005). Brain atrophy rates predict subsequent clinical conversion in normal elderly and amnestic MCI. *Neurology*, 65: 1227–1231.

Jack, C. R., Jr., Slomkowski, M., Gracon, S., Hoover, T. M., Felmlee, J. P., Stewart, K., et al. (2003). MRI as a biomarker of disease progression in a therapeutic trial of milameline for AD. *Neurology*, 60: 253–260.

Jack, C. R., Jr., Weigand, S. D., Shiung, M. M., Przybelski, S. A., O'Brien, P. C., Gunter, J. L., et al. (2007b). Atrophy rates accelerate in amnestic mild cognitive impairment. *Neurology*, 70(19): 1740–1752.

Jack, C. R. Jr., Lowe, V. J., Senjem, M. L., Weigand, S. D., Shiung, M. M., Kemp, B. J., et al. (2007c). 11C PiB and Structural MRI provide complementary information in imaging of AD and amnestic MCI. *Brain*, 131: 665–680.

Jicha, G. A., Parisi, J. E., Dickson, D. W., Johnson, K., Cha, R., Ivnik, R. J., et al. (2006). Neuropathologic outcome of mild cognitive impairment following progression to clinical dementia. *Archives of Neurology*, 63: 674–681.

Kantarci, K., Jack, C. R., Jr., Xu, Y. C., Campeau, N. G., O'Brien, P. C., Smith, G. E., et al. (2001). Mild cognitive impairment and Alzheimer disease: regional diffusivity of water. *Radiology*, 219: 101–107.

Kantarci, K., Petersen, R. C., Boeve, B. F., Knopman, D. S., Weigand, S. D., O'Brien, P. C., et al. (2005). DWI predicts future progression to Alzheimer disease in amnestic mild cognitive impairment. *Neurology*, 64: 902–904.

Kantarci, K., Smith, G. E., Ivnik, R. J., Petersen, R. C., Boeve, B. F., Knopman, D. S., et al. (2002). 1H magnetic resonance spectroscopy, cognitive function, and apolipoprotein E genotype in normal aging, mild cognitive impairment and Alzheimer's disease. *Journal of the International Neuropsychological Society*, 8: 934–942.

Karas, G. B., Burton, E. J., Rombouts, S. A., van Schijndel, R. A., O'Brien, J. T., Scheltens, P., et al. (2003). A comprehensive study of gray matter loss in patients with Alzheimer's disease using optimized voxel-based morphometry. *Neuroimage*, 18: 895–907.

Karas, G. B., Scheltens, P., Rombouts, S. A., Visser, P. J., van Schijndel, R. A., Fox, N. C., et al. (2004). Global and local gray matter loss in mild cognitive impairment and Alzheimer's disease. *Neuroimage*, 23: 708–716.

Kaye, J. A., Swihart, T., Howieson, D., Dame, A., Moore, M. M., Karnos, T., et al. (1997). Volume loss of the hippocampus and temporal lobe in healthy elderly persons destined to develop dementia. *Neurology*, 48: 1297–1304.

Killiany, R. J., Gomez-Isla, T., Moss, M., Kikinis, R., Sandor, T., Jolesz, F., et al. (2000). Use of structural magnetic resonance imaging to predict who will get Alzheimer's disease. *Annals of Neurology*, 47: 430–439.

Killiany, R. J., Hyman, B. T., Gomez-Isla, T., Moss, M. B., Kikinis, R., Jolesz, F., et al. (2002). MRI measures of entorhinal cortex vs hippocampus in preclinical AD. *Neurology*, 58: 1188–1196.

Killiany, R. J., Moss, M. B., Albert, M. S., Sandor, T., Tieman, J., Jolesz, F. (1993). Temporal lobe regions on magnetic resonance imaging identify patients with early Alzheimer's disease. *Archives of Neurology*, 50: 949–954.

Korf, E. S., Wahlund, L. O., Visser, P. J., and Scheltens, P. (2004). Medial temporal lobe atrophy on MRI predicts dementia in patients with mild cognitive impairment. *Neurology*, 63: 94–100.

Krasuski, J. S., Alexander, G. E., Horwitz, B., Daly, E. M., Murphy, D. G., Rapoport, S. I., et al. (1998). Volumes of medial temporal lobe structures in patients with Alzheimer's disease and mild cognitive impairment (and in healthy controls). *Biological Psychiatry*, 43: 60–68.

Laakso, M. P., Lehtovirta, M., Partanen, K., Riekkinen, P. J., and Soininen, H. (2000). Hippocampus in Alzheimer's disease: A 3-year follow-up MRI study. *Biological Psychiatry*, 47: 557–561.

Laakso, M. P., Soininen, H., Partanen, K., Lehtovirta, M., Hallikainen, M., Hanninen, T., et al. (1998). MRI of the hippocampus in Alzheimer's disease: sensitivity, specificity, and analysis of the incorrectly classified subjects. *Neurobiology of Aging*, 19: 23–31.

Le Bihan, D., Breton, E., Lallemand, D., Grenier, P., Cabanis, E., and Laval-Jeantet, M. M. R. (1986). imaging of intravoxel incoherent motions: application to diffusion and perfusion in neurologic disorders. *Radiology*, 161: 401–407.

Lopez, O. L., Jagust, W. J., DeKosky, S. T., Becker, J. T., Fitzpatrick, A., Dulberg, C., et al. (2003). Prevalence and classification of mild cognitive impairment in the Cardiovascular Health Study Cognition Study: part 1. *Archives of Neurology*, 60: 1385–1389.

Lopresti, B. J., Klunk, W. E., Mathis, C. A., Hoge, J. A., Ziolko, S. K., Lu, X., et al. (2005). Simplified quantification of Pittsburgh Compound B amyloid imaging PET studies: a comparative analysis. *Journal of Nuclear Medicine*, 46: 1959–1972.

Markesbery, W. R., Schmitt, F. A., Kryscio, R. J., Davis, D. G., Smith, C. D., and Wekstein, D. R. (2006). Neuropathologic substrate of mild cognitive impairment. *Archives of Neurology*, 63: 38–46.

Marquis, S., Moore, M. M., Howieson, D. B., Sexton, G., Payami, H., Kaye, J. A., et al. (2002). Independent predictors of cognitive decline in healthy elderly persons. *Archives of Neurology*, 59: 601–606.

Meyerhoff, D. J., MacKay, S., Constans, J. M., Norman, D., Van Dyke, C., Fein, G., et al. (1994). Axonal injury and membrane alterations in Alzheimer's disease suggested by in vivo proton magnetic resonance spectroscopic imaging. *Annals of Neurology*, 36: 40–47.

Miller, B. L., Moats, R. A., Shonk, T., Ernst, T., Woolley, S., Ross, B. D. (1993). Alzheimer disease: Depiction of increased cerebral myo-inositol with proton MR spectroscopy. *Radiology*, 187: 433–437.

Parnetti, L., Lowenthal, D. T., Presciutti, O., Pelliccioli, G. P., Palumbo, R., Gobbi, G., et al. (1996). 1H-MRS, MRI-based hippocampal volumetry, and 99mTc-HMPAO-SPECT in normal aging, age-associated memory impairment, and probable Alzheimer's disease. *Journal of the American Geriatric Society*, 44: 133–138.

Parnetti, L., Tarducci, R., Presciutti, O., Lowenthal, D. T., Pippi, M., Palumbo, B., et al. (1997). Proton magnetic resonance spectroscopy can differentiate Alzheimer's disease from normal aging. *Mechanisms of Ageing and Development*, 97: 9–14.

Pennanen, C., Kivipelto, M., Tuomainen, S., Hartikainen, P., Hanninen, T., Laakso, M. P., et al. (2004). Hippocampus and entorhinal cortex in mild cognitive impairment and early AD. *Neurobiology of Aging*, 25: 303–310.

Pennanen, C., Testa, C., Laakso, M. P., Hallikainen, M., Helkala, E. L., Hanninen, T., et al. (2005). A voxel based morphometry study on mild cognitive impairment. *Journal of Neurology, Neurosurgery and Psychiatry*, 76: 11–14.

Petersen, R. C. (2007). Mild cognitive impairment. *Continuum: Lifelong Learning Neurology*, 13: 15–38.

Petersen, R. C., Parisi, J. E., Dickson, D. W., Johnson, K. A., Knopman, D. S., Boeve, B. F., et al. (2006). Neuropathologic features of amnestic mild cognitive impairment. *Archives of Neurology*, 63: 665–672.

Petersen, R. C., Smith, G. E., Ivnik, R. J., Tangalos, E. G., Schaid, D. J., Thibodeau, S. N., et al. (1995). Apolipoprotein E status as a predictor of the development of Alzheimer's disease in memory-impaired individuals. *Journal of American Medical Association*, 273: 1274–1278.

Petersen, R. C., Smith, G. E., Waring, S. C., Ivnik, R. J., Tangalos, E. G., and Kokmen E. (1999). Mild cognitive impairment: Clinical characterization and outcome.. *Archives of Neurology*, 56: 303–308.

Petersen, R. C., Thomas, R. G., Grundman, M., Bennett, D., Doody, R., Ferris, S., et al. (2005). Vitamin E and donepezil for the treatment of mild cognitive impairment. *New England Journal of Medicine*, 352: 2379–2388.

Pike, K. E., Savage, G., Villemagne, V. L., Ng, S., Moss, S. A., Maruff, P., et al. (2007). Beta-amyloid imaging and memory in non-demented individuals: Evidence for preclinical Alzheimer's disease. *Brain*, 130: 2837–2844.

Price, J. C., Klunk, W. E., Lopresti, B. J., Lu, X., Hoge, J. A., Ziolko, S. K., et al. (2005). Kinetic modeling of amyloid binding in humans using PET imaging and Pittsburgh Compound-B. *Journal of Cerebral Blood Flow & Metabolism*, 25: 1528–1247.

Ridha, B. H., Barnes, J., Bartlett, J. W., Godbolt, A., Pepple, T., Rossor, M. N., et al. (2006). Tracking atrophy progression in familial Alzheimer's disease: A serial MRI study. *Lancet Neurology*, 5: 828–834.

Rombouts, S. A., Barkhof, F., Witter, M. P., and Scheltens, P. (2000). Unbiased whole-brain analysis of gray matter loss in Alzheimer's disease. *Neuroscience Letters*, 285: 231–233.

Rowe, C. C., Ng, S., Ackermann, U., Gong, S. J., Pike, K., Savage, G., et al. (2007). Imaging beta-amyloid burden in aging and dementia. *Neurology*, 68: 1718–1725.

Sabbagh, M. N., Shah, F., Reid, R. T., Sue, L., Connor, D. J., Peterson, L. K., et al. (2006). Pathologic and nicotinic receptor binding differences between mild cognitive impairment, Alzheimer disease, and normal aging. *Archives of Neurology*, 63: 1771–1776.

Sandson, T. A., Felician, O., Edelman, R. R., and Warach, S. (1999). Diffusion-weighted magnetic resonance imaging in Alzheimer's disease. *Dementia and Geriatric Cognitive Disorders*, 10: 166–171.

Scahill, R. I., Frost, C., Jenkins, R., Whitwell, J. L., Rossor, M. N., Fox, N. C. (2003). A longitudinal study of brain volume changes in normal aging using serial registered magnetic resonance imaging. *Archives of Neurology*, 60: 989–994.

Scahill, R. I., Schott, J. M., Stevens, J. M., Rossor, M. N., and Fox, N. C. (2002). Mapping the evolution of regional atrophy in Alzheimer's disease: unbiased analysis of fluid-registered serial MRI. *Proceedings of the National Academy of Sciences of the USA*, 99: 4703–4707.

Schott, J. M., Fox, N. C., Frost, C., Scahill, R. I., Janssen, J. C., Chan, D., et al. (2003). Assessing the onset of structural change in familial Alzheimer's disease. *Annals of Neurology*, 53: 181–188.

Schott, J. M., Price, S. L., Frost, C., Whitwell, J. L., Rossor, M. N., and Fox, N. C. (2005). Measuring atrophy in Alzheimer disease: a serial MRI study over 6 and 12 months. *Neurology*, 65: 119–124.

Schuff, N., Amend, D., Ezekiel, F., Steinman, S. K., Tanabe, J., Norman, D., et al. (1997). Changes of hippocampal N-acetyl aspartate and volume in Alzheimer's disease. A proton MR spectroscopic imaging and MRI study. *Neurology*, 49: 1513–1521.

Schuff, N., Amend, D. L., Meyerhoff, D. J., Tanabe, J. L., Norman, D., Fein, G., et al. (1998). Alzheimer disease: Quantitative H-1 MR spectroscopic imaging of frontoparietal brain. *Radiology*, 207: 91–102.

Senjem, M. L., Gunter, J. L., Shiung, M. M., Petersen, R. C., Jack, C. R., Jr. (2005). Comparison of different methodological implementations of voxel-based morphometry in neurodegenerative disease. *Neuroimage*, 26: 600–608.

Shiino, A., Watanabe, T., Maeda, K., Kotani, E., Akiguchi, I., and Matsuda, M. (2006). Four subgroups of Alzheimer's disease based on patterns of atrophy using VBM and a unique pattern for early onset disease. *Neuroimage*, 33: 17–26.

Shonk, T. and Ross, B. D. (1995). Role of increased cerebral myo-inositol in the dementia of Down syndrome. *Magnetic Resonance Medicine*, 33: 858–861.

Shonk, T. K., Moats, R. A., Gifford, P., Michaelis, T., Mandigo, J. C., Izumi, J., et al. (1995). Probable Alzheimer disease: Diagnosis with proton MR spectroscopy. *Radiology*, 195: 65–72.

Silbert, L. C., Quinn, J. F., Moore, M. M., Corbridge, E., Ball, M. J., Murdoch, G., et al. (2003). Changes in premorbid brain volume predict Alzheimer's disease pathology. *Neurology*, 61: 487–492.

Stejskal, E. O. and Tanner, J. E. (1965). Spin Diffusion Measurements: Spin Echoes in the Presence of a Time-Dependent Field Gradient. *Journal of Chemical Physics*, 42: 288–292.

Tedeschi, G., Bertolino, A., Lundbom, N., Bonavita, S., Patronas, N. J., Duyn, J. H., et al. (1996). Cortical and subcortical chemical pathology in Alzheimer's disease as assessed by multislice proton magnetic resonance spectroscopic imaging. *Neurology*, 47: 696–704.

Teipel, S. J., Bayer, W., Alexander, G. E., Zebuhr, Y., Teichberg, D., Kulic, L., et al. (2002). Progression of corpus callosum atrophy in Alzheimer disease. *Archives of Neurology*, 59: 243–248.

Thompson, P. M., Hayashi, K. M., de Zubicaray, G., Janke, A. L., Rose, S. E., Semple, J., et al. (2003). Dynamics of gray matter loss in Alzheimer's disease. *Journal of Neuroscience*, 23: 994–1005.

Trivedi, M. A., Wichmann, A. K., Torgerson, B. M., Ward, M. A., Schmitz, T. W., Ries, M. L., et al. (2006). Structural MRI discriminates individuals with Mild Cognitive Impairment from age-matched controls: A combined neuropsychological and voxel based morphometry study. *Alzheimer's and Dementia*, 2: 296–302.

Visser, P. J., Scheltens, P., Verhey, F. R., Schmand, B., Launer, L. J., Jolles, J., et al. (1999). Medial temporal lobe atrophy and memory dysfunction as predictors for dementia in subjects with mild cognitive impairment. *Journal of Neurology*, 246: 477–485.

Wang, L., Swank, J. S., Glick, I. E., Gado, M. H., Miller, M. I., Morris, J. C., et al. (2003). Changes in hippocampal volume and shape across time distinguish dementia of the Alzheimer type from healthy aging. *Neuroimage*, 20: 667–682.

Whitwell, J. L., Petersen, R. C., Negash, S., Weigand, S. D., Kantarci, K., Ivnik, R. J., et al. (2007a). Patterns of atrophy differ among specific subtypes of mild cognitive impairment. *Archives of Neurology*, 64: 1130–1138.

Whitwell, J. L., Przybelski, S. A., Weigand, S. D., Knopman, D. S., Boeve, B. F., Petersen, R. C., et al. (2007b). 3D maps from multiple MRI illustrate changing atrophy patterns as subjects progress from mild cognitive impairment to Alzheimer's disease. *Brain*, 130: 1777–1786.

Whitwell, J. L., Shiung, M. M., Przybelski, S. A., Weigand, S. D., Knopman, D. S., Boeve, B. F., et al. (2007c). MRI patterns of atrophy associated with progression to AD in amnestic mild cognitive impairment. *Neurology*, 70: 512–520.

Whitwell, J. L., Weigand, S. D., Shiung, M. M., Boeve, B. F., Ferman, T. J., Smith, G. E., et al. (2007d). Focal atrophy in dementia with Lewy bodies on MRI: a distinct pattern from Alzheimer's disease. *Brain*, 130: 708–719.

Winblad, B., Palmer, K., Kivipelto, M., Jelic, V., Fratiglioni, L., Wahlund, L. O., et al. (2004). Mild cognitive impairment–beyond controversies, towards a consensus: report of the International Working Group on Mild Cognitive Impairment. *Journal of Internal Medicine*, 256: 240–246.

Xu, Y., Jack, C. R., Jr., O'Brien, P. C., Kokmen, E., Smith, G. E., Ivnik, R. J., et al. (2000). Usefulness of MRI measures of entorhinal cortex versus hippocampus in AD. *Neurology*, 54: 1760–1767.

Zarow, C., Vinters, H. V., Ellis, W. G., Weiner, M. W., Mungas, D., White, L., et al. (2005). Correlates of hippocampal neuron number in Alzheimer's disease and ischemic vascular dementia. *Annals of Neurology*, 57: 896–903.

Zhang, Y., Schuff, N., Jahng, G. H., Bayne, W., Mori, S., Schad, L., et al. (2007). Diffusion tensor imaging of cingulum fibers in mild cognitive impairment and Alzheimer disease. *Neurology*, 68: 13–19.

Functional Imaging with FDG-PET in Mild Cognitive Impairment

Karl Herholz

Background

FDG-PET has now been available for more than 25 years during which a solid body of scientific evidence has been accumulated demonstrating well defined functional impairment of resting glucose metabolism in AD. This regional metabolic impairment is closely related to the severity, progression and type of cognitive deficits (Herholz, 2006). As the awareness increased that early diagnosis of AD is a desirable goal and practical clinical criteria for mild cognitive impairment (MCI) as a high-risk condition for progression to dementia became available (Petersen and Morris, 2005), FDG-PET studies investigating that stage have been performed. They will be reviewed in this chapter.

Methodological Considerations

Studies are usually performed at resting conditions, defined as a relaxed state without a specific task given in a quiet environment with dimmed light. While there is typically a reasonable standardization of PET equipment and image reconstruction (including corrections for scatter and attenuation) provided by the major vendors, provision and control of these conditions before and after tracer injection and during scans is an important issue that may be difficult to maintain in otherwise busy imaging departments. Studies are performed either with eyes closed or eyes open, which is influencing FDG uptake in occipital cortex and, therefore, needs to be done consistently in all subjects.

Other conditions, such as performance of memory (Duara et al., 1992; Kessler et al., 1991) or attention tasks (Buchsbaum et al., 1990) have been investigated. Results are difficult to interpret as functional networks and activation patterns in dysfunctional brains are altered and compensatory overactivation (Anderson et al., 2007; Head et al., 2007), as well as impaired metabolic activation (Kessler et al., 1991), have been found in affected brain areas. Thus, activation studies have not found wider acceptance as a diagnostic standard, but continue to be actively explored, often using fMRI techniques (Xu et al., 2007).

MCI patients are expected to display alterations that are similar, albeit less intense, to those in patients with manifest AD. In AD, impaired metabolism has consistently been described in posterior association cortices, whereas metabolism in primary sensorimotor cortex, primary visual cortex, striatum, pons and cerebellum is typically intact in AD. The contrast between the regions, the association cortices, and unaffected regions is used in visual interpretation of PET scans and has been expressed as a "metabolic ratio" that can be used as a numerical indicator of the presence of this pattern (Herholz et al., 1993) (Figure 13.1). Recognition of this typical pattern that is obvious from simple FDG uptake images has obviated the somewhat cumbersome need for taking arterial (or arterialized) blood samples to quantify regional cerebral metabolic rates of glucose (rCMRglc), a standard practice in the early years of FDG-PET studies (Wienhard et al., 1985). There is, however, no consensus yet on how to choose an optimal reference region for quantitation of metabolic decrease in affected areas. There may also be clinically relevant factors, such as microvascular changes, that could contribute to metabolic impairment, but do not show regional preference and affect the brain globally (Kwan et al., 1999; Mielke et al., 1992). They will be missed by reliance on the image pattern rather than measuring glucose metabolism. On the other hand, regional changes relative to a reference typically show about half the variability compared to measurements of regional glucose metabolic rates in absolute units and, therefore, provide better sensitivity to detect mild and early regional changes in MCI.

The cerebellum is easy to find and to use as a reference region. It is largely unaffected pathologically and functionally in AD, although crossed cerebellar diaschisis has been noted in advanced AD (Akiyama et al., 1989). The primary motor cortex (McNamara et al., 1987), the thalamus (Minoshima et al., 1995b), vermis cerebelli (Desgranges et al., 1998), and pons (Minoshima et al., 1995a) may be more stable, but are relatively small regions where the variation of region placement may contribute to variability of reference values. Yet, all of them have successfully been used as reference regions in studies discriminating AD patients from controls. Occipital cortex activity depends on whether eyes are open or closed, and generally shows relatively large variability even in controls. It is, therefore, not recommended as a reference region. A composite of major reference regions was used for the "metabolic ratio," providing better discrimination between controls and AD than a single reference region (Herholz et al., 1993). Another common approach is "global scaling" as provided by the popular statistical parametric mapping (SPM) software package (Friston et al., 1995), where cortical activity above a certain specified proportion of the maximum activity is used for scaling. Obviously, this approach is sensitive to bias in cases of widespread cortical hypometabolism, but has successfully been applied to

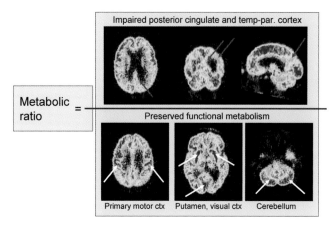

Figure 13–1 Impaired and preserved regional glucose metabolism in AD and the conceptual definition of the "metabolic ratio."

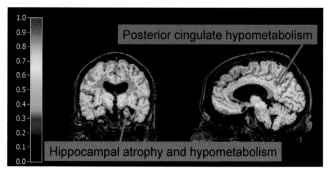

Figure 13–2 PET-MRI fusion demonstrating atrophy and metabolic alterations of beginning AD (MMSE 28) in components of the limbic system. PET data were acquired on a high-resolution research tomograph (HRRT).

MCI (Anchisi et al., 2005) where focal metabolic alterations are likely to have little impact on that global reference. Comparable results across most FDG-PET studies in MCI so far indicate that the choice of the reference region for scaling is not a major confounder, but formal comparisons among procedures have not yet been performed in MCI.

Among those association cortices that are typically affected in AD the posterior cingulate cortex has been identified as being most consistently and intensely impaired (Minoshima, Foster, and Kuhl, 1994). Other association cortices, such as angular gyrus and its vicinity, are also involved early on, but the location of the most intense changes varies considerably among patients and, therefore, causes significant variability in voxel-based data analysis. Thus, impairment of lateral temporo-parietal cortex sometimes appears as being less significant on SPM maps than the mesial posterior cingulate cortex.

Mesial temporal metabolic impairment has been observed as a general feature in patients with memory impairment, including but not limited to patients with MCI and AD (De Santi et al., 2001; Heiss et al., 1992; Mosconi et al., 2005; Nestor et al., 2003; Ouchi et al., 1998). Using a high resolution scanner in mild AD, Jagust et al. (Jagust et al., 1993) demonstrated that patients with mesial temporal lobe hypometabolism have a different neuropsychological profile than those with more severe metabolic impairment in neocortical association cortex. Hippocampal and entorhinal metabolic impairment is difficult to assess visually on standard PET scans because of their small size and lower normal metabolism than most neocortical association cortices, but they can easily be recognized on current high-resolution research scanners (Figure 13.2). Even with standard clinical scanners, it has been demonstrated that an optimized and standardized approach for targeted visual analysis is feasible (Mosconi et al., 2006), and a semi-automated procedure for regional analysis has been developed (Mosconi et al., 2005). The hippocampus frequently is affected by significant atrophy in MCI, and metabolic impairment was observed even after partial volume correction (Mevel et al., 2007). Impairment of hippocampal regions may even be predictive for developing MCI in cognitively normal elderly subjects, as has been demonstrated in a 3-year follow-up study of cognitively normal subjects (de Leon et al., 2001), whereas metabolic impairment of neocortical association areas appears to be more relevant for discriminating AD from MCI (De Santi et al., 2001).

Current image data analysis techniques typically employ spatial transformations to adjust for anatomical variations and to compare regional or voxel values with corresponding regions or voxels in normal control scans. Basically, two approaches have found widespread application for PET. An affine transformation followed by non-linear transformation using discrete cosine basis functions (Ashburner and Friston, 1999) is included in the SPM software package (Wellcome Department of Imaging Neuroscience, London) and a non-linear warping technique was developed as part of the Neurostat Package utilizing stereotactic surface projection (SSP) (Minoshima et al., 1995b). Both are potentially vulnerable to a significant shift of brain areas due to brain atrophy, although the latter has been designed to account for that as far as possible (Ishii et al., 2001). There has been substantial progress in the accuracy and reliability of these techniques (Gholipour et al., 2007). Advanced techniques involve co-registered magnetic resonance images, segmentation of gray and white matter, and cortical flattening (Klein et al., 2008).

Clinical studies require reproducible recognition of regional metabolic impairment. Standard approaches involve visual reading of PET images (with readers blinded to the clinical diagnosis), and voxel-based statistical mapping techniques by SPM or SSP can facilitate the detection focal metabolic abnormalities. From such maps that provide local z or t values, the degree of metabolic reduction within the relevant association areas can be quantified as a number and used for fully objective and automated discrimination between patients and controls (Herholz et al., 2002; Minoshima et al., 1995b). Advanced multivariate pattern recognition techniques of potential use for MCI include the use of neural network classifiers (Kippenhan et al., 1994), pattern extraction techniques from PET sinograms (Sayeed et al., 2002), principal components (Salmon et al., 2009) (Figure 13.3) and partial least-square analysis (Higdon et al., 2004).

The limited spatial resolution of PET studies implies that image data are subject to partial volume effects which have the consequence that atrophy can mimic metabolic reductions. As both can be indicators of neurodegenerative disease, this is usually not a major concern in diagnostic applications. For more accurate quantitation of metabolism, algorithms have been developed to correct for partial volume effects (Aston et al., 2002). They depend on accurate co-registration with high-resolution MRI and gray-white matter segmentation. Even small errors in that process can cause significant bias in results, and they also increase image noise. Thus, their usefulness for clinical studies is limited. A recently developed high-resolution research brain scanner reduces the need for partial volume corrections (Klein et al., 2008), and advanced reconstruction algorithms (Ji-Ho, Anderson, and Mair, 2007) that include resolution recovery may provide alternatives to post-reconstruction PVC in the near future.

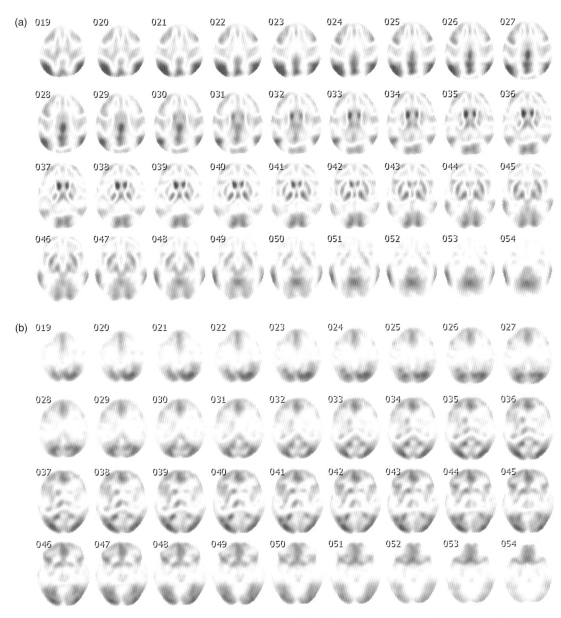

Figure 13–3   The first two principal components describing the variation in FDG-PET data in a mixed sample of normal subjects and AD on a bipolar blue/red scale: The first component (Figure 3A) represents the contrast between metabolic reduction in association areas (blue) and preserved structures (red); the second component (Figure 3B) represents the variation of an anterior/posterior gradient.

Clinical Studies

The first study noting the importance of posterior cingulate hypometabolism in patients with severe memory deficits for predicting progression was performed by Minoshima et al. in 1997 (Minoshima et al., 1997). In that study, eight subjects with memory impairments who later developed dementia were included and it was found that all of them had a significant metabolic impairment of posterior cingulate cortex. While these subjects were not specifically diagnosed as having MCI, their clinical syndromes were similar, if not identical, and clearly supported the idea that Alzheimer-like metabolic lesions could be found in patients suffering from amnesia without the full clinical dementia syndrome. In a European multicenter study, 52 patients with severe memory deficits and MMSE of 24 or better had been followed over

2 years on average (Herholz et al., 1999). Impairment of temporo-parietal cortex (angular gyrus and vicinity) predicted progression of cognitive deficits by 3 MMSE points or more, with 65% sensitivity and 86% specificity (Figure 13.4).

These initial observations were followed by several studies indicating a high predictive power of FDG-PET, with sensitivity and specificity of 70% or higher for predicting rapid progression to dementia (Table 13.1). Data analysis in these longitudinal studies typically was done in retrospect, thus identifying the brain areas that best identified those patients who progressed to dementia. In spite of considerable variability of inclusion criteria and details of data analysis, temporo-parietal and posterior cingulate association cortex consistently emerge as the best target areas for discrimination. The longest follow-up periods so far (3 years) were reported by Berent (Berent et al., 1999) and Arnaiz (Arnaiz et al., 2001) who confirmed the predictive power of temporo-parietal

Table 13–1 Prospective studies in mild cognitive impairment.

Citation	N	Age (years)	Male/female	Entry diagnosis	Follow-up time	Converters	Sensitivity, Specificity	Data analysis	Image scaling	Discriminating brain area
(Berent et al., 1999)	20	70 ± 6	13/7	Isolated memory impairment	3 years	50%	70%, 70%	Neurostat	Thalamus	Association cortex (relative to motor cortex)
(Arnaiz et al., 2001)	20	62 ± 8	12/8	MCI	3 years	45%	75% correct	Logistic regression on ROIs	None	Left temporo-parietal ctx
(Chetelat et al., 2003)	17	70 ± 7	8/9	Amnestic MCI	18 months	41%	100%	SPM99	Global	Right parieto-temporal ctx
(Drzezga et al., 2005)	30	70 ± 8	14/16	MCI (5 amnestic, 25 multiple domain)	16 months	40%	92%, 89%	Neurostat	Not specified	Posterior cingulate ctx
(Anchisi et al., 2005)	48	68 ± 8	25/23	Amnestic MCI	1 year	29%	93%, 82%	SPM99	Global	Bilateral parietal & post. cingulate ctx

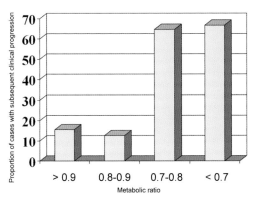

Figure 13–4 Frequency of significant progression (by 3 points on the MMSE scale or more) within 2 years in patients with MCI or beginning dementia (MMSE 24 or higher at entry) is higher in patients with moderate to severe reduction of the metabolic ratio (data from (Herholz et al., 1999)).

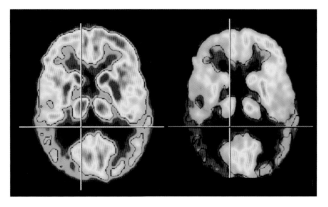

Figure 13–5 Progression of AD: moderate temporo-parietal metabolic impairment at the beginning of clinical dementia (left), which becomes more severe and expands into frontal cortex as the disease progresses (right). Changes are bilateral, but with hemispheric asymmetry that is typically preserved during progression.

hypometabolism. Drzezga (Drzezga et al., 2005) found FDG-PET superior to ApoE4 testing, and Anchisi (Anchisi et al., 2005) demonstrated that a normal FDG-PET in MCI indicates a low chance of progression within 1 year, even if there is a severe memory deficit on neuropsychological testing. Fellgiebel et al. (Fellgiebel et al., 2004) reported a correspondence between elevated tau phosphorylated at threonine 181 protein (p-tau) in cerebrospinal fluid in 14 of 16 MCI patients. At follow-up for 18–24 months four patients converted to dementia, all of whom had pathological FDG-PET and elevated p-tau at entry (Fellgiebel et al., 2007).

The studies cited above typically used reference samples that were based on normal subjects with normal cognition at the time of study. Inevitably, such samples include some subjects who will develop MCI and subsequently AD in the future. Mosconi et al. (Mosconi et al., 2007) demonstrated that using superior normal controls who remained normal for another 4 years increases the sensitivity of FDG-PET to find abnormalities in MCI. In their study all 37 MCI patients studied had significant abnormalities on SSP maps when compared to those superior normal controls. Further research is required to determine the implications of this gain in sensitivity for predicting conversion from MCI to AD. Even at an asymptomatic stage, reduced metabolic rates in temporo-parietal association areas have been observed in individuals at high risk for AD due to family history of AD and possession of the ApoE ε4 allele (Reiman et al., 1996; Small et al., 1995); this abnormality was seen decades before the likely onset of dementia (Reiman et al., 2004). In middle-aged and elderly asymptomatic ApoE ε4-positive individuals temporo-parietal and posterior cingulate rCMRglc declines by about 2% per year (Small et al., 2000). In contrast to these analyses of asymptomatic subject groups, previous studies demonstrating the predictive value of FDG-PET in individual MCI patients used unselected normal controls and will, therefore, have detected only more severe abnormalities. One would, therefore, expect that the degree of abnormality of individuals, when compared to superior controls, will predict the time of dementia-free survival in MCI patients, but that remains to be demonstrated in a prospective study.

Impaired frontal cortical areas appears to be important for progression from MCI to AD. Drzezga et al. (Drzezga et al., 2003) found a significant decline in frontolateral and temporal association cortices associated with that progression. The apolipoprotein ε genotype may also play a role in involving the frontal cortex as carriers of the ApoE4 genotype showed more involvement of anterior cingulate and inferior frontal cortex (Mosconi et al., 2004).

Previous studies in AD have demonstrated that, in general, the severity of metabolic impairments increases not only in the frontal cortex, but in all affected areas while metabolic asymmetries tend to be preserved during progression (Brown et al., 1996; Haxby et al., 1990; Jagust et al., 1988) (Figure 13.5).

Incidence of both MCI and AD heavily depend on patient age while it is less clear whether age has an influence on progression from MCI to AD (DeCarli, 2003; Fleisher et al., 2007). It has also been demonstrated that FDG-PET shows a higher contrast between impairment of association areas and preservation of primary areas and basal ganglia in early onset AD than in late onset AD (Sakamoto et al., 2002). With advancing age, frontal metabolism is reduced most severely in the anterior cingulate and adjacent frontomesial cortex (Pardo et al., 2007). Further studies are needed to evaluate how age interacts with the power of FDG-PET for predicting progression in MCI patients. As yet, studies have mostly looked at patients around age 70 which appears sensible with respect to the higher level of frailty and difficulty of study in older populations, but may not allow accurate predictions for ages 80 and over when the risk for developing AD is highest.

Summary

Assessing regional cerebral glucose metabolism by FDG-PET at resting state is a standard imaging technique to assess cerebral function. An increasing body of evidence indicates that substantial impairment of FDG uptake in temporo-parietal association cortices is a reliable predictor of rapid progression to dementia in MCI patients. Defining target and reference regions, methods for quantitative analysis and other methodological issues that are relevant for using the method in clinical studies are being addressed. Effects of aging, the selection of normal controls, and interaction with age and genetic risk factors are important considerations when designing and interpreting studies.

References

Akiyama, H., Harrop, R., McGeer, P. L., Peppard, R., and McGeer E. G. (1989). Crossed cerebellar and uncrossed basal ganglia and thalamic diaschisis in Alzheimer's disease. *Neurology*, 39: 541–548.

Anchisi, D., Borroni, B., Franceschi, M., Kerrouche, N., Kalbe, E., Beuthien-Beumann, B. et al. (2005). Heterogeneity of brain glucose metabolism in mild cognitive impairment and clinical progression to Alzheimer disease. *Archives of Neurology*, 62: 1728–1733.

Anderson, K. E., Brickman, A. M., Flynn, J., Scarmeas, N., Van Heertum, R., Sackeim, H. et al. (2007). Impairment of nonverbal recognition in Alzheimer disease: A PET O-15 study. *Neurology*, 69: 32–41.

Arnaiz, E., Jelic, V., Almkvist, O., Wahlund, L. O., Winblad, B., Valind, S. et al. (2001). Impaired cerebral glucose metabolism and cognitive functioning predict deterioration in mild cognitive impairment. *Neuroreport*, 12: 851–855.

Ashburner, J. and Friston, K. J. (1999). Nonlinear spatial normalization using basis functions. *Human Brain Mapping*, 7: 254–266.

Aston, J. A., Cunningham, V. J., Asselin, M. C., Hammers, A., Evans, A. C., and Gunn, R. N. (2002). Positron emission tomography partial volume correction: estimation and algorithms. *Journal of cerebral blood flow and metabolism*, 22: 1019–1034.

Berent, S., Giordani, B., Foster, N., Minoshima, S., Lajiness-O'Neill, R., Koeppe, R. et al. (1999). Neuropsychological function and cerebral glucose utilization in isolated memory impairment and Alzheimer's disease. *Journal of Psychiatric Research*, 33: 7–16.

Brown, D. R. P, Hunter, R., Wyper, D. J., Patterson, J., Kelly, R. C., Montaldi, D. et al. (1996). Longitudinal changes in cognitive function and regional cerebral function in Alzheimer's disease: A SPECT blood flow study. *Journal of Psychiatric Research*, 30: 109–126.

Buchsbaum, M. S., Nuechterlein, K. H., Haier, R. J., Wu, J., Sicotte, N., Hazlett, E. et al. (1990). Glucose metabolic rate in normals and schizophrenics during the Continuous Performance Test assessed by positron emission tomography. *The British Journal of Psychiatry*, 156: 216–227.

Chetelat, G., Desgranges, B., de la Sayette, V., Viader, F., Eustache, F., Baron, J. C. (2003). Mild cognitive impairment: Can FDG-PET predict who is to rapidly convert to Alzheimer's disease? *Neurology*, 60: 1374–1377.

de Leon, M. J., Convit, A., Wolf, O. T., Tarshish, C. Y., DeSanti, S., Rusinek, H. et al. (2001). Prediction of cognitive decline in normal elderly subjects with 2-F-18-fluoro-2-deoxy-D-glucose positron-emission tomography (FDG PET). *Proceedings of the National Academy of Sciences of the USA*, 98: 10966–10971.

De Santi, S., de Leon, M. J., Rusinek, H., Convit, A., Tarshish, C. Y., Roche, A. et al. (2001). Hippocampal formation glucose metabolism and volume losses in MCI and AD. *Neurobiology of Aging*, 22: 529–539.

DeCarli C. (2003). Mild cognitive impairment: prevalence, prognosis, aetiology, and treatment. *The Lancet Neurology*, 2: 15–21.

Desgranges, B., Baron, J. C., de, l. S., Petit-Taboue, M. C., Benali, K., Landeau, B. et al. (1998). The neural substrates of memory systems impairment in Alzheimer's disease. A PET study of resting brain glucose utilization. *Brain*, 121: 611–631.

Drzezga, A., Grimmer, T., Riemenschneider, M., Lautenschlager, N., Siebner, H., Alexopoulus, P. et al. (2005). Prediction of individual clinical outcome in MCI by means of genetic assessment and (18)F-FDG PET. *Journal of Nuclear Medicine*, 46: 1625–1632.

Drzezga, A., Lautenschlager, N., Siebner, H., Riemenschneider, M., Willoch, F., Minoshima, S. et al. (2003). Cerebral metabolic changes accompanying conversion of mild cognitive impairment into Alzheimer's disease: A PET follow-up study. *European Journal of Nuclear Medicine and Molecular Imaging*, 30: 1104–1113.

Duara, R., Barker, W. W., Chang, J., Yoshii, F., Loewenstein, D. A., and Pascal, S. (1992). Viability of neocortical function shown in behavioral activation state PET studies in Alzheimer disease. *Journal of Cerebral Blood Flow & Metabolism*, 12: 927–934.

Fellgiebel, A., Scheurich, A., Bartenstein, P., and Muller, M. J. (2007). FDG-PET and CSF phospho-tau for prediction of cognitive decline in mild cognitive impairment. *Psychiatry Research*, 155: 167–171.

Fellgiebel, A., Siessmeier, T., Scheurich, A., Winterer, G., Bartenstein, P., Schmidt, L. G. et al. (2004). Association of elevated phospho-tau levels with Alzheimer-typical 18F-fluoro-2-deoxy-D-glucose positron emission tomography findings in patients with mild cognitive impairment. *Biological Psychiatry*, 56: 279–283.

Fleisher, A. S., Sowell, B. B., Taylor, C., Gamst, A. C., Petersen, R. C. and Thal, L. J., for the Alzheimer's Disease Cooperative S. (2007). Clinical predictors of progression to Alzheimer disease in amnestic mild cognitive impairment. *Neurology*, 68: 1588–1595.

Friston, K. J., Ashburner, J., Poline, J. B., Frith, C. D., Heather, J. D., and Frackowiak, R. S. J. (1995). Spatial registration and normalisation of images. *Human Brain Mapping*, 2: 165–189.

Gholipour, A., Kehtarnavaz, N., Briggs, R., Devous, M., and Gopinath, K. (2007). Brain functional localization: a survey of image registration techniques. *IEEE Transactions on Medical Imaging*, 26: 427–451.

Haxby, J. V., Grady, C. L., Koss, E., Horwitz, B., Heston, L., Schapiro, M. et al. (1990). Longitudinal study of cerebral metabolic asymmetries and associated neuropsychological patterns in early dementia of the Alzheimer type. *Archives of Neurology*, 47: 753–760.

Head, E., Lott, I. T., Patterson, D., Doran, E., and Haier, R. J. (2007). Possible compensatory events in adult Down syndrome brain prior to the development of Alzheimer disease neuropathology: targets for nonpharmacological intervention. *Journal of Alzheimer's Disease*, 11: 61–76.

Heiss, W. D., Pawlik, G., Holthoff, V., Kessler, J., and Szelies, B. (1992). PET correlates of normal and impaired memory functions. [Review]. *Cerebrovascular & Brain Metabolism Reviews*, 4: 1–27.

Herholz, K. (2006). FDG PET: Imaging cerebral glucose metabolism with positron emission tomography. In K. Herholz, D. Perani, C. Morris (eds), *The Dementias—Early Diagnosis and Evaluation* (pp. 229–252). New York: Taylor & Francis.

Herholz, K., Nordberg, A., Salmon, E., Perani, D., Kessler, J., Mielke, R. et al. (1999). Impairment of neocortical metabolism predicts progression in Alzheimer's disease. *Dementia & Geriatric Cognitive Disorders*, 10: 494–504.

Herholz, K., Perani, D., Salmon, E., Franck, G., Fazio, F., Heiss, W. D. et al. (1993). Comparability of FDG PET studies in probable Alzheimer's disease. *Journal of Nuclear Medicine*, 34: 1460–1466.

Herholz, K., Salmon, E., Perani, D., Baron, J. C., Holthoff, V., Frolich, L. et al. (2002). Discrimination between Alzheimer Dementia and Controls by Automated Analysis of Multicenter FDG PET. *Neuroimage*, 17: 302–316.

Higdon, R., Foster, N. L., Koeppe, R. A., DeCarli, C. S., Jagust, W. J., Clark, C. M. et al. (2004). A comparison of classification methods for differentiating fronto-temporal dementia from Alzheimer's disease using FDG-PET imaging. *Statistics in Medicine*, 23: 315–326.

Ishii, K., Willoch, F., Minoshima, S., Drzezga, A., Ficaro, E. P., Cross, D. J. et al. (2001). Statistical brain mapping of 18F-FDG PET in Alzheimer's disease: Validation of anatomic standardization for atrophied brains. *Journal of Nuclear Medicine*, 42: 548–557.

Jagust, W. J., Eberling, J. L., Richardson, B. C., Reed, B. R., Baker, M. G., Nordahl, T. E. et al. (1993). The cortical topography of temporal lobe hypometabolism in early Alzheimer's disease. *Brain Research*, 629: 189–198.

Jagust, W. J., Friedland, R. P., Budinger, T. F., Koss, E., and Ober, B. (1988). Longitudinal studies of regional cerebral metabolism in Alzheimer's disease. *Neurology*, 38: 909–912.

Ji-Ho, C., Anderson, J. M. M., and Mair, B. A. (2007). An accelerated penalized maximum likelihood algorithm for positron emission tomography. *IEEE Transactions on Nuclear Science*, 54: 1648–1659.

Kessler, J., Herholz, K., Grond, M., and Heiss, W. D. (1991). Impaired metabolic activation in Alzheimer's disease: A PET study during continuous visual recognition. *Neuropsychologia*, 29: 229–243.

Kippenhan, J. S., Barker, W. W., Nagel, J., Grady, C., and Duara, R. (1994). Neural-network classification of normal and Alzheimer's disease subjects using high-resolution and low-resolution PET cameras. *Journal of Nuclear Medicine*, 35: 7–15.

Klein, J. C., Herholz, K., Wienhard, K., and Heiss, W.-D. (2008). Cortical Flattening Applied to High-Resolution 18F-FDG PET. *Journal of Nuclear Medicine*, 49: 44–49.

Kwan, L. T., Reed, B. R., Eberling, J. L., Schuff, N., Tanabe, J., Norman, D. et al (1999). Effects of subcortical cerebral infarction on cortical glucose metabolism and cognitive function. *Archives of Neurology*, 56: 809–814.

McNamara, D., Horwitz, B., Grady, C. L. and Rapoport, S. I. (1987). Topographical analysis of glucose metabolism, as measured with positron emission tomography, in dementia of the Alzheimer type: Use of linear histograms. *The International Journal of Neuroscience*, 36: 89–97.

Mevel, K., Desgranges, B., Baron, J. C., Landeau, B., De la Sayette, V., Viader, F. et al. (2007). Detecting hippocampal hypometabolism in Mild Cognitive Impairment using automatic voxel-based approaches. *Neuroimage*, 37: 18–25.

Mielke, R., Herholz, K., Grond, M., Kessler, J., and Heiss, W. D. (1992). Severity of vascular dementia is related to volume of metabolically impaired tissue. *Archives of Neurology*, 49: 909–913.

Minoshima, S., Foster, N. L., and Kuhl, D. E. (1994). Posterior cingulate cortex in Alzheimer's disease [letter]. *Lancet*, 344: 895.

Minoshima, S., Frey, K. A., Foster, N. L., and Kuhl, D. E. (1995a) Preserved pontine glucose metabolism in Alzheimer disease: A reference region for functional brain image (PET) analysis. *Journal of Computer Assisted Tomography*, 19: 541–547.

Minoshima, S., Frey, K. A., Koeppe, R. A., Foster, N. L., and Kuhl, D. E. (1995b) A diagnostic approach in Alzheimer's disease using three-dimensional stereotactic surface projections of fluorine-18-FDG PET. *Journal of Nuclear Medicine*, 36: 1238–1248.

Minoshima, S., Giordani, B., Berent, S., Frey, K. A., Foster, N. L., and Kuhl, D. E. (1997). Metabolic reduction in the posterior cingulate cortex in very early Alzheimer's disease. *Annals of Neurology*, 42: 85–94.

Mosconi, L., De Santi, S., Li, Y., Li, J., Zhan, J., Tsui, W. H. et al. (2006). Visual rating of medial temporal lobe metabolism in mild cognitive impairment and Alzheimer's disease using FDG-PET. *EuropeanJournal of Nuclear Medicine and Molecular Imaging*, 33: 210–221.

Mosconi, L., Perani, D., Sorbi, S., Herholz, K., Holthoff, V., Salmon, E. et al. (2004). Brain metabolism predicts conversion from mild cognitive impairment to dementia in individual carriers of the ApoE E4 allele. *European Journal of Neurology*, 11(Suppl. 2) 27.

Mosconi, L., Tsui, W. H., DeSanti, S., Li, J., Rusinek, H., Convit, A. et al. (2005). Reduced Hippocampal metabolism in MCI and AD: Automated FDG-PET Image Analysis. *Neurology*, 64 1860–1867.

Mosconi, L., Tsui, W. H., Pupi, A., De Santi, S., Drzezga, A., Minoshima, S. et al. (2007). 18F-FDG PET database of longitudinally confirmed healthy elderly individuals improves detection of mild cognitive impairment and Alzheimer's disease. *Journal of Nuclear Medicine*, 48: 1129–1134.

Nestor, P. J., Fryer, T. D., Smielewski, P., and Hodges, J. R. (2003). Limbic hypometabolism in Alzheimer's disease and mild cognitive impairment. *Annals of Neurology*, 54: 343–351.

Ouchi, Y., Nobezawa, S., Okada, H., Yoshikawa, E., Futatsubashi, M., and Kaneko, M. (1998). Altered glucose metabolism in the hippocampal head in memory impairment. *Neurology*, 51: 136–142.

Pardo, J. V., Lee, J. T., Sheikh, S. A., Surerus-Johnson, C., Shah, H., Munch, K. R. et al. (2007). Where the brain grows old: decline in anterior cingulate and medial prefrontal function with normal aging. *NeuroImage*, 35: 1231–1237.

Petersen, R. C. and Morris, J. C. (2005). Mild cognitive impairment as a clinical entity and treatment target. *Archives of Neurology*, 62: 1160–1163; discussion 1167.

Reiman, E. M., Caselli, R. J., Yun, L. S., Chen, K., Bandy, D., Minoshima, S. et al. (1996). Preclinical evidence of Alzheimer's disease in persons homozygous for the epsilon 4 allele for apolipoprotein E. *New England Journal of Medicine*, 334: 752–758.

Reiman, E. M., Chen, K., Alexander, G. E., Caselli, R. J., Bandy, D., Osborne, D. et al. (2004). Functional brain abnormalities in young adults at genetic risk for late-onset Alzheimer's dementia. *Proceedings of the National Academy of Sciences of the United States of America*, 101: 284–289.

Sakamoto, S., Ishii, K., Sasaki, M., Hosaka, K., Mori, T., Matsui, M. et al. (2002). Differences in cerebral metabolic impairment between early and late onset types of Alzheimer's disease. *Journal of the Neurological Sciences*, 200: 27–32.

Salmon, E., Kerrouche, N., Perani, D., Lekeu, F., Holthoff, V., Beuthien-Baumann, B. et al. (2009). On the multivariate nature of brain metabolic impairment in Alzheimer's disease. *Neurobiology of Aging*, 30: 186–197.

Sayeed, A., Petrou, M., Spyrou, N., Kadyrov, A., and Spinks, T. (2002). Diagnostic features of Alzheimer's disease extracted from PET sinograms. *Physics in Medicine and Biology*, 47: 137–148.

Small, G. W., Ercoli, L. M., Silverman, D. H., Huang, S. C., Komo, S., Bookheimer, S. Y. et al. (2000). Cerebral metabolic and cognitive decline in persons at genetic risk for Alzheimer's disease. *Proceedings of the National Academy of Sciences of the United States of America*, 97: 6037–6042.

Small, G. W., Mazziotta, J. C., Collins, M. T., Baxter, L. R., Phelps, M. E., Mandelkern, M. A. et al. (1995). Apolipoprotein E type 4 allele and cerebral glucose metabolism in relatives at risk for familial Alzheimer disease. *The Journal of the American Medical Association*, 273: 942–947.

Wienhard, K., Pawlik, G., Herholz, K., Wagner, R. and Heiss, W. D. (1985). Estimation of local cerebral glucose utilization by positron emission tomography of [18F]2-fluoro-2-deoxy-D-glucose: a critical appraisal of optimization procedures. *Journal of Cerebral Blood Flow & Metabolism*, 5: 115–125.

Xu, G., Antuono, P. G., Jones, J., Xu, Y., Wu, G., Ward, D. et al. (2007). Perfusion fMRI detects deficits in regional CBF during memory-encoding tasks in MCI subjects. *Neurology*, 69: 1650–1656.

Amyloid Imaging and (What is "Normal"?) Aging

William E. Klunk and Chester A. Mathis

Introduction

One could argue that the defining moment for the discovery of Alzheimer's disease (AD) was when Alois Alzheimer, the German psychiatrist with a penchant for relating behavioral syndromes to brain pathology, first linked the profound dementia of his 51-year-old patient, Auguste D., to the presence of a specific pathology in her brain. He described his findings as "tangled bundle[s] of fibrils" and "miliary foci . . . of a peculiar substance" (Alzheimer, 1907). With this description of neurofibrillary tangles and amyloid-beta (Aβ) plaques (the miliary foci), the basis for the characteristic neuropathology that still defines AD 100 years later was born. In an important way, this defining moment in the history of AD was based on imaging plaques and tangles—albeit postmortem imaging performed with a microscope. It is not surprising, then, that when people think of amyloid imaging, there is usually an association with clinical AD. This association is even more understandable given the fact that the diagnosis of AD is usually only verified as "definite AD" at autopsy when a sufficient burden of amyloid plaques alone (Khachaturian, 1985) and CERAD criteria (Mirra et al., 1991), or plaques accompanied by neurofibrillary tangles (NIA/Reagan_Workgroup, 1997) can be demonstrated and associated with a clinical dementia.

However, it should be noted that, in its original context, AD was not a disease of the aged, but was a "presenile" dementia. Alzheimer's mentor, the eminent psychiatrist Emil Kraepelin, went to some lengths to distinguish the disease described by Alzheimer from senile dementia and gave this presenile dementia the eponym of "Alzheimer's disease" (Kraepelin, 1910). It was another psychiatrist before Alzheimer, the Austrian Emil Redlich, who in 1898 was the first to describe "senile" plaques in the brains of two patients with senile dementia (Redlich, 1898). Redlich called these plaques "miliary sclerosis." Thus, the late-onset form of dementia that we now most commonly associate with the term "Alzheimer's disease," might be more correctly called "Redlich's disease." Unfortunately for Redlich, he had no Kraepelin, so Redlich's name is ascribed to "Redlich's syndrome," a rare form of abortive disseminated encephalomyelitis with lesions distributed throughout the brain and the spinal cord (Redlich, 1929). Shortly after the seminal paper by Alzheimer, Oskar Fischer, working under Pick at the German Psychiatric Clinic in Prague, described "miliary necrosis with glandular proliferation of neurofibrils" as "a common alteration of the cortex" in 12 of 16 patients with senile dementia (Fischer, 1907, 1910). Thus, the association of senile dementia with plaques and tangles also was firmly established.

Given the above, it is understandable why amyloid imaging would be associated with AD, but a case can be made that the concept of amyloid imaging should be at least as closely associated with (cognitively normal) aging as it is with dementia. For one thing, amyloid plaques were not originally discovered in the context of dementia. Even before Redlich, plaques were first described in 1892 by the French pathologist Paul Blocq and the Rumanian neurologist Gheorghe Marinescu (while both were working under Charcot) in the postmortem brain of an elderly patient with epilepsy (Blocq and Marinescu, 1892). One hundred and two years later, MacKenzie and Miller (1994) clarified this finding and found amyloid plaques in 10% of nondemented epileptic patients aged 36 to 61 years and documented that the presence of plaques "correlated positively with patient age." The density and distribution of plaques observed by MacKenzie and Miller in nondemented epileptics was the same as that seen in nonepileptic, nondemented individuals, although the age-related incidence of plaques was significantly greater in the epileptics. Thus, the original description of plaques in Blocq and Marinescu's elderly epileptic was in the context of aging, not dementia. It is likely that very few cognitively normal people over the age of 65 came to autopsy in the early 1900s, and that it would be even more unlikely that they would be examined with the specialized histologic stains (postmortem imaging agents) used by Blocq, Redlich, and Alzheimer to visualize amyloid plaques. Had cognitively normal individuals over the age of 65 been frequently studied, it is likely that the association of amyloid plaques with dementia would have been clouded by the appearance of plaques in the nondemented elderly as well.

For example, consider a hypothetical population—approximated from statistics complied by the National Alzheimer's Association (http://www.alz.org/national/documents/Report_2007FactsAndfigures.pdf)—that has a prevalence of AD of ~10% at age 75 and ~20% at age 80 and a maximum prevalence of ~50% (blue squares in Figure 14.1a). To simplify this exercise, we will assume that amyloid pathology begins about 10 years before cognitive symptoms and is necessary and sufficient to cause AD. Of course, the time between the onset of amyloid deposition and the onset of clinical dementia will vary from person to person and the appearance of symptoms will be greatly impacted by the coexistance of other pathologies such as infarcts or Lewy body pathology

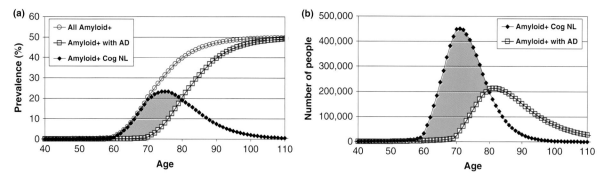

Figure 14–1 Hypothetical population curves showing the prevalence (a) and number of people (b) with amyloid deposition who are either cognitively normal (filled diamonds), have AD (open squares) or a combination of both cognitively normal people and AD patients with amyloid deposition (open circles). The green areas indicate the ages where the prevalence (a) or number of people (b) who are cognitively normal with amyloid is greater than the prevalence or number of people with AD.

(Schneider et al., 2007). We will also ignore the possibility that many people will pass through a period of time when they will carry a diagnosis of mild cognitive impairment (MCI; see below) between their cognitively normal stage and their diagnosis of AD. Although this MCI stage is very important, it extensively complicates this analysis without changing the conclusions. Furthermore, we assume that the death rate of people with amyloid deposits is the same as those without. From this, one could calculate an expected prevalence of all people (whether cognitively normal or with AD) with amyloid-positive scans by simply drawing a new curve shifted 10 years earlier. This prevalence of all amyloid-positive scans would be ~10% at age 65 and ~20% at age 70 in this hypothetical population (red circles in Figure 14.1a). If one then subtracts the prevalence of AD from the total prevalence of amyloid-positive scans, one can get a rough approximation of the prevalence of amyloid-positive scans among individuals without AD in this population. The black diamonds in Figure 14.1a show that we would predict a biphasic distribution of cognitively normal people with amyloid-positive scans that has a peak of ~20% prevalence near age 75. Because there are significantly more people alive during the younger age range, we need to factor in census figures to fully appreciate the impact of this increased prevalence. Using an estimate of the U.S. population across these ages, we can roughly estimate the total number of AD patients (blue squares in Figure 14.1b) and the total number of cognitively normal people with amyloid-positive scans (black diamonds in Figure 14.1b).

This rough analysis suggests that during an age span of almost 20 years from about 60–80 there will be *significantly more cognitively normal individuals with amyloid-positive scans than there are AD patients with amyloid-positive scans*. In fact, the graph in Figure 14.1a predicts that from age ~65–75, the likelihood of finding an amyloid-positive person without AD (10–20% prevalence) will be much higher than the likelihood of finding someone who has AD (<1%–10% prevalence). The graph in Figure 14.1b predicts that the number of cognitively normal people in the U.S. population who are amyloid-positive (~7 000 000) should be much higher than the number of AD patients (~4 500 000). These graphs also predict that by age 90, it will be relatively rare to find a person who is amyloid-positive and cognitively normal, because most people will have converted to clinical AD by this time. This hypothetical model is not intended to be a rigorous epidemiological treatment of the available data and surely is oversimplified. However, the general points about a biphasic distribution of amyloid-positive people without AD and the fact that the size of this amyloid-positive/

cognitively-normal population can rival or exceed the size of the population with AD are likely to withstand more rigorous evaluations. The point to be made is that amyloid imaging is not a tool solely or even primarily for the study of AD, but it may have its most important application to the study of prodromal phases of AD when individuals are still cognitively normal.

In this chapter, we will discuss the application of amyloid imaging to normal aging, MCI, and dementia. We will speculate on the potential strengths and limitations for a variety of uses of amyloid imaging, including clinical diagnosis, preclinical screening, disease monitoring, and surrogate measures of therapeutic agents. First, we will describe the background in which these uses must be judged. This will include the definition of amyloid and the conceptual basis for the design and quantification of amyloid imaging agents as well as the preclinical and postmortem validation of these agents.

Rationale for Studying Amyloid Deposition

Amyloid Deposition in AD and MCI

Given the role that amyloid deposits play in the diagnosis of AD (Khachaturian, 1985; Mirra et al., 1991; NIA/Reagan_Workgroup, 1997), it is clear why one would study amyloid deposition in AD or MCI. MCI is a condition closely related to AD, being characterized by either isolated memory impairment or impairment in several cognitive domains, but not of sufficient severity to meet diagnostic criteria for AD (Petersen et al., 2001). Like AD, MCI is very common and the prevalence increases with age. In community samples, over 19% of subjects ages 65–75 and over 29% of subjects over age 85 were found to meet the criteria for MCI (Lopez et al., 2003). MCI patients convert to AD at a rate of about 10%–15% per year (Larrieu et al., 2002) and MCI may define a prodromal phase of AD (Morris and Price, 2001; Morris et al., 2001; Petersen et al., 2001). Clearly, in vivo identification of amyloid deposition in AD and MCI has important implications for early diagnosis. Perhaps more importantly, the ability to follow an in vivo surrogate marker of amyloid deposition will be critical to the timely development of the new anti-amyloid therapies.

Amyloid Deposition in Normal Aging

The rationale for studying amyloid deposition during normal aging, although perhaps less obvious, is equally compelling. Sometimes it is clearer to use the term "clinically unimpaired" rather than "normal" when referring to elderly individuals who do not meet clinical criteria for either MCI or AD but, as a group, have a broader range of cognitive performance than a group of 20-year-olds. That is, this broad range may not be entirely "normal." There are at least three reasons to relate cognition and amyloid deposition in the clinically unimpaired elderly: (1) definition of the prevalence of amyloid in the clinically unimpaired elderly; (2) determination of whether the greater variability of cognitive performance in the clinically unimpaired elderly (compared to the young) is explained by the presence or absence of amyloid deposition; and (3) assessment of whether clinically unimpaired individuals with substantial amyloid deposition will invariably progress to clinical dementia.

Studies have attempted to address the first two questions with postmortem assessment of amyloid deposition, but there are obvious weaknesses to this approach. First, it is difficult to acquire cognitive testing close to the time of death—when the amyloid assessment is made. The time period between cognitive testing and death can vary by over a year in some studies. Even cognitive testing occurring very close to the time of death is problematic, since any cognitive impairment present could be due to effects of the disease that led to the individual's death. Second, there is an additional selection bias added by the decision to agree to an autopsy. This means that not all of the cognitively assessed group will be represented in the amyloid assessment. Finally, many of these studies involve cognitive testing that was not performed for the specific purposes of the study, but was retrospectively gathered to the best degree possible. Much of the cognitive data available comes from cognitive screening tests such as the Mini-Mental State Exam (MMSE) (Folstein, Folstein, and McHugh, 1975) and not measures that examine the specific components of cognition thought to be particularly affected by aging (e.g., information processing speed, working memory, inhibitory efficiency). Even when longitudinal data on cognitive performance are available (e.g., Davis et al., 1999; Green, Kaye, and Ball, 2000), it is not possible to link an age-related decrease in cognitive performance to an increase in amyloid load (i.e., to establish causality), because amyloid load could only be determined at one time point—after death. All of these factors have hindered attempts to determine the role that amyloid deposition may play in the various cognitive decrements found in the "normal" old. The availability of a technique (i.e., amyloid imaging) that can measure the amyloid load at multiple time points in living individuals who are not close to death is thus a major advantage.

Prevalence and Degree of Amyloid Deposition in Normal Aging

The first reason to study in vivo amyloid deposition in normal aging is to define the prevalence of amyloid deposition in a normal elderly population. Dickson et al. (1992) coined the term "pathological aging" to describe the presence of cerebral amyloid deposition in the nondemented elderly. The prevalence of this pathological aging is extremely difficult to obtain with an autopsy study because of the reasons noted above. Preliminary findings from the "Nun Study" have been reported and suggest that the prevalence of amyloid in the clinically unimpaired elderly may be on the order of 40%, and that the presence of amyloid is correlated with lower scores on several neuropsychological tests of memory function (Wolf et al., 1999). The ability to assess amyloid deposition in living subjects avoids the above difficulties by: (1) allowing precise and detailed definition of cognitive function in healthy individuals within days of the assessment of amyloid deposition, and (2) not requiring a subsequent decision for autopsy which may add a selection bias over and above that incurred in the selection of the group to be cognitively tested.

Price and Morris (1999) have compiled one of the most extensively evaluated groups of clinically unimpaired and very mildly demented subjects clinically evaluated within a year before their death. Very similar findings have been reported by Haroutunian et al. (1998). These studies provide evidence that substantial amyloid deposition occurs in "normal aging." Price and Morris reported the neuropathological findings in 39 clinically unimpaired elderly subjects ages 51–93 and 15 very mildly demented subjects ages 75–95 and compared these to severely demented AD cases. Price and Morris found that all 13 clinically unimpaired cases under the age of 75 had no plaques, whether examined with a sensitive modification of the Bielschowsky stain or with immunohistochemical stains for Aβ. The 26 clinically unimpaired cases over age 75 fell into three categories, unrelated to age (i.e., amyloid deposition did not increase with age in this group). In 8 of the 26 cases (31%), ages 75–88, no plaques could be detected in any region. In 11 cases (42%), ages 75–92, there were a very low number of plaques ($\sim$2/mm^2), all of which were diffuse plaques. In 7 of 26 (27%) clinically unimpaired cases, ages 75–93, there were more numerous plaques, and many were neuritic. Thus 18/26 (69%) cases over age 75 had some evidence of amyloid deposition and over 25% had amyloid deposition typical of AD. Very mildly demented cases showed numbers of plaques that were surprisingly very similar to severely demented AD cases, although the type of plaques changed so that most plaques in severely demented cases were neuritic or cored. A corollary to the observation that patients at the threshold for clinical detection of AD (CDR = 0.5) already have extensive neuropathological changes is the hypothesis that the pathological process of AD must begin significantly before any cognitive change can be clinically detected. Thus Price and Morris suspect that the seven clinically unimpaired cases with numerous plaques may have been preclinical AD (Morris et al., 1996; Price and Morris, 1999). The availability of in vivo amyloid imaging probes such as those described in this chapter would make possible longitudinal imaging studies to test this hypothesis.

Further evidence for preclinical amyloid deposition comes from the study of Down syndrome patients. Having three copies of the Aβ precursor protein gene on chromosome 21, all Down syndrome patients develop amyloid pathology by their 30s or 40s and a large percentage show clinical dementia. Although the time course of amyloid deposition in AD is not known, evidence gained through postmortem study of Down syndrome suggests that amyloid deposition begins over a decade prior to the clinical symptoms of dementia (Hyman, 1992; Hyman, et al., 1995).

Relationship of Age-Related Cognitive Performance Decline to Amyloid Deposition

Identification of amyloid in the normal elderly can address an important question regarding whether the greater variability of cognitive performance in the clinically unimpaired elderly (compared to the young) is explained by the presence or absence of amyloid deposition, as is suggested by some postmortem studies (Wolf et al., 1999). With increasing age, cognitive performance tends to decline in persons who have no obvious neurologic or psychiatric illness—the "normal" old. However, the amount of age-related cognitive performance decline is not uniform across individuals, but rather, there is substantial intersubject variability (Morse, 1993; Rabbitt, 1993), particularly at the lower end of the performance range. This suggests that some older persons experience much greater "subclinical" age-related cognitive dysfunction than do others. This rise in intersubject variability could reflect the increased prevalence in the older population of individuals carrying significant cerebral amyloid loads. Even clinically unimpaired individuals have been shown to have a substantial number of amyloid plaques within their brain (Goldman et al., 2001; Hulette et al., 1998). The role that amyloid plays in producing age-related cognitive impairment in clinically unimpaired older persons is controversial. It is not clear that the amyloid found at autopsy in clinically unimpaired individuals has any relationship to the cognitive performance of these individuals. The few studies that have examined the relation of cognitive performance to the post-mortem presence of amyloid in nondemented older individuals have produced conflicting conclusions. Several studies have used pathological criteria to characterize small groups of clinically unimpaired individuals as having pathologically normal brains or brains with signs of preclinical AD (i.e., "pathological aging" with increased number of diffuse and neuritic plaques and neurofibrillary tangles). Hulette et al. (1998) found that neuritic plaques were relatively common in clinically unimpaired individuals, and those who had them showed a tendency to perform more poorly than those with normal brains on measures of memory and "executive" function. Green, Kaye, and Ball (2000) found that among 19 very old nondemented individuals who came to autopsy, those who had shown some cognitive performance decline (but not dementia) prior to death showed pathological signs of AD including plaques, while those whose cognitive status remained stable did not. In contrast, Goldman et al. (2001) and Davis et al. (1999) found no evidence that nondemented individuals with increased numbers of plaques showed poorer performance or a faster decline in performance than did individuals without plaques.

Information about the cognitive effects of amyloid is important to our understanding of the cognitive effects of the normal aging process. It is possible that the research studies that have contributed to our present knowledge of the cognitive changes associated with normal aging have within their older samples individuals with a substantial amyloid burden. Thus, our understanding of both the nature and severity of the cognitive decrements associated with normal aging may be distorted by the effects of a pathological accumulation of amyloid in a subset of the older population. If it turns out that part of the cognitive impairment currently thought to be intrinsic to normal aging is actually the result of amyloid deposition, this raises the question as to the nature and amount of cognitive dysfunction present in older individuals without elevated amyloid levels. The availability of a biological marker for amyloid (e.g., PET tracers) allows this question to be directly examined. It also makes possible extensive longitudinal cognitive testing to relate to serial measures of amyloid. This will be crucial for examining whether a longitudinal increase in amyloid can eventually lead to MCI or AD. If anti-amyloid therapies do become clinically available, we will need to determine if clinically unimpaired individuals with evidence of a progressive amyloid deposition should be identified and treated.

Do Clinically Unimpaired Individuals with Amyloid Deposition Always Progress to Dementia?

The third reason for studying amyloid deposition in the "normal" elderly is that we do not yet know whether all those who have substantial amyloid deposition without the clinical symptoms of AD will eventually develop clinical AD if they survive for a reasonable period of time (e.g., 10 years). Some investigators have stated that amyloid deposition is responsible for the cognitive impairments seen in AD and that any older individuals with substantial amounts of brain amyloid, even if they presently score in the normal range on cognitive tasks, have preclinical AD (Morris and Price, 2001; Morris et al., 1996, 2001). While there is evidence to support this notion, until now we have not had a tool that would allow the longitudinal studies necessary to effectively test this hypothesis.

Amyloid and the Pathology of AD

The Biochemical Nature of Amyloid

It is important to have a basic understanding of the biochemical nature of the amyloid fibril in order to appreciate the development of the tools for imaging the pathology of AD. Among AD researchers, "amyloid" is most often equated with the Aβ protein, but amyloid is a much more general term. The term amyloid (from the Greek amylon, meaning starch) refers to the "starch-like" staining properties of this substance. This notion is, in turn, derived from Virchow's term, "Cellulose-Frage" used when describing the substance he stained in peripheral tissues with iodine (commonly used to stain cellulose) (Virchow, 1854). Amyloid deposits were soon understood to be composed mainly of protein (Friedreich and Kekulé, 1859), and later shown to exist in a cross beta-sheet fibril conformation (for a review, see Uversky et al. [1999]). All beta-sheet fibrils consist of a regular, repeating, linear array of peptide backbones spaced 4.76 Å apart (Pauling and Corey, 1951). It is this beta-sheet fibrillar nature that forms the structural basis for the interaction of histologic dyes that bind to amyloid deposits in general, without specificity for any particular amyloid protein (Glenner, Eanes, and Page, 1972). Several models have been proposed to explain this binding in molecular terms (Carter and Chou, 1998; Klunk, Pettegrew, and Abraham, 1989; Krebs, Bromley, and Donald, 2005). Beta-sheet specificity appears to be a property of all known in vivo imaging probes for amyloid. The specificity for AD comes from the fact that extensive accumulation of amyloid is largely due to the massive buildup of Aβ. However, AD is often a triple amyloidosis comprised not only of large quantities of Aβ amyloid, but also lesser quantities of amyloid in the form of hyperphosphorylated tau in neurofibrillary tangles and alpha-synuclein in the form of Lewy bodies (Trojanowski and Mattson, 2003). In most cases of AD, the Aβ amyloid component far outweighs the other amyloid components, and it may be that the particular probes used bind inherently better to Aβ or that Aβ presents more available binding sites (Klunk et al., 2003).

Aβ and the Pathophysiology and Neuropathology of AD

Definitive diagnosis of AD relies on the demonstration of amyloid plaques and neurofibrillary tangles at autopsy (Figure 14.2) (Mirra et al., 1991). Amyloid plaques are composed of the 40–42 amino acid–long Aβ peptide (Iwatsubo et al., 1994). Neurofibrillary tangles are mainly composed of a hyperphosphorylated form of the microtubule-associated protein, tau (Goedert, 1993). Aβ also can be found deposited around small arterioles in the form of cerebrovascular amyloid (Roher et al., 1993). Plaques occur earliest in the neocortex, where they are relatively evenly distributed (Thal et al., 2002). Tangles appear first in limbic areas such as the transentorhinal cortex and progress in a predictable topographic pattern to the neocortex (Braak and Braak, 1991).

A growing consensus points to deposition of Aβ plaques as a central event in the pathogenesis of AD. The single most important

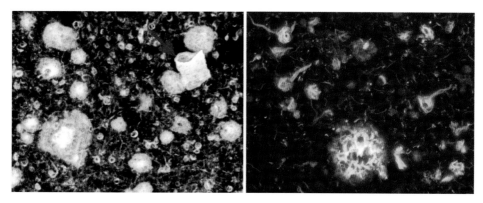

Figure 14–2 (*Left*) Postmortem AD brain tissue stained with the fluorescent Congo red derivative and amyloid fibril stain, X-34(Ikonomovic et al., 2006b; Styren et al., 2000) in frontal cortex (50 μm frozen section) showing multiple Aβ plaques, neurofibrillary tangles, and cerebrovascular amyloid (arrow shows vessel passing obliquely through the section. (*Right*) Entorhinal cortex (8 μm paraffin section) showing multiple tangles and a neuritic plaque.

piece of evidence for this "amyloid cascade hypothesis" of AD is the demonstration that several mutations in the Aβ precursor protein (APP) gene on chromosome 21 cause early onset AD (Hardy and Higgins, 1992). While a very small number of families are affected with this form of AD, the disease is phenotypically very similar to the more common sporadic form of AD, save only for its early age of onset (Lippa et al., 1996). Further genetic support for the amyloid cascade hypothesis comes from the finding that the most common form of autosomal dominant AD, the chromosome 14 mutations, is caused by mutations in the presenilin-1 gene which codes for a protein strongly implicated to be an essential component of the "gamma-secretase" enzyme complex responsible for the C-terminal cleavage of Aβ from its precursor, APP (Xia et al., 2000). In contrast, no mutation in the tau protein has been shown to cause AD. Instead, mutations in tau (chromosome 17) are linked to frontotemporal dementia with Parkinsonism (Goedert, Crowther, and Spillantini, 1998)

It is important to recognize that a sizable body of work existed on the regional distribution of Aβ plaques in postmortem tissue well before the first attempts to image amyloid in vivo. Several investigators, including Mann (1985), Arnold et al. (1991), and Braak and Braak (1997), have performed extensive postmortem studies in efforts to define the cross-sectional, regional distribution and to gain insight into the temporal progression of Aβ plaque deposition in AD. Arnold et al. (1991) mapped the distribution of neurofibrillary tangles and neuritic plaques (amyloid plaques surrounded by dystrophic neurites) in the brains of patients with AD. Compared to neurofibrillary tangles, neuritic plaques were, in general, more evenly distributed throughout the cortex, with the exception of notably fewer neuritic plaques in limbic periallocortex and allocortex (the areas with greatest neurofibrillary tangle density). The cerebellum is notably free of neuritic plaques in AD, although diffuse amyloid deposits which do not label with fibrillar dyes such as Congo red are commonly observed in the cerebellum (Joachim, Morris, and Selkoe, 1989; Yamaguchi et al., 1989).

Braak and colleagues are well known for their neurofibrillary tangle staging system, but they have done extensive work on plaque pathology as well (Braak and Braak, 1997; Thal et al., 2000, 2002). The work of Braak and colleagues can be separted into: (1) a study of Aβ deposition across the entire brain, midbrain, pons, and medulla (Thal et al., 2002); (2) a study of the stages of Aβ deposition across the neocortex (Braak and Braak, 1997); and (3) a detailed study of the stages of Aβ deposition in the temporal lobe

(Thal et al., 2000) (Figure 14.3). Thal et al. (2002) described five "phases" of amyloid plaque deposition across the entire brain. Of course, these postmortem studies are cross-sectional and the temporal pattern of deposition is inferred from patterns of deposition observed in brains with different levels of involvement. For example, if Aβ deposition in region-X is always present when there is deposition in region-Y, but Aβ deposition in region-X can be found in the absence of plaques in region-Y, then it is presumed that deposition in region-X temporally precedes that in region-Y.

Phase-1 is the neocortical phase in which Aβ deposits are found exclusively in the neocortex (Figure 14.3). Although plaques are typically widely distributed in the frontal, parietal, temporal, or occipital neocortex in Phase-1, they typically appear first in the basal neocortex, most frequently in poorly myelinated areas of the anterior temporal and inferior frontal cortex. Braak and Braak (1997) referred to this basal frontotemporal stage as "Stage-A". Braak's group also separately detailed the sequence of Aβ deposits in the temporal lobe (TL) (Thal et al., 2000). In Phase-1, temporal lobe plaques are confined to the basal lateral temporal neocortex (TL-1 stage).

In Phase-2, Aβ deposits can be found in allocortical brain regions including entorhinal cortex, CA1, and the insular cortex (corresponding to the TL-2 stage). Plaques are sometimes seen in the amygdala, the cingulate gyrus, the presubicular region, and the molecular layer of the fascia dentata; and small patches of subpial band-like amyloid appear in the frontal, parietal, temporal, and occipital neocortex (overlapping with the TL-3 stage). All other areas do not show Aβ in this phase.

In Phase-3, Aβ plaques are seen in subcortical regions, including the caudate, putamen, claustrum, basal forebrain nuclei, substantia inominata, thalamus, hypothalamus, lateral habenular nucleus, and white matter just beneath the cortex. In the TL-3 stage, Aβ deposits are found in the molecular layer of the fascia dentata, and bandlike Aβ-deposits occur in the subpial portion of the molecular layer of both the entorhinal region and the temporal neocortex. In addition, confluent lake-like Aβ-deposits appear in the parvopyramidal layer of the presubicular region.

In Phase-4, Aβ deposits can be found in the inferior olivary nucleus, the reticular formation of the medulla oblongata, the substantia nigra, CA4, the central gray of the midbrain, the colliculi superiores and inferiores, and the red nucleus. However, within the inferior olivary nucleus, the reticular formation of the pons and

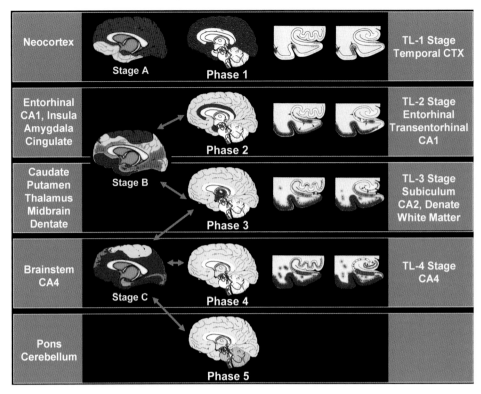

Figure 14–3   Hypothetical sequence of amyloid plaque deposition in the brain. Phases 1–5 shown in the center are based on Thal et al. (2002). Note that at each sequential phase, the new areas of deposition are highlighted in red or pink and previously involved areas are shown cumulatively in yellow. Neocortical stages A-C on the left are based on Braak and Braak (1997). Plaques loads are indicated on a rainbow scale with red indicating the heaviest deposition. Medial temporal lobe stages (TL-1 to TL-4) on the right are shown based on Thal et al. (2000). Deposition is indicated by the density of the red color in the basolateral temporal neocortex, transentorhinal and entorhinal regions, and in the hippocampus at the levels of the anterior entorhinal region (left slice) and of the lateral geniculate body (right slice).

medulla oblongata, and the red nucleus, there are often only one to three plaques in the entire anatomic structure. The TL-4 stage parallels Phase-4 and plaques can be found in CA4 in addition to the other temporal areas listed above.

In Phase-5, Aβ deposits can be found in the reticular formation of the pons, the pontine nuclei, the central and dorsal raphe nuclei, the locus coeruleus, the parabrachial nuclei, the dorsal tegmental nucleus, the reticulotegmental nucleus of the pons, and the cerebellum. In the cerebellum, Aβ most frequently occurs in the molecular layer, and Aβ deposits were never found in the dentate nucleus or other cerebellar nuclei. These cerebellar deposits are very rarely fibrillar and do not typically stain with Congo red or thioflavin-S (Joachim, Morris, and Selkoe, 1989; Yamaguchi et al., 1989).

Progression of neocortical amyloid deposits from Stage-A to Stage-B appears to occur in parallel to Phases-2 and -3. Further progression in the neocortex to Stage-C parallels Phases 3–5.

It should be emphasized that the postmortem models of amyloid deposition discussed above were completed before, and therefore were not influenced by, any in vivo amyloid imaging studies. The patterns described form a basis against which to judge the performance of amyloid imaging tracers. However, several important points that stem from this impressive body of neuropathological data often go unrecognized. First, Aβ deposition starts in the neocortex, not in the medial portions of the temporal lobe. Second, the hippocampus contains smaller amounts of fibrillar Aβ deposits than the surrounding cortical areas, even at later stages. Third, striatal Aβ deposition occurs in 80% of Phase-3 cases and 100% of Phase-4 and Phase-5 cases (Thal et al., 2002). Since *all* of the AD

cases included in the Thal et al. study were in Phases 3–5, this means nearly all their AD cases had striatal amyloid deposition. Extensive amyloid deposition has been reported to occur in the striatum of virtually all AD patients in several prior studies as well. (Braak and Braak, 1990; Brilliant et al., 1997; Suenaga et al., 1990; Wolf et al., 1999). Striatal plaque deposition appears to occur early in the progression of AD pathology and coincides with neocortical pathology and cognitive changes (Wolf et al., 1999). While neuritic elements have been described in ventral striatum (Suenaga et al., 1990), most striatal Aβ deposits are not associated with dystrophic neurites (Brilliant et al., 1992; Suenaga et al., 1990). Despite this poorly understood absence of neuritic changes in the striatum, striatal plaques appear to be fibrillar, as evidenced by the fact that they are stained well by fibril-specific dyes such as the Congo red derivative X-34 (Klunk et al., 2007) and the thioflavin-T derivative 6-CN-BTA-1 (Figure 14.4) (Mathis et al., 2003).

Braak and colleagues proposed a sequential deposition of Aβ, but did not quantify the Aβ load in the various brain areas. Quantification is best done biochemically with enzyme-linked immunosorbant assay (ELISA). Naslund et al. (2000) have used Aβ ELISA analyses to show that frontal cortex contains significantly more Aβ than either the temporal or parietal cortex at CDR stages 0.5–2. Thus the frontal cortex is one of the earliest sites of brain Aβ deposition and typically has the highest concentration of insoluble Aβ deposits of any brain area. The most medial portions of the temporal lobe, such as the hippocampus, typically show lower levels of Aβ deposition, and these occur later than those observed in the neocortex (Braak and Braak, 1997).

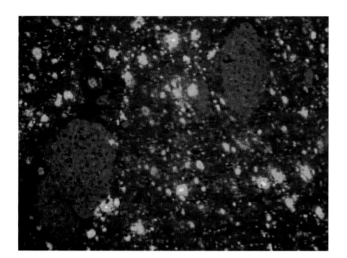

Figure 14–4 Paraffin section from the caudate from an AD brain showing diffuse and compact/cored plaques extensively stained by a highly fluorescent derivative of thioflavin-T, 6-CN-BTA-1.

Principles of Design for Brain Imaging Agents

Considering the description of amyloid given above, the concept of imaging the pathology of AD is really a very simple one: start with a histological dye known to bind specifically to amyloid and chemically modify it so that it: (1) rapidly crosses the blood-brain barrier in large amounts; (2) has high binding affinity and specificity for amyloid; and (3) clears rapidly and completely from all non-amyloid components of the brain (Figure 14.5). There are other more detailed criteria as well, and these have been reviewed

elsewhere (Mathis et al., 2003; Mathis, Wang, and Klunk, 2004a), but a more basic description will be provided here.

Brain Entry

There are certain basic limitations that are inherent to any positron emission tomography (PET) study. The first is that there is a maximum amount of radioactivity that can safely be injected into a human. With appropriate safety margins built in, this means the injected dose of a C-11- or F-18-labeled tracer is typically in the range of 5–20 millicuries (185–740 MBq) of radioactivity. Since the tracer should be highly radioactive (i.e., high specific activity), this dose can be achieved by injecting negligible mass amounts of the "tracer preparation" (<10 µg). Because it is impossible to exclude all sources of the naturally abundant, nonradioactive isotopes (e.g., carbon-12 or fluorine-19) from the radiosynthesis, the tracer preparation is actually a combination of small amounts of the radioactive compound (e.g., <0.1% C-11-tracer) along with much larger amounts of nonradioactive, but otherwise chemically identical, compound (e.g., >99.9% ^{12}C-tracer). Therefore, minimizing the nonradioactive component of the tracer preparation is the key issue for increasing the specific activity and decreasing the mass of injected "tracer preparation." The second limitation is that PET scanner cameras can only detect ~2%–3% of the total radioactivity in their field-of-view (e.g., the brain). Taken together, this means that a certain minimum percentage of injected tracer must enter the brain in order for there to be a detectable signal. This amount can be expressed as the percent injected dose (%ID) per gram of brain (g_{br}) normalized to the total body weight in grams (g_{tot}), or %ID/(g_{br}/g_{tot}). The lower limit of %ID/(g_{br}/g_{tot}) for commonly used radiotracers is 100. Equivalent terms exist in the literature, including percent injected dose index or %IDI, which also has a lower limit of 100 (Klunk

Figure 14–5 Model of tracer entry into the CNS. The physical properties of tracers can cause them to be too large (large red dots), too hydrophilic (blue dots), or too charged (black dots with "±" sign). These tracers traverse the brain vasculature without entering the actual brain parenchyma because they are blocked by the blood-brain barrier (dashed line). Small, neutral, moderately lipophilic compounds (small red dots) cross the blood-brain barrier to different degrees and can interact with target (i.e., amyloid) binding sites. With continuous brain perfusion, unbound tracer should be washed efficiently out of the brain, leaving more bound tracer than free or nonspecifically bound tracer (bottom right). If the affinity of the tracer is poor, the bound tracer can be washed out of the brain too quickly and no detectable target-related signal remains (bottom center). If the tracer itself nonspecifically sticks to non-target binding sites, or if the tracer is metabolized into a derivative that does not wash out of the brain (yellow triangles), then a high nonspecific background can obscure the specific target-related signal (bottom left).

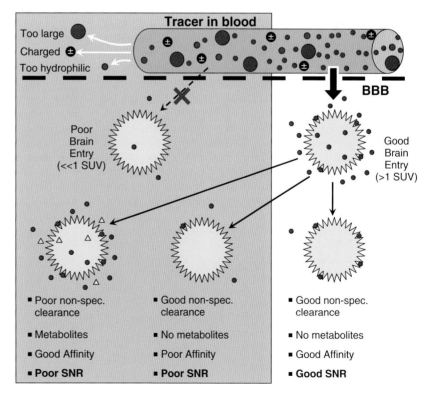

et al., 2002); and %ID*kg/g, in which body weight is expressed in kg and the corresponding lower limit is 0.10 (Mathis et al., 2003). If the value is expressed as a ratio to injected dose instead of a percent, then it becomes the standardized uptake value (SUV) commonly used in nuclear medicine, and the lower limit for brain entry is 1.0. Many reports in the literature do not normalize to body weight, making interpretation more difficult because the threshold is different for each species, depending on the size of the animal. This %ID/g_{br} value would have a threshold of ~4.0 in mice weighing 25 g and ~0.4 in rats weighing 250 g. Without satisfactory initial brain entry, the tracer will not be sufficiently detectable to produce a good signal, and the imaging study will fail. What is more, this criterion refers to the peak brain level and must be attained within minutes after the tracer is injected as a bolus.

The major hurdle preventing tracer molecules from achieving the desired %ID/(g_{br}/g_{tot}) threshold is the blood-brain barrier (BBB). Another factor that can appear to reduce brain entry is rapid active transport out of the brain by the P-glycoprotein ATP-dependent drug efflux pump (Doze et al., 2000). Certain physical characteristics are known to affect the passive exchange of molecules across the BBB. One of these is molecular size. In general, the larger a molecule, the more difficult it is for it to cross the BBB (large red dot in Figure 14.5). Studies suggest that it is best to keep the molecular weight of a tracer below 500 daltons, and compounds above 700 daltons typically have very poor passive diffusion across the BBB (Levin, 1980). Within the optimal range of molecular size, the amount of lipid solubility (lipophilicity) of a molecule becomes a major factor in crossing the BBB. Lipophilicity is usually measured by determining the partitioning of a compound between octanol and aqueous buffer (P_{oct}). This is usually expressed as the $\log_{10}$ of the partition coefficient ($\log P_{oct}$). A compound that partitions equally well into octanol and aqueous buffer in a 1:1 ratio has a $\log P_{oct}$ of 0. A compound that partitions 1000-fold better into the more lipophilic octanol has a $\log P_{oct}$ of 3.0. The effect of lipophilicity on brain entry is biphasic. Compounds that have low lipophilicities (i.e., are hydrophilic; blue dot in Figure 14.5) cannot readily traverse the lipid membranes of the BBB. Compounds that are extremely lipophilic are very sticky and are highly bound to red cell membranes and other lipophilic environments such as plasma proteins, making them less available for brain entry (Dishino et al., 1983; Mathis et al., 2003). The range of $\log P_{oct}$ for good brain entry appears to be ~1–3. The optimum value seems to be near 2 (Gupta, 1989). Ionic charge is another negative factor and both anions and cations cross the BBB very poorly (black dot in Figure 14.5). Organic ions typically have very low lipophilicities, but even when the overall lipophilicity is around 2, organic acids and bases do not passively cross the BBB well.

Brain Clearance

Once enough of the tracer gets into the brain to be detected, then it becomes critical to establish a good signal-to-noise ratio for the target of interest (in this case, the Aβ protein plaque). We will first turn our attention to decreasing the noise. The noise in a PET signal arises from any tracer that is not bound to the target. This non-target-bound tracer pool is typically divided into free tracer and tracer bound (nonspecifically) to sites other than the target. The clearance of free tracer is basically determined by the ease with which the tracer crosses the BBB and the concentration gradient of the tracer across the BBB at any given time. Thus, for a tracer that readily crosses the BBB and is quickly cleared

from the blood by the liver or kidneys, the free component is cleared very quickly.

Clearance of the nonspecifically bound tracer is a bigger problem. The best approach is to administer the tracer in the lowest mass dose possible by keeping the specific activity high (>1 Ci/μmol; >37 GBq/μmol) and design the tracer so that it has few nonspecific binding interactions at these low concentrations of ~1 nM. Nonspecific binding can vary across brain regions, but compounds with similar nonspecific binding properties across all brain regions are preferred to help simplify pharmacokinetic modeling determinations. High nonspecific tracer binding is often a cause of failure for many putative radiotracers. Besides the inherent physical properties of the parent tracer, the formation of metabolites (yellow triangles in Figure 14.5) in the brain or the periphery (which then enter the brain) can produce another source of nonspecific binding.

The acceptable time allowable for clearing the free and nonspecifically bound tracer is dictated by the radioactive half-life of the tracer. Carbon-11 tracers with a 20-minute radioactive half-life must be cleared very quickly before the radioactive signal decays. The clearance half-life for carbon-11 tracers should be under 10 minutes so a good signal-to-noise ratio can be reached before the radioactivity decays beyond detection. With longer lived radioisotopes such as fluorine-18 (109 minutes half-life), correspondingly longer time periods are possible, but in reality the biological clearance of the target-bound tracer usually occurs faster than the radioactive decay.

Specific Signal

Assuming that sufficient radiotracer enters the brain to allow detection and the free and nonspecifically bound tracer clears relatively quickly, then the specific signal or signal-to-noise ratio is determined by the tightness with which the tracer binds to the target and the total concentration of the target in a particular region of interest. The tightness or affinity with which a tracer binds to the target is usually expressed in terms of the dissociation constant (K_d). Differences in the K_d values of ligands are driven mostly by differences in the off-rate from the binding site (Bennett and Yamamura, 1985). It makes sense that a slower off-rate would cause a tracer to hang up longer on its target (red triangles in Figure 14.6), while the free and nonspecifically bound tracer cleared (black circles in Figure 14.6), and thus the signal-to-noise ratio would gradually increase over time until a steady state is reached (open diamonds in Figure 14.6). This phenomenon is readily apparent in the time activity curves of amyloid binding agents when one compares an area with extensive amyloid (e.g., the frontal cortex) to an area with only free and nonspecifically bound tracer, such as the cerebellum (Figure 14.6).

The total concentration of the target is referred to as the B_{max}. In tracer studies, the term B_{max}/K_d determines the ratio of the bound tracer to free tracer and thus sets the maximum signal-to-noise ratio that can be attained. B_{max}/K_d ratios >10 are desirable, but are more necessary in planar imaging than tomography (Eckelman, 1998). The B_{max} for amyloid sites in the cortex can reach over 1 μM, and K_d values are usually <5 nM. However, we do not see signal-to-noise ratio values of 200. This is because B_{max}/K_d considers only the bound:free tracer ratio and does not consider the inevitable in vivo nonspecifically bound tracer levels which can considerably reduce the signal-to-noise ratio. The key point to a specific signal is that, since the B_{max} is set by the biology, the only controllable variables are the affinity and nonspecific binding

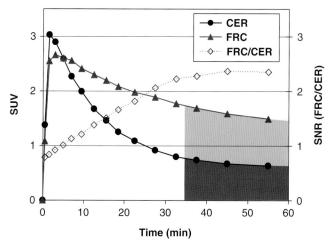

Figure 14–6 Time-activity curves showing the concentration of tracer in a brain area with many target binding sites [(red triangles and frontal cortex ([FRC)]]) or very few target-related binding sites [(black circles and cerebellum [(CER)]]. Also shown is the ratio of tracer in FRC to tracer in CER at each point in time (open diamonds). The shaded gray area represents an integration of the signal in CER from 35–60 minutes post-injection of the tracer. The shaded pink area represents an integration of the signal in the FRC.

of the tracer. The tracer should have the highest possible affinity for the target (i.e., lowest possible K_d) and the lowest possible non-specific binding. Values of K_d above 20 nM often result in the loss of the target-bound tracer along a similar time course as the free and nonspecifically bound tracer.

The simple time-activity curve (TAC) shown in Figure 14.6 nicely depicts all of the requirements for a good imaging agent: (1) the tracer achieves a brain level of >1 SUV quickly after injection; (2) free and nonspecifically bound tracers are cleared quickly from tissue without target (CER); and (3) the affinity of the tracer for the target is sufficiently high to keep the tracer localized in target-laden brain areas (FRC) while other brain areas clear. It is important to keep in mind that the TAC is the "raw material" of a PET study. The time-dependent differentiation of tracer concentration in the target region compared to a reference brain region (sometimes with both adjusted for tracer levels in arterial blood) is the substance from which PET images and quantitative measures are constructed. If a significant difference does not exist at the level of the TAC, then no amount of mathematical analysis will be able to generate a valid difference in the images or quantitative measures of brain retention.

The Radiolabel

Several radionuclides have been used to label amyloid imaging tracers, and these will be mentioned below. It is worth briefly discussing the differences between these various radiolabels. The overarching issue that spawns the use of various tracers is practicality and widespread applicability. Some common radionuclides (iodine-123 and technetium-99m) are specifically suited to single photon emission computed tomography (SPECT), while others (carbon-11 and fluorine-18) are specifically suited to PET. The number of PET scanners is growing quickly, but the numbers are still small relative to SPECT. Although it is difficult to accurately assess the number of PET scanners, the Society of Nuclear Medicine gives an estimate of 1500 PET imaging sites in the U.S. (http://interactive.snm.org/index.cfm?PageID=5571&RPID=969).

These PET scanners are often in large academic medical centers. The number of SPECT scanners is about 10 times that amount (http://www.imagingeconomics.com/issues/articles/MI_2004-06_02.asp). In addition to being more widely accessible, SPECT studies are typically less expensive to perform. On the other hand, PET has often been the preferred research tool because of its superior sensitivity, resolution, and quantitative capabilities. Although iodine-123- and technetium-99m-labeled tracers can both make use of the widespread availability of SPECT, technetium-99m-labeled SPECT tracers are probably the easiest to take into routine use once a good tracer is developed and characterized, because of the simplicity and lower cost of routine tracer production from a technetium-99m generator that is readily available to SPECT facilities. However, because of the large molecular size of the radio-nuclide and the chelator that must be incorporated into the tracer, the initial development of technetium-99m tracers is very challenging, and no promising technetium-99m-labeled amyloid imaging tracers currently exist. Of the common PET radionuclides, the major difference is radioactive half-life. Carbon-11 has a relatively short radioactive half-life of ~20 minutes. However, it is the most versatile radionuclide, since it can be relatively easily incorporated into many organic molecules to be used as imaging agents. A case can be made that the short half-life of carbon-11 makes it the ideal research tool, since it decays quickly enough to allow two or three sequential studies with the same or different tracers within the same imaging session on a single day. Because of its rapid radioactive decay, there also is less radiation exposure with a carbon-11-labeled agent per mCi injected. The major drawback to carbon-11-labeled tracers is the need for an on-site cyclotron for production and immediate use of the carbon-11. Of the 1000 or so PET scanners in the U.S., only a small minority have this on-site capability, but for those that do, carbon-11-labeled tracers hold many advantages. The majority of PET scanner sites rely on external production of fluorine-18 radiotracers (such as [F-18]fluorodeoxyglucose; FDG) by regional cyclotron facilities that distribute the radiotracers to local scanners. The ~110-minute radioactive half-life of fluorine-18 allows distribution within a 2–4-hour travel radius. Thus, the need for a fluorine-18-labeled version of a good carbon-11-labeled tracer is mainly a matter of widening the availability (and thus making the tracer a commercially viable product as well). There are some other advantages to fluorine-18-labeled tracers. For example, the longer half-life allows imaging at longer times after injection, and this may be useful when the optimal signal-to-noise ratio of a tracer is reached more than 90 minutes after injection. Fluorine-18 tracers also can often be labeled at higher specific activities than carbon-11 tracers.

In summary, while the technical quality of an imaging procedure may be optimized with a carbon-11-labeled tracer, the need for widespread availability can still motivate the production of a fluorine-18-labeled version of that tracer. If the sensitivity, resolution, and quantitative capabilities are not critical, then there will be motivation to produce a SPECT tracer (preferably technetium-99m) as well. Both common SPECT radionuclides have relatively long half-lives. Iodine-123 has a 13-hour half-life—allowing widespread distribution—and technetium-99m has a 6-hour half-life. In practice, the 67-hour half-life of the molybdenum-99 "cow" from which the technetium-99m is eluted makes the effective transportation radius of technetium-99m-labeled tracer almost limitless. It is not usually the inherent quality of the imaging data, but the degree of availability that motivates the use of alternate radionuclides to label a given class of imaging tracers.

Basic Principals of In Vivo Quantification (Pharmacokinetic Modeling)

If a tracer successfully meets all of the above requirements, the task of quantification becomes much easier, since there is a large signal with which to work. This section is directed at the nonimager and will include a fairly superficial and sometimes oversimplified handling of the issues of pharmacokinetic modeling. The reader interested in a more rigorous review of the subject should consult more technical treatments of the topic (Carson, 2003; Koeppe, 2002; Price, 2003).

At its most basic level, the data that results from a PET scan might be conceptualized as a series of shipping pallets, each neatly packed with an identical number of small boxes (Figure 14.7). Each box on these shipping pallets is "filled" with a given amount of radioactivity and is coded for its specific position on the pallet. One could uniquely describe one of these boxes in the following way: the box located in the fifth row (R5) of the third column (C3) of the second layer (L2) of the first pallet. We could designate this box as "R5,C3,L2" (Figure 14.7). All the boxes on any one pallet are simultaneously "filled" during the same time interval. Each successive pallet represents an identical arrangement of boxes that were simultaneously "filled" over different, sequential periods of time (e.g., "time frames," such as from 1–3 minutes or 27–33 minutes post injection of the tracer). Thus each box on each pallet can be uniquely defined by: (1) the time frame of the pallet (e.g., 0–1 minute) and (2) the spatial location of the box on the pallet (e.g., R5,C3,L2). In PET, each box would be called a voxel and the entire set of voxels on a pallet would cover the brain as well as some area outside of the brain. Each pallet would represent some portion of time during the entire PET scan.

The PET scanner measures radioactivity emitted from the tracer during defined time periods. The physical position of rings of detector crystals around the head, coupled with a complex mathematical deconvolution of the data (i.e., a volume reconstruction software algorithm) is used to define the location of the voxels and to determine the radioactivity concentration in each voxel. The PET scanner is programmed to repeatedly collect radioactivity data from this array of voxels over discrete time frames, thus, "filling"

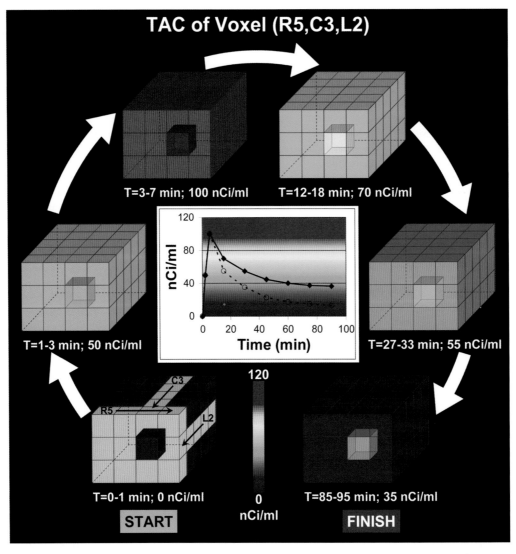

Figure 14–7   Conceptualization of a PET study. See text for explanation. In the $T = 0–1$ minute time frame, row #5, column #3, and layer #2 are highlighted in white. The R5,C3,L2 voxel represents specific binding to target and the other voxels represent free or nonspecifically bound tracer. The radioactivity in voxel R5,C3,L2 is shown in filled diamonds and the radioactivity in all other voxels is represented by the open circles.

multiple time frame "pallets" with voxels of radioactivity concentration data over the course of the entire study (e.g., from 0 to 95 minutes after the intravenous injection of the tracer). When time windows are collected over the entire post-injection period in this manner, the PET data set is called a "dynamic" scan. If the scan is only performed during some latter time period (e.g., beginning 50 minutes after injection and ending at 70 minutes), it is called a "static" scan or "late-summed" scan.

Each voxel can be considered separately across all time frames, or voxels can be grouped into regions of interest (ROIs), that are sometimes called volumes of interest (VOIs). The plot of the radioactivity content (in units of nCi/ml, SUV, etc.) of a voxel or ROI at each time frame generates the TAC for that specific voxel or ROI (Figure 14.7). It is this TAC that forms the basis of most methods of quantification of the PET data.

As mentioned above, the regional distribution of the tracer in the brain is determined by high-affinity, specific binding interactions of the tracer with the target and lower-affinity, nonspecific interactions with other sites. In addition, there is a contribution from the free tracer as it passes through the extracellular space on its way from the arterial to the venous system. Shortly after injection of the tracer, when high levels of tracer are exiting the vascular compartment and entering the brain, the free and nonspecific components dominate and there is little differentiation of tracer concentration across brain regions (Figure 14.7; 0–1, 1–3, and 3–7 minutes time frames). Ideally, as the study progresses and blood levels of tracer fall, the free and nonspecifically bound tracer decreases more rapidly than the specifically bound tracer, and the brain areas with high concentrations of target become differentiated from areas low in target (Figure 14.7; 12–18, 27–33, and 85–95 minutes time frames). It is this differentiation of specific and nonspecific signal that defines the signal-to-noise ratio.

The most thorough and rigorous (and arduous and invasive) approaches to the quantification of PET data employ theoretical mathematical "tracer-kinetic" models of the behavior of ligands in the brain over time. These models are based on "compartments" into which the tracer can equilibrate and rate constants for the movement of tracer from one compartment to another. For example, one model called a "two-tissue compartment, four-parameter" (2T-4k) model would allow a tracer to equilibrate between: (1) the vascular compartment; (2) a tissue compartment containing only specific binding sites (e.g., R5,C3,L2 in Figure 14.7); and (3) a tissue compartment containing both free and nonspecifically bound tracer (e.g., all other "boxes" or voxels in Figure 14.7). Basically, these methods generate theoretical TACs from estimated kinetic rate constants and then iteratively vary the constants (i.e., the "parameters") until the optimal fit of the theoretical TAC and the experimental TAC is obtained. The constants that described the TAC with the optimal fit are used to quantify the amount of tracer in a given voxel or ROI. This concentration is typically expressed as the distribution volume (DV). The ratio of the concentration in the ROI to that of the reference region (such as the cerebellum) is the distribution volume ratio (DVR). A closely related parameter is the binding potential or BP (Mintun et al., 1984). The BP is equal to the DVR minus 1. The importance of this seemingly trivial mathematical conversion can be appreciated in the following example. If a tracer binds to the brain of a subject in such a way as to yield a DVR value of 1.3 at baseline, and if the same subject is imaged with the same tracer at a later date when the number of tracer binding sites has doubled, the new DVR value will be 1.6. Of course, the BP value at baseline would be 0.3 and that at follow-up 0.6. The BP is proportional to the number of binding sites (actually it is proportional to the B_{max}/K_d).

If that tracer binds specifically to amyloid deposits, then the DVR reflects the amyloid load in the voxel or ROI relative to the amount of nonspecifically bound plus free tracer in the reference region. Figure 14.8 shows a "one-tissue two- parameter" (1T-2k) model that allows for only one interaction between the tracer and tissue (i.e., either specific or nonspecific) compared to a 2T-4k model, and the calculated rate constants for each model. It is apparent that the theoretical TAC generated by the 2T-4k model (solid line) fits the experimental TAC (circles) much better than the TAC generated by the 1T-2k model. Compartmental modeling studies are a critically important initial step in the evaluation of a simplified imaging paradigm that could ultimately be translated to the clinic, as these provide a benchmark for selecting, applying, and assessing the performance of the simplified analysis methods.

The "compartmental" approach described above is difficult to routinely apply because of the need for longer scan times and arterial blood collection coupled with HPLC determination of tracer metabolites over the course of the entire study. This is arduous, and the placement and post-scan care of the arterial line represents the most invasive component of PET procedures. Because of this, most researchers and clinicians would like to avoid this approach. However, for every new PET radiotracer, it is important that a compartmental analysis be completed during

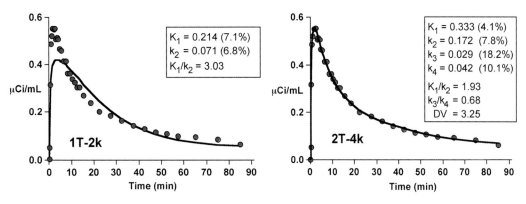

Figure 14–8 Pharmacokinetic model fitting to PET data. The data points represent the same in vivo PET data set fit to two different pharmacokinetic models. On the left, a 1T-2k model is optimized to the data, and the optimal K_1 and k_2 parameters used to generate the solid curve are shown. On the right, a 2T-4K model was used to generate four parameters (K_1, k_2, k_3 and k_4) that define the solid curve on the right. It is visually evident that the curve derived from the 2T-4k model fits the experimental data much better that that derived from the 1T-2k model. (From Price et al., 2005.)

the early stages of human application. This is because it may or *may not* be valid to apply the "simplified" approaches discussed below to a new tracer. The most widely accepted way to validate the use of these simplified methods is to perform both a compartmental and a simplified analysis of the same scan data and show that the simplified method correlates very well with the compartmental approach. "Simplified" reference tissue methods have been developed that substitute the kinetics of the tracer in a reference region (e.g., the cerebellum) for the kinetics in arterial blood in order to define the "input function" of the tracer. Several methods exist (see Price, 2003) and differ in their applicability to reversibly bound tracers (Logan et al., 1990) or irreversibly bound tracers (Gjedde, 1981; Patlak and Blasberg, 1985). These methods typically yield DVR values.

The simplest approach for the quantification of PET data is an integration of the area under a TAC (in units of SUV) over some time window (e.g., 35–60 minutes in Figure 14.6) to yield an average SUV value. An average SUV can be calculated for both target (red plus gray shading in Figure 14.6) and reference regions (gray shading in Figure 14.6). In Figure 14.6 the SUV in the FRC from 35–60 minutes would be ~1.6, and that for the CER would be ~0.7. As can be seen in Figure 14.6, the SUV value is highly dependent on the time window over which it is calculated. It is often useful to go on to calculate a ratio of the SUV value in the target region to the SUV value in the reference region, to control for variations in the amount of tracer injected and the body mass of different subjects, as well as the free and nonspecifically bound tracer in the target region (which is assumed to be equal to that in the reference region). This SUV ratio, or SUVR, can be calculated for several time windows of different length and at different points on the TACs (e.g., 25 minutes from 35–60 minutes or 30 minutes from 60–90 minutes). The FRC:CER SUVR over 35–60 minutes in Figure 14.6 would be ~2.3. The advantage of longer time intervals at earlier times is that there is less noise in the signal, but this comes at the cost of having more free and nonspecifically bound signal in both the target and reference regions, and an equilibrium may not have been reached between the free and specifically bound tracer. The later time intervals have the advantage of having the greatest contribution of specific signal, but tissue clearance and radioactive decay (especially with carbon-11 and its 20-minute half-life) make the signal noisier at later times. With a systematic trial of multiple combinations, an optimal time window can be defined. It is best to choose a time window that falls after an equilibrium state has been reached between free and specifically bound tracer (e.g., after ~40 minutes in Figure 14.6). The SUVR should be fairly equivalent across time windows after steady state has been reached and basically represents the maximum signal-to-noise ratio in the tissue. For amyloid imaging, the cerebellar cortex is usually chosen as the reference region because there are very few fibrillar plaques in this brain area (Joachim, Morris, and Selkoe, 1989; Yamaguchi et al., 1989). The pons is sometimes used for similar reasons (Klunk et al., 2007). However, the kinetics of tracers in white matter are often different from the kinetics in gray matter, making the pons less attractive. The integration approach can technically be employed without generating a full TAC. Thus, the subject may only be in the scanner from 35 to 60 minutes, the scanner collects a single 25-minute time window of data (called a "static" scan rather than a "dynamic" scan), and the average radioactivity in the voxels or ROIs is calculated as the SUV or SUVR. It should be kept in mind that although the full TAC is never generated, the integrated value is based on a specific portion of the full TAC. It is critical to validate this very simple quantitative approach

by comparison to the more rigorous compartment models. Such validation has been performed for only one amyloid imaging PET tracer to date (Lopresti et al., 2005).

Once completed, data from these various analysis approaches can be presented numerically—usually when derived from ROIs—or the numbers can be used to generate "parametric" images: that is, images in which the voxel values are not simply reflective of the raw radioactivity measure for that voxel over some period of time, but reflect a chosen pharmacokinetic parameter for that voxel. Voxels in parametric images can represent DV or DVR values, BP values, SUVR values, or any other calculated parameter. Another common manipulation of the data is to assign a statistical value such as t-values or z-scores to each pixel based on the comparison of a study group and a control group, or even an individual subject to a control group. This technique is usually called statistical parametric mapping (SPM; http://www.fil.ion.bpmf.ac.uk/spm/dox.html) (Clark and Carson, 1993; Friston, Holmes, and Worsley, 1995). Prior to performing SPM, the individual images must be "spatially normalized" to a standard brain template. This process involves subtle moving, splitting/combining, or reshaping (i.e., "warping") of the "real" or "native" voxels so that they exactly match the number and location of the voxels in the standard brain template. This normalization process was first proposed by Fox, Perlmutter, and Raichle (1985) and many approaches have subsequently been devised (Fox, Laird, and Lancaster, 2005).

Pittsburgh Compound-B: The Preclinical Development of an Amyloid Imaging Agent

An example of the preclinical evaluation of amyloid imaging PET tracers can be seen in the development of the thioflavin-T (ThT) derivative, *Pi*ttsburgh Compound-*B*, known as PiB (Klunk et al. 2004), 6-OH-BTA-1 (Mathis et al. 2003), or [N-methyl-C-11]2-(4'-methylaminophenyl)-6-hydroxybenzothiazole (Mathis et al. 2003). There have been hundreds of other compounds reported to be putative amyloid imaging tracers and these have been reviewed elsewhere (Cai, Innis, and Pike, 2007; Mathis, Wang, and Klunk, 2004a). In addition, there have been reports of using high-field magnetic resonance imaging without contrast agents to image amyloid plaques in transgenic mice (Jack et al., 2004, 2005). Since most of these have not been fully evaluated preclinically and the vast majority have not been tested in humans, they will not be discussed here. Those tracers that have been used in published human amyloid imaging studies will be discussed below.

Affinity for Aβ Fibrils and in Vivo Pharmacokinetics in Mice

To appreciate the time scale of tracer development, consider that the first synthetic work aimed at developing ThT derivatives as amyloid PET tracers began in 1999, and the first human study of PiB was performed on February 14, 2002. This time frame may seem somewhat short, but should be put in the context that this three-year period followed a decade of intermittent work on the development of Congo red derivatives as amyloid imaging. Much was learned during the development of the Congo red class of compounds (which includes Chrysamine-G [Klunk, Debnath, and Pettegrew, 1995] and methoxy-X04 [Klunk et al., 2002]) that could be applied to the development of the ThT derivatives. A summary of the development of the Congo red series has been given, and that will not be discussed further here (Mathis, Wang, and Klunk, 2004a).

ThT is a small molecule known to bind to various amyloid proteins when aggregated into a beta-pleated sheet structure (Levine, 1995). After achieving only marginal success with the Congo red derivatives, ThT became an attractive scaffold for amyloid imaging tracer development for several reasons. First, while many histologic dyes are relatively impure mixtures of poorly defined components, ThT is a well-defined, single chemical entity (Figure 14.9). Second, ThT is a small molecule with a molecular weight of just 319 daltons. Third, ThT binds to an entirely separate site on the Aβ fibril than the Congo red compounds, and it was hoped that this diversity would allow the development of better tracers.

Several hundred ThT derivatives have been evaluated in our laboratories over the past 5 years, but Figure 14.9 summarizes the main stages of development that led to the now widely used PET amyloid imaging tracer, PiB. The first step from ThT to 6-Me-BTA-2 was a direct consequence of lessons learned in the Congo red series. That is, charged molecules generally do not enter the brain well through passive diffusion, even when their size and lipophilicity are in the preferred range—and the log P_{oct} of ThT was lower than the preferred range of 1.0–3.0. Removal of the methyl group from the positively charged quaternary heterocyclic nitrogen of the benzothiazolium group of ThT yielded a compound called 6-Me-BTA-2. While this structural alteration was expected to increase brain entry, there was no way to predict the effects of this change on affinity for amyloid. Luckily, the Aβ binding affinity of 6-Me-BTA-2 improved considerably. The inhibition constant (K_i) is a measure of binding affinity closely related to the K_d (Bennett and Yamamura, 1985). Figure 14.9 shows that the K_i of 6-Me-BTA-2 was nearly 10 times better than ThT, although it was not yet near

the goal of <10 nM. The expectation that brain entry would improve was realized with a %IDI value of 78 (very near the goal of 100 %IDI). Unfortunately, the clearance of 6-Me-BTA-2 was very poor, and brain levels actually increased twofold over 30 minutes. The poor clearance indicated that the compound was too lipophilic, and this was consistent with the high log P value of 3.8. The effect of addition or removal of substituents to and from aromatic compounds is fairly predictable because of the work of Hansch and colleagues (Hansch and Leo, 1979). The removal of two methyl groups from 6-Me-BTA-2 yielded the expected drop in log P_{oct} to 2.7 in the compound called BTA-1 (Mathis et al., 2002). Once again, the effect of this structural change on binding affinity was difficult to predict, but once again, the affinity of BTA-1 was improved over 6-Me-BTA-2 to a value near the target affinity. The expected improvement in brain pharmacokinetics was realized by a marked improvement in brain entry to 434 %IDI (well above the target of 100 %IDI) and, more importantly, a marked improvement in brain clearance. When measured in control animals (i.e., wild-type animals without brain amyloid deposits), the clearance of amyloid tracers can be expressed as the ratio of the level of the compound in the brain at 2 minutes to the level of the compound at 30 minutes. This 2':30' ratio was 7.6 for BTA-1 (equivalent to a $t_{1/2}$ of ~9.6 minutes). This compound had essentially met all of the basic requirements of affinity, brain entry, and clearance, and was given serious consideration for human studies. It was, in fact, given the name "Pittsburgh Compound-A" by the Uppsala University PET Centre (see below) during preclinical studies in preparation for human studies. However, the 6-hydroxy derivative of BTA-1, a compound initially known as 6-OH-BTA-1 and eventually named "Pittsburgh Compound-B" or PiB by the

Figure 14–9 Chemical structures, lipophilicity (log P_{oct}), binding affinity (K_i), brain entry (%IDI), and clearance (2':30' ratio) of thioflavin-T, PiB, and intervening derivatives. Numbers in parentheses indicate targets for each parameter.

Compound	logPoct (1–3)	Ki (<10 nM)	%IDI (2') (>100)	2':30' (>5)
Thioflavin-T 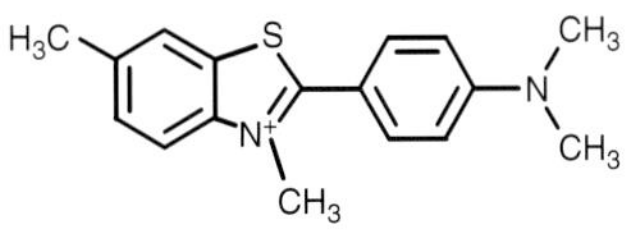	0.57	>500 nM	–	–
6-Me-BTA-2 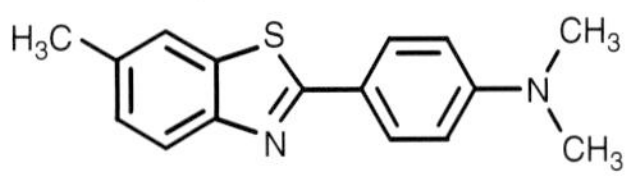	3.8	64 nM	78	0.52
BTA-1 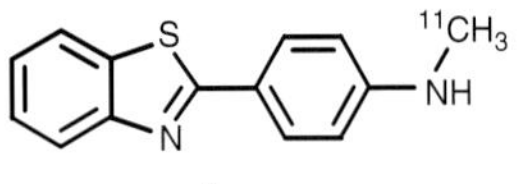	2.7	11 nM	434	7.6
PIB 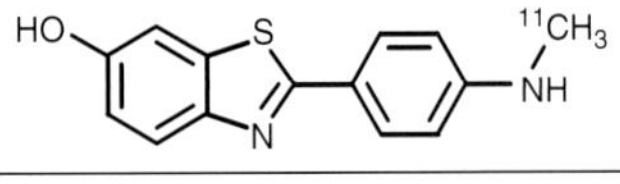	1.2	43 nM	210	12

Uppsala PET Centre, proved to have even better properties in most areas. PiB had a better affinity by most measures, with a K_i of 4.3 nM (below the goal of 10 nM) and a better brain clearance, with a 2':30' ratio of 12 ($t_{1/2}$ ~7.9 minutes). The log P_{oct} was ~1.2. The log P_{oct} and the better clearance were predicted results of the addition of the hydroxyl group. The decreased—but still very good—brain entry also was consistent with the log P_{oct} value near the lower end of the desirable range. Once again, the change in affinity could not be accurately predicted, but was slightly better than that of BTA-1.

Studies in Postmortem AD Brain Tissue

Because of their promising properties, PiB and BTA-1 were subjected to more detailed characterization in preparation for human studies. Some of the earlier studies were performed only with BTA-1, some with both BTA-1 and PiB, and some of the later studies only with PiB. The cross-over studies suggest that findings with BTA-1 are likely to apply equally well to PiB itself. Studies using postmortem AD and control brain tissue showed that BTA-1 and PiB have a high degree of specific binding (>94%) (Klunk et al., 2003). PiB and BTA-1 showed ~tenfold higher levels of binding in areas of postmortem AD brain with heavy Aβ plaque deposits than in the same areas of plaque-free control brain. However, no binding could be detected in AD brain white matter or in brain tissue with large accumulations of neurofibrillary tangles in the absence of plaques (such as entorhinal cortex from Braak stage II nondemented control brain) (Klunk et al., 2003). Furthermore, no significant binding was detected in postmortem neocortical samples from brains with pure DLB Huntington's disease, Pick's disease, motor neuron disease-inclusion dementia, or dementia lacking distinctive histologic features (Klunk et al., 2003). Importantly, the amount of PiB bound to AD brain homogenates quantitatively reflected the Aβ content of the tissue (Klunk et al., 2005). Preliminary histochemical, immunohistological, and biochemical studies of PiB and PiB derivative binding to postmortem AD tissue sections showed that PiB staining co-localizes with Aβ immunohistochemistry (Ikonomovic et al., 2005, 2006a). Plaques that label primarily with antibodies for the either the 40 or the 42 amino acid C-termini of Aβ were labeled by PiB derivatives equally well. PiB staining could be abolished by formic acid pretreatment, indicating that PiB binds to fibrillar, beta-sheet forms of Aβ that are denatured by the formic acid pretreatment. Taken together, these findings suggested that in vivo PiB retention should be fairly specific for fibrillar Aβ amyloid deposits.

In Vivo Pharmacokinetics in Nonhuman Primates

Perhaps the single most important piece of information that resulted in the choice of PiB over BTA-1 for human studies was the comparison of the pharmacokinetic properties of these two compounds in nonhuman primates (Figure 14.10) (Mathis et al., 2003). The logic was to compare PiB and BTA-1 to several PET neuroreceptor ligands that were known to be useful in human studies. The pharmacokinetic behavior of each tracer was compared in the cerebellum—a brain area that has no specific binding sites for any of the tracers. Thus the brain entry and clearance of free plus nonspecifically bound tracer could be directly compared across all compounds. The cerebellar TACs in baboons of [C-11]raclopride, [carbonyl-C-11]WAY100635, [C-11](+)-McN5652, and [F-18]altanserin are compared to those of [C-11]PiB and [C-11]BTA-1 (Figure 14.10). The relatively rapid nonspecific binding clearance rates of [carbonyl-C-11]WAY100635, [C-11]raclopride, and [F-18]-altanserin are important in the success of these PET radioligands for imaging the

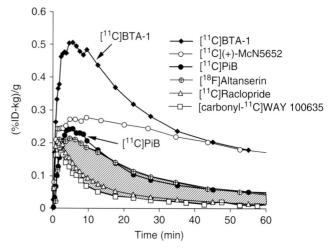

Figure 14–10 Comparison of the entry and clearance of radioactivity in baboon cerebellum of four reference PET radioligands ([C-11]raclopride, [carbonyl-C-11]WAY100635, [C-11](+)-McN5652, and [F-18]altanserin) relative to that for [C-11]BTA-1 and [C-11]PiB. The shaded area is the desired target zone bounded by the cerebellar concentrations of the successful PET neuroreceptor radioligands [F-8]altanserin and [carbonyl-C-11]-WAY100635. [C-11]PiB demonstrated fairly rapid clearance of free and nonspecifically bound radioactivity from baboon cerebellum and was near the upper bound of the target zone, while [C-11]BTA-1 cleared relatively slowly from baboon cerebellum and was clearly out of the zone. (From Mathis et al., 2003.)

serotonin 5-HT1A, dopamine D2, and serotonin 5-HT2A receptor systems (Drevets et al., 1999; Farde et al., 1987, 1988; Pike et al., 1996; Price et al., 2001; Smith et al., 1998). In contrast, the relatively slow in vivo clearance of [C-11]-(+)-McN5652 has limited the usefulness of this radioligand for imaging the serotonin transporter system (Huang et al., 2002; Lopresti et al., 2001). We reasoned that a C-11-labeled amyloid binding tracer with similarly rapid nonspecific binding clearance properties within the range bracketed by [carbonyl-C-11]WAY100635 and [F-18]altanserin might prove useful as an in vivo imaging agent for amyloid plaques—at least from the perspective of clearance of free+nonspecifically bound tracer. The brain clearance properties of [C-11]PiB indicated that the relatively rapid rate of nonspecific clearance of this radiotracer ($t_{1/2} \approx 13$ minutes) was similar to that of other useful PET neuroreceptor imaging agents and those of [C-11]BTA-1 ($t_{1/2} \approx 20$ minutes) were too slow (Figure 14.10).

Two-Photon Imaging Studies in Transgenic Mice

PiB, being a fluorescent compound like the parent ThT, could be studied by two-photon fluorescence microscopy with submicron resolution in the brains of living transgenic mice following peripheral administration (Bacskai et al., 2003). These two-photon studies visually showed that PiB entered the brain quickly and labeled amyloid deposits within minutes. The nonspecific binding was cleared rapidly, whereas specific labeling was prolonged (Figure 14.11). Mice without amyloid (i.e., wild-type mice) showed rapid brain entry and clearance of PiB without any binding. Although studies such as these proved indispensable in documenting the in vivo specific binding behavior of PiB, they required the use of concentrations 1000–10,000 times higher than those used in PET studies.

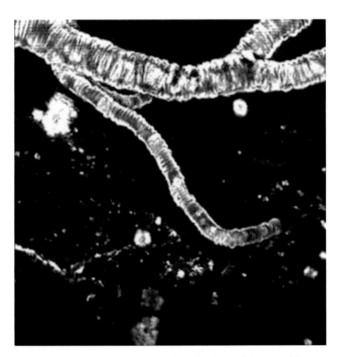

Figure 14–11 Real-time imaging of PiB labeling Aβ deposits (plaques and vascular amyloid) and clearing from the brain of a live, transgenic, Tg2576 mouse. This frame, taken 30 minutes after i.v.IV injection, is a maximum intensity projection of PiB fluorescence within a 3D volume of the brain acquired with a multiphoton microscope. The frame is 615 × 615 μm wide and ~150 μm deep. (From Bacskai et al., 2003.)

MicroPET Studies in Transgenic Mice: the Final Validation or a Return to First Principles?

Because of the high concentrations of PiB required for the two-photon studies, plans were made to use microPET (Cherry, 2001) to validate the tracer pharmacokinetics in transgenic mouse models of amyloid deposition. The PS1/APP mouse was chosen because it develops amyloid burdens well above those in AD brain (Holcomb et al., 1998). In preparation for human studies, a detailed series of experiments was designed to:

1) Determine the TAC of [C-11]PiB after intravenous injection and determine the time at which the largest ratio of [C-11]PiB brain concentration in PS1/APP compared to control mice occurred.

2) Determine whether the enhanced uptake of [C-11]PiB observed in PS1/APP mice was saturable and could be blocked by pretreatment with excess unlabeled PiB.

3) Determine the correlation between [C-11]PiB brain levels in PS1/APP mice (determined ex vivo) and postmortem evaluation of amyloid load by (a) quantitative histologic analysis, (b) measurement of Aβ levels by ELISA, and (c) postmortem [H-3]PiB binding to tissue homogenates.

4) Determine the correlation between [C-11]PiB brain levels in PS1/APP mice (determined in vivo using microPET) and postmortem evaluation of amyloid load by (a) quantitative histologic analysis, (b) measurement of Aβ levels by ELISA, and (c) postmortem [H-3]PiB binding to tissue homogenates.

5) Use the [C-11]PiB/microPET method to determine the natural time course of amyloid deposition in PS/APP mice.

6) Determine the threshold for amyloid detection by the [C-11]PiB/microPET method in PS1/APP mice and the sensitivity and specificity of the [C-11]PiB/microPET in vivo technique.

7) Use the [C-11]PiB/microPET method to quantify amyloid deposition longitudinally for 8 months over the course of a standard immunization therapy protocol begun before or after the initiation of amyloid deposition in PS1/APP mice.

These planned experiments are listed here only to demonstrate a typical approach to verifying the performance and capabilities of a tracer in an animal model as a final validation before the initiation of human studies. Unfortunately, the studies were never completed. Very early in the process, it was discovered that [C-11]PiB retention measured by microPET was no greater in mice with extensive amyloid loads (confirmed postmortem in 12-month-old PS1/APP mice) than in mice with no amyloid deposits. In other words, the extensive amyloid deposits in these transgenic mice could not be detected by microPET with [C-11]PiB (although they had been detectable with two-photon microscopy). This very disappointing result was confirmed by several other groups, and one other group reported these results (Toyama et al., 2005). At this point, it became necessary to return to first principles. The negative in vivo studies were followed up with a series of ex vivo and in vitro experiments to determine the reason for the failure to detect increased PiB retention in the brains of transgenic mice with extensive amyloid deposition (Klunk et al., 2005). Ex vivo brain pharmacokinetic studies confirmed the low in vivo PiB retention observed in microPET experiments. In vitro binding studies showed that PS1/APP brain tissue contained less than one high-affinity ($K_d = 1–2$ nM) PiB binding site per 1000 molecules of Aβ, whereas AD brain contained >500 PiB binding sites per 1000 molecules of Aβ. Synthetic Aβ closely resembled PS1/APP brain in having less than one high-affinity PiB binding site per 1000 molecules of Aβ. Importantly, the characteristics of the few high-affinity PiB binding sites found on synthetic Aβ were very similar to those found in AD brain. That is, in PS1/APP mouse brain and with synthetic Aβ in vitro, there was a low frequency of the type aggregation that produced PiB binding sites, but when these sites were formed, they appeared identical to the sites in AD brain. We hypothesized that differences in the time course of deposition or tissue factors present during deposition led to differences in secondary structure between Aβ deposited in AD brain and either synthetic Aβ or Aβ deposited in PS1/APP mouse brain. While most extensively evaluated in the PS1/APP mouse model, the same failure to detect increased PiB binding was observed in at least three other transgenic mouse models of amyloid deposition. This low number of PiB binding sites appeared to preclude detection of tracer amounts of PiB with microPET. Detectability with two-photon microscopy is most likely based on the facts that: (1) PiB concentrations are 10,000-fold higher, thus saturating all available binding sites, and (2) two-photon microscopy can be used to focus on small brain areas with a high signal-to-noise ratio, thus avoiding partial volume averaging. One might ask, why then not just give more [C-11]PiB in the microPET experiment? The answer is that two-photon microscopy detects the fluorescence of *all* PiB molecules, while microPET detects only the minority of PiB molecules that are radiolabeled. Due to limitations on the availability and use of radioactive PiB, the only way to approach the micromolar levels attained in the two-photon experiment would be to add a relatively small amount of additional radioactive PiB and a relatively large amount of nonradioactive PiB. Adding more nonradioactive

Table 14–1 Biochemical analysis of PS1/APP and human AD brain tissue.

		Aβ1–40	Aβ1–42 (pmol/g wet wt.)	Total Aβ
PS1/APP ($n = 4$)	Insoluble	35 002 ± 21 266	12 838 ± 4453	47 840 ± 25 288
Human AD ($n = 5$)		764 ± 155	1715 ± 265	2479 ± 404
PS1/APP ($n = 4$)	Soluble	1056 ± 302	573 ± 96	1629 ± 380
Human AD ($n = 5$)		5.4 ± 1.9	3.2 ± 0.73	8.6 ± 2.1
PS1/APP ($n = 4$)	% Soluble	3.9 ± 2.7%	4.9 ± 2.5%	4.2 ± 2.6%
Human AD ($n = 5$)		0.73 ± 0.36%	0.19 ± 0.06%	0.36 ± 0.14%

From: Klunk et al. (2005).

PiB would dilute the radioactive signal and might even make the background noise worse. As will be seen below, this would be counterproductive.

Perhaps it should not have been surprising that Aβ aggregated in a test tube (over days) would have different structural characteristics compared to that aggregated in the human brain (perhaps over years). The simple chemical milieu of the in vitro experiment (essentially phosphate-buffered saline and Aβ) is a poor approximation of the complex biochemical milieu of the human brain. X-ray crystallographers are very familiar with the large variety of structural outcomes that can result from even subtle changes in solvent systems. They spend much of their time screening crystals (or often not finding any crystals to screen) that are formed in hundreds or even thousands of different solvent systems and have automated this process with robotics and high-throughput crystal detection systems in efforts to deal with this biological complexity. It may not be equally obvious, but it also should not be surprising that Aβ aggregated in the brain of a mouse under artificial transgenic conditions would be structurally different than that aggregated in human brain. The high levels of soluble Aβ in the transgenic mouse brain (~1600 pmol/g) are much higher than levels found in AD brain (~9 pmol/g) (see table 14.1 from Klunk et al. [2005]). In addition, there is a tenfold higher percentage of soluble Aβ in PS1/APP mouse brain (~4%) than in human brain (~0.4%). This suggests that Aβ aggregation in PS1/APP brain is kinetically driven by the high rate of production of Aβ to some disordered state of Aβ, rather than thermodynamically driven as it may be in human brain to a lower energy and more ordered state of aggregation. This may explain the apparent rapidity of the formation of new Aβ plaques that has been observed over just a few days using two-photon microscopy in transgenic mouse brain (Skoch, Hyman, and Bacskai, 2006). The transgenic mouse brain may be supersaturated with the poorly soluble Aβ peptides that quickly aggregate whenever a seed for aggregation occurs.

Subsequent to the studies by our group (Klunk et al., 2005) and by Toyama et al. (2005), a third group of investigators demonstrated that a small in vivo microPET signal could be detected in transgenic mice if very high specific activity PiB were employed (Maeda et al., 2007). That is, a specific signal could be detected if there was more radioactive PiB per unit mass (recall that most of a "radioactive" sample of PiB or any carbon-11-labeled tracer is composed of nonradioactive compound). An approximately 1.3–1.5-fold higher signal was detected in transgenic APP23 mice over 20 months of age compared to amyloid-free control mice. The specific activity of the PiB (~ 8 Ci/μmol) was about 10 times higher than that used in our studies or the Toyama study. This finding is consistent with theoretical calculations showing that in brains with

extremely low levels of PiB binding sites, the signal-to-noise ratio will be much greater at a specific activity of 8 Ci/μmol than at 0.8 Ci/μmol.

The explanation for this finding is complicated and rests on several principles of ligand binding that are beyond the scope of this chapter. Suffice it to say that using the principles of ligand binding, a theoretical ratio of specific to nonspecific binding can be calculated under conditions in PS1/APP mouse brain and AD brain (Figure 14.12). It is apparent that the signal-to-noise ratio would increase significantly in PS1/APP brain over the range of 0.8–8 Ci/μmol—essentially going from the undetectable range to the detectable range. The same calculation can be performed in the human brain and shows that the optimal signal-to-noise ratio is obtained at a specific activity well below 0.8 Ci/μmol. This is caused by the much higher concentration of tracer binding sites in human AD brain. Thus, increasing the specific activity is not likely to increase the signal-to-noise ratio in AD brain imaging studies. However, higher specific activity could become helpful in subjects with brain amyloid levels near the currently detectable limits.

Despite the initial failures to measure PiB retention in transgenic mice with microPET, PiB was chosen as the lead human amyloid imaging tracer. This decision rested largely on the finding that human brain homogenates had 500 times more PiB binding

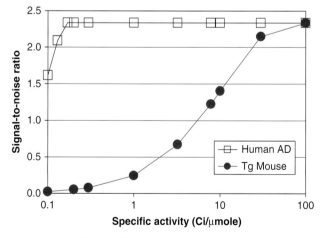

Figure 14–12 Theoretical calculation of the signal-to-noise ratio (SNR) dependence on the specific activity of a radiotracer. When the concentration of binding sites is high (human AD, open squares), there is little change in SNR from 0.2 to 100 Ci/μmole specific activity. When the concentration of binding sites is 1/500th of that as in transgenic mouse brain (Tg mouse, filled circles), there is a marked increase in detectability between 1 and 30 Ci/μmole.

sites per mole of Aβ in the tissue than mouse brain homogenates or equivalent amounts of synthetic Aβ. Several transgenic mouse models produced similar results in several laboratories (Klunk et al., 2005; Toyama et al., 2005). It was believed that these transgenic mouse models of amyloid deposition were simply not good predictors of the behavior of amyloid imaging tracers in human PET studies. Given the good binding characteristics of PiB in postmortem human brain homogenates under near-physiological conditions (Klunk et al., 2005) and the excellent pharmacokinetics of PiB in wild-type mice and nonhuman primates (Mathis et al., 2003), a decision was made to proceed to human studies despite the negative transgenic mouse studies.

Further in vivo studies confirmed that PiB was not metabolized in mice or nonhuman primates in a manner that was likely to complicate amyloid imaging studies in humans (see Figure 14.5) (Mathis et al., 2004b). A complete toxicological evaluation was performed by an independent laboratory in preparation for the human studies and consisted of: (1) acute vascular irritation in rabbits; (2) bacterial reverse mutation assay (Ames test); (3) in vitro mouse lymphoma assay; (4) mammalian erythrocyte micronucleus test; (5) in vitro mammalian chromosome aberration test; (6) expanded acute IV toxicity study in rats; (7) expanded acute IV toxicity study in dogs; and (8) a cardiopulminary study in dogs. This toxicological evaluation verified that PiB showed no significant toxic effects in doses up to 100 times those expected to be used in humans—which was the solubility limit of PiB (Klunk and Mathis [unpublished data]). Radiation dosimetry studies were performed in rodents to predict safe doses for human studies (Stabin et al., 2006). These rodent dosimetry studies were later confirmed in primates (Parsey et al., 2005) and ultimately in humans (Scheinin et al., 2007). In humans, the hepatobiliary and renal systems are the major routes of clearance and excretion, with approximately 20% of the injected radioactivity being excreted into urine. The effective radiation dose was 4.74 mSv/MBq; indicating that the typical clinical doses of PiB have an acceptable effective radiation dose. This dose is comparable with the average exposure expected in other PET brain receptor tracer studies. PiB is rapidly cleared from the body, largely by the kidneys (Scheinin et al., 2007).

Radiotracers Used in Human Amyloid Imaging Studies

The basic principles of brain amyloid radiotracer development described above are useful to keep in mind as one considers the initial attempts to image amyloid deposition in humans. Many of the difficulties encountered can be attributed to problems with size, lipophilicity, specificity, and affinity of the tracers that ultimately lead to poor brain entry, poor retention at specific amyloid target sites, and/or poor brain clearance from nonspecific sites. To date, published data on nine amyloid imaging radiotracer studies have been reported. Table 14.2 lists these agents in the order in which they were applied to human studies along with key pieces of data on the physical properties (logPoct), in vitro pharmacodynamic properties (affinity for Aβ), in vivo pharmacokinetic properties in mice (brain entry and clearance), and finally the specific signal achieved in humans when comparing AD patients to elderly controls. Figure 14.13 shows the chemical structures of the small molecule tracers. Of all the data in table 14.2, the affinity data is the most difficult to compare across studies since differences in methodology (e.g., the radioligand employed) can lead to significant differences in the result.

It is important to keep in mind that this is a rapidly evolving field. For the majority of the newer tracers, definitive studies (and replications) have yet to be performed and published, so current knowledge at the time of publication of this chapter is limited. Over the next few years the landscape of amyloid imaging tracers will undoubtedly change. The seven tracers that have been used in only one small pilot human imaging study will be briefly discussed first. This will be followed by a discussion of [F-18]FDDNP, for which there are three published primary studies and several abstracts of preliminary work. The remainder of this chapter will be devoted largely to a discussion of the more than 25 primary reports and even more published abstracts of human studies using [C-11]PiB.

Radiolabeled Monoclonal Antibody Fragments

The first attempt to noninvasively image brain amyloid deposits in probable AD patients was made using 10H3, a monoclonal antibody Fab fragment targeting the Aβ$_{1-28}$ residues, which was labeled

Table 14–2 Comparison of the properties and performance of amyloid radiotracers studied in humans.

Tracer	Log P_{oct}	Affinity (method)	2 minutes %IDI (mice)	2':30' %IDI Ratio	% Increase AD vs. Control (brain area; method)	Reference
[Tc-99m]10H3[a]	nd[b]	nd[c]	0	nd	~0%	(Majocha et al., 1992) (Friedland et al., 1997)
[F-18]FDDNP	3.9	0.12 nM (K_d; Aβ fibrils)	nd	nd	10% (parietal; DVR)	(Agdeppa et al., 2001) (Small et al., 2006)
[C-11]PiB	1.2	1.4 nM (K_d; AD brain)	210	12	104% (precuneus; DVR)	(Mathis et al., 2003) (Lopresti et al., 2005)
[C-11]SB-13	2.4	2.4 nM (K_d; AD brain)	265	2.7	62% (left frontal; SUVR)	(Ono et al., 2003) (Verhoeff et al., 2004)
[I-123]CQ	Nd	0.45 nM (K_d; Aβ fibrils)	nd	nd	n/a (low brain entry)	(Opazo et al., 2006)
[C-11]BF-227	1.8	4.3 nM (Ki; Aβ fibrils)	~235	5.6	23% (lat. temporal; SUVR)	(Arai et al., 2006) (Kudo et al., 2007)
[I-123]IMPY	2.0	5.3 nM (K_d; AD brain)	~225	11	18% (mean cortical; DV)	(Kung et al., 2004) (Seibyl et al., 2007)
[F-18]AV-1	2.4	6.7 nM (K_i; AD brain)	~180	4.9	42% (mean cortical; DVR)	(Zhang et al., 2005b) (Rowe et al., 2007c)
[F-18]3'F-PiB	1.7	2.2 nM (K_d; AD brain)	312	8.4	73% (precuneus; DVR)	(Mathis et al., 2007)

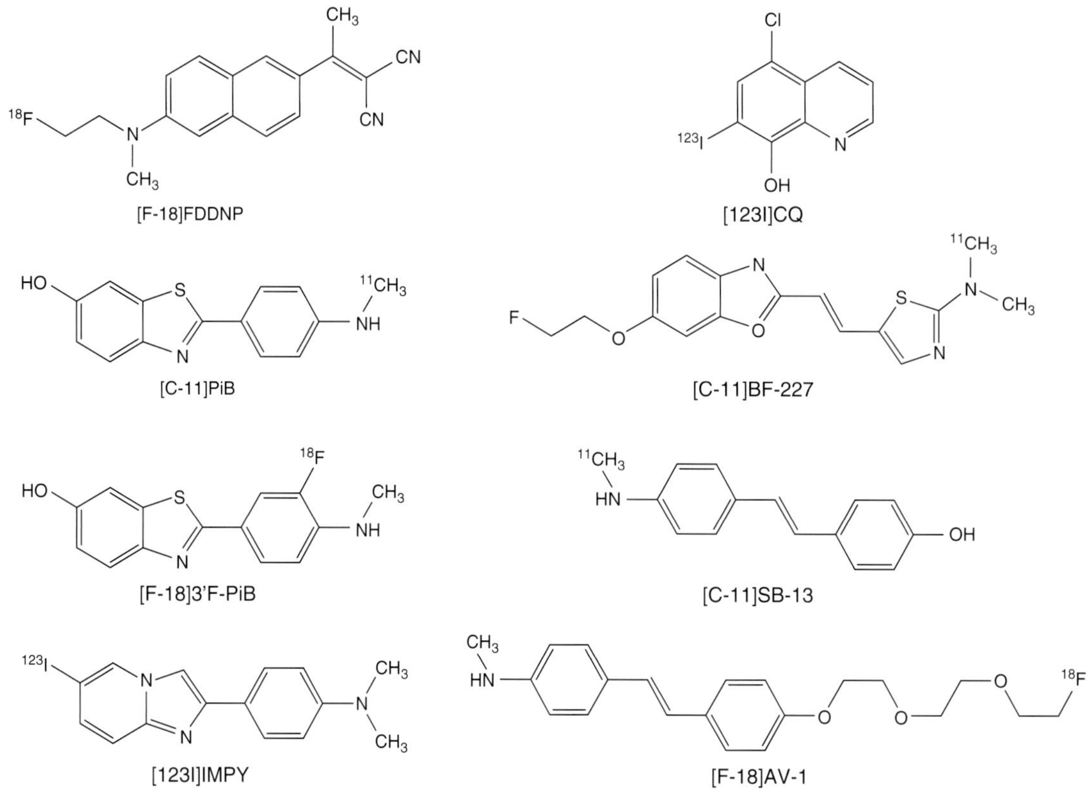

Figure 14–13   Structures of small molecule amyloid radiotracers studied in humans.

with technetium-99m for SPECT imaging (Friedland et al., 1997). While this agent showed specific binding to senile plaques and cerebrovascular amyloid in postmortem tissue sections (Friedland et al., 1994; Majocha et al., 1992), only nonspecific retention in the scalp was observed in human subjects in a manner that did not distinguish AD and control subjects. Preclinical studies showed a lack of entry of [Tc-99m]10H3 into mouse brain, but the strategy was to target cerebrovascular amyloid angiopathy as a marker for brain Aβ amyloidosis, since amyloid deposits around small vessels are very close to the lumen (Mountjoy, Tomlinson, and Gibson, 1982). A major limitation of this approach was the inability of such large molecules to readily enter the brain and achieve concentrations sufficient for detection by standard molecular imaging techniques.

[F-18]FDDNP

[F-18]FDDNP was the second amyloid imaging agent studied in humans. It will be discussed in detail in Section 8 below.

[C-11]PiB

[C-11]PiB was the third tracer studied in humans. It has been extensively studied and will be reviewed in detail in Sections 9–11.

[C-11]SB-13

The fourth tracer to be used in human PET amyloid imaging studies was a stilbene derivative 4-N-methylamino-4'-hydroxystilbene, or SB-13 (Verhoeff et al., 2004). In vitro, [H-3]SB-13 bound specifically and with high affinity ($K_d = 2.4 \pm 0.2$ nM) to cortical homogenates prepared from postmortem brain tissue samples of four patients with a pathological confirmation of AD. In contrast, homogenates of cerebellar and white matter tissues prepared from

both AD or control elderly brain tissue did not represent significant sources of [H-3]SB-13 specific binding. [H-3]SB-13 was shown to have a log P_{oct} of 2.36, and pharmacokinetic studies in rats showed good initial brain entry (~265 %IDI at 2 minutes post injection) and a 2':30' ratio of 2.74 (Ono et al., 2003). In vitro competition binding studies demonstrated comparable potencies in the low nanomolar range ($K_i = 6.9$ nM) for BTA-1 displacement of [H-3]SB-13. FDDNP exhibited less competition with [H-3]SB-13 ($K_i = 294$ nM) as compared to BTA-1. This suggested that benzothiazoles, such as BTA-1 and PiB, share a binding site on the Aβ peptide with SB-13, while FDDNP does not (Kung et al., 2004). [H-3]SB-13 was shown to label Aβ plaques in sections of human AD cortex, but not in control brain. These favorable in vitro properties support the continued investigation of SB-13 as a potential molecular imaging probe for the noninvasive assessment of brain amyloid deposition in human subjects.

SB-13 was labeled with carbon-11 for in vivo investigations in five female AD subjects and six healthy controls using PET (Verhoeff et al., 2004). These same subjects were imaged with PiB, in order to provide a basis of comparison for [C-11]SB-13. Following the injection of [C-11]SB-13, cerebellar time-activity data showed similar retention characteristics between AD patients and controls and this area was used as the reference region. Clearance of cerebellar radioactivity after injection of [C-11]SB-13 was somewhat slower than that observed for PiB in the same subjects, with [C-11]SB-13 exhibiting an approximately 3:1 ratio (from the peak of brain radioactivity to 90 minutes), as compared to an approximately 8:1 ratio for PiB. Increased retention of [C-11]SB-13 was observed in AD subjects compared to controls in cortical areas known to contain significant amyloid deposits in AD, such as the frontal cortex. Across the four cortical areas included in this investigation (frontal, temporal, parietal, occipital), SUVs were determined from 40 to 120 minutes post-injection emission data, and AD cortical averages of [C-11]SB-13 retention were shown to exceed control averages by 44%–75%, with the greatest distinction observed in the left frontal cortex. In the same subjects, the difference in PiB retention between AD subjects and controls was about twice as large as that detected with [C-11]SB-13. PiB retention was increased from 96% to 152% in the AD subjects, and also was maximal in the left frontal cortex. It is likely that the improved distinction between AD and control subjects using PiB is a result of more rapid clearance of nonspecific binding. While the pattern of retention of [C-11]SB-13 appears to mirror that of PiB, the latter provides a greater dynamic range and improved distinction of AD subjects from controls.

[I-123]Clioquinol

The fifth tracer to be used in human amyloid imaging studies was [I-123]Clioquinol ([I-123]CQ). Aβ aggregates in AD are enriched in transition metals such as zinc that mediate assembly. Clioquinol (CQ) targets metal interaction with Aβ. The binding properties of radioiodinated CQ ([I-125]CQ) to different in vitro and in vivo Alzheimer models have been investigated (Opazo et al., 2006). [I-125]CQ (used instead of I-123 for in vitro studies because of its 60-day half-life) showed saturable binding to synthetic Aβ precipitated by Zn(2+) ($K_d = 0.45$ and 1.40 nm for Aβ1–42 and Aβ1–40, respectively), which was fully displaced by free Zn(2+), Cu(2+), the chelator diethylene triamine pentaacetic acid, and partially by Congo red. APP transgenic (Tg2576) mice injected with [I-125]CQ exhibited higher brain retention of tracer compared to non-Tg mice. Autoradiography of brain sections of these animals confirmed selective [I-125]CQ enrichment in the neocortex. Histologically, both thioflavin-S-positive and negative structures were labeled by [I-125]CQ.

A pilot SPECT study of [I-123]CQ in humans showed limited uptake of the tracer into the brain, which did however, appear to be more rapid in AD patients compared to age-matched controls. Opazo et al. suggested that these data support metallated Aβ species as the neuropharmacological target of [I-123]CQ (Opazo et al., 2006). The poor brain entry of [I-123]CQ will prevent it from becoming a useful imaging agent.

[C-11]BF-227

The sixth agent to be reported in human amyloid imaging studies was [N-methyl-C-11]2-(2-[2-dimethylaminothiazol-5-yl]ethenyl)-6-(2-fluoroethoxy)benzoxazole, or [C-11]BF-227 (Arai et al., 2006; Kudo et al., 2007). BF-227 has a log P_{oct} of 1.75 and a good affinity for Aβ1–42 fibrils ($K_i = 4.3$ nM). The K_d in human brain homogenates has not been reported. Good initial brain entry is achieved at 2 minutes post-injection in mice (~235 %IDI), but the 2':30' clearance ratio was only 5:6.

[C-11]BF-227 SUV images in AD patients show increased retention of tracer in 10 AD subjects compared to 11 healthy controls (Kudo et al., 2007) (Figure 14.14). Lateral temporal and parietal cortex showed the greatest retention of [C-11]BF-227 compared to controls, but the increase was only 17%–22.5%. The most notable difference compared to PiB was the relatively low [C-11]BF-227 retention in the frontal cortex of AD subjects. Interestingly, although quantitative postmortem studies show that the frontal cortex contains significantly more Aβ than either the temporal or parietal cortex at CDR stages 0.5–2 (Naslund et al., 2000), frontal [C-11]BF-227 retention was only half that in the

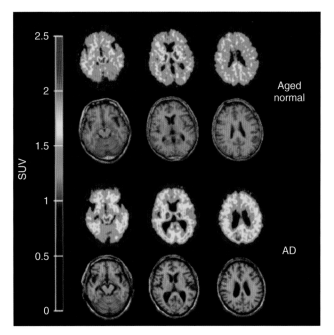

Figure 14–14 SUV images 20–40 minutes post-injection of [C-11]BF-227 in a cognitively normal control (top row) and an AD patient (third row). The respective MR images are shown below the PET images. (From Kudo et al., 2007.)

temporal cortex. This, and the fact that the nonspecific retention of [C-11]BF-227 in the pons of healthy controls (1.67 ± 0.08 SUVR) was far greater than that in the highest cortical area of AD brain, the lateral temporal cortex (1.25 ± 0.06), leaves questions as to whether the regional distribution of [C-11]BF-227 retention faithfully represents the regional distribution of Aβ amyloid.

[I-123]IMPY

Similar to the initial 10H3 antibody tracer, but in contrast to the previous small molecule tracers, the seventh agent evaluated in human amyloid imaging studies, 2-(4'-dimethylaminophenyl)-6-iodoimidazo[1,2-a]pyridine (known as IMPY), was designed to be a single photon emission computed tomography (SPECT) tracer. Kung and colleagues have reported that IMPY has moderate affinity ($K_i = 15$ nM) for synthetic Aβ and autoradiographically labeled plaques in transgenic mouse brain (Zhuang et al., 2003). The K_d measured in human AD brain homogenates was ~threefold better ($K_d = 5.3$ nM) (Kung et al., 2004). Consistent with a log P_{oct} value of 2.0, initial brain entry in mice was very good (~225 %IDI) and brain clearance was excellent (2':30' ratio = 11.1) (Zhuang et al., 2003).

The safety, biodistribution, and dosimetry of [I-123]IMPY was studied in humans and it appears to be a safe radiotracer with appropriate biokinetics for imaging studies in AD patients. Preliminary results of the first human study of [I-123]IMPY have been reported (Clark et al., 2006; Marek et al., 2007; Seibyl et al., 2007). In this study 8 AD patients and 7 healthy controls underwent serial SPECT imaging after either a single bolus injection or a bolus injection followed by multiple mini-bolus injections of [I-123]IMPY. After the single bolus injection 13 serial, dynamic SPECT acquisitions were acquired over 2 hours. During the bolus plus mini-bolus injections, scans were acquired for 90 minutes. In both AD patients and healthy controls uptake and washout of [I-123]IMPY were rapid—with a clearance $t_{1/2}$ of 21.5 minutes for healthy controls and 39.3 minutes for AD subjects ($p = .052$). Preliminary analysis of equilibrium distribution volume showed mean cortical to cerebellar ratios of 1.25 in AD subjects compared to 1.06 in healthy controls. This pilot [I-123]IMPY study demonstrated a small signal difference between AD patients and older healthy controls. The regional patterns of [I-123]IMPY retention did not clearly match the known pattern of amyloid deposition determined through autopsy studies (Braak and Braak, 1997a; Thal et al., 2002).

[F-18]AV-1

The eighth amyloid imaging tracer for which human results have been reported was the tri-polyethylene glycolated compound [F-18](4-[2-(4-[2-(2-[2-fluoroethoxy]-ethoxy)-ethoxy]-phenyl)-vinyl]-phenyl)-methylamine. This compound has been termed AV-1. AV-1 is structurally related to previously reported stilbenes, including [C-11]SB-13 (Kung et al., 2004) and [F-18]FMAPO (Zhang et al., 2005a), and also was developed by Kung and colleagues (Zhang et al., 2005b). In preclinical studies, AV-1 was shown to have a log P_{oct} of 2.41, an initial 2 minutes brain entry of ~180 %IDI and a 2':30' clearance ratio of ~4.9 in mice. The bone uptake at 120 minutes was measurable (~65 %IDI), suggesting there may be in vivo defluorination. The K_i of AV-1 (vs. [I-125]IMPY binding to AD brain homogenates) was 6.7 ± 0.3 nM. For comparison, PiB had a K_i of 2.8 ± 0.5 nM in the same assay. AV-1 showed high contrast plaque labeling in autoradiographic studies of AD brain tissue sections, but no binding studies were reported with AD brain gray matter homogenates (Zhang et al., 2005b).

Preliminary in vivo human AV-1 PET findings have been reported in five mild AD and five control subjects imaged with AV-1 (Rowe et al., 2007b, 2007c). AD subjects showed the greatest AV-1 retention in the precuneus/posterior cingulate and frontal cortex. Controls showed no significant cortical retention. Cerebellum showed no retention in either group. There was significant background in white matter regions. The regional pattern of AV-1 retention was reported to be similar to that of PiB,

suggesting that AV-1 retention is related to Aβ fibrillar amyloid distribution. The main difference between PiB and AV-1 apparent from these preliminary results was a greater degree of nonspecific background retention of AV-1, which led to an appreciably lower effect size for AV-1 when comparing the two subject groups. The mean neocortical AV-1 DVR value for AD subjects was 1.84 ± 0.20, and that of controls was 1.3 ± 0.17 ($p = 0.009$; 42% increase).

[F-18]3'F-PiB

The ninth amyloid imaging tracer for which human results have been reported was the fluorine-18 derivative of PiB, [F-18]2-(3'-fluoro-4'-methylaminophenyl)-6-hydroxybenzothiazole ([F-18]3'F-PiB) (Mathis et al., 2007). The log P_{oct} of [F-18]3'F-PiB is 1.7, which is somewhat higher than that of PiB (1.2), and both bind to homogenates of AD brain with high affinity (K_d PiB = 1.4 nM; K_d [F-18]3'F-PiB = 2.2 nM). The initial brain entry of [F-18]3'F-PiB in mice was excellent (312 %IDI) and the 2':30' clearance ratio of 8.4 was good—although somewhat less than PiB (table 14.2).

The initial human [F-18]3'F-PiB study included three controls and two AD subjects that also were imaged with [C-11]PiB for comparison (Mathis et al., 2007). [F-18]3'F-PiB readily entered the human brain, showing uptake values at 2 minutes that were nearly identical to those of [C-11]PiB in humans. Increased retention of radioactivity following the injection of [F-18]3'F-PiB was observed in cortical areas of AD subjects known to be affected in AD (e.g., precuneus and frontal). [F-18]3'F-PiB showed regional uptake and retention characteristics that closely matched those of [C-11]PiB in cortical brain regions (Figure 14.15). [F-18]3'F-PiB SUVR values (relative to cerebellum) in precuneus and frontal cortex were generally within 10% of [C-11]PiB SUVR values. [F-18]3'F-PiB DVR values in the precuneus of two AD subjects (2.12 ± 0.09) were ~73% higher than that in the three controls (1.22 ± 0.12) and were comparable to [C-11]PiB DVR values measured in the precuneus of the same subjects (AD [C-11]PiB DVR = 2.28 ± 0.15; control [C-11]PiB DVR = 1.15 ± 0.10). Somewhat higher nonspecific retention in

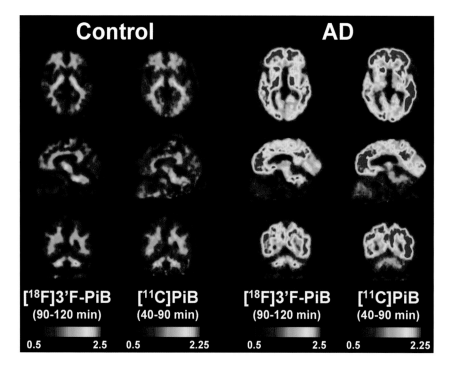

Figure 14–15 Comparison of [F-18]3'F-PiB and [C-11]PiB in the same control (left) and AD subject (right). The transaxial (top), sagittal (middle), and coronal (bottom) SUVR images (relative to cerebellum) were acquired 90–120 minutes post-injection of [F-18]3'F-PiB or 40–90 minutes post-injection of [C-11]PiB.

white matter was observed for [F-18]3'F-PiB relative to [C-11]PiB, especially at shorter times post-injection (40–90minutes), but this did not negatively impact the ability of [F-18]3'F-PiB to identify and quantify cortical Aβ deposits at later times. The optimal time window for signal-to-noise for [F-18]3'F-PiB was 90–120 minutes post-injection compared to an optimal time window of 40–90 minutes for [C-11]PiB (Figure 14.15).

[F-18]FDDNP

The second agent used in efforts to visualize in vivo amyloid deposits was a radiofluorinated derivative of the solvent and viscosity sensitive fluorophore 2- (1-[6-(dimethylamino)-2-naphthyl]ethylidene)malononitrile (DDNP), termed [F-18]FDDNP (Barrio et al., 1999). In vitro characterization of FDDNP demonstrated that it labeled amyloid plaques with high affinity and fluorescently stained both plaques and neurofibrillary tangles at relatively high concentrations (Agdeppa et al., 2001a, 2003; Smid et al., 2006).

Initial human studies in AD patients ($n = 9$) and controls ($n = 7$) showed greater retention of [F-18]FDDNP in frontal, parietal, temporal, and occipital cortices at steady-state (60–120 minutes post-injection). The increased neocortical retention was shown to exceed the reference region (pons) by a margin of 10%–15%. The area of highest retention at equilibrium was a region encompassing the hippocampus/amygdala/entorhinal (h-a-e) cortex region, which was shown to exceed retention in the pons by ~25% (Shoghi-Jadid et al., 2002). Interestingly, autopsy studies (Arnold et al., 1991) showed that neuritic plaques are more densely concentrated in the neocortex, while the mesial temporal lobe structures, including the h-a-e cortex region, contain the fewest neuritic plaques. Neurofibrillary tangles, in contrast, are densely concentrated in the mesial temporal lobe where [F-18]FDDNP retention is greatest (Braak and Braak, 1991). The authors demonstrated significantly higher h-a-e [F-18]FDDNP measures for AD patients as compared to controls, and that [F-18]FDDNP measures were significantly correlated with MMSE (Folstein, Folstein, and McHugh, 1975a).

It has been reported that [F-18]FDDNP can label neurofibrillary tangles in vivo, and it has been speculated that the [F-18]FDDNP signal observed in the medial temporal lobe may at least partly arise from neurofibrillary tangles (Shoghi-Jadid et al., 2002; Small et al., 2006). However, simple in vitro histochemical labeling of neurofibrillary tangles with high concentrations of a fluorescent compound, such as FDDNP, does not necessarily equate to the ability to detect neurofibrillary tangles in vivo with a radiolabeled version of that same compound and PET. This is because the concentrations used in the histochemical staining reaction are ~10,000 times higher than those achieved in vivo and the conditions used for staining and differentiating (washing away free and nonspecifically bound tracer) are typically very non-physiological. Neurofibrillary tangles also have been labeled with [F-18]FDDNP in vitro at relatively low concentrations and then detected autoradiographically (Agdeppa et al., 2003). However, autoradiographic assays do not always predict in vivo detection of neurofibrillary tangles and plaques. This may be because nonphysiological conditions are often used in these assays, much like the histological staining studies. In addition, the spatial resolution and signal-to-noise that can be achieved autoradiographically cannot be achieved during in vivo PET studies. For example, an autoradiographic strategy has been used to successfully label amyloid plaques in vitro using the putative amyloid imaging tracer [I-125] IMPY (Zhuang et al., 2003), but this tracer has not proven useful in vivo (see above). Similarly, a fluorine-18-labeled stilbene has been shown to label plaques in postmortem AD brain sections quite well, but showed no specific binding to homogenates of fresh frozen AD brain tissue (see compound [F-18]**3e** of [Zhang et al., 2005a]). A more convincing strategy to demonstrate that [F-18]FDDNP quantitatively detects neurofibrillary tangles in vivo would be to show a large (e.g., five- to tenfold) increase in [F-18]FDDNP binding to homogenates of postmortem brain tissue rich in neurofibrillary tangles, but without plaques, compared to a brain homogenate without neurofibrillary tangles or plaques. To be even more convincing, this experiment should go on to show a good correlation between the amount of [F-18]FDDNP bound to homogenates from several different "neurofibrillary tangle-pure" brains and the quantitative amount of neurofibrillary tangle-related tau in those same homogenates determined biochemically (e.g., by ELISA). This same strategy has been used both to validate the quantitative assessment of Aβ amyloid by PiB (Klunk et al., 2005) and to show that PiB does *not* detect the neurofibrillary tangle burden in postmortem homogenates (Klunk et al., 2003). Until such confirmatory data is available, claims of in vivo neurofibrillary tangle quantification by any tracer must be considered speculative.

Initial analyses of [F-18]FDDNP PET data were performed using a novel kinetic analysis method, termed the relative residence time (RRT), which relates specific radiotracer binding to the negative net difference between the reciprocal of the tissue clearance constants (k_2) for the reference and target tissues. Very simply put, the RRT is based on the rate of tissue clearance over the whole study rather than a steady-state accumulation at late time points. The result is that the RRT can reflect the clearance of free and nonspecifically bound [F-18]FDDNP during the early portion of the TAC as much or more than specifically bound tracer levels that are best represented during the later, steady-state portion of the TAC. This is readily apparent in the [F-18]FDDNP TACs in Figure 14.16, where it is clear that the equilibrium levels of [F-18]FDDNP are very similar throughout the brain. Furthermore, the equilibrium level in the temporal cortex is identical to that in the occipital cortex, while the RRT value for the temporal cortex (6.14) is nearly 17-fold higher than the RRT in the occipital cortex (0.37). It is evident that the biological basis for this large difference in RRT is not the equilibrium level of tracer specifically bound to amyloid. Rather, the basis for the 17-fold difference in RRT values calculated in temporal and occipital cortex appears to be the higher initial brain level in the occipital cortex and the subsequent more rapid clearance from this area compared to temporal cortex. Several phenomena may play a role in this occurrence, but differences in blood flow to the two brain areas have to be strongly considered as the explanation for both the initial differences in brain entry and the ensuing differences in rate of clearance.

Following this initial analysis, a subsequent analysis of [F-18]FDDNP image data has been reported, comparing 14 AD subjects and 12 controls using both SUVR and Logan DVR approaches computed from 60 to 120 minutes tissue radioactivity concentrations (using the cerebellum as reference). This analysis showed significant differences ($p < 0.001$) in the retention of [F-18]FDDNP between control and AD subjects in regions such as the medial temporal, parietal, and prefrontal cortices; but, as predicted by the [F-18]FDDNP TAC shown above, the magnitude of the signal in the AD subjects did not exceed the control value by more than 15% in any region (Small et al., 2004).

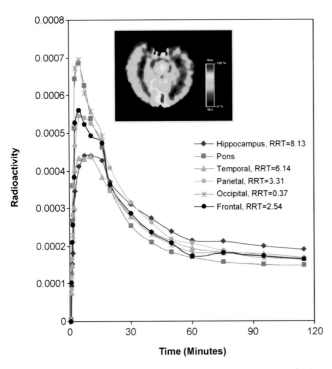

Figure 14–16 Time-activity curves of [F-18]FDDNP in various brain regions of an AD subject. The RRT numbers for each brain area also are shown as an inset. Note that the 16.6-fold difference in RRT between temporal cortex (RRT = 6.14; green triangles) and occipital cortex (RRT = 0.37; orange asterisks) is reflected only in the initial brain entry and clearance, but not at all in the steady-state levels reached after 60 minutes. (From Shoghi-Jadid et al., 2002.)

In another analysis of [F-18]FDDNP imaging in 28 subjects with mild cognitive impairment (MCI; Petersen, 2004), 25 AD subjects and 30 controls utilized the Logan DVR approach (Small et al., 2006). In this study, global DVR values for [F-18]FDDNP (the average of the values for the temporal, parietal, posterior cingulate, and frontal regions) were significantly lower in the control group than in the group with MCI, and the DVR values in the MCI group were lower than in the group with AD. [F-18]FDDNP PET differentiated among the diagnostic groups

better than did [F-18]fluorodeoxyglucose (FDG) PET measures of cerebral metabolism or MRI volume measures (Figure 14.17). The authors concluded that despite considerable overlap between the groups, [F-18]FDDNP PET scanning can "differentiate persons with mild cognitive impairment from those with Alzheimer's disease and those with no cognitive impairment." The mean and standard deviation of the global DVR value in controls was 1.07 ± 0.02; the global DVR in the MCI group was 1.12 ± 0.02 (4.6% higher than controls); and the global DVR value in the AD group was 1.16 ± 0.01 (8.4% higher than control). While the difference between group means was small, the remarkably small biological variation in the subject groups (1%–2% of the mean) resulted in large effect sizes and detection of significant differences.

Although SUVR and DVR analyses of [F-18]FDDNP data have been reported, it should be kept in mind that the applicability of conventional quantitative analysis methodologies, such as compartmental modeling and graphical analyses, to dynamic [F-18]FDDNP PET data remains to be validated. These studies are necessary to fully understand the nature of [F-18]FDDNP retention and to assess the overall sensitivity and specificity of the compound for the detection of AD pathology in vivo.

An independent team of investigators have presented the first direct comparison of [F-18]FDDNP and PiB in the same subjects (Tolboom et al., 2007). Tolboom et al. acquired dynamic 90 minutes PiB and [F-18]FDDNP scans on the same day using the same PET scanner. During both scans, continuous online and discrete manual sampling was performed to derive a metabolite-corrected arterial plasma input curve. Analysis of TACs was performed using the simplified reference tissue model with cerebellum gray matter as reference tissue. Three AD patients, three patients with MCI, and three age-matched normal controls were included in this preliminary study. Tolboom et al. reported that PiB showed good contrast between AD patients and normal controls, as described previously (see below; Klunk et al. 2004). In addition, the range of BP values in MCI patients was broader, probably due to the known heterogeneity of this group (see below) (Lopresti et al., 2005). [F-18]FDDNP provided less contrast between AD patients and normal controls. The PiB BP was in general tenfold higher than the [F-18]FDDNP BP in the same AD patients.

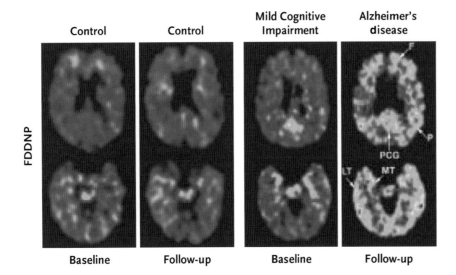

Figure 14–17 Baseline and follow-up (15–35 months) of a cognitively stable control subject (left two columns) and an MCI subject who converted to AD (right two columns) at the level of the parietal (top) or temporal cortex (bottom). A rainbow scale is used to indicate increased [F-18]FDDNP retention (red and yellow areas in the right column). (From Small et al., 2006).

[C-11]PiB

Initial Human Study

[C-11]PiB was the third amyloid imaging tracer to be studied in humans and the first tracer to show a clear correspondence to the known regional distribution of postmortem Aβ amyloid pathology in AD. To date, more [C-11]PiB scans (>2000) have been performed at more sites worldwide (>30) than any other amyloid imaging tracer. These numbers are likely to increase rapidly because of the inclusion of [C-11]PiB imaging in the Alzheimer's Disease Neuroimaging Initiative (Mueller et al., 2005a, 2005b). Because of this, [C-11]PiB is likely to become the benchmark against which newer tracers will be compared.

The first human studies with PiB were a collaboration between the University of Pittsburgh and Uppsala University and were presented in preliminary form in 2002 (Engler et al., 2002), followed by a full report in 2004 (Klunk et al., 2004). This initial study included 16 mild-moderate AD patients, six elderly age-matched controls, and three 21-year-old controls. The young controls were included in the study because of the near certainty that these young subjects would represent true plaque-negative controls. Striking differences in PiB retention were observed between control and AD subjects in brain areas known to contain significant amyloid deposits in AD (e.g., the frontal cortex and the parietal cortex). The control subjects showed rapid entry and clearance of [C-11]PiB from all cortical and subcortical gray matter areas, including the cerebellar cortex (Figure 14.18).

The cerebellum, an area generally lacking fibrillar amyloid plaques in AD, showed nearly identical uptake and clearance of PiB in the cerebellum of HC and AD groups (Figure 14.18a). Subcortical white matter showed relatively lower entry and slower clearance in both HC subjects and AD patients compared to cortical and subcortical gray matter areas (Figure 14.18b). In contrast, the AD patients showed a markedly enhanced retention of PiB compared to HC subjects in areas of the brain known to contain high levels of amyloid deposits in AD (Figures 14.18c–e), such as the parietal and frontal cortices (Arnold et al., 1991; Thal et al., 2002).

The regional distribution of PiB retention was clearly different in AD patients compared to the HC subjects (Figure 14.19). PiB accumulation in AD patients as a group was most prominent in cortical association areas and lower in white matter areas, a pattern consistent with that described in postmortem studies of amyloid deposition in AD brain (Thal et al., 2002). PiB images from HC subjects showed little or no PiB retention in cortical areas, leaving

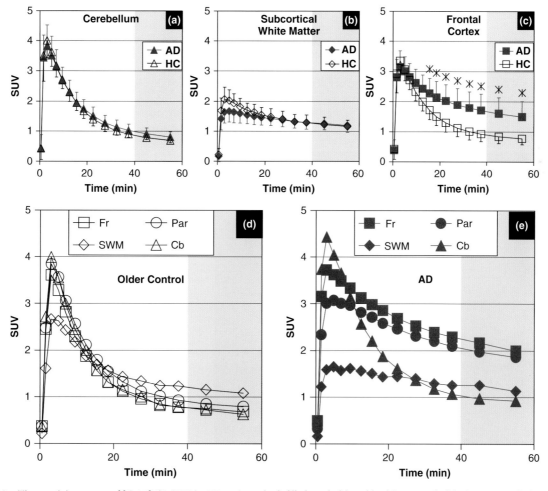

Figure 14–18 Time-activity curves of [C-11]PiB SUV in AD patients (red, filled symbols) and healthy controls (black, open symbols) in two areas without amyloid deposition: cerebellum (Cb; triangles; A) and subcortical white matter (SWM; diamonds; B), and in a brain area with heavy amyloid deposition: frontal cortex (Fr; squares; C). The difference in specific binding signal in the frontal and parietal (Par) cortices between a healthy control and an AD patient is shown in D & E. (From Klunk et al., 2004.)

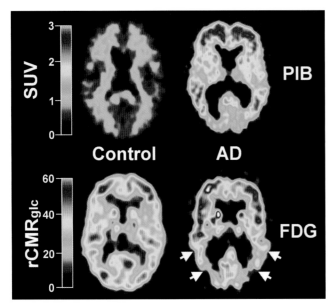

Figure 14–19 [C-11]PiB SUV images of a healthy control subject (left, top) and an AD patient (right, top), and FDG cerebral metabolic images of the same control (bottom, left) and AD patient (bottom, right). Arrows indicate temporoparietal hypometabolism in the AD patient. (From Klunk et al., 2004.)

the subcortical white matter regions highest in relative terms. In absolute terms, the accumulation of PiB in white matter was essentially the same in AD patients and HC subjects (Figure 14.18b). A series of three-dimensional representations of PiB retention superimposed on the MRI of a mild AD patient provides a sense of the regional distribution of PiB retention (Figure 14.20).

The marked difference between PiB retention in the AD patients and the HC subjects is apparent throughout most of the forebrain. Frontal cortex was widely affected in the AD patient, but intense PiB retention also was observed in precuneus/posterior cingulate, temporal, and parietal cortices and in the striatum. The occipital cortex was often affected as well. Lateral temporal cortex appeared to have greater PiB accumulation than mesial temporal areas. Consistent with previous reports of extensive amyloid deposition in the striatum of virtually all AD patients (Braak and Braak, 1990; Brilliant et al., 1997; Suenaga et al., 1990; Wolf et al., 1999), the striatum was found to have significantly higher PiB retention in AD patients than in HC subjects. Cerebellar cortex showed little PiB retention and was similar in AD patients and HC subjects. In general, the observed pattern of PiB retention in AD subjects was found to be consistent with the pattern of amyloid plaque deposition described in postmortem studies of the AD brain (Arnold et al., 1991; Thal et al., 2002). PiB retention typically predominated in the frontal cortex, but it should be noted that the frontal cortex did not always show the highest PiB retention in a given subject, and mean levels of frontal PiB retention exceeded parietal levels by less than 10%.

Given the fact that previous postmortem studies have repeatedly shown that the clinical diagnosis of AD is not 100% specific (i.e., some clinically diagnosed AD patients do not have $A\beta$ deposits at autopsy) and that a significant number of clinically unimpaired elderly are found to have $A\beta$ deposits (Haroutunian et al., 1998; Price and Morris, 1999), it was no surprise that there was not an exact match between clinical diagnosis and PiB retention in this initial study. Three AD subjects had levels of PiB retention in cortical regions typical of controls. These atypical AD patients had high MMSE scores (28–29) and showed no significant deterioration over the 2–4 year follow-up period prior to the PiB study (i.e., MMSE remained 28–29). Other mild AD patients with

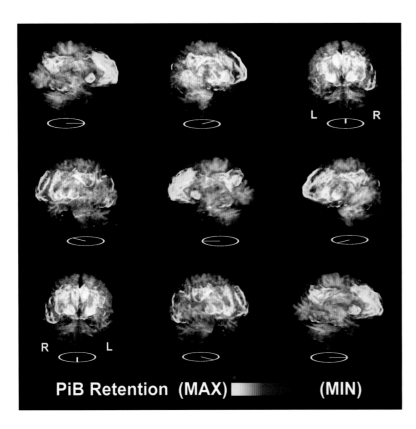

Figure 14–20 Three-dimesional representation of PiB retention (in color) superimposed on this mild AD patient's MR scan (grayscale). Note the characteristic pattern of retention in medial, basal, and dorsolateral frontal cortex, anterior-ventral striatum, precuneous (medial parietal), parietal, and lateral temporal cortex. Also note the lack of retention in cerebellum and brainstem. The scale for PiB is set to accentuate the highest areas of deposition, and low levels of PiB retention in other cortical areas are not visible here.

similar clinical profiles showed typical AD-like changes in PiB retention and rCMRglc. It was unclear whether PiB was simply insensitive to the amount of amyloid deposits in the brains of these three atypical AD patients with MMSE scores of 28–29, or whether PiB imaging had correctly identified subjects without amyloid deposits in whom the clinical diagnosis of AD was incorrect and could/would not be confirmed by postmortem evaluation. In the elderly control group, the oldest subject (76 years old) consistently showed the highest cortical PiB retention and the lowest cortical rCMRglc. This subject had not expressed any subjective memory complaints and performed within the normal range on the neuropsychological test battery except for difficulty copying a complex cube. This type of case, which could be described as an asymptomatic amyloid-positive case, highlights the issue of specificity versus early detection. One possibility could be that a high PiB signal was obtained in the absence of amyloid deposits (i.e., a false-positive). If this finding does represent the true presence of amyloid in an asymptomatic individual, the question becomes whether substantial amyloid deposition can be found as part of the "normal" aging process in subjects who will never develop AD (Morris et al., 1996), or whether increased amyloid deposition is always a sign of preclinical AD (Goldman et al., 2001; Morris and Price, 2001; Schmitt et al., 2000). The ability to longitudinally follow PiB retention as an in vivo measure of amyloid deposition provides a new tool through which we may be able to answer this question in a manner that postmortem studies cannot.

Engler et al. (2006) provided some insight into the clinical history of the three atypical AD patients and the high-PiB control in a two-year follow-up study. In the study, all three of the low-PiB AD subjects were classified as MCI—although it is not clear if this was by clinicians blinded to the PiB PET results. Engler et al. state, "Their clinical symptoms may have a different pathological basis than Alzheimer's disease." Nevertheless, as Engler and colleagues note, further follow-up will be required to definitively diagnose these subjects. With regard to the oldest control, who showed PiB retention in the "low AD" range at baseline, Engler et al. report that this subject showed no change in cognition or rCMRglc over the follow-up period, and showed either slight (temporal and parietal) or no increases in PiB retention (frontal and striatum). This could be consistent with a false-positive result if PiB retention follows a fairly rapid course, or it could be consistent with a true positive if PiB retention begins long before clinical symptoms and follows a fairly lengthy course (see below). As in the case of the three atypical AD patients, more time will be needed to answer this question with certainty.

Since the initial PiB PET study (Klunk et al., 2004), several studies using PiB in AD patients and control subjects have confirmed these findings (Archer et al., 2006; Buckner et al., 2005; Edison et al., 2006; Fagan et al., 2006, 2007; Kemppainen et al., 2006; Lopresti et al., 2005; Mintun et al., 2006; Nelissen et al., 2007; Pike et al., 2007; Price et al., 2005; Rowe et al., 2007a; Ziolko et al., 2006).

Two-Year Follow-Up of the Original PiB Cohort

Understanding the natural history of amyloid deposition is of great importance for advancing our knowledge of the pathophysiology of AD—both during the clinically apparent phase as well as during the antecedent preclinical phase (Goldman et al., 2001). Awareness of the natural history of amyloid deposition also will be necessary to interpret experimental anti-amyloid drug studies that might extend over a year or more. Postmortem studies cannot, of course, directly assess the progression of amyloid deposition in an individual over time, and attempts to deduce the natural history by comparing a

series of postmortem cases with different clinical severities and amyloid loads have significant limitations (Hyman and Gomez-Isla, 1997). Nevertheless, several very extensive postmortem studies have provided useful information (Braak and Braak, 1997; Thal et al., 2002). For example, although some degree of correlation has been reported between plaque load (Cummings et al., 1996; Parvathy et al., 2001) or Aβ levels (Naslund et al., 2000) and measures of cognition, it is generally believed that neither the number nor the total area of neocortical plaques correlate well with cognitive deficits before death (Braak and Braak, 1998; Terry et al., 1991). We must keep this background in mind as we interpret the study by Engler et al. (2006) in which the first longitudinal study of Aβ amyloid deposition in living subjects is reported—a two-year follow-up of the original PiB study cohort discussed above (Klunk et al., 2004, 2006). Remarkably, Engler and colleagues succeeded in rescanning all 16 of the original subjects who had a clinical diagnosis of AD 1.5–2.5 years after the baseline PiB scan. They also rescanned the one control who showed evidence of high PiB retention in the baseline study. Thirteen of these subjects also had baseline and repeat FDG scans.

Engler and colleagues did not find increases in PiB retention (and presumably amyloid deposition) over the two-year follow-up. Instead, their two primary findings were: (1) PiB retention showed no significant change over the 2 ± 0.5 years of follow-up, and (2) the regional cerebral metabolism rate for glucose (rCMRglc; indexed by FDG-PET) fell an additional 20% from baseline. Since cognition typically worsens steadily over time in AD, and since postmortem amyloid deposits do not correlate well with cognition (Braak and Braak, 1998; Terry et al., 1991), the lack of progression in PiB retention is not unexpected. Several considerations make these findings less straightforward, and this has been discussed in detail elsewhere (Klunk et al., 2006).

The difference between changes in group averages and trajectories of individual subjects requires special consideration in this study. Engler et al. do compare subgroups of AD patients (four who had significant cognitive decline and nine who were clinically stable). Although PiB retention was higher in the declining group at baseline and follow-up, Engler et al. did not find any difference in interval change in PiB retention between these groups. In the areas of highest PiB retention (frontal and posterior cingulate/precuneus) they report a slight increase in the AD-Stable group and small decrements in the AD-Progressive group. However, Engler et al. might have taken greater advantage of their longitudinal data by discussing the changes in individual subjects. For example, they did not directly report the *trajectories* of PiB retention and rCMRglc for individual subjects over time, but these data can be determined from their Figure 14.2 and are shown below (Figure 14.21).

It is apparent that most subjects (7 of 13) show *both* a small increase in PiB retention and a more substantial decrease in metabolism over time. This appears to be hidden in the grouped analyses by relatively large decreases in PiB retention in four subjects (3, 5, 7, and 15). The paradoxical changes in subjects 5 and 15 (decreased PiB retention and increased metabolism) are difficult to explain, as both changes are contrary to that expected in AD. However, the decreases in PiB retention, coupled with decreases in metabolism in subjects 3 and 7, may relate to the phenomenon previously described in Down syndrome and AD. A prior study indicated that Aβ deposits *decline* late in the course of AD in Down syndrome (Wegiel et al., 1999), and another suggested that the same phenomenon may occur in sporadic AD (Hyman, Marzloff, and Arriagada, 1993). Thus, it is intriguing that subjects 3 and 7, who had the most advanced disease at baseline and who also

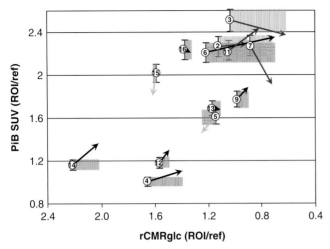

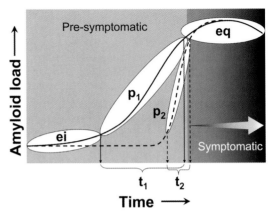

Figure 14–21 Individual trajectories of PiB retention and rCMRglc in the parietal cortex of the 13 subjects with both baseline and follow-up PiB and FDG imaging data. Increasing PiB retention (i.e., worsening disease) is shown on the y-axis in the units used by Engler et al. Decreasing metabolism (i.e., worsening disease) is shown on an inverted scale on the x-axis. The numbers in circles correspond to the individual subjects from the Engler et al. study and represent the baseline PiB and FDG values; the arrows point toward the follow-up values. The shaded rectangles indicate the 4.1% test/re-test variability of PiB-PET in the parietal lobe. Red arrows (and orange rectangles) indicate the four clinically-declining AD subjects (2, 3, 7 and 11). All other subjects were clinically stable, but green arrows emphasize the two subjects (5 and 15) with paradoxical improvements in both PiB retention (decreased) and cerebral metabolism (increased). Subjects 2, 13, and 16 showed essentially no change in PiB retention, but the other subjects showed changes greater than to be expected from test/re-test variability alone.

Figure 14–22 Hypothetical schematic of the progression of amyloid deposition over time from the very early initiation (ei) phase, to the continuously progressive (p) phase, and finally to the late equilibrium (eq) phase. Relatively long (p_1 & t_1) and brief (p_2 & t_2) progressive phases are shown. Symptoms are not evident until the equilibrium (eq) phase, but the cascade of pathological events that leads to these symptoms (i.e., neurofibrillary pathology and synapse loss) is initiated during the progressive phase (p). (From Klunk et al., 2006.)

showed significant cognitive worsening over the two-year follow-up, were the only subjects who had both decreased PiB retention and rCMRglc.

Consequently, interpretation of amyloid changes over time must take into account the status of any particular subject relative to the full spectrum of amyloid changes that may occur in AD. Figure 14.22 shows a schematic of three hypothetical phases of Aβ amyloid deposition: (1) very early initiation (ei), (2) continuously progressive (p), and (3) late equilibrium/symptomatic (eq). The study by Engler et al. suggests that these mild-moderate AD patients are in the late equilibrium phase, because most subjects show small increases in amyloid load, some are stable, and the two more advanced subjects show declining amyloid loads. The continuously progressive phase (p) must exist, and PiB PET may be well-suited to track it, but when in the clinical course of AD will we find it? A second question is how long does the progressive phase last? Will it be a decade or more (e.g., p_1 and t_1 in Figure 14.22) or just a few years (e.g., p_2 and t_2). Preliminary data suggest that most subjects with mild cognitive impairment (MCI) have levels of PiB retention equal to that of AD patients (see below). Therefore, these MCI subjects may already be in the equilibrium phase (Lopresti et al., 2005; Price et al., 2005). If this is true, we must look for the progressive phase among asymptomatic subjects. Mintun et al. (2006) have recently shown that asymptomatic subjects can be identified with levels of PiB retention that are intermediate between those typically observed in normal controls and clinically diagnosed AD patients (see below). It will be very important to document the natural history of amyloid deposition in these subjects.

The Engler et al. (2006) study is a landmark description of the natural history of amyloid deposition in living subjects, although many other issues still remain for future longitudinal studies. It reminds us that neither the clinical course nor the pathology of AD progresses in a simple, linear fashion from beginning to end, but that both are highly variable. Any interpretation of changes over time must be made from the perspective of where a given patient stands in the disease process. Further, these results imply that in order for an anti-amyloid therapy to be shown to be effective in altering the natural course of amyloid deposition, it cannot simply stabilize amyloid load in symptomatic AD patients, but must reduce amyloid load. The stability in group average PiB retention and the ~5% test-retest variability mean that in order to detect the effect of an anti-amyloid therapy by PiB PET in symptomatic AD patients, the therapy will probably need to induce *at least* a 10%–15% decrease in amyloid load. From a clinical perspective as well, a decrease in amyloid load of 10%–15% or more will likely be necessary in order to achieve meaningful clinical effects, so the detection threshold of amyloid imaging is not likely to be a limiting factor.

Validation of Quantitative Pharmacokinetics Analysis Methods for PiB PET

Compartmental Modeling and Logan Graphical Analysis With Arterial Blood Data

More recent human PiB studies have extended the initial proof-of-concept study of Klunk et al. (2004) by including magnetic resonance (MR) image co-registration for region-of-interest placement, 90 minutes of PET emission data acquisition, arterial input function determination, metabolite correction, and conventional protein-ligand binding compartmental analyses (Price et al., 2005). These arterial-based analyses found that the PiB PET data were generally well described by a 2-tissue 4-parameter (2T-4k) compartmental model that assumed negligible radiotracer occupancy of the binding sites and reversible in vivo kinetics. Although the 2T-4k approach proved to be the compartmental model that best described the observed PET data, inherent difficulties in regions with low signal (e.g., most areas in control brain or the cerebellum in AD brain) occasionally resulted in spurious estimates of the measures of PiB retention in these regions. Therefore, the DVR measure (see above) of PiB retention was determined using another pharmacokinetic method called the "Logan graphical analysis method." The use of 90 minutes of emission data and an arterial input function (ART90) showed lower intersubject variability than 2T-4k measures, though the methods were strongly correlated (r ~0.9) across all regions-of-interest. Twofold differences between control and AD ART90 DVR measures were detected in the areas of highest amyloid deposition. The ART90 method also yielded stable results with test-retest reliability of about 7% across primary areas of interest. For these reasons ART90 was selected over the 2T-4k compartmental model as the benchmark method for the analysis of PiB PET data (Price et al., 2005) and was the method against which the simplified methods discussed below were compared.

Simplified Assessments of Brain Amyloid Using [C-11]PiB

While the ART90 method may involve a simplification of the data analysis methodology in that estimates of DVR are obtained by a simple linear regression of graphical variables, implementation of the method remains tedious because of the need for collection of 90 minutes of emission data and an arterial line used to collect blood for determination of the levels of PiB and its metabolites across the entire study. In addition to subject inconvenience and discomfort, the actual determination of PiB and PiB metabolites is not trivial because of the rapid metabolism in blood (Price et al., 2005). This adds further difficulty to the ART90 method. To make the use of PiB more feasible in a wider range of applications, it would be advantageous to identify yet more simplified methods of analysis that provide outcome measure estimates that compare well to ART90 and allow simpler methods of data acquisition (e.g., omission of arterial blood collection and shortened scan times).

Recent work has compared simplified methods and analyses for in vivo assessments of brain amyloid deposition using PiB PET imaging (Lopresti et al., 2005, 2006). The simplifications examined included: (1) shortening the scan period from 90 to 60 minutes (i.e., ART90 and ART60); (2) substitution of actual arterial blood collection and metabolite correction with an image-derived arterial input function from a volume-of-interest defined over the carotid artery and a population-based metabolite correction; (3) replacing arterial input altogether with a completely image-driven analysis method based on the kinetics of the tracer in the cerebellum (i.e., cerebellar input), such as the non-invasive Logan analysis (CER60 and CER90); and (4) use of a late single-scan measure of the radioactivity distribution (SUVR60 and SUVR90). Within each level of simplification, performance was compared to the benchmark quantitative method, ART90, and was assessed by four criteria: (a) fidelity of regional rank order; (b) test-retest variability; (c) correlation between the simplified method and ART90 outcome measures; and (d) Cohen's effect size.

When compared to controls, all simplified methods yielded similarly significant increases ($p < 0.001$) in PiB retention in brain regions of AD subjects known to contain high levels of amyloid deposits, although the performance of the simplified methods varied in terms of the evaluation criteria. While analysis methods that used 90 minutes of emission data performed better across the evaluation criteria than those employing only 60 minutes, most 60-minute scan methods proved useful. Across all simplified methods of analysis, the regional rank order of PiB retention in AD subjects was identical to that described for 2T-4k and ART90, with the most PiB retention observed in posterior cingulate gyrus/precuneus, followed by anterior cingulate gyrus, frontal cortex, and parietal cortex. The MCI subjects showed levels of PiB retention in brain that ranged from control levels to AD levels. This was an expected finding, considering the heterogeneous pathologic substrates of MCI previously described in postmortem studies.

The noninvasive Logan graphical analysis method using cerebellum as reference (CER90 and CER60) showed the lowest test-retest variability of any method examined (<5% across regions). The CER90 and CER60 methods also are fairly easy to implement. Parametric DVR images determined using CER90 showed an essentially identical pattern of PiB retention to that determined using the ART90 method in both control and AD subjects (Figure 14.23).

The SUV-based methods are the simplest in terms of implementation and execution, and the SUVR60 method requires only 20 minutes of PET scanner time for data collection (40–60 minutes interval). Both SUVR90 and SUVR60 performed very well in terms of the established evaluation criteria, and showed the greatest dynamic range, mean difference, and effect sizes between AD and control subject groups (Cohen effect size = 6.9).

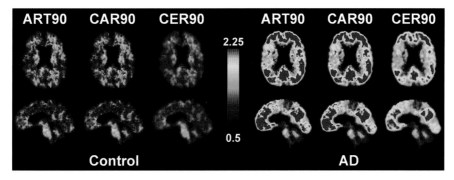

Figure 14–23 Parametric DVR images from one control and one AD patient calculated by three different methods. In the ART90 method, tracer levels actually measured in arterial plasma samples are employed as the input function used to calculate the DV values from 90 minutes of scan data (ART90). In the Car90 method, arterial tracer levels are estimated from ROI drawn over the carotid arteries on the scan and then used as the input function. In the CER90 method, average tracer levels in a cerebellar cortex reference region are employed as the input function used to calculate the PiB retention measure. The CER90 method inherently normalizes the DV in all voxels to that in the cerebellar reference region and thus results in DV ratio (i.e., DVR) values. In the ART90 and CAR90 methods, the DV of each voxel can then be expressed as a ratio to the average DV value calculated for the cerebellar reference ROI to determine the DVR value. (From Lopresti et al., 2006.)

Reference Tissue Models

Although the CER90 Logan graphical method described above can be generally defined as a "reference tissue" approach, the classic "Reference Tissue Model" (RTM) approach to pharmacokinetic modeling uses a compartmental approach, but the use of an arterial line is avoided by substitution of a reference tissue TAC for the arterial TAC as the "input function" (Blomqvist et al., 1989; Cunningham et al., 1991). As was mentioned above for the arterial compartmental modeling approach, a disadvantage of the RTM can be its poor performance in brain areas with very low specific binding, such as cortical areas of the control brain in amyloid imaging studies. A simplified reference tissue model (SRTM) that also uses a compartmental approach, but requires fewer parameters (three vs. four or more) was developed to overcome these disadvantages and improve performance at the voxel level (Gunn et al., 1997; Lammertsma and Hume, 1996). Unfortunately, the standard SRTM was found to work least well with PiB data by Lopresti et al. (2005), and similar problems have been reported with other tracers (Suzuki et al., 2005; Verhoeff et al., 2004). Improved approaches to the RTM have employed simultaneous fitting to multiple ROIs to minimize the effect of low-signal ROIs fit in isolation (Buck et al., 1996) and higher-order models (i.e., more compartments) (Wu and Carson, 2002). Zhou et al., have used such an RTM approach for the analysis of PiB data (Zhou et al. 2007). They showed that an RTM method using three parameters and simultaneous fitting of ROIs was a robust compartmental modeling approach that could be useful in [C-11]PiB PET studies to detect early markers of AD where specific ROIs with high amyloid loads can been identified.

Voxel-Based Methods

In addition to the region-of-interest–based methods discussed above, voxel-based methods have been applied to the analysis of PiB data (Kemppainen et al., 2006; Ziolko et al., 2006). As the name implies, voxel-based methods perform any of the calculations described above on every voxel individually, rather than groups of voxels in ROIs (i.e., each voxel becomes an ROI). An advantage of voxel-based methods is that analyses are done across the whole brain, so no area with an interesting finding would be ignored, as could happen in an ROI analysis if that area was not included as part of a chosen ROI. A disadvantage of voxel-based methods is increased noise, since the noise-averaging that occurs when multiple voxels are combined into an ROI is not applicable at the single voxel level.

Ziolko et al. generated parametric images of PiB retention (over 90 minutes post-injection) using the Logan graphical analysis with cerebellar data as input (CER90 DVR) (Ziolko et al., 2006). Ten AD patients and 11 controls were compared using parametric (SPM) and nonparametric (SnPM) statistical methods with family-wise error (FWE) and false discovery rate (FDR) corrections. PiB results were consistent with previous regional results; AD subjects showed highly significant retention in frontal, parietal, temporal, and posterior cingulate cortices (FDR-corrected $p < 1.4e{-}10$). PiB analyses were of high statistical significance and a large spatial extent. Additionally, the PiB analyses retained significance after both FWE and FDR corrections. These results indicate that voxel-based methods will be useful for future larger longitudinal studies of amyloid deposition that could improve AD diagnosis and anti-amyloid therapy assessment.

Kemppainen et al. (2006) used a voxel-based analysis method to identify brain regions with significant increases in PiB retention in 17 AD vs. 11 healthy control subjects, indicative of increased amyloid accumulation in these regions. Parametric images were computed by calculating a region-to-cerebellum ratio (SUVR) over 60–90 minutes in each voxel. Group differences in PiB retention were analyzed with statistical parametric mapping (SPM) and automated region-of-interest (ROI) analysis. As previously seen with the ROI methods, SPM showed increased retention ($p < 0.001$) in the frontal, parietal, and lateral temporal cortices, as well as in the posterior cingulate and the striatum. No significant differences in uptake were found in the primary sensory and motor cortices, primary visual cortex, thalamus, and medial temporal lobe.

Selecting a Preferred Analysis Method for a Specific Study

The selection of a "method-of-choice" will depend upon the nature of the particular application. The simplified methods discussed above all provided outcomes that compared well to the ART90 method, and overall the similarities were greater than the differences between methods. Nevertheless, each method has certain advantages and disadvantages for specific purposes.

Scan duration

In general, it appears that all methods that use 90 minutes of data consistently outperform the corresponding method using only the first 60 minutes. Acquisition of these data requires a full 90-minute dynamic scan for CER90, but all of the data necessary for the SUVR90 analysis can be obtained by having the subject in the scanner during a 50-minute (i.e., 40–90 minutes) time window. The comparable performance of the SUVR60 method using the 20-minute (40–60 minutes) window suggests that it may be possible to optimize/shorten the 40–90 minutes window even further without loss of performance. This fact has now been put to use in the Alzheimer's Disease Neuroimaging Initiative (ADNI), which has adopted a SUVR approach using data from 50–70 minutes post-injection. This 50–70-minute time period has been shown to achieve an optimal correlation to the ART90 method (McNamee et al., 2009). This may be especially important for the study of severe AD patients who may not be able to tolerate a full 90 minutes of emission data acquisition. In addition to the shorter scan time, other advantages of the SUVR method include simplicity of application (making it more applicable to routine clinical studies), superior effect size (up to 6.9, depending on the brain region), very good test-retest reproducibility (~5%), and a large dynamic range. A disadvantage shared by the SUVR and CER methods is the greater influence of any inaccuracies contributed by the cerebellar data used as reference. This would be particularly apparent if there was detectable amyloid deposition in the cerebellum.

Cross-sectional Intergroup Comparisons

In the primary cortical areas-of-interest, all methods demonstrated the ability to distinguish AD and control subjects without any overlap between groups. Although the exploratory calculations yielded greatest effect sizes for the SUV-based methods (6.9 for posterior cingulate gyrus [PCG]), the CER methods yielded similar effect sizes of ~6.5. Cohen (1998) defined any effect size greater than 0.8 to be considered "large." To put this in another perspective, using a parametric test of significance (2-tailed t-test), these effect sizes correspond to a highly significant difference between the AD and control group mean values with a p value of <0.0000001.

Longitudinal Studies

Another type of comparison study is one in which longitudinal examinations of PiB retention are made in the same subject to study the natural history of disease progression or the response to anti-amyloid therapies. In this instance, it is desirable to have the most reliable repeat measure possible, in order to be sensitive to what could potentially be small changes in the degree of amyloid deposition or clearance between serial examinations. This may be an important consideration when planning a longitudinal study using PiB, where one would expect the differences in PiB retention between serial examinations to be small; or a study which focused on early MCI or normal aging, where there would be the expectation of a lower specific binding signal compared to AD. The cerebellar methods CER90 and CER60 have shown the lowest test-retest variability, and this makes CER90 an attractive method for detecting small effects of experimental anti-amyloid therapies over time, particularly in cases with low levels of amyloid deposition that must ultimately be the principle target of these therapies. However, as noted above for the use of [C-11]PiB in ADNI, practical considerations such as scanner availability and subject throughput may necessitate shorter scan times and the 20-minute SUVR methods have proven to be acceptable alternatives (McNamee et al., 2009).

Postmortem Validation of [C-11]PiB

From the initial report, it has been noted that the regional distribution of [C-11]PiB retention correlates well with the known postmortem distribution of Aβ amyloid pathology (Klunk et al., 2004). This is an important first step that must be made by all amyloid imaging tracers, but it is critical that this is followed by in vivo-to-postmortem correlations in individual subjects as the autopsy tissue becomes available. There have been two such reports on subjects imaged with [C-11]PiB; an atypical case with prominent Lewy body and vascular amyloid pathology (Bacskai et al., 2007), and a case with typical AD pathology (Ikonomovic et al., 2008).

The Bacskai et al. report (2007) described the postmortem finding of a patient who carried a clinical diagnosis of dementia with Lewy Bodies (DLB) and died after a subdural hematoma. A PiB PET study was performed on this 78-year-old man two years after he received a diagnosis of DLB. The PiB scan showed marked retention in association neocortical regions (Figure 14.24).

Areas affected included the posterior cingulate, precuneus, posterior parietal, middle and inferior temporal, insular, and lateral and orbital frontal cortices. Formal cognitive testing performed after the PiB scan revealed global cognitive and functional impairments: MMSE = 25 and CDR = 1.0, against a background of above average intelligence (AmNART EIQ = 116). The subject died of complications following surgical evacuation of a traumatic subdural hematoma three months after the PiB scan, and an autopsy was performed. Microscopic examination confirmed the diagnosis of DLB, the Braak DLB stage being 4/6 (Braak et al., 2003). There were plentiful Lewy bodies in the substantia nigra with marked neuronal loss; there were Lewy bodies in the entorhinal region as well as in the cingulate and temporal neocortices. Neuropathological findings characteristic of AD also were present, with moderate numbers of neurofibrillary tangles in temporal and parietal cortices as well as in limbic regions, including the amygdala and basal forebrain; rare tangles were seen in the occipital cortex. The Braak tangle stage was IV/VI (Braak and Braak, 1991). There were several forms of Aβ pathology including: (1) severe bilateral cerebral amyloid angiopathy (CAA); (2) moderate diffuse plaques, frequent in the visual cortex but infrequent elsewhere by immunohistochemistry; and (3) rare cored plaques by immunohistochemistry, but prominent cored plaques by PiB histochemistry. The overall frequency of plaques was low and met CERAD criteria for "possible AD" (Mirra et al., 1991). Taking the tangles into consideration along with the plaques, the findings were consistent with

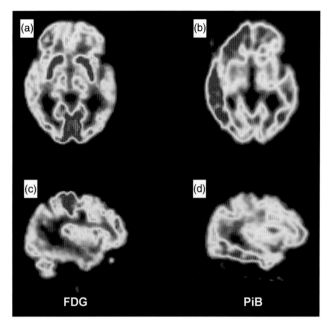

Figure 14–24 PET images from a 78-year-old patient with dementia. FDG (A) and PiB (B) PET images at the level of the striatum. Red areas represent higher metabolism of FDG and higher PiB retention. There is diffuse hypometabolism and PiB retention in frontal and temporal cortices. Regions with relatively normal metabolism, such as striatum and medial occipital cortex, demonstrate relatively less PiB retention. Evidence of a known subdural effusion occurring in the interval between FDG and PiB imaging is seen in the right frontal convexity of the PiB image. C and D,: coregistered left parasagittal FDG (C) and PiB (D) images at the level of the insula. In this view, PiB retention is greatest in the inferior temporal gyrus, and there is relative sparing of the primary sensorimotor cortex where FDG uptake is highest. (From Bacskai et al., 2007.)

an "intermediate likelihood of dementia due to AD," based on NIA-Reagan criteria (NIA/Reagan_Workgroup, 1997; Newell et al., 1999), also consistent with coexistent Lewy body disease. Soluble and insoluble Aβ40 and Aβ42 were biochemically measured in frontal, parietal, and cingulate regions and compared with measures of PiB binding in the homogenates, and with in vivo measures of PiB retention obtained with PET. Together, the biochemical and histological data demonstrated that positive PET imaging of PiB in life reflected the presence of amyloid pathology.

A second autopsy study was performed on a typical, late-stage AD case studied with PiB 10 months prior to death (DeKosky et al., 2007; Ikonomovic et al., 2008). A 64-year-old female with severe AD (MMSE = 1 at the time of PiB PET and MR imaging), enrolled in the University of Pittsburgh Alzheimer's Disease Research Center, was followed clinically for one year. Her apolipoprotein-E genotype was 3/4. Dementia symptoms were first recorded 8 years prior to her death. At autopsy, the brain weighed 1070 grams and upon gross examination was unremarkable except for cortical and hippocampal atrophy and minimal atherosclerosis of the circle of Willis. The neuropathological diagnosis by CERAD criteria (Mirra et al., 1991) was "definite AD," and the Braak stage was V/VI (Braak and Braak, 1991). There were no cortical or brainstem Lewy bodies (assessed by α-synuclein immunohistochemistry), no obvious neuronal loss in the cerebral cortex, and minimal cortical gliosis. There were no infarcts in subcortical or cortical structures. Immunohistochemical analysis using antibodies generated against Aβ demonstrated frequent areas of neuropil staining and mild amyloid angiopathy. Bielschowsky staining of frequent senile plaques and neurofibrillary tangles was observed in all neocortical areas; this was confirmed with immunohistochemistry using the anti-phosphotau antibody clone AT8.

The MRI scan showed prominent central and hippocampal atrophy and the PiB PET scan showed typical PiB retention in frontal, precuneus, temporal, and parietal cortices and striatum (Figure 14.25a). Frozen samples were collected from the right hemisphere by a standard autopsy protocol and these brain areas were mapped onto corresponding ROIs on the MRI and PiB PET scans. Aβ42 levels were determined in the frozen postmortem brain

tissue by ELISA and correlated to in vivo PiB DVR measures of amyloid load (Figure 14.25b). There was a close correlation ($r = 0.79$) between in vivo PiB retention (DVR) and the level of Aβ42 in the tissue ($p < 0.0002$).

Applications of Human Amyloid Imaging

(What Is) Normal Aging?

As stated in the introduction to this chapter, if we accept the commonly held concepts that: (1) the prevalence of AD increases with age, doubling in ~5 year increments (Evans et al., 1989; Katzman, 1976); (2) everyone who develops AD develops amyloid deposition prior to the onset of clinical symptoms; and (3) the time between onset of amyloid deposition and clinical AD is ~10 years (Hyman et al., 1995), then the graphs in Figure 14.1 predict that there will be a considerable age span during which amyloid deposition is more frequently found in clinically unimpaired people than in AD patients (green areas in Figure 14.1). This model predicts that between ages 65 and 85 about 20% of all people who do not have clinical AD will be amyloid-positive. In addition, in the sections above detailing the rationale for studying cognitively normal people with amyloid imaging, arguments were made that it will be important to actually test the hypothetical model of Figure 14.1 to: (1) determine the prevalence of amyloid-positivity in cognitively normal people; (2) determine whether the variability in cognitive performance that is detectable even prior to dementia is related to amyloid deposition; and (3) determine whether cognitively normal individuals with substantial amyloid deposition will invariably progress to clinical dementia. There is not yet enough longitudinal data to address the third issue, but several investigations have begun to address the first two. Thus, amyloid imaging is a tool that is being increasingly applied to the study of normal aging and may ultimately find a larger application for this purpose than for the study of AD per se.

Definitions of Cutoffs

The first issue to address in the application of amyloid imaging to clinically unimpaired people is how we determine whether someone has an "abnormal" amyloid load. It is critical to keep in mind that although we use the dichotomous terms amyloid-positive and amyloid-negative (or PiB-positive/PiB-negative, or high PiB/low PiB, etc.) that *amyloid load is a continuous variable*. In a given brain region, an individual could conceivably have no plaques, one plaque, ten plaques, hundreds or thousands of plaques. Perhaps less than 10 plaques will not be detectable. Hundreds of plaques may give a questionable signal while thousands of plaques may give an unambiguous signal. That is, as with any analytical technique, there will be a threshold for detection. We currently do not know what this threshold will be for PiB PET. In patients with clinical dementia, the presence or absence of amyloid does appear more dichotomous, because by the time a person is symptomatic, if they have amyloid deposition at all, they usually have extensive deposits. This is usually the case with MCI as well. MCI subjects typically appear very "AD-like" or "control-like," although one occasionally finds MCI subjects with intermediate levels of amyloid deposition (see below). The group that best displays the continuous nature of amyloid load is the clinically unimpaired elderly group. In this group, we find convincingly amyloid-negative scans, infrequent AD-like scans, and intermediate scans that test our ability to discriminate the earliest signs of amyloid deposition. Even within groups of AD and

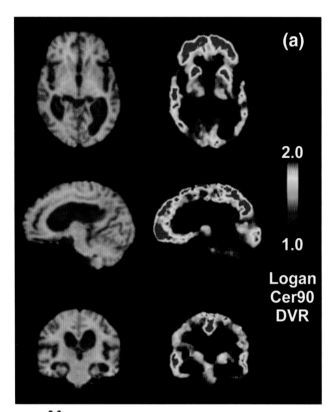

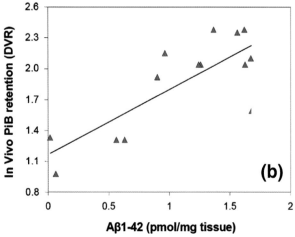

Figure 14–25 (a) MRI and PiB PET images of a 64 y/o-year-old woman with severe AD who came to autopsy 10 months after this PiB study shown in transaxial (top), sagittal (center), and coronal views (bottom). (b) Correlation between the in vivo measure of PiB retention (CER90 DVR) and the amount of Aβ in homogenates of brain regions matched to the PiB ROIs.

MCI subjects that are all clearly amyloid-positive, there exists a continuous distribution of amyloid deposition. Therefore, as we discuss cutoffs for "amyloid-positivity" below, the continuous nature of the amyloid load will result in gray zones in which there will be a mixture of true amyloid-positive and true amyloid-negative subjects that overlap, simply because of the inherent variability of any biological measurement such as PiB retention. The larger the dynamic range (i.e., the span from the lowest amyloid-negative to the highest amyloid-positive case) of a tracer, the fewer the number of subjects that will fall into this gray zone.

Defining the cutoffs between amyloid-positivity and amyloid-negativity is an evolving field; and currently, each group has independently defined their own cutoff values for the specific amyloid measure used in their study. For the PiB studies discussed below, one must keep in mind that the absolute value of these cutoffs will differ depending on whether the analysis method results in a DVR or a SUVR measure (SUVR typically being higher). Within each of those two subdivisions, the absolute value of the cutoffs will differ depending on the reference region used (usually cerebellum, but sometimes pons). The absolute value of the cutoffs will differ depending on the length of the data set used to calculate the DVR (e.g., 60 or 90 minutes of data), or the time window for the SUVR (e.g., 40–60 minutes or 50–70 minutes). Another factor that will affect the absolute value of the cutoff is whether or not the data was atrophy-corrected using MRI (Price et al., 2005). Thus, while each group is likely to report a slightly different absolute cutoff value, if two groups studied the same cohort they should identify the same amyloid-positive subjects, regardless of their particular analysis method. That is, whatever the cutoff measure used, it is important that the field as a whole becomes consistent with regard to which subjects are defined as amyloid-positive (or "high amyloid" or "high PiB") and which are defined as amyloid-negative.

In addition to the objective differences in analysis methods, there also are subjective differences in the decision of where to draw the cutoff line. Some groups have chosen a natural break in the continuity of their control data as the cutoff. However, as more and more amyloid-positive cognitively normal subjects are added, this natural break-point tends to become obscured and the data forms more of a continuum. Other groups have used the range of amyloid measures found in younger (aged 20–40) controls to define the amyloid-negative range, since it would be highly unlikely that these younger people would have amyloid deposition. Still other groups have used visual reads to determine which subjects had regional patterns of PiB retention that suggest true amyloid deposition and used this to determine the upper limit of "normal." This approach may not be sensitive enough to pick up subjects in the earliest stages of amyloid deposition and may miss cases that start asymmetrically in one or two brain areas. This brings up the issue of which brain area or areas to use in defining abnormality. One could base amyloid-positivity on one or two typically high PiB areas (e.g., frontal cortex or precuneus), or a global measure could be used. The latter could miss focal amyloid deposition, but should focal deposition in one unusual area (e.g., occipital lobe) constitute an amyloid-positive scan? Some groups have used statistical approaches to define "clusters" of cases likely to be amyloid-positive or amyloid-negative. Villemagne et al. (2008) have used a receiver-operating-characteristic (ROC) analysis to distinguish amyloid-positive and amyloid-negative cases, but this analysis is dependent on the distribution of PiB retention observed in an AD cohort. Aizenstein et al. (2008) used an approach that is independent of an AD cohort and defines the amyloid-negative control range in a completely objective manner by iteratively excluding statistical outliers. The objectivity of these approaches is appealing and will likely prove useful. In the end, the definition of amyloid-negative may have to be refined retrospectively after 5–10 years of follow-up. That is, we will make our best guess at which subjects are true amyloid-negatives and then retroactively exclude anyone who clearly becomes amyloid-positive over time (or perhaps anyone who becomes cognitively impaired). Whatever the final outcome, it is important to keep in mind that the definition of amyloid-positivity is evolving and at present is somewhat unique to each center that is performing amyloid imaging studies.

Amyloid Imaging Studies in Normal Aging

Prevalence of Amyloid Deposition in Normal Aging

In a sense, every amyloid imaging study to date has had a component of a normal aging study in it if it included cognitively normal controls. As stated above in the section describing the initial PiB study, one of the nine cognitively normal controls (and the eldest of the six controls above age 59) showed evidence of amyloid deposition (Klunk et al., 2004). In the study of Lopresti et al. (2005) two of the eight controls (65 ± 16 years) showed elevated PiB retention. We have had the opportunity to study both of these controls for a period of 2 years and have demonstrated increasing levels of PiB retention in both of them despite stable and normal cognition (Figure 14.26) (Klunk et al., 2007).

Figure 14–26 Two PiB PET DVR images of a cognitively normal elderly control at baseline and 24 months later. Note the early frontal PiB retention on the baseline scan and the clear increase in this and other brain areas at 24 months. The white outlines are taken from the co-registered MRI scans.

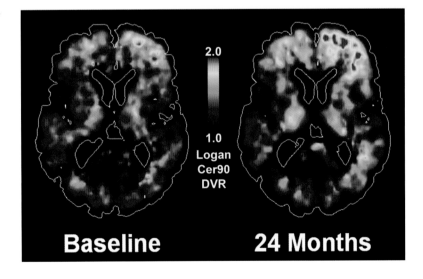

Mintun et al. (2006) designed a study to specifically investigate whether abnormal PiB binding occurs in clinically normal individuals, prior to the development of cognitive changes. They studied 41 nondemented subjects (65.3 ± 16.13, range 20–86 years). Twenty nondemented subjects were similarly aged with the AD subjects; these 20 had a mean age of 77.4 ± 5.24 years (range 66–86 years). They found four of the 20 older nondemented subjects had elevated cortical PiB values (20% of the older group). As a group, these four amyloid-positive controls had PiB retention that was not significantly different from that in AD subjects. Two of these four nondemented subjects had PiB retention, both visually and quantitatively, that was indistinguishable from the AD subjects. Similarly, Rowe et al. (2007a) studied 27 elderly cognitively normal controls (72.6 ± 6.9 years) with PiB. They found six of their controls (22%) showed high cortical PiB retention despite normal neuropsychological scores. In a subsequent study with many of the same subjects, the Melbourne group found 7 of 30 cognitively normal elderly (23%) showing evidence of amyloid deposition on PiB scans (Villemagne et al., 2008).

In our current series in Pittsburgh, 16 of 62 (26%) subjects between the ages of 61 and 89 have evidence of amyloid deposition on PiB PET (Aizenstein et al., 2008). Interestingly, of the 13 subjects 80 or above, only 2 (15%) show evidence of amyloid deposition. While these numbers are too small to constitute substantial evidence, they are consistent with the model that suggests the prevalence of amyloid positivity will be lower above age 80 than in the 70–80-year-old age range (see Figure 14.1). As a group, these early amyloid imaging studies in controls suggest a 20%–25% prevalence of amyloid-positivity in cognitively normal people aged 65–85.

Although the discussion above emphasizes the ~25% prevalence of PiB retention in the clinically unimpaired elderly, it is important to keep this finding in perspective. These early-stage amyloid-positive control subjects are not usually "AD-like" in the sense that MCI subjects often have PiB scans that are AD-like. That is, the amyloid-positive, cognitively normal elderly are usually easily distinguished from AD and amyloid-positive MCI patients. Figure 14.27a shows mean, sagittal DVR images from 29 amyloid-negative elderly subjects, nine amyloid-positive elderly subjects, and nine AD patients (Aizenstein et al., 2008). It is clear that, on average, the amyloid-positive clinically unimpaired elderly have

considerably less PiB retention than the AD subjects. However, the distribution is very similar. That is, rather than showing non-specific accumulation, there is a pattern of retention that is similar to the regional distribution of PiB retention observed in AD patients. Figure 14.27b shows difference images obtained by subtracting the three groups from each other. It can be seen that the amyloid-positive clinically unimpaired subjects differ from the amyloid-negative group with respect to increased PiB retention in the frontal, anterior cingulate, precuneus, lateral temporal, and parietal cortices and striatum. These are the same areas in which the AD patients exceed the controls, albeit to a much greater degree (Figure 14.27b, right). This regional pattern of PiB retention in amyloid-positve controls is similar to that observed in AD, but the level of PiB retention is not AD-like. In fact, the AD patients exceed the amyloid-positive elderly (Figure 14.27b, center) by a greater degree than the amyloid-positive elderly exceed the amyloid-negative group (Figure 14.27b, left).

This concept is very apparent in the quantitative data. Figure 14.27c shows a global average of PiB retention in six brain areas that are typically increased in AD patients (frontal, anterior cingulate, precuneus, lateral temporal, and parietal cortices and striatum). Of the 23 AD patients and 54 elderly controls studied, 12 clinically unimpaired controls (~22%) fall into the amyloid-positive range that was determined by a statistical outlier approach (red rectangle in Figure 14.27c) (Aizenstein et al. 2008). The distinction between AD patients and controls is very clear; there is only one low-PiB AD case that overlaps the amyloid-positive control range. The dotted line represents a cutoff with 96% sensitivity and 100% specificity for the discrimination of AD patients from controls. Ng et al. (2007a) have reported very similar findings in a group of 25 controls and 15 AD patients. Despite the presence of amyloid-positive cases in the control group, only one low-PiB AD case overlapped with the upper end of the control group.

It should be noted that not all PiB PET studies have reported amyloid deposition in their control groups. Edison et al. (2006) studied 14 controls (64.8 ± 6.2 years) and none showed clear increased PiB retention, although one was marginally higher than the rest of the group. Similarly, Kemppainen et al. (2006) studied 14 elderly control subjects (65.6 ± 7.2 years) and there was a suggestion of elevated PiB retention in only one. It is not clear whether

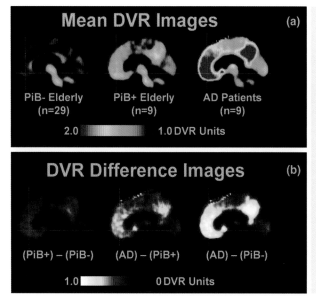

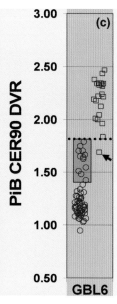

Figure 14–27 (a) Mean DVR images of 29 amyloid-negative clinically unimpaired subjects (left), 9 amyloid-positive clinically unimpaired subjects (center), and 9 AD patients (right). (b) Difference images obtained by subtracting the amyloid-negative mean image from either the amyloid-positive elderly mean (left) or the AD patient mean (right), or by subtracting the amyloid-positive mean image from the AD mean image (center). Adapted from (Aizenstein et al. (2008). (c) PiB retention in 54 clinically unimpaired elderly controls (red circles) and 23 AD patients (blue squares). The red rectangle indicates the amyloid-positive range determined by a statistical outlier approach (Aizenstein et al. 2008). GBL6 refers to the average PiB retention in frontal, anterior cingulate, precuneus, lateral temporal and parietal cortices, and striatum. The dotted line represents a cutoff with 96% sensitivity and 100% specificity for the discrimination of AD patients from controls.

there was any effort in the Edison or Kemppainen studies to exclude amyloid-positive controls. Depending on the question to be asked, it may be appropriate to exclude amyloid-positive controls from specific analyses, but this should be clearly stated. For example, Klunk et al. (2007) excluded amyloid-positive controls in an effort to define a group of amyloid-negative controls for comparison to subjects who carried mutations that cause early-onset familial AD.

One is tempted to downplay the significance of finding in vivo evidence for early amyloid deposition in cognitively normal subjects by pointing out the fact that many autopsy studies have previously shown a similar prevalence of amyloid deposition in cognitively normal elderly (Haroutunian et al., 1998; Price and Morris, 1999; Wolf et al., 1999). However, the importance of verifying these postmortem findings in the *living* brain should not be ignored. Consider the fact that two-photon microscopy has shown that new plaques form in vivo in transgenic mice over a period of days (Garcia-Alloza et al., 2006). It is not known how quickly this can happen (i.e., hours vs. days), since imaging was performed at weekly intervals, but it is a fairly rapid event. In addition, in transgenic mice, plaques appear to reach their final size relatively quickly after formation and then remain a stable size, neither growing, nor shrinking (Christie et al., 2001). Thus it appears that plaques form quickly and bloom to their final size quickly in what might be considered an explosive or "popcorn" fashion. Thus it is not inconceivable that the metabolic insults suffered by the brain after death could set up a chain of events that could lead to the rapid postmortem formation of plaques. That is, it is important to show that the postmortem amount and distribution of Aβ plaques is not a postmortem artifact. The transgenic mouse studies just mentioned have already provided evidence that this is not the case in the mouse model (Christie et al., 2001), but it is equally important to show that evidence of amyloid deposition can be found in the living human brain, especially in cognitively normal people. These in vivo amyloid imaging human studies leave little doubt that the accumulation of Aβ deposits in cognitively normal people is a real phenomenon, and they set the stage to determine the eventual significance and clinical outcome of asymptomatic amyloid deposition.

Amyloid and Cognition: A Broader View

Cause and Effect: In addition to determining the prevalence of amyloid deposition in the clinically unimpaired elderly, another motivation for amyloid imaging is to determine the cognitive effects of amyloid deposition in these nondemented individuals. That is, does amyloid deposition in a given brain area have a demonstrable effect on the function of that specific brain area, and is that effect proportional to the amount of amyloid deposited? This sort of cause-and-effect approach is classical in behavioral neurology, with roots in the study of the clinical and neuropsychological sequelae of acute brain insults such as strokes and traumatic brain injury.

Mintun et al. (2006) reported that the psychometric performances of the four amyloid-positive nondemented individuals in their study did not differ as a group from those of the 16 amyloid-negative nondemented individuals age 60 years or older. Rowe et al. (2007a) reported that the cognitive performance of the controls with high cortical PiB retention ($n = 6$) in their study was not significantly different than that of those without evidence of high PiB retention ($n = 21$). The mean MMSE was 29 for both groups and all subjects performed within the expected range for age and education on neuropsychological tasks. They reported a minor and nonsignificant reduction in performance on several cognitive tests

in those with high PiB retention (Rowe et al., 2007a). Aizenstein et al. (2008) reported no significant difference in neurocognitive performance among the 9 of 43 elderly controls who showed increased PiB retention. Thus a significant amyloid load can be present in the brain of some individuals with little or no cognitive effect. This finding was certainly predicted by postmortem studies that reported amyloid deposition in subjects that were cognitively normal prior to death (Haroutunian et al., 1998; Price and Morris, 1999; Wolf et al., 1999), and the lack of a tight correlation between amyloid load and cognition extends into clinicopathological studies performed in AD patients (Braak and Braak, 1998; Terry et al., 1991). But again, it is very important to reproduce this finding in vivo in situations where subjects can be tested in good health at times very close to the imaging study. Much more important, these in vivo amyloid imaging studies can follow the subjects over time to determine the ultimate significance of amyloid deposition in a cognitively normal person.

More recently, more extensive cognitive assessments have been performed on clinically unimpaired subjects who are studied with amyloid imaging. Pike et al. (2007) focused on episodic memory impairment, since this is an early and prominent sign of AD, and examined the relationship between episodic memory and Aβ burden in nondemented persons and in AD. They used PiB PET to study 31 AD patients, 33 MCI patients, and 32 clinically unimpaired subjects. They found 22% of their clinically unimpaired subjects to have increased cortical PiB retention. They found a significant correlation between impaired episodic memory performance and PiB retention, both in MCI patients and the clinically unimpaired group, but *not* in the AD group. This relationship was less robust for nonmemory cognitive domains. Similarly, Forsberg et al. (2007) found episodic memory to be negatively correlated with PiB retention in their sample of 21 MCI subjects. Villemagne et al. (2008) took a somewhat different approach by using PiB PET to study 34 elderly subjects who entered an aging study showing no cognitive impairment 6–10 years earlier. Of these 34, 10 (29%) showed cognitive decline on follow-up and 7 of the 10 (70%) were amyloid-positive. Only 4 (17%) of the 24 cognitively stable subjects were amyloid-positive. Even more interesting, three of the 10 decliners now met the criteria for MCI and one met the criteria for AD, and these "converters" represented four of the five highest levels of PiB retention of the 34 subjects.

The relationship between amyloid load and cognitive performance has also been investigated during the clinical course of AD. Klunk et al. (2004) reported a nonsignificant trend towards higher PiB retention in AD patients with lower MMSE scores. Engler et al. (2006) reported a negative correlation ($P = 0.018$) between scores on the Rey Auditory Verbal Learning (RAVL) test and PiB retention in the parietal cortex in their two-year follow-up study. Rowe et al. (2007a) found that both the CDR and the MMSE correlated with neocortical DVR when all subjects (control, AD, and other dementias) were pooled, but there was no correlation in any group when analyzed separately. For example, in the AD group, there was no correlation between PiB DVR and MMSE score or with specific domains of cognitive function such as episodic memory. Likewise, as stated above, Pike et al. (2007) found no correlation between PiB retention and episodic memory in AD patients. Edison et al. (2006) investigated the association between brain amyloid load in Alzheimer disease (AD) measured by PiB PET and cognition. In 19 AD patients and 14 controls, higher cortical amyloid load correlated with lower scores on facial and word recognition tests (Warrington test). Thus, like the previous postmortem studies (Braak and Braak, 1998; Terry et al., 1991), these in vivo amyloid imaging studies found only weak correlations between amyloid deposition and cognitive ability.

One explanation for the weak relationship between amyloid pathology and degree of cognitive impairment may lie in the cognitive reserve hypothesis. The cognitive reserve hypothesis suggests that some individuals, either for genetic or environmental reasons, have brains that can better withstand pathological changes than others (Roe et al., 2007). Thus, the expression of clinical impairment is an interplay between causative pathology and physiological resistance to cellular injury. Education is often taken as a surrogate of cognitive reserve either because highly educated individuals have facilitated the development of reserve mechanisms (environmental) or those genetically endowed with high reserve have better success in the educational environment. Kemppainen et al. (2008) have compared high- and low-education patients with mild AD who were matched for clinical severity on MMSE (26.2 ± 1.3 in the high group and 25.0 ± 2.1 in the low group; $p = 0.23$). There were some small but statistically significant differences between the groups on tests such as WMS-R logical memory II and WAIS-R similarities, with the high-education group performing better. The 12 high-education patients differed in PiB retention from the 13 low-education AD patients due to increased PiB retention in the lateral frontal cortex. The high-education AD patients also showed lower metabolism in the temporoparietal region. Kemppainen et al. interpreted the more advanced pathological and functional brain changes in high-education patients with mild AD to be in accordance with the brain cognitive reserve hypothesis (Kemppainen et al., 2008).

Action and Reaction: The straightforward cause-and-effect thinking—born out of the study of stroke, brain injury, and electrical stimulation of the cortex (e.g., a stroke in Broca's area results in an expressive aphasia)—may not apply to the deposition of Aβ in normal aging and AD. Some have concluded that this means that Aβ deposits have little causal association to the cognitive impairments seen in AD (Terry et al., 1991)—although some revisions to this conclusion have been made (Terry, 2001). However, it is possible that another paradigm may need to be adopted for slowly-evolving insults to the brain such as the accumulation of Aβ. Since Aβ deposition appears to begin a decade or more before clinical symptoms, there is clearly considerable time for adaptive brain reactions to occur. The brain is clearly able to adapt to other slowly evolving insults as evidenced by the asymptomatic nature of many large meningiomas (Olivero, Lister, and Elwood, 1995). Thus, functional defects expected in a given brain area because of amyloid deposition in that brain area may be masked by an adaptive reorganization of function to other brain areas or within that brain area.

Nelissen et al. (2007) have posed the interesting hypothesis that postmortem measures of Aβ amyloid deposition correlate only weakly with cognitive dysfunction before death, because functional reorganization forms a critical intermediary step between Aβ amyloid-associated brain injury and clinical disease expression. To test this hypothesis, they studied 15 patients with mild AD and 16 cognitively intact controls with a combination of functional magnetic resonance imaging (fMRI) and PiB PET. The fMRI design had two factors: task (associative-semantic vs. visuoperceptual judgement) and input-modality (written words vs. pictures). They found that the posterior third of the left superior temporal sulcus (STS) showed a lower fMRI response in AD patients during the associative-semantic compared with the visuoperceptual task. Response amplitude correlated inversely with PiB retention in that region (i.e., a direct cause-and-effect model). They found a substantially different functional pattern contralaterally. The fMRI response

in the right posterior STS during the associative-semantic versus the visuoperceptual task was higher in AD than in controls. Accuracy on the Boston Naming test correlated positively with the degree to which AD patients were able to recruit the right STS. PiB uptake in the right STS did not correlate with naming accuracy. Nelissen et al. suggested that a functional reorganization of the language system occurs in response to Aβ-related brain injury in early-stage AD and determines the degree of anomia more than Aβ load per se does.

A related concept to keep in mind when analyzing the effect of Aβ deposition on brain function is that the deposition of Aβ may exert its major effect at distant sites. Two independent groups have shown that neuritic processes are markedly dystrophic and swollen near fibrillar plaques in transgenic mice (Brendza et al., 2005; D'Amore et al., 2003), and similar postmortem findings have been described in AD (Knowles et al., 1999). Thus, neurites extending into or out of an amyloid-containing brain area could be structurally and functionally compromised. This means Aβ deposits in one area could disrupt the function of brain areas that send or receive projections from that brain area. There is some preliminary in vivo evidence to suggest that amyloid deposition in the neocortex is associated with decreased activation of the medial temporal lobe measured with functional magnetic resonance imaging (fMRI) (Sperling et al., 2007).

Buckner et al. (2005) have put forth a hypothesis about how the deposition of amyloid could not only affect brain activity, but be a result of activity in certain brain systems such as the "default network" (Raichle and Snyder, 2007). Buckner and colleagues explored AD and antecedent factors associated with AD using amyloid imaging and unbiased measures of longitudinal atrophy in combination with reanalysis of previous metabolic and functional studies across five in vivo imaging methods. Convergence of effects was seen in posterior cortical regions, including posterior cingulate, retrosplenial, and lateral parietal cortex. These regions were active in default states in young adults and also showed amyloid deposition in older adults with AD. They hypothesize that lifetime cerebral metabolism associated with regionally specific default activity predisposes cortical regions to AD-related changes, including amyloid deposition, metabolic disruption, and atrophy. Buckner et al. suggested that these cortical regions may be part of a network with the medial temporal lobe whose disruption contributes to memory impairment (Buckner et al. 2005).

MCI

The first amyloid imaging study to include MCI patients was reported by Price et al. (2005) and later expanded by Lopresti et al. (2005). In the Lopresti et al. study, 10 MCI patients were compared to AD patients and control subjects. From this very first amyloid imaging study of MCI, it became clear that individual MCI subjects—with cognitive impairments that were intermediate between controls and AD patients—seldom had PiB retention intermediate between controls and AD patients. Only two of the 10 MCI patients had PiB retention that fell between the control and AD ranges (e.g., MCI-2 in Figure 14.28). Five of the ten MCI subjects had PiB retention that was largely indistinguishable from the AD patients (e.g., MCI-3 in Figure 14.28), and three MCI patients had no evidence of PiB retention (e.g., MCI-1 in Figure 14.28). These findings have held as the Pittsburgh MCI cohort has increased in numbers. Currently 58% of the 24 MCI subjects studied with PiB PET are amyloid-positive. Similarly, Rowe et al. (2007a) studied 9 subjects with mild cognitive impairment (MCI) using PiB PET. They reported that subjects with MCI presented either an "AD-like" (60%) or normal pattern of PiB retention.

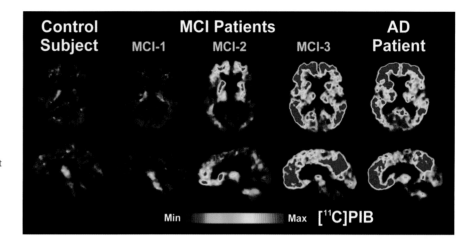

Figure 14–28   PiB PET DVR images in a normal elderly control (far left), three different MCI subjects (center images), and a mild AD patient (far right). MCI-1 has control-like levels of PiB retention, MCI-3 has AD-like levels of PiB retention, and MCI-2 is intermediate.

Kemppainen et al. (2007) studied 13 patients with amnestic MCI and 14 control subjects with PiB PET. An SPM analysis showed that, as a group, patients with MCI had significantly higher PiB retention vs. control subjects in the frontal, parietal, and lateral temporal cortices as well as in the posterior cingulate/precuneus. The SPM results were supported by the automated ROI analysis in which MCI patients (as a group) showed increased PiB retention in the frontal cortex, posterior cingulate/precuneus, parietal, and lateral temporal cortices and striatum. Individually, in the frontal cortex and posterior cingulate/precuneus, 8 of 13 patients (62%) with MCI had PiB retention more than 2 standard deviations above the control mean. As noted above, the MCI subjects that had at least one Apo-E ε4 allele tended to have higher PiB retention than MCI subjects without Apo-E ε4.

Pike et al. (2007) reported that amyloid-positivity varied greatly between MCI subtypes. They found all six nonamnestic MCI participants in their study had a "PiB-negative" scan, whereas 18 (75%) of the amnestic MCI subgroup were "PiB-positive." They hypothesized that the etiology of the cognitive problems in the nonamnestic group might include depression, dementia where Aβ deposition is not a feature (e.g., frontotemporal dementia), or they may prove to be part of the 5%–10% who have stable MCI, or the 20% who revert to apparent normality (Busse et al., 2006; Gauthier et al., 2006). Small et al. (2006) did not distinguish amyloid-positive and amyloid-negative subgroups within their MCI cohort using [F-18]FDDNP.

Several concepts evolve from these observations. The first concept has treatment implications. If MCI patients who are destined for AD already have a nearly maximal amyloid load, then this mild clinical state already represents a fairly severe stage of pathology. The implication of this is that if future anti-amyloid therapies prove, as expected, to be optimally effective if begun at the earliest stages of pathology, then it may be necessary to detect amyloid deposition even before the first symptoms of MCI become apparent, i.e., at a presymptomatic stage.

Secondly, the near-maximal amyloid loads observed in many MCI patients suggest that the period of greatest change in amyloid load occurs pre-symptomatically. Put another way, if one wishes to study the natural history of amyloid deposition during the period of the most rapid increases in brain amyloid levels, one should be studying cognitively normal control subjects in the 60–80-year-old age range (see above).

The third concept relates to diagnostic considerations. MCI is a clinical syndrome and does not necessarily imply an etiology. It is most often considered a prodromal form of AD, but it also can be an early stage of other dementias such as vascular dementia with Lewy bodies, or cognitive impairment associated with psychiatric or medical conditions (Petersen and Morris, 2005). Over long periods of follow-up, many MCI patients convert to AD, but many do not. In a longitudinal study of 134 MCI cases followed for 4 or more years, Hansson et al. (2006) reported that 43% developed clinical AD, 42% remained cognitively stable (but could, of course, develop AD in the future), and 15% developed other dementias (mostly vascular). Similar findings have been reported in a community-based cohort (Larrieu et al., 2002). Thus it is very difficult to determine which MCI subjects are destined to develop AD. It will be very important to follow the amyloid-positive and amyloid-negative MCI cases to determine if amyloid positivity can predict conversion to AD.

Forsberg et al. (2007) have reported significant progress in this area. Twenty-one patients diagnosed with MCI (mean age 63.3 ±7.8 years) were studied with PiB PET, as well as assessment of cognitive function and CSF biomarkers. The mean cortical PiB retention for the MCI patients was intermediate compared to cognitively normal controls and AD patients, but closer inspection of the data shows that 12/21 (57%) of the MCI subjects fell into the typical AD range and the other 9/21 (43%) were distributed near the control range. Seven MCI patients who converted to AD an average of 8.1 ± 6.0 months later showed significantly higher PiB retention compared to nonconverting MCI patients and HC. When viewed in terms of baseline amyloid-positivity, all 7 MCI-to-AD converters were amyloid-positive at baseline and 9 of the 14 nonconverters were amyloid-negative. As a group, the PiB retention in MCI converters was comparable to AD patients (Figure 14.29). Correlations were observed in the MCI patients between PiB retention and CSF Aβ(1–42), total Tau, and episodic memory, respectively. This study is especially impressive given that, even though 7 of 12 (58%) amyloid-positive MCI patients, compared to 0 of 9 amyloid-negative MCI patients, converted to AD, the follow-up period was less than one year on average and the expectation would be that more of the amyloid-positive MCI patients would convert over the next few years.

Amyloid Deposition in Early-Onset, Autosomal Dominant, Familial AD (eoFAD)

In order to explore the natural history of preclinical amyloid deposition in people at high risk for AD, Klunk et al. (2007) used PiB PET to study 10 subjects from two unrelated families, carrying

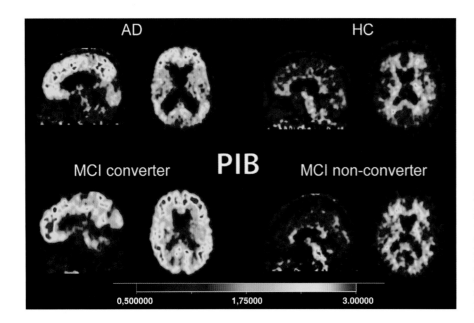

Figure 14–29 PiB PET images of an AD patient (top, left), a cognitively normal elderly control (top, right), an MCI subject who later converted to clinical AD (bottom, left), and an MCI subject who retained the diagnosis of MCI one year later (bottom, right). MCI subject images were from baseline when the diagnosis was MCI for both subjects. (From Forsberg et al., 2007.)

two different presenilin-1 (PS1) mutations (namely, C410Y and A426P). Non-carrier controls from both kindreds ($n = 2$) also were studied with PiB PET and compared with sporadic AD subjects ($n = 12$) and controls from the general population ($n = 18$). Unexpectedly, all 10 PS1 mutation carriers showed a strikingly similar, focal deposition of amyloid that appeared to begin in the striatum (Figure 14.30). The data currently available from sporadic AD patients, MCI patients, and cognitively normal older subjects who show low levels of PiB retention do not suggest that amyloid deposition typically begins in the striatum early in the course of sporadic AD (Mintun et al., 2006). In these older subjects, the earliest deposition in appears to be in the frontal cortex and the precuneus/posterior cingulate region (Mintun et al., 2006). These same areas showed small increases in most of the PS1 mutation carriers in this study.

Postmortem evaluation of tissue from two parents of PS1-C410Y subjects in this study confirmed extensive striatal amyloid deposition, along with typical cortical deposition. The postmortem pattern of amyloid deposition in PS1 mutation carriers with clinical dementia has been reported to be very similar to the pattern observed in sporadic AD (Lippa et al., 1996). Another postmortem study suggested that PS1 mutation carriers have similar loads of $A\beta_{40}$-containing plaques and greater loads of $A\beta_{42(43)}$-containing plaques in their frontal cortex compared to sporadic AD cases (Mann et al., 2001). Both of these previous studies included deceased individuals from the PS1-C410Y kindred included in this study. However, neither of these studies included the striatum in their analysis. Our limited analysis of striatal and nearby cortical tissue from two deceased parents of subjects in the current in vivo study suggests that the number of plaques in the cortex never reaches the level observed in the striatum of PS1-C410Y mutation carriers.

Remes et al. (2008) recently studied 49-year-old and 60-year-old siblings from a Finnish family with autosomal dominant dementia and frequent cerebral amyloid angiopathy and intracerebral hemorrhages due to an APP locus duplication (Remes et al., 2004; Rovelet-Lecrux et al., 2007). Similar to the findings of Klunk et al. (2007), PiB retention was highest in the striatum (up to 280% of the control mean), and the overall pattern of increased PiB retention was different from that seen in sporadic AD. However, PiB retention also was markedly increased in the posterior

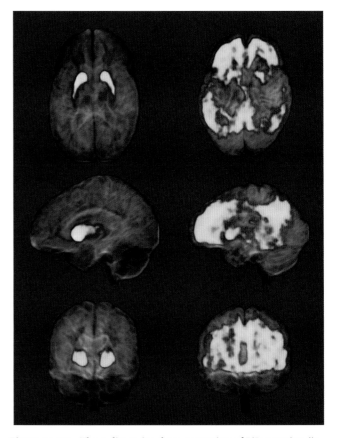

Figure 14–30 Three-dimensional representation of PiB retention (in color) superimposed on the MRI scan (grayscale) of an asymptomatic carrier of a presenilin-1 mutation (left) and a mild AD patient (right). The top views are transaxial, the center views are sagittal, and the bottom views are coronal. Note the focal nature of the striatal PiB retention in the presenilin-1 mutation carrier compared to the typical late-onset AD pattern on the right. Striatal deposition is present in the late-onset AD patient, but this is never as extensive as that in the presenilin-1 carrier.

cingulate/precuneus of these two subjects and was marginally increased in other cortical brain areas.

Taking the data from these studies together with the previous postmortem studies, we can hypothesize a natural history of amyloid deposition in the PS1-C410Y mutation carriers. In these individuals, amyloid deposition appears to begin in the striatum before the mid-30s—at least 10 years before the onset of symptoms. Amyloid deposition in the striatum progresses rapidly and may reach an early plateau. Sometime after the striatal amyloid becomes well-established, neocortical amyloid deposition begins in a pattern that is similar to that seen in the first stages of sporadic AD. By the time of death, the neocortical amyloid pathology reaches or exceeds that typical for sporadic AD, but never reaches the density observed in the striatum of these mutation carriers. It may be that cognitive symptoms do not occur in PS1-C410Y mutation carriers until neocortical plaque pathology becomes substantial (and perhaps neurofibrillary tangle pathology as well). In the PS1-A426P mutation carriers, it is more difficult to form a hypothesis about the natural history of amyloid deposition because of the absence of postmortem tissue from late-stage cases up to this point in time.

It is not yet known whether these two PS1 mutation kindreds are representative of eoFAD mutation carriers in general. To date, there is one other report of amyloid imaging using PiB in a symptomatic patient with eoFAD. Theuns et al. (2006) reported widespread retention of PiB, typical of that observed in sporadic AD, in a 57-year-old patient (MMSE of 18) with a novel K724N mutation in the C-terminal intracytosolic fragment of APP. The subject showed no disproportionate PiB retention in the striatum. Although the regional distribution of amyloid deposition in this APP-K724N mutation carrier prior to the onset of symptoms is not known, the typical sporadic AD-like pattern of amyloid deposition in this subject raises the question of whether other eoFAD carriers will show the early striatal amyloid deposition observed in this study, or will they have a course similar to that of subjects with late-onset AD.

Although the focal nature and very early appearance of this striatal pathology was surprising in these eoFAD cases, the postmortem presence of striatal amyloid in sporadic AD has been previously described (see neuropathology section above). Extensive amyloid deposition has been reported to occur in the striatum and thalamus of virtually all AD patients (Braak and Braak, 1990; Brilliant et al., 1997; Suenaga et al., 1990; Thal et al., 2002), and we observed substantial PiB retention in the striatum of sporadic AD patients in our previous in vivo studies (Klunk et al., 2004; Price et al., 2005). While neuritic plaques have been observed in ventral striatum (Suenaga et al., 1990), most striatal plaques are not neuritic (Brilliant et al., 1997; Suenaga et al., 1990). Despite this poorly understood paucity of neuritic changes in the striatum, striatal plaques appear to be fibrillar as evidenced by the fact that they are stained well by the fibril-specific Congo red derivative, X-34 (Styren et al., 2000). Our postmortem study of the two parents of PS1-C410Y carriers included in this study also revealed marked subcortical amyloid deposits; although by the time of death, cortical amyloid deposits had become extensive as well (Lippa et al., 1996). However, as observed in the present in vivo PiB study, the postmortem striatal deposits were disproportionately high in the PS1-C410Y mutation carriers.

In addition to the lack of neuritic dystrophy, striatal amyloid deposits in both sporadic AD and eoFAD (despite being fibrillar) are not typically associated with cell loss and do not cause extrapyramidal symptoms early in the clinical course. However, Parkinsonism has been reported in C410Y mutation carriers late in the course of the disease (Mann et al., 2001). This is reminiscent

of the lack of tissue reaction observed around the diffuse plaques observed in the cerebellum. However, while the lack of toxic effects of cerebellar amyloid may be due simply to lack of extensive β-sheet conformation (Styren, Kamboh, and DeKosky, 1998), another explanation must be sought for the lack of apparent amyloid toxicity in the striatum where the deposits are largely fibrillar. The presence or absence of tissue factors and the type of neurons and circuitry present may explain the differences in tissue reactivity to Aβ deposits between cortical areas and the striatum. A full understanding of these factors may provide important clues for the development of therapies that could help protect cortical neurons from the toxic effects of Aβ.

It will be important to address the cause of the very early amyloid deposition in the striatum of the PS1 mutation carriers. While the reason is not yet known, we have also seen disproportionate retention of PiB in the striatum of an APP mutation carrier and a nondemented Down syndrome subject (unpublished observations), although both of these cases had more cortical involvement than any of the PS1 mutation carriers included in this report. These early-onset forms of AD all share overproduction of Aβ (particularly the 42 amino acid form) as a proposed mechanism of Aβ deposition (Younkin, 1997), whereas decreased clearance might be more important in late-onset AD (Whitaker et al., 2003). It may be that the cellular milieu of the striatum is particularly prone to amyloid deposition under conditions of overproduction. Although the relevance to human AD is not known, it should be noted that striatal amyloid deposition has been described in a PS1/APP double transgenic mouse model (Perez et al., 2005).

FTLD

Frontotemporal lobar dementia (FTLD) is pathologically distinct from AD in that it is a non-Aβ dementia (Taniguchi et al., 2004). However, the clinical presentations of these dementias overlap, and differential diagnosis can be challenging. Thus, although Aβ pathology should not be present in FTLD, amyloid imaging can be a useful tool in ruling out or ruling in AD pathology in unclear cases. Rabinovici et al. (2007) used amyloid imaging to discriminate AD from FTLD. They studied 7 AD patients, 12 FTLD patients, and 8 cognitively normal controls with PiB PET and FDG. PiB DVR images were visually rated by a blinded investigator as positive or negative for cortical PiB, and FDG images were rated as consistent with AD or FTLD. They found all patients with AD (7/7) had positive PiB scans by visual inspection, while 8/12 patients with FTLD and 7/8 controls had negative PiB scans. Of the four "PiB-positive" patients with FTLD, two had FDG scans that suggested AD, and two had FDG scans suggestive of FTLD (Figure 14.31). They concluded that amyloid imaging could help discriminate AD from FTLD, but point out that pathologic correlation is needed to determine whether patients with PiB-positive FTLD represent false positives, comorbid FTLD/AD pathology, or AD pathology mimicking an FTLD clinical syndrome.

Drzezga et al. (2008) have reported results of a study of patients with semantic dementia (SD; a relatively rare clinical syndrome, assigned to the group of FTLDs). Their goal was to determine whether differences between AD and SD can be found by means of in vivo amyloid-plaque imaging using PiB PET, and whether this would be complementary to information obtained by measurement of cerebral glucose metabolism with FDG PET. Eight AD and 8 SD patients were diagnosed using established clinical criteria, matched for gender, age, and overall degree of cognitive impairment. Drzezga et al. found characteristic patterns of hypometabolism in AD (bilateral temporoparietal and frontal cortex). In SD, they found typical

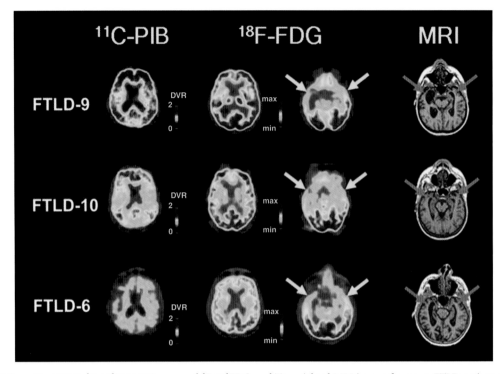

Figure 14–31 PIB-positive FTLD. [C-11]PIB DVR, summed [F-18]FDG, and T1-weighted MRI images from two FTLD patients with positive [C-11]PIB scans, and a third SemD patient with a negative [C-11]PIB scan (FTLD-6, an 81-year-old male). Orange arrows highlight anterior temporal atrophy noted on MRI, and yellow arrows point to anterior temporal hypometabolism seen on [F-18]FDG scans. Images are presented in neurological orientation. (From Rabinovici et al., 2007.)

temporal (left > right) and minor frontal mesial hypometabolism. Significantly stronger cortical retention of PiB was observed in all patients with AD (bilateral temporoparietal, frontal, posterior cingulate cortex, and precuneus) than in those with SD, extending the differences found in FDG-PET between the groups. No significant cortical PiB retention was found in SD. Overall, the differences in PiB retention between AD and SD were more extensive than differences in cerebral metabolism determined by FDG

(Figure 14.32). They concluded that, "These findings support the notion that SD can be diagnosed in vivo as a separate entity from AD using amyloid plaque imaging. In general, amyloid plaque PET may complement neuropsychological assessment regarding reliable differential diagnosis of AD and FTLD dementias based on characterization of underlying pathology and may improve the definition of individual prognosis and the selection of patients for scientific trials" (Drzezga et al., 2008).

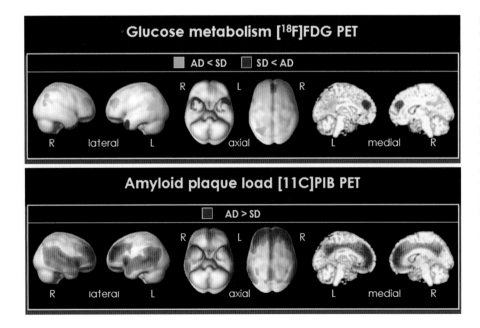

Figure 14–32 Statistical group comparison of [F-18]FDG PET and [C-11]PIB PET findings in AD and SD patients. (Top) Differences in hypometabolism between the patient groups. Lower metabolism in AD is displayed in green, lower metabolism in SD is displayed in red. (Bottom) Differences in amyloid plaque deposition between the patient groups. Higher plaque load in AD displayed in red. There were no areas in which plaque load was greater in SD compared to AD. Views from left to right: right lateral, left lateral, caudal, cranial, left medial, and right medial (results projected on a smooth average MRI template, medial aspects on SPM96 template). (Adapted from Drzezga et al., 2008.)

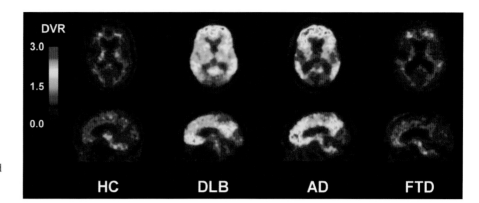

Figure 14–33 PiB PET DVR images of a typical healthy control (HC), a typical AD patient, and a PiB-positive DLB patient, and a PiB-negative FTLD (or FTD) patient. (From Rowe et al., 2007a.)

Rowe et al. (2007a) included 6 FTLD subjects in a PiB PET study. In contrast to 17/17 AD patients who were amyloid-positive, increased PiB retention was absent in all 6 FTLD patients.

Engler et al. (2008) studied 10 patients with clinically diagnosed FTLD with PiB PET. PiB retention in the FTLD subjects was compared with PiB retention in 17 AD patients and 8 healthy controls, defined as being PiB-negative. The 8 FTLD patients showed significantly lower PiB retention than the AD patients in frontal, parietal, temporal, and occipital cortices, and in the putamen. The PiB uptake in these FTLD patients as a group did not differ significantly from the controls in any region. However, two of the 10 FTLD patients showed PiB retention similar to AD patients. Engler et al. concluded that, "PiB could potentially aid in differentiating between FTLD and AD."

DLB

Dementia with Lewy bodies (DLB) is an entity that has significant clinical and pathological overlap with AD (McKeith 2006). At one extreme, pure DLB shows extensive deposition of α-synuclein in the form of intracellular Lewy bodies and "Lewy neurites" (Dickson, 2002), but no significant Aβ pathology. Preliminary evidence suggests that PiB does not bind to α-synuclein deposits in detectable amounts (Fodero-Tavoletti et al., 2006; Klunk et al., 2003), so amyloid imaging can play a similar role in DLB as that discussed above for FTLD, in that it can rule in or rule out the presence of significant Aβ pathology. The interpretation of findings will be different, since there are commonly mixed AD and DLB pathologies in both clinical AD and DLB, but identification of "pure DLB" in the absence of Aβ pathology is an important goal. Rowe et al. (2007a) included 10 cases of DLB in a PiB PET amyloid imaging study. Cortical PiB binding was markedly elevated in every AD subject ($n = 17$) regardless of disease severity. Most DLB subjects also showed increased PiB binding, similar in distribution to AD (Figure 14.33); however, the degree of binding was generally lower and more variable in DLB subjects, ranging from control-like to AD-like (Figure 14.34). PiB binding did not correlate with dementia severity in AD or DLB. Several DLB subjects had little evidence of amyloid deposition (Figure 14.34). PiB scans were not able to reliably distinguish DLB from AD other than in cases with no or very low cortical PiB retention. In the DLB subjects, high neocortical PiB retention (especially in precuneus/posterior cingulate) correlated with shorter time between the onset of cognitive impairment and the development of diagnostic clinical features.

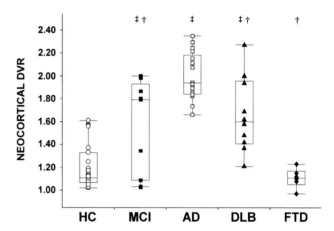

Figure 14–34 Box and whisker plots displaying median and 1st and 99th percentiles of neocortical Aβ burden as quantified by [C-11]PiB DVR for AD (open squares), DLB(filled triangles), FTD (filled diamonds), MCI (filled squares), and healthy controls (HC; open circles). †Significant results for MCI, DLB, and FTD vs. AD ($p < 0.05$). ‡Significant results vs. controls ($p < 0.05$). (From Rowe et al., 2007a.)

Parkinson's Disease

Vascular Aβ deposition is common in Parkinson's disease, and amyloid plaques are often found in Parkinson's disease with dementia (Jellinger, 2003; Mastaglia et al., 2003). In addition, α-synuclein, the major component of the Lewy bodies found in Parkinson's disease, forms amyloid fibrils (Conway, Harper, and Lansbury, 2000). Although preclinical data suggest that PiB does not bind to α-synuclein deposits in the absence of Aβ deposits (Fodero-Tavoletti et al., 2006; Klunk et al., 2003), this raises the question of whether PiB retention would commonly be found in Parkinson's disease. Johansson et al. (2008) have studied five cognitively normal, early stage Parkinson's disease patients with PiB PET and compared these results to 16 patients with AD and six healthy controls from a previous study. They found that PiB retention was not significantly increased in these early stage Parkinson's disease patients compared to healthy controls, but suggest that studies of more advanced Parkinson's disease patients may show different results.

Maetzler et al. (2008) have used PiB PET to study 10 Parkinson's disease with dementia (PDD) subjects and compared the PDD subjects to control and AD subjects. They found 2 of the 10 PDD subjects to have PiB retention indistinguishable from AD patients, while the other 8 were very similar to controls. They found a very small elevation of PiB retention in the brainstem (mesencephalon and pons) of the PiB-negative PDD subjects, and an increased brainstem:precuneus ratio. They suggested that this may be due to PiB binding to α-synuclein deposits, but this is highly doubtful given the in vitro findings that showed the PiB does not bind to homogenates of postmortem DLB brain tissue unless Aβ plaques are present (Fodero-Tavoletti et al., 2007). Furthermore, Johansson et al. found no evidence of increased PiB retention in the pons of five nondemented PD subjects in which extensive brainstem α-synuclein pathology would surely be present (Johansson et al., 2008).

Cerebral Amyloid Angiopathy (CAA)

In addition to deposition in the form of plaques, Aβ is found deposited around arterioles in AD cortex and meninges in over 80% of cases (Jellinger, 2002). CAA can be found in the absence of dementia and is frequently associated with strokes (Maia, Mackenzie, and Feldman, 2007). The strokes and the amyloid angiopathy are typically most frequently located in the occipital lobe (Attems et al., 2007; Rosand et al., 2005). The distinction between AD and CAA is even more blurred than that between AD and DLB—especially when one considers the potential overlap of CAA without dementia and prodromal AD in an amyloid-positive, cognitively normal person. Nevertheless, CAA appears to be a distinct clinical entity and can be seen in early-onset hereditary forms, including those due to mutations in the amyloid precursor protein (Zhang-Nunes et al., 2006). Accordingly, Johnson et al. (2007) evaluated PiB PET as a potential noninvasive method for detection of CAA in six nondemented subjects diagnosed with probable CAA, 15 healthy control subjects, and nine patients with probable AD. They found that all CAA and AD subjects were PiB-positive, both by distribution volume ratio measurements and by visual inspection of PiB PET images. Global cortical PiB retention was significantly increased in CAA relative to healthy control subjects but was lower in CAA than in AD subjects. The occipital-to-global PiB ratio, however, was significantly greater in CAA than in AD subjects—consistent with the known predilection of CAA for the occipital lobe (Figure 14.35).

Atypical Presentations of AD

In addition to overlap between the typical clinical syndrome of AD with FTLD, DLB, and CAA, AD can sometimes present in an atypical manner consisting of slowly progressive focal cortical syndromes (Galton et al., 2000). Here again, amyloid imaging could potentially be useful for determining the presence or absence of Aβ pathology in these unusual cases. Ng et al. (2007b) explored the presence and topography of Aβ deposits using PiB PET in 15 healthy controls, 10 patients with Alzheimer disease, one patient with primary progressive aphasia (PPA), and one patient with posterior cortical atrophy (PCA). The retention of PiB was compared among the different groups using statistical parametric mapping. Both patients with atypical dementia had a similar PiB binding pattern to AD, although PiB retention was higher on the left cerebral hemisphere in the patient with PPA and higher in the occipital cortex in the patient with PCA. That is, PiB retention was higher in brain areas that are associated with the particular clinical symptoms. Ng et al. concluded that the presence of distinctive focal PiB retention patterns could be demonstrated in these two patients with atypical onset of dementia. They suggested that PiB "has the potential to facilitate differential diagnosis of dementia and identify patients who could benefit from specific therapeutic strategies aimed at beta amyloid reduction."

Depression

Late-life depression is a risk factor for persistent MCI and future dementia. Two meta-analyses suggest that late-life depression approximately doubles an individual's risk of developing dementia (Jorm, 2001; Ownby et al., 2006). It is not known with certainty whether this increase in dementia is mediated through an increase in AD pathology, or through mechanisms unrelated to AD, such as vascular pathology. A preliminary study by Butters et al. (2007) investigated the relationships among late-life depression and MCI that persisted after antidepressant therapy, with two imaging approaches: PiB PET and volumetric MRI of white matter hyperintensities (to assess vascular pathology). Butters et al. studied 11 recently remitted late-life depression subjects (72.2 ± 5.2 years). Nine presented and were treated in a depression clinic and seven of these were found to meet criteria for a diagnosis of MCI. The

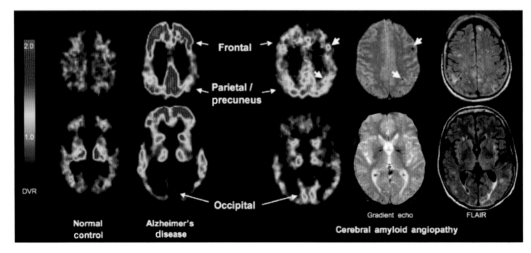

Figure 14–35   PiB PET DVR images at two transaxial levels from a PiB-negative normal control subject (left), an AD patient (second from left), and a patient with CAA (PET and MRIs on the right). Compared with AD and controls, CAA subjects had an intermediate level of global PiB retention, but compared with AD, CAA subjects had relatively increased occipital retention. Microbleeds seen in this CAA patient, shown in coregistered gradient echo magnetic resonance images, at times appear proximal to foci of amyloid deposition (small arrows). (From Johnson et al., 2007.)

remaining two presented with MCI to an AD research clinic and were found to have a history of mid-life-onset depression. PiB retention in the frontal, parietal, and posterior cingulate/precuneus cortices was variable across late-life depression subjects in a manner similar to that described above for never-depressed MCI subjects (Lopresti et al., 2005; Pike et al., 2007; Price et al., 2005; Rowe et al., 2007a). That is, approximately half of the depressed-recovered MCI subjects had AD-like levels of PiB retention. White matter hyperintensity volume also was variable, but was significantly greater in the late-life depression subjects versus controls. While this preliminary study needs to be greatly expanded before any firm conclusion can be reached, these early results suggest that both amyloid and vascular pathology may play synergistic roles in the increased prevalence of dementia observed following late-life depression. It may be that depression is frequently the presenting symptom of this combined pathology.

PiB and Prion Diseases

The human prion diseases (spongiform encephalopathies) include Creutzfeldt-Jakob disease (CJD) and "new variant" CJD, Gerstmann-Straussler-Scheinker syndrome, and kuru (Kretzschmar, 1993). They are progressive neurodegenerative illnesses with dementia and ataxia. The typical neuropathological changes consist of spongiform degeneration, amyloid plaques composed not of Aβ but prion protein (PrP), gliosis, and nerve cell loss. The distribution of plaques is distinct from that in AD, particularly because prion plaques are usually concentrated in the cerebellum, an area typically devoid of fibrillar Aβ plaques in AD. Mutations of the prion protein gene are associated with heritable human prion disease. These forms of heritable prion disease often have clinical and neuropathological changes not typical of any known variant of human prion disease.

Boxer et al. (2007) compared two brothers (35 and 41 years old) who were ultimately found to be concordant for a 6 octapeptide repeat insertion mutation (6-OPRI) in the gene that codes for PrP. The younger brother was initially diagnosed with early-onset AD after a 3-year history of progressive memory loss, and both brothers were said to have "similar clinical syndromes." Both had similar FDG scans judged to be typical for AD because of the regional pattern of cerebral hypometabolism. Their father had died at age 47, apparently without a confirmed diagnosis, after a 10-year history of progressive dementia. Since there is considerable overlap in the clinical presentations of early-onset dementia (EOD) caused by prion and AD gene mutations, a major motivation for this study was to determine if amyloid imaging could be helpful in the differential diagnosis of EOD. The younger brother underwent amyloid imaging with FDDNP (Shoghi-Jadid et al., 2002) at UCLA, and the older brother was imaged with PiB (Klunk et al., 2004) at the Lawrence Berkeley National Laboratory.

The 35-year-old brother's FDDNP scan was read as "intermediate" between controls and AD, with asymmetric (right > left) FDDNP retention. The highest FDDNP values were in the medial temporal and parietal lobes. The FDDNP retention pattern was noted to be of "lesser intensity and in a pattern different from that typically found in AD." The 41-year-old brother had a control-like (i.e., normal) pattern on his PiB scan.

The conclusion drawn from the authors' review of the two imaging studies was that, "Although not performed in the same subject, the PiB and FDDNP results suggest that FDDNP has a greater binding affinity for PrP-amyloid than PiB" (Boxer et al., 2007). However, when one critically considers the data presented, along with the known neuropathology of this PrP gene mutation,

one must question whether the FDDNP signal was related to PrP-amyloid deposition at all. The most significant problem was the discordance between the regional pattern of FDDNP retention described in this study and the known regional distribution of PrP-amyloid pathology. This is true both for 6-OPRI kindreds in general, and, more importantly, for the postmortem pathology of the 41-year-old, who died while the Boxer et al. paper was being written. The authors point out that previous studies showed 6-OPRI kindreds to have variable cortical spongiosis with or without diffuse PrP-amyloid deposition in the cerebellar molecular layer (Vital et al., 1998). Postmortem PrP immunohistochemical examination of the brain of the 41-year-old brother demonstrated the presence of prominent PrP-amyloid deposition in the cerebellar, greater than in the cerebral cortex. The pathology clearly indicates that if FDDNP or PiB were binding to PrP-amyloid pathology, the signal should be highest in the cerebellum. Not only was increased FDDNP retention not observed in the cerebellum, but the retention in the cerebellum was so low that the authors used this region as their reference tissue.

As stated above in the section on pharmacokinetic modeling, the binding of a tracer in the brain is proportional to the BP or the total concentration of binding sites (B_{max}) divided by the affinity of the tracer for that binding site (K_d). Therefore, the detectability of a given amyloid protein is related to the concentration of the amyloid in the brain and the affinity of the amyloid imaging tracer for that particular amyloid. It has been shown (and discussed above) that PiB does not detect neurofibrillary tangles (Klunk et al., 2003) or α-synuclein (Fodero-Tavoletti et al., 2006; Klunk et al., 2003). The study by Boxer et al. suggests that neither PiB nor FDDNP can detect the amount and type of PrP amyloid deposited in this 6-OPRI mutation kindred.

Direct Comparison of PiB and FDDNP

Tolboom et al. (2007) have presented the first preliminary evidence on the direct comparison of [F-18]FDDNP and PiB in the same subjects. They acquired dynamic 90-minute PiB and [F-18]FDDNP scans on the same day using the same PET scanner. During both scans, continuous online and discrete manual sampling was performed to derive a metabolite-corrected arterial plasma input curve. Analysis of TACs was performed using the simplified reference tissue model with cerebellum gray matter as reference tissue. Three AD patients, three patients with MCI, and three age-matched normal controls were included in this preliminary study. Tolboom et al. reported that PiB showed good contrast between AD patients and normal controls, as described previously (Klunk et al., 2004). In addition, the range of BP values in MCI patients was broader, probably due to the known heterogeneity of this group (Lopresti et al., 2005). [F-18]FDDNP provided less contrast between AD patients and normal controls. The PiB BP was in general tenfold higher than the [F-18]FDDNP BP in the *same* AD patients.

Amyloid Imaging Compared to Other Biomarkers

Amyloid Imaging and Apolipoprotein-E Genotype

It has been reported that the presence of an apolipoprotein-E ε4 (Apo-E4) allele is associated with increased amyloid deposition in AD (Ohm et al., 1995; Pirttila et al., 1997), however, the relationship between Apo-E4 and postmortem amyloid load is complex and not always observed (Berg et al., 1998). Klunk et al., (2004) found no effect of Apo-E genotype on PiB retention in any brain area of AD patients. Furthermore, there was no trend toward increased PiB retention in the AD patients with two ε4 alleles ($n = 6$) compared with the AD patients who had no ε4 alleles ($n = 8$). Rowe et al. (2007a) found that, with all subjects combined (controls, AD, and other dementias), the presence of an Apo-E ε4 allele was associated with higher PiB binding, but within groups there was no significant difference. Kemppainen et al. (2007) studied 13 patients with amnestic MCI and found that MCI subjects that had at least one APOE ε4 allele tended to have higher PiB retention than MCI subjects without APOE ε4. Thus, if Apo-E ε4 does cause increased Aβ deposition, it is often not detectable by PiB PET, except perhaps at early clinical stages.

PiB and FDG

In the initial PiB PET study, the largest and only significant ($p < 0.02$; Bonferroni corrected) difference in glucose metabolism (determined with FDG PET) between AD patients and control subjects was observed in the parietal cortex. The relative differences in metabolic rate between AD patients and HC subjects were in general smaller (e.g., 41% in parietal cortex) than the relative differences in PiB retention (e.g., 94% in frontal cortex). An inverse correlation between PiB retention and glucose metabolism was observed in most cortical areas, but this trend reached significance only in the parietal cortex ($p < 0.001$; Bonferroni corrected). The lack of correlation between PiB and glucose metabolism in the frontal cortex suggests that Aβ deposition alone is not sufficient to *locally* reduce cerebral metabolism. However, since glucose metabolism primarily reflects metabolic activity in synapses, we must keep in mind that the effect of Aβ deposition in a given brain region may be most evident in the terminal fields of axons projecting out of that region. The two-year follow-up of these same subjects found no significant difference in PiB retention between baseline and follow-up, while a significant ($p < 0.01$) 20% decrease in metabolic rate was observed in cortical brain regions. A significant negative correlation between metabolic rate and PiB retention was again observed in the parietal cortex in the Alzheimer patients at follow-up. This follow-up study suggests that measurement of cerebral metabolism with FDG is better suited to tracking brain changes during the clinically apparent stage of AD than is PiB.

Ziolko et al. (2006) evaluated statistical methods for the assessment of group differences in PiB retention, and compared these results to FDG studies of glucose metabolism performed in the same subjects, on the same day. PET studies were performed in 10 mild to moderate AD and 11 control subjects. Parametric images of PiB and FDG retention were compared using parametric (SPM) and nonparametric (SnPM) statistical methods with familywise error (FWE) and false discovery rate (FDR) corrections. PiB results were consistent with previous regional results, as AD subjects showed highly significant retention in frontal, parietal, temporal, and precuneus/posterior cingulate cortices (FDR-corrected $p < 0.0000000002$). FDG results showed regions of marginally significant decreases in uptake in AD subjects in the frontal, parietal, temporal, and precuneus/posterior cingulate cortices (FDR-corrected $p < 0.1$), consistent with previous studies (Herholz et al., 2002; Silverman et al., 2001). Relative to FDG, the PiB analyses were of greater statistical significance and larger spatial extent. Additionally, the PiB analyses retained significance after both FWE and FDR corrections.

Edison et al. (2006) investigated the association between brain amyloid load in AD (measured by PiB) and regional cerebral glucose metabolism (rCMRGlc) measured by FDG in 12 subjects with AD and eight controls. Parametric images of PiB binding and rCMRGlc were interrogated with an ROI atlas and statistical parametric mapping. AD subjects showed twofold increases in mean PiB binding in cingulate, frontal, temporal, parietal, and occipital cortical areas. Mean levels of temporal and parietal rCMRGlc were reduced by 20% in AD and these correlated with mini-mental scores, immediate recall, and recognition memory test for words. Higher PiB uptake correlated with lower rCMRGlc in temporal and parietal cortices, but the high frontal amyloid load detected by PiB PET in AD in the face of spared glucose metabolism was interpreted by Edison et al. to suggest that amyloid plaque formation may not be directly responsible for neuronal dysfunction in this disorder.

Forsberg et al. (2007) studied 21 patients diagnosed with MCI with PiB and FDG PET, as well as assessment of cognitive function and CSF sampling. Seven MCI patients that later at clinical follow-up converted to AD (8.1 ± 6.0 [S.D.] months) showed significantly higher PiB retention compared to nonconverting MCI patients. However, there was no significant difference in rCMRglc between MCI patients and healthy controls in any cortical brain region.

Rabinovici et al. (2007) performed both FDG and PiB scans on 6 clinically diagnosed AD patients and 11 clinically diagnosed FTLD patients. The results of the PET visual reads done for their study by a blinded reader are shown in Table 14.3. All seven patients with AD demonstrated cortical PiB retention on visual inspection (i.e., a "PiB-positive" scan), while 8/12 patients with FTLD and 7/8 controls did not (PiB-negative scan). Visual reads of FDG PET scans agreed with the clinical diagnosis in 5/6 patients with AD and 8/11 patients with FTLD (table 14.2). PiB and FDG suggested the same diagnosis (PiB-positive scan and FDG consistent with AD, or PiB-negative scan and FDG consistent with FTLD) in 13/17 patients. In 3/4 cases in which there was a discrepancy, the FDG scan suggested FTLD, while the PiB scan was positive. A second blinded reader agreed with the primary visual read on 19/19 patient PiB scans (kappa = 1.00) and 15/17 FDG scans (kappa = 0.76). Both disparate FDG reads occurred in FTLD patients: one who was PiB-positive (read as AD by the primary reader and FTLD by the second reader), and one who was PiB-negative (primary read FTLD, second read AD). Rabinovici et al. noted that these findings suggest that "in a dementia population, PiB visual interpretations (which depend on determining the presence or absence of tracer activity in cortex) are highly reproducible, more so than visual reads of F-18-FDG scans, which rely on the interpretation of occasionally ambiguous patterns" (Rabinovici et al., 2007).

Ng et al. (2007a) compared a visual assessment to a quantitative assessment of PiB and FDG PET data for the detection of Alzheimer's disease compared to cognitively intact controls. Their goal was to explore the clinical potential of amyloid imaging for the diagnosis of AD by comparison of the accuracy of visual reading of PiB images with quantitative analysis and FDG images. They studied 15 AD patients (age 71.1 ± 11.3 years) and 25 clinically

Table 14.3   Visual reads (by primary reader) of PET scans.

PET read	Clinical AD		Clinical FTLD		Controls	
	PiB(+)	PiB(−)	PiB(+)	PiB(−)	PiB(+)	PiB(−)
FDG-AD	5	0	2	1	0	0
FDG-FTLD	1	0	2	6	0	0
FDG-N/A	1	0	0	1	1	7
Total	7	0	4	8	1	7

From (Rabinovici et al., 2007).

unimpaired subjects (age 71.9 ± 6.82 years) with PiB PET and FDG PET. PiB images (SUVR-cerebellum from 40 to 70 minutes) and FDG images (SUVR-cerebellum from 60 to 80 minutes) were rated separately by two readers as normal, possible AD, or probable AD. Quantitative analyses used the DVR of frontal cortex, parietotemporal cortex, posterior cingulate/precuneus, and caudate nucleus for PiB, and SUVR of parietotemporal cortex and posterior cingulate/precuneus for FDG (with cerebellum as the reference for both). Visual agreement between readers was excellent for PiB (kappa = 0.90) and good for FDG (kappa = 0.56). Based on the clinical diagnosis, Ng et al. found PiB was more accurate than FDG both on visual reading (accuracy 90% vs. 70%) and ROC analysis (95% vs. 83%). Ng et al. concluded that the visual analysis of PiB images appears more accurate than visual reading of FDG for identification of AD and had accuracy similar to quantitative analysis of a 90-minute dynamic scan. They point out that the accuracy of PiB PET is limited by the existence of PiB-positive controls in any elderly cohort of clinically unimpaired subjects, and that longitudinal follow-up will be required to determine if this represents detection of preclinical AD. If one looks at this study simply from the perspective of detecting a pathological signal in subjects who have AD, then both readers rated 15/15 AD patients as "Probable AD" from the PiB scans, but only rated 10 (experienced reader) or 11 (newly trained reader) of the 15 AD patients as "Probable AD" from the FDG scan.

PiB and MRI

Archer et al. (2006) determined the relationship between cerebral amyloid plaque load determined with PiB, and rates of cerebral atrophy in AD. They correlated PiB PET findings with volumetric MRI measurements in nine subjects with mild to moderate AD and found a significant, positive correlation between rates of whole brain atrophy and whole brain and regional PiB uptake.

PiB and Cerebrospinal Fluid (CSF) Aβ

Soluble Aβ peptide is found in the CSF of AD patients and controls (Motter et al., 1995; Nitsch et al., 1995; Pirttila et al., 1994). Although there is considerable overlap, CSF Aβ42 is lower in AD patients than controls and this is thought to be related to sequestration in parenchymal and vascular Aβ deposits (Pirttila et al., 1996). In MCI patients, a combination of high CSF total-tau and low CSF Aβ42 measures at baseline yielded a sensitivity of 95% and a specificity of 83% for prediction of conversion to AD over a 4–6-year period (hazard ratio 17.7) (Hansson et al., 2006). The extensive overlap between CSF Aβ42 levels in AD patients and controls has hampered the use of this biomarker as a diagnostic test, but autopsy follow-up studies have suggested that part of the problem may be incorrect clinical diagnosis, i.e., low CSF Aβ and high CSF tau may be a better reflection of CNS pathology than the correlations with clinical diagnosis reveal (Galasko et al., 1998). Fagan et al. have reported two studies comparing CSF Aβ42 levels and PiB retention (Fagan et al., 2006, 2007). In their first report, they compared the in vivo brain amyloid load determined using PiB PET with CSF Aβ42 and tau measures in clinically characterized research subjects. They found that the subjects fell into two non-overlapping groups: those with positive PiB retention had the lowest CSF Aβ42 level, and those with negative PiB retention had the highest CSF Aβ42 level. No relation was observed between PiB retention and CSF Aβ40, tau, phospho-tau(181), plasma Aβ40, or plasma Aβ42. Importantly, PiB retention and CSF Aβ42 did not consistently correspond with clinical diagnosis; three cognitively normal subjects were PiB-positive with low CSF Aβ42, suggesting

the presence of amyloid in the absence of cognitive impairment (i.e., preclinical AD). Fagan et al. suggested that these findings indicate that brain amyloid deposition results in low CSF Aβ42, and that amyloid imaging and CSF Aβ42 may potentially serve as antecedent biomarkers of (preclinical) AD.

In the second study, Fagan et al. (2007) investigated the ability of CSF measures to discriminate early-stage AD (defined by clinical criteria and the presence/absence of brain amyloid) from nondemented aging and to assess whether these biomarkers can predict future dementia in cognitively normal individuals. They studied 139 community-dwelling volunteers aged 60–91 years and clinically judged as cognitively normal (Clinical Dementia Rating [CDR], 0) or having very mild (CDR, 0.5) or mild (CDR, 1) AD dementia. Consistent with previous studies, they found that individuals with very mild or mild AD had reduced mean levels of CSF Aβ42 and increased levels of CSF tau and phosphorylated tau(181). The CSF Aβ42 level corresponded with the presence or absence of brain amyloid (determined with PiB PET) in demented and nondemented individuals. That is, all PiB-positive subjects had low CSF Aβ42 (red symbols in Figure 14.36) and all PiB-negative subjects had higher levels of CSF Aβ42 (green symbols in Figure 14.36). However, in both studies, the cutoff between low and normal levels of CSF Aβ42 was very narrow and the PiB PET imaging provided a much clearer distinction between PiB-positive and PiB-negative groups. This study holds important implications for the use of CSF Aβ42 and PiB PET as screening tools for amyloid deposition in asymptomatic individuals, and this will be discussed below.

Forsberg et al. (2007) measured CSF Aβ1–42, total tau and phosphor-tau in 21 patients diagnosed with MCI (mean age 63.3 ± 7.8 years) who also were studied with PiB PET. They found significant negative correlations between CSF Aβ1–42 and PiB retention in the frontal cortex and posterior cingulate/precuneus (Figure 14.37). Nonsignificant negative correlations also were observed between CSF Aβ1–42 and PiB retention in the temporal and parietal cortex. Similarly, nonsignificant positive correlations were observed between CSF total and phosphor-tau and PiB retention in frontal, temporal, and parietal cortices and posterior cingulate/precuneus.

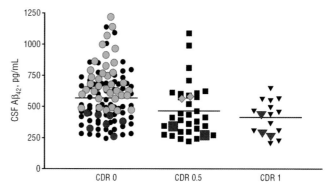

Figure 14–36 Cerebrospinal fluid (CSF) Aβ42 levels as a function of CDR score and cortical amyloid. Fifty subjects were imaged with PiB PET. CDR scores and diagnoses were determined by blinded clinicians. There are 2 classifications of subjects with a CDR of 0.5: the green diamonds indicate PIB– and non–AD dementia at follow-up. Red squares indicate PIB+ and AD dementia. Any symbol in green indicates PIB– subjects. Any symbol in red indicates PIB+ subjects. Black symbols represent subjects who did not undergo a PiB scan. (From Fagan et al., 2007.)

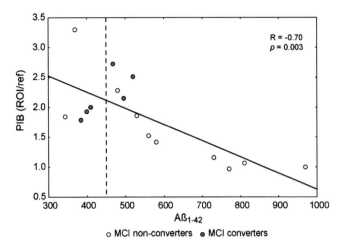

Figure 14–37 Correlation between PIB retention in posterior cingulate/precuneus and Aβ1–42 levels. MCI patients who converted to AD are indicated with filled circles. The cutoff for abnormal CSF Aβ1–42 is < 450 pg/ml in this study. (From Forsberg et al., 2007.)

Looking to the Future

The following statement appeared in the initial human PiB PET study and remains true today (Klunk et al., 2004):

"As the technology of amyloid imaging moves forward, it will be important to avoid the circular reasoning inherent in the association of amyloid deposition with both the diagnosis and the cause of AD. Therefore, at the outset, it may be best to not equate amyloid deposition to clinical diagnosis. Rather than as a method of diagnosis, it might be best to first think of PiB retention more fundamentally as a method to detect and quantify brain β-amyloidosis, a term first used in reference to AD by Glenner (1983). Several basic, unbiased questions then can be asked regarding (1) the correlation of β-amyloidosis with clinical diagnosis; (2) the natural history of β-amyloidosis and its onset relative to clinical symptoms of dementia; and (3) the ability of β-amyloidosis to serve as a surrogate marker of efficacy for antiamyloid therapeutics."

It is with this philosophy in mind, that we will consider the potential uses and limitations of PiB PET.

Clinical Diagnosis—Pushing the Envelope

The term "Alzheimer's disease" has both clinical definitions (DSM-IV, 1995; McKhann et al., 1984) and neuropathological definitions (Khachaturian, 1985; Mirra et al., 1991, NIA/Reagan_Workgroup, 1997). One can have a clinical syndrome consistent with AD without AD pathology. Likewise, one can have AD pathology without a clinical dementia. The term "Definite AD" implies the simultaneous existence of both clinical and pathological AD (McKhann et al., 1984). A finding of AD neuropathology at autopsy in a cognitively normal person is not a "neuropathological false positive" for AD; it is simply a discovery of a pathologic change without a clinical correlate. Similarly, the failure to find AD neuropathology in a clinically "Probable AD" patient is not a "neuropathological false negative" for AD; it is simply a demonstration that this case is not Definite AD. Likewise, if used with correct expectations, amyloid imaging cannot give false positives or false negatives for AD, because amyloid imaging cannot be expected to do more than identify the presence or absence of β-amyloidosis. False positives could occur with amyloid imaging

if there appeared to be in vivo amyloid deposition and postmortem examination showed there was no amyloid present. False negatives could likewise occur if the in vivo amyloid imaging technique was not sufficiently sensitive to detect the true presence of amyloid. However, these are false positives and negatives for β-amyloidosis, *not* for AD. Some have called the detection of Aβ deposition in cognitively normal controls "false positives" because a PiB-positive result was obtained in a subject without AD. This logic presumes that amyloid imaging—in isolation from any clinical data—can detect clinical diagnosis. This is an unreasonable expectation. Figure 14.1 predicts that during certain age ranges, there are more clinically unimpaired individuals with amyloid-positive scans than there are AD patients. One cannot use an amyloid imaging scan in isolation to give a clinical diagnosis. The clinician and neuropsychologist must play a role in the interpretation of amyloid imaging studies.

From the Ng et al. visual assessment study (2007a) and the FTLD study of Rabinovici et al. (2007) that were discussed above, it is clear that amyloid imaging can help identify the presence of AD pathology in symptomatic subjects and thus may be a diagnostic tool in these impaired subjects. However, it is equally clear from the 20%–25% prevalence of amyloid-positivity in clinically unimpaired elderly, that amyloid-positivity cannot be equated with clinical symptomatology. That is, since amyloid imaging detects brain β-amyloidosis and not clinical AD, one cannot expect to use this technology to separate clinical AD patients from clinically unimpaired patients. Therefore, studies that calculate "diagnostic accuracy rates" from comparing amyloid imaging to clinical diagnosis such as the one by Ng et al. (2007a), carry an inherent degree of "inaccuracy" in the clinically unimpaired elderly control cases—even when the clinical diagnoses are defined in highly experienced clinical research centers. Some subjects in any relatively large group of cognitively normal elderly controls will be amyloid-positive. With further longitudinal studies, we may learn that these clinically unimpaired amyloid-positive cases have preclinical AD, but that does not equate to saying that a positive PiB scan in a preclinical AD patient is correct in the context of detecting clinical AD (at least not in the way AD is currently defined in terms of symptomatology).

The potential clinical use of amyloid imaging is not likely to be the separation of cognitively normal controls from MCI or AD patients. An amyloid-positive PiB scan looks the same in an MCI patient as it does in an AD patient. Even some controls can have levels of amyloid deposition that look the same as AD cases. If amyloid imaging becomes a useful clinical tool, it will more likely be in the context of the three following categories:

1) Ruling in or ruling out AD from the differential diagnosis of a subject with a clinical dementia that does not fall easily into any one diagnostic category (e.g., distinguishing AD from FTLD or pure DLB).

2) Segregating MCI subjects into AD and non-AD subsets. First, however, longitudinal studies must show that amyloid deposition in clinically defined MCI patients leads to dementia.

3) Presymptomatic diagnosis of AD. This is the most challenging and controversial. Much more longitudinal data would be necessary before any such use should be contemplated. However, such a presymptomatic diagnostic tool may be a critical part of pulling together early and effective treatment strategies for AD.

In research centers, the clinical diagnosis of AD is confirmed by pathology 85%—90% of the time (Gearing et al., 1995; Lopez et al., 2000), although the accuracy is lower in community settings. One could argue that current clinical diagnosis in research centers is adequately accurate and there is no need for imaging or other biomarkers. This may be true if we are satisfied with maintaining the status quo of accurately diagnosing individuals with symptomatic AD. However, a recent therapeutic trial strongly hints that waiting to diagnose and treat in the symptomatic period of AD may doom anti-amyloid strategies to failure. Autopsy reports on four cases from the AN-1792 trial support the concept that anti-Aβ immunotherapy can remove Aβ deposits from the human brain (Bombois et al., 2007; Ferrer et al., 2004; Masliah et al., 2005; Nicoll et al., 2003). However, non-Aβ pathology (neurofibrillary tangles, cell loss, etc.) remained in these cases and the overall clinical response seen in the AN-1792 immunotherapy trial was modest in the face of apparently good clearance of Aβ deposits (Gilman et al., 2005). Another report showed elevated soluble Aβ in two of the postmortem cases (Patton et al., 2006). This suggests that, to attain its optimal clinical effect, anti-amyloid therapy may need to be initiated at the very earliest stages of amyloid deposition, prior to extensive neurofibrillary changes, synapse loss, and neuronal death. In order to achieve this goal, it may be necessary to start anti-amyloid therapy at preclinical stages. Thus, the status quo may not be sufficient to lead us to effective therapies for AD and is very unlikely to lead us to effective preventative treatments; and a real need exists for antecedent biomarkers for preclinical stages of AD.

Although, for most people, thorough clinical evaluations in AD research centers are no more accessible and no less costly than a PET scan, PET is not likely to become a first-line screening tool for everyone over age 60. We must also keep in mind that until a truly effective treatment exists, it is very hard to justify widespread screening for amyloid pathology in cognitively normal people. Hopefully, effective treatments will be available in the near future. How then should amyloid imaging be used as a screening tool? It may make sense to use another less expensive and more accessible biomarker as a first-line screen. The data discussed above suggests CSF Aβ42, or another biomarker that correlates with amyloid imaging, could fill this role. One can envision first performing a primary screen with CSF Aβ42. With further study, we may find that almost everyone with Aβ42 lower than a certain cutoff will be amyloid-positive. It may not make sense to perform amyloid imaging on these people, since we can be sure they will be amyloid-positive—unless we want a baseline before a treatment to determine the effect of that treatment. We also may find that almost everyone with a CSF Aβ42 level above a different cutoff is amyloid-negative and will not need amyloid imaging to confirm this. However, there is likely to be a substantial number of cases in the indeterminate range for CSF Aβ42, and these are the subjects who might benefit most from amyloid imaging as a secondary, higher resolution screening tool.

Surrogate Marker—Considerations Regarding Soluble and Insoluble Aβ

Increasing evidence suggests soluble oligomers of Aβ, at low or sub-nanomolar concentrations, are an important toxic species (Haass and Selkoe, 2007; Lesne et al., 2006). For the purpose of this discussion, we will assume that soluble oligomers are the *only* toxic form of Aβ, and that monomers and fibrils/plaques are inert (although this assumption is not likely to be true). Amyloid imaging with the existing tracers cannot detect soluble oligomers either because of low binding affinity or the low concentration of oligomers. Even if they could, this signal would be swamped by the presence of hundreds or thousands times higher concentrations of insoluble plaque Aβ. Does this make amyloid imaging useless as a surrogate marker of efficacy for anti-amyloid therapies, since reduction of oligomers would be the key to therapeutic success?

Certainly, it would be desirable to have a PET tracer that was specific for soluble oligomers and sensitive enough to detect them. However, such a tracer may not be possible to develop. Before dismissing the usefulness of imaging insoluble amyloid, one should consider the basic principle of chemical equilibrium. There is every reason to believe that Aβ monomers, oligomers, and insoluble fibrils are in equilibrium in the same way as a moderately soluble chemical, and crystals of that chemical would be in equilibrium in a test tube. If one decants the supernatant solution and adds pure buffer to the crystals, soon there will be more soluble chemical in the solution. If one does this repeatedly, the crystals will become depleted and the concentration of chemical in solution will fall as well. It is likely, and existing evidence discussed below suggests, that the same sort of equilibrium exists among monomeric, oligomeric, and fibrillar Aβ.

Plaques have been suggested to be a potential detoxifying mechanism, since the concentration of soluble oligomers would be decreased as Aβ is shunted away from oligomers and into plaques. Since we are assuming that soluble oligomers are the only toxic species, then one must grant that it is better to have 99% of the CNS Aβ in a less toxic plaque form than to have 100% in the toxic oligomeric form. However, this is *not* to say that it is good to have plaques in the brain. Postmortem analyses of senile plaques reveal numerous dystrophic processes in their vicinity (Knowles et al., 1999). D'Amore et al. (2003) have used in vivo multiphoton microscopy of a transgenic mouse model of AD to simultaneously image senile plaques and nearby neuronal processes. Imaging of three-dimensional volumes in the vicinity of plaques revealed subtle changes in neurite geometry in or near *diffuse* plaques. By contrast, marked disruptions in neurite morphology, including dystrophic neurites immediately surrounding plaques as well as major alterations in neurite trajectories, were seen in association with thioflavin-S-positive fibrillar plaques. Nearly half of all labeled processes that came within 50 microns of a thioflavin-S-positive plaque were altered, suggesting a fairly large "halo" of neuropil alterations that extend beyond the discrete border of a thioflavin-S plaque (D'Amore et al., 2003). Since our discussion allows only toxic oligomers to effect this neuritic damage, then we must postulate that Aβ plaques are surrounded by a concentration gradient of oligomers. The most likely reason for this would be an equilibrium between the plaque Aβ and the surrounding oligomeric Aβ. Otherwise, diffusion of the soluble oligomers should destroy any spatial gradient of toxicity around plaques. This is supported by evidence that the amount of soluble Aβ is correlated with the number of plaques (Parvathy et al., 2001).

A recent paper suggests that oligomers and fibrils are formed through different mechanisms and oligomers do not go on to form insoluble amyloid fibrils (Necula et al., 2007). Even if this is true, both oligomers and fibrils must be in equilibrium with monomers, so fibrils and oligomers come into equilibrium with each other through the monomeric intermediate.

Therefore plaques could be considered as good, bad, or neutral, depending on the situation. During the early stages of plaque deposition, when active synthesis of monomeric Aβ begins to outpace clearance, shunting monomers or oligomers into plaques may be a beneficial event. The fact that only ~1% of Aβ remains soluble in AD brain and ~99% is deposited in plaques could be protective. At the point of equilibrium (probably achieved early in the course of clinical AD), plaque load no longer increases (see Engler et al. [2006]), and therefore plaque deposition no longer serves as a buffer to lower soluble Aβ. At this point, the presence of plaques may have a neutral effect. However, when our goal is to decrease oligomeric Aβ by either decreasing production of Aβ (e.g., secretase inhibitors) or increasing clearance of Aβ (immunotherapy), then the regeneration of the small monomeric and oligomeric pools of Aβ from the much larger plaque pool of Aβ would be very detrimental. In this situation, plaques become the equivalent of a toxic waste dump of leaking barrels beside a pond contaminated with the toxin contained in those barrels. One could pump the pond dry and refill it, but the toxic leak would keep it contaminated until the barrels themselves were removed. An equivalent situation is likely to apply to any therapy that is directed at decreasing oligomeric Aβ. In order to have more than a transient effect, it is likely that anti-oligomer treatments will have to shift the entire Aβ equilibrium towards clearance of all forms of Aβ (monomers, oligomers, and fibrils). The finding that the use of an oligomer-specific antibody to achieve reduction or immunoneutralization of soluble Aβ oligomers in the cortex of Tg2576 mice was accompanied by a > 50% reduction in plaque burden (determined by % plaque area) is consistent with this equilibrium theory. Even in this discussion in which oligomeric Aβ was defined to be the only toxic form of Aβ (although other forms are likely to carry some toxicity), we can see that removal of plaques is likely to serve as a surrogate marker of efficacy.

What Amyloid Imaging Can and Cannot Be Expected to Do

As with most new technologies, there is an initial period of excess in both skepticism and optimism. Eventually, the realities of what the technology can and cannot achieve become clear. The naturally skeptical begin to accept certain capabilities and the naturally optimistic begin to acknowledge that certain capabilities are not likely to be realized. We are certainly in this sorting-out phase with amyloid imaging. Clearly, amyloid imaging cannot replace a good clinical evaluation. Similarly, amyloid imaging provides information complementary to the structural information from MRI or the functional information obtained from fMRI or FDG PET and will not replace these valuable imaging tools. As we gain more experience in many centers around the world with well over 2000 scans safely performed, the "cans" and "cannots" of amyloid imaging come more into focus. The following list shows our *predictions* of what is reasonable to expect from amyloid imaging. Note that in many cases, much more experimental evidence is required to support the uses that we currently think could prove possible in the future. We understand that many points on this list are speculative and controversial. We hope that this will stimulate research that will provide definitive evidence either for or against these speculations.

Reasonable Expectations for Amyloid Imaging

Diagnostic/Screening Uses

Amyloid imaging can detect brain amyloid pathology, *not* clinical status. Therefore, amyloid imaging:

a. Cannot diagnose *clinical* AD in the absence of clinical/neuropsychological information or in a cognitively normal individual.

b. Cannot be used to distinguish between the clinical diagnoses of AD, MCI, or "cognitively-normal-but-amyloid-positive"

based on qualitative or quantitative differences in the scan results.

However, since amyloid imaging can clarify the pathological underpinnings of clinical cognitive impairment, amyloid imaging:

c. Can detect AD pathology in a cognitively normal or cognitively impaired individual.

d. Can determine if an MCI patient is amyloid-positive or amyloid-negative and, therefore, may be able to determine if an MCI subject has, or is likely to develop, AD.

e. Can determine if a clinical dementia syndrome that is atypical for AD is accompanied by AD pathology and is, therefore, likely to be an atypical presentation of AD.

f. Can likely rule out AD as a cause of a clinical dementia syndrome in an amyloid-negative patient and focus attention on diagnoses other than AD (e.g., FTLD, pure DLB, vascular dementia, prion, etc.).

g. Can distinguish patterns of amyloid deposition that may be suggestive of CAA.

h. May be able to predict high risk for AD in a cognitively normal person.

In addition, amyloid imaging:

i. Can be widely applied through the use of F-18 PET tracers or SPECT tracers.

Drug Development

Amyloid imaging:

a. Is *not* likely to be able to detect the effect of a drug that decreases amyloid production without resulting in a net decrease in amyloid load in AD patients, since amyloid load appears to plateau.

b. Can likely detect amyloid lowering drug effects (if clearance is at least 10%–15%).

c. Can define amyloid-positive treatment groups, including amyloid-positive clinically unimpaired subjects for anti-amyloid prevention trials.

d. Can likely monitor the efficacy of amyloid-reducing treatment in individual subjects.

Pathophysiology

Amyloid imaging:

a. Can determine if pathological amyloid deposition exists in a subject's brain.

b. Can detect compact and diffuse plaques and CAA.

c. Cannot detect neurofibrillary tangles or Lewy Bodies or Lewy Neurites in vivo.

d. Cannot image the low concentrations of oligomers that exist along with high concentrations of fibrillar deposits with the current beta-sheet imaging tracers.

e. Cannot stage severity of AD or accurately follow progression over time during the clinical phase of AD.

f. Can likely follow the progression of prodromal AD during the presymptomatic period.

g. Can delineate and compare the natural history of amyloid deposition in typical AD and in early-onset forms (FAD, Down syndrome, etc.).

Conclusion

Amyloid plaques were first described by Blocq and Marinescu in the brain of an elderly patient with epilepsy (Blocq and Marinescu 1892). It was only later that Alzheimer associated plaques and tangles with early-onset dementia. Thus the original description of amyloid plaques was more in the context of aging than AD. The opening premise to this chapter was that amyloid imaging should not be synonymous with imaging AD but has at least equal applicability to the study of aging. Of course, amyloid imaging will find many applications in the study—and hopefully treatment—of AD. However, one thing that is already becoming clear from amyloid imaging studies is how early the full burden of plaques seems to accumulate, often by the time a patient develops MCI. This finding brings with it the challenge to define the earliest evidence of plaque accumulation, and this is very likely to be in the clinically unimpaired elderly. We will need to understand the significance of asymptomatic brain β-amyloidosis. Does it lead to sub-clinical cognitive deficits? Does it lead to AD? If good anti-amyloid therapies can be developed, should they be started at this preclinical stage? Perhaps most importantly, if amyloid deposition can be reversed at this early stage, can AD be prevented? The current paradigm of diagnosing and treating AD during the clinically symptomatic period may not lead us to the treatment success we desire. This may require a new paradigm for the pre-symptomatic period of AD. Amyloid imaging may have its most important application in the detection and longitudinal follow-up of this prodromal state. It may lead to a new definition of what is "normal" aging.

References

Agdeppa, E. D., Kepe, V., Liu, J., Small, G. W., Huang, S. C., Petric, A. et al. (2003). 2-Dialkylamino-6-acylmalononitrile substituted naphthalenes (DDNP analogs): Novel diagnostic and therapeutic tools in Alzheimer's disease. *Molecular Imaging and Biology*, 5: 404–417.

Agdeppa, E. D., Kepe, V., Liu, J., Flores-Torres, S., Satyamurthy, N., Petric, A. et al. (2001). Binding characteristics of radiofluorinated 6-dialkylamino-2-naphthylethylidene derivatives as positron emission tomography imaging probes for beta-amyloid plaques in Alzheimer's disease. *The Journal of Neuroscience*, 21: RC189.

Aizenstein, H. J., Nebes, R. D., Saxton, J. A., Price, J. C., Mathis, C. A., Tsopelas, N. D. et al. (2008). Amyloid deposition is frequent and often is not associated with significant cognitive impairment in the elderly. *Archives of Neurology*, 65: 1509–1517.

Alzheimer, A. (1907). Über eine eigenartige Erkrankung der Hirnrinde. *Allgemeine Zeitschrift für Psychiatrie und Psychisch-Gerichtliche Medizin*, 64: 146–148.

Arai, H., Okamura, N., Furukawa, K., Maruyama, M., Furumoto, S., Narita, T. et al. (2006). [^{11}C]-BF-227 and PET to visualize amyloid in Alzheimer's disease patients. *Alzheimer's & Dementia*, 2: S312.

Archer, H. A., Edison, P., Brooks, D. J., Barnes, J., Frost, C., Yeatman, T. et al. (2006). Amyloid load and cerebral atrophy in Alzheimer's disease: An 11C-PIB positron emission tomography study. *Annals of Neurology*, 60: 145–147.

Arnold, S. E., Hyman, B. T., Flory, J., Damasio, A. R., and Van Hoesen, G. W. (1991). The topographical and neuroanatomical distribution of neurofibrillary tangles and neuritic plaques in the cerebral cortex of patients with Alzheimer's disease. *Cerebral Cortex*, 1: 103–116.

Attems, J., Quass, M., Jellinger, K. A., and Lintner, F. (2007). Topographical distribution of cerebral amyloid angiopathy and its effect on cognitive decline are influenced by Alzheimer disease pathology. *Journal of Neurology Sciences*, 257: 49–55.

Bacskai, B. J., Hickey, G. A., Skoch, J., Kajdasz, S. T., Wang, Y., Huang, G. F. et al. (2003). Four-dimensional multiphoton imaging of brain entry, amyloid binding, and clearance of an amyloid-beta ligand in transgenic mice. *Proceedings of the National Academy of Sciences of the USA*, 100: 12462–12467.

Bacskai, B. J., Frosch, M. P., Freeman, S. H., Raymond, S. B., Augustinack, J. C., Johnson, K. A. et al. (2007). Molecular imaging with Pittsburgh Compound B confirmed at autopsy: A case report. *Archives of Neurology* 64: 431–434.

Barrio, J. R., Huang, S. C., Cole, G. M., Satyamurthy, N. M., Petric, A., Phelps, M. E. et al. (1999). PET imaging of tangles and plaques in Alzheimer's disease with a highly hydrophilic probe. *Journal of Labelled Compounds & Radiopharmaceuticals* 42:S194–S195.

Bennett, J. P. and Yamamura, H. I. (1985). Neurotransmitter, hormone, or drug receptor binding methods. In H. I. Yamamura, S. J. Enna, and M. J. Kuhar (eds), *Neurotransmitter Receptor Binding*, 2 Ed. (pp. 61–89). New York: Raven Press.

Berg, L., McKeel, D. W. J., Miller, J. P., Storandt, M., Rubin, E. H., Morris, J. C. et al. (1998). Clinicopathologic studies in cognitively healthy aging and Alzheimer's disease: Relation of histologic markers to dementia severity, age, sex, and apolipoprotein E genotype. *Archives of Neurology* 55: 326–335.

Blocq, P. and Marinescu, G. (1892). Sur les lésions et la pathogénie de l'épilepsie dite essentielle. *Sem Méd*, 12: 445–446.

Blomqvist, G., Pauli, S., Farde, L., Eriksson, L., Persson, A., and Halldin, C. (1989). Dynamic models of reversible ligand binding. In C. Beckers, A. Goffinet, and A. Bol (eds), *Clinical Research and Clinical Diagnosis* (pp. 35–44). Dardrecht, The Netherlands: Kluwer Academic Publishers.

Bombois, S., Maurage, C. A., Gompel, M., Deramecourt, V., Mackowiak-Cordoliani, M. A., Black, R. S. et al. (2007). Absence of beta-amyloid deposits after immunization in Alzheimer disease with Lewy body dementia. *Archives of Neurology*, 64: 583–587.

Boxer, A. L., Rabinovici, G. D., Kepe, V., Goldman, J., Furst, A. J., Huang, S. C. et al. (2007). Amyloid imaging in distinguishing atypical prion disease from Alzheimer disease. *Neurology*, 69: 283–290.

Braak, H. and Braak, E. (1990). Alzheimer's disease: striatal amyloid deposits and neurofibrillary changes. *Journal of Neuropathology and Experimental Neurology*, 49: 215–224.

Braak, H. and Braak, E. (1991). Neuropathological staging of Alzheimer-related changes. *Acta Neuropathologica (Berlin)*, 82: 239–259.

Braak, H. and Braak, E. (1997). Frequency of stages of Alzheimer-related lesions in different age categories. *Neurobiology of Aging*, 18: 351–357.

Braak, H. and Braak, E. (1998). Evolution of neuronal changes in the course of Alzheimer's disease. *Journal of Neural Transmission. Supplementum*, 53: 127–140.

Braak, H., Del Tredici, K., Rub, U., de Vos, R. A., Jansen Steur, E. N., and Braak, E. (2003). Staging of brain pathology related to sporadic Parkinson's disease. *Neurobiology of Aging*, 24: 197–211.

Brendza, R. P., Bacskai, B. J., Cirrito, J. R., Simmons, K. A., Skoch, J. M., Klunk, W. E. et al. (2005). Anti-Abeta antibody treatment promotes the rapid recovery of amyloid-associated neuritic dystrophy in PDAPP transgenic mice. The *Journal of Clinical Investigation*, 115: 428–433.

Brilliant, M., Elble, R. J., Ghobrial, M., and Struble, R. G. (1992). Distribution of amyloid in the brainstem of patients with Alzheimer disease. *Neuroscience Letters*, 148: 23–26.

Brilliant, M. J., Elble, R. J., Ghobrial, M., and Struble, R. G. (1997). The distribution of amyloid beta protein deposition in the corpus striatum of patients with Alzheimer's disease. *Neuropathology and Applied Neurobiology*, 23: 322–325.

Buck, A., Westera, G., vonSchulthess, G. K., and Burger, C. (1996). Modeling alternatives for cerebral carbon-11-iomazenil kinetics. *Journal of Nuclear Medicine*, 37: 699–705.

Buckner, R. L., Snyder, A. Z., Shannon, B. J., LaRossa, G., Sachs, R., Fotenos, A. F. et al. (2005). Molecular, structural, and functional characterization of Alzheimer's disease: Evidence for a relationship between default activity, amyloid, and memory. *The Journal of Neuroscience*, 25: 7709–7717.

Busse, A., Hensel, A., Guhne, U., Angermeyer, M. C., and Riedel-Heller, S. G. (2006). Mild cognitive impairment: Long-term course of four clinical subtypes. *Neurology*, 67: 2176–2185.

Butters, M. A., Meltzer, C. C., Aizenstein, H. J., Price, J. C., Mathis, C. A., Klunk, W. E. et al. (2007). White matter hyperintensities, amyloid, and cognition in late-life depression. *Journal of the International Neuropsychological Society,* 13(Suppl. S1): 180.

Cai, L., Innis, R. B., and Pike, V. W. (2007). Radioligand development for PET imaging of beta-amyloid (Abeta)—current status. *Current Medicinal Chemistry,* 14: 19–52.

Carson, R. (2003). Tracer kinetic modeling in PET. In P. E. Valk, D. L. Bailey, D. W. Townsend, and M. N. Maisey (eds), *Positron Emission Tomography: Basic Science and Clinical Practice* (pp. 147–179). London: Springer.

Carter, D. B. and Chou, K. C. (1998). A model for structure-dependent binding of Congo red to Alzheimer beta-amyloid fibrils. *Neurobiology of Aging,* 19: 37–40.

Cherry, S. R. (2001). Fundamentals of positron emission tomography and applications in preclinical drug development. *Journal of Clinical Pharmacology,* 41: 482–491.

Christie, R. H., Bacskai, B. J., Zipfel, W. R., Williams, R. M., Kajdasz, S. T., Webb, W. W. et al. (2001). Growth arrest of individual senile plaques in a model of Alzheimer's disease observed by in vivo multiphoton microscopy. *The Journal of Neuroscience,* 21: 858–864.

Clark, C. and Carson, R. (1993). Analysis of covariance in statistical parametric mapping. *Journal of Cerebral Blood Flow Metabolism,* 13: 1038–1040.

Clark, C. M., Newberg, A. B., Watson, M., Wintering, N. A., Skovronsky, D. M., and Kung, H. F. (2006). Imaging amyloid with I^{123} IMPY SPECT. *Alzheimer's and Dementia,* 2: S342.

Cohen, J. (1988). *Statistical Power Analyses for the Behavioral Sciences,* 2nd Ed. Hillsdale, NJ: Lawrence Erlbaum Associates.

Conway, K. A., Harper, J. D., and Lansbury, P. T., Jr. (2000). Fibrils formed in vitro from alpha-synuclein and two mutant forms linked to Parkinson's disease are typical amyloid. *Biochemistry,* 39: 2552–2563.

Cummings, B. J., Pike, C. J., Shankle, R., and Cotman, C. W. (1996). Beta-amyloid deposition and other measures of neuropathology predict cognitive status in Alzheimers disease. *Neurobiology of Aging,* 17: 921–933.

Cunningham, V. J., Hume, S. P., Price, G. R., Ahier, R. G., Cremer, J. E., and Jones, A. K. (1991). Compartmental analysis of diprenorphine binding to opiate receptors in the rat in vivo and its comparison with equilibrium data in vitro. *Journal of Cerebral Blood Flow and Metabolism,* 11: 1–9.

D'Amore, J. D., Kajdasz, S. T., McLellan, M. E., Bacskai, B. J., Stern, E. A., and Hyman, B. T. (2003). In vivo multiphoton imaging of a transgenic mouse model of Alzheimer disease reveals marked thioflavine-S-associated alterations in neurite trajectories. *Journal of Neuropathology and Experimental neurology,* 62: 137–145.

Davis, D. G., Schmitt, F. A., Wekstein, D. R., and Markesbery, W. R. (1999). Alzheimer neuropathologic alterations in aged cognitively normal subjects. *Journal of Neuropathology and Experimental Neurology,* 58: 376–388.

DeKosky, S. T., Mathis, C. M., Price, J. C., Ikonomovic, M. D., Hamilton, R. L., Abrahamson, E. E. et al. (2007). Correlation of regional *in vivo* Pittsburgh compound-B (PIB) retention with in vitro PIB, Aβ levels, and amyloid plaque density: Validation of PIB-PET in postmortem human brain. *Alzheimer's & Dementia,* 3: S105.

Dickson, D. W. (2002). Dementia with Lewy bodies: Neuropathology. *Journal of Geriatric Psychiatry and Neurology,* 15: 210–216.

Dickson, D. W., Crystal, H. A., Mattiace, L. A., Masur, D. M., Blau, A. D., Davies, P. et al. (1992). Identification of normal and pathological aging in prospectively studied nondemented elderly humans. *Neurobiology of Aging,* 13: 179–189.

Dishino, D. D., Welch, M. J., Kilbourn, M. R., and Raichle, M. E. (1983). Relationship between lipophilicity and brain extraction of C-11-labeled radiopharmaceuticals. *Journal of Nuclear Medicine,* 24: 1030–1038.

Doze, P., Van, W. A., Elsinga, P. H., Hendrikse, N. H., and Vaalburg, W. (2000). Enhanced cerebral uptake of receptor ligands by modulation of P-glycoprotein function in the blood-brain barrier. *Synapse,* 36: 66–74.

Drevets, W. C., Frank, E., Price, J. C., Kupfer, D. J., Holt, D., Greer, P. J. et al. (1999). PET imaging of serotonin 1A receptor binding in depression. *Biological Psychiatry,* 46: 1375–1387.

Drzezga, A., Grimmer, T., Henriksen, G., Stangier, I., Perneczky, R., Diehl-Schmid, J. et al. (2008). Imaging of amyloid plaques and cerebral glucose metabolism in semantic dementia and Alzheimer's disease. *Neuroimage,* 39: 619–633.

DSM-IV. (1995). *DSM-IV Diagnostic and Statistical Manual of Mental Disorders,* (3rd Ed.). Washington D.C.: American Psychiatric Association.

Eckelman, W. C. (1998). Sensitivity of new radiopharmaceuticals. *Nuclear Medicine and Biology,* 25: 169–173.

Edison, P., Archer, H. A., Hinz, R., Hammers, A., Pavese, N., Tai, Y. F. et al. (2006). Amyloid, hypometabolism, and cognition in Alzheimer disease. An [11C]PIB and [18F]FDG PET study. *Neurology,* 68: 501–508.

Engler, H., Santillo, A. F., Wang, S. X., Lindau, M., Savitcheva, I., Nordberg, A. et al. (2008). In vivo amyloid imaging with PET in frontotemporal dementia. *European Journal of Nuclear Medicine and Molecular Imaging,* 35: 100–106.

Engler, H., Forsberg, A., Almkvist, O., Blomquist, G., Larsson, E., Savitcheva, I. et al. (2006). Two-year follow-up of amyloid deposition in patients with Alzheimer's disease. *Brain,* 129: 2856–2866.

Engler, H., Nordberg, A., Blomqvist, G., Bergström, M., Estrada, S., Barletta, J. et al. (2002). First human study with a benzothiazole amyloid-imaging agent in Alzheimer's disease and control subjects. *Neurobiology of Aging,* 23(1S): S429.

Evans, D. A., Funkenstein, H. H., Albert, M. S., Scherr, P. A., Cook, N. R., Chown, M. J. et al. (1989). Prevalence of Alzheimer's disease in a community population of older persons. Higher than previously reported. *The Journal of the American Medical Association,* 262: 2551–2556.

Fagan, A. M., Roe, C. M., Xiong, C., Mintun, M. A., Morris, J. C., and Holtzman, D. M. (2007). Cerebrospinal fluid tau/beta-amyloid(42) ratio as a prediction of cognitive decline in nondemented older adults. *Archives of Neurology,* 64: 343–349.

Fagan, A. M., Mintun, M. A., Mach, R. H., Lee, S. Y., Dence, C. S., Shah, A. R. et al. (2006). Inverse relation between in vivo amyloid imaging load and cerebrospinal fluid Abeta(42) in humans. *Annals of Neurology,* 59: 512–519.

Farde, L., Halldin, C., Stone-Elander, S., and Sedvall, G. (1987). PET analysis of human dopamine receptor subtypes using 11C-SCH 23390 and 11C-raclopride. *Psychopharmacology (Berlin),* 92: 278–284.

Farde, L., Pauli, S., Hall, H., Eriksson, L., Halldin, C., Hogberg, T. et al. (1988). Stereoselective binding of 11C-raclopride in living human brain—a search for extrastriatal central D2-dopamine receptors by PET. *Psychopharmacology (Berlin),* 94: 471–478.

Ferrer, I., Boada, R., Sanchez, G., Rey, M. J., and Costa-Jussa, F. (2004). Neuropathology and pathogenesis of encephalitis following amyloid-beta immunization in Alzheimer's disease. *Brain Pathology,* 14: 11–20.

Fischer, O. (1907). Miliare Nekrosen mit drusigen Wucherungen der Neurofibrillen, eine regelmässige Veränderung der Hirnrinde bei seniler Demenz. *Monatsschrift für Psychiatrie und Neurologie,* 22: 361–372.

Fischer, O. (1910). Die presbyophrene Demenz, deren anatomische Grundlage und klinische Abgrenzung. *Zeitschrift für die gesamte Neurologie und Psychiatrie,* 3: 371–471.

Fodero-Tavoletti, M., Cappai, R., Krause, S., Lippoldt, A., Foster, L., Leone, L. et al. (2006). In vitro characterization of PIB binding to α-synuclein. *Alzheimer's and Dementia,* 2: S333–S334.

Fodero-Tavoletti, M. T., Smith, D. P., McLean, C. A., Adlard, P. A., Barnham, K. J., Foster, L. E. et al. (2007). In vitro characterization of Pittsburgh compound-B binding to Lewy bodies. *The Journal of Neuroscience,* 27: 10365–10371.

Folstein, M., Folstein, S., and McHugh, P. R. (1975a). Mini-mental state: A practical method for grading the cognitive state of patients for the clinician. *Journal of Psychiatric Research,* 12: 189–198.

Forsberg, A., Engler, H., Almkvist, O., Blomquist, G., Hagman, G., Wall, A. et al. (2007). PET imaging of amyloid deposition in patients with mild cognitive impairment. *Neurobiology of Aging.* doi: 10.1016/j.neurobiolaging.2007.03.029.

Fox, P. T., Perlmutter, J. S., and Raichle, M. E. (1985). A stereotactic method of anatomical localization for positron emission tomography. *Journal of Computer Assisted Tomography,* 9: 141–153.

Fox, P. T., Laird, A. R., and Lancaster, J. L. (2005). Coordinate-based voxel-wise meta-analysis: dividends of spatial normalization. Report of a virtual workshop. *Human Brain Mapping*, 25: 1–5.

Friedland, R. P., Majocha, R. E., Reno, J. M., Lyle, L. R., and Marotta, C. A. (1994). Development of an anti-A beta monoclonal antibody for *in vivo* imaging of amyloid angiopathy in Alzheimer's disease. *Molecular Neurobiology*, 9: 107–113.

Friedland, R. P., Kalaria, R., Berridge, M., Miraldi, F., Hedera, P., Reno, J. et al. (1997). Neuroimaging of vessel amyloid in Alzheimer's disease. *Annals of the New York Academy of Sciences*, 826: 242–247.

Friedreich, N. and Kekulé, A. (1859). Zur amyloidfrage. *Virchows Archiv für pathologische Anatomie*, 16: 50–65.

Friston, K. J., Holmes, A. P., and Worsley, K. J. (1995). Statistical parametric mapping in functional imaging: A general linear approach. *Human Brain Mapping*, 2: 189–210.

Galasko, D., Chang, L., Motter, R., Clark, C. M., Kaye, J., Knopman, D. et al. (1998). High cerebrospinal fluid tau and low amyloid beta42 levels in the clinical diagnosis of Alzheimer disease and relation to apolipoprotein E genotype. *Archives of Neurology*, 55: 937–945.

Galton, C. J., Patterson, K., Xuereb, J. H., and Hodges, J. R. (2000). Atypical and typical presentations of Alzheimer's disease: a clinical, neuropsychological, neuroimaging and pathological study of 13 cases. *Brain*, 123(Pt. 3): 484–498.

Garcia-Alloza, M., Robbins, E. M., Zhang-Nunes, S. X., Purcell, S. M., Betensky, R. A., Raju, S. et al. (2006). Characterization of amyloid deposition in the APPswe/PS1dE9 mouse model of Alzheimer disease. *Neurobiology of Disease*, 24: 516–524.

Gauthier, S., Reisberg, B., Zaudig, M., Petersen, R. C., Ritchie, K., Broich, K. et al. (2006). Mild cognitive impairment. *Lancet*, 367: 1262–1270.

Gearing, M., Mirra, S. S., Hedreen, J. C., Sumi, S. M., Hansen, L. A., and Heyman, A. (1995). The Consortium to Establish a Registry for Alzheimer's Disease (CERAD). Part X. Neuropathology confirmation of the clinical diagnosis of Alzheimer's disease. *Neurology*, 45: 461–466.

Gilman, S., Koller, M., Black, R. S., Jenkins, L., Griffith, S. G., Fox, N. C. et al. (2005). Clinical effects of Ab immunization (AN1792) in patients with AD in an interrupted trial. *Neurology*, 64: 1553–1562.

Gjedde, A. (1981). High- and low-affinity transport of D-glucose from blood to brain. *Journal of Neurochemistry*, 36: 1463–1471.

Glenner, G. G. (1983). Alzheimer's disease. The commonest form of amyloidosis. *Archives of Pathology and Laboratory Medicine*, 107: 281–282.

Glenner, G. G., Eanes, E. D., and Page, D. L. (1972). The relation of the properties of Congo red-stained amyloid fibrils to the β-conformation. *The Journal of Histochemistry and Cytochemistry*, 20: 821–826.

Goedert, M. (1993). Tau protein and the neurofibrillary pathology of Alzheimer's disease. *Trends in Neurosciences*, 16: 460–465.

Goedert, M., Crowther, R. A., and Spillantini, M. G. (1998). Tau mutations cause frontotemporal dementias. *Neuron*, 21: 955–958.

Goldman, W. P., Price, J. L., Storandt, M., Grant, E. A., McKeel, D. W., Jr., Rubin, E. H. et al. (2001). Absence of cognitive impairment or decline in preclinical Alzheimer's disease. *Neurology*, 56: 361–367.

Green, M. S., Kaye, J. A., and Ball, M. J. (2000). The Oregon brain aging study: Neuropathology accompanying healthy aging in the oldest old. *Neurology*, 54: 105–113.

Gunn, R. N., Lammertsma, A. A., Hume, S. P., and Cunningham, V. J. (1997). Parametric imaging of ligand-receptor binding in PET using a simplified reference region model. *Neuroimage*, 6: 279–287.

Gupta, S. P. (1989). QSAR studies on drugs acting at the central nervous system. *Chemical Reviews*, 89: 1765–1800.

Haass, C. and Selkoe, D. J. (2007). Soluble protein oligomers in neurodegeneration: lessons from the Alzheimer's amyloid beta-peptide. *Nature Reviews. Molecular Cell Biology*, 8: 101–112.

Hansch, C. and Leo, A. (1979). *Substituent Constants for Correlation Analysis in Chemistry and Biology*. New York: John Wiley & Sons.

Hansson, O., Zetterberg, H., Buchhave, P., Londos, E., Blennow, K., and Minthon, L. (2006). Association between CSF biomarkers and incipient Alzheimer's disease in patients with mild cognitive impairment: A follow-up study. *Lancet Neurology*, 5: 228–234.

Hardy, J. A. and Higgins, G. A. (1992). Alzheimer's disease: The amyloid cascade hypothesis. *Science*, 256: 184–185.

Haroutunian, V., Perl, D., Purohit, D., Marin, D., Khan, K., Lantz, M. et al. (1998). Regional distribution of neuritic plaques in the nondemented elderly and subjects with very mild Alzheimer's disease. *Archives of Neurology*, 55: 1185–1191.

Herholz, K., Salmon, E., Perani, D., Baron, J. C., Holthoff, V., Frolich, L. et al. (2002). Discrimination between Alzheimer dementia and controls by automated analysis of multicenter FDG PET. *Neuroimage*, 17: 302–316.

Holcomb, L., Gordon, M. N., McGowan, E., Yu, X., Benkovic, S., Jantzen, P. et al. (1998). Accelerated Alzheimer-type phenotype in transgenic mice carrying both mutant amyloid precursor protein and presenilin 1 transgenes. *Nature Medicine*, 4: 97–100.

Huang, Y., Hwang, D. R., Narendran, R., Sudo, Y., Chatterjee, R., Bae, S. A. et al. (2002). Comparative evaluation in nonhuman primates of five PET radiotracers for imaging the serotonin transporters: [11C]McN 5652, [11C]ADAM, [11C]DASB, [11C]DAPA, and [11C]AFM. *Journal of Cerebral Blood Flow and Metabolism*, 22: 1377–1398.

Hulette, C. M., Welsh-Bohmer, K. A., Murray, M. G., Saunders, A. M., Mash, D. C., McIntyre, L. M. (1998). Neuropathological and neuropsychological changes in "normal" aging. *Journal of Neuropathology and Experimental Neurology*, 57: 1168–1174.

Hyman, B. T. (1992). Down syndrome and Alzheimer disease. Progress in Clinical and Biological Research, 379: 123–142.

Hyman, B. T. and Gomez-Isla, T. (1997). The natural history of Alzheimer neurofibrillary tangles and amyloid deposits. *Neurobiology of Aging*, 18: 386–387; discussion 389–392.

Hyman, B. T., Marzloff, K., and Arriagada, P. V. (1993). The lack of accumulation of senile plaques or amyloid burden in Alzheimer's disease suggests a dynamic balance between amyloid deposition and resolution. *Journal of Neuropathology and Experimental Neurology*, 52: 594–600.

Hyman, B. T., West, H. L., Rebeck, G. W., Lai, F., and Mann, D. M. (1995). Neuropathological changes in Down's syndrome hippocampal formation. Effect of age and apolipoprotein E genotype. *Archives of Neurology*, 52: 373–378.

Ikonomovic, M. D., Abrahamson, E. E., Isanski, B. A., DeKosky, S. T., Raji, C., Debnath, M. L. et al. (2005). Histological characterization of PIB binding to amyloid plaques in Alzheimer's disease. *Alzheimer's & Dementia: The Journal of the Alzheimer's Association*, 1: 38.

Ikonomovic, M. D., Abrahamson, E. E., Hope, C. E., Paljug, W. R. Isanski, B. A. Debnath, M. L. et al. (2006a). Correlation analysis of the histofluorescence of an analogue of Pittsburgh Compound-B and Aβ peptide levels in Alzheimer's disease. *Alzheimer's & Dementia: The Journal of the Alzheimer's Association*, 2: S352.

Ikonomovic, M. D., Abrahamson, E. E., Isanski, B. A., Debnath, M. L., Mathis, C. A., Dekosky, S. T. et al. (2006b). X-34 labeling of abnormal protein aggregates during the progression of Alzheimer's disease. *Methods in Enzymology*, 412: 123–144.

Ikonomovic, M. D., Klunk, W. E., Abrahamson, E. E., Mathis, C. A., Price, J. C., Tsopelas, N. D. et al. (2008). Postmortem correlates of in vivo PiB-PET amyloid imaging in a typical case of Alzheimer's disease. *Brain*, 131: 1630–1645.

Iwatsubo, T., Odaka, A., Suzuki, N., Mizusawa, H., Nukina, N., and Ihara, Y. (1994). Visualization of A beta 42(43) and A beta 40 in senile plaques with end-specific A beta monoclonals: evidence that an initially deposited species is A beta 42(43). *Neuron*, 13: 45–53.

Jack, C. R., Jr., Garwood, M., Wengenack, T. M., Borowski, B., Curran, G. L., Lin, J. et al. (2004). In vivo visualization of Alzheimer's amyloid plaques by magnetic resonance imaging in transgenic mice without a contrast agent. *Magnetic Resonance in Medicine*, 52: 1263–1271.

Jack, C. R., Jr., Wengenack, T. M., Reyes, D. A., Garwood, M., Curran, G. L., Borowski, B. J. et al. (2005). In vivo magnetic resonance microimaging of individual amyloid plaques in Alzheimer's transgenic mice. *The Journal of Neuroscience*, 25: 10041–10048.

Jellinger, K. A. (2002). Alzheimer disease and cerebrovascular pathology: an update. *Journal of Neural Transmission*, 109: 813–836.

Jellinger, K. A. (2003). Prevalence of Alzheimer lesions in Parkinson's disease. *Movement Disorders*, 18: 1207–1208.

Joachim, C. L., Morris, J. H., and Selkoe, D. J. (1989). Diffuse senile plaques occur commonly in the cerebellum in Alzheimer's disease. *American Journal of Pathology*, 135: 309–319.

Johansson, A., Savitcheva, I., Forsberg, A., Engler, H., Långström, B., Nordberg, A. et al. (2008). [^{11}C]-PIB imaging in patients with Parkinson's disease: Preliminary results. *Parkinsonism and Related Disorders*, 14: 345–347.

Johnson, K. A., Gregas, M., Becker, J. A., Kinnecom, C., Salat, D. H., Moran, E. K. et al. (2007). Imaging of amyloid burden and distribution in cerebral amyloid angiopathy. *Annals of Neurology*, 62: 229–234.

Jorm, A. F. (2001). History of depression as a risk factor for dementia: an updated review. *The Australian and New Zealand Journal of Psychiatry*, 35: 776–781.

Katzman, R. (1976). Editorial: The prevalence and malignancy of Alzheimer disease. A major killer. *Archives of Neurology*, 33: 217–218.

Kemppainen, N. M., Aalto, S., Karrasch, M., Nagren, K., Savisto, N., Oikonen, V. et al. (2008). Cognitive reserve hypothesis: Pittsburgh Compound B and fluorodeoxyglucose positron emission tomography in relation to education in mild Alzheimer's disease. *Annals of Neurology*, 63: 112–118.

Kemppainen, N. M., Aalto, S., Wilson, I. A., Nagren, K., Helin, S., Bruck, A. et al. (2006). Voxel-based analysis of PET amyloid ligand [11C]PIB uptake in Alzheimer disease. *Neurology*, 67: 1575–1580.

Kemppainen, N. M., Aalto, S., Wilson, I. A., Nagren, K., Helin, S., Bruck, A. et al. (2007). PET amyloid ligand [11C]PIB uptake is increased in mild cognitive impairment. *Neurology*, 68: 1603–1606.

Khachaturian, Z. S. (1985). Diagnosis of Alzheimer's disease. *Archives of Neurology*, 42: 1097–1105.

Klunk, W. E., Pettegrew, J. W., and Abraham, D. J. (1989). Quantitative evaluation of Congo red binding to amyloid-like proteins with a beta-pleated sheet conformation. *The Journal of Histochemistry and Cytochemistry*, 37: 1273–1281.

Klunk, W. E., Debnath, M. L., and Pettegrew, J. W. (1995). Chrysamine-G binding to Alzheimer and control brain: Autopsy study of a new amyloid probe. *Neurobiology of Aging*, 16: 541–548.

Klunk, W. E., Mathis, C. A., Price, J. C., Lopresti, B. J., and DeKosky, S. T. (2006) Scientific Commentary: Two-year follow-up of amyloid deposition in patients with Alzheimer's disease. *Brain*, 129: 2805–2807.

Klunk, W. E., Bacskai, B. J., Mathis, C. A., Kajdasz, S. T., McLellan, M. E., Frosch, M. P. et al. (2002). Imaging Abeta plaques in living transgenic mice with multiphoton microscopy and methoxy-X04, a systemically administered Congo red derivative. *Journal of Neuropathology and Experimental Neurology*, 61: 797–805.

Klunk, W. E., Wang, Y., Huang, G. F., Debnath, M. L., Holt, D. P., Shao, L. et al. (2003). The binding of 2-(4'-methylaminophenyl)benzothiazole to postmortem brain homogenates is dominated by the amyloid component. *The Journal of Neuroscience*, 23: 2086–2092.

Klunk, W. E., Lopresti, B. J., Ikonomovic, M. D., Lefterov, I. M., Koldamova, R. P., Abrahamson, E. E. (2005). Binding of the positron emission tomography tracer Pittsburgh compound-B reflects the amount of amyloid-beta in Alzheimer's disease brain but not in transgenic mouse brain. *The Journal of Neuroscience*, 25: 10598–10606.

Klunk, W. E., Engler, H., Nordberg, A., Wang, Y., Blomqvist, G., Holt, D. P. et al. (2004). Imaging brain amyloid in Alzheimers disease with Pittsburgh Compound-B. *Annals of Neurology*, 55: 306–319.

Klunk, W. E., Price, J. C., Mathis, C. A., Tsopelas, N. D., Lopresti, B. J., Ziolko, S. K. et al. (2007). Amyloid deposition begins in the striatum of presenilin-1 mutation carriers from two unrelated pedigrees. *The Journal of Neuroscience*, 27: 6174–6184.

Knowles, R. B., Wyart, C., Buldyrev, S. V., Cruz, L., Urbanc, B., Hasselmo, M. E. et al. (1999). Plaque-induced neurite abnormalities: implications for disruption of neural networks in Alzheimer's disease. *Proceedings of the National Academy of Sciences of the USA*, 96: 5274–5279.

Koeppe, R. (2002). Data analysis and image processing. In R. Wahl and J. Buchanan (eds), *Principles and Practice of Positron Emission Tomography* (pp. 65–99). Philadelphia: Lippincott Williams & Wilkins.

Kraepelin, E. (1910). *Psychiatrie: Ein Lehrbuch für Studierende und Ärzte*. 8th Ed. (pp 593–632). Leipzig: Barth.

Krebs, M. R., Bromley, E. H., and Donald, A. M. (2005). The binding of thioflavin-T to amyloid fibrils: localisation and implications. *Journal of Structural Biology*, 149: 30–37.

Kretzschmar, H. A. (1993). Neuropathology of human prion diseases (spongiform encephalopathies). [Review]. *Developments in Biological Standardization*, 80: 71–90.

Kudo, Y., Okamura, N., Furumoto, S., Tashiro, M., Furukawa, K., Maruyama, M. et al. (2007) 2-(2-[2-Dimethylaminothiazol-5-yl]ethenyl)-6-(2-[fluoro]ethoxy)benzoxazole: a novel PET agent for in vivo detection of dense amyloid plaques in Alzheimer's disease patients. *Journal of Nuclear Medicine*, 48: 553–561.

Kung, M. P., Hou, C., Zhuang, Z. P., Skovronsky, D., and Kung, H. F. (2004). Binding of two potential imaging agents targeting amyloid plaques in postmortem brain tissues of patients with Alzheimer's disease. *Brain Research*, 1025: 98–105.

Lammertsma, A. A., and Hume, S. P. (1996). Simplified reference tissue model for PET receptor studies. *Neuroimage*, 4: 153–158.

Larrieu, S., Letenneur, L., Orgogozo, J. M., Fabrigoule, C., Amieva, H., Le Carret, N. et al. (2002). Incidence and outcome of mild cognitive impairment in a population-based prospective cohort. *Neurology*, 59: 1594–1599.

Lesne, S., Koh, M. T., Kotilinek, L., Kayed, R., Glabe, C. G., Yang, A. et al. (2006). A specific amyloid-beta protein assembly in the brain impairs memory. *Nature*, 440: 352–357.

Levin, V. A. (1980). Relationship of octanol/water partition coefficient and molecular weight to rat brain capillary permeability. *Journal of Medicinal Chemistry*, 23: 682–684.

Levine, H., 3rd (1995). Thioflavin T interaction with amyloid b-sheet structures. *Amyloid-International Journal of Experimental & Clinical Investigation*, 2: 1–6.

Lippa, C. F., Saunders, A. M., Smith, T. W., Swearer, J. M., Drachman, D. A., Ghetti, B. et al. (1996). Familial and sporadic Alzheimer's disease: Neuropathology cannot exclude a final common pathway. *Neurology*, 96: 406–412.

Logan, J., Fowler, J. S., Volkow, N. D., Wolf, A. P., Dewey, S. L., Schlyer, D. J. et al. (1990). Graphical analysis of reversible radioligand binding from time-activity measurements applied to [N-^{11}C-methyl]-(-)-cocaine PET studies in human subjects. *Journal of Cerebral Blood Flow and Metabolism*, 10: 740–747.

Lopez, O. L., Becker, J. T., Klunk, W., Saxton, J., Hamilton, R. L., Kaufer, D. I. et al. (2000). Research evaluation and diagnosis of probable Alzheimer's disease over the last two decades: I. *Neurology*, 55: 1854–1862.

Lopez, O. L., Jagust, W. J., DeKosky, S. T., Becker, J. T., Fitzpatrick, A., Dulberg, C. et al. (2003). Prevalence and classification of mild cognitive impairment in the cardiovascular health study cognition study. *Archives of Neurology*, 60: 1385–1389.

Lopresti, B. J., Price, J. C., Mathis, C. A., and Klunk, W. E. (2006). Quantitative assessments of amyloid deposition in vivo using PET and [C-11]PIB: progress toward a methodologic simplification. In Vellas, B., Grundman, M., Feldman, H and Fitten, L. J. (eds), *Research and Practice in Alzheimer's Disease* (pp. 251–264). Paris: Serdi.

Lopresti, B. J., Mathis, C. A., Price, J. C., Villemagne, V. L., Meltzer, C. C., Holt, D. P. et al. (2001). Serotonin transporter binding in vivo: further examination of [11C]-McN5652. In A. E. Gjedde (ed.), *Molecular and Pharmacological Brain Imaging with Positron Emission Tomography* (pp. 265–271). San Diego: Academic press.

Lopresti, B. J., Klunk, W. E., Mathis, C. A., Hoge, J. A., Ziolko, S. K., Lu, X. et al. (2005). Simplified quantification of Pittsburgh compound B amyloid imaging PET studies: A comparative analysis. *Journal of Nuclear Medicine*, 46: 1959–1972.

MacKenzie, I. R. and Miller, L. A. (1994). Senile plaques in temporal lobe epilepsy. *Acta Neuropathologica (Berlin)* 87: 504–510.

Maeda, J., Ji, B., Irie, T., Tomiyama, T., Maruyama, M., Okauchi, T. et al. (2007). Longitudinal, quantitative assessment of amyloid, neuroinflammation, and anti-amyloid treatment in a living mouse model of

Alzheimer's disease enabled by positron emission tomography. *The Journal of Neuroscience,* 27: 10957–10968.

Maetzler, W., Reimold, M., Liepelt, I., Solbach, C., Leyhe, T., Schweitzer, K. et al. (2008). [11C]PIB binding in Parkinson's disease dementia. *Neuroimage,* 39: 1027–1033.

Maia, L. F., Mackenzie, I. R., and Feldman, H. H. (2007). Clinical phenotypes of Cerebral Amyloid Angiopathy. *Journal of the Neurological Sciences,* 257: 23–30.

Majocha, R. E., Reno, J. M., Friedland, R. P., VanHaight, C., Lyle, L. R., and Marotta, C. A. (1992). Development of a monoclonal antibody specific for beta/A4 amyloid in Alzheimer's disease brain for application to in vivo imaging of amyloid angiopathy. *Journal of Nuclear Medicine,* 33: 2184–2189.

Mann, D. M., Pickering-Brown, S. M., Takeuchi, A., and Iwatsubo, T. (2001). Amyloid angiopathy and variability in amyloid beta deposition is determined by mutation position in presenilin-1-linked Alzheimer's disease. *The American Journal of Pathology,* 158: 2165–2175.

Mann, D. M. A. (1985). The neuropathology of Alzheimer's disease: A review with pathogenetic, aetiological and therapeutic considerations. *Mechanisms of Ageing and Development,* 31: 213–255.

Marek, K., Jennings, D., Tamagnan, G., Koren, A., Skovronsky, D., and Seibyl, J. (2007). IMPY imaging in Alzheimer's disease and healthy controls. *Alzheimer's & Dementia,* 3: S112.

Masliah, E., Hansen, L., Adame, A., Crews, L., Bard, F., Lee, C. et al. (2005). Ab vaccination effects on plaque pathology in the absence of encephalitis in Alzheimer disease. *Neurology,* 64: 129–131.

Mastaglia, F. L., Johnsen, R. D., Byrnes, M. L., and Kakulas, B. A. (2003). Prevalence of amyloid-beta deposition in the cerebral cortex in Parkinson's disease. *Movement Disorders,* 18: 81–86.

Mathis, C. A., Wang, Y., and Klunk, W. E. (2004a). Imaging beta-amyloid plaques and neurofibrillary tangles in the aging human brain. *Current Pharmaceutical Design,* 10: 1469–1492.

Mathis, C. A., Wang, Y., Holt, D. P., Huang, G. F., Debnath, M. L., and Klunk, W. E. (2003). Synthesis and evaluation of 11C-labeled 6-substituted 2-arylbenzothiazoles as amyloid imaging agents. *Journal of Medicinal Chemistry,* 46: 2740–2754.

Mathis, C. A., Holt, D., Wang, Y. M., Huang, G. F., Debnath, M., Shao, L. et al. (2004b). Species-dependent formation and identification of the brain metabolites of the amyloid imaging agent [C-11]PIB. *Neurobiology of Aging,* 25: S277–S278.

Mathis, C. A., Lopresti, B., Mason, N., Price, J., Flatt, N., Bi, W. et al. (2007). Comparison of the amyloid imaging agents [F-18]3'-F-PIB and [C-11]PIB in Alzheimer's disease and control subjects. *Journal of Nuclear Medicine,* 48: 56P.

Mathis, C. A., Bacskai, B. J., Kajdasz, S. T., McLellan, M. E., Frosch, M. P., Hyman, B. T. et al. (2002). A lipophilic thioflavin-T derivative for positron emission tomography (PET) imaging of amyloid in brain. *Bioorganic & Medicinal Chemistry Letters,* 12: 295–298.

McKeith, I. G. (2006). Consensus guidelines for the clinical and pathologic diagnosis of dementia with Lewy bodies (DLB): Report of the Consortium on DLB International Workshop. *Journal of Alzheimers Disease,* 9: 417–423.

McKhann, G., Drachman, D., Folstein, M., Katzman, R., Price, D., and Stadlan, E. M. (1984). Clinical diagnosis of Alzheimer's disease: Report of the NINCDS-ADRDA work group under the auspices of the Department of Health and Human Services Task Force on Alzheimer's disease. *Neurology,* 34: 939–944.

McNamee, R. L., Yee, S. H., Price, J. C., Klunk, W. E., Rosario, B., Weissfeld, L. et al. (2009). Consideration of optimal time window for Pittsburgh Compound B PET summed uptake measurements. *Journal of Nuclear Medicine,* 50: 348–355.

Mintun, M. A., Raichle, M. E., Kilbourn, M. R., Wooten, G. F., and Welch, M. J. (1984). A quantitative model for the in vivo assessment of drug binding sites with positron emission tomography. *Annals of Neurology,* 15: 217–227.

Mintun, M. A., Larossa, G. N., Sheline, Y. I., Dence, C. S., Lee, S. Y., Mach, R. H. et al. (2006). [11C]PIB in a nondemented population: Potential antecedent marker of Alzheimer disease. *Neurology,* 67: 446–452.

Mirra, S. S., Heyman, A., McKeel, D., Sumi, S. M., Crain, B. J., Brownlee, L. M. et al. (1991). The Consortium to Establish a Registry for Alzheimer's Disease (CERAD). Part II. Standardization of the neuropathologic assessment of Alzheimer's disease. *Neurology,* 41: 479–486.

Morris, J. C. and Price, A. L. (2001). Pathologic correlates of nondemented aging, mild cognitive impairment, and early-stage Alzheimer's disease. *Journal of Molecular Neuroscience,* 17: 101–118.

Morris, J. C., Storandt, M., McKeel, D. W., Jr., Rubin, E. H., Price, J. L., Grant, E. A. et al. (1996). Cerebral amyloid deposition and diffuse plaques in "normal" aging: Evidence for presymptomatic and very mild Alzheimer's disease. *Neurology,* 46: 707–719.

Morris, J. C., Storandt, M., Miller, J. P., McKeel, D. W., Price, J. L., Rubin, E. H. et al. (2001). Mild cognitive impairment represents early-stage Alzheimer disease. *Archives of Neurology,* 58: 397–405.

Morse, C. K. (1993). Does variability increase with age? An archival study of cognitive measures. *Psychology and Aging,* 8: 156–164.

Motter, R., Vigo-Pelfrey, C., Kholodenko, D., Barbour, R., Johnson-Wood, K., Galasko, D. et al. (1995). Reduction of beta-amyloid peptide42 in the cerebrospinal fluid of patients with Alzheimer's disease. *Annals of Neurology,* 38: 643–648.

Mountjoy, C. Q., Tomlinson, B. E., and Gibson, P. H. (1982). Amyloid and senile plaques and cerebral blood vessels. A semi-quantitative investigation of a possible relationship. *Journal of the Neurological Sciences,* 57: 89–103.

Mueller, S. G., Weiner, M. W., Thal, L. J., Petersen, R. C., Jack, C. R., Jagust, W. et al. (2005a). Ways toward an early diagnosis in Alzheimer's disease: The Alzheimer's Disease Neuroimaging Initiative (ADNI). *Alzheimer's Dementia,* 1: 55–66.

Mueller, S. G., Weiner, M. W., Thal, L. J., Petersen, R. C., Jack, C., Jagust, W. et al. (2005b). The Alzheimer's disease neuroimaging initiative. *Neuroimaging clinics of North America,* 15: 869–877.

Naslund, J., Haroutunian, V., Mohs, R., Davis, K. L., Davies, P., Greengard, P. et al. (2000). Correlation between elevated levels of amyloid beta-peptide in the brain and cognitive decline. *The Journal of the American Medical Association,* 283: 1571–1577.

Necula, M., Kayed, R., Milton, S. and Glabe, C. G. (2007). Small molecule inhibitors of aggregation indicate that amyloid beta oligomerization and fibrillization pathways are independent and distinct. *The Journal of Biological Chemistry,* 282: 10311–10324.

Nelissen, N., Vandenbulcke, M., Fannes, K., Verbruggen, A., Peeters, R., Dupont, P. et al. (2007). Abeta amyloid deposition in the language system and how the brain responds. *Brain,* 130: 2055–2069.

Newell, K. L., Hyman, B. T., Growdon, J. H., and Hedley-Whyte, E. T. (1999). Application of the National Institute on Aging (NIA)-Reagan Institute criteria for the neuropathological diagnosis of Alzheimer's disease. *Journal of Neuropathology and Experimental Neurology,* 58: 1147–1155.

Ng, S., Villemagne, V. L., Berlangieri, S., Lee, S. T., Cherk, M., Gong, S. J. et al. (2007a). Visual assessment versus quantitative assessment of 11C-PIB PET and 18F-FDG PET for detection of Alzheimer's disease. *Journal of Nuclear Medicine,* 48: 547–552.

Ng, S. Y., Villemagne, V. L., Masters, C. L., and Rowe, C. C. (2007b). Evaluating atypical dementia syndromes using positron emission tomography with carbon 11 labeled pittsburgh compound B. *Archives of Neurology,* 64: 1140–1144.

NIA/Reagan_Workgroup, (1997). Consensus recommendations for the postmortem diagnosis of Alzheimer's disease. The National Institute on Aging, and Reagan Institute Working Group on Diagnostic Criteria for the Neuropathological Assessment of Alzheimer's Disease. *Neurobiology of Aging,* 18: S1–S2.

Nicoll, J. A., Wilkinson, D., Holmes, C., Steart, P., Markham, H., and Weller, R. O. (2003). Neuropathology of human Alzheimer disease after immunization with amyloid-B peptide: A case report. *Nature Medicine,* 9: 448–452.

Nitsch, R. M., Rebeck, G. W., Deng, M., Richardson, U. I., Tennis, M., Schenk, D. B. et al. (1995). Cerebrospinal fluid levels of amyloid beta-protein in Alzheimer's disease: inverse correlation with severity of dementia and effect of apolipoprotein E genotype. *Annals of Neurology,* 37: 512–518.

Ohm, T. G., Kirca, M., Bohl, J., Scharnagl, H., Gross, W., and Marz, W. (1995). Apolipoprotein E polymorphism influences not only cerebral senile plaque load but also Alzheimer-type neurofibrillary tangle formation. *Neuroscience*, 66: 583–587.

Olivero, W. C., Lister, J. R., and Elwood, P. W. (1995). The natural history and growth rate of asymptomatic meningiomas: A review of 60 patients. *Journal of Neurosurgery*, 83: 222–224.

Ono, M., Wilson, A., Nobrega, J., Westaway, D., Verhoeff, P., Zhuang, Z. P. et al. (2003). 11C-labeled stilbene derivatives as Abeta-aggregate-specific PET imaging agents for Alzheimer's disease. *Nuclear Medicine and Biology*, 30: 565–571.

Opazo, C., Luza, S., Villemagne, V. L., Volitakis, I., Rowe, C., Barnham, K. J. et al. (2006). Radioiodinated clioquinol as a biomarker for beta-amyloid: Zn complexes in Alzheimer's disease. *Aging Cell*, 5: 69–79.

Ownby, R. L., Crocco, E., Acevedo, A., John, V., and Loewenstein, D. (2006). Depression and risk for Alzheimer disease: Systematic review, meta-analysis, and metaregression analysis. *Archives of General Psychiatry*, 63: 530–538.

Parsey, R. V., Sokol, L. O., Belanger, M. J., Kumar, J. S., Simpson, N. R., Wang, T. et al. (2005). Amyloid plaque imaging agent [C-11]-6-OH-BTA-1: biodistribution and radiation dosimetry in baboon. *Nuclear Medicine Communications*, 26: 875–880.

Parvathy, S., Davies, P., Haroutunian, V., Purohit, D. P., Davis, K. L., Mohs, R. C. et al. (2001). Correlation between Abetax-40-, Abetax-42-, and Abetax-43-containing amyloid plaques and cognitive decline. *Archives of Neurology*, 58: 2025–2032.

Patlak, C. S. and Blasberg, R. G. (1985). Graphical evaluation of blood-to-brain transfer constants from multiple- time uptake data. Generalizations. *Journal of Cerebral Blood Flow and Metabolism*, 5: 584–590.

Patton, R. L., Kalback, W. M., Esh, C. L., Kokjohn, T. A., Van Vickle, G. D., Luehrs, D. C. et al. (2006). Amyloid-beta peptide remnants in AN-1792-immunized Alzheimer's disease patients: a biochemical analysis. *The American Journal of Pathology*, 169: 1048–1063.

Pauling, L. and Corey, R. B. (1951). The pleated sheet, a new layer configuration of polypeptide chains. *Proceedings of the National Academy of Sciences of the USA*, 37: 251–256.

Perez, S. E., Lazarov, O., Koprich, J. B., Chen, E. Y., Rodriguez-Menendez, V., Lipton, J. W. et al. (2005). Nigrostriatal dysfunction in familial Alzheimer's disease-linked APPswe/PS1DeltaE9 transgenic mice. *The Journal of Neuroscience*, 25: 10220–10229.

Petersen, R. C. (2004). Mild cognitive impairment as a diagnostic entity. *Journal of the Internal Medicine*, 256: 183–194.

Petersen, R. C. and Morris, J. C. (2005). Mild cognitive impairment as a clinical entity and treatment target. *Archives of Neurology*, 62: 1160–1163.

Petersen, R. C., Stevens, J. C., Ganguli, M., Tangalos, E. G., Cummings, J. L., and DeKosky, S. T. (2001). Practice parameter: early detection of dementia: mild cognitive impairment (an evidence-based review). Report of the Quality Standards Subcommittee of the American Academy of Neurology. *Neurology*, 56: 1133–1142.

Pike, K. E., Savage, G., Villemagne, V. L., Ng, S., Moss, S. A., Maruff, P. et al. (2007). β-Amyloid imaging and memory in nondemented individuals: Evidence for preclinical Alzheimer's disease. *Brain*, 130: 2837–2844.

Pike, V. W., McCarron, J. A., Lammertsma, A. A., Osman, S., Hume, S. P., Sargent, P. A. et al. (1996). Exquisite delineation of 5-HT1A receptors in human brain with PET and [carbonyl-11 C]WAY-100635. *European Journal of Pharmacology*, 301: R5–R7.

Pirttila, T., Kim, K. S., Mehta, P. D., Frey, H., and Wisniewski, H. M. (1994). Soluble amyloid beta-protein in the cerebrospinal fluid from patients with Alzheimer's disease, vascular dementia and controls. *Journal of the Neurological Sciences*, 127: 90–95.

Pirttila, T., Mehta, P. D., Soininen, H., Kim, K. S., Heinonen, O., Paljarvi, L. et al. (1996). Cerebrospinal fluid concentrations of soluble amyloid beta- protein and apolipoprotein E in patients with Alzheimer's disease: Correlations with amyloid load in the brain. *Archives of Neurology*, 96: 189–193.

Pirttila, T., Soininen, H., Mehta, P. D., Heinonen, O., Lehtimaki, T., Bogdanovic, N. et al. (1997). Apolipoprotein E genotype and amyloid load in Alzheimer disease and control brains. *Neurobiology of Aging*, 18: 121–127.

Price, J. C. (2003). Principles of tracer kinetic analysis. *Neuroimaging Clinics of North America*, 13: 689–704.

Price, J. C., Lopresti, B. J., Meltzer, C. C., Smith, G. S., Mason, N. S., Huang, Y. et al. (2001). Analyses of [(18)F]altanserin bolus injection PET data. II: Consideration of radiolabeled metabolites in humans. *Synapse*, 41: 11–21.

Price, J. C., Klunk, W. E., Lopresti, B. J., Lu, X., Hoge, J. A., Ziolko, S. K. et al. (2005). Kinetic modeling of amyloid binding in humans using PET imaging and Pittsburgh Compound-B. *Journal of Cerebral Blood Flow and Metabolism*, 25: 1528–1547.

Price, J. L. and Morris, J. C. (1999). Tangles and plaques in nondemented aging and "preclinical" Alzheimer's disease. *Annals of Neurology*, 45: 358–368.

Rabbitt, P. (1993). Does it all go together when it goes? The Nineteenth Bartlett Memorial Lecture. *The Quarterly Journal of Experimental Psychology A*, 46: 385–434.

Rabinovici, G. D., Furst, A. J., O'Neil, J. P., Racine, C. A., Mormino, E. C., Baker, S. L. et al. (2007). 11C-PIB PET imaging in Alzheimer disease and frontotemporal lobar degeneration. *Neurology*, 68: 1205–1212.

Raichle, M. E. and Snyder, A. Z. (2007). A default mode of brain function: A brief history of an evolving idea. *Neuroimage*, 37: 1083–1090.

Redlich, E. (1898). Über miliare Sklerose der Hirnrinde bei seniler Atrophie. *Jahrbucher Psychiatrica et Neurologica*, 17: 208–216.

Redlich, E. (1929). Über abortive Formen der Encephalomyelitis disseminata. *Deutsche Medizinische Wochenschrift*, 55: 562–563.

Remes, A. M., Finnila, S., Mononen, H., Tuominen, H., Takalo, R. Herva, R. et al. (2004). Hereditary dementia with intracerebral hemorrhages and cerebral amyloid angiopathy. *Neurology*, 63: 234–240.

Remes, A. M., Laru, L., Tuominen, H., Aalto, S., Kemppainen, N., Mononen, H. et al. (2008). 11C-PIB-PET amyloid imaging in patients with APP locus duplication. *Archives in Neurology*, 65: 540–544.

Roe, C. M., Xiong, C., Miller, J. P. and Morris, J. C. (2007). Education and Alzheimer disease without dementia: support for the cognitive reserve hypothesis. *Neurology*, 68: 223–228.

Roher, A. E., Lowenson, J. D., Clarke, S., Woods, A. S., Cotter, R. J., Gowing, E. et al. (1993). beta-Amyloid-(1–42) is a major component of cerebrovascular amyloid deposits: implications for the pathology of Alzheimer disease. *Proceedings of the National Academy of Sciences of the USA*, 90: 10836–10840.

Rosand, J., Muzikansky, A., Kumar, A., Wisco, J. J., Smith, E. E., Betensky, R. A. et al. (2005). Spatial clustering of hemorrhages in probable cerebral amyloid angiopathy. *Annals of Neurology*, 58: 459–462.

Rovelet-Lecrux, A., Frebourg, T., Tuominen, H., Majamaa, K., Campion, D., and Remes, A. M. (2007). APP locus duplication in a Finnish family with dementia and intracerebral haemorrhage. *Journal of Neurology, Neurosurgery, and Psychiatry*, 78: 1158–1159.

Rowe, C. C., Ng, S., Ackermann, U., Gong, S. J., Pike, K., Savage, G. et al. (2007a). Imaging beta-amyloid burden in aging and dementia. *Neurology*, 68: 1718–1725.

Rowe, C. C., Ng, S., Mulligan, R. S., Ackermann, U., Browne, W., O'Keefe, G. et al. (2007b). Initial results from human studies of a novel F-18 PET ligand for brain beta-amyloid imaging. *Alzheimer's & Dementia*, 3: S173–S174.

Rowe, C. C., Ng, S., Mulligan, R. S., Ackermann, U., Browne, W., O'Keefe, G. et al. (2007c). First results from human studies of a novel F-18 PET ligand for brain b-amyloid imaging. *Journal of Nuclear Medicine*, 48: 57P.

Scheinin, N. M., Tolvanen, T. K., Wilson, I. A., Arponen, E. M., Nagren, K. A., and Rinne, J. O. (2007). Biodistribution and radiation dosimetry of the amyloid imaging agent 11C-PIB in humans. *Journal of Nuclear Medicine*, 48: 128–133.

Schmitt, F. A., Davis, D. G., Wekstein, D. R., Smith, C. D., Ashford, J. W., and Markesbery, W. R. (2000). "Preclinical" AD revisited: neuropathology of cognitively normal older adults. *Neurology*, 55: 370–376.

Schneider, J. A., Arvanitakis, Z., Bang, W., and Bennett, D. A. (2007). Mixed brain pathologies account for most dementia cases in community-dwelling older persons. *Neurology*, 69: 2197–2204.

Seibyl, J., Jennings, D., Koren, A., Skovronsky, D., Tamagnan, G., and Marek, K. (2007). Clinical evaluation of 123-I IMPY as a beta-amyloid imaging biomarker in Alzheimer's subjects and controls. *Journal of Nuclear Medicine*, 48: 57.

Shoghi-Jadid, K., Small, G. W., Agdeppa, E. D., Kepe, V., Ercoli, L. M., Siddarth, P. et al. (2002). Localization of neurofibrillary tangles and beta-amyloid plaques in the brains of living patients with Alzheimer disease. *The American Journal of Geriatric Psychiatry*, 10: 24–35.

Silverman, D. H., Small, G. W., Chang, C. Y., Lu, C. S., Kung De Aburto, M. A., Chen, W. et al. (2001). Positron emission tomography in evaluation of dementia: Regional brain metabolism and long-term outcome. *The Journal of the American Medical Association* 286: 2120–2127.

Skoch, J., Hyman, B. T., and Bacskai, B. J. (2006). Preclinical characterization of amyloid imaging probes with multiphoton microscopy. *Journal of Alzheimer's Disease*, 9: 401–407.

Small, G., Kepe, V., Huang, S. C., Ercoli, L., Siddarth, P., Miller, K. et al. (2004). Plaque and tangle brain imaging using [F-18]FDDNP PET differentiates Alzheimer's disease, mild cognitive impairment and older controls. *Neuropsychopharmacology*, 29: S8.

Small, G. W., Kepe, V., Ercoli, L. M., Siddarth, P., Bookheimer, S. Y., Miller, K. J. et al. (2006). PET of brain amyloid and tau in mild cognitive impairment. *The New England Journal of Medicine*, 355: 2652–2663.

Smid, L. M., Vovko, T. D., Popovic, M., Petric, A., Kepe, V., Barrio, J. R. et al. (2006). The 2,6-disubstituted naphthalene derivative FDDNP labeling reliably predicts Congo red birefringence of protein deposits in brain sections of selected human neurodegenerative diseases. *Brain Pathology*, 16: 124–130.

Smith, G., Price, J., Lopresti, B., Huang, Y., Simpson, N., Holt, D. et al. (1998). Test-retest variability of serotonin 5-HT$_{2A}$ receptor binding measured with positron emission tomography (PET) and [^{18}F]altanserin in the human brain. *Synapse*, 30: 380–393.

Sperling, R., Laviolette, P., White, E., Gregas, M., Moran, E., Rentz, D. et al. (2007). Neocortical amyloid deposition associated with decreased medial temporal lobe fMRI activation. *Neurology*, 68: A329.

Stabin, M. G., Peterson, T. E., Holburn, G. E., and Emmons, M. A. (2006). Voxel-based mouse and rat models for internal dose calculations. *Journal of Nuclear Medicine*, 47: 655–659.

Styren, S. D., Kamboh, M. I., and DeKosky, S. T. (1998). Expression of differential immune factors in temporal cortex and cerebellum: the role of alpha-1-antichymotrypsin, apolipoprotein, E., and reactive glia in the progression of Alzheimer's disease. *The Journal of Comparative Neurology*, 396: 511–520.

Styren, S. D., Hamilton, R. L., Styren, G. C., and Klunk, W. E. (2000). X-34, a fluorescent derivative of Congo red: A novel histochemical stain for Alzheimer's disease pathology. *The Journal of Histochemistry and Cytochemistry*, 48: 1223–1232.

Suenaga, T., Hirano, A., Llena, J. F., Yen, S. H., and Dickson, D. W. (1990). Modified Bielschowsky stain and immunohistochemical studies on striatal plaques in Alzheimer's disease. *Acta Neuropathologica (Berlin)*, 80: 280–286.

Suzuki, A., Tashiro, M., Kimura, Y., Mochizuki, H., Ishii, K., Watabe, H. et al. (2005). Use of reference tissue models for quantification of histamine H1 receptors in human brain by using positron emission tomography and [^{11}C]doxepin. *Annals of Nuclear Medicine*, 19: 425–433.

Taniguchi, S., McDonagh, A. M., Pickering-Brown, S. M., Umeda, Y., Iwatsubo, T., Hasegawa, M. et al. (2004). The neuropathology of frontotemporal lobar degeneration with respect to the cytological and biochemical characteristics of tau protein. *Neuropathology and Applied Neurobiology*, 30: 1–18.

Terry, R. D. (2001). An honorable compromise regarding amyloid in Alzheimer disease. *Annals of Neurology*, 49: 684.

Terry, R. D., Masliah, E., Salmon, D. P., Butters, N., DeTeresa, R., Hill, R. et al. (1991). Physical basis of cognitive alterations in Alzheimer's disease: Synapse loss is the major correlate of cognitive impairment. *Annals of Neurology*, 30: 572–580.

Thal, D. R., Rub, U., Orantes, M., and Braak, H. (2002). Phases of Aß-deposition in the human brain and its relevance for the development of AD. *Neurology*, 58: 1791–1800.

Thal, D. R., Rub, U., Schultz, C., Sassin, I., Ghebremedhin, E., Del Tredici, K. et al. (2000). Sequence of Abeta-protein deposition in the human medial temporal lobe. *Journal of Neuropathology and Experimental Neurology*, 59: 733–748.

Theuns, J., Marjaux, E., Vandenbulcke, M., Van Laere, K., Kumar-Singh, S., Bormans, G. et al. (2006). Alzheimer dementia caused by a novel mutation located in the APP C-terminal intracytosolic fragment. *Human Mutation*, 27: 888–896.

Tolboom, N., Yaqub, M., van der Flier, W., Boellaard, R., Luurtsema, G., Windhorst, B. et al. (2007). Imaging beta amyloid deposition in vivo: Quantitative comparison of [^{18}F]FDDNP and [^{11}C]PIB. *Journal of Nuclear Medicine*, 48: 57P.

Toyama, H., Ye, D., Ichise, M., Liow, J. S., Cai, L., Jacobowitz, D. et al. (2005). PET imaging of brain with the beta-amyloid probe, [^{11}C]6-OH-BTA-1, in a transgenic mouse model of Alzheimer's disease. *European Journal of Nuclear Medicine and Molecular Imaging*, 32: 593–600.

Trojanowski, J. Q. and Mattson, M. P. (2003). Overview of protein aggregation in single, double, and triple neurodegenerative brain amyloidoses. *Neuromuscular Disorders*, 4: 1–6.

Uversky, V. N., Talapatra, A., Gillespie, J. R., and Fink, A. L. (1999). Protein deposits as the molecular basis of amyloidosis. Part I. Systemic amyloidoses. *Medical Science Monitor*, 5: 1001–1012.

Verhoeff, N. P., Wilson, A. A., Takeshita, S., Trop, L., Hussey, D., Singh, K. et al. (2004). In-vivo imaging of Alzheimer disease beta-amyloid with [11C]SB-13 PET. *The American Journal of Geriatric Psychiatry*, 12: 584–595.

Villemagne, V. L., Pike, K. E., Darby, D., Maruff, P., Savage, G., Ng, S. et al. (2008). Abeta deposits in older nondemented individuals with cognitive decline are indicative of preclinical Alzheimer's disease. *Neuropsychologia*, 46: 1688–1697.

Virchow, R. (1854). Zur cellulose-frage. *Archiv für pathologische Anatomie und Physiologie und für klinische Medizin*, 6: 416–426.

Vital, C., Gray, F., Vital, A., Parchi, P., Capellari, S., Petersen, R. B. et al. (1998). Prion encephalopathy with insertion of octapeptide repeats: the number of repeats determines the type of cerebellar deposits. *Neuropathology and Applied Neurobiology*, 24: 125–130.

Wegiel, J., Wisniewski, H. M., Morys, J., Tarnawski, M., Kuchna, I., Dziewiatkowski, J. et al. (1999). Neuronal loss and beta-amyloid removal in the amygdala of people with Down syndrome. *Neurobiology of Aging*, 20: 259–269.

Whitaker, C., Eckman, C., Almeida, C., Feinstein, D., Atwood, C., Eckman, E. et al. (2003). Live discussion: Amyloid-beta degradation: the forgotten half of Alzheimer's disease. 12 September 2002. *Journal of Alzheimer's Disease*, 5: 491–497.

Wolf, D. S., Gearing, M., Snowdon, D. A., Mori, H., Markesbery, W. R., and Mirra, S. S. (1999). Progression of regional neuropathology in Alzheimer disease and normal elderly: findings from the Nun study. *Alzheimer Disease and Associated Disorders*, 13: 226–231.

Wu, Y. and Carson, R. E. (2002). Noise reduction in the simplified reference tissue model for neuroreceptor functional imaging. *Journal of Cerebral Blood Flow and Metabolism*, 22: 1440–1452.

Xia, W., Ostaszewski, B. L., Kimberly, W. T., Rahmati, T., Moore, C. L., Wolfe, M. S. et al. (2000). FAD mutations in presenilin-1 or amyloid precursor protein decrease the efficacy of a gamma-secretase inhibitor: evidence for direct involvement of PS1 in the gamma-secretase cleavage complex. *Neurobiology of Disease*, 7: 673–681.

Yamaguchi, H., Hirai, S., Morimatsu, M., Shoji, M., and Nakazato, Y. (1989). Diffuse type of senile plaques in the cerebellum of Alzheimer-type dementia demonstrated by beta protein immunostain. *Acta Neuropathologica*, 77: 314–319.

Younkin, S. G. (1997). The APP and PS1/2 mutations linked to early onset familial Alzheimer's disease increase the extracellular concentration of A beta 1–42 (43). *Rinsho Shinkeigaku—Clinical Neurology*, 37: 1099.

Zhang-Nunes, S. X., Maat-Schieman, M. L., van Duinen, S. G., Roos, R. A., Frosch, M. P., and Greenberg, S. M. (2006). The cerebral beta-amyloid angiopathies: hereditary and sporadic. *Brain Pathology*, 16: 30–39.

Zhang, W., Oya, S., Kung, M. P., Hou, C., Maier, D. L., and Kung, H. F. (2005a). F-18 stilbenes as PET imaging agents for detecting beta-amyloid plaques in the brain. *Journal of Medicinal Chemistry,* 48: 5980–5988.

Zhang, W., Oya, S., Kung, M. P., Hou, C., Maier, D. L., and Kung, H. F. (2005b). F-18 Polyethyleneglycol stilbenes as PET imaging agents targeting Abeta aggregates in the brain. *Nuclear Medicine and Biology,* 32: 799–809.

Zhou, Y., Resnick, S. M., Ye, W., Fan, H., Holt, D. P., Klunk, W. E. et al. (2007). Using a reference tissue model with spatial constraint to quantify [11C]Pittsburgh compound B PET for early diagnosis of Alzheimer's disease. *Neuroimage,* 36: 298–312.

Zhuang, Z. P., Kung, M. P., Wilson, A., Lee, C. W., Plossl, K., Hou, C. et al. (2003). Structure-activity relationship of imidazo[1,2-a]pyridines as ligands for detecting beta-amyloid plaques in the brain. *Journal of Medicinal Chemistry,* 46: 237–243.

Ziolko, S. K., Weissfeld, L. A., Klunk, W. E., Mathis, C. A., Hoge, J. A., Lopresti, B. J. et al. (2006). Evaluation of voxel-based methods for the statistical analysis of PIB PET amyloid imaging studies in Alzheimer's disease. *Neuroimage,* 33: 94–102.

Differential Diagnosis of Dementia Using Functional Neuroimaging

Eric Salmon, Fabienne Collette, and Gaëtan Garraux

Introduction

Functional imaging with positron emission tomography (PET) and single photon emission computed tomography (SPECT) has been used for more than 25 years to assist clinicians in the diagnosis of dementia. Measurements of cerebral blood flow (CBF), cerebral metabolic rate of oxygen (CMRO2) and cerebral metabolic rate of glucose (CMRGlu) are considered markers of regional brain function, linked to regional synaptic activity. If a distinction between brain function and structure is important, a parallel analysis of both imaging modalities may be particularly interesting (De Santi et al., 2001).

The distribution pattern of decreased cerebral activity essentially provides phenotypic information concerning the dementia processes. A first remark is that the sensitivity of neuroimaging for local brain pathology is not absolute (not 100%), and we certainly lack information on cases where a mismatch occurs. A second remark is that regional cerebral activity is not specific for the underlying pathology. This explains why new markers of specific pathologies (such as amyloid deposition in Alzheimer's disease) need to be assessed if we want to improve the accuracy of the technique for identifying precise dementia types.

In the following paragraphs, we will concentrate on the information obtained with functional imaging to help in the differential diagnosis of dementia. We will first provide a few methodological considerations on the available data, and then review the literature that compared functional neuroimaging between groups of patients with dementia.

Methodological Considerations

The clinician knows that the exact diagnosis of a dementia syndrome is difficult. Several studies showed that even the pathological diagnosis (the definite diagnosis) may be uncertain, due to a variable density of specific lesions or because of a combination of several potentially causal brain lesions in the same patient (Ince, 2001). Consequently, it is important to emphasize that only few neuroimaging studies have included a significant sample of pathologically confirmed diagnoses (Silverman et al., 2001). For example, one such SPECT study gathered CBF images in 43 patients with

Alzheimer's disease (AD) and in 11 non-AD demented subjects (Bonte et al., 1997). Sensitivity of functional imaging for the (definite) diagnosis of AD was 86%, specificity was 73%, positive predictive value reached 92% and negative predictive value was 57%. Such a study gives values that define the use of functional imaging in the differential diagnosis of dementias.

The method of analysis of neuroimaging data is quite variable. Studies reported visual analysis, regions-of-interest (ROI), voxel-based and multivariate analysis. Visual analysis may rest on criteria that are too strict (for example, bilateral posterior decrease in activity to characterize AD), and may suffer from the absence of a statistical "cut-off." ROI methods depend on the *a priori* interest of the researcher. Compared to visual assessment of functional images, the use of a semi-quantitative ROI method does not depend (or depends less) on the experience of the investigator (Staffen et al., 1997). In the later study, sensitivity levels found by visual assessment of SPECT perfusion scans were similar to those found by the ROI method: visual 49% versus ROI 47% for MCI, while for AD, visual assessment was 75% and ROI evaluation 73%. Voxel-based analysis may provide an advantage to assess mid-line regions that are not always easy to delineate (Foster et al., 2007). For example, a voxel-based program (3D-SSP) was used to analyze the posterior cingulate gyrus and precuneus in early AD patients and elderly controls, with global mean normalization (Imabayashi et al., 2004) (see Figure 15.1 for a corresponding SPM analysis). Voxel-based analysis demonstrated 86% accuracy for discriminating AD from control participants, while visual inspection showed a relatively low diagnostic accuracy of about 74%. Both ROI and voxel-based analyses frequently use "activity ratios," comparing regional activity to a "reference" (such as global mean in the above study) to take the important interindividual variability in global cerebral activity into account. There is, for example, an important debate concerning impaired activity in the hippocampus of AD patients and choosing an appropriate reference region may be one step to highlight medial temporal involvement in the disease. Multivariate analyses can combine the global aspect of visual analysis with statistical constraints, but published data are still scarce.

Correcting brain activity for local atrophy might be of interest when this allows increasing the difference between populations. In most cases, however, the improvement in discrimination is limited, or even diminished. For example, when AD patients with a visual

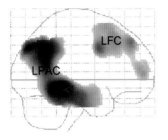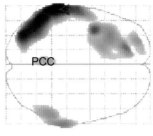

Figure 15–1 Voxel-based analysis (Statistical Parametric Mapping) showing brain areas with significant reduction of glucose metabolism in AD. Glass brain representation. LPAC: lateral posterior association cortices; PCC: posterior cingulate cortex; LFC: lateral frontal cortex.

variant (AD-vs) were compared to elderly controls and to an AD population without prominent visual impairment, correction for atrophy did not modify the distinction, and AD-vs showed a significant decrease in metabolism in visual association areas compared to the reference AD group (Bokde et al., 2001).

Medications should be taken into account. This concerns drugs regulating blood glucose (for FDG-PET), anti-parkinsonian agents (for studies of the nigrostriatal pathway), but also sedatives that can decrease the global brain activity of the patient.

The ultimate limitations for the diagnostic usefulness of functional imaging are the heterogeneity of dementia (for example, the different stages or the subtypes of a similar disease), the probability of combined pathologies, and essentially the fact that the measured brain activity reflects a phenotype more than a specific pathology. The last point is well illustrated by corticobasal degeneration (CBD). Functional imaging is quite useful to detect metabolic impairment related to the classical type of this syndrome, which is clinically characterized by an asymmetrical movement disorder (Garraux et al., 2000), whereas non-classical presentations with progressive aphasia or with frontal type dementia may not be correctly diagnosed as CBD, using functional imaging of brain activity. In keeping with this statement, a study confirmed that a voxel-based method of analysis, Statistical Parametric Mapping (SPM) is "capable of producing meaningful significance maps of individual patients in a routine clinical environment" (Barnes et al., 2000; Signorini et al., 1999). But the authors insisted on the fact that interpreting functional imaging patterns in dementia is more difficult than the initial identification of abnormalities.

An interesting meta-analysis was previously published on 48 SPECT studies selected from 1985 to 2002 (Dougall, Bruggink, and Ebmeier, 2004b). Diagnostic comparison groups included vascular dementia (VaD; 13 studies), frontotemporal dementia (FTD; 7 studies), healthy elderly volunteers (27 studies), and non-dementia patients (13 studies). The pooled weighted sensitivity and specificity of functional imaging in discriminating clinically defined AD from VaD were 71% and 76%, respectively. The pooled weighted sensitivity and specificity of CBF images in differentiating AD from FTD were 71% and 78%, respectively. These calculated percentages for differential diagnosis are interesting because most published values of sensitivity and specificity are obtained by comparing a given dementia with a population of elderly healthy controls. In another study, a large population of 363 demented patients was prospectively studied for a few years, and patients were classified into disease groups according to established clinical criteria (Talbot et al., 1998). The degree to which different SPECT patterns obtained at the time of inclusion provided arguments for the diagnosis was determined by calculating the likelihood ratios for

pairwise disease group comparisons. Bilateral posterior decrease in brain activity was found to significantly increase the odds of a patient having AD, as opposed to VaD or FTD. Bilateral anterior hypoperfusion significantly increased the odds of a patient having FTD as opposed to AD, VaD, or Lewy body disease (LBD). "Patchy" CBF changes significantly increased the odds of a patient having VaD as opposed to AD. This study allowed delineating conditions that were best distinguished by SPECT images.

In the following paragraphs, we will review studies that frequently compared two dementia conditions (ideally matched for clinical severity on global scales). This is a frequent situation, since functional imaging is essentially used to provide arguments for a given diagnosis that is suspected by a clinical assessment. We will briefly mention the activity pattern observed in each dementia compared to elderly controls, but we will mainly concentrate on the differential diagnosis.

Impaired Cerebral Activity Pattern Observed in Alzheimer's Disease

Initial studies with SPECT reported the accuracy of different cerebral activity patterns for the diagnosis of AD. The predictive probability of AD was 82% when a bilateral temporo-parietal decrease in activity was observed, and it was 77% when a bilateral temporo-parietal pattern was associated with an additional (mainly frontal) defect (Holman et al., 1992). The predictive values were only 57% with unilateral temporo-parietal defects (since the pattern could also be found in vascular dementia, Parkinson's disease and dementia, and primary progressive aphasia), 43% with hypoperfusion limited to the frontal regions, 18% with other large defects or with normal distribution of perfusion, and 0% with multiple small cortical defects. Unilateral involvement of posterior associative cortices was considered as not contributory to the diagnosis of AD; however, it was later considered as an important argument to predict evolution to AD in patients with isolated memory impairment (Herholz et al., 1999). In another study gathering 58 AD patients and 20 controls, and including 17 patients with VaD, the sensitivity of a bilateral temporo-parietal hypoperfusion pattern for the diagnosis of AD was only 20%, with a specificity of 80% (Bergman et al., 1997). This report suggested that involvement of association cortices might extend beyond temporo-parietal regions in AD. The authors calculated that, with a 50% prevalence of AD in a memory clinic, the positive and the negative predictive value was about 30%. We will later discuss the use of functional imaging to distinguish AD from VaD, but the results may be partly explained by clinical SPECT studies reporting bilateral posterior hypoperfusion in 75% of AD patients, but also in 45% of non-AD demented patients, in patients with Parkinson's disease and dementia, in more than 15% of VaD patients and in a few other conditions (Kuwabara et al., 1990; Masterman et al., 1997). Importantly, the usefulness of CBF-SPECT was assessed in 49 patients with pathological confirmation (Bonte et al., 2006). For the diagnosis of AD (with or without Lewy bodies), sensitivity was 87%; specificity, 89%; positive predictive value, 93%; negative predictive value, 81%; accuracy, 88%, and likelihood ratio, 8.2%.

By comparison with those contradictory SPECT studies that relied on visual analysis of lateral cortical defects only, voxel-based analysis of decreased metabolism in posterior cingulate and precuneus measured with PET provided 82% accuracy for the early diagnosis of AD compared to controls (Imabayashi et al., 2004). The usefulness of FDG-PET was recently evaluated in 44 subjects

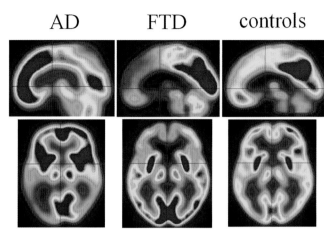

AD   FTD   controls

Figure 15–2 Mean FDG-PET images of patients with Alzheimer's disease (AD), frontotemporal dementia (FTD) and control are displayed according to sagittal (top) and transverse (bottom) sections. The sagittal views demonstrate decreased activity in posterior cingulate cortex (PCC) in AD and in anterior cingulate cortex (ACC) in FTD. The transverse sections show reduced metabolism predominant in posterior associative cortices in AD and in frontal regions in FTD.

with autopsy confirmation obtained after 5 years (Jagust et al., 2007). The authors performed a visual analysis, but took posterior cingulate hypometabolism into account (see Figure 15.2). PET's sensitivity for diagnosing AD was 84% and specificity was 74%, the values being higher than clinical evaluation. Positive and negative predictive values were 81% and 78%, respectively. PET added valuable information to initial clinical evaluation for predicting AD pathology.

Multivariate analytic techniques (that take into account all the voxels in an image simultaneously) might identify diagnostic patterns that are not captured by univariate methods (that take into account each voxel or each ROI independently). CBF images measured with PET scans were acquired during rest in 17 probable mild AD subjects, 16 control subjects and 23 subjects with minimal to mild cognitive

impairment (MCI), but no dementia (Scarmeas et al., 2004). Expert clinical reading had low success in discriminating AD and controls. There were no significant mean CBF differences among groups in traditional univariate SPM or region of interest (ROI) analyses. A covariance pattern was identified whose mean expression was significantly higher in the AD as compared to controls. There was significant overlap, however, and depending on the cut-off value, sensitivity and specificity reached 79% and 81%, or 94% and 63%, respectively. Sites of decreased concomitant flow in AD were found in cingulate, inferior parietal lobule, middle and inferior frontal, supramarginal and precentral gyri, whereas increased concomitant flow included insula, cuneus, pulvinar, lingual, fusiform, superior occipital and parahippocampal gyri. The covariance analysis-derived pattern was then prospectively applied to the MCI subjects. Consistent with the concept of questionable dementia, subjects with a Clinical Dementia Rating score of 0.5 had a significantly higher mean covariance AD pattern expression than elderly controls (Scarmeas et al., 2004). Similarly, a method for pattern recognition (neural network classifier) has been used to classify perfusion patterns obtained with 120 standardized cortical ROIs. The area under the receiver operating characteristic (ROC) curve was 0.93 ± 0.04 to discriminate patients with AD from healthy controls (Chan et al., 1994).

Specific tracers have been used to characterize impaired cholinergic neurotransmission (Kuhl et al., 1999) or brain amyloid deposits in AD (Klunk et al., 2004) and they are discussed in Chapter 14. Few reports have appeared concerning the differential diagnosis properties of these tracers, and we lack large population studies to know the relative sensitivity and specificity of those exams. In a preliminary study, PET and 11C-MP4A was used to measure regional acetylcholine esterase (AChE) activity (reflecting cholinergic pathways integrity) in four non-demented subjects and four AD patients; the findings were compared with measurements of blood flow (CBF) and glucose metabolism (Herholz et al., 2000). Initial tracer extraction was closely related to CBF. AChE activity was reduced significantly in all brain regions in demented subjects (see Figure 15.3), whereas reductions in metabolism and CBF were more limited to temporo-parietal association areas. Interesting

Figure 15–3 PET study with 11C-MP4A measuring regional acetylcholine esterase activity (cholinergic pathway). Parametric images of enzyme activity show decreased cortical cholinergic activity in Alzheimer's disease. (Courtesy of Karl Herholz, University of Cologne, Germany).

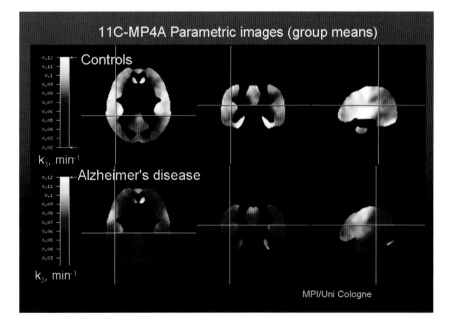

results were obtained with tracers targeting amyloid senile plaques and tau neurofibrillary tangles, the neuropathological hallmarks of AD that accumulate in some brain regions even in the pre-dementia stage of the disease (Small et al., 2006b). PET examinations were performed with a molecule that binds to plaques and tangles in vitro (18FDDNP) and with 18FDG in 25 AD patients, 28 MCI subjects, and 30 healthy controls. Most of them underwent magnetic resonance imaging (MRI). Global values for pathological FDDNP-PET binding (average of the values for the temporal, parietal, posterior cingulate, and frontal regions) were lower in the control group than in the group with MCI, and the values for binding in the MCI group were lower than in the AD group. When comparing the AD group with the MCI group, the accuracy (area under the curve or AUC) for FDDNP global binding (0.98) was significantly greater than the accuracy for FDG-PET global metabolism (0.87), FDG posterior cingulate metabolism (0.82), FDG parietal metabolism (0.80), or MRI medial temporal volume (0.62). Note that the comparison of the AUC between the FDG and MRI studies also showed a significant difference in favor of functional imaging. For the comparison between the MCI group and the control group, the AUC for FDDNP global binding (0.95) was significantly greater than those for FDG-PET global metabolism (0.77), FDG posterior cingulate metabolism (0.74), FDG parietal metabolism (0.70), or MRI medial temporal volume (0.64). The authors reported that initial FDDNP studies in FTD show binding in frontal and temporal regions, but not in parietal regions, suggesting that FDDNP labels regional tau tangles and might differentiate frontotemporal dementia from AD according to the binding patterns (Small, Kepe, and Barrio, 2006a).

In summary, functional imaging of regional CBF or metabolism provides good sensitivity for the diagnosis of AD. In expert centers, different methods to analyze data give similar results, but multivariate analyses provide the best regional information for diagnostic purposes. The posterior cingulate cortex, the medial temporal structures and the posterior and lateral associative cortices are key regions to examine for an early diagnosis (Chetelat et al., 2005; Johnson et al., 1998). The specificity of CBF or metabolic data is modest, and we will consider similarities and differences between cerebral activity patterns from various dementias later in this chapter. Markers of specific brain lesions may certainly improve the accuracy of AD diagnosis, but a general remark is that pathological confirmation is required in large cohorts to validate the diagnostic efficiency of functional imaging with any tracer.

Differentiating AD and Depression

Depression is not always easy to characterize in elderly subjects, and it is frequently accompanied by cognitive impairment. Under clinical routine conditions, SPECT perfusion images were obtained in 23 patients with AD, 17 patients with geriatric depression and 12 age-matched controls (Stoppe et al., 1995). Semiquantitative analysis (cortical/cerebellar ratios) of eight different ROIs revealed that the population of depressed subjects exhibited perfusion values between the AD and control group. The difference between the "depression" and AD groups was most prominent in the left parieto-occipital region (see Figure 15.4). SPM was also used to compare cerebral perfusion measured in 39 elderly depressed patients as well as 15 AD patients and 11 healthy volunteers (Ebmeier et al., 1998). Patients with "late-onset"

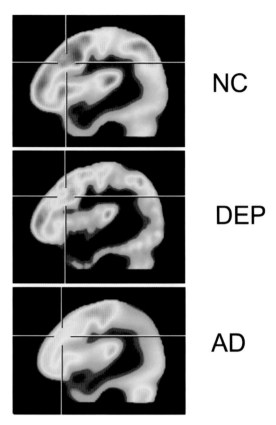

Figure 15–4 Mean FDG-PET images in controls (NC) and patients with major depression (DEP) or Alzheimer's disease (AD). The lateral sagittal view shows that parieto-occipital metabolism is lower in AD than in NC and DEP. (European research program NEST-DD).

depression showed reductions in temporal lobe perfusion compared with "early-onset" depression and controls. AD patients had the expected reduced perfusion in the temporo-parietal and prefrontal cortex, as well as in basal ganglia, compared with healthy controls. Compared with depressed patients, they showed a relative hypoperfusion in temporo-parietal cortex only. This difference was more pronounced between AD patients and patients with early-onset depression, compared to patients with late-onset depression. The results supported a vulnerability hypothesis, which predicts that patients with late-onset depression will show more brain changes than patients with an early onset of depression. In another study, z-scores for the lateral parietal, lateral temporal, bilateral precuneus and bilateral posterior cingulate gyrus were significantly reduced in AD patients compared with a group of patients with major depression (Hanada et al., 2006). In the reverse comparison, the z-scores for the lateral frontal, left thalamus and bilateral medial frontal regions were significantly lower in the major depression group than in the AD patients. All patients were classified into the appropriate categories using discriminant analysis and z-scores of frontal and parietal regions.

In summary, appropriate analyses of functional imaging do allow differentiating AD from depression in elderly subjects. Moreover, the interest of longitudinal functional imaging was also highlighted, since worsening of rCBF impairment (over 18 months) favored the diagnosis of neurodegenerative dementia, whereas improvement in rCBF was mainly observed in psychiatric conditions (Golan et al., 1996).

Can Functional Imaging Distinguish AD from Vascular Dementia?

In pioneering studies, mean global CBF was shown to be decreased significantly in both AD and vascular dementia (VaD) compared to controls (Abe et al., 1996). The pattern of VaD was shown to consist of scattered areas with reduction of metabolism typically extending over cortical and subcortical structures (Mielke and Heiss, 1998). This was quite different from the pattern observed in probable AD, characterized by hypometabolism in temporo-parietal and frontal association areas, but relative preservation of primary cortical areas, basal ganglia and cerebellum. The total volume of hypometabolic regions was related to severity of dementia and did not differ between AD and VaD, even in patients with small lacunar infarcts. The two groups of patients were found to be significantly different concerning the frequency of occurrence of bilateral perfusion deficits in posterior associative cortices (Gemmell et al., 1987). Twenty-three of 36 patients with clinical AD and 25 of 33 patients with clinical multiple infarct dementia (MID) had SPECT patterns compatible with the clinical diagnosis. SPECT distinguished AD from MID in the majority (80%) of cases (Launes et al., 1991). In another study, perfusion SPECT images of 19 AD patients, eight MID, three FTD, five other dementias and 22 healthy controls were visually assessed (Honda et al., 2002). The area under the ROC curve was calculated for between group comparisons. Mean accuracy of SPECT was 0.71 for dementia vs. controls, 0.61 for AD vs. controls, and 0.67 for AD vs. MID. Dementia severity was quite variable, and the authors noted that considerable inter-observer variation was present in CBF-SPECT interpretation.

The brain imaging criteria for subcortical ischemic vascular dementia (SIVD) is said to incorporate two clinical entities, the lacunar state and Binswanger's disease. Changes in regional CBF were investigated in a study including 12 SIVD patients with predominant white matter lesions, 13 patients with predominant lacunar infarctions and 17 controls (Shim et al., 2006). SPM was used to analyze CBF-SPECT images, and a common reduction of normalized CBF was observed in the bilateral thalami, the anterior cingulate gyri, the superior temporal gyri, the caudate head and the left parahippocampal gyrus for both subtypes of vascular dementia compared to the control group. The study suggested that the two subsets of SIVD might have a common CBF pattern. This is consistent with the idea that the subcortical subtype of vascular cognitive impairment is relatively homogeneous, in terms of clinical pattern, natural history, response to treatment and prognosis (Alvarez-Sauco et al., 2005; Baezner and Daffertshofer, 2003).

All the previous univariate voxel-based analyses ignored the functional correlations among regions. A voxel-based multivariate technique was applied to a large FDG-PET data of 153 subjects, one-third each being probable subcortical VaD, probable AD and normal controls (Kerrouche et al., 2006). Principal component (PC) analysis was applied and PCs were used as feature vectors in a canonical variate analysis to generate canonical variates (CVs), that is, linear combinations of PC scores. The first two CVs efficiently separated the groups. CV(1) separated VaD from AD with 100% accuracy, whereas CV(2) separated controls from demented subjects with 72% sensitivity and 96% specificity. Images depicting CVs showed that lower metabolism differentiating VaD from AD mainly concerned the deep gray nuclei, cerebellum, primary cortices, middle temporal gyrus, and anterior cingulate gyrus, whereas lower metabolism in AD versus VaD concerned mainly the hippocampal region and orbitofrontal, posterior cingulate, and posterior parietal cortices (Figure 15.5).

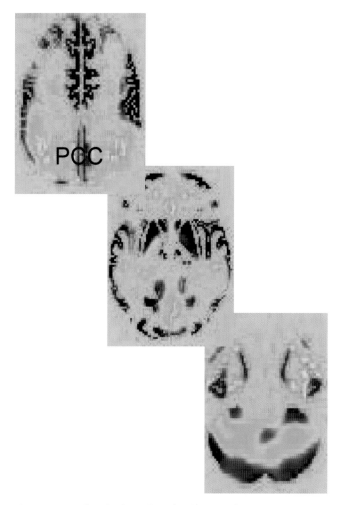

Figure 15–5 Three brain sections showing PCA discrimination between vascular dementia (black and blue) and Alzheimer's disease (red and yellow). The upper section shows predominant involvement of posterior cingulate cortex in AD and anterior cingulate cortex in VaD. The middle section shows decreased activity in basal ganglia in VaD. The lower section shows metabolic imparment in medial and lateral temporal cortex in AD, and in cerebellum in VaD. (Courtesy of Nacer Kerrouche, European research program NEST-DD).

In summary, both MID and subcortical VaD can be distinguished from AD, and multivariate analyses are particularly adequate to pick up the differential multi-regional involvement observed in the diseases.

AD and Hydrocephalus

It may be difficult to differentiate brain atrophy occurring in AD from hydrocephalus. A pioneering study reported that AD subjects demonstrated bilateral temporo-parietal hypometabolism while normal pressure hydrocephalus subjects showed globally diminished cerebral metabolism (Jagust, Friedland, and Budinger, 1985). There is also a frequent decrease in thalamic activity in hydrocephalus. Accordingly, a case report described the story of a patient who was confirmed to have AD by a biopsy performed during a shunt operation for hydrocephalus (Jeong et al., 2004). She was followed for four years using neuropsychological tests and PET. Her clinical symptoms remained improved for 2.5 years and then declined. When the PET data obtained after 1 year were compared to the presurgical PET image, increased activity was shown in the bilateral frontal area, basal ganglia, and thalamus, which may reflect brain regions associated with the improvement of hydrocephalus. When PET images obtained after one year and four years were contrasted, a decrease in activity was demonstrated in bilateral temporo-parietal area and the posterior cingulate gyrus, reflecting brain regions associated with the aggravation of AD.

AD Versus Lewy Body Dementia

Lewy body dementia (LBD) might be the second most common cause of degenerative dementia after AD. Clinical premortem diagnosis of LBD relies upon the International Consensus Criteria (Weisman and McKeith, 2007). The typical presentation of dementia in LBD combines cortical and subcortical cognitive impairments, with worse visuospatial and executive dysfunction, but less memory impairment than AD. Core clinical features of LBD include fluctuating attention, recurrent visual hallucinations, and parkinsonism. An accurate differential diagnosis between LBD and AD could improve the therapeutic handling of LBD patients, made difficult due to their supersensitivity to neuroleptic treatment, their REM sleep behavior disorder and the difficult treatment of their hallucinations.

Functional imaging has first been used to assess brain perfusion and metabolism in this pathology. For example, cerebral perfusion patterns were compared in 34 patients presenting with a probable diagnosis of LBD, and in 28 AD subjects (Pasquier et al., 2002). Tracer distribution was quantified using ROIs in eight symmetrical paired zones and expressed as a perfusion index (ratio of regional over cerebellum uptake). A comparison of findings in the LBD and AD groups demonstrated significant differences in mean perfusion indexes in the right and left occipital regions (lower values in LDB), and left medial temporal region (reduced values in AD). LBD was correctly identified in 22 patients (a relatively poor sensitivity of 65%) while AD was correctly identified in 20 patients (specificity of 71%). In the LBD group, right and left occipital perfusion indexes were high (0.95 or more) in all eight non-hallucinating patients, while bilateral occipital hypoperfusion was observed in 15 of the 26 patients (58%) with visual hallucinations. Accordingly, in another study, AD and LBD groups differed only in occipital perfusion and SPECT measures (occipital and medial temporal) and correctly classified 69% of all subjects, with a poor 65% sensitivity and a good 87% specificity for LBD against AD and control subjects (Lobotesis et al., 2001). In an FDG-PET study where the authors used a metabolic ratio of 0.92 in the visual association cortex as a cut-off (mean-2 SD of normal control subjects), a small population of seven LBD patients could be distinguished from 11 AD subjects with a sensitivity of 86% and a specificity of 91% (Higuchi et al., 2000). Similarly, other authors found that the relative occipital CMRglc (normalized to the sensorimotor CMRglc) was a useful measure for the differential diagnosis of LBD ($n = 12$) from AD ($n = 12$). The sensitivity and specificity were 92% when using the minimal value of the normalized occipital CMRglc in the control group as the cut-off point (Ishii et al., 1998a). Those studies suggest that FDG-PET might be efficient to distinguish LBD and AD when ROIs are used, but the samples reported in PET studies are small, and might not be representative of the general population of patients.

Voxel-based methods have been used to analyze functional images in LBD series. For example, differences in rCBF between AD

subjects, LBD patients and healthy volunteers were investigated using SPM (Colloby et al., 2002). Forty-eight AD, 23 LBD and 20 age-matched control subjects were enrolled. Applying a height threshold of $P < 0.001$ uncorrected, significant perfusion deficits in the parietal and frontal brain regions were observed in both AD and LBD groups, compared with the control subjects. In addition, significant temporal perfusion deficits were identified in the AD subjects, whereas the LBD patients had deficits in the occipital region. Comparison of dementia groups yielded hypoperfusion in both the parietal and occipital brain regions in LBD compared with AD. In another study, SPECT data on 20 patients with LBD and 75 patients with AD were analyzed using 3D SSP, i.e., three-dimensional stereotactic surface projections (Shimizu et al., 2005). The LBD group showed a significant CBF reduction in the temporo-parietal, frontal lobe and posterior cingulate, similar to the CBF pattern in the AD group, but regional CBF in the medial and lateral occipital lobes decreased significantly in patients with LBD, compared with patients with AD. Receiver operating characteristic analysis revealed that regional CBF measurement of the medial occipital lobe, including the cuneus and lingual gyrus, yielded a good sensitivity of 85% and a specificity of 85% in discriminating LBD from AD. When different methods of analysis were directly compared in another report, the area under the ROC curve for an automatic diagnosis system based on 18FDG-PET and 3D-SSP was 0.77, while the mean area under the ROC curve for visual inspection by experts and beginners was 0.76 and 0.65, respectively (Kono et al., 2007). In summary, voxel-based methods provide information similar to visual analysis or ROI technique applied by experienced clinicians. The observation of an occipital reduction of activity may help to differentiate LBD from AD, but values for diagnostic accuracy remain modest, around 80% (see Figure 15.6).

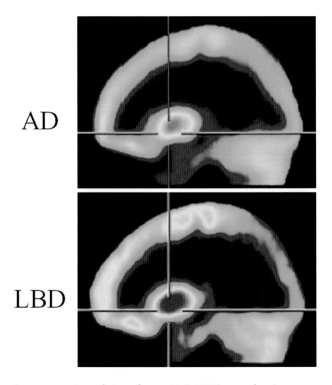

Figure 15–6 Lateral view of mean FDG-PET images showing preferential hypometabolism in the superior occipital gyrus in Lewy body dementia (LBD) compared to AD. (European research program NEST-DD).

The distinction between LBD and Parkinson's disease with dementia remains a matter of debate (Lippa et al., 2007). Several studies have been performed in Parkinsonian patients with dementia. Regional cerebral perfusion was evaluated in 30 Parkinsonian patients with ($n = 15$) or without ($n = 15$) dementia, 19 AD patients and 13 control subjects (Spampinato et al., 1991). Perfusion was measured in the frontal, parietal, temporal and occipital cortex, and values were expressed as cortical/cerebellar activity ratios. Regional CBF ratios in non-demented Parkinsonian patients did not differ from controls, whereas in patients with Parkinson's disease and dementia (PDD) a significant reduction was found in the parietal, temporal and occipital cortex. Tracer uptake ratios were significantly reduced in all regions in the AD group. Thus, PDD and AD shared a common pattern of marked posterior hypoperfusion. Such an observation explains the relatively poor specificity of functional imaging measurements of brain activity for the diagnosis of AD, because specificity is highly dependent on the populations entered in the study. In another study, FDG-PET images obtained in nine normal subjects, nine PDD patients and nine AD patients were analyzed with 3D-SSP (Vander Borght et al., 1997). PDD and AD showed global glucose metabolic reduction with similar regional accentuation involving the lateral parietal, lateral temporal and lateral frontal association cortices and posterior cingulate cortex in comparison to normal controls. When comparing between PDD and AD, however, PDD showed greater metabolic reduction in the visual cortex and relatively preserved metabolism in the medial temporal cortex. Subsequently, CBF images obtained in six patients with LBD, seven patients with PDD, 21 patients with PD, 12 patients with AD and 12 control subjects were analyzed with 3D-SSP (Mito et al., 2005). As expected, cerebral perfusion was decreased in the occipital lobe of the LBD patients, compared with the AD patients. More interestingly, LBD and PDD showed a similar cerebral perfusion reduction pattern at the lateral parietal association, and lateral temporal association and precuneus on SPECT using pixel-by-pixel comparison, although greater perfusion reduction was observed in LBD than in PDD. In a similar study, CBF images gathered in 31 cognitively intact subjects with PD, in 34 PDD subjects, in 37 healthy controls, in 32 AD patients and in 15 LBD subjects were analyzed with SPM (Firbank et al., 2003). The precuneus and inferior lateral parietal regions showed a perfusion deficit in PDD, similar to the pattern observed in LBD. In comparison, AD showed a perfusion deficit in the mid-line parietal region, in a more anterior and inferior location than in PDD, involving the posterior cingulate as well as the precuneus.

Markers of the dopaminergic system have been used to improve the distinction between LBD and AD. Using IBZM to label striatal dopaminergic receptors, LBD patients had significantly lower caudate/putamen ratios (95% confidence intervals: LBD 0.893-0.965) than either controls or AD patients (controls 1.031-1.168, AD 0.972-1.175) (Walker et al., 1997). In LBD, the postsynaptic side has not been studied extensively as presynaptic markers have been much more frequently used.

The integrity of the nigro-striatal presynaptic dopaminergic system has been thoroughly assessed with FP-CIT-SPECT (a marker of presynaptic dopaminergic transporters). In 27 patients with LBD, 17 AD patients, 19 drug naive patients with PD and 16 controls, the occipital cortex was used as a reference, and ratios for the caudate nucleus and the anterior and posterior putamen of both hemispheres were calculated (Walker et al., 2002). Both LBD and PD patients had significantly lower uptake of radioactivity than patients with AD and controls in the caudate

nucleus and the anterior and posterior putamen. Similarly, presynaptic dopaminergic integrity was studied with FP-CIT in 164 older subjects, 33 healthy older control subjects, 34 AD, 23 LBD, 38 PD and 36 with PD and dementia (O'Brien et al., 2004). Significant reductions in FP-CIT binding occurred in the caudate and anterior and posterior putamen in subjects with LBD compared with AD subjects and controls. Dopaminergic transporter loss in LBD was of similar magnitude to that seen in PD, but with a flatter rostrocaudal (caudate-putamen) gradient, while the greatest loss in all three areas was seen in those who had PDD. Both ROI analysis and visual ratings provided good (but not complete!) separation between LBD and AD patients (for ROI: sensitivity, 78%; specificity, 94%; positive predictive value, 90%). The technique did not separate subjects with LBD, PD, and PDD. In another large study, patients with clinical diagnoses of probable ($n = 94$) or possible ($n = 57$) LBD or non-LBD dementia ($n = 147$) were studied with FP-CIT-SPECT (McKeith et al., 2007). Three readers, unaware of the clinical diagnosis, classified the images as normal or abnormal by visual inspection. Abnormal scans had a mean sensitivity of 78% for detecting clinical probable LBD, with specificity of 90% for excluding non-LDB dementia, which was predominantly due to AD. A mean value of 86% was achieved for overall diagnostic accuracy, 82% for positive predictive value, and 87% for negative predictive value. Inter-reader agreement for rating scans as normal or abnormal was high. Those values are fair, and they support a revision of the International Consensus Criteria for LBD with a recommendation that low binding to dopaminergic transporters on nigro-striatal projections, measured with SPECT or PET imaging, be included as a suggestive feature for diagnosis. However, the specificity of the technique is not optimal even for AD. Moreover, all data were obtained in clinical populations, and the accuracy of a clinical diagnosis (taken as "gold standard" in the previous studies) is recognized to be limited in LBD.

In one study, postmortem confirmation of the diagnosis was obtained in 11 LBD patients (7 Lewy body variant of AD [LBVAD] and 4 pure diffuse Lewy body disease [DLBD]) and in 10 definite AD patients, who had ante-mortem FDG-PET imaging (Minoshima et al., 2001). Autopsy-confirmed AD and LBD patients showed significant metabolic reductions involving parietotemporal association, posterior cingulate, and frontal association cortices. Only LBD patients showed significant metabolic reductions in the occipital cortex, particularly in the primary visual cortex, which distinguished LBD versus AD with 90% sensitivity and 80% specificity. Multivariate analysis revealed that occipital metabolic changes in LBD were independent from those in the adjacent parieto-temporal cortices.

In the absence of a study reporting diagnostic accuracy of presynaptic dopaminergic imaging in an autopsy confirmed population of LBD patients, it is interesting to consider studies that combined FP-CIT and perfusion SPECT imaging. In such a combined study comprising 20 patients with probable LBD and 24 with probable AD, a significantly lower ratio of specific (bilateral caudate nucleus, putamen) to nonspecific (occipital cortex) FP-CIT binding was observed in LBD, compared to AD (Ceravolo et al., 2003). Perfusion data (SPM analysis) showed a significant decrease in temporo-parietal blood flow in AD versus LBD, whereas in LBD a significant occipital hypoperfusion was observed compared to AD. In another report, the utility of occipital lobe perfusion in the diagnosis of LBD was assessed using the FP-CIT findings obtained in the same patients as a "gold standard" (Kemp et al., 2007). Eighty-four consecutive patients underwent both HMPAO-SPECT and FP-CIT-SPECT as part of their routine investigations for suspected

LBD. Thirty-nine of the 84 FP-CIT scans were abnormal, suggesting a (surprisingly low) prevalence of 44% of patients with LBD in this series. In those patients classified as LBD, 28% of HMPAO SPECT scans demonstrated occipital hypoperfusion. In patients with a dementia other than LBD, 31% of patients also demonstrated occipital hypoperfusion. The authors concluded that occipital lobe hypoperfusion, as demonstrated by HMPAO SPECT in patients with suspected LBD, does not appear to either rule in, or rule out, the diagnosis. Such a study providing very poor sensitivity value for the clinical diagnosis of LBD essentially demonstrates the need for large multicenter studies with pathological confirmation.

Fifty-two patients (7 with a clinical diagnosis of FTD, 25 with AD and 20 with LBD) and 19 control subjects underwent both (11)C-DTBZ (a marker of dopaminergic synaptic vesicles) and FDG-PET scans (Koeppe et al., 2005). DTBZ scans provided maps of K1 (CBF pattern) and DV (distribution volume of the tracer bound to synaptic vesicles). Using FDG-PET or DTBZ-K1 (that gave very similar images), regression analysis provided the same regions as best discriminators: the parietal cortex for differentiating controls from all dementia (FTD/AD/LBD); the anterior and posterior cingulate for distinguishing FTD versus AD/DLB, and occipital and anterior cingulate for differentiating AD versus DLB. Discriminant analysis demonstrated that DTBZ-K1 and FDG-PET yielded similar levels of sensitivity and specificity for differentiating the subjects in this study, reaching 90% and 80%, respectively, when all dementias were compared to controls, or 75% sensitivity and 60% to 70% specificity when AD/DLB were contrasted to FTD. Including DTBZ-DV (in the putamen) in addition to either DTBZ-K1 or FDG-PET improved discrimination between DLB and AD groups (sensitivity, 90% and specificity, 96%). Combining cortical activity and measure of nigro-striatal projections appears to be a very elegant way to differentiate AD from LBD.

Postmortem studies have shown that cholinergic forebrain neuronal losses in Parkinson's disease with dementia (PDD) are equal to or greater than those in AD. PET AChE imaging was used to compare 12 AD patients, 14 PDD subjects, 11 PD without dementia and 10 controls (Bohnen et al., 2003). Compared with controls, mean cortical AChE activity was lowest in patients with PDD (-20%), followed by patients with Parkinson's disease without dementia (-13%). Mean cortical AChE activity was relatively preserved in patients with AD (-9%), except for regionally selective involvement of the lateral temporal cortex.

Another approach, cardiac MIBG imaging, was used to assess early disturbances of the cardiac sympathetic nervous system in LBD patients ($n = 11$), compared to nine probable AD patients (Estorch et al., 2006). Planar anterior images of the thorax were acquired at 15 minutes (early study) and four hours (late study) after tracer injection. Myocardial MIBG activity was quantified by means of a comparison with the nonspecific activity observed around the heart, in the mediastinum. A heart-to-mediastinum ratio >1.8 was considered normal. Patients with LBD showed decreased cardiac MIBG uptake compared to AD subjects, both in the early phase (1.34 ± 0.27 vs. 1.84 ± 0.22), and in the late study (1.22 ± 0.23 vs. 1.73 ± 0.08). A scintigraphy with [(123)I]MIBG was further combined with orthostatic tests and cardiac examinations in 14 patients with LBD and 14 AD patients (Yoshita, Taki, and Yamada, 2001). Orthostatic hypotension was seen in 13 LBD patients and in four AD patients. In all patients with LBD, the heart to mediastinum ratio of MIBG uptake was pathologically decreased in both early and delayed images, independently of the duration of disease and the importance of autonomic failure. All

patients with AD had normal MIBG uptake in the heart regardless of duration of disease and autonomic failure. In a subsequent study, cardiac sympathetic denervation was examined using myocardial MIBG scintigraphy in 37 patients with LBD (seven without and 30 with parkinsonism), 42 patients with AD, and 10 normal elderly controls (Yoshita et al., 2006). The heart-to-mediastinum uptake of myocardial MIBG uptake was decreased in the LBD groups versus the AD group and control population, while no differences were found between the AD and control groups or between the LBD patients with or without parkinsonism. In discriminating between LBD and AD, the delayed heart-to-mediastinum ratio had a sensitivity of 100%, a specificity of 100%, and a positive predictive value of 100% at a cut-off value of 1.68. In a combined study, medial occipital perfusion was significantly decreased in a LBD group, compared with an AD group. The mean heart/mediastinum ratio of MIBG uptake was also significantly lower in the LBD than in the AD group. Although functional imaging failed to demonstrate significant hypoperfusion in the medial occipital lobe in five patients with LBD, marked reduction of MIBG uptake was found in all LBD patients. ROC analysis revealed that MIBG myocardial scintigraphy enabled more accurate discrimination than brain perfusion between LBD and AD (Hanyu et al., 2006). Those results are certainly interesting, but we need information on the specificity of the technique when other parkinsonian syndromes with autonomic dysfunction are considered. MIBG myocardial scintigraphy was performed in 25 patients with PD, 15 patients with striatonigral degeneration (SND), 14 patients with progressive supranuclear palsy (PSP) and 20 control subjects (Yoshita, 1998). The mean value of heart/mediastinum ratio in patients with PD was significantly lower than those with SND, PSP, or controls. However, the mean value of heart/mediastinum ratio in SND with orthostatic hypotension was lower than that in SND without hypotension.

In summary, many studies have shown the clinical interest of functional imaging to help in the differential diagnosis between LBD and AD. Lesions of the substantia nigra constitute a pathological landmark of LBD and not of AD (Ceravolo et al., 2004). The demonstration of a loss of integrity of the nigro-striatal dopaminergic terminals with functional imaging is certainly a diagnostic marker of LBD. We just lack studies that would provide values for the diagnostic accuracy of the technique in pathologically proven cases. There is one such study in a small population that reported 90% sensitivity and 80% specificity when metabolic decrease in occipital regions is used for differential diagnosis of LBD and AD (Minoshima et al., 2001). Few studies provided a direct comparison of diverse methods (brain perfusion or metabolism vs. measures of nigro-striatal dopaminergic integrity or myocardial autonomic dysfunction), but none used pathological verification as a gold standard. Finally, so far functional imaging cannot differentiate PDD from LBD.

Differential Diagnosis of Parkinsonian Syndromes with Dementia

Patients with early to mid-stage Huntington's disease (HD) evaluated with FDG-PET showed lower metabolism in both caudate and putamen in comparison with a group of normal volunteers (Berent et al., 1988). But in another report, neuroimaging lacked sufficient sensitivity and specificity, since the appropriate diagnostic can easily be reached by DNA sequencing on a blood sample (Appollonio et al., 1997).

FDG-PET was performed in 11 non-demented PD patients with advanced disease and 10 age-matched controls (Berding et al., 2001). Significant regional reductions of glucose uptake were found in the parietal, frontal, temporal cortex, and caudate nucleus of PD subjects. The authors suggested that caution is mandatory if FDG-PET is being used to differentiate advanced PD from Parkinson's disease and dementia (PDD) and PSP where similar reductions are seen. SPM was used to compare FDG-PET obtained in 20 PSP patients, six FTD patients and a group of healthy controls (Garraux et al., 1999). In PSP compared to healthy subjects, a subcortico-frontal metabolic impairment included both motor and cognitive neural networks (Figure 15.7). When comparing FTD to controls, glucose uptake was reduced in dorsolateral and ventrolateral pre-frontal cortices, in frontopolar and anterior cingulate regions, in anterior temporal, right inferior parietal cortex, and bilateral striatum (see Figure 15.2). Finally, FTD showed more severe striato-frontal metabolic impairment than PSP, while mesencephalo-thalamic involvement was only observed in PSP. SPM was also used to compare FDG-PET images in 22 patients with the classical form of corticobasal degeneration (CBD) syndrome, 46 healthy subjects and 21 patients with PSP (Garraux et al., 2000). In comparison with controls, the metabolic impairment in CBD was asymmetrically distributed in the putamen, thalamus, precentral, lateral premotor and supplementary motor areas, dorsolateral prefrontal cortex, and the anterior part of the inferior parietal lobe including the intraparietal sulcus (see Figure 15.7). When PSP was compared with CBD, metabolic impairment predominated in the mid-brain,

anterior cingulate and orbitofrontal regions. The reverse contrast showed more premotor/SMA and parietal involvement in CBD (Hosaka et al., 2002). Moreover, in a study of CBF-SPECT obtained in 12 PSP and 12 CBD patients, an asymmetry index of rCBF was significantly higher in CBD patients compared with PSP patients in all cortical regions and in the basal ganglia (Zhang et al., 2001). Note that little is known on the interest of functional imaging in the differential diagnosis of CBD patients having predominant cognitive features.

Sensitivity values were provided in another study, where 135 parkinsonian patients were referred for FDG-PET to determine whether their diagnosis could be made accurately based upon their scans (Eckert et al., 2005). Imaging-based diagnosis was obtained by visual assessment of the individual scans and by computer-assisted interpretation. The results were compared with two-year follow-up clinical assessments made by independent movement disorders specialists who were blinded to the original PET findings. Computer assessment agreed with clinical diagnosis in 92.4% of all subjects (98% early PD, 92% late PD, 96% MSA, 85% PSP, 90% CBD, 86% healthy control subjects). Concordance of visual inspection with clinical diagnosis was achieved in 85.4% of the patients scanned (88% early PD, 97% late PD, 76% MSA, 60% PSP, 91% CBD, 91% healthy control subjects). A multivariate procedure was used in a study that compared rCBF-SPECT obtained in 21 CBD and 20 PD patients (Kreisler et al., 2005). A factorial discriminant analysis (FDA) was performed on 26 ROIs and asymmetry indices of 13 pairs of ROIs. FDA performed using the full set of parameters classified all the patients correctly. The most discriminating ROIs were the temporo-insular, temporo-parietal, and frontal medial regions.

SPECT was used to measure changes in striatal dopamine D2 receptor binding in a small sample comprising seven PD patients, six PSP patients and eight normal controls (Oyanagi et al., 2002). A voxel-by-voxel method provided parametric images of the D2 ligand binding potential. SPM indicated that D2 receptor density in the striatum of PSP patients was significantly lower than that of PD patients and normal controls. However, specific striatal dopamine D2 receptor binding using IBZM-SPECT, as calculated by a basal ganglia to frontal cortex ratio (BG/FC), was reduced in five PSP patients, but normal in three other patients (Arnold et al., 1994). On structural MRI, these three patients exhibited multiple hyperintense white matter lesions. This pilot study with IBZM-SPECT for in vivo imaging of striatal dopamine D2 receptors was said to support published neuropathological findings that clinical signs of PSP appeared to be due to heterogeneous neuropathology.

The pattern of presynaptic dopaminergic degeneration was studied with betaCIT-SPECT in 18 patients with probable MSA, eight patients with PSP, four patients with CBD, 48 patients with PD and 14 control subjects (Pirker et al., 2000). Overall, striatal binding was significantly reduced in MSA (-51% of normal mean), PSP (-60%), CBD (-35%), and PD (-58%), without overlap with control values. Asymmetry of striatal beta-CIT binding was significantly increased in patients with CBD and PD, as compared with control subjects. Although asymmetry seemed to be less pronounced in MSA and PSP than in PD, this was not statistically significant. Putamen-caudate nucleus ratios were significantly reduced (as compared with control subjects) in patients with PD, MSA, and PSP, but not with CBD. In most patients, it was not possible to differentiate parkinsonian disorders from PD with this method. The pattern of dopamine transporter loss was also assessed with SPECT in the striatum of 10 controls, 20 patients with PD, and nine with PSP (Im et al., 2006). A ratio of caudate,

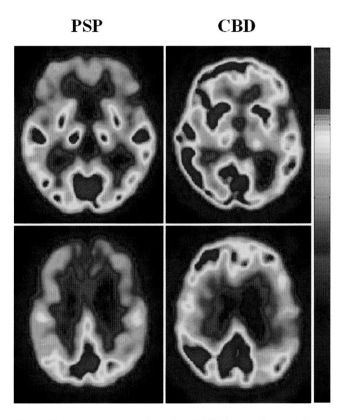

PSP   **CBD**

Figure 15–7 Transverse sections of FDG-PET images illustrate the metabolic distribution in progressive supranuclear palsy (PSP) and the classical form of corticobasal degeneration (CBD). PSP has decreased activity in bilateral frontal regions and caudate nucleus, whereas an asymmetric reduction of metabolism in parietal and frontal cortex, striatum and thalamus is characteristic of CBD.

anterior putamen and posterior putamen versus occipital uptake was calculated. Values were significantly reduced in all striatal ROIs of PD and PSP patients, compared with controls. The reduction was greater in posterior putamen (78%) than in caudate (56%) in PD, while it was similar (75%) in all regions in PSP. The reduction patterns of uptake were significantly different between PD and PSP groups. Accordingly, FP-CIT–SPECT was obtained in 21 PD patients, 15 PSP patients and 20 age-matched healthy controls (Filippi et al., 2006). A ratio of striatal to nonspecific occipital binding was calculated. The asymmetry index for the whole striatum was also calculated for PD and PSP. Compared to healthy controls, the dopamine transporters density in caudate and putamen was significantly reduced both in Parkinson's disease (−43%, −49%, contralaterally to the most affected side; −37%, −41%, ipsilaterally) and in PSP (−57%, −59%, contralaterally; −57%, −59%, ipsilaterally). Values were significantly lower in PSP patients than in PD group. The asymmetry index was significantly higher in PD than in PSP, but with an overlap between the two groups. Loss of integrity of both the pre- and postsynaptic sides of the nigro-striatal dopaminergic pathway in PSP is illustrated in figure 15.8.

SPM was used to analyze Beta-CIT pictures acquired in 14 patients with PSP, 17 with PD, 15 with MSA, and 13 healthy control subjects (Seppi et al., 2006). All patients showed a significant decrease in striatal beta-CIT uptake without any overlap with the control group. Patients with MSA and PSP could not be distinguished, but they showed an additional reduction in brain stem beta-CIT signal compared with controls and patients with PD. Interestingly, mid-brain beta-CIT uptake discriminated atypical parkinsonian disorders from PD with an overall correct classification of 91%.

One study investigated whether combined perfusion and dopamine transporters imaging can aid in the differential diagnosis of parkinsonian disorders (Van Laere et al., 2006). One–hundred-twenty-nine patients were studied retrospectively: 24 MSA (multiple system atrophy), 12 PSP (progressive supranuclear palsy), eight

LBD, 27 ET (essential tremor), and 58 IPD (idiopathic Parkinson's disease). Diagnosis was based on established clinical criteria after follow-up of 5.5 ±3.8 years in an academic specialist movement disorders clinic. Group characterization was done using a categorical voxel-based design and, second, a predefined volume-of-interest approach along cortical and subcortical structures, including striatal asymmetry and antero-posterior indices. Stepwise forward discriminant analysis was performed and cross-validity was tested using a classical leave-one-out procedure. Characteristic patterns for perfusion and dopamine transporter imaging were found for all pathologies. In the parkinson-plus population, MSA, PSP, and LBD could be discriminated in 100% of the cases. When including IPD, discrimination accuracy was 82.4%. FP-CIT-SPECT as a single technique was able to discriminate between ET and all other neurodegenerative forms with an accuracy of 93.0%, but inclusion of perfusion information augmented this slightly to 97.4%. As already pointed out for another study (Koeppe et al., 2005), combining cortical activity and measure of striato-nigral projections appears to be a very elegant way to differentiate pathologies with parkinsonism and dementia.

Brain acetylcholinesterase activity was measured with PET in 16 patients with Parkinson's disease (PD), 12 patients with progressive supranuclear palsy (PSP), and 13 age-matched controls (Shinotoh et al., 1999). In PD patients, there was a significant reduction (−17%) of cerebral cortical AChE activity compared with normal controls, whereas there was only a nonsignificant reduction (−10%) of activity in PSP patients. However, there was a prominent reduction (−38%) of thalamic AChE activity in PSP patients compared with normal controls, whereas there was only a nonsignificant reduction (−13%) of thalamic activity in PD patients. When the thalamic–to-cerebral–cortical-activity ratio was taken for each subject, PD and PSP could be separated.

In summary, parkinsonian syndrome with dementia, such as PSP and CBD, may be distinguished using functional imaging. However, there are very few reports with pathological confirmation, while many studies highlighted the heterogeneity of pathological presentation of CBD and PSP.

Metabolic Pattern in FTD versus AD

Frontotemporal dementia (FTD) is clinically characterized by predominant social and behavioral impairment and the early diagnosis is difficult. FTD is suggested to be among the three more frequent degenerative dementias.

Early comparisons showed that reduced uptake in the posterior cerebral hemispheres was characteristic of AD, while selective anterior hemisphere abnormalities characterized both FTD and PSP (Testa et al., 1988). Necropsy examinations were performed in three patients with the clinical features of PSP in whom PET had demonstrated predominantly frontal hypometabolism (Foster et al., 1992). In two of these patients the diagnosis of PSP was confirmed pathologically, and no morphological abnormalities were found in the cerebral cortex. The third patient had extensive cortical and subcortical neuronal loss and gliosis without neurofibrillary tangles, consistent with the diagnosis of progressive subcortical gliosis (PSG), a form of FTD. Even in retrospect no unique clinical neurological abnormality or finding on laboratory investigation could be identified that distinguished this latter patient from those with pathologically confirmed PSP. The authors concluded that PSG and PSP may be indistinguishable during life, and necropsy confirmation is needed for definite diagnosis. FTD

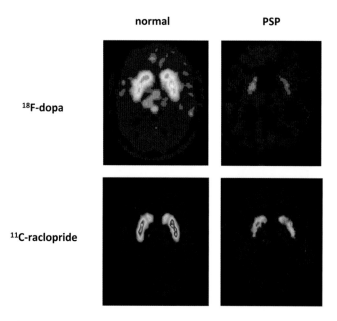

normal   **PSP**

18F-dopa

11C-raclopride

Figure 15–8   Transverse sections showing decreased uptake of (presynaptic) 18Fdopa, and decreased binding of (postsynaptic) 11C-raclopride in the dopaminergic nigro-striatal pathway of a patient with PSP. (Courtesy of David Brooks, Hammersmith Imanet and Imperial College London).

patients showed lower blood flow in the frontal cortex than AD, depressive subjects and controls (Alexander et al., 1995). The sensitivity and specificity of SPECT was reported to be 89% and 79%, respectively for AD, and 56% and 79%, respectively, for FTD (Velakoulis and Lloyd, 1998). In 25 pathologically confirmed cases of FTD, SPECT images obtained at initial evaluation were visually rated by an experienced blinded nuclear medicine consultant and compared with those of 31 patients with pathologically proven AD (McNeill et al., 2007). A reduction in frontal CBF was more common in FTD and was of diagnostic value (sensitivity, 0.80; specificity, 0.65, and likelihood ratio (LR), 2.25). A pattern of bilateral frontal CBF reduction without the presence of associated bilateral parietal CBF change was diagnostically more accurate (sensitivity, 0.80; specificity, 0.81, and LR, 4.13). In this study, diagnostic categorization (FTD or AD) on the basis of SPECT alone was disappointingly less accurate than clinical diagnosis (based on neurology and detailed neuropsychological evaluation). However, one patient with FTD was initially clinically misdiagnosed as AD, owing to the lack of availability of full neuropsychological assessment, and SPECT correctly diagnosed this patient, providing a diagnostic gain of 4%. Switching from SPECT to FDG-PET, a recent study emphasized the benefit of adding FDG-PET assessment to clinical decision for reaching differential diagnosis between FTD and AD (Foster et al., 2007). Six dementia experts provided FTD or AD diagnosis based on clinical scenarios and FDG-PET, in patients with pathological verification (31 AD and 14 FTD). Inter-rater reliability was greater for FDG-PET visual analysis (transaxial images or SSP projections) than for clinical assessment. Accuracy of the diagnostic decision based on SSP projection was 89.6%, sensitivity for FTD was 73%, and sensitivity for AD was 97.6%. Importantly, the addition of FDG-PET to clinical scenarios increased diagnostic accuracy and confidence for both AD and FTD. In another study, the metabolism was significantly lower in 21 clinically diagnosed FTD patients, compared to 21 probable AD subjects not only in the orbital gyri, anterior cingulate gyri, middle and superior frontal gyri and left inferior frontal gyrus, but also in the hippocampi, anterior temporal lobes, basal ganglia and thalami (Ishii et al., 1998b) (see Figure 15.2). This suggested that multivariate comparisons might improve the distinction between both conditions, and we will now review several reports following the logic of multiple comparisons.

Values characterizing diagnostic accuracy were obtained in a stepwise logistic regression analysis that identified the severity of bifrontal hypoperfusion as the most significant contributing parameter to classify AD versus FTD with SPECT (Pickut et al., 1997). A predictive model correctly classified 81% of the FTD group, but only 74% of the AD subjects. A CBF-SPECT study was performed in 16 patients with FTD, 27 with early-onset AD, 25 with late-onset AD, 19 with subcortical white matter dementia and 28 normal controls (Sjogren et al., 2000). In FTD patients, the medial superior frontal gyrus, near the frontal pole, was found to be the region with the most reduced rCBF values. An anterior-to-posterior rCBF ratio (medial superior frontal gyrus/ medial temporal lobes) was calculated, which significantly separated the FTD group from the other dementia groups and controls with a good sensitivity of 87% and a specificity of at least 78%. Arterial spin labelling (ASL) MRI was also used to compare brain perfusion in 21 patients with FTD, 24 patients with AD, and 25 control subjects (Du et al., 2006). All subjects had also T1-weighted structural images. ASL-MRI detected a pattern of hypoperfusion in right frontal regions in patients with FTD vs.

control subjects. FTD had higher perfusion than AD in the parietal regions and posterior cingulate. Adding frontal perfusion to gray matter atrophy significantly improved the classification of FTD from normal aging to 74%, and adding parietal perfusion to gray matter atrophy significantly improved the classification of FTD from AD to 75%. More interestingly, combining frontal and parietal lobe perfusion further improved the classification of FTD from AD to 87%. A factorial discriminant analysis further helped in the classification of CBF-SPECT images (Charpentier et al., 2000). Five variables were selected: right median frontal, left lateral frontal, left temporo-parietal, left temporo-parietal-occipital activity, and MMSE. One-hundred percent of patients with FTD were correctly classified by the decision rule (20/20 patients), as were 90% of patients with AD (18/20). However, when data reduction techniques were performed on the entire functional images, using principal components analysis (PCA) and partial least-squares (PLS), and combined with linear discriminant analysis (LDA), quadratic (QDA) or logistic regression (LR) to classify subjects as having AD or FTD, the methods achieved a diagnostic accuracy (as assessed by leave-one-out cross-validation) that was similar to visual ratings by expert raters (Higdon et al., 2004). Methods using PLS appeared to be more successful, and averaging or using VOI data was recommended. More precisely, the different studies reviewed above suggest that one might get better differential diagnosis accuracy by assessing activity in more specific brain regions.

For example, the posterior cingulate sign was evaluated for the differential diagnosis between AD and FTD (Bonte et al., 2004). CBF-SPECT images of 20 patients with clinically confirmed or autopsy-proven (10 patients) AD and 20 patients with clinically confirmed or autopsy-proven (7 patients) FTD were compared with images of 20 elderly healthy control subjects using SPM. Sixteen of 20 patients with AD showed the posterior cingulate sign in the form of significant blood flow reductions, while one of 20 patients with FTD showed the posterior cingulate sign. However, that patient's illness subsequently evolved into AD. In the same vein, the ventromedial prefrontal and anterior cingulate cortex were shown to be the most affected regions in FTD (Salmon et al., 2003), and a recent MRI study reported that the annual rate of cingulate atrophy rates discriminated perfectly between FTD and controls (Barnes et al., 2007).

PET-amyloid imaging was also used for differential diagnostic purposes. All AD patients (7/7) had positive (11)C-PIB scans by visual inspection, while eight out of 12 patients with FTD and seven of eight controls had negative scans (Rabinovici et al., 2007). Of the four PIB-positive patients with FTD, two had FDG-PET scans that suggested AD, and two had FDG-PET scans suggestive of fronto-temporal lobar degeneration (FTLD). Mean uptake values were higher in AD than in FTLD in whole brain, lateral frontal, precuneus, and lateral temporal cortex, while values in FTLD did not significantly differ from controls. It is important to note that those results are different from data obtained with 18FDDNP-PET, using a molecule that binds to both plaques and tangles (Small et al., 2006b).

In summary, functional imaging allows differentiating between FTD and AD, and an efficient strategy consists of selecting precise regions known to be selectively affected by one or the other disease process. New imaging techniques that target specific brain lesions are of great interest in diseases where the underlying brain pathology is heterogeneous (Jackson and Lowe, 1996), and an effort should be made to get autopsy confirmation in a series of patients studied with functional imaging.

Semantic Dementia, Nonfluent Primary Progressive Aphasia and AD

The clinical presentation in frontotemporal dementia (FTD) reflects the distribution of the pathologic changes (Hodges, 2001). Three major clinical syndromes can be identified. In the frontal variant of FTD, changes in social behavior reflect orbital and medial frontal lobe pathology. In semantic dementia, there is a breakdown in the conceptual database which underlies language production and comprehension, along with deficits in nonverbal semantic knowledge; patients show asymmetric rostral and lateral temporal atrophy with relative sparing of the hippocampal formation (Adlam et al., 2006). In nonfluent primary progressive aphasia, the phonologic and syntactic components of language are affected in association with left peri-sylvian involvement (Amici et al., 2006). Note that the exercise of differential diagnosis is difficult with nonfluent PPA, which constitutes a syndrome, and can evolve to FTD or CBD (Kertesz et al., 2003), but also to AD (De Oliveira, Castro, and Bittencourt, 1989; Galton et al., 2000; Greene et al., 1996) (see Figure 15.9).

FDG-PET images of 14 patients comprising the clinical prototypes of FTLD (FTD, SD and PPA) were compared to 15 patients with early-onset AD (EOAD). A voxel-based group comparison

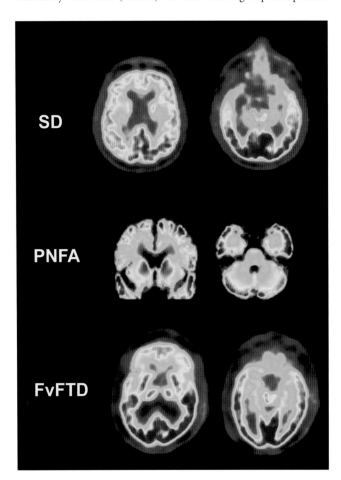

Figure 15–9 Sections of FDG-PET images showing predominant left temporal involvement in semantic dementia (SD), left peri-sylvian (mainly frontal) metabolic impairment in progressive nonfluent aphasia (PNFA), and frontal / anterior temporal involvement in the frontal variant of frontotemporal dementia (fvFTD). (Courtesy of William Jagust, University of California, Berkeley).

identified metabolic impairment in the bilateral ventromedial frontal area, the left anterior insula and inferior frontal cortex in FTLD, compared to EOAD patients (Ibach et al., 2004). The authors suggested that the a priori heterogeneous prototypes of FTLD (FTD, SD, PPA) might share common ground and be distinguishable as an entire group from EOAD. However, such a conclusion would have been stronger with a "random effect" analysis rather than a comparison of mean metabolic values in the groups. Effectively, CBF-SPECT was assessed in eight patients with a nonfluent form of progressive aphasia, and eight with a fluent form of progressive aphasia, compared to 16 healthy volunteers (Newberg et al., 2000). The most prominent deficit in the nonfluent group was found in the left dorsolateral prefrontal region, and differed from the most prominent deficits in the group with fluent aphasia, found in the left temporal and parietal cortex. Slightly different regions were involved in reports on nonfluent PPA. When FDG-PET images of 10 (nonfluent) PPA patients and 10 AD patients were compared using SPM, a decrease in metabolism was observed in the left anterior insula (Nestor et al., 2003). However, in another small sample of five PPA, 10 AD patients and 10 normal subjects (Zahn et al., 2005), group comparisons revealed left anterior lateral temporal abnormalities in PPA in comparison to normal subjects. AD patients showed more limited hypometabolism within the same area. In addition, left lateral parietal abnormalities were demonstrated in both PPA and AD. PPA and AD patients differed significantly with respect to the frequency of medial temporal lobe and posterior cingulate/precuneus involvement.

CBF-SPECT images were obtained in patients with AD, FTD, PPA and SD. Principal component (PC) analysis was performed and three PCs explained 86% of the variation in rCBF indices (regional versus cerebellar activity) between all subjects. The first PC appeared to reflect the average cortical rCBF value and separated patient groups from normal controls, but failed to distinguish between patient groups. The second PC reflected anterior-posterior asymmetry and separated AD from all three forms of FTLD. This PC also separated FTD and SD from controls, but failed to distinguish between FTD, PA and SD. The third PC reflected left-right asymmetry and separated PPA from all other groups (Talbot et al., 1995).

In summary, AD can be distinguished from SD and PPA using functional imaging, but the distinction using CBF or metabolism will probably depend on the stage of the disease. In early cases with PPA, the use of specific markers of amyloid might help in the differentiation.

Creutzfeldt Jakob Disease

Functional imaging in Creutzfeldt-Jakob disease (CJD) may demonstrate a heterogeneous decrease in activity throughout the brain, differing from patterns observed in common degenerative types of dementia (Aharon-Peretz et al., 1995). However, a nonspecific metabolic decrease in the left cerebral hemisphere and the right cerebellum was also reported (Bavis et al., 2003). The summary is that activity patterns are very heterogeneous in CJD, and that we lack population studies to illustrate differences with other dementia types. Interestingly, CBF was measured in 11 patients with Gerstmann-Straussler-Scheinker syndrome caused by Pro102Leu mutation in PRNP. The 3D stereotactic surface projection (SSP) method detected abnormalities in five patients early on during the course of the illness. SPECT findings showed diffusely decreased CBF, described as a mosaic pattern, with the lowest perfusion noted in the occipital lobes and with relative preservation of cerebellar activity (Arata et al., 2006). Those studies suggest an absence of specificity in the brain distribution of prion pathology.

Conclusions

Potential new therapies for the treatment of AD demand early and accurate diagnosis. Although clinical evaluation is generally sufficient when the disease is well established, we reviewed studies that demonstrate that functional neuroimaging can be helpful in detecting the earliest changes of AD, or to differentiate AD from the other forms of dementia.

However, this conclusion has been previously challenged. A retrospective audit of HMPAO-SPECT scans was undertaken to assess the utility of brain perfusion imaging in a cohort of young cognitively impaired patients in whom diagnostic uncertainty remained after standard clinical and neuropsychological assessment and structural brain imaging. SPECT scans were assessed by five raters (two neurologists and three nuclear medicine specialists) on two occasions six months apart, first without any clinical data and second with brief pertinent clinical information. SPECT diagnoses were compared with clinical diagnoses subsequently established by the two neurologists with access to all clinical, neuropsychological and neuroimaging data. Despite reasonable intra- and inter-rater reliability, diagnostic accuracy ranged from 32% to 58% only. SPECT scan normality or abnormality in blind and informed viewings gave respective sensitivities of 77% and 71%, specificities of 44% and 38%, positive predictive values of 88% and 87% and negative predictive values of 27% and 18%. However, calculating pairwise disease group comparisons, likelihood ratios (LR) suggested some diagnostic gain in differentiating AD from 'not AD' (LR 5.63), and mainly AD versus FTD/focal pathology, which constitute an important aspect of functional imaging (Doran et al., 2005).

In another report, the current clinical practice for interpreting CBF-SPECT images was examined by having 16 experts evaluate the appearance of SPECT images in patients with probable AD, patients with major depressive episodes, and healthy volunteers (Dougall, Nobili, and Ebmeier, 2004a). The experts rated diagnostic criteria of scan appearance according to their individual diagnostic practices. Experts were nuclear medicine specialists, psychiatrists and physicists taking part in a European multicenter collaborative project. They examined 158 perfusion scans, and then the same perfusion scans together with statistical parametric maps (SPMs). The sensitivity of the experts' diagnostic judgments was significantly and negatively correlated with the importance they attributed to reduced regional perfusion in the parietal lobes. A corresponding positive correlation was observed for diagnostic specificity against depressed and healthy volunteers. Similar results were observed with SPMs, where in addition the area under the ROC curve was significantly reduced with raters' increased diagnostic reliance on frontal lobe perfusion deficits. Sensitivity was greater with SPM for patients younger than 70 years and with dementia severity. The more importance experts placed on parietal (symmetrical) perfusion deficits, the less sensitive and the more specific their diagnostic judgment was.

A general recommendation when using functional imaging for differential diagnosis of dementia would be to rely on clusters of brain regions characteristically involved in each disorder rather than a single "pattern." In the example of AD, this would mean focusing attention on posterior cingulate cortex and precuneus, and on medial temporal structures in addition to posterior and lateral associative cortices. A second recommendation would be to combine information. Appropriate interpretation of functional imaging cannot be made without information concerning structural imaging. Some uncertainties concerning specificity of functional imaging for the diagnostic of AD may be eliminated if clinicians observe parkinsonian signs, for example. Moreover, an important message from the studies reviewed in this chapter is the added value of combining CBF or metabolic evaluation and a more specific assessment of the integrity of the nigro-striatal dopaminergic system or the presence of amyloid deposits, for example.

References

Abe, S., Hanyu, H., Arai, H, Iwamoto, T, and Takasaki, M. (1996). Cerebral hemodynamics in patients with dementia]. *Nippon Ronen Igakkai Zasshi*, 33: 95–104.

Adlam, A. L., Patterson, K., Rogers, T. T., Nestor, P. J., Salmond, C. H., Acosta-Cabronero, J. et al. (2006). Semantic dementia and fluent primary progressive aphasia: two sides of the same coin? *Brain*, 129: 3066–3080.

Aharon-Peretz, J., Peretz, A., Hemli, J. A., Honigman, S., and Israel, O. (1995). SPECT diagnosis of Creutzfeld-Jacob disease. *Journal of Nuclear Medicine*, 36: 616–617.

Alexander, G. E., Prohovnik, I., Sackeim, H. A., Stern. Y., and Mayeux, R. (1995). Cortical perfusion and gray matter weight in frontal lobe dementia. *The Journal of Neuropsychiatry and Clinical Neurosciences*, 7: 188–196.

Alvarez-Sauco, M., Molto-Jorda, J. M., Morera-Guitart, J., Frutos-Alegria, M. T., and Matias-Guiu Guia, J. (2005). An update on the diagnosis of vascular dementia. *Revista de Neurologia*, 41: 484–492.

Amici, S., Gorno-Tempini, M. L., Ogar, J. M., Dronkers, N. F., and Miller, B. L. (2006). An overview on Primary Progressive Aphasia and its variants. *Behavioural Neurology*, 17: 77–87.

Appollonio, I., Frisoni, G. B., Curto, N., Trabucchi, M., and Frattola, L. (1997). Which diagnostic procedures in the elderly? The case of late-onset Huntington's disease. *Journal of Geriatric Psychiatry and Neurology*, 10: 39–46.

Arata, H., Takashima, H., Hirano, R., Tomimitsu, H., Machigashira, K., Izumi, K. et al. (2006). Early clinical signs and imaging findings in Gerstmann-Straussler-Scheinker syndrome (Pro102Leu). *Neurology*, 66: 1672–1678.

Arnold, G., Tatsch, K., Oertel, W. H., Vogl, T., Schwarz, J., Kraft, E. et al. (1994). Clinical progressive supranuclear palsy: differential diagnosis by IBZM-SPECT and MRI. *Journal of Neural Transmission. Supplementum*, 42: 111–118.

Baezner, H. and Daffertshofer, M. (2003). Subcortical vascular encephalopathy. *Therapeutische Umschau. Revue thérapeutique*, 60: 541–552.

Barnes, A., Lusman, D., Patterson, J., Brown, D., and Wyper, D. (2000). The use of statistical parametric mapping (SPM96) as a decision aid in the differential diagnosis of dementia using 99mTc-HMPAO SPECT. *Behavioural Neurology*, 12: 77–86.

Barnes, J., Godbolt, A. K., Frost, C., Boyes, R. G., Jones, B. F., Scahill, R. I. et al. (2007). Atrophy rates of the cingulate gyrus and hippocampus in AD and FTLD. *Neurobiology of Aging*, 28: 20–28.

Bavis, J., Reynolds, P., Tegeler, C., and Clark, P. (2003). Asymmetric neuroimaging in Creutzfeldt-Jakob disease: A ruse. *Journal of Neuroimaging*, 13: 376–379.

Berding, G., Odin, P., Brooks, D. J., Nikkhah, G., Matthies, C., Peschel, T. et al. (2001). Resting regional cerebral glucose metabolism in advanced Parkinson's disease studied in the off and on conditions with [(18)F]FDG-PET. *Movement Disorders*, 16: 1014–1022.

Berent, S., Giordani, B., Lehtinen, S., Markel, D., Penney, J. B., Buchtel, H. A. et al. (1988). Positron emission tomographic scan investigations of Huntington's disease: Cerebral metabolic correlates of cognitive function. *Annals of Neurology*, 23: 541–546.

Bergman, H., Chertkow, H., Wolfson, C., Stern, J., Rush, C., Whitehead, V. et al. (1997). HM-PAO (CERETEC) SPECT brain scanning in the diagnosis of Alzheimer's disease. *Journal of the American Geriatrics Society*, 45: 15–20.

Bohnen, N. I., Kaufer, D. I., Ivanco, L. S., Lopresti, B., Koeppe, R. A., Davis, J. G. et al. (2003). Cortical cholinergic function is more severely affected in parkinsonian dementia than in Alzheimer disease: an in vivo positron emission tomographic study. *Archives of Neurology*, 60: 1745–1748.

Bokde, A. L., Pietrini, P., Ibanez, V., Furey, M. L., Alexander, G. E., Graff-Radford, N. R. et al. (2001). The effect of brain atrophy on cerebral hypometabolism in the visual variant of Alzheimer disease. *Archives of Neurology*, 58: 480–486.

Bonte, F. J., Harris, T. S., Hynan, L. S., Bigio, E. H., and White, C. L., 3rd. (2006). Tc-99m HMPAO SPECT in the differential diagnosis of the dementias with histopathologic confirmation. *Clinical Nuclear Medicine*, 31: 376–378.

Bonte, F. J., Harris, T. S., Roney, C. A., and Hynan, L. S. (2004). Differential diagnosis between Alzheimer's and frontotemporal disease by the posterior cingulate sign. *Journal of Nuclear Medicine*, 45: 771–774.

Bonte, F. J., Weiner, M. F., Bigio, E. H., and White, C. L., 3rd. (1997). Brain blood flow in the dementias: SPECT with histopathologic correlation in 54 patients. *Radiology*, 202: 793–797.

Ceravolo, R., Volterrani, D., Gambaccini, G., Bernardini, S., Rossi, C., Logi, C. et al. (2004). Presynaptic nigro-striatal function in a group of Alzheimer's disease patients with parkinsonism: Evidence from a dopamine transporter imaging study. *Journal of Neural Transmission*, 111: 1065–1073.

Ceravolo, R., Volterrani, D., Gambaccini, G., Rossi, C., Logi, C., Manca, G. et al. (2003). Dopaminergic degeneration and perfusional impairment in Lewy body dementia and Alzheimer's disease. *Neurological Sciences*, 24: 162–163.

Chan, K. H., Johnson, K. A., Becker, J. A., Satlin, A., Mendelson, J., Garada, B. et al. (1994). A neural network classifier for cerebral perfusion imaging. *Journal of Nuclear Medicine*, 35: 771–774.

Charpentier, P., Lavenu, I., Defebvre, L., Duhamel, A., Lecouffe, P., Pasquier, F. et al. (2000). Alzheimer's disease and frontotemporal dementia are differentiated by discriminant analysis applied to (99m)Tc HmPAO SPECT data. *Journal of Neurology, Neurosurgery, and Psychiatry*, 69: 661–663.

Chetelat, G., Eustache, F., Viader, F., De La Sayette, V., Pelerin, A., Mezenge, F. et al. (2005). FDG-PET measurement is more accurate than neuropsychological assessments to predict global cognitive deterioration in patients with mild cognitive impairment. *Neurocase*, 11: 14–25.

Colloby, S. J., Fenwick, J. D., Williams, E. D., Paling, S. M., Lobotesis, K., Ballard, C. et al. (2002). A comparison of (99m)Tc-HMPAO SPECT changes in dementia with Lewy bodies and Alzheimer's disease using statistical parametric mapping. *European Journal of Nuclear Medicine and Molecular Imaging*, 29: 615–622.

De Oliveira, S. A., Castro, M. J., and Bittencourt, P. R. (1989). Slowly progressive aphasia followed by Alzheimer's dementia: a case report. *Arquivos De neuro-Psiquiatria*, 47: 72–75.

De Santi, S., de Leon, M. J., Rusinek, H., Convit, A., Tarshish, C. Y., Roche, A. et al. (2001). Hippocampal formation glucose metabolism and volume losses in MCI and AD. *Neurobiology of Aging*, 22: 529–539.

Doran, M., Vinjamuri, S., Collins, J., Parker, D., and Larner, A. J. (2005). Single-photon emission computed tomography perfusion imaging in the differential diagnosis of dementia: a retrospective regional audit. *International Journal of Clinical Practice*, 59: 496–500.

Dougall, N., Nobili, F., and Ebmeier, K. P. (2004a). Predicting the accuracy of a diagnosis of Alzheimer's disease with 99mTc HMPAO single photon emission computed tomography. *Psychiatry Research*, 131: 157–168.

Dougall, N. J., Bruggink, S., and Ebmeier, K. P. (2004b). Systematic review of the diagnostic accuracy of 99mTc-HMPAO-SPECT in dementia. *The American Journal of Geriatric Psychiatry*, 12: 554–570.

Du, A. T., Jahng, G. H., Hayasaka, S., Kramer, J. H., Rosen, H. J., Gorno-Tempini, M. L. et al. (2006). Hypoperfusion in frontotemporal dementia and Alzheimer disease by arterial spin labeling MRI. *Neurology*, 67: 1215–1220.

Ebmeier, K. P., Glabus, M. F., Prentice, N., Ryman, A., and Goodwin, G. M. (1998). A voxel-based analysis of cerebral perfusion in dementia and depression of old age. *Neuroimage*, 7: 199–208.

Eckert, T., Barnes, A., Dhawan, V., Frucht, S., Gordon, M. F., Feigin, A. S. et al. (2005). FDG PET in the differential diagnosis of parkinsonian disorders. *Neuroimage*, 26: 912–921.

Estorch, M., Camacho, V., Fuertes, J., Rodriguez-Revuelto, A., Hernandez, M. A., Flotats, A. et al. (2006). Dementia with Lewy bodies and Alzheimer's disease: differential diagnosis by cardiac sympathetic innervation MIBG imaging. *Revista Española de Medicina Nuclear*, 25: 229–235.

Filippi, L., Manni, C., Pierantozzi, M., Brusa, L., Danieli, R., Stanzione, P. et al. (2006). 123I-FP-CIT in progressive supranuclear palsy and in Parkinson's disease: a SPECT semiquantitative study. *Nuclear Medicine Communications*, 27: 381–386.

Firbank, M. J., Colloby, S. J., Burn, D. J., McKeith, I. G., and O'Brien, J. T. (2003). Regional cerebral blood flow in Parkinson's disease with and without dementia. *Neuroimage*, 20: 1309–1319.

Foster, N. L., Gilman, S., Berent, S., Sima, A. A., D'Amato, C., Koeppe, R. A. et al. (1992). Progressive subcortical gliosis and progressive supranuclear palsy can have similar clinical and PET abnormalities. *Journal of Neurology, Neurosurgery, and Psychiatry*, 55: 707–713.

Foster, N. L., Heidebrink, J. L., Clark, C. M., Jagust, W. J., Arnold, S. E., Barbas, N. R., et al. (2007). FDG-PET improves accuracy in distinguishing frontotemporal dementia and Alzheimer's disease. *Brain*, 2007; 130: 2616–2635.

Galton, C. J., Patterson, K., Xuereb, J. H., Hodges, J. R. (2000). Atypical and typical presentations of Alzheimer's disease: a clinical, neuropsychological, neuroimaging and pathological study of 13 cases. *Brain*, 123(Pt. 3): 484–498.

Garraux, G., Salmon, E., Degueldre, C., Lemaire, C., Laureys, S., and Franck, G. (1999). Comparison of impaired subcortico-frontal metabolic networks in normal aging, subcortico-frontal dementia, and cortical frontal dementia. *Neuroimage*, 10: 149–162.

Garraux, G., Salmon, E., Peigneux, P., Kreisler, A., Degueldre, C., Lemaire, C. et al. (2000). Voxel-based distribution of metabolic impairment in corticobasal degeneration. *Movement Disorders*, 15: 894–904.

Gemmell, H. G., Sharp, P. F., Besson, J. A., Crawford, J. R., Ebmeier, K. P., Davidson, J. et al. (1987). Differential diagnosis in dementia using the cerebral blood flow agent 99mTc HM-PAO: A SPECT study. *Journal of Computer Assisted Tomography*, 11: 398–402.

Golan, H., Kremer, J., Freedman, M., and Ichise, M. (1996). Usefulness of follow-up regional cerebral blood flow measurements by single-photon emission computed tomography in the differential diagnosis of dementia. *Journal of Neuroimaging*, 6: 23–28.

Greene, J. D., Patterson, K., Xuereb, J., and Hodges, J. R. (1996). Alzheimer disease and nonfluent progressive aphasia. *Archives of Neurology*, 53: 1072–1078.

Hanada, K., Hosono, M., Kudo, T., Hitomi, Y., Yagyu, Y., Kirime, E. et al. (2006). Regional cerebral blood flow in the assessment of major depression and Alzheimer's disease in the early elderly. *Nuclear Medicine Communications*, 27: 535–541.

Hanyu, H., Shimizu, S., Hirao, K., Kanetaka, H., Iwamoto, T., Chikamori, T. et al. (2006). Comparative value of brain perfusion SPECT and [(123)I]MIBG myocardial scintigraphy in distinguishing between dementia with Lewy bodies and Alzheimer's disease. *European Journal of Nuclear Medicine and Molecular Imaging*, 33: 248–253.

Herholz, K., Bauer, B., Wienhard, K., Kracht, L., Mielke, R., Lenz, M. O. et al. (2000). In-vivo measurements of regional acetylcholine esterase activity in degenerative dementia: comparison with blood flow and glucose metabolism. *Journal of Neural Transmission*, 107: 1457–1468.

Herholz, K., Nordberg, A., Salmon, E., Perani, D., Kessler, J., Mielke, R. et al. (1999). Impairment of neocortical metabolism predicts progression in Alzheimer's disease. *Dementia and Geriatric Cognitive Disorders*, 10: 494–504.

Higdon, R., Foster, N. L., Koeppe, R. A., DeCarli, C. S., Jagust, W. J., Clark, C. M. et al. (2004). A comparison of classification methods for differentiating fronto-temporal dementia from Alzheimer's disease using FDG-PET imaging. *Statistics in Medicine*, 23: 315–326.

Higuchi, M., Tashiro, M., Arai, H., Okamura, N., Hara, S., Higuchi, S. et al. (2000). Glucose hypometabolism and neuropathological correlates in brains of dementia with Lewy bodies. *Experimental Neurology*, 162: 247–256.

Hodges, J. R. (2001). Frontotemporal dementia (Pick's disease): Clinical features and assessment. *Neurology*, 56: S6–S10.

Holman, B. L., Johnson, K. A., Gerada, B., Carvalho, P. A., and Satlin, A. (1992). The scintigraphic appearance of Alzheimer's disease: A prospective study using technetium-99m-HMPAO SPECT. *Journal of Nuclear Medicine*, 33: 181–185.

Honda, N., Machida, K., Hosono, M., Matsumoto, T., Matsuda, H., Oshima, M. et al. (2002). Interobserver variation in diagnosis of dementia by brain perfusion SPECT. *Radiation Medicine*, 20: 281–289.

Hosaka, K., Ishii, K., Sakamoto, S., Mori, T., Sasaki, M., Hirono, N. et al. (2002). Voxel-based comparison of regional cerebral glucose metabolism between PSP and corticobasal degeneration. *Journal of the Neurolgical Sciences*, 199: 67–71.

Ibach, B., Poljansky, S., Marienhagen, J., Sommer, M., Manner, P., and Hajak G. (2004). Contrasting metabolic impairment in frontotemporal degeneration and early onset Alzheimer's disease. *Neuroimage*, 23: 739–743.

Im, J. H., Chung, S. J., Kim, J. S., and Lee, M. C. (2006). Differential patterns of dopamine transporter loss in the basal ganglia of progressive supranuclear palsy and Parkinson's disease: analysis with [((123)I]IPT single photon emission computed tomography. *Journal of the Neurological Sciences*, 244: 103–109.

Imabayashi, E., Matsuda, H., Asada, T., Ohnishi, T., Sakamoto, S., Nakano, S. et al. (2004). Superiority of 3-dimensional stereotactic surface projection analysis over visual inspection in discrimination of patients with very early Alzheimer's disease from controls using brain perfusion SPECT. *Journal of Nuclear Medicine*, 45: 1450–1457.

Ince, G. (2001). Pathological correlates of late-onset dementia in a multicentre, community-based population in England and Wales. Neuropathology Group of the Medical Research Council Cognitive Function and Aging Study (MRC CFAS). *Lancet*, 357: 169–175.

Ishii, K., Imamura, T., Sasaki, M., Yamaji, S., Sakamoto, S., Kitagaki, H. et al. (1998a). Regional cerebral glucose metabolism in dementia with Lewy bodies and Alzheimer's disease. *Neurology*, 51: 125–130.

Ishii, K., Sakamoto, S., Sasaki, M., Kitagaki, H., Yamaji, S., Hashimoto, M. et al. (1998b). Cerebral glucose metabolism in patients with frontotemporal dementia. *Journal of Nuclear Medicine*, 39: 1875–1878.

Jackson, M. and Lowe J. (1996). The new neuropathology of degenerative frontotemporal dementias. *Acta Neuropathologica (Berlin)*, 91: 127–134.

Jagust, W., Reed, B. R., Mungas, D., Ellis, W., and DeCarli C. (2007). What does fluorodeoxyglucose PET imaging add to a clinical diagnosis of dementia? *Neurology*, (in press).

Jagust, W. J., Friedland, R. P., and Budinger, T. F. (1985). Positron emission tomography with [18F]fluorodeoxyglucose differentiates normal pressure hydrocephalus from Alzheimer-type dementia. *Journal of Neurology, Neurosurgery, and Psychiatry*, 48: 1091–1096.

Jeong, Y., Chin, J., Tae, W. S., Hong, S. B., Kim, S. E., Suh, Y. L. et al. (2004). Serial positron emission tomography findings in a patient with hydrocephalic dementia and Alzheimer's disease. *Journal of Neuroimaging*, 2004; 14: 170–175.

Johnson, K. A., Jones, K., Holman, B. L., Becker, J. A., Spiers, P. A., Satlin, A. et al. (1998). Preclinical prediction of Alzheimer's disease using SPECT. *Neurology*, 50: 1563–1571.

Kemp, P. M., Hoffmann, S. A., Tossici-Bolt, L., Fleming, J. S., and Holmes, C. (2007). Limitations of the HMPAO SPECT appearances of occipital lobe perfusion in the differential diagnosis of dementia with Lewy bodies. *Nuclear Medicine Communications*, 28: 451–456.

Kerrouche, N., Herholz, K., Mielke, R., Holthoff, V., and Baron, J. C. (2006). 18FDG PET in vascular dementia: differentiation from Alzheimer's disease using voxel-based multivariate analysis. *Journal of Cerebral Blood Flow and Metabolism*, 26: 1213–1221.

Kertesz, A., Davidson, W., McCabe, P., Takagi, K., and Munoz, D. (2003). Primary progressive aphasia: diagnosis, varieties, evolution. *Journal of the International Neuropsychological Society*, 9: 710–719.

Klunk, W. E., Engler, H., Nordberg, A., Wang, Y., Blomqvist, G., Holt, D. P. et al. (2004). Imaging brain amyloid in Alzheimers disease with Pittsburgh Compound-B. *Annals of Neurology*, 55: 306–319.

Koeppe, R. A., Gilman, S., Joshi, A., Liu, S., Little, R., Junck, L. et al. (2005). 11C-DTBZ and 18F-FDG PET measures in differentiating dementias. *Journal of Nuclear Medicine*, 46: 936–944.

Kono, A. K., Ishii, K., Sofue, K., Miyamoto, N., Sakamoto, S., and Mori E. (2007). Fully automatic differential diagnosis system for dementia with Lewy bodies and Alzheimer's disease using FDG-PET and 3D-SSP. *European Journal of Nuclear Medicine and Molecular Imaging*, 34: 1490–1497.

Kreisler, A., Defebvre, L., Lecouffe, P., Duhamel, A., Charpentier, P., Steinling, M. et al. (2005). Corticobasal degeneration and Parkinson's disease assessed by HmPaO SPECT: The utility of factorial discriminant analysis. *Movement Disorders*, 20: 1431–1438.

Kuhl, D. E., Koeppe, R. A., Minoshima, S., Snyder, S. E., Ficaro, E. P., Foster, N. L. et al. (1999). In vivo mapping of cerebral acetylcholinesterase activity in aging and Alzheimer's disease. *Neurology*, 52: 691–699.

Kuwabara, Y., Ichiya, Y., Otsuka, M., Tahara, T., Fukumura, T., Gunasekera, R. et al. (1990). Differential diagnosis of bilateral parietal abnormalities in I-123 IMP SPECT imaging. *Clinical Nuclear Medicine*, 15: 893–899.

Launes, J., Sulkava, R., Erkinjuntti, T., Nikkinen, P., Lindroth, L., Liewendahl, K. et al. (1991). 99Tcm-HMPAO SPECT in suspected dementia. *Nuclear Medicine Communications*, 12: 757–765.

Lippa, C. F., Duda, J. E., Grossman, M., Hurtig, H. I., Aarsland, D., Boeve, B. F. et al. (2007). DLB and PDD boundary issues: diagnosis, treatment, molecular pathology, and biomarkers. *Neurology*, 68: 812–819.

Lobotesis, K., Fenwick, J. D., Phipps, A., Ryman, A., Swann, A., Ballard, C. et al. (2001). Occipital hypoperfusion on SPECT in dementia with Lewy bodies but not AD. *Neurology*, 56: 643–649.

Masterman, D. L., Mendez, M. F., Fairbanks, L. A., and Cummings, J. L. (1997). Sensitivity, specificity, and positive predictive value of technetium 99-HMPAO SPECT in discriminating Alzheimer's disease from other dementias. *Journal of Geriatric Psychiatry and Neurology*, 10: 15–21.

McKeith, I., OBrien, J., Walker, Z., Tatsch, K., Booij, J., Darcourt, J. et al. (2007). Sensitivity and specificity of dopamine transporter imaging with 123I-FP-CIT SPECT in dementia with Lewy bodies: a phase III, multicentre study. *Lancet Neurology*, 6: 305–313.

McNeill, R., Sare, G. M., Manoharan, M., Testa, H. J., Mann, D. M., Neary, D. et al. (2007). Accuracy of single-photon emission computed tomography in differentiating frontotemporal dementia from Alzheimer's disease. *Journal of Neurology, Neurosurgery, and Psychiatry*, 78: 350–355.

Mielke, R., and Heiss, W. D. (1998). Positron emission tomography for diagnosis of Alzheimer's disease and vascular dementia. *Journal of Neural Transmission. Supplementum*, 53: 237–250.

Minoshima, S., Foster, N. L., Sima, A. A., Frey, K. A., Albin, R. L., and Kuhl, D. E. (2001). Alzheimer's disease versus dementia with Lewy bodies: cerebral metabolic distinction with autopsy confirmation. *Annals of Neurology*, 50: 358–365.

Mito, Y., Yoshida, K., Yabe, I., Makino, K., Hirotani, M., Tashiro, K. et al. (2005). Brain 3D-SSP SPECT analysis in dementia with Lewy bodies, Parkinson's disease with and without dementia, and Alzheimer's disease. *Clinical Neurology and Neurosurgery*, 107: 396–403.

Nestor, P. J., Graham, N. L., Fryer, T. D., Williams, G. B., Patterson, K., Hodges, J. R. (2003). Progressive non-fluent aphasia is associated with hypometabolism centred on the left anterior insula. *Brain*, 126: 2406–2418.

Newberg, A. B., Mozley, P. D., Sadek, A. H., Grossman, M., and Alavi A. (2000). Regional cerebral distribution of [Tc-99m] hexylmethylpropylene amineoxine in patients with progressive aphasia. *Journal of Neuroimaging*, 10: 162–168.

O'Brien, J. T., Colloby, S., Fenwick, J., Williams, E. D., Firbank, M., Burn, D. et al. (2004). Dopamine transporter loss visualized with FP-CIT SPECT in the differential diagnosis of dementia with Lewy bodies. *Archives of Neurology*, 61: 919–925.

Oyanagi, C., Katsumi, Y., Hanakawa, T., Hayashi, T., Thuy, D. D., Hashikawa, K. et al. (2002). Comparison of striatal dopamine D2 receptors in Parkinson's disease and progressive supranuclear palsy patients using [123I] iodobenzofuran single-photon emission computed tomography. *Journal of Neuroimaging*, 12: 316–324.

Pasquier, J., Michel, B. F., Brenot-Rossi, I., Hassan-Sebbag, N., Sauvan, R., Gastaut, J. L. (2002). Value of (99m)Tc-ECD SPET for the diagnosis of dementia with Lewy bodies. *European Journal of Nuclear Medicine and Molecular Imaging*, 29: 1342–1348.

Pickut, B. A., Saerens, J., Marien, P., Borggreve, F., Goeman, J., Vandevivere, J. et al. (1997). Discriminative use of SPECT in frontal lobe-type dementia versus (senile) dementia of the Alzheimer's type. *Journal of Nuclear Medicine*, 38: 929–934.

Pirker, W., Asenbaum, S., Bencsits, G., Prayer, D., Gerschlager, W., Deecke, L. et al. (2000). [123I]beta-CIT SPECT in multiple system atrophy, progressive supranuclear palsy, and corticobasal degeneration. *Movement Disorders*, 15: 1158–1167.

Rabinovici, G. D., Furst, A. J., O'Neil, J. P., Racine, C. A., Mormino, E. C., Baker, S. L. et al. (2007). 11C-PIB PET imaging in Alzheimer disease and frontotemporal lobar degeneration. *Neurology*, 68: 1205–1212.

Salmon, E., Garraux, G., Delbeuck, X., Collette, F., Kalbe, E., Zuendorf, G. et al. (2003). Predominant ventromedial frontopolar metabolic impairment in frontotemporal dementia. *Neuroimage*, 20: 435–440.

Scarmeas, N., Habeck, C. G., Zarahn, E., Anderson, K. E., Park, A., Hilton, J. et al. (2004). Covariance PET patterns in early Alzheimer's disease and subjects with cognitive impairment but no dementia: Utility in group discrimination and correlations with functional performance. *Neuroimage*, 23: 35–45.

Seppi, K., Scherfler, C., Donnemiller, E., Virgolini, I., Schocke, M. F., Goebel, G. et al. (2006). Topography of dopamine transporter availability in progressive supranuclear palsy: a voxelwise [123I]beta-CIT SPECT analysis. *Archives of Neurology*, 63: 1154–60.

Shim, Y. S., Yang, D. W., Kim, B. S., Shon, Y. M., and Chung, Y. A. (2006). Comparison of regional cerebral blood flow in two subsets of subcortical ischemic vascular dementia: Statistical parametric mapping analysis of SPECT. *Journal of the Neurological Sciences*, 250: 85–91.

Shimizu, S., Hanyu, H., Kanetaka, H., Iwamoto, T., Koizumi, K., and Abe K. (2005). Differentiation of dementia with Lewy bodies from Alzheimer's disease using brain SPECT. *Dementia and Geriatric Cognitive Disorders*, 20: 25–30.

Shinotoh, H., Namba, H., Yamaguchi, M., Fukushi, K., Nagatsuka, S., Iyo, M., et al. (1999). Positron emission tomographic measurement of acetylcholinesterase activity reveals differential loss of ascending cholinergic systems in Parkinson's disease and progressive supranuclear palsy. *Annals of Neurology*, 46: 62–69.

Signorini, M., Paulesu, E., Friston, K., Perani, D., Colleluori, A., Lucignani, G. et al. (1999). Rapid assessment of regional cerebral metabolic abnormalities in single subjects with quantitative and nonquantitative [18F]FDG PET: A clinical validation of statistical parametric mapping. *Neuroimage*, 9: 63–80.

Silverman, D. H., Small, G. W., Chang, C. Y., Lu, C. S., Kung De Aburto, M. A., Chen, W. et al. (2001). Positron emission tomography in evaluation of dementia: Regional brain metabolism and long-term outcome. *The Journal of the American Medical Association*, 286: 2120–2127.

Sjogren, M., Gustafson, L., Wikkelso, C., and Wallin A. (2000). Frontotemporal dementia can be distinguished from Alzheimer's disease and subcortical white matter dementia by an anterior-to-posterior rCBF-SPET ratio. *Dementia and Geriatric Cognitive Disorders*, 11: 275–285.

Small, G. W., Kepe, V., and Barrio, J. R. (2006a). Seeing is believing: neuroimaging adds to our understanding of cerebral pathology. *Current Opinion in Psychiatry*, 19: 564–569.

Small, G. W., Kepe, V., Ercoli, L. M., Siddarth, P., Bookheimer, S. Y., Miller, K. J., et al. (2006b). PET of brain amyloid and tau in mild cognitive impairment. *The New England Journal of Medicine*, 355: 2652–2663.

Spampinato, U., Habert, M. O., Mas, J. L., Bourdel, M. C., Ziegler, M., de Recondo, J. et al. (1991). (99mTc)-HM-PAO SPECT and cognitive impairment in Parkinson's disease: a comparison with dementia of the Alzheimer type. *Journal of Neurology, Neurosurgery, and Psychiatry*, 54: 787–792.

Staffen, W., Trinka, E., Iglseder, B., Pilz, P., Homann, N., and Ladurner G. (1997). Clinical and diagnostic findings in a patient with Creutzfeldt-Jakob disease (type Heidenhain). *Journal of Neuroimaging*, 7: 50–54.

Stoppe, G., Staedt, J., Kogler, A., Schutze, R., Kunert, H. J., Sandrock, D. et al. (1995). 99mTc-HMPAO-SPECT in the diagnosis of senile dementia of Alzheimer's type—a study under clinical routine conditions. *Journal of Neural Transmission. General Section*, 99: 195–211.

Talbot, P. R., Lloyd, J. J., Snowden, J. S., Neary, D., and Testa, H. J. (1998). A clinical role for 99mTc-HMPAO SPECT in the investigation of dementia? *Journal of Neurology, Neurosurgery, and Psychiatry*, 64: 306–313.

Talbot, P. R., Snowden, J. S., Lloyd, J. J., Neary, D., and Testa, H. J. (1995). The contribution of single photon emission tomography to the clinical differentiation of degenerative cortical brain disorders. *Journal of Neurology*, 242: 579–586.

Testa, H. J., Snowden, J. S., Neary, D., Shields, R. A., Burjan, A. W., Prescott, M. C. et al. (1988). The use of [99mTc]-HM-PAO in the diagnosis of primary degenerative dementia. *Journal of Cerebral Blood Flow and Metabolism*, 8: S123–S126.

Van Laere, K., Casteels, C., De Ceuninck, L., Vanbilloen, B., Maes, A., Mortelmans, L. et al. (2006). Dual-tracer dopamine transporter and perfusion SPECT in differential diagnosis of parkinsonism using template-based discriminant analysis. *Journal of Nuclear Medicine*, 47: 384–392.

Vander Borght, T., Minoshima, S., Giordani, B., Foster, N. L., Frey, K. A., Berent, S. et al. (1997). Cerebral metabolic differences in Parkinsons and Alzheimers diseases matched for dementia severity. *Journal of Nuclear Medicine*, 38: 797–802.

Velakoulis, D. and Lloyd, J. H. (1998). The role of SPECT scanning in a neuropsychiatry unit. *The Australian and New Zealand Journal of Psychiatry*, 32: 511–522.

Walker, Z., Costa, D. C., Janssen, A. G., Walker, R. W., Livingstone, G., Katona, C. L. (1997). Dementia with lewy bodies: a study of post-synaptic dopaminergic receptors with iodine-123 iodobenzamide single-photon emission tomography. *European Journal of Nuclear Medicine*, 24: 609–614.

Walker, Z., Costa, D. C., Walker, R. W., Shaw, K., Gacinovic, S., Stevens, T. et al. (2002). Differentiation of dementia with Lewy bodies from Alzheimer's disease using a dopaminergic presynaptic ligand. *Journal of Neurology, Neurosurgery, and Psychiatry*, 73: 134–140.

Weisman, D. and McKeith, I. (2007). Dementia with Lewy bodies. *Seminars in Neurology*, 27: 42–47.

Yoshita, M. (1998). Differentiation of idiopathic Parkinson's disease from striatonigral degeneration and progressive supranuclear palsy using iodine-123 meta-iodobenzylguanidine myocardial scintigraphy. *Journal of Neurological Sciences*, 155: 60–67.

Yoshita, M., Taki, J., and Yamada, M. (2001). A clinical role for [(123)I]MIBG myocardial scintigraphy in the distinction between dementia of the Alzheimer's-type and dementia with Lewy bodies. *Journal of Neurology, Neurosurgery, and Psychiatry*, 71: 583–588.

Yoshita, M., Taki, J., Yokoyama, K., Noguchi-Shinohara, M., Matsumoto, Y., Nakajima, K. et al. (2006). Value of 123I-MIBG radioactivity in the differential diagnosis of DLB from AD. *Neurology*, 66: 1850–1854.

Zahn, R., Buechert, M., Overmans, J., Talazko, J., Specht, K., Ko, C. W. et al. (2005). Mapping of temporal and parietal cortex in progressive nonfluent aphasia and Alzheimer's disease using chemical shift imaging, voxel-based morphometry and positron emission tomography. *Psychiatry Research*, 140: 115–131.

Zhang, L., Murata, Y., Ishida, R., Saitoh, Y., Mizusawa, H., and Shibuya H. (2001). Differentiating between progressive supranuclear palsy and corticobasal degeneration by brain perfusion SPET. *Nuclear Medicine Communications*, 22: 767–772.

16

MRI and the Differential Diagnosis of Dementia

António J. Bastos-Leite and Philip Scheltens

Introduction

Structural neuroimaging with either computed tomography (CT) or magnetic resonance (MR) imaging is recommended for the initial evaluation of patients with dementia (Knopman et al., 2001), and is being increasingly used to support the clinical diagnosis beyond the traditional exclusionary approach (Scheltens et al., 2002).

Alzheimer's disease (AD) is the most common cause of dementia, with prevalence rates higher than 40% at the age of 85 (Evans et al., 1989), but a large proportion of patients with dementia have a combination of different types of pathology in the brain (Esiri et al., 1999; Heyman et al., 1998; Holmes et al., 1999; Hulette et al., 1997; Ince et al., 1991; Kalaria and Ballard, 1999; Lim et al., 1999; MRC CFAS, 2001; Snowdon et al., 1997). Vascular dementia (VaD), dementia with Lewy bodies (DLB), Parkinson disease with dementia (PDD), frontotemporal lobar degeneration (FTLD), and some rare atypical parkinsonian syndromes are the other most well-known causes of dementia next to AD.

Although there are established clinical criteria for the diagnosis of diseases causing dementia (McKeith et al., 1996; McKhann et al., 1984; Neary et al., 1998; Roman et al., 1993), the definite diagnosis was always believed to be histopathological. However, there are considerable discrepancies between different postmortem pathological criteria that render postmortem diagnosis less a "gold standard" than previously assumed (Nagy et al., 1998; Polvikoski et al., 2001). Clinical information is always needed for a correct classification and should always lead the diagnostic process. Next to this, neuroimaging plays a very useful role by helping to depict underlying pathology (see Chapter 3 for a discussion of the Neuropathology of Aging).

Currently, brain atrophy and cerebrovascular disease are the two most important characteristics in the evaluation of dementia by means of structural neuroimaging. MR is currently the preferred imaging modality for dementia. T1-weighted images (T1-WI) are needed to detect brain atrophy, especially in the medial temporal lobe, for which coronal high-resolution images are required. For the detection of cerebrovascular pathology, the MR imaging protocol should also include axial T2-weighted images (T2-WI), axial fluid-attenuated inversion recovery (FLAIR) or proton density-weighted images (PD-WI), and axial gradient-echo T2*-weighted images (T2*-WI). T2*-WI are particularly useful in detecting microbleeds (Bastos Leite, Scheltens, and Barkhof, 2004a).

Alzheimer's Disease

Because neuropathological changes underlying late-onset AD first occur in the medial temporal lobe (Braak and Braak, 1991), structural neuroimaging in AD has been focused on the detection of medial temporal lobe atrophy (MTA), particularly of the hippocampus, parahippocampal gyrus (including the entorhinal cortex), and amygdala. MR and CT are indeed sensitive to MTA in AD (de Leon et al., 1989; Kido et al., 1989; Seab et al., 1988), correlating with Alzheimer pathology at postmortem (Bobinski et al., 2000; Davis et al., 1995). MTA can be assessed by using visual rating scales (Scheltens et al., 1992a), linear measurements of temporal lobe structures (Bastos-Leite et al., 2006a; Frisoni et al., 1996; Jobst et al., 1992), and volumetry of the hippocampus (Jack et al., 1992). The most well-known visual rating scale for MTA (Scheltens et al., 1992a) is based on the evaluation of the choroidal fissure width, the temporal horn width, and the hippocampal height (Table 16.1) using coronal high resolution T1-WI perpendicular to the long axis of the temporal lobe (Figure 16.1). It is easily applicable in clinical practice, but slightly observer-dependent (Scheltens et al., 1995). MTA scores of 2 or less are not frequently associated with dementia (Barkhof et al., 2007). The fimbriosubicular distance is a linear measurement that enables evaluation of the hippocampal sulcus width (Figure 16.2), and complements the visual rating scale for MTA (Bastos-Leite et al., 2006a). Linear measurements of the temporal horn width can be used in routine clinical settings, and have the advantage of being applicable both to CT and MR (Frisoni et al., 1996, 2002). Volumetric analyses are time-consuming and therefore not well-suited for clinical practice (Wahlund et al., 1999).

Besides the existence of MTA, the most important structural imaging feature of AD is the progression of hippocampal atrophy. Jack et al. (1998) have found a yearly decline in hippocampal volume that is approximately 2.5 times greater in patients with AD than in normal-aged subjects, and a relation that exists between memory loss and hippocampal damage across the spectrum from normal aging to dementia (Petersen et al., 2000). Visual rating scales are relatively insensitive to changes of hippocampal volume over time. In addition, the corresponding neuroanatomical changes may be too mild, diffuse, or topographically complex to be detected even by manually traced measurements of regions of interest. New serial volumetric imaging techniques developed in the past few years

Table 16–1   Visual rating scale for medial temporal lobe atrophy.

Score	Width of Choroidal Fissure	Width of Temporal Horn	Height of Hippocampus
0	Normal	Normal	Normal
1	↑	Normal	Normal
2	↑↑	↑	↓
3	↑↑↑	↑↑	↓↓
4	↑↑↑	↑↑↑	↓↓↓

↑ = increased, ↓ = decreased. Reproduced with permission of Scheltens et al. (1992a).

represent an added value in identifying the progression of MTA (Barnes et al., 2007; Crum et al., 2001; Ridha et al., 2007). Additionally, they can be used to detect neocortical changes (Fox et al., 2001).

Global brain volume changes can be accurately determined cross-sectionally by using voxel-based morphometry (VBM)—a voxel-wise, fully automated, and unbiased technique that enables comparisons of the local brain tissue concentration between groups of subjects (Ashburner and Friston, 2000). Besides the typical volume loss occurring in temporal lobe structures, VBM shows that patients with AD have global cortical atrophy (with relative sparing of the sensorimotor cortex, occipital poles, and cerebellum), as well as atrophy of the caudate nuclei and medial thalami (Karas et al., 2003).

AD typically occurs in elderly patients, but it may also develop at earlier ages, either sporadically or as a familial autosomal dominant inherited disorder. Patients with early-onset AD tend to present with complaints other than memory impairment, which apparently reflects a different distribution of the underlying pathology. In fact, patients with early-onset sporadic AD have greater neocortical atrophy at the temporoparietal junction, but less hippocampal atrophy, than patients with late-onset AD (Frisoni et al., 2005). Disproportionate precuneus atrophy (Figure 16.3) is also more prominent in patients with early-onset sporadic AD (Karas et al., 2007).

Alzheimer's Disease with Cerebrovascular Disease and Other Pathologies

The most frequent combination of brain pathology in dementia is that which occurs between degenerative and vascular pathology (Esiri et al., 1999; Heyman et al., 1998; Holmes et al., 1999; Hulette et al., 1997; Kalaria and Ballard, 1999; Lim et al., 1999; MRC CFAS, 2001; Snowdon et al., 1997), but there are also combinations among different types of degenerative pathology—namely between Alzheimer pathology and Lewy bodies (Holmes et al., 1999; Ince et al., 1991; Lim et al., 1999). Additional pathologies in AD can lower the threshold for dementia or increase its severity, and may represent an independent target for treatment.

Neuroimaging is very useful for the diagnosis of both large and small-vessel disease. Small-vessel disease is frequently not suspected clinically (Lopez et al., 1995; Massoud et al., 2000) and more often associated with dementia than large-vessel disease (Esiri, 2000). White and deep gray matter hyperintensities on T2-WI, FLAIR images, and PD-WI are generally considered as a surrogate marker of ischemic small-vessel disease

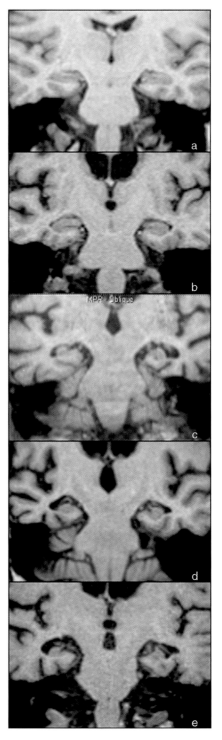

Figure 16–1   Coronal high-resolution T1-weighted images perpendicular to the long axis of the temporal lobe, showing the different degrees of medial temporal lobe atrophy (MTA), according to the visual rating scale proposed by Scheltens et al. (1992c): (a) absence of atrophy (MTA = 0); (b) minimal atrophy (MTA = 1); (c) mild atrophy on the right side (MTA = 2); severe atrophy on the left (MTA = 4); (d) moderate atrophy (MTA = 3); and (e) severe atrophy (MTA = 4).

in elderly subjects (Fazekas et al., 1987; Scheltens et al., 1992b) (see also Chapter 17). An example of a lacune is shown in Figure 16.4.

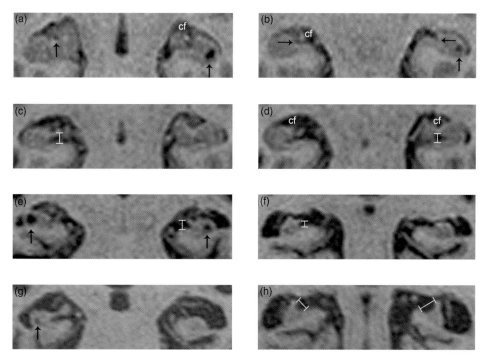

Figure 16–2 Magnified coronal high-resolution T1-weighted images (T1-WI) of the hippocampal region.

A and B: Coronal T1-WI of a 68-year old nondemented control showing discrete enlargement of the choroidal fissures (CF), suggesting grade 1 medial temporal lobe atrophy (MTA), and hippocampal cavities bilaterally (vertical arrows). Note that both hippocampal sulci are not enlarged (horizontal arrows).

C and D: Coronal T1-WI of a 54-year old patient with Alzheimer's disease (AD) showing enlargement of the hippocampal sulcus, measured between the fimbria and the subiculum (vertical measurement overlays), and enlargement of the choroidal fissures (CF) (MTA, grade 1).

E and F: Coronal T1-WI of a 76-year old patient with AD showing enlargement of the hippocampal sulcus (vertical measurement overlays), moderate to severe MTA (grade 3) and hippocampal cavities bilaterally (vertical arrows).

G and H: Coronal T1-WI of a 93-year old patient with AD showing severe MTA (grade 4), and a small hippocampal cavity on the right side (vertical arrow). Note that the fimbria appears laterally displaced. This displacement contributes to an increase of the fimbriosubicular distance (oblique measurement overlays).

Figure 16–3 Voxel-based mophometry clusters showing areas of brain atrophy in patients with early-onset sporadic Alzheimer's disease. The region with more pronounced atrophy (in orange-red) corresponds to the precuneus (courtesy of Giorgos Karas).

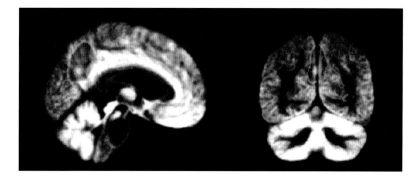

Dementia with Lewy Bodies and Parkinson's Disease with Dementia

Dementia with Lewy bodies (DLB) is currently considered the second most common type of degenerative dementia, and is characterized by an often rapidly progressive clinical syndrome, including fluctuations in cognitive functioning and spontaneous "parkinsonism." The precise nosological relationship between DLB, AD, and Parkinson's disease with dementia (PDD) are not yet completely clarified (McKeith et al., 1996, 2004). When fully developed, DLB and PDD overlap both clinically and pathologically. If the previous history is unknown, patients with each of these disorders may be indistinguishable (Emre, 2003; McKeith et al., 2004).

Structural MR imaging studies involving patients with DLB have focused on the differential diagnosis between DLB and other types of dementia. Studies comparing patients with DLB, AD, VaD, and healthy elderly controls have found that, although MTA is more frequent and severe in all dementia groups than in controls, patients with DLB have significantly lower MTA scores and larger temporal lobe, hippocampal, and amygdala volumes than those with AD. Therefore, in spite of the absence of a specific pattern of brain atrophy in DLB, the absence of MTA may be a useful finding to differentiate patients with DLB from

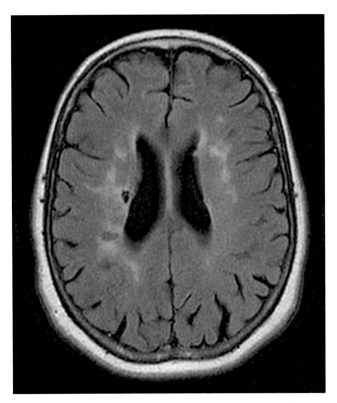

Figure 16–4 Axial fluid-attenuated inversion recovery image of a patient with vascular cognitive impairment showing a right-sided lacune within an area of high signal intensity next to the ventricle.

patients with AD (Barber et al., 1999, 2000; Burton et al., 2002). Conversely, atrophy of the putamen is a feature suggestive of DLB, but not of AD (Cousins et al., 2003). Very recently, a pattern of relatively focused atrophy of the midbrain, hypothalamus, and substantia innominata was also observed in patients with DLB (Whitwell et al., 2007), which may better reflect the distribution of the underlying pathology.

Whereas PDD was claimed not to be associated with a specific pattern of MR imaging abnormalities (Huber et al., 1989), Laakso et al. (1996) have found severe hippocampal atrophy in patients with PDD, which is surprising considering the aforementioned resemblance between PDD and DLB. One explanation for this finding may be that the included patients with PDD had coexistent Alzheimer's pathology. However, more recent studies have suggested that the pattern of gray matter volume loss in PDD is different from AD, and more closely resembles the pattern of atrophy observed in DLB (Burton et al., 2004), but there are still discrepancies concerning the severity of brain atrophy between studies comparing PDD with DLB (Beyer et al., 2007; Burton et al., 2004).

Frontotemporal Lobar Degeneration

Frontotemporal lobar degeneration (FTLD) accounts for a substantial proportion of cases with primary degenerative dementia occurring before the age of 65 years. Clinical criteria proposed by Neary et al. (1998) discern three main prototypic syndromes—frontotemporal dementia (FTD), progressive nonfluent aphasia (PNFA), and semantic dementia (SD), also known as progressive

fluent aphasia or a temporal variant of FTLD. In addition to the sporadic form, there are also familial cases of FTLD, often linked to chromosome 17 abnormalities.

Neuroimaging studies in patients with clinical and pathological diagnosis of FTLD may show a pattern of marked anterior temporal and frontal atrophy, resulting in the so-called "knife edge" appearance and dilatation (ballooning) of the temporal and frontal horns of the lateral ventricles (Figure 16.5), in some cases associated with predominantly frontal white matter changes (Knopman et al., 1989; Larsson et al., 2000). Characteristically, FTLD primarily affects the temporal pole, but relatively spares the posterior part of the hippocampus (Laakso et al., 2000).

Asymmetric atrophy is also a distinctive feature of FTLD—particularly of SD and PNFA. Selective inferolateral and anterior left temporal lobe atrophy is characteristic of SD. In PNFA, atrophy appears to be more diffuse and involves the left frontal and perisylvian structures (Abe et al., 1997; Chan et al., 2001; Hodges, 2001; Hodges and Patterson, 1996). One variant of FTLD affecting the right temporal lobe presents with progressive prosopagnosia (Hodges, 2001).

Because hypoperfusion or hypometabolism may precede volume loss, the previously mentioned patterns of atrophy may not be found in early cases. Therefore, functional studies are useful to detect FTLD at an early stage of disease progression (Rombouts et al., 2003) (See also Chapter 15).

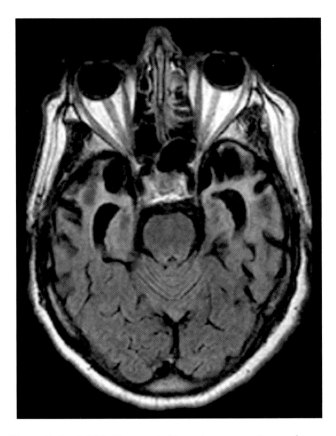

Figure 16–5 Axial fluid-attenuated inversion recovery image of a patient with frontotemporal dementia, showing severe anterior temporal lobe atrophy with a "knife edge" appearance, dilatation of the temporal horns of the lateral ventricles, and anterior temporal subcortical hyperintensity.

Dementia and Atypical Parkinsonian Syndromes

Characteristic findings on routine MR imaging can contribute to the identification of atypical parkinsonian syndromes (Savoiardo et al., 1989; Schrag et al., 2000) associated with dementia (Grimes et al., 1999; Litvan et al., 1996). Asymmetric atrophy involving the posterior frontal and parietal regions contralateral to the clinically most-affected side occurs in the vast majority of patients with corticobasal degeneration (CBD). Mild signal changes on FLAIR and PD-WI in the atrophic cortex have been described in some of these patients. Despite the existence of pathological changes in the basal ganglia, MR imaging abnormalities of these structures were almost never reported (Savoiardo, Grisoli, and Girotti, 2000).

Midbrain atrophy (Figure 16.6) and diffuse hyperintensity on T2-WI in the mesencephalic tegmentum and tectum occur in progressive supranuclear palsy (PSP), due to predominance of tau pathology in these regions (Aiba et al., 1997; Yagishita and Oda, 1996). Midbrain atrophy can be simply and accurately assessed by measuring the antero-posterior diameter of the midbrain on axial T2-WI or T1-WI. Midbrain atrophy is considered to be present when the anteroposterior diameter of the mesencephalon is <15 mm (Schrag et al., 2000; Warmuth-Metz et al., 2001), but visual inspection using sagittal T1-WI should also be done, because when there is midbrain atrophy, the mesencephalic caudo-cranial dimension is reduced and the floor of the third ventricle appears more superiorly concave than normal (Savoiardo et al., 1989, 2000)—a shape that resembles the bill of a hummingbird (Kato et al., 2003). Besides infratentorial abnormalities, VBM and serial volumetric imaging studies have also shown a distinct pattern of mesio-frontal atrophy in PSP (Brenneis et al., 2004; Paviour et al., 2004).

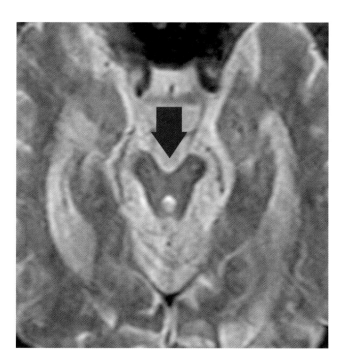

Figure 16–6   Axial T2-weighted image showing midbrain atrophy (arrow) and the consequent dilatation of the cerebral aqueduct.

Vascular Dementia

VaD is the second most common type of dementia (Roman et al., 2002). The most specific diagnostic criteria for VaD are the National Institute of Neurological Disorders and Stroke (NINDS)-Association Internationale pour la Recherche et l'Enseignement en Neurosciences (AIREN) criteria. These criteria emphasize the heterogeneity of both clinical syndromes and pathological subtypes of VaD, the need to establish a temporal relation between stroke and the onset of dementia, and the importance of brain imaging to support clinical findings (Roman et al., 1993). Because the NINDS-AIREN criteria consider structural neuroimaging crucial for the diagnosis of VaD, operational definitions for the radiological part of these criteria were proposed, both in terms of topography and severity of lesions (Table 16.2) (van Straaten et al., 2003).

The main clinicopathological subtypes of VaD are large-vessel and small-vessel disease (Roman et al., 2002), the latter being more prevalent (Esiri, 2000). Large-vessel VaD results from vascular lesions located in strategic regions of the brain, such as the hippocampus, paramedian thalamus, and the thalamocortical networks. Small-vessel VaD may either result from multiple subcortical lacunar infarcts, bilateral thalamic lesions, or from diffuse white matter lesions. Subcortical ischemic small-vessel VaD is currently recognized as the most broad and homogeneous subtype of VaD (Erkinjuntti et al., 2000). Binswanger's disease and cerebral autosomal dominant arteriopathy with subcortical infarcts and leucoencephalopathy (CADASIL) are examples of clinical entities representing subcortical ischemic small-vessel VaD. Cerebral amyloid angiopathies (CAA) are considered to be subtypes of cortical-subcortical small-vessel disease, but they have associated large-vessel pathology as well. Both CADASIL and some forms of CAA have a genetic basis (Roman et al., 2002). Finally, deep venous thrombosis and dural arteriovenous fistulae are vascular abnormalities that may rarely cause venous hypertensive encephalopathy or bilateral thalamic congestion, and lead to dementia (Hurst et al., 1998; Krolak-Salmon et al., 2002; Tanaka et al., 1999).

T2-weighted MR sequences are far more sensitive for depicting cerebrovascular disease than CT (Wahlund et al., 2001), although CT was found to be more specific than MR in predicting subsequent symptomatic cerebrovascular disease (Lopez et al., 1995). In addition, the sensitivity of T2-WI for depicting thalamic lesions is superior to FLAIR and, given the well-known clinical relevance of these lesions, FLAIR should not be used as the only T2-weighted sequence to detect thalamic lesions in patients suspected of having VaD (Bastos Leite et al., 2004b).

Infarcts may either be complete or incomplete. Complete infarcts correspond to areas of tissue destruction, whereas incomplete infarcts may only represent demyelination and edema. Hypointensity on T1-WI usually represents tissue destruction, and may thus be considered as a surrogate marker for complete infarcts. Therefore, lesions hyperintense on T2-WI and isointense on T1-WI may just correspond to demyelination (Fazekas et al., 1991; Udaka, Sawada, and, Kameyam, 2002). FLAIR has the additional advantage of easily identifying cystic lesions (Barkhof and Scheltens, 2002), and the combination of FLAIR with T1-WI may be useful in differentiating the more aggressive lesions from those that might have less power to cause cognitive impairment.

Complete infarcts of deep small vessels are defined as lacunar infarcts, and some authors consider this definition also dependent on size (from 2–3 to 15–20 mm in diameter) (Fisher, 1982; Loeb, 1995; Roman et al., 2002). Enlarged perivascular (Virchow-Robin)

Table 16–2   Operational definitions for the imaging guidelines of the National Institute of Neurological Disorders and Stroke (NINDS)—Association Internationale pour la Recherche et l'Enseignement en Neurosciences (AIREN) Criteria for Vascular Dementia (VaD).

Topography

Large-vessel stroke—arterial territorial infarct involving the cortical gray matter

- Anterior cerebral artery (ACA)—only bilateral ACA infarcts are sufficient to meet the NINDS-AIREN criteria
- Posterior cerebral artery (PCA)—infarcts in the PCA territory can only be included when they involve the following regions:

  1. Paramedian thalamus
  2. Inferior medial temporal lobe

- Association areas—a middle cerebral artery (MCA) infarct needs to involve the following regions:

  1. Parietotemporal (e.g., angular gyrus)
  2. Temporo-occipital

- Watershed territories—an infarct occurring in a watershed territory (between MCA and ACA or between MCA and PCA) needs to involve the following regions:

  1. Superior frontal region
  2. Parietal region

Small-vessel disease

- Ischemic pathology resulting from occlusion of small perforating arteries may become apparent as white matter lesions or as deep small-vessel infarcts (e.g., lacunar infarcts):

  1. White matter lesions
  2. Multiple basal ganglia, thalamic, and frontal white matter lacunar infarcts—the criteria are met when there are at least two lacunar infarcts in the basal ganglia, thalamus or internal capsule, and at least two lacunar infarcts in the frontal white matter
  3. Bilateral thalamic lesions

Severity

- Large-vessel disease of the dominant hemisphere—if there is a large-vessel infarct, the criteria are only met when the infarct is located in the dominant hemisphere. In the absence of clinical information, the left hemisphere is considered dominant
- Bilateral large-vessel hemispheric strokes—the infarct located in the non-dominant hemisphere should involve an area listed under topography. The infarct located in the dominant hemisphere does not need to meet the topography criteria
- Extensive white matter lesions or leukoencephalopathy involving at least ¼ of the total white matter. Extensive white matter lesions are considered to involve at least ¼ of the total white matter when they are confluent—grade 3 in the age-related white matter changes (ARWMC) scale (Wahlund et al., 2001)—in at least two regions, and beginning confluent—grade 2 in the ARWMC scale—in two other regions. A lesion is considered confluent when it measures >20 mm or it consists of ≥2 smaller lesions fused by connecting bridges

Fulfillment of radiological criteria for probable VaD

- Large-vessel disease—a lesion must be scored in at least one subsection of both topography and severity (both the topography and severity criteria should be met)
- Small-vessel disease—for white matter lesions, both the topography and severity criteria should be met; for multiple lacunar infarcts and bilateral thalamic lesions, only the topography criterion is sufficient

Modified with permission of van Straaten et al. (2003).

spaces correspond to extensions of the subarachnoid space around small vessels. Misclassification of different cystic lacunar infarcts and enlarged Virchow-Robin spaces may therefore occur, but most of the enlarged Virchow-Robin spaces measure <2 mm and normally surround perforating arteries entering the striatum at the anterior perforated substance (Bokura et al., 1998; Braffman et al., 1988). Their appearance in large numbers reflects focal brain atrophy around blood vessels and may lead to the so-called *état criblé*, especially in the basal ganglia (Awad et al., 1986; Braffman et al., 1988; Poirier and Derouesne, 1985) (see Figure 16.7). Moreover, the association of enlarged Virchow-Robin spaces and white matter lesions with cognitive impairment occurs (Maclullich et al., 2004), and widening of Virchow-Robin spaces can be considered to be a measure of focal atrophy (Barkhof, 2004).

As previously mentioned, white and deep gray matter hyperintensities on T2-WI, FLAIR images, and PD-WI are generally considered to be a surrogate marker of ischemic small-vessel disease in elderly subjects (Fazekas et al., 1987; Scheltens et al., 1992b). Since the occurrence of white matter hyperintensities (WMH) increases progressively with age, they are usually referred to as age-related white matter changes. Moreover, they are associated with vascular risk factors, as well as with other types of cerebrovascular disease (Breteler et al., 1994; Lindgren et al., 1994; Longstreth, et al., 1996). Since the original visual rating scale of Fazekas et al. (1987), several others have been proposed for rating WMH. Currently, the most complete is that proposed by Wahlund et al. (2001), applicable both to CT and MR imaging. However, recently published vascular cognitive impairment harmonization standards recommend volumetric measurements—normalized for head size and taking into account gender effects—to quantify WMH (Hachinski et al., 2006). According to the NINDS-AIREN criteria, white matter changes alone may be sufficient to cause dementia when at least one quarter of the white matter is involved (Roman et al., 1993). Although this proportion has been defined arbitrarily, it is in accordance with the finding that only severe white matter disease is associated with cognitive dysfunction (Boone et al., 1992). Extensive and diffuse white matter changes affecting predominantly deep and periventricular white matter, but relatively sparing the U-fibers, occur in Binswanger disease (Roman et al., 2002).

In patients with CADASIL, diffuse white matter signal changes involving the U-fibers occur mainly in the temporal, temporopolar, and frontal regions (Figure 16.8) (Auer et al., 2001;

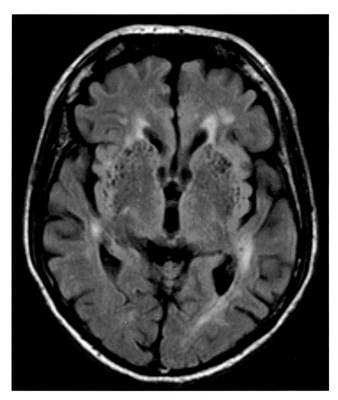

Figure 16–7 Axial fluid-attenuated inversion recovery image showing the typical état criblé in the basal ganglia.

Such a relation may be expected when patients are young and it is unlikely they have associated Alzheimer's pathology—when cognitive functions are normal before stroke, impaired immediately after, and do not worsen over time, when vascular lesions are located in strategic regions, and when well-defined vasculopathies known to cause dementia are proven, such as CADASIL or CAA (Leys et al., 1999; Pasquier and Leys, 1997). In other circumstances, it is possible that both degenerative and vascular pathology may contribute to cognitive impairment. A study of a large sample of patients fulfilling the NINDS-AIREN criteria, rigorously screened for fulfillment of the corresponding radiological criteria according to operational definitions, have shown that more than half of the patients with VaD have considerable MTA—a neuroimaging finding suggestive of degenerative pathology. In addition, the study has shown that both MTA and large-vessel disease contribute to global cognitive impairment, whereas the effect of small-vessel disease contributes only to executive dysfunction (Bastos-Leite et al., 2007). Another study of a subsample of the same population has shown that approximately 10% of patients fulfilling diagnostic criteria for VaD have midbrain atrophy, which was found to be associated with cognitive impairment even after correction for abnormalities representing degenerative and vascular supratentorial pathology (Bastos Leite et al., 2006b). It is conceivable that midbrain atrophy represents concomitance of degenerative pathology (Parvizi et al., 2000), and that its occurrence in the periaqueductal gray matter may explain the association with cognitive impairment by disruption of mesencephalic connections and neurotransmitter systems.

Figure 16–8 Axial fluid-attenuated inversion recovery images of a patient with cerebral autosomal dominant arteriopathy with subcortical infarcts and leukoencephalopathy (CADASIL). The images show diffuse white matter hyperintensities involving the U-fibers, mainly in the temporal, temporopolar, and frontal regions.

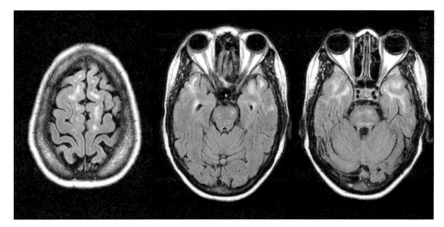

Skehan, Hutchinson, and MacErlaine, 1995; Yousry et al., 1999). Microbleeds, defined by some authors as hypointense foci (<5 mm) on T2-WI or gradient-echo T2*-WI (Fazekas et al., 1999; Offenbacher et al., 1996) are present in a considerable proportion of these patients, as well as in patients with CAA (Greenberg, Finklestein, and Schaefer, 1996; Lesnik Oberstein et al., 2001). However, the most typical feature of CAA is the occurrence of cortical-subcortical (lobar) hemorrhages (Greenberg, Finklestein, and Schaefer, 1996; Knudsen et al., 2001).

Given that vascular and degenerative pathology frequently coexist (Esiri et al., 1999; Heyman et al., 1998; Holmes et al., 1999; Hulette et al., 1997; Kalaria and Ballard, 1999; Lim et al., 1999; MRC CFAS, 2001; Snowdon et al., 1997), the causal relation between vascular lesions alone and dementia is not always clear.

Clinical Usefulness of MR Imaging in Other Types of Dementia

Multiple sclerosis (MS) is the most common inflammatory demyelinating disease, and occurs mainly in young people, but it may lead to cognitive dysfunction due to accumulation of white matter lesions, occurrence of cortical and juxtacortical lesions, and brain atrophy (Lazeron et al., 2000, 2005). The pattern of white matter signal abnormalities on MR is very useful for the differentiation between ischemic lesions and inflammatory demyelinating lesions. The most specific MR diagnostic criteria for MS were proposed by Barkhof et al. (1997), and a modification of them is currently included as part of the guidelines from the International Panel on the diagnosis of MS (McDonald et al., 2001). MR is also very useful for the diagnosis of other disorders that may lead to dementia and primarily affect white matter, such as herpes simplex encephalitis, human immunodeficiency virus encephalitis, and progressive multifocal leukoencephalopathy (Valk, Barkhof, and Scheltens, 2002).

MR may still show specific imaging patterns of atrophy or signal abnormalities in other disorders. Atrophy of the striatum, most conspicuous on visual inspection in the caudate nucleus, is typical of Huntington's disease (Valk, Barkhof, and Scheltens, 2002), although putaminal atrophy is a better predictor of disease onset in presymptomatic subjects (Harris et al., 1999). Rapidly progressive brain atrophy, as well as striatal and cortical hyperintensity on FLAIR, PD-WI, or T2-WI preceded by signal abnormalities on diffusion-weighted imaging (DWI) occur in patients with Creutzfeldt-Jakob disease (Collie et al., 2001; Demaerel et al., 1999; Finkenstaedt et al., 1996; Tribl et al., 2002). Additionally, in the new variant of Creutzfeldt-Jakob disease, bilateral hyperintensity of the pulvinar is a very specific imaging finding (Zeidler et al., 2000).

Normal pressure hydrocephalus (NPH) is a rare disorder that, even more rarely, allegedly causes dementia (Bradley, 2000). MR is the correct imaging modality to evaluate the pulsatile motion of cerebrospinal fluid (CSF) in the cerebral aqueduct—either visually, as a low intensity signal on T2-WI (flow void), or using quantitative phase-contrast measurements. In NPH, both flow void and phase-contrast measurements are increased due to reduced ventricular compliance (Barkhof et al., 1994; Bradley Kortman, and Burgoyne, 1986), and it seems that only when they are prominently increased there is prediction of a positive response to shunt therapy (Bradley et al., 1991a, 1996). Given the frequent coexistence of NPH with deep and periventricular white matter ischemic changes (Bradley, 2001; Bradley et al., 1991b), it is matter of controversy whether NPH alone represents a true disease entity causing dementia.

Limitations of the Existing Data and Future Perspectives

MR studies performed to investigate the value of MTA for the differential diagnosis of dementia did not find unequivocal results. O'Brien et al. (1997) carried out a study to determine the specificity of hippocampal atrophy for the differentiation between AD and other conditions associated with cognitive impairment, such as VaD and major depression. They have found that MTA ratings were useful to differentiate patients with AD from patients with other types of dementia. Conversely, Laakso et al. (1996) have found that hippocampal atrophy was not specific for differentiating patients with AD from patients with VaD or PDD, although they could not rule out the coexistence of Alzheimer's pathology in patients with VaD or PDD. Barber et al. (1999, 2000) have found different degrees of hippocampal atrophy occurring in AD, VaD, and DLB—the most severe in AD and the less severe in DLB. And although there was a trend toward less atrophy in DLB compared with VaD, no significant volumetric difference between these two groups was observed. Finally, within the FTLD subtypes, there are marked differences in the pattern of hippocampal atrophy—FTD and SD show bilateral hippocampal atrophy. In SD, the left hippocampus is smaller, even compared with patients with AD; and in PNFA, no significant hippocampal atrophy occurs (van de Pol et al., 2006).

The previously mentioned results may reflect, in part, the heterogeneity of the corresponding populations concerning disease severity; but may also reflect combinations of different types of pathology, and even differences in the distribution of pathology. In the future, it is expected that molecular imaging techniques will detect neuropathology before the occurrence of considerable brain atrophy, either by means of positron emission tomography, single photon emission computed tomography, or even with MR microscopy. Functional neuroimaging techniques may also detect the consequences of the underlying pathology at a microscopic level, which probably will help to identify persons at risk of developing dementia and reach earlier diagnoses, as well as better monitor the potential benefit of treatment.

References

Abe, K., Ukita, H., and Yanagihara, T. (1997). Imaging in primary progressive aphasia. *Neuroradiology*, 39: 556–559.

Aiba, I., Hashizume, Y., Yoshida, M., Okuda, S., Murakami, N., and Ujihira, N. (1997). Relationship between brainstem MRI and pathological findings in progressive supranuclear palsy—study in autopsy cases. *Journal of the Neurological Sciences*, 152: 210–217.

Ashburner, J. and Friston, K. J. (2000). Voxel-based morphometry—the methods. *Neuroimage*, 11: 805–821.

Auer, D. P., Putz, B., Gossl, C., Elbel, G., Gasser, T., and Dichgans, M. (2001). Differential lesion patterns in CADASIL and sporadic subcortical arteriosclerotic encephalopathy: MR imaging study with statistical parametric group comparison. *Radiology*, 218: 443–451.

Awad, I. A., Johnson, P. C., Spetzler, R. F., and Hodak, J. A. (1986). Incidental subcortical lesions identified on magnetic resonance imaging in the elderly. II. Postmortem pathological correlations. *Stroke*, 17: 1090–1097.

Barber, R., Gholkar, A., Scheltens, P., Ballard, C., and McKeith, I. G. (1999). O'Brien JT. Medial temporal lobe atrophy on MRI in dementia with Lewy bodies. *Neurology*, 52: 1153–1158.

Barber, R., Ballard, C., McKeith, I. G., and Gholkar, A. (2000). O'Brien JT. MRI volumetric study of dementia with Lewy bodies: A comparison with AD and vascular dementia. *Neurology*, 54: 1304–1309.

Barkhof, F., Kouwenhoven, M., Scheltens, P., Sprenger, M., Algra, P., and Valk, J. (1994). Phase-contrast cine MR imaging of normal aqueductal CSF flow. Effect of aging and relation to CSF void on modulus MR. *Acta Radiologica*, 35: 123–130.

Barkhof, F., Filippi, M., Miller, D. H., Scheltens, P., Campi, A., Polman, C. H. et al. (1997). Comparison of MRI criteria at first presentation to predict conversion to clinically definite multiple sclerosis. *Brain*, 120(Pt. 11): 2059–2069.

Barkhof, F. and Scheltens, P. (2002). Imaging of white matter lesions. *Cerebrovascular Diseases*, 13(Suppl. 2): 21–30.

Barkhof, F. (2004). Enlarged Virchow-Robin spaces: do they matter? *Journal of Neurology, Neurosurgery, and Psychiatry*, 75: 1516–1517.

Barkhof, F., Polvikoski, T. M., van Straaten, E. C. et al. (2007). The significance of medial temporal lobe atrophy: a postmortem MRI study in the very old. *Neurology*, 69: 1521–1527.

Barnes, J., Lewis, E. B., Scahill, R. I. et al. (2007). Automated measurement of hippocampal atrophy using fluid-registered serial MRI in AD and controls. *Journal of Computer Assisted Tomography*, 31: 581–587.

Bastos Leite, A. J., Scheltens, P., and Barkhof, F. (2004a). Pathological aging of the brain: an overview. *Topics in Magnetic Resonance Imaging*, 15: 369–389.

Bastos Leite, A. J., van Straaten, E. C., Scheltens, P., Lycklama, G., and Barkhof, F. (2004b). Thalamic lesions in vascular dementia: low sensitivity of fluid-attenuated inversion recovery (FLAIR) imaging. *Stroke*, 35: 415–419.

Bastos-Leite, A. J., van Waesberghe, J. H., Oen, A. L., van der Flier, W. M. Scheltens, P., and Barkhof, F. (2006a). Hippocampal sulcus width and cavities: comparison between patients with Alzheimer disease and nondemented elderly subjects. *AJNR. American Journal of Neuroradiology*, 27: 2141–2145.

Bastos Leite, A. J., van der Flier, W. M., van Straaten, E. C., Scheltens, P., and Barkhof, F. (2006b). Infratentorial abnormalities in vascular dementia. *Stroke*, 37: 105–110.

Bastos-Leite, A. J., van der Flier, W. M., van Straaten, E. C., Staekenborg, S. S, Scheltens, P., and Barkhof, F. (2007). The contribution of medial temporal lobe atrophy and vascular pathology to cognitive impairment in vascular dementia. *Stroke*, 38: 3182–3185.

Beyer, M. K., Larsen, J. P., and Aarsland, D. (2007). Gray matter atrophy in Parkinson disease with dementia and dementia with Lewy bodies. *Neurology*, 69: 747–754.

Bobinski, M., de Leon, M. J., Wegiel, J. et al. (2000). The histological validation of post mortem magnetic resonance imaging-determined hippocampal volume in Alzheimer's disease. *Neuroscience*, 95: 721–725.

Bokura, H., Kobayashi, S., and Yamaguchi, S. (1998). Distinguishing silent lacunar infarction from enlarged Virchow-Robin spaces: A magnetic resonance imaging and pathological study. *Journal of Neurology*, 245: 116–122.

Boone, K. B., Miller, B. L., Lesser, I. M. et al. (1992). Neuropsychological correlates of white-matter lesions in healthy elderly subjects. A threshold effect. *Archives of Neurology*, 49: 549–554.

Braak, H. and Braak, E. (1991). Neuropathological stageing of Alzheimer-related changes. *Acta Neuropathologica*, 82: 239–259.

Bradley, W. G. (2000). Normal pressure hydrocephalus: New concepts on etiology and diagnosis. *AJNR. American Journal of Neuroradiology*, 21: 1586–1590.

Bradley, W. G. (2001). Normal pressure hydrocephalus and deep white matter ischemia: Which is the chicken, and which is the egg? *American Journal of Neuroradiology*, 22: 1638–1640.

Bradley, W. G., Jr., Kortman, K. E. and Burgoyne, B. (1986). Flowing cerebrospinal fluid in normal and hydrocephalic states: Appearance on MR images. *Radiology*, 159: 611–616.

Bradley, W. G., Jr., Scalzo, D., Queralt, J., Nitz, W. N., Atkinson, D. J., and Wong, P. (1996). Normal-pressure hydrocephalus: Evaluation with cerebrospinal fluid flow measurements at MR imaging. *Radiology*, 198: 523–529.

Bradley, W. G., Jr., Whittemore, A. R., Kortman, K. E. et al. (1991a). Marked cerebrospinal fluid void: Indicator of successful shunt in patients with suspected normal-pressure hydrocephalus. *Radiology*, 178: 459–466.

Bradley, W. G., Jr., Whittemore. A. R., Watanabe, A. S., Davis, S. J., Teresi, L. M., and Homyak, M. (1991b). Association of deep white matter infarction with chronic communicating hydrocephalus: Implications regarding the possible origin of normal-pressure hydrocephalus. *American Journal of Neuroradiology*, 12: 31–39.

Braffman, B. H., Zimmerman, R. A., Trojanowski, J. Q., Gonatas, N. K., Hickey, W. F., and Schlaepfer, W. W. (1988). Brain MR: Pathologic correlation with gross and histopathology. 1. Lacunar infarction and Virchow-Robin spaces. *AJR. American Journal of Roentgenology*, 151: 551–558.

Brenneis, C., Seppi, K., Schocke, M., Benke, T., Wenning, G. K., and Poewe, W. (2004). Voxel based morphometry reveals a distinct pattern of frontal atrophy in progressive supranuclear palsy. *Journal of Neurology, Neurosurgery, and Psychiatry*, 75: 246–249.

Breteler, M. M., van Swieten, J. C., Bots, M. L. et al. (1994). Cerebral white matter lesions, vascular risk factors, and cognitive function in a population-based study: the Rotterdam Study. *Neurology*, 44: 1246–1252.

Burton, E. J., Karas, G., Paling, S. M. et al. (2002). Patterns of cerebral atrophy in dementia with Lewy bodies using voxel-based morphometry. *Neuroimage*, 17: 618–630.

Burton, E. J., McKeith, I. G., Burn, D. J., Williams, E. D., and O'Brien, J. T. (2004). Cerebral atrophy in Parkinson's disease with and without dementia: A comparison with Alzheimer's disease, dementia with Lewy bodies and controls. *Brain*, 127: 791–800.

Chan, D., Fox, N. C., Scahill, R. I. et al. (2001). Patterns of temporal lobe atrophy in semantic dementia and Alzheimer's disease. *Annals of Neurology*, 49: 433–442.

Collie, D. A., Sellar, R. J., Zeidler, M., Colchester, A. C., Knight, R., and Will, R. G. (2001). MRI of Creutzfeldt-Jakob disease: Imaging features and recommended MRI protocol. *Clinical Radiology*, 56: 726–739.

Cousins, D. A., Burton, E. J., Burn, D., Gholkar, A., McKeith, I. G., and O'Brien, J. T. (2003). Atrophy of the putamen in dementia with Lewy bodies but not Alzheimer's disease: an MRI study. *Neurology*, 61: 1191–1195.

Crum, W. R., Scahill, R. I., and Fox, N. C. (2001). Automated hippocampal segmentation by regional fluid registration of serial MRI: Validation and application in Alzheimer's disease. *Neuroimage*, 13: 847–855.

Davis, P. C., Gearing, M., Gray, L. et al. (1995). The CERAD experience, Part VIII: Neuroimaging-neuropathology correlates of temporal lobe changes in Alzheimer's disease. *Neurology*, 45: 178–179.

de Leon, M. J., George, A. E., Stylopoulos, L. A., Smith, G., and Miller, D. C. (1989). Early marker for Alzheimer's disease: the atrophic hippocampus. *Lancet*, 2: 672–673.

Demaerel, P., Heiner, L., Robberecht, W., Sciot, R., and Wilms, G. (1999). Diffusion-weighted MRI in sporadic Creutzfeldt-Jakob disease. *Neurology*, 52: 205–208.

Emre, M. (2003). Dementia associated with Parkinson's disease. *Lancet Neurology*, 2: 229–237.

Erkinjuntti, T., Inzitari, D., Pantoni, L. et al. (2000). Research criteria for subcortical vascular dementia in clinical trials. *Journal of Neural Transmission. Supplementum*, 59: 23–30.

Esiri, M. M., Nagy, Z., Smith, M. Z., Barnetson, L., and Smith, A. D. (1999). Cerebrovascular disease and threshold for dementia in the early stages of Alzheimer's disease. *Lancet*, 354: 919–920.

Esiri, M. M. (2000). Which vascular lesions are of importance in vascular dementia? *Annals of the New York Academy of Sciences*, 903: 239–243.

Evans, D. A., Funkenstein, H. H., Albert, M. S. et al. (1989). Prevalence of Alzheimer's disease in a community population of older persons. Higher than previously reported. *The Journal of the American Medical Association*, 262: 2551–2556.

Fazekas, F., Chawluk, J. B., Alavi, A., Hurtig, H. I., and Zimmerman, R. A. (1987). MR signal abnormalities at 1.5 T in Alzheimer's dementia and normal aging. *American Journal of Roentgenology*, 149: 351–356.

Fazekas, F., Kleinert, R., Offenbacher, H. et al. (1991). The morphologic correlate of incidental punctate white matter hyperintensities on MR images. *American Journal of Neuroradiology*, 12: 915–921.

Fazekas, F., Kleinert, R., Roob, G. et al. (1999). Histopathologic analysis of foci of signal loss on gradient-echo T2*-weighted MR images in patients with spontaneous intracerebral hemorrhage: evidence of microangiopathy-related microbleeds. *American Journal of Neuroradiology*, 20: 637–642.

Finkenstaedt, M., Szudra, A., Zerr, I. et al. (1996). MR imaging of Creutzfeldt-Jakob disease. *Radiology*, 199: 793–798.

Fisher, C. M. (1982). Lacunar strokes and infarcts: A review. *Neurology*, 32: 871–876.

Fox, N. C., Crum, W. R., Scahill, R. I., Stevens, J. M., Janssen, J. C., and Rossor, M. N. (2001). Imaging of onset and progression of Alzheimer's disease with voxel-compression mapping of serial magnetic resonance images. *Lancet*, 358: 201–205.

Frisoni, G. B., Beltramello, A., Weiss, C., Geroldi, C., Bianchetti, A., and Trabucchi, M. (1996). Linear measures of atrophy in mild Alzheimer disease. *American Journal of Neuroradiology*, 17: 913–923.

Frisoni, G. B., Geroldi, C., Beltramello, A. et al. (2002). Radial width of the temporal horn: A sensitive measure in Alzheimer disease. *American Journal of Neuroradiology*, 23: 35–47.

Frisoni, G. B., Testa, C., Sabattoli, F., Beltramello, A., Soininen, H., and Laakso, M. P. (2005). Structural correlates of early and late onset Alzheimer's disease: Voxel based morphometric study. *Journal of Neurology, Neurosurgery, and Psychiatry*, 76: 112–114.

Greenberg, S. M., Finklestein, S. P., and Schaefer, P. W. (1996). Petechial hemorrhages accompanying lobar hemorrhage: detection by gradient-echo MRI. *Neurology*, 46: 1751–1754.

Grimes, D. A., Lang, A. E., and Bergeron, C. B. (1999). Dementia as the most common presentation of cortical-basal ganglionic degeneration. *Neurology*, 53: 1969–1974.

Hachinski, V., Iadecola, C., Petersen, R. C. et al. (2006). National Institute of Neurological Disorders and Stroke-Canadian Stroke Network vascular cognitive impairment harmonization standards. *Stroke*, 37: 2220–2241.

Harris, G. J., Codori, A. M., Lewis, R. F., Schmidt, E., Bedi, A., and Brandt, J. (1999). Reduced basal ganglia blood flow and volume in presymptomatic, gene-tested persons at-risk for Huntington's disease. *Brain*, 122(Pt. 9): 1667–1678.

Heyman, A., Fillenbaum, G. G., Welsh-Bohmer, K. A. et al. (1998). Cerebral infarcts in patients with autopsy-proven Alzheimer's disease: CERAD, part XVIII. Consortium to Establish a Registry for Alzheimer's Disease. *Neurology*, 51: 159–162.

Hodges, J. R. and Patterson, K. (1996). Nonfluent progressive aphasia and semantic dementia: A comparative neuropsychological study. *Journal of the International Neuropsychological Society*, 2: 511–524.

Hodges, J. R. (2001). Frontotemporal dementia (Pick's disease): Clinical features and assessment. *Neurology*, 56: S6–S10.

Holmes, C., Cairns, N., Lantos, P., and Mann, A. (1999). Validity of current clinical criteria for Alzheimer's disease, vascular dementia and dementia with Lewy bodies. *The British Journal of Psychiatry*, 174: 45–50.

Huber, S. J., Shuttleworth, E. C., Christy, J. A., Chakeres, D. W., Curtin, A., and Paulson, G. W. (1989). Magnetic resonance imaging in dementia of Parkinson's disease. *Journal of Neurology, Neurosurgery, and Psychiatry*, 52: 1221–1227.

Hulette, C., Nochlin, D., McKeel, D. et al. (1997). Clinical-neuropathologic findings in multi-infarct dementia: a report of six autopsied cases. *Neurology*, 48: 668–672.

Hurst, R. W., Bagley, L. J., Galetta, S. et al. (1998). Dementia resulting from dural arteriovenous fistulas: The pathologic findings of venous hypertensive encephalopathy. *American Journal of Neuroradiology*, 19: 1267–1273.

Ince, P., Irving, D., MacArthur, F., and Perry, R. H. (1991). Quantitative neuropathological study of Alzheimer-type pathology in the hippocampus: comparison of senile dementia of Alzheimer type, senile dementia of Lewy body type, Parkinson's disease and non-demented elderly control patients. *Journal of Neurological Sciences*, 106: 142–152.

Jack, C. R., Jr., Petersen, R. C., O'Brien, P. C., and Tangalos, E. G. (1992). MR-based hippocampal volumetry in the diagnosis of Alzheimer's disease. *Neurology*, 42: 183–188.

Jack, C. R., Jr., Petersen, R. C., Xu, Y. et al. (1998). Rate of medial temporal lobe atrophy in typical aging and Alzheimer's disease. *Neurology*, 51: 993–999.

Jobst, K. A., Smith, A. D., Szatmari, M. et al. (1992). Detection in life of confirmed Alzheimer's disease using a simple measurement of medial temporal lobe atrophy by computed tomography. *Lancet*, 340: 1179–1183.

Kalaria, R. N. and Ballard, C. (1999). Overlap between pathology of Alzheimer disease and vascular dementia. *Alzheimer Disease and Associated Disorders*, 13(Suppl. 3): S115–S123.

Karas, G. B., Burton, E. J., Rombouts, S. A. et al. (2003). A comprehensive study of gray matter loss in patients with Alzheimer's disease using optimized voxel-based morphometry. *Neuroimage*, 18: 895–907.

Karas, G., Scheltens, P., Rombouts, S. et al. (2007). Precuneus atrophy in early-onset Alzheimer's disease: a morphometric structural MRI study. *Neuroradiology*, 49: 967–976.

Kato, N., Arai, K., and Hattori, T. (2003). Study of the rostral midbrain atrophy in progressive supranuclear palsy. *Journal of the Neurological Sciences*, 210: 57–60.

Kido, D. K., Caine, E. D., LeMay, M., Ekholm, S., Booth, H., and Panzer, R. (1989). Temporal lobe atrophy in patients with Alzheimer disease: A CT study. *American Journal of Neuroradiology*, 10: 551–555.

Knopman, D. S., Christensen, K. J., Schut, L. J. et al. (1989). The spectrum of imaging and neuropsychological findings in Pick's disease. *Neurology*, 39: 362–368.

Knopman, D. S., DeKosky, S. T., Cummings, J. L. et al. (2001). Practice parameter: diagnosis of dementia (an evidence-based review). Report of the Quality Standards Subcommittee of the American Academy of Neurology. *Neurology*, 56: 1143–1153.

Knudsen, K. A, Rosand, J., Karluk, D., and Greenberg, S. M. (2001). Clinical diagnosis of cerebral amyloid angiopathy: Validation of the Boston criteria. *Neurology*, 56: 537–539.

Krolak-Salmon, P., Montavont, A., Hermier, M., Milliery, M., and Vighetto, A. (2002). Thalamic venous infarction as a cause of subacute dementia. *Neurology*, 58: 1689–1691.

Laakso, M. P., Partanen, K., Riekkinen, P. et al. (1996). Hippocampal volumes in Alzheimer's disease, Parkinson's disease with and without dementia, and in vascular dementia: An MRI study. *Neurology*, 46: 678–681.

Laakso, M. P., Frisoni, G. B., Kononen, M. et al. (2000). Hippocampus and entorhinal cortex in frontotemporal dementia and Alzheimer's disease: a morphometric MRI study. *Biological Psychiatry*, 47: 1056–1063.

Larsson, E., Passant, U., Sundgren, P. C. et al. (2000). Magnetic resonance imaging and histopathology in dementia, clinically of frontotemporal type. *Dementia and Geriatric Cognitive Disorders*, 11: 123–134.

Lazeron, R. H., Langdon, D. W., Filippi, M. et al. (2000). Neuropsychological impairment in multiple sclerosis patients: the role of (juxta)cortical lesion on FLAIR. *Multiple Sclerosis*, 6: 280–285.

Lazeron, R. H., Boringa J. B., Schouten, M. et al. (2005). Brain atrophy and lesion load as explaining parameters for cognitive impairment in multiple sclerosis. *Multiple Sclerosis*, 11: 524–531.

Lesnik Oberstein, S. A., van den, B. R., van Buchem, M. A. et al. (2001). Cerebral microbleeds in CADASIL. *Neurology*, 57: 1066–1070.

Leys, D., Erkinjuntti, T., Desmond, D. W. et al. (1999). Vascular dementia: the role of cerebral infarcts. *Alzheimer's Disease and Associated Disorders*, 13(Suppl. 3): S38–S48.

Lim, A., Tsuang, D., Kukull, W. et al. (1999). Clinico-neuropathological correlation of Alzheimer's disease in a community-based case series. *Journal of the American Geriatrics Society*, 47: 564–569.

Lindgren, A., Roijer, A., Rudling, O. et al. (1994). Cerebral lesions on magnetic resonance imaging, heart disease, and vascular risk factors in subjects without stroke. A population-based study. *Stroke*, 25: 929–934.

Litvan, I., Agid, Y., Calne, D. et al. (1996). Clinical research criteria for the diagnosis of progressive supranuclear palsy (Steele-Richardson-Olszewski syndrome): Report of the NINDS-SPSP international workshop. *Neurology*, 47: 1–9.

Loeb, C. (1995). Dementia due to lacunar infarctions: A misnomer or a clinical entity? *European Neurology*, 35: 187–192.

Longstreth, W. T., Jr., Manolio, T. A., Arnold, A. et al. (1996). Clinical correlates of white matter findings on cranial magnetic resonance imaging of 3301 elderly people. The Cardiovascular Health Study. *Stroke*, 27: 1274–1282.

Lopez, O. L., Becker, J. T., Jungreis, C. A. et al. (1995). Computed tomography—but not magnetic resonance imaging—identified periventricular white-matter lesions predict symptomatic cerebrovascular disease in probable Alzheimer's disease. *Archives of Neurology*, 52: 659–664.

Maclullich, A. M., Wardlaw, J. M., Ferguson, K. J., Starr, J. M., Seckl, J. R., and Deary, I. J. (2004). Enlarged perivascular spaces are associated with cognitive function in healthy elderly men. *Journal of Neurology, Neurosurgery, and Psychiatry*, 75: 1519–1523.

Massoud, F., Devi, G., Moroney, J. T. et al. (2000). The role of routine laboratory studies and neuroimaging in the diagnosis of dementia: A clinicopathological study. *Journal of the American Geriatrics Society*, 48: 1204–1210.

McDonald, W. I., Compston, A., Edan, G. et al. (2001). Recommended diagnostic criteria for multiple sclerosis: Guidelines from the International Panel on the diagnosis of multiple sclerosis. *Annals of Neurology*, 50: 121–127.

McKeith, I. G., Galasko, D., Kosaka, K. et al. (1996). Consensus guidelines for the clinical and pathologic diagnosis of dementia with Lewy bodies (DLB): Report of the consortium on DLB international workshop. *Neurology*, 47: 1113–1124.

McKeith, I., Mintzer, J., Aarsland, D. et al. (2004). Dementia with Lewy bodies. *Lancet Neurology*, 3: 19–28.

McKhann, G., Drachman, D., Folstein, M., Katzman, R., Price, D., and Stadlan, E. M. (1984). Clinical diagnosis of Alzheimer's disease: Report of the NINCDS-ADRDA Work Group under the auspices of Department of Health and Human Services Task Force on Alzheimer's Disease. *Neurology*, 34: 939–944.

MRC CFAS. (2001). Pathological correlates of late-onset dementia in a multi-centre, community-based population in England and Wales. *Lancet*, 357: 169–175.

Nagy, Z., Esiri, M. M., Joachim, C. et al. (1998). Comparison of pathological diagnostic criteria for Alzheimer disease. *Alzheimer's Disease and Associated Disorders*, 12: 182–189.

Neary, D., Snowden, J. S., Gustafson, L. et al. (1998). Frontotemporal lobar degeneration: A consensus on clinical diagnostic criteria. *Neurology*, 51: 1546–1554.

O'Brien, J. T., Desmond, P., Ames, D., Schweitzer, I., Chiu, E., and Tress, B. (1997). Temporal lobe magnetic resonance imaging can differentiate Alzheimer's disease from normal ageing, depression, vascular dementia and other causes of cognitive impairment. *Psychological Medicine*, 27: 1267–1275.

Offenbacher, H., Fazekas, F., Schmidt, R., Koch, M., Fazekas, G., and Kapeller, P. (1996). MR of cerebral abnormalities concomitant with primary intracerebral hematomas. *American Journal of Neuroradiology*, 17: 573–578.

Parvizi, J., Van Hoesen, G. W., and Damasio, A. (2000). Selective pathological changes of the periaqueductal gray matter in Alzheimer's disease. *Annals of Neurology*, 48: 344–353.

Pasquier, F. and Leys, D. (1997). Why are stroke patients prone to develop dementia? *Journal of Neurology*, 244: 135–142.

Paviour, D. C., Schott, J. M., Stevens, J. M. et al. (2004). Pathological substrate for regional distribution of increased atrophy rates in progressive supranuclear palsy. *Journal of Neurology, Neurosurgery, and Psychiatry*, 75: 1772–1775.

Petersen, R. C., Jack, C. R., Jr., Xu, Y. C., et al. (2000). Memory and MRI-based hippocampal volumes in aging and AD. *Neurology*, 54: 581–587.

Poirier, J. and Derouesne, C. (1985). The concept of cerebral lacunae from 1838 to the present. *Revista De Neurologia (Paris)*, 141: 3–17.

Polvikoski, T., Sulkava, R., Myllykangas, L. et al. (2001). Prevalence of Alzheimer's disease in very elderly people: a prospective neuropathological study. *Neurology*, 56: 1690–1696.

Ridha, B. H., Barnes, J., van de Pol, L. A. et al. (2007). Application of automated medial temporal lobe atrophy scale to Alzheimer disease. *Archives of Neurology*, 64: 849–854.

Roman, G. C., Tatemichi, T. K., Erkinjuntti, T. et al. (1993). Vascular dementia: Diagnostic criteria for research studies. Report of the NINDS-AIREN International Workshop. *Neurology*, 43: 250–260.

Roman, G. C., Erkinjuntti, T., Wallin, A., Pantoni, L., and Chui, H. C. (2002). Subcortical ischaemic vascular dementia. *Lancet Neurology*, 1: 426–436.

Rombouts, S. A., van Swieten, J. C., Pijnenburg, Y. A., Goekoop, R., Barkhof, F., and Scheltens, P. (2003). Loss of frontal fMRI activation in early frontotemporal dementia compared to early AD. *Neurology*, 60: 1904–1908.

Savoiardo, M., Strada, L., Girotti, F. et al. (1989). MR imaging in progressive supranuclear palsy and Shy-Drager syndrome. *Journal of Computer Assisted Tomography*, 13: 555–560.

Savoiardo, M., Grisoli, M., and Girotti, F. (2000). Magnetic resonance imaging in CBD, related atypical parkinsonian disorders, and dementias. In I. Litvan, C. G. Goetz, and A. E. Lang (eds), *Corticobasal Degeneration and Related Disorders* (pp. 197–208). Philadelphia: Lippincott Williams & Wilkins.

Scheltens, P., Leys, D., Barkhof, F. et al. (1992a). Atrophy of medial temporal lobes on MRI in "probable" Alzheimer's disease and normal ageing: Diagnostic value and neuropsychological correlates. *Journal of Neurology, Neurosurgery, and Psychiatry*, 55: 967–972.

Scheltens, P., Barkhof, F., Valk, J. et al. (1992b). White matter lesions on magnetic resonance imaging in clinically diagnosed Alzheimer's disease. Evidence for heterogeneity. *Brain*, 115(Pt. 3): 735–748.

Scheltens, P., Launer, L. J., Barkhof, F., Weinstein, H. C., and van Gool, W. A. (1995). Visual assessment of medial temporal lobe atrophy on magnetic resonance imaging: interobserver reliability. *Journal of Neurology*, 242: 557–560.

Scheltens, P., Fox, N., Barkhof, F., and De Carli, C. (2002). Structural magnetic resonance imaging in the practical assessment of dementia: beyond exclusion. *Lancet Neurology*, 1: 13–21.

Schrag, A., Good, C. D., Miszkiel, K. et al. (2000). Differentiation of atypical parkinsonian syndromes with routine MRI. *Neurology*, 54: 697–702.

Seab, J. P., Jagust, W. J., Wong, S. T., Roos, M. S., Reed, B. R., and Budinger, T. F. (1988). Quantitative NMR measurements of hippocampal atrophy in Alzheimer's disease. *Magnetic Resonance in Medicine*, 8: 200–208.

Skehan, S. J., Hutchinson, M., and MacErlaine, D. P. (1995). Cerebral autosomal dominant arteriopathy with subcortical infarcts and leukoencephalopathy: MR findings. *American Journal of Neuroradiology*, 16: 2115–2119.

Snowdon, D. A., Greiner, L. H., Mortimer, J. A., Riley, K. P., Greiner, P. A., and Markesbery, W. R. (1997). Brain infarction and the clinical expression of Alzheimer disease. The Nun Study. *The Journal of the American Medical Association*, 277: 813–817.

Tanaka, K., Morooka, Y., Nakagawa, Y., and Shimizu, S. (1999). Dural arteriovenous malformation manifesting as dementia due to ischemia in bilateral thalami. A case report. *Surgical Neurology*, 51: 489–493.

Tribl, G. G., Strasser, G., Zeitlhofer, J. et al. (2002). Sequential MRI in a case of Creutzfeldt–Jakob disease. *Neuroradiology*, 44: 223–226.

Udaka, F., Sawada, H., and Kameyama, M. (2002). White matter lesions and dementia: MRI-pathological correlation. *Annals of the New York Academy of Sciences*, 977: 411–415.

Valk, J., Barkhof, F., and Scheltens, P. (2002). *Magnetic Resonance in Dementia*. Berlin: Springer.

van de Pol, L. A., Hensel, A., van der Flier, W. M. et al. (2006). Hippocampal atrophy on MRI in frontotemporal lobar degeneration and Alzheimers disease. *Journal of Neurology, Neurosurgery, and Psychiatry*, 77: 439–442.

van Straaten, E. C., Scheltens, P., Knol, D. L. et al. (2003). Operational definitions for the NINDS-AIREN criteria for vascular dementia: an interobserver study. *Stroke*, 34: 1907–1912.

Wahlund, L. O., Julin, P., Lindqvist, J., and Scheltens, P. (1999). Visual assessment of medial temporal lobe atrophy in demented and healthy control subjects: correlation with volumetry. *Psychiatry Research*, 90: 193–199.

Wahlund, L. O., Barkhof, F., Fazekas, F. et al. (2001). A new rating scale for age-related white matter changes applicable to MRI and CT. *Stroke*, 32: 1318–1322.

Warmuth-Metz, M., Naumann, M., Csoti, I., and Solymosi, L. (2001). Measurement of the midbrain diameter on routine magnetic resonance imaging: A simple and accurate method of differentiating between Parkinson disease and progressive supranuclear palsy. *Archives of Neurology*, 58: 1076–1079.

Whitwell, J. L., Weigand, S. D., Shiung, M. M. et al. (2007). Focal atrophy in dementia with Lewy bodies on MRI: A distinct pattern from Alzheimer's disease. *Brain*, 130: 708–719.

Yagishita, A. and Oda, M. (1996). Progressive supranuclear palsy: MRI and pathological findings. *Neuroradiology*; 38(Suppl. 1): S60–S66.

Yousry, T. A., Seelos, K., Mayer, M. et al. (1999). Characteristic MR lesion pattern and correlation of T1 and T2 lesion volume with neurologic and neuropsychological findings in cerebral autosomal dominant arteriopathy with subcortical infarcts and leukoencephalopathy (CADASIL). *American Journal of Neuroradiology*, 20: 91–100.

Zeidler, M., Sellar, R. J., Collie, D. A. et al. (2000). The pulvinar sign on magnetic resonance imaging in variant Creutzfeldt-Jakob disease. *Lancet*, 355: 1412–1418.

17

White Matter Hyperintensities in Aging and Dementia

Adriane Mayda, Mitsuhiro Yoshita, and Charles DeCarli

Introduction

Growth in the number of individuals over 65 years of age in the world is unprecedented. For example, nearly 20% of the population in Italy is over age 65 (Kinsella and Velkoff, 2001). In the United States, approximately 330 individuals per hour turn 60 and as many as 78 million will turn 65 by 2011 (U.S. Census Bureau, 2007), resulting in a near doubling of the population age 65 and older by 2030 (Kinsella and Velkoff, 2001). The percentage of individuals over age 65 is increasing even more rapidly in developing countries (Kinsella and Velkoff, 2001). It is, therefore, timely to consider diseases associated with aging, such as cognitive impairment.

Complaints of cognitive impairment, particularly memory loss, are common to older individuals (Cutler and Grams, 1988). Cross-sectional epidemiological studies suggest linear age-related decline in memory performance, although remarkable differences in individual trajectories of decline exist (Wilson et al., 2002). These data have been used to suggest that the results of at least some of the studies of cognitive aging may be contaminated by the inclusion of individuals with incipient disease (Wilson et al., 2002).

While Alzheimer's disease (AD) is clearly the major cause of cognitive impairment among the elderly (Ferri et al., 2005; Ganguli et al., 2000; Hebert et al., 2004), current evidence suggests that an individual's lifetime risk for cerebrovascular disease (CVD) may be similar or even higher than AD (Seshadri et al., 2006), and these two diseases commonly occur in the same individual (Schneider et al., 2007). Although stroke is the hallmark clinical sign of CVD, it is important to recognize that the full spectrum of CVD includes clinically asymptomatic cerebral infarction, white matter hyperintensities (WMH), and even accelerated brain atrophy (Decarli, 2004) that are common to advancing age among cognitively normal community dwelling individuals (Decarli, Massaro et al., 2005) (Figure 17.1). Interestingly, these clinically silent brain lesions result in subtle impairments of cognitive function (Gunning-Dixon and Raz, 2000) similar to those cognitive changes associated with "healthy" aging (West, 1996).

Over the past 10–20 years, cognitive neuroscience, assisted by the use of functional magnetic resonance imaging (fMRI), has substantially advanced our knowledge of cognitive systems, offering new theories about cognitive aging (Cabeza, 2002; Grady, 2000; Grady et al., 2006). These studies, however, have focused primarily on cortical gray-matter function. Recent advances in magnetic resonance imaging (MRI), such as the introduction of diffusion tensor imaging (DTI) and improvements in computer algorithms relating to anatomical mapping of cerebral white matter (DeCarli et al., 2005; Wen and Sachdev, 2004), have led to a renewed interest in the role of axonal connectivity as it relates to cognitive systems and aging (Sullivan and Pfefferbaum, 2006). Approaches that combine fMRI with DTI and other measures of white matter pathology enable a unique "neural systems" approach to the study of human cognition. Although such studies are as yet relatively uncommon (Nordahl et al., 2006), there is much future promise to this approach.

In this chapter, we review current scientific evidence regarding the impact of white matter changes—particularly white matter hyperintensities (WMH)—on cognition with aging, and in the setting of cognitive impairment syndromes such as mild cognitive impairment (MCI) and Alzheimer's disease (AD). Before we discuss the specifics of these findings, however, we will briefly review current concepts regarding the importance of white matter integrity and neural systems function.

Functional Anatomy of Cerebral White Matter

As we note in our introduction, research on brain-behavior relationships has historically stressed the importance of the cerebral cortex and subcortical gray matter for cognitive processing. Recent evidence, however, indicates that, as an essential component of extended neural networks in the brain, the integrity of cerebral white matter tracts are also critical for many higher-order cognitive processes including attention, executive functioning, nonverbal/visual-spatial processing, and generalized processing speed (Gunning-Dixon and Raz, 2000). Although the relationship between cerebral white matter and cognition has yet to be fully explored, Geschwind's seminal works linked isolated injury of cerebral white matter to a variety of neurobehavioral disorders over four decades ago (Geschwind, 1965a). Clinical evidence of the effects of white matter disconnection can be observed in patients with conduction aphasia, in which a lesion of the arcuate fasciculus uncouples Broca's area from Wernicke's area, leading to poor verbal repetition skills (Geschwind, 1965b). Although data from these patients clearly support white matter disconnection leading to dysfunction, recent evidence suggests that even the asymptomatic disruption of white matter may lead to subtle cognitive impairments. The advent of MRI has facilitated the investigation of detailed functional specialization of cerebral white matter and considerably advanced our understanding of the importance of distributed neural systems.

Spectrum of Cerebral Vascular Disease

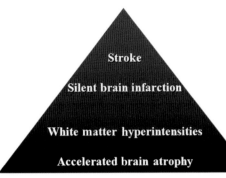

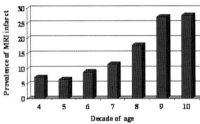

Figure 17–1 Spectrum of cerebrovascular disease. Vascular brain injury can be viewed as a pyramid of severity with the less common clinical manifestation (stroke) at the peak. Conversely, cerebral infarction, detected by MRI is extremely common, reaching a prevalence of nearly 30% after the 8th decade of life.

In recent years, the way we think about brain mechanisms underlying complex cognitive, behavioral, and even motor processes has moved from a localization approach that attempts to attribute one function to one locus, to a more global circuits approach that investigates the contribution of distributed neural networks to function (Goldman-Rakic, 1988; Mesulam, 1990). This paradigm shift includes the realization that disconnection of white matter tracts may be just as effective in producing functional impairment as lesions in gray matter. Functions attributable to the frontal lobes may be of particular importance to this disconnection hypothesis because of the extensive reciprocal connections of the frontal lobe to subcortical areas as well as the parietal, temporal, and occipital lobes (Miller and Asaad, 2002).

Of particular interest to cognitive aging and dementia are the cognitive effects of the disruption of frontal-subcortical circuits thought to be involved in executive function, especially the dorsolateral prefrontal cortex (DLPFC) (Alexander et al., 1986). Five parallel frontal-subcortical circuits form closed anatomical loops, originating and ending in the frontal cortex and traveling through the caudate nucleus, globus pallidus, and thalamus (Cummings, 1995, 1998). Disruption of this circuit at any point can result in behavioral deficits associated with DLPFC dysfunction, such as implicit learning and memory. Function of this system may also degrade with age. For example, Aizenstein et al. (2006) found that elderly adults had reduced striatal (putamen) activation in an implicit learning task relative to young controls, supporting the theory that changes in this network of regions is related to cognitive aging. Age-related differences in DLPFC may affect episodic memory performance, as well. Results from neuroimaging studies find that the DLPFC implements processes critical for organizing items in working memory (Blumenfeld and Ranganath, 2006), and that DLPFC connections to the hippocampus are important for long-term memory storage (Ranganath, 2006).

Another potentially important circuit that may be disrupted by age-related increases in white matter abnormalities is the prefrontal-parietal circuit described by Goldman-Rakic (1987). Reciprocal anatomical connections between prefrontal cortex and posterior parietal cortex are thought to play a role in visual-spatial processing, attend to selective stimuli, and hold visual-spatial information online; therefore, disruption of this circuit could potentially affect visual processing and working memory. Research on the anatomic specificity of white matter abnormalities as they relate to these particular systems is ongoing, but WMH frequency mapping (DeCarli, Fletcher et al., 2005; Wen and Sachdev, 2004) and DTI have the potential to further our understanding of the specific white-matter systems that may be affected by age and disease (Figure 17.2). Understanding the importance of white matter connections that subserve widely distributed neural systems may significantly impact our concepts of how aging and asymptomatic vascular brain injury adversely impact cognitive function. In the next section, we explore data relating to changes in cerebral white matter associated with auspiciously "normal" cognitive aging.

Aging and Cerebral White Matter

Advancing age has profound effects on the anatomy, neurochemistry, and physiology of the brain. Age-related anatomical brain differences include atrophy, ventricular, and sulcal enlargement, increased white matter hyperintensities (WMH) and clinically asymptomatic cerebral infarctions (Decarli, Massaro et al., 2005; Yue et al., 1997). Changes at the cellular level involve region-specific neuronal cell loss, dendritic degeneration, and synapse loss (Uylings and de Brabander, 2002). In addition to these changes in brain structure, there are consistent age-related differences in cognitive performance, although individual performance varies considerably (Rapp and Amaral, 1992; Wilson et al., 2002). Aging does not inevitably lead to diminished cognitive performance because multiple co-occurring causal mechanisms are probably involved, as well as individual differences in response to these processes (Buckner, 2005; Wilson et al., 2002). Recent evidence indicates lifetime risks for hypertension, atherosclerosis, and cerebrovascular disease are high (Seshadri et al., 2006; Vasan et al., 2002) and

Template Based Mapping of WMH and DTI

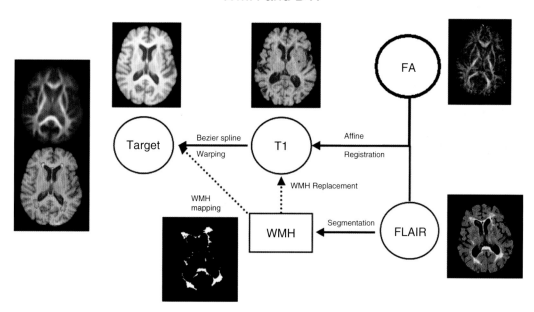

Figure 17–2 Improved imaging methods that map cerebral white matter abnormalities (white matter hyperintensities) as illustrated in this figure offer unique opportunities to explore the anatomical relationship between white matter injury and specific cognitive systems.

associated with subtle alterations in cognitive performance among nondemented older individuals (Elias et al., 2004). The same vascular risk factors are also associated with increased WMH burden (Jeerakathil et al., 2004). We hypothesize that clinically silent small-vessel cerebrovascular disease is a contributing factor to normal age-related declines in brain structure and function, possibly through disruption of the frontal-subcortical circuits described previously. We further hypothesize that preservation of these circuits in the absence of white matter abnormalities are important for the maintained compensatory cognitive function apparent in successful aging. Before we address specific evidence for the effect of white matter changes on cognition, we must review age-related differences in cognitive function that will then be compared to differences in cognitive performance associated with cerebral white matter injury.

Cognitive Changes with Age

Behavioral studies indicate that even normal healthy adults show declines in performance on many cognitive tasks, such as those that tap working memory, encoding and retrieval of episodic memory, prospective memory, and such executive functions as attentional capacity (Grady and Craik, 2000). Currently, many theories attempt to explain normal age-related decline in memory such as those attributing memory weaknesses to failure of strategic processing, deficits in semantic processing, problems in the utilization of context, or changes in basic mechanisms underlying all aspects of cognition (Light, 1996). Much of the current evidence supports the latter theory, named the "resource deficit hypothesis," which states that age-related impairments in cognition are mediated by changes in one or more fundamental processes that participate in a variety of domains. Potential mediators of this age-related deficit in memory-dependent domains include changes in attention, working memory, inhibition, and/or processing speed. Work by Salthouse seems to suggest that both working memory capacity and

general cognitive slowing appear to account for substantial portions of age-related variability in memory and other cognitive areas (Light, 1996; Salthouse, 2000).

Frontal Lobe Aging Hypothesis

Age-related declines are most striking in measures of frontal lobe function with behavioral studies indicating that older individuals exhibit deficits in executive control processes dependent on prefrontal cortex (PFC) function (West, 1996). Cognitive impairments in older adults are comparable (though milder) to those in patients with frontal lobe damage (Moscovitch and Winocur, 1995). Volumetric studies indicate that prefrontal cortex is selectively decreased in elderly individuals (Raz et al., 1997), and functional neuroimaging evidence suggests that successful cognitive performance in elderly individuals is associated with spared prefrontal activation (Cabeza, 2002) (Figure 17.3). This evidence lends support to the frontal lobe aging hypothesis, which states that age-related cognitive deficits are mediated by PFC dysfunction. To maintain normal cognitive function despite these deficits in executive function, older individuals may require more extensive prefrontal resources to succeed at a given task. For example, recent evidence suggests that the aging brain responds to age-related changes in anatomy and physiology by reorganizing its functions to maintain normal cognitive function. Cabeza (2002) has reported that, under similar conditions, prefrontal activity during cognitive processes tends to be less lateralized in older adults than younger adults. This model is referred to as HAROLD (Hemispheric Asymmetry Reduction in OLDer adults) and has been supported by functional neuroimaging evidence from domains of episodic memory, semantic memory, working memory, perception, and inhibitory control. Age-related increases in neural recruitment, therefore, may play a compensatory role in the brain or reflect a difficulty in recruiting specialized neural systems known as dedifferentiation or nonselective recruitment. Though these theories are not

Regional Brain Aging

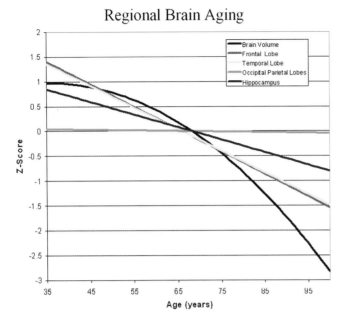

Figure 17–3 Graphic representation of average age-related differences for various brain regions illustrating the heterogeneous nature of brain aging. In particular, frontal and temporal lobe cortices decline linearly in volume with advancing age. Loss of frontal cortex volume has been postulated to contribute the age related cognitive differences (frontal aging hypothesis).

mutually exclusive, evidence of improved cognitive performance with increased bilateral involvement in older adults suggests that this is a compensatory mechanism. For example, Reuter-Lorenz et al. (2000) reported that older adults who display a pattern of bilateral activation were faster in a verbal working-memory task than those who did not display the pattern. However, little is currently known about the mechanism of this age-related change in PFC function.

It has been suggested by Rypma et al. (2000) that working memory decline with normal aging can be accounted for by age-related changes in DLPFC. They report that older adults have reduced activity in DLPFC during memory retrieval as compared to young adults. They also show that young adults have increased activity in DLPFC as reaction time (RT) increases, whereas the opposite is true for older adults such that slower elderly adults have reduced DLPFC activity (Rypma et al., 2005). Salthouse and others have suggested that reductions in processing speed are related to decreases in the overall efficiency of cognitive processing (Salthouse, 1996), which could explain these results. It has been further suggested that behavioral declines could result from an age-related decrease in neural efficiency, which in turn leads to slowing and then a degradation in the quality of the information encoded, maintained, and available for retrieval (Rypma and D'Esposito, 2000; Rypma et al., 2005). This idea is also shared by Cerella who proposed a "disconnection hypothesis" based on the notion that cognitive task performance required transmission across a vast array of interconnected nodes. The fewer number of nodes there are across which information is transmitted, the more direct the processing paths will be, and the quicker information will be processed. Reductions in the integrity of direct-processing links between nodes requires the use of more indirect links for successful task performance (Cerella, 1990). However, the precise mechanism of this speed-cognition relation is not well-understood.

Injury to white matter tracts connecting PFC with its anatomical targets is one possible mechanism for explaining some of the age-related working memory decline and slowing. In a recent meta-analysis, Gunning-Dixon and Raz (2000) showed that the presence and extent of age-related alterations in the cerebral white matter are related to processing speed, executive function, and explicit (immediate and delayed) memory, but not general indices of intelligence (fluid or crystallized) or fine-motor functioning. In the following section, we review current evidence related to the association between age-related reductions in white matter integrity and the cognitive changes commonly ascribed to advancing age.

Aging and White Matter Integrity

Magnetic resonance diffusion tensor imaging (DTI) of the brain is a noninvasive in vivo method for characterizing the integrity of anatomical connections, and provides a quantitative assessment of white matter microstructure. This section focuses on results from studies of normal aging and WMH using DTI to investigate age-related reductions in white matter tissue integrity and cognition. First, we will briefly summarize current concepts of DTI. Second, we provide a summary of DTI findings in normal aging, followed by summaries of DTI findings in subjects with WMH, and (finally) a brief review of the limited data relating DTI findings to cognitive function in normal aging.

Diffusion is the translational movement of molecules induced by Brownian random motion. MRI is sensitive to water self-diffusion, as spins undergoing a random diffusion motion in the presence of magnetic field gradients accumulate different randomly distributed phase shifts. In biological tissue, the self-diffusion of water molecules is not free but hindered and restricted by the presence of various barriers. By introducing spatial magnetic field gradients, it is possible to obtain MR sequences that are sensitive to the diffusivity of water along a chosen direction, obtaining diffusion-weighted image (DWI). The diffusivity of water in white matter is hindered mostly by axonal membranes, and by myelin sheaths. In axonal bundles, the diffusivity of water is therefore much larger along the direction of the bundle in comparison to other directions (Beaulieu, 2002). The diffusion coefficient measured in the human brain by MRI is generally dependent upon the directionality. In tracts of parallel fibers, diffusion occurs along the direction of the fibers. The extent of restricted freedom of movement is called "anisotropy." In the DTI, it is possible to derive the mean diffusivity (MD) and various measures of diffusion anisotropy, such as fractional anisotropy (FA) (Basser and Jones, 2002; Pierpaoli and Basser, 1996). DTI data contain information about the principal direction of diffusion in a voxel. This information is encoded by the eigenvalues and eigenvectors of the diffusion tensor. Tractography algorithms make it possible to delineate white matter fiber bundles of the brain using this information.

Image quantification is generally performed over a region of interest (ROI) by calculating the mean values of MD and FA (or other indices derived from the diffusion tensor). Specification of the anatomical location of the putative between group differences is therefore a precondition. The major problem with the ROI approach is the inability to attribute changes to a specific tract within regions containing two or more white matter tracts. Also, the manual definition of a ROI for the entire length of a tract is rarely achieved. Further, the conventional ROI approach is time-consuming and has poor statistical accuracy due to the high degree of intra and intersubject variation of the fractional anisotropy values, even within a highly homogeneous tract (Kanaan et al., 2006). More recently, some investigators have started using voxel-based analysis (VBA) (Medina et al., 2006; Xie et al., 2006) and DTI-based, tract-specific measurements (TSM) (Taoka et al., 2006). VBA is an operator-independent approach that allows the analysis of the entire brain volume without a priori hypothesis regarding the anatomical location of between-group differences. FA or MD images in each subject are registered into a standard space, and then voxel-wise statistics are carried out to detect regional difference between populations or to find areas that correlated with covariate of interest. This can be very useful as exploratory analysis, especially where white matter changes are diffuse. The accuracy and utility of VBA is still a matter of debate (Jones et al., 2005). This is especially true for areas surrounding the cerebral ventricles because coregistration of low resolution, high-contrast FA maps may generate significant misregistration using conventional registration algorithms and partial volume artifacts in regions of high and low anisotropy. The accurate localization of differences to specific tracts is also difficult because data are often heavily smoothed as part of the preprocessing (Figure 17.4). This results in low-resolution parametric maps from which to infer group differences. Anatomical identification of regions exhibiting significant group differences can be difficult because clusters of voxels will not typically lie neatly within a single tract. TSM allows testing of between-group differences within a specific tract. TSM overcomes some of the limitation of ROI and VBA analysis (e.g., better anatomical localization of the single tracts, analysis throughout the almost entire length of the bandle), but has a number of problems including operator-dependent placement of regions from which the tracking starts, and difficulties in resolving the crossing or meeting of different fibers.

The main correlates of aging are reduced diffusional anisotropy, reflecting rarefaction of directionally oriented axonal membranes, and increased mean diffusivity, reflecting rarefaction of cellular membranes and other structures hindering diffusion. A number of studies have reported age-related reduction of FA in the corpus callosum (Abe et al., 2002; Bhagat and Beaulieu, 2004; Nusbaum et al., 2001; O'Sullivan et al., 2001; Pfefferbaum et al., 2000; Sullivan et al., 2001, 2006). Other areas have also been investigated. Age-related decline in white matter anisotropy has been detected in the anterior cingulum and middle frontal gyrus (Pfefferbaum and Sullivan, 2005). Others have reported reduced FA in left and right pericallosal regions and in the centrum

semiovale (Pfefferbaum et al., 2000; Sullivan et al., 2001) in sub-cortical white matter, superior frontal gyrus, superior temporal gyrus, supra marginal gyrus, and in the postcentral gyrus (Bhagat and Beaulieu, 2004). Nusbaum et al. (2001) reported reduced FA in the internal capsule and frontal and parietal subcortical white matter. Interestingly, several authors reported anterior-posterior gradients in the age-related reduction of FA (Head et al., 2004; O'Sullivan, Jones et al., 2001; Pfefferbaum et al., 2000; Salat et al., 2005; Sullivan et al., 2001, 2006). Sullivan et al. (2001) confirmed that the age-related disproportional reduction of FA was seen in frontal regions when compared to posterior regions. Moreover, no age-related differences were found in the splenium, as opposed to the genu of the corpus callosum (Bhagat and Beaulieu, 2004; Jones et al., 1999). While reduced FA is well established, particularly for anterior regions, findings concerning MD appear more variable. Chun et al. (2000) reported a general age-related increase of MD, especially in periventricular regions. Bhagat et al. (2004) reported increased MD in the genu and splenium of the corpus callosum, in the internal and external capsule, and in the centrum semiovale. Their findings are essentially in line with those reported in the above study that reported an anterior-posterior gradient existing also for MD (Abe et al., 2002; O'Sullivan, Jones et al., 2001). When compared to the age-related reduction of FA, the increase in MD generally tends to have weaker significance. On the other hand, the lack of significant age-related changes, with the exception of lateral ventricular regions, were reported using subjects that included 80 individuals whose ages ranged from 20 to 85 years (Helenius et al., 2002). Taken collectively, the reduction in FA is more pronounced than the increase in MD, although the underlying measurement technique is essentially the same for both.

As noted, WMH increase in prevalence and extent with advancing age and the presence of cerebrovascular risk factors. A number of studies have measured DTI and MTR parameters separately in WMH or leukoaraiosis (the presence of reduced tissue contrast seen by computed x-ray tomography). In general, these studies find that white matter integrity is further compromised in WMH as compared to surrounding normal-appearing white matter. Jones et al. (1999) performed quantitative assessment using MD and FA maps. In regions where macroscopic lesions were detectable, they observed a characteristic pattern of increased MD and reduced FA, which was different from that observed in patients with cerebral infarctions. FA was remarkably low in both patients with

DTI Tract Tracing: Thalamo-Cortical Connections

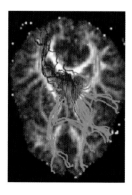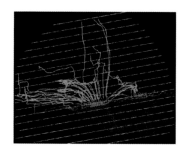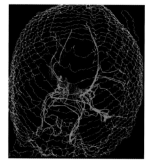

Figure 17–4 Example of white matter tract tracing based on diffusion tensor imaging (DTI). This approach will likely advance current knowledge in the relationship between white matter injury and cognition.

leukoaraiosis and infarcts as compared to controls. Conversely, MD values were higher, not only in both groups compared to controls, but also in patients with necrotic infarcts as compared to patients with leukoaraiosis. Other authors focused on changes in the normal-appearing white matter of patients with WMH (O'Sullivan et al., 2004; O'Sullivan, Summers et al., 2001). Using ROI analysis, O'Sullivan et al. (2004) demonstrated increased MD and reduced FA in the normal-appearing white matter of patients with leukoaraiosis compared to healthy controls (O'Sullivan, Summers et al., 2001), while Fazekas et al. (2005) found an approximate reduction of 10% in MTR of WMH compared with normal-appearing white matter in 198 cognitively normal subjects aged between 52 and 87 years. In addition to this, Taylor et al. (2007) showed that greater anterior white matter lesion volumes were associated with higher diffusivity and lower anisotropy in the white matter of the dorsolateral prefrontal cortex. Such data indicate that normal-appearing white matter in subjects with WMH may not be as intact as that in subjects without such lesions, and that subtle reductions in white matter integrity, as measured by DTI or MTR, may be associated with widespread negative effects on cognition beyond the region of obvious WMH using conventional MRI (Figure 17.5).

There are relatively few studies of DTI and cognitive function in aging, although two excellent reviews exist (Malloy et al., 2007; Sullivan and Pfefferbaum, 2006). Both reviews note that research in this area to date is relatively limited, but a small number of studies have found significant associations between various DTI measures and cognition. For example, Madden et al. (2004) found a significant relationship between FA in the splenium of the corpus callosum and reaction time (RT) to a choice reaction time task for young subjects. A similar relationship was also found with the anterior limb of the internal capsule of older subjects. In contrast,

Correlations with Age, FA and WMH

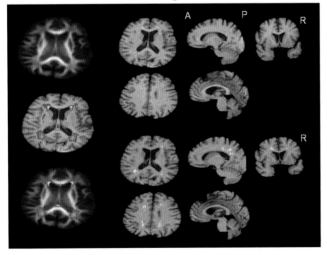

Figure 17–5 Example of age-related differences in fractional anisotropy and prevalent WMH. The three images in the left column are examples of average FA, prevalent WMH superimposed on a 3-dimensional anatomical image and prevalent WMH superimposed on the average FA image. The series of images to the right are examples of significant associations between age and FA values after adjusting for WMH. Many of the previously reported age-related differences in FA—in particular frontal FA—are clearly associated with WMH, although wide-spread differences in FA in "normal appearing white matter" also occur suggesting more diffuse effects.

another study showed a similar relationship between choice reaction time and the genu of the corpus callosum (Sullivan et al., 2001). Given these inconsistencies and age-related differences in reaction time, and their impact on cognitive function (Salthouse, 1988, 1993), the importance of these results in specific cognitive processes is not clear.

In two additional studies, O'Sullivan et al. (2001, 2004) examined DTI differences with age to differences in simple and complex attention and general intelligence. The initial study consisted of a small number of subjects (10 young and 20 older) and found that a measure of executive function (Trail Making Test, Part B minus Part A) was significantly correlated with mean diffusivity in an ROI that included anterior white matter and the genu of the corpus callosum. Verbal fluency was correlated with FA in an ROI of middle white matter that included mostly frontal and temporal, as well as periventricular white matter. These correlations remained significant after accounting for age, sex, white matter volume, premorbid IQ estimate, and general cognitive functioning. A second study of individuals with lacunar infarction and extensive WMH found significant relationships between mean diffusivity in normal-appearing periventricular white matter and performance on the Wisconsin Card Sorting test (O'Sullivan et al., 2004), but did not report relationships between cognition and DTI measures of abnormal white matter. In addition, the authors did not account for the potential independent effects of lacunes. Although the studies just reviewed find strong relationships between regional FA and cognition, other studies find significant relationships between DTI measures and motor speed, but not cognition (Fazekas et al., 2005).

Sullivan et al. (2006) propose an interesting hypothesis that the integrity of cerebral white matter may be an important component in retaining compensation of cognitive function with age (Cabeza, 2002). This is similar to the hypothesis put forward in the introductory sections of this chapter, and fits well with the results of Nordahl et al. (2006), although direct, comparative analyses of WMH, DTI, and prefrontal function have yet to be reported. In fact, many of the studies described above failed to look simultaneously at voxel-based WMH and DTI measures, making direct comparison of these two modalities less clear. Moreover, repeated studies of WMH showing significant relationships with other frontal-mediated tasks or cerebral metabolism noted above have yet to be performed. One hypothesis could be that DTI measures may be less sensitive to cognition in areas where WMH are extensive, but may give new insights into information processing in areas where WMH are less common (Sullivan and Pfefferbaum, 2006).

In conclusion, WMH occur in a considerable proportion of healthy elderly subjects. The presence and nature of these lesions, however, and their relationship with aging and cognitive decline remain controversial. Previous studies suggest that white matter injury is primarily related to ischemic events due to small vessel pathology (Pantoni, 2002). Other pathological correlates include decreases in myelinated axons (Bronge et al., 2002; Grafton et al., 1991; Meier-Ruge et al., 1992) and gliosis (Grafton et al., 1991; Takao et al., 1999). DTI has the ability to detect subtle changes in brain tissue. Still, the true nature of the tissue alterations underlying changes in FA is currently unknown. Especially for the study of older subjects, it is important to clarify the relationship between WMH, FA, or MD and their impact on cognitive ability. Future studies that can compare these measures directly or can longitudinally examine the evolution of regional FA and WMH are clearly needed.

Cerebrovascular Disease, WMH and Cognitive Aging

Many studies of aging have not taken into account the effect of white-matter abnormalities. It is important to consider this effect as a contributing factor recognizing that cerebrovascular disease (CVD), as measured by WMH, is prevalent in the elderly population and may have a profound effect on cognition. Thus, varying contributions of white-matter lesions may contaminate studies of aging. Some studies have attempted to control for white-matter lesions by excluding subjects with cerebrovascular risk factors (Rosen et al., 2002) or those on any type of prescription medications (Rypma and D'Esposito, 2000), but this may not be an exhaustive exclusion and is certainly not a representative sample of the aging population. Therefore, more studies are needed that take the effect of WMH on cognitive aging into account. In this section, we focus primarily on available evidence that links CVD to WMH and reduced cognitive performance in otherwise healthy, older individuals.

WMH are white abnormalities that appear as high-signal intensity in deep or periventricular white matter on T2-weighted MR images due to increased water content and degeneration of macromolecule structures within areas of damaged white matter. WMH are common, and increase in prevalence and severity with advancing age (Breteler et al., 1994; de Leeuw et al., 2001; Decarli, Massaro et al., 2005; Wen and Sachdev, 2004), even in the absence of clinically relevant cognitive impairment. The underlying pathology is nonspecific and includes multiple types of injury to white matter, such as myelin loss, gliosis, and neuropil atrophy (Bronge, 2002). WMH are strongly associated with stroke risk factors (Jeerakathil et al., 2004). Neuropathological studies have shown substantial age-related disturbances in white matter as evidenced by demyelination, deterioration, and axonal loss (Kemper, 1994).

A number of epidemiological studies show strong associations between elevations in mid-life blood pressure and the prevalence of later-life cognitive impairment and dementia (Elias et al., 1993, 2004; Elias, M. F. et al., 1995; Elias, P. K. et al., 1995; Launer et al., 1995). The mechanisms by which cerebrovascular risk factors (CVRFs) lead to cognitive impairment remain unclear, but a number of cross-sectional epidemiological studies, as well as longitudinal prospective studies, suggest that CVRF-related brain changes are associated with these cognitive changes (Figure 17.6).

Large epidemiological studies, while sometimes limited in the extent of cognitive testing available, consistently show moderate associations between brain atrophy or WMH volumes and diminished cognitive impairment (Breteler, 2000; de Groot et al., 1998, 2000; Longstreth et al., 1996; Longstreth et al., 2000; Ott et al., 1996). A number of smaller, cross-sectional studies consistently suggest deficits in tests of attention and mental processing (Boone et al., 1992; Breteler, 1994; DeCarli et al., 1995; Schmidt et al., 1995), although impairments in memory and general intelligence are also seen (Breteler et al., 1994; DeCarli et al., 1995). A number of these studies also show a threshold effect, where extensive amounts of WMH are necessary before cognitive impairments are seen (Boone et al., 1992; DeCarli et al., 1995; Schmidt et al., 1995).

Two studies from the Cardiovascular Health Study have examined the relationship between cognitive impairment and clinically silent cerebral infarction (Longstreth et al., 1998; Price et al., 1997). While Price et al. (1997) focused primarily on the neurological manifestations of silent cerebral infarcts, they noted a

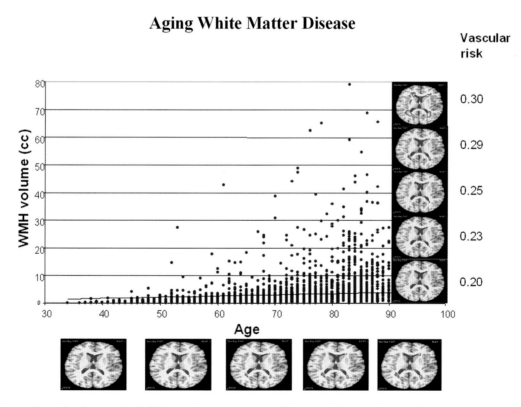

Figure 17–6 Age and vascular disease related differences in WMH extent and location. The series of images below the x-axis summarize age-related differences, whereas the images to the right summary the impact of vascular disease. Much of later-life variability in WMH may reflect concomitant vascular risk.

Longitudinal Blood Pressure Measures

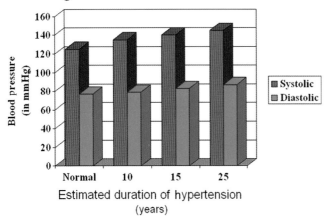

Figure 17–7 Mean systolic and diastolic blood pressure in relation to the duration of hypertension. While diastolic blood pressure is relatively well-controlled for subjects with long-standing hypertension, systolic blood pressure appears to increase with duration of disease. These data suggest that current treatments of systolic hypertension may be less than ideal.

significant increase in the number of individuals with a history of memory loss amongst those with silent cerebral infarction. Longstreth et al. (1998) examined cognitive function in more detail and noted a significant association between silent cerebral infarctions and diminished performances on the modified Mini-Mental State Examination (MMSE) and the Digit-Symbol Substitution Test (DSS). These findings are remarkably similar to the previously reported effect of WMH on cognition (Longstreth et al., 1996). Findings from these studies have been confirmed in another large population-based study (Vermeer et al., 2002, 2003).

Unfortunately, these studies did not examine the impact of lifetime cerebrovascular risk on brain structure and cognition (Figure 17.7). Results from the NHLBI Twin Study, however, confirm the suspected link between CVRFs, brain injury, and decline in cognitive performance over time (Swan et al., 1998). Lifetime

patterns of systolic blood pressure were significantly associated with differences in brain atrophy, WMH volume, and 10-year changes in MMSE and DSS scores (Swan et al., 1998) (Figure 17.8).

Importantly, however, even after correcting for age, education, baseline cognitive performance, and incident cerebrovascular disease, there were strongly significant associations between WMH volume, DSS, the Benton Visual Retention Test (BVRT), and a Verbal Fluency Test (VFT). Significant associations between brain volume and 10-year differences in MMSE, DSS, and VFT were also found. These results suggest that the cognitive changes associated with elevations in mid-life blood pressure may be mediated by the brain injury induced by prolonged elevations of blood pressure (and possibly other CVRFs). A follow-up study of the same subjects explored the pattern of cognitive changes in association with mid-life blood pressure patterns more carefully (Swan et al., 2000). Cognitive tests selected for this study fell into the two broad functional categories of memory and psychomotor speed. Subjects with combined brain atrophy and WMH were significantly older and had a higher prevalence of CVRFs (Swan et al., 2000), and performed more poorly on all tests of psychomotor speed even after correcting for age, educational achievement, and incident cerebro-vascular disease, whereas group differences on memory tests were small. These results confirm the notion that the cognitive changes associated with CVRFs generally impact frontal executive functioning (Swan et al., 2000) (Figure 17.9).

Longitudinal studies offer the advantage of examining lifetime CVRF influences on brain behavior relationships. Unfortunately, these studies have generally focused on older individuals (Swan et al., 1998, 2000), while epidemiological studies show that the impact of CVRFs—especially diabetes and hypertension—may occur at a considerably younger age (Knopman et al., 2001). Seshadri et al. (2004) examined the relationship between stroke risk factors, brain volume, and cognition in a younger group of individuals with an average age of 62 years. Age-corrected differences in brain volume were significantly and positively associated with performance on tests of attention and executive function (e.g., Trails A and B), new learning (e.g., paired associates), and visual-spatial function (e.g., delayed visual reproduction and Hooper visual organization test), but not with performance on

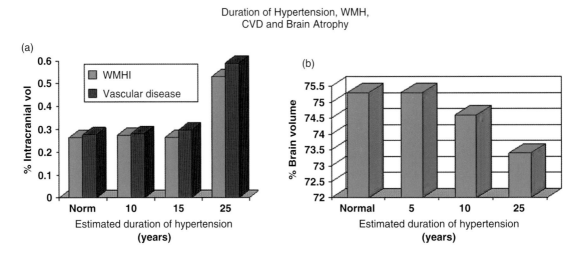

Figure 17–8 (**a**). Relationship between WMH and vascular disease seen on MRI (WMH+MRI infarction) and hypertension duration. A clear increase in vascular brain injury occurs for those individuals with the longest duration of hypertension. (**b**). Relationship between brain volume and hypertension duration. It also clear that those individuals with the longest duration of hypertension have the lowest percent brain volume.

Cognitive Performance and History of Hypertension

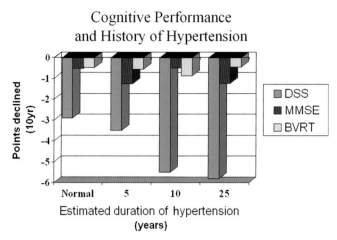

Figure 17–9 Relationship between duration of hypertension and yearly change in cognition. A significant linear effect can be seen with the digit symbol substitution test, a measure of executive function. It is hypothesized that the brain changes associated with hypertension mediate these cognitive changes. DSS denotes digit symbol substitution; MMSE denotes mini-mental status examination; BVRT denotes Benton visual retention task.

tests of verbal memory or naming. While these results are consistent with those of Swan et al. (2000), they suggest that the impact of CVRFs on brain structure and function may begin shortly after mid-life. A follow-up study examining the impact of WMH on the same cohort had similar findings (Au et al., 2006).

In summary, subtle cognitive deficits in community dwelling, essentially normal individuals are associated with CVRFs, and appear to be mediated by CVRF-related brain injury. This process begins relatively early in life, because cognitive impairment and brain injury are present to some degree even in individuals 60 years of age or younger. Frontal lobe-mediated cognitive domains of attention, concentration, and psychomotor speed are most affected in subjects free of dementia or stroke (Au et al., 2006). The relationship between frontal lobe impairments in normal aging and WMH has yet to be fully explored, but research indicates that WMH have a selective effect on the frontal lobes' structure and function. In these studies, the presence of WMH was significantly associated with decreased frontal lobe N-acetylaspartate (NAA) levels and glucose metabolism (DeCarli et al., 1995; Schuff et al., 2003; Tullberg et al., 2004). Other studies show strong correlations between memory impairment and future cognitive decline in patients with dementia and WMH (Reed et al., 2000, 2001).

A recent study by Nordahl et al. (2006) sought to directly examine the relationship between WMH and prefrontal cortex (PFC) activity in a group of cognitively normal elderly individuals during an episodic retrieval and a verbal working-memory task—two tasks in which age-related changes in PFC activity have been observed (Grady, 2000; Tisserand and Jolles, 2003). Moreover, WMH were quantified from structural MRI to examine the effects of both global WMH and regional dorsal PFC WMH on task-related activity in the PFC, as well as in areas that are functionally related to the PFC during episodic and working-memory task performance. To investigate the effect of WMH on PFC activity, the authors first identified regions of interest based on task-related BOLD activation, and then correlated WMH volumes with the magnitude of the activation within these regions. Two major

hypotheses were tested: 1) global white-matter degeneration would result in reduced activation in the PFC during each of the memory tasks, and 2) regional white-matter degeneration within the dorsal PFC would result in reduced activation in areas that interact with dorsal PFC in a task-specific manner.

Subjects for this study consisted of 15 cognitively normal individuals (4 male/11 female) over the age of 65 (range: 66-86). Importantly, individuals in this study were not preselected for presence or absence of WMH, but were selected on the basis of normal cognitive ability. In this respect, this sample is comparable to samples used in other functional neuroimaging studies of normal aging. The subjects performed the episodic-memory and the verbal-maintenance tasks as previously reported (Nordahl et al., 2005).

All subjects performed at a high level of accuracy on the cognitive tasks. Although whole-brain WMH severity was not significantly correlated with performance on immediate recall, it was significantly correlated with performance on delayed recall. WMH volumes were not correlated with performance on the verbal maintenance tasks.

Analyses of fMRI activity during each task were performed to test the two previously stated hypotheses. The first hypothesis tested correlations between global WMH severity and PFC activation, and the second hypothesis tested correlations between WMH severity within dorsal PFC and activation in other cortical areas activated during each task. To test the prediction that global WMH severity was negatively correlated with the magnitude of activation in PFC regions, dorsal and ventral PFC regions of interest (ROIs) were delineated based on group-averaged activations, and mean parameter estimates for each ROI were correlated with total WMH volume.

During episodic memory performance, total WMH volume was negatively correlated with ventral ($r = -.545$, $p = .034$) PFC activity, with a similar trend apparent in the right dorsal ($r = -.496$, $p = .059$) PFC. To test the prediction that dorsal PFC WMH may be associated with decreased recruitment of other brain regions that are functionally related to PFC, the authors correlated measures of dorsal PFC WMH severity with parameter estimates of activation in other regions that are recruited during episodic retrieval. Previous functional imaging studies suggest that in addition to dorsal and ventral PFC activity, episodic retrieval is also associated with medial temporal lobe (MTL), anterior cingulate (BA 24/32), posterior cingulate (BA 23/29/30), and posterior parietal (BA 40) cortex activity (see (Buckner and Wheeler, 2001; Cabeza and Nyberg, 2000; Desgranges et al., 1998; Tisserand and Jolles, 2003). Dorsal PFC WMH volume was strongly negatively correlated with activations in dorsal and left ventral PFC, with a similar trend evident in right ventral PFC. In addition, dorsal PFC WMH volumes were also strongly and negatively correlated with activation in bilateral MTL, anterior cingulate cortex (ACC) (BA 32), and right parietal cortex (BA 7/40) activity. To a lesser extent, there was also an association with posterior cingulate cortex activity (BA 23/29/31).

Similar, but even stronger, activation of dorsal and ventral PFC were seen during the verbal maintenance tasks. Whole-brain WMH volumes were negatively correlated with left and right dorsal PFC activations. In addition, whole brain WMH volume was negatively correlated with ventral PFC activations, but these effects did not quite reach statistical significance. Analysis of regions outside the PFC was also performed. Specifically, the authors were interested in ACC (BA 24/32) and posterior parietal cortex (BA 7/40), two areas that are commonly activated during working memory tasks (see Smith and Jonides, 1999). Dorsal PFC WMH were significantly and negatively correlated with bilateral dorsal and ventral PFC activations, and also with the ACC and left parietal cortex. A similar correlation was observed in the right parietal cortex, but was not statistically significant.

These results strongly suggest that WMH disrupts the functional integrity of a widely distributed memory system involving parietal, dorsal lateral prefrontal, anterior cingulate, and hippocampal regions (Baddeley, 2003). Although the exact pathophysiology by which WMH may affect this system requires further research, it is clear that disruption of specific pathways must be involved. As noted above, these might include connections between the dorsolateral prefrontal cortex and their subcortical targets (Alexander et al., 1986), the long cortico-cortical connections between prefrontal and posterior parietal cortex (Burruss et al., 2000; Cavada and Goldman-Rakic, 1989a, 1989b; Cummings, 1993; Selemon and Goldman-Rakic, 1988; Tekin and Cummings, 2002), or the prefrontal, retrosplenial, hippocampal circuit (Morris et al., 1999; Petrides and Pandya, 1999). Current research in our laboratory is systematically exploring these various pathways using diffusion-tensor imaging. We hypothesize that those pathways directly involved in memory system dysfunction by WMH will sshow reduced FA that is more highly correlated with memory-task performance and cognitive activation than regional WMH indicating the specificity of the identified white-matter bundles.

These separate lines of evidence coalesce to create a body of evidence that asymptomatic vascular brain injury results in subtle frontal lobe dysfunction and cognitive impairments assumed to relate to frontal lobe function, which are often ascribed to "normal cognitive aging" (West, 1996). These findings suggest that "normal cognitive aging" may be, in part, the consequence of asymptomatic CVD—an area of study that we are currently pursuing in our laboratory.

Given that episodic memory performance involves coordination between dorsolateral prefrontal cortex-mediated working memory and hippocampus-mediated consolidation, it would not be surprising to find associations between vascular disease and mild cognitive impairment (MCI) (DeCarli et al., 2001; Lopez et al., 2003). In a later section, we describe data from our laboratory, giving evidence for the existence of a vascular form of MCI. Before we discuss the influence of WMH on cognitive impairment in MCI and AD, however, we review recent neuropathological evidence relating to the pathophysiology of WMH in these disorders.

Pathology of WMH

Although a host of studies have reported pathological associations with WMH (please see DeCarli and Scheltens, 2002 for exhaustive review), most of these studies have focused on postmortem imaging of fixed tissues. A recent study by Jagust et al. (2008) correlated regional neuropathological findings with in vivo MRI imaging of 93 individuals who were followed longitudinally to death. Each subject received standardized MRI sequence acquisition, as well as analysis of WMH, brain, hippocampus and infarct volumes. WMH volumes were log transformed to normalize variance. These measures were compared to a systematic neuropathological survey that included a newly developed scale to assess the neuropathological features of cerebrovascular disease (Chui et al., 2006).

In univariate analyses against log WMH, positive correlations were noted between WMH and AD and CVD pathology, as well as

hippocampal sclerosis. All pathological variables of CVD (cystic infarction, lacunar infarction, microscopic infarction, cortical infarction, subcortical infarctions, and white matter incomplete infarctions) were positively correlated with log WMH. Secondary analysis also revealed that the extent of cerebrovascular arteriosclerosis was also positively associated with WMH ($\beta = 0.13$, SE = 0.03, p-value = 0.0002). No significant relationship between CAA and log WMH was found in the sample as a whole, although there was a weak trend in the high AD path group ($r = 0.16$, $p = 0.30$; no significant interaction). In the final multivariate model for log WMH, age at death and the extent of white matter incomplete infarction explained 32% of the variance in log WMH. Of note, the extent of arteriosclerosis was positively associated with log WMH at a marginally significant level ($\beta = 0.07$, SE = 0.04, $p = 0.059$) after adjustment for age at death and extent of incomplete white-matter infarction. Importantly, there was no association between WMH and indices of Alzheimer pathology supporting the notion that these are two distinct processes. From these results, the authors note that they cannot state with certainty whether the pathological "incomplete infarction" (pallor, demyelination, and axonal loss) that was found to be associated with WMH reflects CVD and not Wallerian degeneration. However, the latter was deemed to be less likely in view of the lack of association between WMH and AD pathology. They conclude, "In the setting of progressive cognitive impairment in late-life, this study suggests that WMH is associated with vascular disease, and complete and incomplete infarction, and is thus a more specific finding than previously supposed."

Given evidence that WMH are likely independent of AD pathology, we now examine data related to the impact of WMH in two of the most common cognitive impairment syndromes—amnestic MCI (aMCI) and dementia.

WMH and Memory Performance in MCI

Recent work suggests that the extent of WMH is increased in individuals with MCI (DeCarli et al., 2001; Lopez et al., 2003; Yoshita et al., 2006). In a recent study, Nordahl et al. (2005) used WMH as a marker for small vessel CVD severity—to identify and contrast two groups of subjects with aMCI. In this study, the authors proposed that WMH related to small vessel CVD might play a role in the episodic memory impairment characteristic of aMCI. The authors predicted that WMH might compromise executive control processes that are critical for working memory, which in turn may lead to episodic memory deficits and a diagnosis of aMCI. This hypothesis was based on the preposition that if information cannot be actively maintained and manipulated at an immediate or short-term level, impairments in consolidation and retrieval could occur (Blumenfeld and Ranganath, 2006; Ranganath et al., 2003). Thus, whereas hippocampal dysfunction may be associated with isolated episodic memory impairments, small-vessel CVD may lead to a distinct pattern of deficits that includes both episodic-memory impairment and deficits in executive control processes.

To test their hypothesis, the authors examined a group of individuals who were clinically diagnosed with aMCI, and used MRI to stratify the subjects into two subgroups: (1) those with severe WMH without hippocampal atrophy (MCI-WMH), and (2) those with severe hippocampal atrophy without extensive WMH (MCI-HA). Cognitive performance for each of these groups was compared to a group of age-matched control subjects. Importantly, these specific subgroups of aMCI subjects were selected to isolate the different mechanisms by which WMH and HA may lead to episodic memory impairment in MCI (Figure 17.10). Although CVD and AD pathology often co-occur, the nature of the interaction is unclear and complex to study due to the difficulty of disentangling the two in standard clinical samples. Thus, a highly selected sample was studied to investigate the separate roles that each type of brain lesion may play in producing memory impairment.

The study was divided into two parts. First, the authors compared the performance of aMCI patients and controls on the neuropsychological tests that were used to diagnose aMCI according to standard criteria (Petersen et al., 1999). This explored whether standard neuropsychological tests used widely in clinical practice would differ between the two MCI groups. Second, the authors compared the performance of these subjects on a battery of behavioral tasks used widely in the cognitive neuroscience literature. This second series of tasks was designed to explore the different cognitive mechanisms that underlie memory loss in aMCI. The battery included an episodic-memory task, two working-memory tasks, and a version of the continuous performance test (CPT) (see Nordahl et al., 2005 for complete details). The authors predicted that both groups of MCI participants would show deficits on the episodic-memory task, but that the MCI-WMH group would show additional impairments on the working memory tasks and on the CPT consistent with the hypothesized deficits in frontal function associated with WMH.

Results showed that, by design, MCI-HA individuals had significantly smaller hippocampi than MCI-WMH, whereas MCI-WMH did not differ from healthy controls with regard to hippocampal volume. Conversely, MCI-WMH had significantly

higher WMH volumes than MCI-HA, which also did not differ from control volumes. The two MCI groups were equally impaired on all episodic-memory tests relative to controls: WMS-R Logical Memory I & II, and MAS List Learning, Immediate Recall and Delayed Recall (Nordahl et al., 2005). The two MCI groups did not differ from each other or in terms of controls on other neuropsychological tasks such as the Digit Span or Boston Naming. There were, however, striking differences in performance on all of the working-memory tasks, including the n-back and verbal and spatial variants of the item-recognition task, where the MCI-HA group performed similar to normal controls, but the MCI-WMH performed significantly more poorly. Further testing of executive control using the CPT revealed that MCI-WMH subjects had poorer attention and committed more impulsive errors than MCI-HA or normal controls. In addition, WMH volumes were inversely associated with performance on these tasks (Figure 17.11).

This study was designed to test the hypothesis that among individuals diagnosed with aMCI, small vessel CVD and hippocampal dysfunction give rise to different profiles of cognitive deficits (Nordahl et al., 2005). Results revealed that, although these two groups were virtually indistinguishable on standard neuropsychological tests administered at the time of diagnosis of MCI, more detailed testing revealed reliable differences between the two subgroups of MCI subjects. Whereas MCI-HA patients exhibited relatively specific episodic-memory impairment, MCI-WMH patients exhibited deficits on episodic memory, working memory, and attentional control tasks. These findings suggest that MCI-WMH subjects, in contrast to MCI-HA subjects, suffered from impaired executive control processes that affect a wide variety of cognitive domains.

Although episodic memory has historically been linked to the hippocampus and surrounding cortices (as noted above),

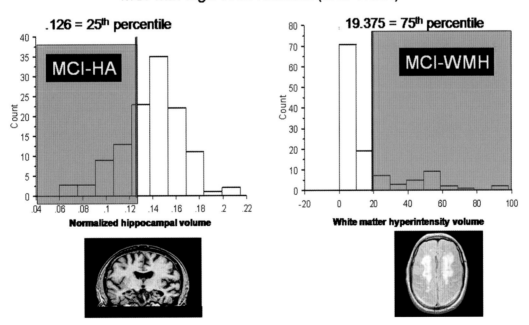

Figure 17–10 Methods used to define the two subclasses of mild cognitive impairment (MCI) with MRI examples. Please see text for complete description.

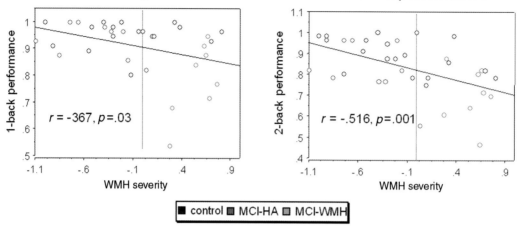

Figure 17–11 Association between WMH volume and performance on a test of executive function among cognitively normal individuals and individuals with the two MCI subtypes. These results show that WMH contributes to impairments in executive function in a continuous fashion across all individuals independent of cognitive category, although the impact is greatest among the MCI-WMH subgroup.

evidence from neuropsychological and neuroimaging studies suggest that the PFC plays a critical role in implementing executive control processes that contribute to normal episodic-memory function (Blumenfeld and Ranganath, 2006; Ranganath et al., 2003). In this study, MCI-WMH subjects were impaired not only on episodic memory tasks, but also on a battery of working-memory tasks in both verbal and spatial domains, as well as an attentional-control task. The author's interpretation of the data was that episodic-memory failure in MCI-WMH subjects was secondary to a more general impairment in executive control processes.

The authors conclude by hypothesizing that WMH may reflect a disruption of the white-matter tracts that connect dorsolateral prefrontal cortex (DLPFC) with its targets. Disruption of these neural circuits could lead to deficits in executive control processes that impact a wide range of cognitive domains, including episodic memory. As discussed previously, multiple neural circuits exist that, if disrupted, might lead to the findings described above. For example, lesions affecting connections between the DLPFC and its subcortical targets (Alexander et al., 1986), or lesions affecting the long cortico-cortical connections between prefrontal and posterior parietal cortex (Cavada and Goldman-Rakic, 1989a, 1989b; Selemon and Goldman-Rakic, 1988), would be expected to result in impaired working memory and executive-control processes (Burruss et al., 2000; Cummings, 1993; Tekin and Cummings, 2002). Disconnection of the prefrontal, retrosplenial, hippocampal circuit may also give rise to deficits observed (Morris et al., 1999; Petrides and Pandya, 1999).

If CVD, as manifested by WMH, leads to deficits in executive-control processes, then MCI subjects with extensive WMH might be expected to have more severe cognitive deficits and develop dementia more rapidly. Unfortunately, the results of a number of studies are mixed (DeCarli et al., 2004; Rossi et al., 2007; Wolf et al., 2000). Inconsistencies in the results may reflect subject selection and various other technical difficulties. Importantly, the most recent study by Rossi et al. (2007) was most similar to the Nordahl et al. (2005) study in that subjects were stratified according to both the extent of hippocampal atrophy and WMH severity. The results of this study show that

individuals with both hippocampal atrophy and extensive WMH have the greatest likelihood of progressing to dementia over a brief period of observation.

WMH in Dementia

In the previous sections, we reviewed evidence that CVD-related brain injury leads to subtle cognitive impairments in otherwise healthy older individuals and, when sufficient, may even lead to clinically significant cognitive impairment, such as MCI. In this section, we critically review available data relating the role of WMH to clinical dementia (Figure 17.12).

The relative impact of CVD on dementia occurrence has a long and debatable history (Brust, 1988; O'Brien, 1988). While there is a well-developed literature with regard to dementia after stroke (Henon et al., 2001; Moroney et al., 1996, 1997a, 1997b; Tatemichi, 1990; Tatemichi et al., 1990, 1992, 1995a, 1995b), it is quite common to identify individuals who have a slowly progressive dementing illness, multiple vascular risk factors, and extensive WMH using brain imaging. The impact of this asymptomatic CVD brain injury on dementia incidence remains unclear, but accumulating evidence suggests that CVD-related brain injury may significantly increase the likelihood of developing dementia, possibly through an additive interaction with AD (Esiri et al., 1999; Jagust, 2001; Schneider et al., 2003; Schneider et al., 2004; Snowdon et al., 1997).

Increased WMH burden is found in patients with dementia of the Alzheimer's type (Barber et al., 1999; Fazekas et al., 1996; McDonald et al., 1991; Mirsen et al., 1991; Scheltens et al., 1992, 1995; Waldemar et al., 1994; Yoshita et al., 2006). While some studies find significant relationships between WMH and certain cognitive functions or dementia severity (Bondareff et al., 1988, 1990; Diaz et al., 1991; Harrell et al., 1991; Kertesz et al., 1990; Ott et al., 1997; Stout et al., 1996; Yoshita et al., 2006), other studies do not (Barber et al., 1999; Bennett et al., 1992, 1994; Brilliant et al., 1995; DeCarli et al., 1995; Doody et al., 1998; Fazekas et al., 1987, 1996; Kozachuk et al., 1990; Leys et al., 1990; Lopez et al., 1992, 1995; Marder et al., 1995; McDonald et al., 1991; Mirsen et al., 1991; Scheltens et al., 1992, 1995; Schmidt, 1992; Starkstein et al.,

Regional Atrophy and WMH in NL, MCI and AD

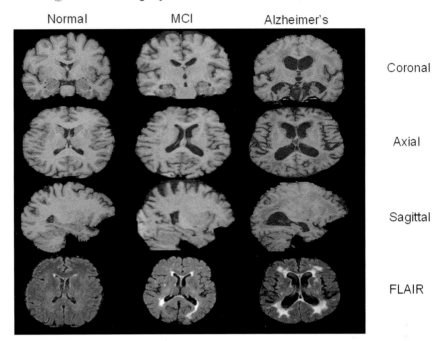

Figure 17–12 MRI examples of differences in brain atrophy and WMH amongst representative images from cognitively normal, MCI and dementia patients. Both regional atrophy and increase in WMH are associated with progressive cognitive impairment.

1997; Teipel et al., 1998; Wahlund et al., 1994). Differences in study populations and the heterogeneity of white-matter changes may explain the inconsistency among these studies. For example, selection of AD patients without vascular risk factors may result in excluding individuals with extensive WMH (Kozachuk et al., 1990), thereby minimizing their effects. In patients with CVD and dementia, small subcortical infarcts also frequently accompany WMH (Caplan, 1995; Roman, 1987), obscuring the independent effects that WMH confer to the dementia (Bennett et al., 1994).

Recently, new methods have been developed that allow for anatomical mapping of WMH (DeCarli et al., 2005; Wen and Sachdev, 2004) that may offer more explicit assessment of the impact of WMH on cognition (Figure 17.13). One study using this technology (Yoshita et al., 2006) evaluated the anatomical distribution of WMH among a group of cognitively normal MCI and AD patients. A total of 87 individuals were studied, nearly equally divided among the three cognitive groups. The prevalence of vascular risk factors, such as hypertension, was also determined. The results found a significant rostral-to-caudal progression of WMH in association with cognitive ability, with all three groups having WMH in the anterior periventricular areas, but MCI extending to the mid-portion of the periventricular region and AD patients having significantly more WMH posteriorly. Post-hoc analyses revealed two patterns of WMH distribution. Among individuals with vascular risk factors, periventricular WMH was significantly increased, while there was a localized increase of WMH in posterior regions in association with increasing cognitive impairment. Multiple regression analysis found these two spatial distributions to be independent, although both were more prevalent in the demented group. These findings raised the possibility that WMH may result from both degenerative and vascular processes, and both may contribute to the cognitive disability associated with dementia. These data suggest, like the pathological literature (Schneider et al., 2003, 2004), that CVD may serve as a risk factor for expressed dementia in association with AD.

Contrasting results come from another series of MRI studies (Mungas et al., 2001, 2002, 2005). In these studies, individuals with memory impairment, WMH, and lacunar infarction consistent with subcortical ischemic disease were enrolled in a longitudinal study. MRI results found that the volumes of cortical gray matter and hippocampus were the strongest predictors of cognitive impairment and cognitive decline as compared to quantitative measures of infarct volume or WMH. Another study of the same cohort also showed that memory impairment and hippocampal volume were the strongest predictors of progression from MCI to dementia (DeCarli et al., 2004). These data suggest that, in a cohort of individuals recruited through a memory disorders clinic, even if allowed to have evidence of subcortical vascular brain injury, AD pathology remains the predominate etiology of cognitive impairment. These results, however, contrast somewhat with epidemiological studies (Kuller et al., 2003; Vermeer et al., 2003; Wu et al., 2002), where WMH and brain infarction are significantly associated with dementia—sometimes in an additive fashion (Wu et al., 2002). Such differences could result from differences in methodology (most MRI analysis of large cohorts are qualitative) or sample selection, as these cohorts are unselected and, therefore, may have higher degrees of CVD or less AD pathology. Newer imaging tools, such as brain amyloid imaging (Mathis et al., 2005), may prove extremely helpful in determining the extent of concurrent AD pathology, thereby allowing for accurate estimation of the relative contributions of both CVD and AD pathologies to cognition across the spectrum of cognitive ability.

Conclusion

The relationship between cognitive impairment and WMH remains poorly understood. Newer methods, however, may enable a more anatomically specific analysis of WMH that could provide important new insights regarding the impact of white-matter injury on neural systems and widely distributed cognitive

Distribution of High Frequency WMH

Anterior   Posterior

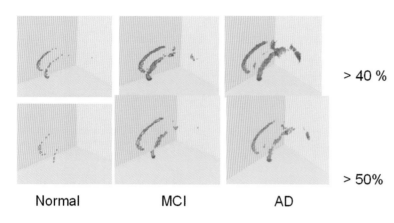

> 40 %

> 50%

Normal   MCI   AD

Figure 17–13 Spatial distribution of WMH from cognitively normal, MCI and dementia subjects indicating the anterior to posterior progression of WMH with increasing cognitive impairment. Images reveal anatomical distribution where either 40% or 50% of subjects have WMH at a particular location.

Role of AD and WMH in Cognition

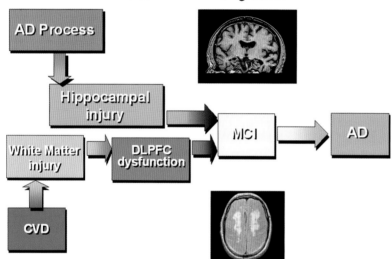

Figure 17–14 Model of possible biological mechanisms whereby cerebrovascular disease (as manifest by WMH) and AD pathologies contribute to MCI and subsequent development of AD dementia.

functions. Given that WMH and associated CVRFs are so prevalent and play a role in producing cognitive impairment (DeCarli et al., 1995), understanding the role they play in the aging brain is essential (Figure 17.14). This is especially important since the presence of WMH is often undetected because it is clinically silent in many individuals. Because white-matter abnormalities resulting from CVD are both preventable and treatable by changes in lifestyle or medication, understanding these mechanisms could lead to interventions that serve to slow age-related cognitive changes. Cognitive impairment, CVD, and their effects on health and well-being will continue to be a major public health concern as the elderly population continues to grow as a proportion of the population (US Census Bureau, 2004).

References

Abe, O., Aoki, S., Hayashi, N., Yamada, H., Kunimatsu, A., Mori, H. et al. (2002). Normal aging in the central nervous system: quantitative MR diffusion-tensor analysis. *Neurobiology of Aging*, 23(3): 433–441.

Aizenstein, H. J., Butters, M. A., Clark, K. A., Figurski, J. L., Andrew Stenger, V., Nebes, R. D. et al. (2006). Prefrontal and striatal activation in elderly subjects during concurrent implicit and explicit sequence learning. *Neurobiology of Aging*, 27(5): 741–751.

Alexander, G. E., DeLong M. R., Strick, P. L. (1986). Parallel organization of functionally segregated circuits linking basal ganglia and cortex. *Annual Review of Neuroscience*, 9: 357–381.

Au, R., Massaro, J. M., Wolf, P. A., Young, M. E., Beiser, A., Seshadri, S. et al. (2006). Association of white matter hyperintensity volume with decreased cognitive functioning: The Framingham Heart Study. *Archives of Neurology*, 63(2): 246–250.

Baddeley, A. (2003). Working memory: Looking back and looking forward. *Nature Reviews. Neuroscience* 4(10): 829–839.

Barber, R., Scheltens, P., Gholkar, A., Ballard, C., McKeith, I., Ince, P. et al. (1999). White matter lesions on magnetic resonance imaging in dementia with Lewy bodies, Alzheimer's disease, vascular dementia, and normal aging. *Journal of Neurology, Neurosurgery and Psychiatry*, 67: 66–72.

Basser, P. J. and Jones, D. K. (2002). Diffusion-tensor MRI: Theory, experimental design and data analysis—a technical review. *NMR in Biomedicine*, 15(7–8): 456–467.

Beaulieu, C. (2002). The basis of anisotropic water diffusion in the nervous system—a technical review. *NMR in Biomedicine* 15(7–8): 435–455.

Bennett, D. A., Gilley, D. W., Wilson, R. S., Huckman, M. S., Fox, J. H. (1992). Clinical correlates of high signal lesions on magnetic resonance imaging in Alzheimer's disease. *Journal of Neurology*, 239(4): 186–190.

Bennett, D. A., Gilley, D. W., Lee, S., Cochran, E. J. (1994). White matter changes: Neurobehavioral manifestations of Binswanger's disease and clinical correlates in Alzheimer's disease. *Dementia*, 5(3–4): 148–152.

Bhagat, Y. A. and Beaulieu, C. (2004). Diffusion anisotropy in subcortical white matter and cortical gray matter: Changes with aging and the role of CSF-suppression. *Journal of Magnetic Resonance Imaging*, 20(2): 216–227.

Blumenfeld, R. S. and Ranganath, C. (2006). Dorsolateral prefrontal cortex promotes long-term memory formation through its role in working memory organization. *Journal of Neuroscience*, 26(3): 916–925.

Bondareff, W., Raval, J., Colletti, P. M., Hauser, D. L. (1988). Quantitative magnetic resonance imaging and the severity of dementia in Alzheimer's disease. *The American Journal of Psychiatry*, 145: 853–856.

Bondareff, W., Raval, J., Woo, B., Hauser, D. L., Colletti, P. M. (1990). Magnetic resonance imaging and the severity of dementia in older adults. *Archives of General Psychiatry*, 47: 47–51.

Boone, K. B., Miller, B. L., Lesser, I. M., Mehringer, C. M., Hill, E., and Berman, N. (1992). Cognitive deficits with white-matter lesions in healthy elderly. *Archives of Neurology*, 49: 549–554.

Breteler, M. M. (2000). Vascular involvement in cognitive decline and dementia. Epidemiologic evidence from the Rotterdam Study and the Rotterdam Scan Study. *Annals of the New York Academy of Sciences*, 903(11 Suppl. 5): 457–465.

Breteler, M. M., Claus, J. J., Grobbee, D. E., Hofman, A. (1994). Cardiovascular disease and distribution of cognitive function in elderly people: The Rotterdam Study. *British Medical Journal*, 308(6944): 1604–1608.

Breteler, M. M., van Amerongen, N. M., van Swieten, J. C., Claus, J. J., Grobbee, D. E., van Gijn, J. et al. (1994). Cognitive correlates of ventricular enlargement and cerebral white matter lesions on MRI: The Rotterdam Study. *Stroke*, 25: 1109–1115.

Brilliant, M., Hughes, L., Anderson, D., Ghobrial, M., Elble, R. (1995). Rarefied white matter in patients with Alzheimer disease. *Alzheimer's Disease and Associated Disorders*, 9: 39–46.

Bronge, L. (2002). Magnetic resonance imaging in dementia. A study of brain white matter changes. *Acta radiologica. Supplementum*, 428: 1–32.

Bronge, L., Bogdanovic, N., Wahlund, L. O. (2002). Postmortem MRI and histopathology of white matter changes in Alzheimer brains. A quantitative, comparative study. *Dementia and Geriatric Cognitive Disorders*, 13(4): 205–212.

Brust, J. C. M. (1988). Vascular dementia is overdiagnosed. *Archives of Neurology*, 45: 799–801.

Buckner, R. L. (2005). Three principles for cognitive aging research. In R. Cabeza, L. Nyberg and D. Park (eds), *Cognitive Neuroscience of Aging* (pp. 267–285). New York: Oxford University Press.

Buckner, R. L. and Wheeler, M. E. (2001). The cognitive neuroscience of remembering. *Nature Reviews. Neuroscience*. 2(9): 624–634.

Burruss, J. W., Hurley, R. A., Taber, K. H., Rauch, R. A., Norton, R. E., Hayman, L. A. (2000). Functional neuroanatomy of the frontal lobe circuits. *Radiology*, 214(1): 227–230.

Cabeza, R. (2002). Hemispheric asymmetry reduction in older adults: The HAROLD model. *Psychology and Aging*, 17(1): 85–100.

Cabeza, R. and Nyberg, L. (2000). Imaging cognition II: An empirical review of 275 PET and fMRI studies. *Journal of Cognitive Neuroscience*, 12(1): 1–47.

Caplan, L. R. (1995). Binswanger's disease-revisited. *Neurology*, 45: 626–633.

Cavada, C. and Goldman-Rakic, P. S. (1989a). Posterior parietal cortex in rhesus monkey: I. Parcellation of areas based on distinctive limbic and sensory corticocortical connections. *The Journal of Comparative Neurology*, 287(4): 393–421.

Cavada, C. and Goldman-Rakic, P. S. (1989b). Posterior parietal cortex in rhesus monkey: II. Evidence for segregated corticocortical networks linking sensory and limbic areas with the frontal lobe. *The Journal of Comparative Neurology*, 287(4): 422–445.

Cerella, J. (1990). Aging and information processing rate. In J. Birren and K. Schaie (eds), *Handbook of the Psychology of Aging*. San Diego: Academic Press.

Chui, H. C., Zarow, C., Mack, W. J., Ellis, W. G., Zheng, L., Jagust, W. J. et al. (2006). Cognitive impact of subcortical vascular and Alzheimer's disease pathology. *Annals of Neurology*, 60(6): 677–687.

Chun, T., Filippi, C. G., Zimmerman, R. D., Ulug, A. M. (2000). Diffusion changes in the aging human brain. *AJNR. American Journal of Neuroradiology*, 21(6): 1078–1083.

Cummings, J. L. (1993). Frontal-subcortical circuits and human behavior. *Archives of Neurology*, 50(8): 873–880.

Cummings, J. L. (1995). Anatomic and behavioral aspects of frontal-subcortical circuits. In J. Grafman and K. J. Holyoak (eds), *Annals of the New York Academy of Sciences* (Vol. 769, pp. 1–13) New York: The New York Academy of Sciences.

Cummings, J. L. (1998). Frontal-subcortical circuits and human behavior. *Journal of Psychosomatic Research*, 44(6): 627–628.

Cutler, S. J. and Grams, A. E. (1988). Correlates of self-reported everyday memory problems. *Journal of Gerontology: Social Sciences*, 43: S82–S90.

de Groot, J. C., de Leeuw, F. E., Breteler, M. M. (1998). Cognitive correlates of cerebral white matter changes. *Journal of Neural Transmission. Supplementum*, 53(1): 41–67.

de Groot, J. C., de Leeuw, F. E., Oudkerk, M., van Gijn, J., Hofman, A., Jolles, J. et al. (2000). Cerebral white matter lesions and cognitive function: The Rotterdam Scan Study [see comments]. *Annals of Neurology*, 47(2): 145–151.

de Leeuw, F. E., de Groot, J. C., Achten, E., Oudkerk, M., Ramos, L. M., Heijboer, R. et al. (2001). Prevalence of cerebral white matter lesions in elderly people: A population based magnetic resonance imaging study. The Rotterdam Scan Study. *Journal of Neurology, Neurosurgery, and Psychiatry*, 70(1): 9–14.

Decarli, C. (2004). Vascular factors in dementia: An overview. *Journal of the Neurological Sciences*, 226(1–2): 19–23.

DeCarli, C., Fletcher, E., Ramey, V., Harvey, D., Jagust, W. J. (2005). Anatomical mapping of white matter hyperintensities (WMH): Exploring the relationships between periventricular WMH, deep WMH, and total WMH burden. *Stroke*, 36(1): 50–55.

DeCarli, C., Massaro, J., Harvey, D., Hald, J., Tullberg, M., Au, R. et al. (2005). Measures of brain morphology and infarction in the framingham heart study: Establishing what is normal. *Neurobiology of Aging*, 26(4): 491–510.

DeCarli, C., Miller, B. L., Swan, G. E., Reed, T., Wolf, P. A., Carmelli, D. (2001). Cerebrovascular and brain morphologic correlates of mild cognitive impairment in the National Heart, Lung, and Blood Institute Twin Study. *Archives of Neurology*, 58(4): 643–647.

DeCarli, C., Mungas, D., Harvey, D., Reed, B., Weiner, M., Chui, H. et al. (2004). Memory impairment, but not cerebrovascular disease, predicts progression of MCI to dementia. *Neurology*, 63(2): 220–227.

DeCarli, C., Murphy, D. G., Tranh, M., Grady, C. L., Haxby, J. V., Gillette, J. A. et al. (1995). The effect of white matter hyperintensity volume on brain structure, cognitive performance, and cerebral metabolism of glucose in 51 healthy adults. *Neurology*, 45(11): 2077–2084.

DeCarli, C. and Scheltens, P. (2002). Structural Brain Imaging. In T. Erkinjuntti and S. Gauthier (eds), *Vascular Cognitive Impairment* (pp. 433–459). London: Martin Dunitz, LTD.

Desgranges, B., Baron, J. C., Eustache, F. (1998). The functional neuroanatomy of episodic memory: The role of the frontal lobes, the hippocampal formation, and other areas. *Neuroimage*, 8(2): 198–213.

Diaz, J. F., Merskey, H., Hachinski, V. C., Lee, D. H., Boniferro, M., Wong, C. J. et al. (1991). Improved recognition of leukoaraiosis and cognitive impairment in Alzheimer's disease. *Archives of Neurology*, 48(10): 1022–1025.

Doody, R. S., Massman, P. J., Mawad, M., Nance, M. (1998). Cognitive consequences of subcortical magnetic resonance imaging changes in Alzheimer's disease: comparison to small vessel ischemic vascular dementia. *Neuropsychiatry, Neuropsychology, and Behavioral Neurology*, 11: 191–199.

Elias, M. F., D'Agostino, R. B., Elias, P. K., Wolf, P. A. (1995). Neuropsychological test performance, cognitive functioning, blood pressure, and age: The Framingham Heart Study. *Experimental Aging Research*, 21(4): 369–391.

Elias, M. F., Sullivan, L. M., D'Agostino, R. B., Elias, P. K., Beiser, A., Au, R. et al. (2004). Framingham stroke risk profile and lowered cognitive performance. *Stroke*, 35(2): 404–409.

Elias, M. F., Wolf, P. A, D'Agostino, R. B., Cobb, J., and White, L. R. (1993). Untreated blood pressure level is inversely related to cognitive functioning: the Framingham Study. *American Journal of Epidemiology*, 138: 353–364.

Elias, P. K., D'Agostino, R. B., Elias, M. F., Wolf, P. A. (1995). Blood pressure, hypertension, and age as risk factors for poor cognitive performance. *Experimental Aging Research*, 21(4): 393–417.

Esiri, M. M., Nagy, Z., Smith, M. Z., Barnetson, L., Smith, A. D. (1999). Cerebrovascular disease and threshold for dementia in the early stages of Alzheimer's disease. *Lancet*, 354(9182): 919–920.

Fazekas, F., Chawluk, J. B., Alavi, A., Hurtig, H. I., Zimmerman, R. A. (1987). MR signal abnormalities at 1.5 T in Alzheimer's dementia and normal aging. *American Journal of Neuroradiology*, 8: 421–426.

Fazekas, F., Kapeller, P., Schmidt, R., Offenbacher, H., Payer, F., Fazekas, G. (1996). The relation of cerebral magnetic resonance signal hyperintensities to Alzheimer's disease. *Journal of the Neurological Sciences*, 142(1–2): 121–125.

Fazekas, F., Ropele, S., Enzinger, C., Gorani, F., Seewann, A., Petrovic, K. et al. (2005). MTI of white matter hyperintensities. *Brain*, 128(Pt. 12): 2926–2932.

Ferri, C. P., Prince, M., Brayne, C., Brodaty, H., Fratiglioni, L., Ganguli, M. et al. (2005). Global prevalence of dementia: A Delphi consensus study. *Lancet*, 366(9503): 2112–2117.

Ganguli, M., Dodge, H. H., Chen, P., Belle, S., DeKosky, S. T. (2000). Ten-year incidence of dementia in a rural elderly US community population: The MoVIES Project. *Neurology*, 54(5): 1109–1116.

Geschwind, N. (1965a). Disconnexion syndromes in animals and man. I. *Brain*, 88(2): 237–294.

Geschwind, N. (1965b). Disconnexion syndromes in animals and man. II. *Brain*, 88(3): 585–644.

Goldman-Rakic, P. S. (1987). Circuitry of the frontal association cortex and its relevance to dementia. *Archives of Gerontology and Geriatrics*, 6(3): 299–309.

Goldman-Rakic, P. S. (1988). Topography of cognition: Parallel distributed networks in primate association cortex. *Annual Review of Neuroscience*, 11: 137–156.

Grady, C. L. (2000). Functional brain imaging and age-related changes in cognition. *Biological Psychology*, 54(1–3): 259–281.

Grady, C. L. and Craik, F. I. (2000). Changes in memory processing with age. *Current Opinion in Neurobiology*, 10(2): 224–231.

Grady, C. L., Springer, M. V., Hongwanishkul, D., McIntosh, A. R., Winocur, G. (2006). Age-related changes in brain activity across the adult lifespan. *Journal of Cognitive Neuroscience*, 18(2): 227–241.

Grafton, S. T., Sumi, S. M., Stimac, G. K., Alvord, E. C., Jr., Shaw, C. M., Nochlin, D. (1991). Comparison of postmortem magnetic resonance imaging and neuropathologic findings in the cerebral white matter. *Archives of Neurology*, 48(3): 293–298.

Gunning-Dixon, F. M. and Raz, N. (2000). The cognitive correlates of white matter abnormalities in normal aging: A quantitative review. *Neuropsychology*, 14(2): 224–232.

Harrell, L. E., Duvall, E., Folks, D. G., Duke, L., Bartolucci, A., Conboy, T. et al. (1991). The relationship of high-intensity signals on magnetic resonance images to cognitive and psychiatric state in Alzheimer's disease. *Archives of Neurology*, 48: 1136–1140.

Head, D., Buckner, R. L., Shimony, J. S., Williams, L. E., Akbudak, E., Conturo, T. E. et al. (2004). Differential vulnerability of anterior white matter in nondemented aging with minimal acceleration in dementia of the Alzheimer type: Evidence from diffusion tensor imaging. *Cerebral Cortex*, 14(4): 410–423.

Hebert, L. E., Scherr, P. A., Bienias, J. L., Bennett, D. A., Evans, D. A. (2004). State-specific projections through 2025 of Alzheimer disease prevalence. *Neurology*, 62(9): 1645.

Helenius, J., Soinne, L., Perkio, J., Salonen, O., Kangasmaki, A., Kaste, M. et al. (2002). Diffusion-weighted MR imaging in normal human brains in various age groups. *American Journal of Neuroradiology*, 23(2): 194–199.

Henon, H., Durieu, I., Guerouaou, D., Lebert, F., Pasquier, F., Leys, D. (2001). Poststroke dementia: incidence and relationship to prestroke cognitive decline. *Neurology*, 57(7): 1216–1222.

Jagust, W. (2001). Untangling vascular dementia. *Lancet*, 358(9299): 2097–2098.

Jagust, W. J., Zheng, L., Harvey, D. J., Mack, W. J., Vinters, H. V., Weiner, M. W. et al. (2008). Neuropathological basis of magnetic resonance images in aging and dementia. *Annals of Neurology*, 63(1): 72-80.

Jeerakathil, T., Wolf, P. A., Beiser, A., Massaro, J., Seshadri, S., D'Agostino, R. B. et al. (2004). Stroke risk profile predicts white matter hyperintensity volume: The Framingham Study. *Stroke*, 35(8): 1857–1861.

Jones, D. K., Lythgoe, D., Horsfield, M. A., Simmons, A., Williams, S. C., Markus, H. S. (1999). Characterization of white matter damage in ischemic leukoaraiosis with diffusion tensor MRI. *Stroke*, 30(2): 393–397.

Jones, D. K., Symms, M. R., Cercignani, M., Howard, R. J. (2005). The effect of filter size on VBM analyses of DT-MRI data. *Neuroimage*, 26(2): 546–54.

Kanaan, R. A., Shergill, S. S., Barker, G. J., Catani, M., Ng, V. W., Howard, R. et al. (2006). Tract-specific anisotropy measurements in diffusion tensor imaging. *Psychiatry Research* 146(1): 73–82.

Kemper, T. (1994). Neuroanatomical and neuropathological changes during aging and in dementia. In M. Albert and E. Knoepfel (eds), *Clinical Neurology of Aging* (pp. 3–67). New York, Oxford University Press.

Kertesz, A., Polk, M., Carr, T. (1990). Cognition and white matter changes on magnetic resonance imaging in dementia. *Archives of Neurology*, 47: 387–391.

Kinsella, K. and Velkoff, V. A. (2001). *An Aging World: 2001* (p. 190). Washington, D.C.: U.S Census Bureau.

Knopman, D., Boland, L. L., Mosley, T., Howard, G., Liao, D., Szklo, M. et al. (2001). Cardiovascular risk factors and cognitive decline in middle-aged adults. *Neurology*, 56(1): 42–48.

Kozachuk, W. E., DeCarli, C., Schapiro, M. B., Wagner, E. E., Rapoport, S. I., Horwitz, B. (1990). White matter hyperintensities in dementia of Alzheimer's type and in healthy subjects without cerebrovascular risk factors: a magnetic resonance imaging study. *Archives of Neurology*, 47: 1306–1310.

Kuller, L. H., Lopez, O. L., Newman, A., Beauchamp, N. J., Burke, G., Dulberg, C. et al. (2003). Risk factors for dementia in the cardiovascular health cognition study. *Neuroepidemiology*, 22(1): 13–22.

Launer, L. J., Masaki, K., Petrovich, H., Foley, D., and Havlik, R. J. (1995). The association between mid-life blood pressure levels and late-life cognitive function. The Honolulu-Asia Aging Study. *The Journal of the American Medical Association*, 274(1846–1851).

Leys, D., Soetaert, G., Petit, H., Fauquette, A., Pruvo, J. P., Steinling, M. (1990). Periventricular and white matter magnetic resonance imaging hyperintensities do not differ between Alzheimer's disease and normal aging. *Archives of Neurology*, 47: 524–527.

Light, L. L. (1996). Memory and Aging. In E. L. Bjork and R. A. Bjork (eds), *Memory* (pp. 443–490). San Diego: Academic Press.

Longstreth, W. T., Jr., Arnold, A. M., Manolio, T. A., Burke, G. L., Bryan, N., Jungreis, C. A. et al. (2000). Clinical correlates of ventricular and sulcal size on cranial magnetic resonance imaging of 3301 elderly people. The Cardiovascular Health Study. Collaborative Research Group. *Neuroepidemiology*, 19(1): 30–42.

Longstreth, W. T., Jr., Bernick, C., Manolio, T. A., Bryan, N., Jungreis, C. A., Price, T. R. (1998). Lacunar infarcts defined by magnetic resonance imaging of 3660 elderly people: The Cardiovascular Health Study. *Archives of Neurology*, 55(9): 1217–1225.

Longstreth, W. T., Jr., Manolio, T. A., Arnold, A., Burke, G. L., Bryan, N., Jungreis, C. A. et al. (1996). Clinical correlates of white matter findings on cranial magnetic resonance imaging of 3301 elderly people. The Cardiovascular Health Study [see comments]. *Stroke*, 27(8): 1274–1282.

Lopez, O. L., Becker, J. T., Jungreis, C. A., Rezek, D., Estol, C., Boller, F. et al. (1995). Computed tomography-but not magnetic resonance imaging-identified periventricular white-matter lesions predict symptomatic cerebrovascular disease in probable Alzheimer's disease. *Archives of Neurology*, 52: 659–664.

Lopez, O. L., Becker, J. T., Rezek, D., Wess, J., Boller, F., Reynolds, C. F. I. et al. (1992). Neuropsychiatric correlates of cerebral white-matter radiolucencies in probable Alzheimer's disease. *Archives of Neurology*, 49: 828–834.

Lopez, O. L., Jagust, W. J., Dulberg, C., Becker, J. T., DeKosky, S. T., Fitzpatrick, A. et al. (2003). Risk factors for mild cognitive impairment in the cardiovascular health study cognition study: part 2. *Archives of Neurology*, 60(10): 1394–1399.

Madden, D. J., Whiting, W. L., Huettel, S. A., White, L. E., MacFall, J. R., Provenzale, J. M. (2004). Diffusion tensor imaging of adult age differences in cerebral white matter: relation to response time. *Neuroimage*, 21(3): 1174–1181.

Malloy, P., Corrcia, S., Stebbins, G., Laidlay, D. H. (2007). Neuroimaging of white matter in aging and dementia. *The Clinical Neuropsychologist*, 21: 73–109.

Marder, K., Richards, M., Bello, J., Bell, K., Sano, M., Miller, L. et al. (1995). Clinical correlates of Alzheimer's disease with and without silent radiographic abnormalities. *Archives of Neurology*, 52: 146–151.

Mathis, C. A., Klunk, W. E., Price, J. C., DeKosky, S. T. (2005). Imaging technology for neurodegenerative diseases: progress toward detection of specific pathologies. *Archives of Neurology*, 62(2): 196–200.

McDonald, W. M., Krishnan, K. R., Doraiswamy, P. M., Figiel, G. S., Husain, M. M., Boyko, O. B. (1991). Magnetic resonance findings in patients with early-onset Alzheimer's disease. *Biological Psychiatry*, 29: 799–810.

Medina, D., DeToledo-Morrell, L., Urresta, F., Gabrieli, J. D., Moseley, M., Fleischman, D. et al. (2006). White matter changes in mild cognitive impairment and AD: A diffusion tensor imaging study. *Neurobiology of Aging*, 27(5): 663–672.

Meier-Ruge, W., Ulrich, J., Bruhlmann, M., Meier, E. (1992). Age-related white matter atrophy in the human brain. *Annals of the New York Academy of Sciences*, 673: 260–269.

Mesulam, M. M. (1990). Large-scale neurocognitive networks and distributed processing for attention, language, and memory. *Annals of Neurology*, 28(5): 597–613.

Miller, E. K. and Asaad, W. F. (2002). The prefrontal cortex, conjunction and cognition. In J. Grafman (ed), *Handbook of Neuropsychology* (Vol. 7: The Frontal Lobes). St. Louis: Elsevier.

Mirsen, T. R., Lee, D. H., Wong, C. J., Diaz, J. F., Fox, A. J., Hachinski, V. C. et al. (1991). Clinical correlates of white-matter changes on magnetic resonance imaging scans of the brain. *Archives of Neurology*, 48(10): 1015–1021.

Moroney, J. T., Bagiella, E., Desmond, D. W., Paik, M. C., Stern, Y., Tatemichi, T. K. (1996). Risk factors for incident dementia after stroke. Role of hypoxic and ischemic disorders. *Stroke*, 27(8): 1283–1289.

Moroney, J. T., Bagiella, E., Desmond, D. W., Paik, M. C., Stern, Y., Tatemichi, T. K. (1997a). Cerebral hypoxia and ischemia in the pathogenesis of dementia after stroke. *Annals of the New York Academy of Sciences*, 826(3): 433–436.

Moroney, J. T., Bagiella, E., Tatemichi, T. K., Paik, M. C., Stern, Y., Desmond, D. W. (1997b). Dementia after stroke increases the risk of long-term stroke recurrence. *Neurology*, 48(5): 1317–1325.

Morris, R., Pandya, D. N., Petrides, M. (1999). Fiber system linking the mid-dorsolateral frontal cortex with the retrosplenial/presubicular region in the rhesus monkey. *The Journal of Comparative Neurology*, 407(2): 183–192.

Moscovitch, M. and Winocur, G. (1995). Frontal lobes, memory, and aging. *Annals of the New York Academy of Sciences*, 769: 119–150.

Mungas, D., Harvey, D., Reed, B. R., Jagust, W. J., DeCarli, C., Beckett, L. et al. (2005). Longitudinal volumetric MRI change and rate of cognitive decline. *Neurology*, 65(4): 565–571.

Mungas, D., Jagust, W. J., Reed, B. R., Kramer, J. H., Weiner, M. W., Schuff, N. et al. (2001). MRI predictors of cognition in subcortical ischemic vascular disease and Alzheimer's disease. *Neurology*, 57(12): 2229–2235.

Mungas, D., Reed, B. R., Jagust, W. J., DeCarli, C., Mack, W. J., Kramer, J. H. et al. (2002). Volumetric MRI predicts rate of cognitive decline related to AD and cerebrovascular disease. *Neurology*, 59(6): 867–873.

Nordahl, C. W., Ranganath, C., Yonelinas, A. P., Decarli, C., Fletcher, E., Jagust, W. J. (2005). Different mechanisms of episodic memory failure in mild cognitive impairment. *Neuropsychologia*, 43(11): 1688–1697.

Nordahl, C. W., Ranganath, C., Yonelinas, A. P., DeCarli, C., Reed, B. R., Jagust, W. J. (2006). White matter changes compromise prefrontal cortex function in healthy elderly individuals. *Journal of Cognitive Neuroscience*, 18(3): 418–429.

Nusbaum, A. O., Tang, C. Y., Buchsbaum, M. S., Wei, T. C., Atlas, S. W. (2001). Regional and global changes in cerebral diffusion with normal aging. *AJNR. American Journal of Neuroradiology*, 22(1): 136–142.

O'Brien, M. D. (1988). Vascular dementia is underdiagnosed. *Archives of Neurology*, 45: 797–798.

O'Sullivan, M., Jones, D. K., Summers, P. E., Morris, R. G., Williams, S. C., Markus, H. S. (2001). Evidence for cortical "disconnection" as a mechanism of age-related cognitive decline. *Neurology*, 57(4): 632–638.

O'Sullivan, M., Jones, D. K., Summers, P. E., Morris, R. G., Williams, S. C. R., Markus, H. S. (2004). Diffusion tensor MRI correlates with executive dysfunction in patients with ischaemic leukoaraiosis. *Journal of Neurology, Neurosurgery, and Psychiatry*, 75(3): 441–447.

O'Sullivan, M., Morris, R. G., Huckstep, B., Jones, D. K., Williams, S. C., Markus, H. S. (2001). Normal-appearing white matter in ischemic leukoaraiosis: a diffusion tensor MRI study. *Neurology*, 57(12): 2307–2310.

O'Sullivan, M., Summers, P. E., Jones, D. K., Jarosz, J. M., Williams, S. C., Markus, H. S. (1996). Association of diabetes mellitus and dementia: the Rotterdam Study. *Diabetologia*, 39(11): 1392–1397.

Ott, A., Stolk, R. P., Hofman, A., van Harskamp, F., Grobbee, D. E., Breteler, M. M. (1997). A SPECT imaging study of MRI white matter hyperintensity in patients with degenerative dementia. *Dementia and Geriatric Cognitive Disorders*, 8: 348–354.

Ott, B. R., Faberman, R. S., Noto, R. B., Rogg, J. M., Hough, T. J., Tung, G. A. et al. (1999). Mild cognitive impairment: clinical characterization and outcome. *Archives of Neurology*, 56(3): 303–308.

Pantoni, L. (2002). Pathophysiology of age-related cerebral white matter changes. *Cerebrovascular Diseases*, 13(Suppl. 2): 7–10.

Petrides, M. and Pandya, D. N. (1999). Dorsolateral prefrontal cortex: comparative cytoarchitectonic analysis in the human and the macaque brain and corticocortical connection patterns. *The European Journal of Neuroscience*, 11(3): 1011–1036.

Pfefferbaum, A. and Sullivan, E. V. (2005). Disruption of brain white matter microstructure by excessive intracellular and extracellular fluid in alcoholism: evidence from diffusion tensor imaging. *Neuropsychopharmacology*, 30(2): 423–432.

Petersen, R. C., Smith, G. E., Waring, S. C., Ivnik, R. J., Tangalos, E. G., Kokmen, E. (2000). Age-related decline in brain white matter anisotropy measured with spatially corrected echo-planar diffusion tensor imaging. *Magnetic Resonance in Medicine*, 44(2): 259–268.

Pierpaoli, C. and Basser, P. J. (1996). Toward a quantitative assessment of diffusion anisotropy. *Magnetic Resonance in Medicine*, 36(6): 893–906.

Pfefferbaum, A., Sullivan, E. V., Hedehus, M., Lim, K. O., Adalsteinsson, E., Moseley, M. (1997). Silent brain infarction on magnetic resonance imaging and neurological abnormalities in community-dwelling older adults. The Cardiovascular Health Study. CHS Collaborative Research Group. *Stroke*, 28(6): 1158–1164.

Price, T. R., Manolio, T. A., Kronmal, R. A., Kittner, S. J., Yue, N. C., Robbins, J. et al. (2003). Prefrontal activity associated with working memory and episodic long-term memory. *Neuropsychologia*, 41(3): 378–389.

Ranganath, C. (2006). Working memory for visual objects: Complementary roles of inferior temporal, medial temporal, and prefrontal cortex. *Neuroscience*, 139(1): 277–289.

Ranganath, C., Johnson, M. K., D'Esposito, M. (1997). Selective aging of the human cerebral cortex observed in vivo: Differential vulnerability of the prefrontal gray matter. *Cerebral Cortex*, 7(3): 268–282.

Rapp, P. R. and Amaral, D. G. (1992). Individual differences in the cognitive and neurobiological consequences of normal aging. *Trends in Neurosciences*, 15(9): 340–345.

Reed, B. R., Eberling, J. L., Mungas, D., Weiner, M., Jagust, W. J. (2000). Memory failure has different mechanisms in subcortical stroke and Alzheimer's disease. *Annals of Neurology*, 48(3): 275–284.

Reed, B. R., Eberling, J. L., Mungas, D., Weiner, M. W., Jagust, W. J. (2001). Frontal lobe hypometabolism predicts cognitive decline in patients with lacunar infarcts. *Archives of Neurology*, 58: 493–497.

Reuter-Lorenz, P. A., Jonides, J., Smith, E. E., Hartley, A., Miller, A., Marshuetz, C. et al. (2000). Age differences in the frontal lateralization of verbal and spatial working memory revealed by PET. *Journal of Cognitive Neuroscience*, 12(1): 174–187.

Roman, G. C. (1987). Senile dementia of the Binswanger type: A vascular form of dementia in the elderly. *The Journal of the American Medical Association*, 258: 1782–1788.

Rosen, A. C., Prull, M. W., O'Hara, R., Race, E. A., Desmond, J. E., Glover, G. H. et al. (2002). Variable effects of aging on frontal lobe contributions to memory. *Neuroreport*, 13(18): 2425–2428.

Rossi, R., Geroldi, C., Bresciani, L., Testa, C., Binetti, G., Zanetti, O. et al. (2007). Clinical and neuropsychological features associated with structural imaging patterns in patients with mild cognitive impairment. *Dementia and Geriatric Cognitive Disorders*, 23(3): 175–183.

Rypma, B., Berger, J. S., Genova, H. M., Rebbechi, D., D'Esposito, M. (2005). Dissociating age-related changes in cognitive strategy and neural efficiency using event-related fMRI. *Cortex*, 41(4): 582–594.

Rypma, B. and D'Esposito, M. (2000). Isolating the neural mechanisms of age-related changes in human working memory. *Nature Neuroscience*, 3(5): 509–515.

Salat, D. H., Tuch, D. S., Greve, D. N., van der Kouwe, A. J., Hevelone, N. D., Zaleta, A. K. et al. (2005). Age-related alterations in white matter microstructure measured by diffusion tensor imaging. *Neurobiology of Aging*, 26(8): 1215–1227.

Salthouse, T. A. (1988). The role of processing resources in cognitive aging. In M. L. Howe and C. J. Brainerd (eds), *Cognitive Development in Adulthood: Progress in Cognitive Development Research* (pp. 185–239). New York: Springer-Verlag.

Salthouse, T. A. (1993). Speed mediation of adult age differences in cognition. *Developmental Psychology*, 29: 722–738.

Salthouse, T. A. (1996). The processing-speed theory of adult age differences in cognition. *Psychological Review*, 103(3): 403–428.

Salthouse, T. A. (2000). Aging and measures of processing speed. *Biological Psychology*, 54(1–3): 35–54.

Scheltens, P., Barkhof, F., Valk, J., Algra, P. R., van der Hoop, R. G., Nauta, J. et al. (1992). White matter lesions on magnetic resonance imaging in clinically diagnosed Alzheimer's disease: Evidence for heterogeneity. *Brain*, 115: 735–748.

Scheltens, P., Barkhof, F., Leys, D., Wolters, E. C., Ravid, R., Kamphorst, W. (1995). Histopathologic correlates of white matter changes on MRI in Alzheimer's disease and normal aging. *Neurology*, 45: 883–888.

Schmidt, R. (1992). Comparison of magnetic resonance imaging in Alzheimer's disease, vascular dementia and normal aging. *European Neurology*, 32: 164–169.

Schmidt, R., Fazekas, F., Koch, M., Kapeller, P., Augustin, M., Offenbacher, H. et al. (1995). Magnetic resonance imaging cerebral abnormalities and neuropsychologic test performance in elderly hypertensive subjects. A case-control study. *Archives of Neurology*, 52(9): 905–910.

Schneider, J. A., Arvanitakis, Z., Bang, W., Bennett, D. A. (2007). Mixed brain pathologies account for most dementia cases in community-dwelling older persons. *Neurology*, 69(24): 2197–2204.

Schneider, J. A., Wilson, R. S., Cochran, E. J., Bienias, J. L., Arnold, S. E., Evans, D. A. et al. (2003). Relation of cerebral infarctions to dementia and cognitive function in older persons. *Neurology*, 60(7): 1082–1088.

Schneider, J. A., Wilson, R. S., Bienias, J. L., Evans, D. A., Bennett, D. A. (2004). Cerebral infarctions and the likelihood of dementia from Alzheimer disease pathology. *Neurology*, 62(7): 1148–1155.

Schuff, N., Capizzano, A. A., Du, A. T., Amend, D. L., O'Neill, J., Norman, D. et al. (2003). Different patterns of N-acetylaspartate loss in subcortical ischemic vascular dementia and AD. *Neurology*, 61(3): 358–364.

Selemon, L. D. and Goldman-Rakic, P. S. (1988). Common cortical and subcortical targets of the dorsolateral prefrontal and posterior parietal cortices in the rhesus monkey: Evidence for a distributed neural network subserving spatially guided behavior. *The Journal of Neuroscience*, 8(11): 4049–4068.

Seshadri, S., Beiser, A., Kelly-Hayes, M., Kase, C. S., Au, R., Kannel, W. B. et al. (2006). The lifetime risk of stroke: estimates from the Framingham Study. *Stroke*, 37(2): 345–350.

Seshadri, S., Wolf, P. A., Beiser, A., Elias, M. F., Au, R., Kase, C. S. et al. (2004). Stroke risk profile, brain volume, and cognitive function: The Framingham Offspring Study. *Neurology*, 63(9): 1591–159.

Smith, E. E. and Jonides, J. (1999). Storage and executive processes in the frontal lobes. *Science*, 283(5408): 1657–1661.

Snowdon, D. A., Greiner, L. H., Mortimer, J. A., Riley, K. P., Greiner, P. A., Markesbery, W. R. (1997). Brain infarction and the clinical expression of Alzheimer disease. The Nun Study. *The Journal of the American Medical Association*, 277(813–817).

Starkstein, S. E., Sabe, L., Vazquez, S., Di Lorenzo, G., Martinez, A., Petracca, G. et al. (1997). Neuropsychological, psychiatric, and cerebral perfusion correlates of leukoaraiosis in Alzheimer's disease. *Journal of Neurology, Neurosurgery, and Psychiatry*, 63: 66–73.

Stout, J. C., Jernigan, T. L., Archibald, S. L., Salmon, D. P. (1996). Association of dementia severity with cortical gray matter and abnormal white matter volumes in dementia of the Alzheimer type. *Archives of Neurology*, 53: 742–749.

Sullivan, E. V., Adalsteinsson, E., Hedehus, M., Ju, C., Moseley, M., Lim, K. O. et al. (2001). Equivalent disruption of regional white matter microstructure in ageing healthy men and women. *Neuroreport*, 12(1): 99–104.

Sullivan, E. V., Adalsteinsson, E., Pfefferbaum, A. (2006). Selective age-related degradation of anterior callosal fiber bundles quantified in vivo with fiber tracking. *Cerebral Cortex*, 16(7): 1030–1039.

Sullivan, E. V. and Pfefferbaum, A. (2006). Diffusion tensor imaging and aging. *Neuroscience and Biobehavioral Reviews*, 30(6): 749–761.

Swan, G. E., DeCarli, C., Miller, B. L., Reed, T., Wolf, P. A., Jack, L. M. et al. (1998). Association of midlife blood pressure to late-life cognitive decline and brain morphology. *Neurology*, 51(4): 986–993.

Swan, G. E., DeCarli, C., Miller, B. L., Reed, T., Wolf, P. A., Carmelli, D. (2000). Biobehavioral characteristics of nondemented older adults with subclinical brain atrophy. *Neurology*, 54(11): 2108–2114.

Takao, M., Koto, A., Tanahashi, N., Fukuuchi, Y., Takagi, M., Morinaga, S. (1999). Pathologic findings of silent hyperintense white matter lesions on MRI. *Journal of Neurological Sciences*, 167(2): 127–131.

Taoka, T., Iwasaki, S., Sakamoto, M., Nakagawa, H., Fukusumi, A., Myochin, K. et al. (2006). Diffusion anisotropy and diffusivity of white matter tracts within the temporal stem in Alzheimer disease: evaluation of the "tract of interest" by diffusion tensor tractography. *American Journal of Neuroradiology*, 27(5): 1040–1045.

Tatemichi, T. K. (1990). How acute brain failure becomes chronic: A view of the mechanisms of dementia related to stroke. *Neurology*, 40: 1652–1659.

Tatemichi, T. K., Desmond, D. W., Mayeux, R. et al. (1992). Dementia after stroke: Baseline frequency, risks, and clinical features in a hospitalized cohort. *Neurology*, 42: 1185–1193.

Tatemichi, T. K., Desmond, D. W., Prohovnik, I. (1995a). Strategic infarcts in vascular dementia. A clinical and brain imaging experience. *Arzneimittel-Forschung*, 45(3A): 371–385.

Tatemichi, T. K., Desmond, D. W., Prohovnik, I., Eidelberg, D. (1995b). Dementia associated with bilateral carotid occlusions: Neuropsychological and haemodynamic course after extracranial to intracranial bypass surgery. *Journal of Neurology, Neurosurgery and Psychiatry*, 58(5): 633–636.

Tatemichi, T. K., Foulkes, M. A., Mohr, J. P. et al. (1990). Dementia in stroke survivors in the stroke data bank cohort. Prevalence, incidence, risk factors, and computed tomographic findings. *Stroke*, 21: 858–866.

Taylor, W. D., Bae, J. N., MacFall, J. R., Payne, M. E., Provenzale, J. M., Steffens, D. C. et al. (2007). Widespread effects of hyperintense lesions on cerebral white matter structure. *American Journal of Roentgenology*, 188(6): 1695–1704.

Teipel, S. J., Hampel, H., Alexander, G. E., Schapiro, M. B., Horwitz, B., Teichberg, D. et al. (1998). Dissociation between corpus callosum atrophy and white matter pathology in Alzheimer's disease. *Neurology*, 51: 1381–1385.

Tekin, S. and Cummings, J. L. (2002). Frontal-subcortical neuronal circuits and clinical neuropsychiatry: An update. *Journal of Psychosomatic Research*, 53(2): 647–654.

Tisserand, D. J. and Jolles, J. (2003). On the involvement of prefrontal networks in cognitive ageing. *Cortex*, 39(4–5): 1107–1128.

Tullberg, M., Fletcher, E., DeCarli, C., Mungas, D., Reed, B. R., Harvey, D. J. et al. (2004). White matter lesions impair frontal lobe function regardless of their location. *Neurology*, 63(2): 246–253.

US Census Bureau. (2004). U.S. Interim Projections by Age, Sex, Race, and Hispanic Origin. from http://www.census.gov/ipc/www/usinterimproj/natprojtab02a.pdf.

US Census Bureau. (2007, 08/09/2007). Newsroom.

Uylings, H. B. and de Brabander, J. M. (2002). Neuronal changes in normal human aging and Alzheimer's disease. *Brain and Cognition*, 49(3): 268–276.

Vasan, R. S., Beiser, A., Seshadri, S., Larson, M. G., Kannel, W. B., D'Agostino, R. B. et al. (2002). Residual lifetime risk for developing hypertension in middle-aged women and men: The Framingham Heart Study. *The Journal of the American Medical Association*, 287(8): 1003–1010.

Vermeer, S. E., Koudstaal, P. J., Oudkerk, M., Hofman, A., Breteler, M. M. (2002). Prevalence and risk factors of silent brain infarcts in the population-based Rotterdam Scan Study. *Stroke*, 33(1): 21–25.

Vermeer, S. E., Prins, N. D., den Heijer, T., Hofman, A., Koudstaal, P. J., Breteler, M. M. (2003). Silent brain infarcts and the risk of dementia and cognitive decline. *The New England Journal of Medicine*, 348(13): 1215–1222.

Wahlund, L., O., Basun, H., Almkvist, O., Andersson-Lundman, G., Julin, P., Saaf, J. (1994). White matter hyperintensities in dementia: does it matter? *Magnetic Resonance Imaging*, 12(3): 387–394.

Waldemar, G., Christiansen, P., Larsson, H. B., Hogh, P., Laursen, H., Lassen, N. A. et al. (1994). White matter magnetic resonance hyperintensities in dementia of the Alzheimer type: Morphological and regional cerebral blood flow correlates. *Journal of Neurology, Neurosurgery and Psychiatry*, 57: 1458–1465.

Wen, W. and Sachdev, P. (2004). The topography of white matter hyperintensities on brain MRI in healthy 60- to 64-year-old individuals. *Neuroimage*, 22(1): 144–154.

Wen, W. and Sachdev, P. S. (2004). Extent and distribution of white matter hyperintensities in stroke patients: The Sydney Stroke Study. *Stroke*, 35(12): 2813–2819.

West, R. L. (1996). An application of prefrontal cortex function theory to cognitive aging. *Psychological Bulletin*, 120(2): 272–292.

Wilson, R. S., Beckett, L. A., Barnes, L. L., Schneider, J. A., Bach, J., Evans, D. A. et al. (2002). Individual differences in rates of change in cognitive abilities of older persons. *Psychology and Aging*, 17(2): 179–193.

Wolf, H., Ecke, G. M., Bettin, S., Dietrich, J., Gertz, H. J. (2000). Do white matter changes contribute to the subsequent development of dementia in patients with mild cognitive impairment? A longitudinal study. *International Journal of Geriatric Psychiatry*, 15(9): 803–812.

Wu, C. C., Mungas, D., Petkov, C. I., Eberling, J. L., Zrelak, P. A., Buonocore, M. H. et al. (2002). Brain structure and cognition in a community sample of elderly Latinos. *Neurology*, 59(3): 383–391.

Xie, S., Xiao, J. X., Gong, G. L., Zang, Y. F., Wang, Y. H., Wu, H. K. et al. (2006). Voxel-based detection of white matter abnormalities in mild Alzheimer disease. *Neurology*, 66(12): 1845–1849.

Yoshita, M., Fletcher, E., Harvey, D., Ortega, M., Martinez, O., Mungas, D. M. et al. (2006). Extent and distribution of white matter hyperintensities in normal aging, MCI, and AD. *Neurology*, 67(12): 2192–2198.

Yue, N. C., Arnold, A. M., Longstreth, W. T., Jr., Elster, A. D., Jungreis, C. A., O'Leary, D. H. et al. (1997). Sulcal, ventricular, and white matter changes at MR imaging in the aging brain: data from the cardiovascular health study [see comments]. *Radiology*, 202(1): 33–39.

18

Functional MRI Studies in Aging and Early Alzheimer's Disease: Predicting Clinical Decline

Reisa Sperling

Keywords: functional MRI; hippocampus; memory; mild cognitive impairment; Alzheimer's disease

Alzheimer's disease (AD) is characterized by an insidious progression of episodic memory impairment that typically begins years prior to the time a clinical diagnosis is established. Similarly, postmortem reports and studies of subjects at genetic risk for AD suggest that the pathophysiological process of AD has been set in motion years (if not decades) before the severity of symptoms warrants a clinical diagnosis. The long prodromal phase of AD provides a tantalizing opportunity to detect early alterations in brain structure and function, at a point when potential disease-modifying therapies would likely be most efficacious. Despite tremendous advances in understanding the basic pathobiology involved in AD, we still lack a detailed understanding of exactly how the pathology of AD translates into the emergent clinical syndrome of memory loss and other domains of cognitive impairment. Neuroimaging, particularly a combination of molecular, structural, and functional imaging techniques, has the potential to illuminate the "black box" that remains between the pathophysiological process of AD and the clinical course of the disease, and ultimately to provide an accurate and early diagnostic index. A number of promising imaging techniques, many of which are covered in other chapters in this book, are being studied in aging and early AD. This chapter will focus on use of task-related functional magnetic resonance imaging (fMRI) to investigate the neural underpinnings of memory impairment in early AD, the detection of early functional alterations in subjects at risk for AD, and the prediction of subsequent clinical decline.

Potential of Functional Imaging

Increasingly, evidence from laboratory and animal studies suggests that AD may manifest initially as "synaptic failure" (Selkoe, 2002; Walsh and Selkoe, 2004). Functional imaging techniques—in particular, those that study brain activity during cognitive processes—have the potential to detect the earliest impact of the pathophysiological process of AD on the functional integrity of neural networks. Structural imaging, with volumetric magnetic resonance imaging, is presumably quite sensitive to the loss of neurons and surrounding neuropil, but this process may occur relatively late

in the pathologic cascade of AD. By the time of very mild clinical dementia, there is already significant neuronal loss in specific medial temporal lobe (MTL) structures (Gomez-Isla et al., 1996). It is likely that these neurons would show evidence of dysfunction prior to cell death. Functional imaging techniques that observe the brain at rest, such as 18-flurodeoxyglucose (FDG), positron emission tomography (PET), perfusion MRI (Alsop, Detre, and Grossman, 2000; Johnson, 2005), and resting state fMRI (Greicius et al., 2004; Rombouts et al., 2005b) have shown evidence of regional abnormalities in early AD and may prove valuable in predicting subsequent decline in at-risk subjects. To detect brain dysfunction in individuals with very subtle cognitive impairment, and even asymptomatic individuals with early pathology of AD, we may need to employ more sensitive measures that probe the brain during exactly the types of cognitive processes that will become clinically impaired as the disease progresses. To borrow an analogy from the field of cardiology, exercise or pharmacological "stress tests" are thought to be more sensitive in detecting occult coronary artery disease than resting electrocardiograms. Similarly, task-related functional MRI might be considered a "brain stress test," which may be able to detect alterations in the brain's functional capacity prior to detection of neuronal loss or even evidence of dysfunction at rest.

Physiological Basis of fMRI

The fMRI technique most widely used to investigate neural activity is based on imaging of the blood oxygen level dependent (BOLD) contrast (Ogawa et al., 1990). This endogenous contrast is thought to be generated by changing ratios of oxygenated hemoglobin to deoxygenated hemoglobin, which is a natural paramagnetic substance in capillary beds and larger blood vessels subserving neural tissue. Whereas FDG-PET measures glucose metabolism thought to reflect neuronal synaptic activity, BOLD fMRI is considered to reflect the integrated synaptic activity of neurons as measured by MRI signal modulation due to changes in blood flow, blood volume, and blood oxyhemoglobin/deoxyhemoglobin ratio (Logothetis, 2001). Thus, it is important to remember that BOLD fMRI is an indirect measure of neuronal activity; however, this technique may provide an important "window" into the neural underpinnings of complex cognitive processes.

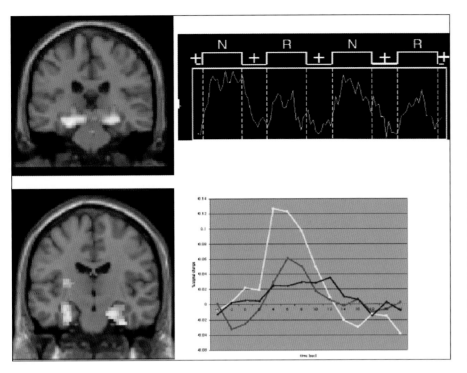

Figure 18–1 Functional MRI data during a face-name encoding paradigm. The top left figure demonstrates a statistical parametric map (SPM) of the hippocampus showing greater MR signal response to novel (N) face-name pairs compared to repeated (R) face-name pairs in a block design fMRI paradigm. The top right shows a representative time course of the MR signal in the block design paradigm, with marked increased in signal during novel blocks compared to blocks of visual fixation (+) or repeated blocks. The bottom left demonstrates significant hippocampal activation for an event-related face-name paradigm comparing successful vs. failed encoding. The bottom right graph shows the MR signal change in the right hippocampus for those face-name pairs correctly remembered with high confidence (yellow line), low confidence (pink line), or forgotten (blue line).

In addition, BOLD fMRI is almost always reported as a "relative measure," comparing the MR signal during one task to a control task or "baseline condition." Typically, fMRI experiments compare the MRI signal during one cognitive condition (e.g., memory encoding) to a control task (e.g., viewing familiar stimuli) or to a passive baseline condition (e.g., visual fixation). This can be done in a "block design" paradigm (see Figure 18.1) in which stimuli of each cognitive condition are grouped together in blocks lasting 20–40 s, or in "event-related" paradigms in which single stimuli from several different conditions are interspersed. The peak hemodynamic response is typically observed 4–6 s after the stimulus onset. Comparisons between conditions are often performed using a voxel-wise approach, with analytic toolboxes such as Statistical Parametric Mapping (SPM). This approach allows the investigation of fMRI activity within the entire brain, accounting for the issue of multiple comparisons between several thousand voxels. Both increases in BOLD signal in one condition relative to another, hitherto referred to as "fMRI activation," and decreases in BOLD signal in that condition, hitherto referred to as "fMRI deactivation," can be detected. Deactivations or negative BOLD responses have been shown to reflect task-related decreases in neuronal activity below levels detected during spontaneous activity (Shmuel et al., 2006), but it remains unclear whether this phenomenon is due to specific inhibitory influences.

Unfortunately, there is no absolute determination of fMRI signal at "baseline." Even resting fMRI scans primarily investigate the correlations between regional MR signal over time, rather than absolute measurements of MR signal at rest. Arterial spin labeling (ASL) perfusion fMRI techniques may provide a more robust baseline measurement of perfusion (but task-related) fMRI studies utilizing ASL techniques still rely on the "subtraction" of MR signal in one condition versus another. The combination of multiple imaging modalities—particularly perfusion MR, FDG-PET, and task-related BOLD fMRI—may prove valuable in elucidating whether the observed functional changes in patient populations relate primarily to alterations in "baseline" function vs. the neural requirements of the cognitive task, or perhaps to a combination of both factors.

An early concern regarding fMRI studies in aging and AD was that altered BOLD signals might merely reflect a global decoupling of the hemodynamic response resulting from age-related changes in the vascular system, as a few studies have demonstrated fMRI alterations in sensorimotor areas in both cognitively normal older and AD patients (Buckner et al., 2000; D'Esposito et al., 1999; Rombouts et al., 2005a) (See also Chapter 2 for a discussion of this issue). Importantly, multiple studies have now demonstrated that even patients with mild-to-moderate clinical AD can generate a "normal" BOLD response in many brain regions that is quite similar in magnitude and extent to age-matched normal older control subjects, and that the fMRI alterations are regionally specific to the required memory task (Machulda et al., 2003; Sperling et al., 2003a).

Neural Networks Supporting Normal Memory Function in Young and Older Controls

One of the most fruitful applications to date of fMRI in cognitive neuroscience has been to elucidate the brain networks that support memory processes in normal individuals. Multiple fMRI studies using a "subsequent memory" paradigm have demonstrated that greater fMRI activity during encoding in specific brain regions is associated with the likelihood of subsequent successful retrieval of the information (Brewer et al., 1998; Chua et al., 2007; Kirchhoff et al., 2000; Sperling et al., 2003b; Wagner et al., 1998). Not surprisingly, regions within the MTL, as well as the left inferior prefrontal cortex, have consistently demonstrated this subsequent memory effect. Several pharmacological fMRI experiments have demonstrated decreased activation in the hippocampus and prefrontal regions with the administration of medications that impair memory performance, such as benzodiazepines and anticholinergics (Schon et al., 2005; Sperling et al., 2002). Taken together, these fMRI experiments suggest that activation of specific neural structures are related to memory performance, and that these fMRI paradigms might be particularly useful in probing memory function in early Alzheimer's disease.

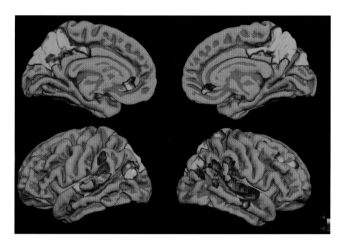

Figure 18–2 The default network, a set of regions which demonstrate higher fMRI activity during rest compared to challenging cognitive tasks. In this group fMRI data map, regions in blue demonstrate greater MR signal during rest (visual fixation) compared to novel face-name encoding.

Our own fMRI work has focused primarily on associative memory processes—in particular, face-name associations. Converging evidence suggests that one primary role of the hippocampal formation in episodic encoding is to form new associations between previously unrelated items of information (Eichenbaum, 1996; Squire and Zola-Morgan, 1991). Learning the names of new individuals we encounter can be thought of as a particularly difficult cross-modal, noncontextual, paired associate memory task, which may be particularly useful in detecting the earliest memory

impairment in AD (Fowler et al., 2002; Gallo et al., 2004; Morris et al., 1991). Difficulty remembering proper names is the most common memory complaint of older individuals visiting memory clinics (Leirer et al., 1990; Zelinski and Gilewski, 1988). Multiple fMRI studies have recently reported that associative memory paradigms produce robust activation of the anterior hippocampal formation (Kirwan and Stark, 2004; Small et al., 2001; Zeineh et al., 2003), and our own fMRI studies in young subjects using a face-name associative encoding task have confirmed these findings (Sperling et al., 2001, 2002, 2003b).

Also of interest is the consistent finding that a specific set of brain regions actually deactivate (i.e., demonstrate a decrease in BOLD activity with the task) during successful memory formation (Daselaar, Prince, and Cabeza, 2004). These regions—in particular, lateral parietal and medial parietal regions, including the precuneus and posterior cingulate—are central components of the "default-mode network" (see Figure 18.2) characterized by Raichle and colleagues in a series of both PET and fMRI studies (Fox et al., 2005; Raichle, 2001).

These parietal regions demonstrate significant connectivity with the hippocampus in resting-state network analyses (Greicius et al., 2003; Vincent et al., 2006). Recent work has also noted an overlap of these medial and lateral parietal regions with a "retrospenial memory system" that typically activates during memory retrieval tasks (Buckner et al., 2005; Wheeler and Buckner, 2004). Interestingly, our own work in cognitively normal young and older adults also suggests that the degree to which individuals can deactivate this network during encoding is strongly related to their subsequent memory performance (Miller et al., 2008b; Sperling, 2007) (see Figure 18.3). Thus, our current hypothesis is that successful memory formation requires coordinated and reciprocal activation in the hippocampal-based memory

Figure 18–3 Group fMRI data (top) maps with MR signal time courses (bottom) for young and elderly controls show hippocampal activation (left) and precuneus deactivation (right) during the successful encoding of face-name pairs ($p < 0.005$). Low performing elderly controls failed to deactivate the precuneus and demonstrated increased hippocampal and prefrontal activation for successful but not failed encoding trials, perhaps as a compensatory response to failure of default network activity.

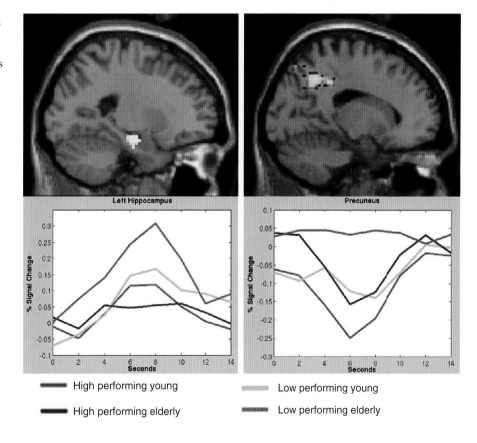

High performing young
High performing elderly
Low performing young
Low performing elderly

system, and deactivation in the retrosplenial memory system. Furthermore, we postulate that the degree of deactivation at encoding will predict the degree of activation during retrieval, but these fMRI experiments are ongoing in young and older subjects.

fMRI Studies in Patients with Clinically Diagnosed Alzheimer's Disease

Not surprisingly, given the salience of memory dysfunction in early AD, the majority of fMRI studies in AD to date have focused on episodic memory tasks (Dickerson et al., 2005; Golby et al., 2005; Gron et al., 2002; Hamalainen et al., 2007; Kato, Knopman, and Liu, 2001; Machulda et al., 2003; Pariente et al., 2005; Remy, 2005; Rombouts et al., 2000; Small et al., 1999; Sperling et al., 2003a). These studies have employed a variety of unfamiliar visual stimuli, including faces (Pariente, 2005; Rombouts, 2005a, Small et al., 1999; face-name pairs (Sperling, 2003 #980), scenes (Golby et al., 2005), line drawings (Hamalainen et al., 2007; Rombouts et al., 2000), geometric shapes (Kato, Knopman, and Liu, 2001), and verbal stimuli (Remy et al., 2005). These studies have consistently found evidence of decreased activation in AD patients compared to healthy older control groups during the encoding of novel stimuli—particularly, in medial temporal lobe (MTL) structures including the hippocampus and parahippocampus. Our own work, using the block-design face-name paradigm, has found that AD patients demonstrate significantly less hippocampal activation in the "novel vs. repeated" comparison than normal older controls (Dickerson, 2005; Sperling, 2003a). Recently, we have investigated the activation during repeated stimuli in AD and found that AD patients continue to demonstrate increased activation to stimuli that are highly familiarized to normal older controls (Pihlajamaki et al., 2008). This finding may explain the sensitivity of novel vs. repeated contrasts, and suggests that failure of repetition suppression may be a sensitive marker of AD-related hippocampal dysfunction (Johnson et al., 2004). Interestingly, several fMRI studies, including our own, have also found evidence of increased neocortical activation in AD compared to controls, particularly in frontal and parietal regions, which may represent a compensatory process in the setting of hippocampal failure (Grady et al., 2003; Pariente et al., 2005; Remy et al., 2005; Sperling, 2003a).

More recently, several groups have also reported alterations in the pattern of deactivation in AD patients (Buckner et al., 2005; Greicius et al., 2004; Lustig et al., 2003; Petrella et al., 2006; Rombouts et al., 2005a). These alterations in deactivation occur in the default mode network (Raichle et al., 2001). As recently noted by Buckner et al. (Buckner et al., 2005), the regions involved in the "default mode network" are strikingly similar to those regions that typically demonstrate evidence of fibrillar amyloid deposition binding with Pittsburgh Compound B (PIB) in PET studies in AD (Klunk et al., 2004), as well as to the pattern of hypometabolism found on FDG PET studies of AD patients (Alexander et al., 2002; Meltzer et al., 1996; Silverman et al., 2001) and subjects who are at-risk for AD; (Jagust et al., 2006; Reiman et al., 2004; Small et al., 2000) and of hypoperfusion on resting MR perfusion studies in AD (Alsop, Detre, and Grossman, 2000; Johnson et al., 2005). This default-mode network has demonstrated alterations at rest and in block-design fMRI paradigms in aging and AD (Greicius et al., 2004; Lustig et al., 2003).

Our own recent fMRI work suggests that the alterations in hippocampal activation and parietal deactivation over the course of MCI and AD are strongly correlated (Celone, 2006). Similarly, resting state fMRI data has demonstrated alterations in parietal and hippocampal connectivity in MCI and AD (Greicius et al., 2004). Thus, converging evidence suggests that a distributed memory network is disrupted by the pathophysiological process of AD, which includes both medial temporal lobe systems and medial and lateral parietal regions involved in default-mode activity. Future studies to probe alterations in connectivity between these system, which combine fMRI with other techniques such as diffusion tensor imaging, may prove particularly valuable in elucidating the early functional alterations in AD (Wierenga and Bondi, 2007).

fMRI Alterations in Mild Cognitive Impairment

If fMRI is going to prove to be a valuable tool in early detection, it is critical to demonstrate functional alterations in subjects at-risk for AD prior to the stage of clinical dementia. Mild cognitive impairment is often thought to represent a transitional stage between normal aging and mild AD (Petersen, 2004), but includes a very heterogeneous set of individuals. MCI is a significant risk factor for AD, with estimates as high as 15%–18% annual risk of conversion to clinical AD, but both autopsy and amyloid imaging studies suggest that a substantial proportion of MCI subjects do not have AD pathology as the cause of their clinical syndrome of memory impairment (Kemppainen, 2007; Petersen et al., 2006). There is also marked variability in the criteria used to define MCI in these research studies, although recently, some standardized criteria have been developed and implemented in large-scale clinical trials and imaging studies (Grundman, 2004).

Relatively few fMRI studies have been published to date in MCI subjects. The results have been quite variable, with nearly half of the published studies reporting decreased activation in MCI, and the other half reporting evidence of increased activation in MCI compared to normal subjects. These studies have also included a very broad definition of MCI, including a wide range of degree of cognitive impairment. This chapter will begin with a brief review of the studies that found evidence of decreased activation in cognitively impaired subjects. Small et al. (1999) reported a subset of memory impairment subjects who demonstrated hypoactivation similar to that of AD patients, with another group of impaired subjects who demonstrated entorhinal and hippocampal activation that was similar to controls, and had decreased activation in the subiculum. In comparison to older controls, Machulda et al. (2003) found that MTL activation was decreased to a similar degree in patients with MCI and AD patients during a picture-encoding task. Petrella et al. (2006) found no differences between MCI and controls in MTL activation during an associative encoding paradigm. During the forced-choice recognition retrieval task in this study, decreased left hippocampal activation was seen in MCI as compared to controls; however, this finding was no longer present when memory performance accuracy was included as a covariate in the analysis. One of our own studies also found evidence of decreased MTL activation during face-name encoding in subjects who were thought to be in late stages of MCI with significant functional impairment as assessed by a high Clinical Dementia Rating Sum of Box (CDR-SB) score (Celone et al., 2006; Morris, 1993). Johnson et al. (2006b) found right hippocampal hypoactivation in MCI patients as compared to controls during a recognition paradigm for novel (compared to previously-learned) items. In an earlier study, Johnson et al. (2004) also found that MCI patients failed to show the same slope of decreasing hippocampal activation with stimulus repetition seen in control subjects, suggesting that there was disruption of the adaptive or habituating response to familiar stimuli in MCI. Figure 18.4 illustrates the findings from these three studies by Johnson et al., all of which demonstrated significantly decreased MTL activation in MCI subjects compared to age-matched controls.

MCI

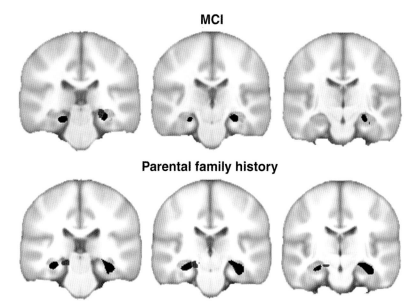

Parental family history

Figure 18–4 Composite figure summarizing results from Johnson and colleagues in three studies comparing MCI subjects to older controls (top row) and two studies in subjects with a family history of AD to age-matched controls without a family history (bottom row). The areas shown in blue, red, and green represent regions showing decreased MTL activation in the MCI subjects and familial subjects compared to controls.

Turning to the fMRI studies that have reported increased MTL activation in MCI patients, Hamalainen et al. (2007) found that MCI subjects had greater activation as compared to older controls in the hippocampus and parahippocampal gyrus during a visual object-encoding paradigm. Importantly, these MCI subjects performed the fMRI memory paradigm relatively well, at an intermediate range between the controls and the AD group. There are also several studies from our own group showing evidence of increased fMRI activation, particularly in very mildly impaired MCI subjects. The initial study used a scene-encoding fMRI paradigm in 32 subjects across a range of clinical impairment as assessed by CDR-SB (Dickerson, 2004b). Interestingly, we found evidence of positive correlation between the degree of clinical impairment and the extent of activation in the posterior hippocampus and parahippocampal regions such that subjects with more impairment had a greater extent of MTL activation. Despite this paradoxical finding in the fMRI activation, we observed a negative correlation with volume in the MTL such that subjects with greater clinical impairment had smaller hippocampal volume. A multivariate analysis showed that increasing impairment (CDR-SB) was related to older age, *decreased* volume of the left hippocampus, and *increased* extent of activation in the right parahippocampal gyrus. Better performance on the post-scan recognition memory test was also correlated with greater MTL activation, but also with larger MTL volume. At clinical follow-up two years later, those subjects with greater MTL activation were more likely to demonstrate clinical decline (the longitudinal study is reviewed in more detail in the section on clinical prediction).

Two of our studies with the face-name encoding paradigm have also shown evidence of increased MTL activation, particularly in MCI subjects who were at the very mild end of the impairment continuum, as assessed by CDR-SB, MMSE, and neuropsychological test performance. The first study compared activation in these very mild MCI subjects to controls and mild AD patients (Dickerson, 2005b). Compared with older controls, the MCI subjects showed a greater extent of hippocampal activation, and only minimal atrophy of the hippocampus. These very mild MCI subjects also performed in the same range as the control group on post-scan memory tests. The AD patients had smaller MTL volumes, decreased activation in these regions, and performed below the

normal control group on the post-scan memory test. Across all the subjects in the three groups, post-scan memory task performance correlated with extent of activation in the hippocampus. In our second study with the face-name paradigm, which included a subset of subjects from the first study, we utilized independent component analyses to explore the alterations in larger memory networks in older controls: two groups of MCI subjects—one on the milder end and one on the more impaired end—and a group of mild AD patients (Celone et al., 2006). We again found evidence of greater activation in the very mild MCI (vMCI) subjects compared to controls, particularly in the MTL (see Figure 18.5). As mentioned above, we also found significantly decreased activation in the significantly impaired MCI (sMCI) group, which was at levels similar to AD. These alterations in MTL activation were significantly related to changes we observed in the default network, particularly in the medial and lateral parietal regions. We also found that greater activation in the MTL and greater deactivation in the parietal regions was related to performance on the post-scan memory test.

There have also been a few fMRI studies in MCI subjects that have employed event-related designs that can better control for the effects of memory performance, as the stimuli can be divided on the basis of successful vs. failed memory processes. Kircher et al. (2007) found that MCI subjects activated the left hippocampus and surrounding cortical regions to a greater degree than control subjects, even though the MCI performed similarly to controls on the fMRI memory paradigm. In an event-related verbal memory retrieval task, Heun et al. (2007) also found evidence of increased activation in MCI subjects as compared to normal older controls when specifically examining successful retrieval trials.

The published fMRI data in MCI is inconclusive to say the least; however, there may be some consistent findings across these studies. It is likely that at least some of the variability in fMRI data from MCI subjects relates to the level of the subjects' clinical impairment and to their ability to perform the memory task utilized in the paradigm. In general, the less-impaired MCI subjects—as assessed by their CDR or neuropsychological performance—perform better on the fMRI memory tasks and have shown evidence of greater activation. Thus, we have hypothesized that MTL "hyperactivation" early in the course of MCI might

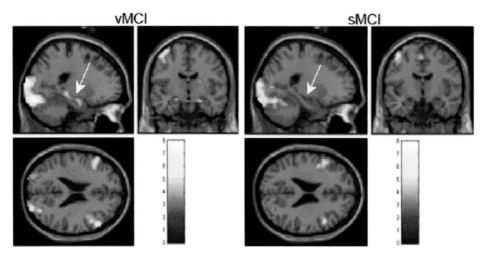

Figure 18–5 Group fMRI data from 15 very mildly impaired MCI (vMCI) and 12 significantly impaired MCI (sMCI) subjects on a face-name encoding task. The vMCI subjects showed evidence of hippocampal "hyperactivation" compared to controls. The sMCI subjects showed significantly decreased hippocampal activation at levels similar to those seen in mild AD patients.

play a compensatory role in maintaining memory performance in the setting of early AD pathology. Furthermore, the location of the hyperactivation within the MTL seems to be specific to the memory task demands of the paradigm—that is, the associative memory tasks have shown greater activation in MCI in the anterior hippocampus, while scene-encoding tasks have demonstrated greater activation in MCI in posterior hippocampus and parahippocampal regions. Both of the event-related studies published to date in MCI subjects (Heun et al., 2007; Kircher et al., 2007) found evidence of increased activation in MCI when controlling for behavioral measures—namely, memory success vs. failure. The concept of compensation, and other potential explanations for the observed "hyperactivation," is discussed in more detail later in the chapter. Studies with more impaired MCI subjects who are closer to the AD patients on the clinical spectrum, and who fail to perform well on the memory task, have demonstrated decreased MTL activation. Thus, we have postulated that at later stages of MCI—at the point of significant neuronal loss—individuals can no longer compensate, resulting in decreased MTL activation and clinically apparent memory impairment heralding incipient AD. These findings have led us to hypothesize there is an "inverse U-shaped curve" to the trajectory of MTL activation, which begins very early in the course of prodromal AD (see Figure 18.6). However, it is clear that additional research is needed to clarify the contribution of performance and clinical status (as well as other factors) to the complex pattern of functional alterations observed in MCI subjects.

fMRI Studies in Asymptomatic Subjects at Genetic Risk for AD

Asymptomatic individuals with genetic risk factors for AD, such as carriers of the apolipoprotein E epsilon 4 (ApoE ε4) allele or autosomal dominant mutations such as presenilin-1, are particularly valuable subjects to assess with functional imaging. This topic is reviewed in more detail in Chapter 9, but will be briefly discussed here, as it is very relevant to the "compensatory hyperactivation" hypothesis. Bookheimer et al. (2000) reported that despite equivalent performance on a verbal paired-associate task, cognitively intact ApoE ε4 carriers showed significantly greater fMRI activation—particularly prominent in bilateral MTL regions as compared to noncarriers. Subsequent studies stratified by the

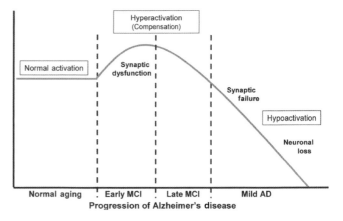

Figure 18–6 Hypothetical model of the trajectory of fMRI activation over the course of prodromal AD. Hyperactivation may occur early in the pathophysiological course of AD, at a point when individuals are still able to compensate and perform memory tasks. At the point of late MCI, there is already synaptic failure and neuronal loss, associated with hippocampal hypoactivation and clinically apparent memory impairment.

ApoE ε4 genotype have been somewhat mixed in their results, with several studies also reporting greater activation in ApoE ε4 carriers (Bondi et al., 2005; Fleisher et al., 2005; Han et al., 2007; Smith et al., 2002; Wishart, 2004), but there have also been a similar number of studies finding evidence of decreased activation in ApoE ε4 carriers (Borghesani et al., 2007; Lind, 2006a, 2006b; Mondadori et al., 2007; Smith, 1999; Trivedi et al., 2006). Individuals with other genetic risk factors for AD have also been studied with fMRI. Haier et al. (2003) reported FDG-PET evidence of *increased* MTL activation (hypermetabolism) during cognitive tasks in nondemented Down's syndrome patients. A recent fMRI study by Mondadori et al. (2006) also found evidence of increased activation that was specific to the episodic memory paradigm in a young asymptomatic carrier of the presenilin 1 mutation. The Mondadori study also reported evidence of decreased fMRI activation in a middle-aged presenilin-1 mutation carrier who fulfilled the criteria for amnestic MCI and likely had a more advanced stage of AD-related neuropathology. This study parallels the findings across the continuum of impairment in MCI subjects discussed above, and again suggests that there may be a nonlinear trajectory of fMRI activation that evolves over the course of prodromal AD (Sperling, 2007) (see Figure 18.6). Interestingly, despite the discrepant results reported across the genetic groups in the above studies, and the variety of memory paradigms examining both encoding and retrieval processes, nearly all of these studies have found evidence that greater MTL activation is related to performance on the respective memory tasks. Thus, the disparate findings may relate to the interaction between ability to perform the task and presence of genetic risk factors.

In addition, there have been several studies of individuals with a positive family history of AD, but not necessarily with an identified gene. These studies have also found somewhat discrepant results regarding increased vs. decreased activation in at-risk subjects. A large study by Bassett et al. (2006) found evidence of *increased* fMRI activation in the frontal and temporal lobes— including the hippocampus—during memory encoding in asymptomatic offspring of autopsy-confirmed AD patients, as compared to a control group without a family history. Although a large percentage of the offspring possessed at least one copy of the ApoE ε4 allele, the increased activation was found to be unrelated to this genetic risk. Johnson et al. (2006a) have conducted two large fMRI studies comparing asymptomatic middle-aged adults (mean age 55) who have a parent clinically diagnosed with sporadic AD and matched controls without parental history of AD. Both of these studies—one an encoding task and one a metamemory task— demonstrated *decreased* hippocampal activation in the family risk group (see Figure 18.4). Interestingly, although there was no main effect of ApoE genotype seen in these studies, the group with a negative family history but who did possess an ApoE epsilon 4 allele showed the *greatest* hippocampal activation. Interestingly, this group also performed at the highest accuracy in the recognition task, however all subjects of these middle-aged subjects performed extremely well. These studies, which stratify subjects by familial history, suggest that there may be a complicated interaction between ApoE and other genetic risk factors that influence hippocampal activation.

Similar to the discrepant findings in MCI, the reports of genetic at-risk and familial at-risk subjects have been quite variable. There is somewhat of an emergent theme that MTL activation is driven primarily by the memory task performance, which may interact with family history or specific genetic risk factors, and presumably early AD pathology. Longitudinal fMRI studies of these at-risk subjects, ideally in combination with amyloid and FDG-PET imaging, should help to disambiguate the findings from the cross-sectional studies and improve our understanding of the sequence of change on imaging markers.

The Conundrum of Hyperactivation: Is More Always Better?

As multiple studies have reported evidence of hyperactivation in subjects at-risk for neurodegenerative diseases, a fundamental and not yet resolved question in the field of fMRI and memory is whether or not more activation is better or worse. In young subjects, numerous "subsequent memory" studies (Brewer et al., 1998; Strange et al., 2002; Wagner et al., 1998), including our own (Chua et al., 2007; Dickerson et al., 2007; Sperling et al., 2003b) clearly suggest that increased MTL activation predicts successful memory performance. However, increased regional brain activation may also reflect greater task difficulty, increased "cognitive work" (Grady, 1996; Reuter-Lorenz, 2002), or differences in cognitive processing strategy (Kirchhoff and Buckner, 2006; Mandzia, 2004). It is difficult to accurately assess whether at-risk subject groups find memory tasks more challenging than they would in the absence of early pathology.

It is also clear that not all hyperactivation is beneficial. Studies of normal aging have indicated evidence of compensatory recruitment to maintain performance (Cabeza, 2002) and "nonselective recruitment," which does not benefit task performance (Logan et al., 2002). Functional imaging studies across a variety of neurological and psychiatric disorders suggest that task-related regional brain hyperactivation may be a common neural response to physiological stress or injury, as evidence of hyperactivation has been reported in Huntington's disease (Rosas, Feigin, and Hersch, 2004), Parkinson's disease (Monchi, 2004), cerebrovascular disease (Cao, 1999; Cramer et al., 1997; Nhan et al., 2004), multiple sclerosis (Filippi et al., 2004; Morgen et al., 2004; Reddy et al., 2000; Wishart et al., 2004), traumatic brain injury (McAllister et al., 1999), HIV (Ernst et al., 2002), alcoholism (Desmond et al., 2003), and schizophrenia (Callicott, 2003).

Although in many of the above studies hyperactivation was associated with the relative preservation of performance on the task, it may also reflect evidence of the underlying neuropathological process or a pathophysiological response that is not necessarily compensatory. Recent electrophysiological data from transgenic mouse models suggest that amyloid plaques may alter axonal morphology, resulting in desynchronized transmission of postsynaptic potentials, and requiring increased levels of stimulation for successful information propagation (Stern et al., 2004). Postmortem studies have reported abnormal cholinergic sprouting and dystrophic neurites associated with elevated levels of A-beta 1-42 in patients with AD (Masliah et al., 2003), and increased presence of neuronal growth markers in the parallel with early AD neuropathology in Down's syndrome patients (Head, 2003). It has even been postulated that AD results from neuroplasticity mechanisms gone awry (Mesulam, 1999). In postmortem tissue from patients with MCI, cholinergic markers are upregulated within the hippocampus and prefrontal cortices, nicely paralleling our fMRI data and suggesting that the cholinergic system itself shows evidence of compensatory response during the early stages of AD pathology (DeKosky et al., 2002). It is also possible that hyperactivation is related primarily to alterations in baseline cerebral perfusion. Because fMRI is a relative measure, it is possible that the increased activation reflects a relative increase from a lower baseline (see Wierenga and Bondi, 2007 for detailed discussion of this issue). This is less likely, however, to explain all of the studies finding evidence of hyperactivation, as many of these paradigms utilized contrasts (novel vs. repeated, or successful vs. failed memory trials), which do not rely on a baseline or low-level condition for comparison.

As mentioned above, several of the studies in genetically at-risk subjects (Bookheimer et al., 2000; Mondadori, 2006; Smith et al., 2002), and our own studies in very mildly impaired MCI subjects (Celone, 2006; Dickerson, 2005), have suggested that the hyperactivation is apparent in the at-risk group despite an equivalent level of performance on the tasks. This is suggestive that the increased activation is compensatory and required to achieve a similar level of performance in the setting of early pathology. Compensation may be manifested as greater regional brain activity (hyperactivation) in the same network engaged by control subjects, or possibly recruitment of additional networks to maintain task performance (Stern et al., 2000); Becker, 1996 #295; Backman, 1999 #306; Grady et al., 2003 #1276; Pariente et al., 2005 #1558).

The increased use of event-related fMRI paradigms that can isolate the neural activity associated with successful vs. failed memory processes should shed light on this conundrum. Specifically, if the hyperactivation is seen only during successful encoding trials, it is likely that, indeed, it is an effective compensatory mechanism. Alternatively, if the hyperactivation is seen for both successful and failed encoding trials, it represents either ineffectual attempts at compensation or a manifestation of the underlying pathophysiological process. The two event-related studies in MCI published to date both suggest that the hyperactivation was particularly apparent in successful encoding or successful retrieval trials, providing some additional support for the compensatory hypothesis (Heun et al., 2006; Kircher et al., 2007).

Prediction of Subsequent Cognitive Decline

Very few longitudinal studies involving fMRI have been published to date, but a few studies have presented clinical follow-up data on subjects imaged with fMRI at baseline. Interestingly, several of these studies suggest that "hyperactivation" at the time of initial imaging was associated with higher likelihood of subsequent cognitive decline (Bookheimer et al., 2000; Dickerson et al., 2004a; Miller et al., 2008b). One study in ApoE episilon 4 carriers found that decreased activation in a parietal region was predictive of subsequent memory decline; however, MTL activation was not discussed in this study (Lind et al., 2006a). Bookheimer et al. (2000) found that increased extent of fMRI activation in the left hemisphere, including the MTL, was predictive of memory decline in ApoE 4 carriers. In our initial scene-encoding fMRI study in MCI subjects, we found that those individuals who subsequently declined over the 2.5-year period of clinical follow-up actually demonstrated significantly *greater* MTL activation at baseline as compared to those MCI subjects who remained clinically stable (Dickerson et al., 2004b). The increased activation was particularly evident in the posterior hippocampus and parahippocampal gyrus, which were specifically engaged in the scene-encoding paradigm utilized in our initial fMRI studies. We have now completed additional clinical follow-up over 4 years in 25 of the subjects in the original sample (Miller et al., 2008b). Over the 4-year follow-up interval, these subjects demonstrated a wide range of cognitive decline, with some remaining quite stable and others progressing to dementia (change in CDR-SB ranging from 0 to 4.5). The degree of cognitive decline was predicted by hippocampal activation at the time of baseline scanning, with greater hippocampal activation predicting greater decline ($p < 0.05$) (see Figure 18.7). This finding was present even after controlling for baseline degree of impairment (CDR-SB), age, education, and hippocampal volume.

We have recently completed longitudinal fMRI studies in a group of 51 older individuals, across a range of cognitive impairment, imaged with alternate forms of the face-name paradigm at baseline, and with a 2-year follow-up (Sperling et al., 2008). Preliminary analyses indicate that subjects who remained cognitively normal over the 2 years demonstrated no evidence of change in activation, whereas the subjects who demonstrated significant cognitive decline demonstrated a decrease in activation—specifically, in the right hippocampal formation. Interestingly, we again observed that those subjects who declined had greater hippocampal activation at baseline, and that the amount of hyperactivation at baseline correlated with both loss of hippocampal signal and amount of clinical decline over the 2 years. Thus, although we have hypothesized that hippocampal hyperactivation may be compensatory, it may also be a harbinger of impending hippocampal failure.

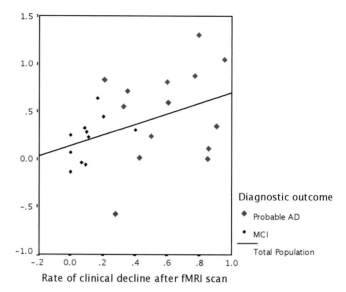

Figure 18–7   Greater hippocampal activation at the time of baseline fMRI scanning predicts greater cognitive decline over the following 5 years. Y axis shows parameter estimates (representing % signal change) of differential hippocampal activation for the novel vs. repeated contrast. X axis shows estimated rate of change in CDR sum-of-boxes score per year over 5 years after baseline fMRI scan. Black triangles indicate participants who remained classified as MCI at follow-up; red triangles indicate participants who were diagnosed with probable Alzheimer's disease during the follow-up interval. Adapted from (Miller et al., 2008b).

Pharmacological fMRI in AD Clinical Trials: Prediction of Subsequent Improvement?

One of the greatest potential benefits of fMRI may be in "proof of concept" clinical trials of novel therapeutic agents for the treatment of AD. There are a large number of promising therapies entering clinical trials; however, there have also been several very large Phase III trials that have failed to demonstrate any benefit. These Phase III trials in AD patients typically require hundreds of subjects per arm, and run a minimum of 18 months. Structural imaging techniques are increasingly included as outcome measures in these longer clinical trials, but it is unclear whether volumetric MRI will be useful in early trials of shorter duration. In addition, at least one large clinical trial of an immunotherapeutic agent demonstrated a paradoxical finding of increased rate of brain atrophy being related to positive clinical response (Fox et al., 2004). This paradoxical finding might relate to removal of amyloid, or possibly the inflammatory response associated with the immunotherapy, but it is unclear whether these smaller brains were actually "working better," as suggested by a post-hoc analysis of some of the memory test measures. The addition of functional imaging techniques—such as FDG-PET and both resting and task-related fMRI—might be very useful in early-stage clinical trials for detecting a signal of efficacy and perhaps even to predict subsequent clinical response (Dickerson and Sperling, 2005).

To bring this promise to fruition, however, a great deal of work to validate fMRI as a surrogate marker for use in clinical trials remains to be done. A number of these validation studies are ongoing in our laboratory, including longitudinal studies to assess test-retest reliability, both within and across scanner platforms. We have also recently published a study investigating the relationship of fMRI activation in AD patients during our face-name paradigm to

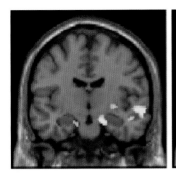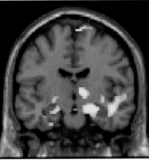

Figure 18–8 fMRI data from an individual AD patient, a 74-year-old woman, at baseline (left) and 12 weeks post-infusion (right) with a monoclonal antibody against amyloid-beta 1-42.

performance on standardized memory measures used in clinical trials, such as the ADAS-Cog (Diamond et al., 2007). We found that greater fMRI activation in inferior prefrontal and left temporal regions was significantly correlated with performance on the ADAS-Cog, as well as other verbal memory measures, even when accounting for atrophy in these regions.

We have had the opportunity to perform some pilot fMRI studies in early clinical trials of potential disease-modifying agents. It is too early to know whether these drugs will prove efficacious in slowing the progression of AD, however we have found some tantalizing evidence that increased fMRI activation over time is related to clinical improvement in some of these individuals. Figure 18.8 demonstrates the fMRI data in an individual AD patient from a placebo-controlled, blinded Phase I study of a monoclonal antibody against amyloid-beta 1-42. This AD patient shows a typical pattern of hippocampal hypoactivation at baseline, and demonstrated a marked increase in activation on repeat fMRI scanning 12 weeks after infusion. This patient was later revealed to have been randomized to active treatment, and showed a subsequent positive clinical response, remaining at an MMSE above her baseline level for over 1 year.

Although individual cases like this are intriguing, larger scale, placebo-controlled pharmacologic fMRI studies are clearly needed to assess whether fMRI can track and ultimately predict long-term clinical response. Several fMRI studies in MCI and AD patients with FDA-approved medications, such as cholinesterase inhibitors, have demonstrated evidence of increased fMRI activation on treatment; however, none of these studies were conducted with a double-blind, randomized, placebo-controlled design (Goekoop et al., 2004; Rombouts et al., 2002; Saykin, 2004).

Summary and Future Directions of Research

In summary, fMRI has shown evidence of specific alterations in memory networks that may be able to differentiate the process of normal aging from early AD. The fMRI studies in patients with clinically diagnosed AD have consistently demonstrated decreased activation in MTL structures during the encoding of new information. The studies in subjects at-risk for AD—both genetically at-risk and MCI subjects—have yielded quite variable results to date, with nearly equal numbers of studies reporting decreased and increased activation in at-risk subjects compared to control groups. We have postulated that these variable results relate to where subjects fall on the continuum of prodromal AD, and to their ability to perform the fMRI paradigm. Interestingly, the finding that increased activation is related to better performance is a consistent finding across these

at-risk studies, and the finding of hyperactivation seems to be specific to those at-risk subjects who are able to perform the memory tasks well. Very little longitudinal fMRI work has been published to date, but a few studies suggest that the pattern of fMRI activation at baseline may predict the likelihood of subsequent cognitive decline in these at-risk subjects.

The recent advances in the in vivo detection of amyloid with PET imaging (Klunk, 2004; Small, 2006) (see Chapter 14) provide a unique opportunity to study brain function in nondemented individuals who have varying levels of amyloid burden. Longitudinal studies that combine amyloid imaging with functional and structural MRI, and perhaps FDG-PET, should prove particularly valuable in elucidating the earliest functional alterations related to the process of AD, and ultimately developing imaging markers that can accurately predict the clinical course years prior to the onset of dementia.

Acknowledgements

This manuscript represents the work of many individuals who have contributed to our own studies and to my thoughts on this topic—in particular, Dorene Rentz, Psy.D., Brad Dickerson, M.D.; Maija Pihlajamaki, M.D., Ph.D.; Kim Celone; Saul Miller; Pete LaViolette; Kelly O'Keefe; Amy DeLuca; Jacqueline O'Brien; Eli Diamond, M.D.; Julie Bates, Ph.D.; Bruce Rosen, M.D.; Douglas Greve, Ph.D., Ali Atri, M.D., Ph.D., Keith Johnson, M.D.; Deborah Blacker, M.D., Sci.D., Dennis Selkoe, M.D., and Marilyn Albert, Ph.D. I would especially like to acknowledge Kim Celone Saul Miller, Brad Dickerson, M.D., and Sterling Johnson, Ph.D., who kindly contributed figures of their work for this chapter.

References

Alexander, G. E., Chen, K., Pietrini, P., Rapoport, S. I., and Reiman, E. M. (2002). Longitudinal PET evaluation of cerebral metabolic decline in dementia: A potential outcome measure in Alzheimer's disease treatment studies. *The American Journal of Psychiatry*, 159: 738–745.

Alsop, D. C., Detre, J. A., and Grossman, M. (2000). Assessment of cerebral blood flow in Alzheimer's disease by spin-labeled magnetic resonance imaging. *Annals of Neurology*, 47: 93–100.

Backman, L., Andersson, J. L., Nyberg, L., Winblad, B., Nordberg, A., Almkvist, O. (1999). Brain regions associated with episodic retrieval in normal aging and Alzheimer's disease. *Neurology*, 52: 1861–1870.

Bassett, S. S., Yousem, D. M., Cristinzio, C., Kusevic, I., Yassa, M. A., Caffo, B. S. et al. (2006). Familial risk for Alzheimer's disease alters fMRI activation patterns. *Brain*, 129: 1229–1239.

Becker, J. T., Mintun, M. A., Aleva, K., Wiseman, M. B., Nichols, T., Dekosky, S. T. (1996). Alterations in functional neuroanatomical connectivity in Alzheimer's disease. Positron emission tomography of auditory verbal short-term memory. *Annals of the New York Academy of Sciences*, 777: 239–242.

Bondi, M. W., Houston, W. S., Eyler, L. T.,and Brown, G. G. (2005). fMRI evidence of compensatory mechanisms in older adults at genetic risk for Alzheimer disease. *Neurology*, 64: 501–508.

Bookheimer, S. Y., Strojwas, M. H., Cohen, M. S, Saunders, A. M, Pericak-Vance, M. A. Mazziotta, J. et al. (2000). Patterns of brain activation in people at risk for Alzheimer's disease. *The New England Journal of Medicine*, 343: 450–456.

Borghesani, P. R., Johnson, L. C., Shelton, A. L., Peskind, E. R., Aylward, E. H., Schellenberg, G. D. et al. (2007). Altered medial temporal lobe responses during visuospatial encoding in healthy APOE*4 carriers. *Neurobiology of Aging*, 29: 981–991.

Brewer, J. B., Zhao, Z., Desmond, J. E., Glover, G. H., and Gabrieli, J. D (1998). Making memories: brain activity that predicts how well visual experience will be remembered. *Science*, 281: 1185–1187.

Buckner, R. L., Koutstaal, W., Schacter, D. L., and Rosen, B. R. (2000). Functional MRI evidence for a role of frontal and inferior temporal cortex in amodal components of priming. *Brain*, 123(3): 620–640.

Buckner, R. L., Snyder, A. Z., Shannon, B. J., LaRossa, G., Sachs, R., Fotenos A. F. et al. (2005). Molecular, structural, and functional characterization of Alzheimer's disease: Evidence for a relationship between default activity, amyloid, and memory. *The Journal of Neuroscience*, 25: 7709–7717.

Cabeza, R., Anderson, N. D., Locantore, J. K., and McIntosh, A. R. (2002). Aging gracefully: Compensatory brain activity in high-performing older adults. *Neuroimage*, 17: 1394–1402.

Callicott, J. H., Egan, M. F., Mattay, V. S., Bertolino, A., Bone, A. D., Verchinksi, B. et al. (2003). Abnormal fMRI response of the dorsolateral prefrontal cortex in cognitively intact siblings of patients with schizophrenia. *The American Journal of Psychiatry*, 160: 709–719.

Cao, Y., Vikingstad, E. M., George, K. P., Johnson, A. F., and Welch, K. M. (1999) Cortical language activation in stroke patients recovering from aphasia with functional MRI. *Stroke*, 30: 2331–2340.

Celone, K. A., Calhoun, V. D., Dickerson, B. C, Atri, A., Chua, E. F., Miller, S. L. et al. (2006). Alterations in memory networks in mild cognitive impairment and Alzheimer's disease: An independent component analysis. *The Journal of Neuroscience*, 26: 10222–10231.

Chua, E. F., Schacter, D. L. R., Giovannetti, E. and Sperling, R. A. (2007). Evidence for a specific role of the anterior hippocampal region in successful associative encoding. *Hippocampus*, 17(11): 1071–1080.

Cramer, S. C., Nelles, G., Benson, R. R., Kaplan, J. D., Parker, R. A., Kwong, K. K. et al. (1997). A functional MRI study of subjects recovered from hemiparetic stroke. *Stroke*, 28: 2518–2527.

D'Esposito, M., Zarahn, E., Aguirre, G. K. and Rypma, B. (1999). The effect of normal aging on the coupling of neural activity to the bold hemodynamic response. *Neuroimage*, 10: 6–14.

Daselaar, S. M., Prince, S. E., and Cabeza, R. (2004). When less means more: Deactivations during encoding that predict subsequent memory. *Neuroimage*, 23: 921–927.

DeKosky, S. T., Ikonomovic, M. D., Styren, S. D., Beckett, L., Wisniewski, S., Bennett, D. A. et al. (2002). Upregulation of choline acetyltransferase activity in hippocampus and frontal cortex of elderly subjects with mild cognitive impairment. *Annals of Neurology*, 51: 145–155.

Desmond, J. E., Chen, S. H., DeRosa, E., Pryor, M. R., Pfefferbaum, A., and Sullivan, E. V. (2003). Increased frontocerebellar activation in alcoholics during verbal working memory: An fMRI study. *Neuroimage*, 19: 1510–1520.

Diamond, E. L., Miller, S., Dickerson, B. C., Atri, A., DePeau, K., Fenstermacher, E. et al. (2007). Relationship of fMRI activation to clinical trial memory measures in Alzheimer disease. *Neurology*, 69: 1331–1341.

Dickerson, B. C. and Sperling, R. A. (2005). Neuroimage biomarkers for clinical trials of disease modifying therapies in Alzheimer's disease. *NeuroRx: The Journal of the American Society for Experimental NeuroTherapeutics*, 2: 348–360.

Dickerson, B. C., Miller, S. L., Greve, D. N., Dale, A. M., Albert, M. S., Schacter, D. L. et al. (2007). Prefrontal-hippocampal-fusiform activity during encoding predicts intraindividual differences in free recall ability: An event-related functional-anatomic MRI study. *Hippocampus*, 17: 1060–1070.

Dickerson, B. C., Salat, D. H., Bates, J. F., Atiya, M., Killiany, R. J., Greve, D. N. et al. (2004a). Medial temporal lobe function and structure in mild cognitive impairment. *Annals of Neurology*, 56: 27–35.

Dickerson, B. C., Salat, D., Bates, J. F., Atiya, M., Killiany, R., Greve, D. et al. (2004b). MRI measures of medial temporal lobe function and structure in questionable Alzheimer's disease. *Annals of Neurology*, 56(1): 27–35.

Dickerson, B. C., Salat, D., Greve, D., Chua, E. R., Giovannetti, E., Rentz, D. et al. (2005). Increased hippocampal activation in mild cognitive impairment compared to normal aging and AD. *Neurology*, 65: 404–411.

Eichenbaum, H., Schoenbaum, G., Young, B., and Bunsey, M. (1996). Functional organization of the hippocampal memory system. *Proceedings of the National Academy of Sciences of the USA*, 93: 13500–13507.

Ernst, T., Chang, L., Jovich, J., Ames, N., and Arnold, S. (2002). Abnormal brain activation on functional MRI in cognitively asymptomatic HIV patients. *Neurology*, 59: 1343–1349.

Filippi, M., Rocca, M. A., Mezzapesa, D. M., Falini, A., Colombo, B., Scotti, G. et al. (2004). A functional MRI study of cortical activations associated with object manipulation in patients with MS. *Neuroimage*, 21: 1147–1154.

Fleisher, A. S., Houston, W. S., Eyler, L. T., Frye, S., Jenkins, C., Thal, L. J. et al. (2005). Identification of Alzheimer disease risk by functional magnetic resonance imaging. *AMA Archives of Neurology*, 62: 1881–1888.

Fowler, K. S., Saling, M. M., Conway, E. L., Semple, J. M., and Louis, W. J. (2002). Paired associate performance in the early detection of DAT. *Journal of the International Neuropsychological Society*, 8: 58–71.

Fox, M. D., Snyder, A. Z., Vincent, J. L., Corbetta, M., Van Essen, D. C., and Raichle, M. E. (2005). The human brain is intrinsically organized into dynamic, anticorrelated functional networks. *Proceedings of the National Academy of Sciences of the USA*, 102: 9673–9678.

Fox, N. C., Black, R., Gilman, S., Rossor, M. N., Griffith, S., Jenkins, L. et al. (2004). Effects of amyloid-beta immunotherapy (an 1792) on MRI measures of brain, ventricle, and hippocampal volumes in Alzheimer's Disease. In *The Ninth International Conference on Alzheimer's Disease and Related Disorders*. Washington, D.C.

Gallo, D. A., Sullivan, A. L., Daffner, K. R., Schacter, D. L., and Budson, A. E. (2004). Associative recognition in Alzheimer's disease: evidence for impaired recall-to-reject. *Neuropsychology*, 18: 556–563.

Goekoop, R., Rombouts, S. A., Jonker, C., Hibbel, A., Knol, D. L., Truyen, L. et al. (2004). Challenging the cholinergic system in mild cognitive impairment: A pharmacological fMRI study. *Neuroimage*, 23: 1450–1459.

Golby, A., Silverberg, G., Race, E., Gabrieli, S., O'Shea, J., Knierim, K. et al. (2005). Memory encoding in Alzheimer's disease: An fMRI study of explicit and implicit memory. *Brain*, 128: 773–787.

Gomez-Isla, T., Price, J. L., McKeel, D. W., Jr., Morris, J. C., Growdon, J. H., and Hyman, B. T. (1996). Profound loss of layer II entorhinal cortex neurons occurs in very mild Alzheimer's disease. *The Journal of Neuroscience*, 16: 4491–4500.

Grady, C. L. (1996). Age-related changes in cortical blood flow activation during perception and memory. *Annals of the New York Academy of Sciences*, 777: 14–21.

Grady, C. L, McIntosh, A. R, Beig, S., Keightley, M. L., Burian, H., and Black, S. E. (2003). Evidence from functional neuroimaging of a compensatory prefrontal network in Alzheimer's disease. *The Journal of Neuroscience*, 23: 986–993.

Greicius, M. D., Krasnow, B., Reiss, A. L., and Menon, V. (2003). Functional connectivity in the resting brain: A network analysis of the default mode hypothesis. *Proceedings of the National Academy of Sciences of the USA*, 100: 253–258.

Greicius, M. D., Srivastava, G., Reiss, A. L., and Menon, V. (2004). Default-mode network activity distinguishes Alzheimer's disease from healthy aging: evidence from functional MRI. *Proceedings of the National Academy of Sciences of the USA*, 101: 4637–4642.

Gron, G., Bittner, D., Schmitz, B., Wunderlich, A. P., and Riepe, M. W. (2002). Subjective memory complaints: objective neural markers in patients with Alzheimer's disease and major depressive disorder. *Annals of Neurology*, 51: 491–498.

Grundman, M., Petersen, R. C., Ferris, S. H., Thomas, R. G., Aisen, P. S., Bennett, D. A. et al. (2004). Mild cognitive impairment can be distinguished from Alzheimer disease and normal aging for clinical trials. *AMA Archives of Neurology*, 61: 59–66.

Haier, R. J, Alkire, M. T., White, N. S., Uncapher, M. R., Head, E., Lott, I. T. et al. (2003). Temporal cortex hypermetabolism in Down syndrome prior to the onset of dementia. *Neurology*, 61: 1673–1679.

Hamalainen, A., Pihlajamaki, M., Tanila, H., Hanninen, T., Niskanen, E., Tervo, S. et al. (2007). Increased fMRI responses during encoding in mild cognitive impairment. *Neurobiology of Aging*, 28: 1889–1903.

Han, S. D., Houston, W. S., Jak, A. J., Eyler, L. T., Nagel, B. J., Fleisher, A. et al. (2007). Verbal paired-associate learning by APOE genotype in nondemented older adults: fMRI evidence of a right hemispheric compensatory response. *Neurobiology of Aging*, 28: 238–247.

Head, E., Lott, I. T., Hof, P. R., Bouras, C., Su, J. H., Kim, R. et al. (2003). Parallel compensatory and pathological events associated with tau pathology in middle aged individuals with Down syndrome. *Journal of Neuropathology and Experimental Neurology*, 62: 917–926.

Heun, R., Freymann, K., Erb, M., Leube, D. T., Jessen, F., Kircher, T. T. et al. (2006). Successful verbal retrieval in elderly subjects is related to concurrent hippocampal and posterior cingulate activation. *Dementia and Geriatric Cognitive Disorders*, 22: 165–172.

Heun, R., Freymann, K., Erb, M., Leube, D. T., Jessen, F., Kircher, T. T. et al. (2007). Mild cognitive impairment (MCI) and actual retrieval performance affect cerebral activation in the elderly. *Neurobiology of Aging*, 28: 404–413.

Jagust, W., Gitcho, A., Sun, F., Kuczynski, B., Mungas, D., and Haan, M. (2006). Brain imaging evidence of preclinical Alzheimer's disease in normal aging. *Annals of Neurology*, 59: 673–681.

Johnson, N. A., Jahng, G. H., Weiner, M. W., Miller, B. L., Chui, H. C., Jagust, W. J. et al. (2005). Pattern of cerebral hypoperfusion in Alzheimer disease and mild cognitive impairment measured with arterial spin-labeling MR imaging: initial experience. *Radiology* 234: 851–859.

Johnson, S. C., Baxter, L. C., Susskind-Wilder, L., Connor, D. J., Sabbagh, M. N. et al. (2004). Hippocampal adaptation to face repetition in healthy elderly and mild cognitive impairment. *Neuropsychologia* 42: 980–989.

Johnson, S. C., Schmitz, T. W., Trivedi, M. A., Ries, M. L., Torgerson, B. M., Carlsson, C. M. et al. (2006a). The influence of Alzheimer disease family history and apolipoprotein E epsilon4 on mesial temporal lobe activation. *The Journal of Neuroscience*, 26: 6069–6076.

Johnson, S. C., Schmitz, T. W., Moritz, C. H., Meyerand, M. E., Rowley, H. A., Alexander, A. L. et al. (2006b). Activation of brain regions vulnerable to Alzheimer's disease: The effect of mild cognitive impairment. *Neurobiology of Aging*, 27: 1604–1612.

Kato, T., Knopman, D., and Liu, H. (2001). Dissociation of regional activation in mild AD during visual encoding: A functional MRI study. *Neurology*, 57: 812–816.

Kempainnen, N. M., Aalto, S., Wilson, I. A., Nagren, K., Helin, S., Bruck, A. et al. (2007). PET amyloid ligand [11C]PIB uptake is increased in mild cognitive impairment. *Neurology* 68: 1603–1606.

Kircher, T. T., Weis, S., Freymann, K., Erb, M., Jessen, F., Grodd, W. et al. (2007). Hippocampal activation in patients with mild cognitive impairment is necessary for successful memory encoding. *Journal of Neurology, Neurosurgery, and Psychiatry*, 78: 812–818.

Kirchhoff, B. A. and Buckner, R. L. (2006). Functional-anatomic correlates of individual differences in memory. *Neuron*, 51: 263–274.

Kirchhoff, B. A., Wagner, A. D., Maril, A., and Stern, C. E. (2000). Prefrontal-temporal circuitry for episodic encoding and subsequent memory. *The Journal of Neuroscience*, 20: 6173–6180.

Kirwan, C. B. and Stark, C. E. (2004). Medial temporal lobe activation during encoding and retrieval of novel face-name pairs. *Hippocampus*, 14: 919–930.

Klunk, W. E., Engler, H., Nordberg, A., Wang, Y., Blomqvist, G., Holt, D. P. et al. (2004). Imaging brain amyloid in Alzheimer's disease with Pittsburgh Compound-B. *Annals of Neurology*, 55: 306–319.

Leirer, V. O., Morrow, D. G., Sheikh, J. I., and Pariante, G. M. (1990). Memory skills elders want to improve. *Experimental Aging Research*, 16: 155–158.

Lind, J., Ingvar, M., Persson, J., Sleegers, K., Van Broeckhoven, C., Adolfsson, R. et al. (2006a). Parietal cortex activation predicts memory decline in apolipoprotein E-epsilon4 carriers. *Neuroreport*, 17: 1683–1686.

Lind, J., Larsson, A., Persson, J., Ingvar, M., Nilsson, L. G., Backman, L. et al. (2006b). Reduced hippocampal volume in non-demented carriers of the apolipoprotein E epsilon4: Relation to chronological age and recognition memory. *Neuroscience Letters*, 396: 23–27.

Logan, J. M., Sanders, A. L., Snyder, A. Z., Morris, J. C., and Buckner, R. L. (2002). Under-recruitment and nonselective recruitment: Dissociable neural mechanisms associated with aging. *Neuron*, 33: 827–840.

Logothetis, N. K., Pauls, J., Augath, M., Trinath, T., and Oeltermann, A. (2001). Neurophysiological investigation of the basis of the fMRI signal. *Nature*, 412: 150–157.

Lustig, C., Snyder, A. Z., Bhakta, M., O'Brien, K. C., McAvoy, M., Raichle, M. E. et al. (2003). Functional deactivations: change with age and dementia of the Alzheimer type. *Proceedings of the National Academy of Sciences of the USA*, 100: 14504–14509.

Machulda, M. M., Ward, H. A., Borowski, B., Gunter, J. L., Cha, R. H., O'Brien, P. C. et al. (2003). Comparison of memory fMRI response among normal, MCI, and Alzheimer's patients. *Neurology*, 61: 500–506.

Mandzia, J. L., Black, S. E., McAndrews, M. P., Grady, C., and Graham, S. (2004). fMRI differences in encoding and retrieval of pictures due to encoding strategy in the elderly. *Human Brain Mapping*, 21: 1–14.

Masliah, E., Alford, M., Adame, A., Rockenstein, E., Galasko, D., Salmon, D. et al. (2003). Abeta1-42 promotes cholinergic sprouting in patients with AD and Lewy body variant of AD. *Neurology*, 61: 206–211.

McAllister, T. W., Saykin, A. J., Flashman, L. A., Sparling, M. B., Johnson, S. C., Guerin, S. J. et al. (1999). Brain activation during working memory 1 month after mild traumatic brain injury: a functional MRI study. *Neurology*, 53: 1300–1308.

Meltzer, C. C., Zubieta, J. K., Brandt, J., Tune, L. E., Mayberg, H. S., and Frost, J. J. (1996). Regional hypometabolism in Alzheimer's disease as measured by positron emission tomography after correction for effects of partial volume averaging. *Neurology*, 47: 454–461.

Mesulam, M. M. (1999). Neuroplasticity failure in Alzheimer's disease: bridging the gap between plaques and tangles. *Neuron*, 24: 521–529.

Miller, S. L., Fenstermacher, E., Bates, J., Blacker, D., Sperling, R. A., and Dickerson, B. C. (2008a). Hippocampal activation in adults with mild cognitive impairment predicts subsequent cognitive decline. *Journal of Neurology, Neurosurgery, and Psychiatry*, 79: 630–635.

Miller, S. L., Celone, K., DePeau, K., Diamond, E., Dickerson, B. C., Rentz, D. et al. (2008b). Age-related memory impairment associated with loss of parietal deactivation but preserved hippocampal activation. *Proceedings of the National Academy of Sciences of the USA*, 105: 2181–2186.

Monchi, O., Petrides, M., Doyon, J., Postuma, R. B., Worsley, K., and Dagher, A. (2004). Neural bases of set-shifting deficits in Parkinson's disease. *The Journal of Neuroscience*, 24: 702–710.

Mondadori, C. R., Buchmann, A., Mustovic, H., Schmidt, C. F., Boesiger, P., Nitsch, R. M. et al. (2006). Enhanced brain activity may precede the diagnosis of Alzheimer's disease by 30 years. *Brain*, 129: 2908–2922.

Mondadori, C R, de Quervain, D. J., Buchmann, A., Mustovic, H., Wollmer, M. A., Schmidt, C. F. et al. (2007). Better memory and neural efficiency in young apolipoprotein E epsilon4 carriers. *Cerebral Cortex*, 17: 1934–1947.

Morgen, K., Kadom, N., Sawaki, L., Tessitore, A., Ohayon, J., McFarland, H. et al. (2004). Training-dependent plasticity in patients with multiple sclerosis. *Brain*, 127: 2506–2517.

Morris, J. C. (1993). The Clinical Dementia Rating (CDR): Current version and scoring rules. *Neurology*, 43: 2412–2414.

Morris, J. C., McKeel, D. W., Jr., Storandt, M., Rubin, E. H., Price, J. L., Grant, E. A. (1991). Very mild Alzheimer's disease: informant-based clinical, psychometric, and pathologic distinction from normal aging [see comments]. *Neurology*, 41: 469–478.

Nhan, H., Barquist, K., Bell, K., Esselman, P., Odderson, I. R., and Cramer, S. C. (2004). Brain function early after stroke in relation to subsequent recovery. *Journal of Cerebral Blood Flow and Metabolism*, 24: 756–763.

Ogawa, S, Lee, T. M., Nayak, A. S. Glynn, P. (1990). Oxygenation-sensitive contrast in magnetic resonance image of rodent brain at high magnetic fields. *Magnetic Resonance in Medicine*, 14: 68–78.

Pariente, J., Cole, S., Henson, R., Clare, L., Kennedy, A., Rossor, M. et al. (2005). Alzheimer's patients engage an alternative network during a memory task. *Annals of Neurology*, 58: 870–879.

Petersen, R. C. (2004). Mild cognitive impairment as a diagnostic entity. *Journal of Internal Medicine*, 256: 183–194.

Petersen, R. C., Parisi, J. E., Dickson, D. W., Johnson, K. A., Knopman, D. S., Boeve, B. F. et al. (2006). Neuropathologic features of amnestic mild cognitive impairment. *Archives of Neurology*, 63: 665–672.

Petrella, J., Krishnan, S., Slavin, M., Tran, T. T., Murty, L., and Doraiswamy, P. (2006). Mild Cognitive Impairment: Evaluation with 4-T Functional MR Imaging. *Radiology*, 240: 177–186.

Pihlajamaki, M., Depeau, K. M., Blacker, D., and Sperling, R. A. (2008). Impaired medial temporal repetition suppression is related to failure of parietal deactivation in Alzheimer disease. *The American Journal of Geriatric Psychiatry: Official Journal of the American Association for Geriatric Psychiatry*, 16: 283–292.

Raichle, M. E., MacLeod, A. M., Snyder, A. Z., Powers, W. J., Gusnard, D. A., and Shulman, G. L. (2001). A default mode of brain function. *Proceedings of the National Academy of Sciences of the USA*, 98: 676–682.

Reddy, H., Narayanan, S., Matthews, P. M., Hoge, R. D., Pike, G. B., Duquette, P. et al. (2000). Relating axonal injury to functional recovery in MS. *Neurology*, 54: 236–239.

Reiman, E. M., Chen, K., Alexander, G. E., Caselli, R. J., Bandy, D., Osborne, D. et al. (2004). Functional brain abnormalities in young adults at genetic risk for late-onset Alzheimer's dementia. *Proceedings of the National Academy of Sciences of the USA*, 101: 284–289.

Remy, F., Mirrashed, F., Campbell, B., and Richter, W. (2005). Verbal episodic memory impairment in Alzheimer's disease: A combined structural and functional MRI study. *Neuroimage*, 25: 253–266.

Reuter-Lorenz, P. (2002). New visions of the aging mind and brain. *Trends in Cognitive Sciences*, 6: 394.

Rombouts, S. A., Barkhof, F., Van Meel, C. S., and Scheltens, P. (2002). Alterations in brain activation during cholinergic enhancement with rivastigmine in Alzheimer's disease. *Journal of Neurology, Neurosurgery, and Psychiatry*, 73: 665–671.

Rombouts, S. A., Goekoop, R., Stam, C. J., Barkhof, F., and Scheltens, P. (2005a). Delayed rather than decreased BOLD response as a marker for early Alzheimer's disease. *Neuroimage*, 26: 1078–1085.

Rombouts, S. A., Barkhof, F., Goekoop, R., Stam, C. J., and Scheltens, P. (2005b). Altered resting state networks in mild cognitive impairment and mild Alzheimer's disease: an fMRI study. *Human Brain Mapping*, 26: 231–239.

Rombouts, S. A., Barkhof, F., Veltman, D. J., Machielsen. W. C., Witter, M. P., Bierlaagh, M. A. et.al. (2000). Functional MR imaging in Alzheimer's disease during memory encoding. *American Journal of Neuroradiology*, 21: 1869–1875.

Rosas, H. D., Feigin, A. S., and Hersch, S. M. (2004). Using advances in neuroimaging to detect, understand, and monitor disease progression in Huntington's disease. *NeuroRx: The Journal of the American Society for Experimental NeuroTherapeutics*, 1: 263–272.

Saykin, A. J., Wishart, H. A., Rabin, L. A., Flashman, L. A., McHugh, T. L., Mamourian, A. C. et al. (2004). Cholinergic enhancement of frontal lobe activity in mild cognitive impairment. *Brain*, 127: 1574–1583.

Schon, K., Atri, A., Hasselmo, M. E., Tricarico, M. D., LoPresti, M. L., and Stern, C. E. (2005). Scopolamine reduces persistent activity related to long-term encoding in the parahippocampal gyrus during delayed matching in humans. *The Journal of Neuroscience*, 5: 9112–9123.

Selkoe, D. J. (2002). Alzheimer's disease is a synaptic failure. *Science*, 298: 789–791.

Shmuel, A., Augath, M., Oeltermann, A., and Logothetis, N. K. (2006). Negative functional MRI response correlates with decreases in neuronal activity in monkey visual area V1. *Nature Neuroscience*, 9: 569–577.

Silverman, D. H., Small, G. W., Chang, C. Y., Lu, C. S., Kung De Aburto, M. A., Chen, W. et al. (2001). Positron emission tomography in evaluation of dementia: Regional brain metabolism and long-term outcome. *The Journal of the American Medical Association*, 286: 2120–2127.

Small, G. W., Kepe, V., Ercoli, L. M., Siddarth, P., Bookheimer, S. Y., Miller, K. J. et al. (2006). PET of brain amyloid and tau in mild cognitive impairment. *The New England Journal of Medicine*, 355: 2652–2663.

Small, G. W., Ercoli, L. M., Silverman, D. H., Huang, S. C., Komo, S., Bookheimer, S. Y. et al. (2000). Cerebral metabolic and cognitive decline in persons at genetic risk for Alzheimer's disease. *Proceedings of the National Academy of Sciences of the USA*, 97: 6037–6042.

Small, S. A., Perera, G. M., DeLaPaz, R., Mayeux, R., and Stern, Y. (1999). Differential regional dysfunction of the hippocampal formation among elderly with memory decline and Alzheimer's disease. *Annals of Neurology*, 45: 466–472.

Small, S. A., Nava, A. S., Perera, G. M., DeLaPaz, R., Mayeux, R., and Stern, Y. (2001). Circuit mechanisms underlying memory encoding and retrieval in the long axis of the hippocampal formation. *Nature Neuroscience*, 4: 442–449.

Smith, C. D., Andersen, A. H., Kryscio, R. J., Schmitt. F. A., Kindy. M. S., Blonder, L. X. et al. (1999). Altered brain activation in cognitively intact individuals at high risk for Alzheimer's disease. *Neurology*, 53: 1391–1396.

Smith, C. D., Andersen, A. H., Kryscio, R. J., Schmitt, F. A., Kindy, M. S., Blonder, L. X. et al. (2002). Women at risk for AD show increased parietal activation during a fluency task. *Neurology*, 58: 1197–1202.

Sperling, R. (2007). Functional MRI studies of associative encoding in normal aging, mild cognitive impairment, and Alzheimer's disease. *Annals of the New York Academy of Sciences*, 1097: 146–155.

Sperling, R., Bates, J., Chua, E., Cocchiarella, A., Schacter, D. L., Rosen, B. et al. (2003a). fMRI studies of associative encoding in young and elderly controls and mild AD patients. *Journal of Neurology, Neurosurgery, and Psychiatry*, 74: 44–50.

Sperling, R. A., Bates, J., Cocchiarella, A., Schacter, D., Rosen, B., and Albert, M. (2001). Encoding Novel Face-Name Associations: A functional MRI Study. *Human Brain Mapping*, 14: 129–139.

Sperling, R., Chua, E., Cocchiarella, A., Rand-Giovannetti, E., Poldrack, R., Schacter, D. L. et al. (2003b). Putting names to faces: Successful encoding of associative memories activates the anterior hippocampal formation. *Neuroimage*, 20: 1400–1410.

Sperling, R. A., O'Brien, J., O'Keefe, K., DeLuca, A., LaViolette, P., Bakkour, A. et al. (2008). Longitudinal fMRI demonstrates loss of hippocampal activation over the course of MCI. *Neurology*, 70: A445.

Sperling, R. A., Greve, D., Dale, A., Killiany, R., Rosen, B., Holmes, J. et al. (2002). fMRI detection of pharmacologically induced memory impairment. *Proceedings of the National Academy of Sciences*, 99: 455–460.

Squire, L. R. and Zola-Morgan, S. (1991). The medial temporal lobe memory system. *Science*, 253: 1380–1386.

Stern, E. A., Bacskai, B. J., Hickey, G. A., Attenello, F. J., Lombardo, J. A., and Hyman, B. T. (2004). Cortical synaptic integration *in vivo* is disrupted by amyloid-beta plaques. *The Journal of Neuroscience*, 24: 4535–4540.

Stern, Y., Moeller, J. R., Anderson, K. E., Luber, B., Zubin, N. R., DiMauro, A. A. et al. (2000). Different brain networks mediate task performance in normal aging and AD: Defining compensation. *Neurology*, 55: 1291–1297.

Strange, B. A., Otten, L. J., Josephs, O., Rugg, M. D., and Dolan, R. J. (2002). Dissociable human perirhinal, hippocampal, and parahippocampal roles during verbal encoding. *The Journal of Neuroscience*, 22: 523–528.

Trivedi, M. A., Schmitz, T. W., Ries, M. L., Torgerson, B. M., Sager, M. A., Hermann, B. P. et al. (2006). Reduced hippocampal activation during episodic encoding in middle-aged individuals at genetic risk of Alzheimer's disease: A cross-sectional study. *BMC medicine*, 4: 1.

Vincent, J. L., Snyder, A. Z., Fox, M. D., Shannon, B. J., Andrews, J. R., Raichle, M. E. et al. (2006). Coherent spontaneous activity identifies a hippocampal-parietal memory network. *Journal of Neurophysiology*, 96: 3517–3531.

Wagner, A. D., Schacter, D. L., Rotte, M., Koutstaal, W., Maril, A., Dale, A. M. et al. (1998). Building memories: remembering and forgetting of verbal experiences as predicted by brain activity. *Science*, 281: 1188–1191.

Walsh, D. M. and Selkoe, D. J. (2004). Deciphering the molecular basis of memory failure in Alzheimer's disease. *Neuron*, 44: 181–193.

Wheeler, M. E. and Buckner, R. L. (2004). Functional-anatomic correlates of remembering and knowing. *Neuroimage*, 21: 1337–1349.

Wierenga, C. E. and Bondi, M. W. (2007). Use of functional magnetic resonance imaging in the early identification of Alzheimer's disease. *Neuropsychology Review*, 17: 127–143.

Wishart, H. A., Saykin, A. J., McDonald, B. C., Mamourian, A. C., Flashman, L. A., Schuschu, K. R. et al. (2004). Brain activation patterns associated with working memory in relapsing-remitting MS. *Neurology*, 62: 234–238.

Zeineh, M. M., Engel, S. A., Thompson, P. M., and Bookheimer, S. Y. (2003). Dynamics of the hippocampus during encoding and retrieval of face-name pairs. *Science*, 299: 577–580.

Zelinski, E. M. and Gilewski, M. J. (1988). Assessment of memory complaints by rating scales and questionnaires. *Psychopharmacology Bulletin*, 24: 523–529.

19

MRI as a Surrogate Marker in Clinical Trials in Alzheimer's Disease

Frank Jessen and Harald Hampel

Introduction

Due to the ever-increasing number of elderly people in Europe, Northern America, Japan, India, and China, as well as many other countries worldwide, the dramatically growing projected future prevalence of dementia is a devastating threat to all major socio-economic systems. Since Alzheimer's disease (AD) is the most common cause of dementia, it has become the one of the primary development target areas, facilitated by large-scale investments by the pharmaceutical industry besides cancer, cardiovascular disease, and stroke. As a consequence of intense drug development efforts, there are currently more than 30 novel compounds already in Phase I , II, and III trials. Over the last couple of decades, substantial knowledge about the pathophysiology of AD has emerged, and several of these therapeutic compounds aim at modification of the disease process. Based on past guideline recommendations of regulatory authorities such as Federal Food and Drug Administration (FDA) in the United States and the European Agency for the Development of Medical Products (EMEA), the primary outcome measures in clinical AD trials to date are neuropsychological and psychometric test batteries of cognition, clinical ratings, and assessments of daily functioning. These measures directly reflect the drug-related benefit for the patient and the caregivers. However, the cognitive performance and clinical status of patients with dementia fluctuates, and the reliability of the applied instruments is frequently limited by the dependency on raters and caregiver's information. Currently, with the development of novel disease-modifying agents, there is a strong need for indicators of the biological disease process that underlie clinical symptoms. These biomarkers should facilitate early clinical pre-dementia and even preclinical disease detection, be able to monitor disease progression, and mirror the effects of drugs on disease activity. Over the last decade, substantial progress in biomarker development has been made. The rapidly advancing field of structural, metabolic, functional, and molecular neuroimaging is most promising for delivering biomarkers, which fulfills these requirements. High-resolution structural MRI, in combination with innovative data -processing techniques, has so far provided the best researched and most matured biomarker candidates for AD. A large and ever-growing body of literature has provided reliable and valid evidence that distinct patterns and rates of brain atrophy are detectable at early disease stages in AD, and characterize disease progression. With regard to drug development, a biomarker becomes particularly meaningful, if the effects of interventions on this biomarker are closely associated with relevant clinical outcomes. In this case, a biomarker may serve as a true surrogate marker.

Definition of a Surrogate Marker

According to the definition by regulatory agencies such as FDA or EMEA, a surrogate marker is a laboratory or clinical measurement that is used in clinical trials as a substitute for a clinically meaningful endpoint (Broich, 2007; Temple, 1999) (see Table 19.1). The rationale for surrogate marker use can be greater convenience in measuring this marker than the clinical outcome, more reliability of the surrogate marker measurement itself than the clinical endpoint, shortening of clinical trials, or reduction of sample size. In the case of AD, a surrogate marker should distinguish between affected patients and healthy subjects, be associated with AD pathology, mirror disease progression, and predict clinically meaningful outcomes such as cognition and the ability to function in daily living. The need for reliable prediction of the effect of an intervention on a clinical outcome by the surrogate markers rather than just an association of the marker with an outcome—and the requirement that the effect on the clinical outcome should be explained by the effect of the intervention on the surrogate marker—makes surrogate marker validation particularly challenging (Fleming and DeMets, 1996). In the following chapter, we will provide an in-depth discussion of the literature on structural MRI in AD regarding these issues to define its role as a surrogate marker candidate in clinical AD trials.

Cross-sectional MRI Studies in AD

When addressing the suitability of a biological indicator as a surrogate marker candidate, the first issue is to define the typical alterations of this marker in association with the disease. Therefore, we will summarize the main data of cross-sectional MRI studies in AD and highlight the most consistent findings. Since the MRI

Table 19–1   Definition of a Surrogate Marker in Therapeutic Trials (Temple, 1999).

- Laboratory measurement or physical sign
- Substitute for a clinically meaningful endpoint (i.e. a direct measure of how a patient feels, functions, or survives)
- Predictor the effect of the therapy

literature in AD is extensive, this overview cannot cover all published materials, however we will summarize the key findings. Like in most complex system neurodegenerative disease, the neuropathology of AD is hypothesized to follow a specific spatio/temporal pattern that has been described by several authors (Braak and Braak, 1991; Delacourte et al., 1999) While the amyloid deposition appears to be more diffusely spread within cortical areas, hyperphosphorylation of the tau protein and neurofibrillary tangle (NFT) formation, as well as the neurodegenerative process, seem to initiate and then spread from the transentorhinal and entorhinal region via the limbic system in areas such as the hippocampus and the medial temporal lobe (MTL) to the cortex. Since pyramidal cells that interconnect distinct regions of the brain are primary affected by NFT, widespread dysfunction in cortical association areas is a consequence of NFT formation in the MTL neurons. Denervation of these cortical regions might, in turn, promote local NFT formation and neurodegeneration (Smith, 2002). The temporal cascade of these events also reflects the sequence of symptoms in the course of the AD.

Due to its most prominent role in early AD, numerous MRI studies searched for structural changes in the MTL. Accordingly, early studies already identified atrophy of the hippocampus (see Figures 19.1 and 19.2) and neighboring structures in AD in comparison with healthy elderly subjects (e.g., Kesslak, Nalcioglu, and Cotman, 1991; Seab et al., 1988). While initial studies investigated only small groups of patients, subsequent reports replicated the pilot data in larger samples. Laakso et al. (1998) measured hippocampal volumes in 160 participants. They reported a correct diagnostic classification of 92% of AD cases in comparison with healthy controls, solely based on hippocampal volume. Jack et al. (1997) reported a reduction of the mean of -1.75 SD in very mild and -2.22 SD in moderate AD patients ($n = 94$) in comparison with control subjects ($n = 126$). The authors highlighted that the hippocampal volume performed best of all medial temporal lobe volumes measured in the discrimination of AD and healthy subjects. Recent studies confirmed that that no other region of the MTL, including the entorhinal cortex, is superior to the hippocampus in discriminating between AD patients and healthy controls (Pennanen et al., 2004; Teipel et al., 2006; Xu et al., 2000).

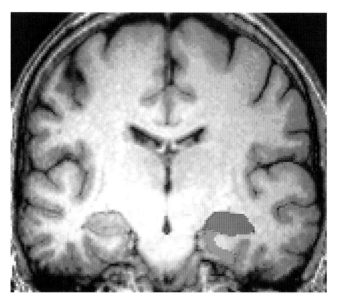

Figure 19–2   Entorhinal cortex volumetry. Coronal section through the medial temporal lobe showing the location of the hippocampus *(red)* and the entorhinal cortex *(green)* With kind permission from Springer Science and Business Media (Teipel et al, 2008).

While the majority of volumetric MRI studies in AD used manual tracing to measure the hippocampus and neighbouring structures (see Figures 19.1 amd 19.2), a number of recent studies have used user-independent automated methods. With these, grey matter reduction of the medial temporal lobe was confirmed (e.g., Busatto et al., 2003; Hirata et al., 2005; Karas et al., 2003). Three-dimensional (3D) deformation-based approaches further identified specific volume reductions in the CA1 region and the subiculum of the hippocampus (Frisoni et al., 2006; Scher et al., 2007; Wang, L. et al., 2006), which is in agreement with the primary histopathological affection of the regions by AD (e.g., Corder et al., 2000). Mueller et al. (2007), however, analyzed hippocampal subfields at higher field strengths (4 Tesla), and showed that the dentate gyrus is the first and most significant indicator for AD, and not area CA1 (in which changes were related to aging, but not specifically to AD).

Age in general is an important confound in the study of hippocampal volume in AD (Jack et al., 1997; van den Pol et al., 2006). Therefore, age transformation of hippocampal volume increases the diagnostic accuracy of hippocampal and medial temporal lobe volume in the discrimination between AD and controls (Hampel et al., 2002).

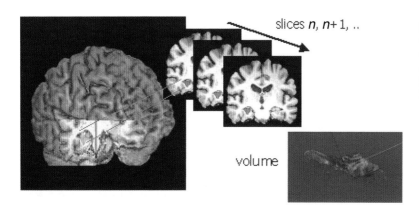

Figure 19–1   Manual measurement of hippocampus volume. The ROI is manually defined in consecutive slices covering the hippocampus. The volume then is determined from summing all voxels contained in the ROI across all slices. With kind permission from Springer Science and Business Media (Teipel et al., 2008).

The atrophy in AD is not restricted to the MTL, but rather spreads throughout the entire limbic system (Callen et al., 2001; Copenhaver et al., 2006), including the cingulate gyrus (see Figures 19.3 and 19.4) (Jones et al., 2006; Miller et al., 2003), even in early disease stages.

A significant advance of computational neuroscience has been the development of whole brain hypothesis-free data analysis techniques. These have revealed widespread atrophy beyond the MTL and the limbic system in AD. Grey matter volume reduction was observed particularly in the cingulate gyrus and the frontal and parietal lobes, but also in subcortical structures like the caudate nucleus and the thalamus. Sensorimotor areas, the occipital lobe, and the cerebellum are mostly spared (Karas et al., 2003; Thompson et al., 2001).

Some groups have particularly focused on the integrity of the corpus callosum as an indirect measure of neocortical neurodegeneration and structural interhemispheric connectivity. A reduction of the area of the corpus callosum has been consistently reported in a number of independent studies (Chaim et al., 2007; Hampel et al., 1998; Thomann et al., 2006; Wang, P. J. et al., 2006).

Of particular interest in the investigation of the primarily neuropathologically based cholinergic deficit hypothesis in AD are recent MRI findings demonstrating reductions of the substantia innominata as the origin of cholinergic innervation of the cortex (Hanyu et al., 2005). This finding has been extended further by Teipel et al. (2005), showing grey matter reduction in the anteromedial and anterolateral N. basalis of Meynert to correlate with atrophy of neocortical areas receiving cholinergic projections (see Figure 19.5).

Whereas most previous studies have focused on univariate analysis of regions of interest or image voxels, recent studies have applied multivariate techniques for pattern identification of disease-specific morphometric changes. With these approaches, spatially correlated patterns of atrophic changes can be detected and used for classification of individuals. Methods for pattern recognition, including principal component analysis (PCA) (see Figure 19.6) (Chen et al., 2004; Teipel, Born et al., 2007; Teipel, Stahl et al., 2007) or support vector machine algorithms (SVM) (Lao et al., 2004), have been successfully applied to differentiating AD patients from elderly healthy controls. Longitudinal changes as small as 0.04% of brain volume can be successfully detected based on PCA (Chen et al., 2004). When using the subspace of voxels that best discriminates AD patients from healthy subjects, the prediction of conversion to dementia in mild cognitive impairment (MCI) achieves an accuracy of 80% . However, these methods need to be still validated in larger samples of patients to determine the robust spatial patterns of volumetric or shape-related changes that allow reliable diagnostic classification. Other multivariate techniques, such as independent component analysis (ICA), that are more sensitive toward localized changes may be capable of detecting relatively isolated atrophy, especially at early stages of the disease. Such techniques, however, have so far only been applied for analysis of task-related changes in brain function without diagnostic application (McKeown et al., 1998). This is to outline the future perspectives that come with the fast development of MR-related hardware and software, allowing refined data post-processing and analysis of structural MRI.

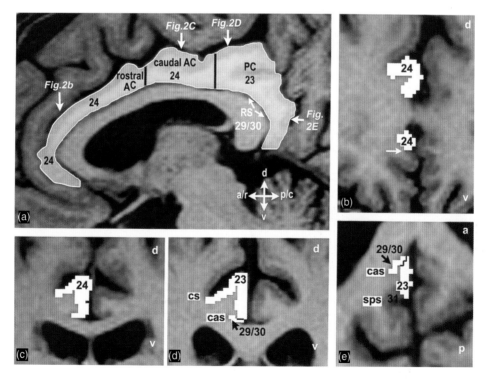

Figure 19–3   Changes in early Alzheimer's disease in various sub-regions of the cingulate gyrus. The cingulate gyrus has been divided into various sub-regions as illustrated. The sub-regions reflect approximately the Brodmann areas. Rostral AC indicates the cingulate gyrus anterior to the anterior-commissure (AC); the caudal AC is the subregion of the cingulate gyrus between the anterior commissure and posterior commissure. The sub-region RS corresponds with Brodmann areas 29 and 30 and is located in the depth of the callosal sulcus and does not appear on the medial surface of the cingulate gyrus. Sub-region PC was approximately defined as similar to Brodmann area 23. This is Figure 19.2 from Jones et al., (2006). With kind permission from Oxford University Press (Jones et al., 2006).

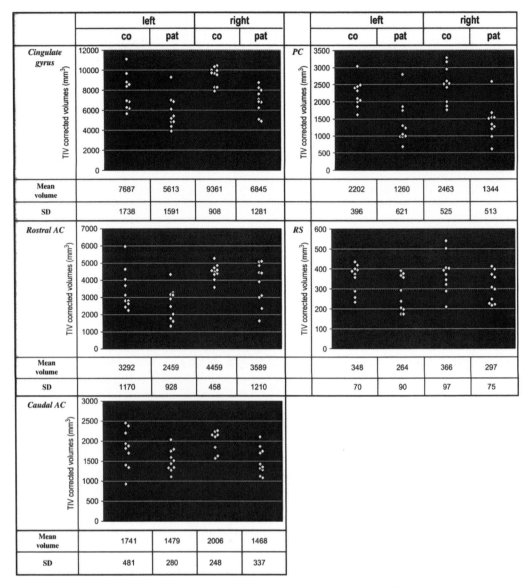

	left co	left pat	right co	right pat		left co	left pat	right co	right pat
Cingulate gyrus					**PC**				
Mean volume	7687	5613	9361	6845		2202	1260	2463	1344
SD	1738	1591	908	1281		396	621	525	513
Rostral AC					**RS**				
Mean volume	3292	2459	4459	3589		348	264	366	297
SD	1170	928	458	1210		70	90	97	75
Caudal AC									
Mean volume	1741	1479	2006	1468					
SD	481	280	248	337					

Figure 19–4 Volumetric differences between AD patients and controls in the various sub-regions of the cingulate gyrus (see Figure 19.3). Mean volumes are displayed as TIV-corrected geometric mean volumes. This is Figure 19.3 from Jones et al., (2006). With kind permission from Oxford University Press (Jones et at., 2006).

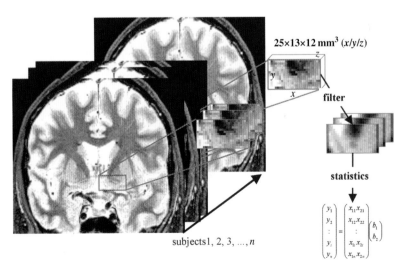

25×13×12 mm³ (x/y/z)

filter

statistics

$$\begin{pmatrix} y_1 \\ y_2 \\ \vdots \\ y_i \\ y_n \end{pmatrix} = \begin{pmatrix} x_{11} x_{21} \\ x_{12} x_{22} \\ \vdots \\ x_{1i} x_{2i} \\ x_{1n} x_{2n} \end{pmatrix} \begin{pmatrix} b_1 \\ b_2 \end{pmatrix}$$

subjects 1, 2, 3, ..., n

Figure 19–5 Image regression analysis of basal forebrain atrophy in AD. Proton density weighted MRI scans are spatially transformed into standard space. Then a square ROI is placed on the substantia innominata (the area of the cholinergic basal forebrain) according to the middle of the anterior commissure. Signal intensity within the *square* ROI is extracted from each scan and after smoothing subjected to a univariate voxelwise statistics. With kind permission from Springer Science and Business Media (Teipel et al., 2008).

(a)

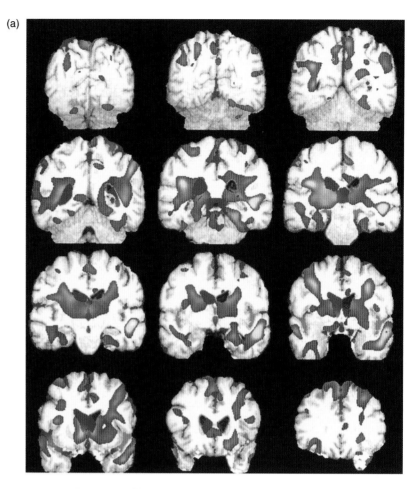

(b)

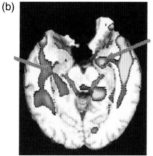

Figure 19–6 Projection of the significant component of the canonical images of CSF and brain maps into voxel space—coronal sections. The canonical images for CSF and brain in voxel space projected on the rendered coronal sections (a) and on an axial slice through the long axis of the hippocampus (b) of the T1-weighted template brain. Red to yellow: components of the canonical image of brain that are reduced in AD relative to controls. Blue to green: components of the canonical image of CSF that are increased in AD relative to controls. The green arrows point to the right and left hippocampus formation on the axial slice that has been reconstructed parallel to the long axis of the hippocampus. Reprinted with kind permission from (Teipel et al., 2007). Copyright © 2007 Elsevier. All right reserved.

Overall, there is accumulating evidence that structural MRI provides reliable images of a distinct pattern of atrophy and grey matter loss that reflect the spatial distribution of neurodegeneration reported in post-mortem histopathological studies. Thus, cross-sectional MRI is clearly capable of describing the core characteristics of the disease. In the next section of this chapter, we will discuss studies that have directly linked MRI with post-mortem data.

Correlation of MRI Findings with Post-mortem Data

A crucial issue in defining the potential role of a surrogate marker candidate is the association of the marker with the pathophysiological process of the disease. AD is primarily characterized by an accumulation of Aß peptide with subsequent extracellular amyloid plaques formation, hyperphosphorylation and intracellular

aggregation of tau protein (neurofibrillary tangles, NFTs), and progressing neurodegeneration. At present, none of these microstructural features can be directly visualized by MRI in living AD patients. However, MRI measures have been linked to post-mortem features of AD and other indicators of pathology, like CSF parameters and amyloid deposition detection with PET.

In an early study inspired by the Consortium to establish a registry for Alzheimer's Disease (CERAD), the imaging data of 20 AD patients (CT: $n = 11$; MRI: $n = 9$) were visually rated according to a set of scales. The authors reported a correlation between the rating of the size of the temporal horn on brain images with neuropathological evidence for hippocampal atrophy (Kendall's tau: 0.45, $p = 0.046$). The mean interval between neuroimaging and death in that study was 2.6 years (Davis et al., 1995).

In a study of 67 individuals, including patients with different dementia etiologies and nondemented subjects, Jack et al. (2002) reported a significant correlation of antemortem hippocampal

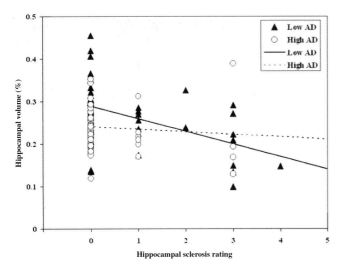

Figure 19–7 Relation between pathologically measured hippocampal sclerosis and magnetic resonance measured hippocampal volume for two groups of subjects defined by the extent of Alzheimer's disease (AD) pathology using a median split. *Triangles* denote low AD; *circles* denote high AD; *solid line* denotes low AD; *dotted line* denotes high AD. Reprinted with permission from (Jagust et al., 2008). Copyright © 2008 John Wiley & Sons, Inc. All right reserved.

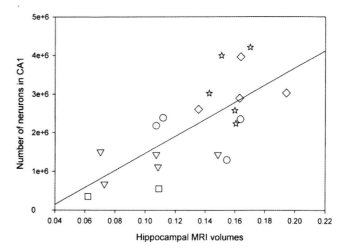

Figure 19–8 Estimated number of neurons in cornu ammonis 1 region of the hippocampus (CA1) is strongly correlated with the volume of the hippocampus determined from magnetic resonance imaging. *Stars* indicate healthy control subjects; *circles* indicate cognitively impaired not meeting criteria for Alzheimer's disease (AD); *triangles* indicate AD; *squares* indicate AD with hippocampal sclerosis; and *diamonds* indicate ischemic vascular dementia. MRI = magnetic resonance imaging. Reprinted with permission from (Zarow et al., 2005). Copyright © 2005 John Wiley & Sons, Inc. All right reserved.

volume on MRI and Braak stages ($r = -0.39, p < 0.001$). The mean interval between MRI and death was 1.8 years. In addition, hippocampal atrophy may be associated with other pathological processes such as hippocampal sclerosis (Jagust et al., 2008), illustrating the complexity of the relationship between hippocampal atrophy and neuropathology. In a study with 93 autopsied brains that included Alzheimer's disease patients, cardio-vascular dementia patients and healthy subjects it was found that hippocampal sclerosis and hippocampal volume varied according to the extent of AD pathology: hippocampal sclerosis (see Figure 19.7) has a stronger and significant effect in the group with low AD pathology (Spearman's $r = -0.44; p = 0.002$), but a weak and non-significant effect in the group with high AD pathology (Spearman's $r = -0.1; p = 0.52$) (interaction $p = 0.075$). Hippocampal sclerosis scores and Braak stage were not correlated with one another ($r = -0.01; p = 0.90$), and there was no association between a Braak and Braak stage $\geq$IV and the presence of hippocampal sclerosis ($\chi[2] = 0.90; p = 0.34$) (Jagust et al., 2008).

Csernansky et al. (2004) showed a correlation of NFT density in the hippocampus and antemortem hippocampal volume (left: $r = -0.62, p = 0.03$; right: $-0.55, p = 0.06$) in a group of 10 AD patients and two controls (mean interval between MRI and death of 2.2 years). There was no significant correlation between the number of amyloid plaques in the hippocampus with hippocampal volume on an MRI (left: $r = -0.49, p = 0.10$; right: $-0.32, p = 0.30$), but the number of plaques did correlate with total brain volume ($r = -0.68, p = 0.01$). The correlation of antemortem hippocampal volume on MRI and postmortem NFT density in the hippocampus was further confirmed by Silbert et al. (2003) in a sample of 24 demented subjects ($R^2 = 0.247, p < 0.05$) with a mean interval between last MRI and death of 3 years. Ventricular volume was associated with cortical load of amyloid plaques ($R^2 = 0.262, p < 0.05$). This study is of particular relevance because it obtained longitudinal MRI prior to death. In this study, the rate of longitudinal volume reduction of the hippocampus was not associated with hippocampal NFT. However, ventricular enlargement over

time was related to cortical NFT ($R^2 = 0.451, p < 0.01$) and amyloid plaque ($R^2 = 0.458, p < 0.01$) burden.

In a group of 20 subjects, including patients with AD, vascular dementia, mixed dementia, and cognitive impairment not meeting operationalized clinical criteria for AD plus healthy controls, Zarow et al. (2005) reported a high correlation of hippocampal volume on MRI with neuronal counts in the CA1 region of the hippocampus ($r = 0.72; p < 0.001$) and with the volume of CA1 ($r = 0.54, p < 0.02$), but not with neuronal number and volume of CA2 (see Figures 19.8 and 19.9). The interval between neuroimaging and death in that study was 2.6 years.

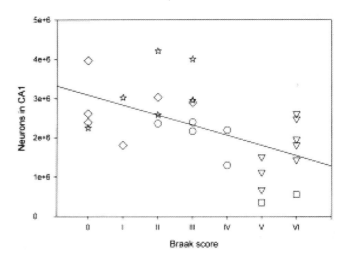

Figure 19–9 Number of neurons in cornu ammonis 1 region of the hippocampus (CA1) versus Braak score. *Stars* indicate healthy control subjects; *circles* indicate cognitively impaired not meeting criteria for Alzheimer's disease (AD); *triangles* indicate AD; *squares* indicate AD with hippocampal sclerosis; and *diamonds* indicate ischemic vascular dementia. Reprinted with permission from (Zarow et al., 2005). Copyright © 2005 John Wiley & Sons, Inc. All right reserved.

A small number of studies have performed postmortem MRIs prior to histology. Bobinski et al. (2000) used this approach in 11 AD patients and four healthy comparison subjects. First they reported a high correlation of MRI-derived and histologically-derived sub-volumes of the hippocampus. Further, they found high correlations of volumes on MRI and neuronal cell counts in the hippocampus ($r = 0.90$, $p < 0.001$) and the hippocampus/subiculum subvolumes ($r = 0.84$, $p < 0.001$).

In a sample of 56 subjects, including demented, cognitively impaired, and nonimpaired individuals, Gosche et al. (2002) reported that postmortem MRI hippocampal volume significantly predicts the presence of the neuropathological criteria of AD ($p < 001$). In nondemented subjects, the hippocampal volume was a better predictor of the presence of the neuropathological criteria of AD than episodic memory. In nondemented subjects, Braak Stage 1 and 2 could be distinguished from Braak Stage 3 and 4 by hippocampal volume on an MRI. In cognitively unimpaired subjects, Braak Stage 2 could even be distinguished from Braak Stage 1.

In a study on white matter lesions in AD, Bronge et al. (2002) correlated white matter hyperintensities on postmortem MRI with a neuropathological count of white matter lesions in six AD cases. They observed a correlation of percentage of white matter lesions between MRI and pathology of $r^2 = 0.71$ ($p < 0.001$), with pathology systematically identifying more lesions than MRI.

Indirect indicators of AD pathology have also been related to MRI measures in AD. Schröder et al. (1997) reported significant correlations of the volumes of the temporal lobes in 17 AD patients with the CSF measures of Aß1-42 ($r = 0.48$) and total Aß4 ($r = 0.046$). Hampel et al. (2005) showed a correlation of hippocampal volume and CSF concentrations of phosphorylated tau protein 231 (pTau231) in 22 patients with mild to moderate AD ($p < 0.001$). Significantly increased concentrations of CSF pTau231 correlated with rate of hippocampal change over time assessed by volumetric MRI (left: $p < 0.001$; right: $p = 0.02$). Antemortem CSF pTau231 correlated in turn with the postmortem assessed mediotemporal and neocortical NFT count in AD patients (Buerger et al., 2006).

In one study, Schonknecht et al. (2003) failed to observe a significant correlation of total CSF tau protein with either whole brain, frontal lobe, temporal lobe, or amygdale-hippocampus measures in 88 AD subjects. However, total tau is considered to be a nonspecific marker of neurodegeneration, while phosphorylated tau is considered specific for for AD.

Finally, recent studies correlated amyloid load measures determined by PET with MRI-based measures of brain structure. Archer et al. (2006) used ^{11}C-PIB-PET to visualize cerebral amyloid deposition, and reported a correlation of whole brain atrophy with ^{11}C-PIB uptake. Small et al. (2006) used FDDNP PET to measure amyloid and NFT in AD patients, subjects with MCI, and controls. The authors reported a correlation of global FDDNP uptake with medial temporal lobe volume ($r = -0.28$; $p = 0.02$), and ventricular size ($r = 0.36$; $p = 0.002$).

To summarize the current state of the literature, there is solid evidence that MRI measures are correlated with the histopathological features of AD. The evidence at present suggests that hippocampal volume on MRI particularly reflects hippocampal NFT load and neuropathological Braak stages. Whole brain measures seem to reflect cortical amyloid and NFT load.

Correlation of Cross-sectional MRI Findings with Clinical Variables in AD

A surrogate marker must be a correlate of a clinically relevant feature of the disease. AD is characterized by progressive cognitive and functional impairment. Thus, atrophy on MRI should correlate with cognitive performance, and functional abilities to serve as a surrogate marker.

A number of studies in AD patients have investigated the association of MRI measures with disease severity. Early studies revealed a significant correlation of overall disease stage and brain structure. Murphy et al. (1993) reported a significant correlation of the Mini-Mental-State Examination (MMSE) with total brain volume in AD patients ($r = 0.53$). Stout et al. (1996) also reported a significant correlation of grey matter volume with dementia severity measures (MMSE: $r = 0.38$; Dementia Rating Scale: $r = 0.34$). In that study, there was also an inverse correlation with white matter volume and dementia severity (MMSE: $r = -0.45$; DRS: $r = -0.41$). Black et al. (2000) found a correlation between corpus callosum volume and the MMSE in AD patients ($r = 0.39$).

In later studies, Teipel et al. (2003) showed that medial temporal lobe measures discriminate between healthy subjects and patients with mild and moderate AD better than corpus callosum measures, which is a marker of cortical neuronal density. In severely demented patients, however, the discriminative power, expressed by receiver-operating curves (ROC), was not different between both measures. This indicates that the neurodegeneration spreads from medial-temporal areas to cortical areas as the disease and the clinical symptoms progress, which is in agreement with neuropathological studies.

In novel study using 3D cortical mapping techniques, Apostolova et al. (2006) reported a correlation between MMSE scores and grey matter volume in the entorhinal and parahippocampal region, the precuneus, the superior parietal lobe, and the subgenual cingulate/orbitofrontal cortex. Significant correlations were also seen in the bilateral temporal, medial frontal, left angular gyrus, and supramagrinal gyrus. In a similar study, Baxter et al. (2006) found a correlation of the MMSE with grey matter volume in the temporal lobes, and additionally with the cognitive subscale of the Alzheimer's Disease Assessment scale (ADAScog) in the frontal region.

In addition to global measures, several studies have correlated individual domains of cognition with MRI measures. The most frequently examined cognitive domain is episodic memory. In an early study in 14 AD patients, Wahlund et al. (1993) found a correlation of CSF space of the basal part of the brain and of the relative volume of the lateral ventricles with episodic memory. Petersen et al. (2000) examined the association of several cognitive tasks with the volume of medial temporal lobe measures in 94 AD patients and 126 control subjects. They reported a prediction of episodic memory performance by hippocampal volume—in particular, in the AD patients. Other studies investigated the role of the amygdala in memory impairment in AD. Mizuno et al. (2000) showed a correlation of the volume of the amygdala with memory performance in 46 AD patients ($r = 0.5$ -0.6). Mori et al. (1997) reported that the volume of the right amygdala predicts visual memory, while the volume of the subiculum predicts verbal memory. Basso et al. (2006) found a correlation of a memory-orientation task with the amygdala volumes ($r = -0.4$, $p = 0.002$), but not with the hippocampal volume in 56 AD patients. Mori et al. (1999) found a particular correlation of the amygdala volume with emotional memory. The association of different MTL volumes with memory performance in AD has been found by several other groups (Deweer et al., 1995; Fama et al., 1997; Kohler et al., 1998; Laasko et al., 1995; Mauri et al., 1998; Pantel et al., 2004 ; Sencakova et al., 2001; van der Flier et al., 2005).

There is evidence for a material-specific difference in correlation of memory performance with either the right or the left hippocampus. Cahn et al. (1998) reported that the right hippocampal volume in AD patients correlates with face memory performance, while the left correlates with verbal memory. Stout et al. (1999) also identified a correlation of MTL structures with memory performance, but additionally observed a correlation of the thalamic volume with memory performance in 27 AD patients. Beyond episodic memory, Sencakova et al. (2001) found a correlation of several other cognitive domains with hippocampal volume.

Whole brain analysis revealed the association of various cognitive domains with different brain regions. Naming difficulties have been related to left lateral temporal cortex and left anterior cingulate gyrus volumes (Grossman et al., 2004). Praxia has been shown to correlate with grey matter volume in the left temporoparietal region (Pantel et al., 2004). Inferior-temporal volume loss has been associated with visual constructive impairment (Boxer et al., 2003). Fama et al. (2000) found a correlation of nonverbal fluency with frontal gray matter. Similarly, Duarte et al. (2006) found a correlation of executive functions with frontal grey matter. Performance in attention tasks have also been related to grey matter volume of the frontal lobe (Fama et al., 1997).

In summary, there is strong evidence for an inverse relationship of total brain volume and the cognitive impairment in AD, reflecting the decline of function with progressive neurodegeneration. With regard to specific cognitive domains, the best evidence is available for the correlation of memory performance with volumes of MTL structures—in particular, the hippocampus and the amygdala. The reported correlation coefficients vary roughly between 0.3 and 0.6. Furthermore, there is evidence for a correlation of frontal lobe volume with measures of executive functions and attention. Several other domains have been investigated in single studies, or in a small number of studies, and require further investigations. Overall, structural MRI measures—in particular, whole brain volume and measures of MTL structures—are associated with clinically characteristic symptoms of the disease, which is one basic requirement for a surrogate marker.

Longitudinal MRI Studies in AD

A surrogate marker, to be applied in clinical trials as an indicator of drug effects on disease progression, should capture longitudinal changes that characterize the disease process. In structural MRI, atrophy is the indicator of the disease process. Below we will review the data on longitudinal progression rates of atrophy in AD.

As in cross-sectional studies, MTL structures and (in particular) the hippocampus have been subject of several longitudinal studies. Jack et al. (1998) reported an annual rate of hippocampal volume reduction in 24 AD patients of 3.98% (SD 1.92), while elderly control subjects ($n = 24$) showed an annual volume reduction of 1.55% (SD 1.38). In the identical sample, the temporal horn showed an annual increase of 14.87% (SD 8.47) in AD patients as compared to 6.15% (SD 7.69) in healthy elderly. The two MRI scans in this study were at least 12 months apart. In a later study, Jack et al. (2000) reported an annual hippocampal volume decline of 3.5% (SD 1.8) in 28 AD. The same group reported an annual atrophy rate of 3.0% (SD 4.5) to 3.6% (SD 3.2) in 64 AD patients,

depending on the speed of decline. In comparison, stable control subjects showed an annual hippocampal atrophy progression of 1.4% (SD 1.2) (Jack et al., 2004). Laasko et al. (2000) followed 27 AD patients over three years and found a 8.3% volume reduction of the hippocampus in this period of time (on average) as compared with 3.0% in eight control subjects. Du et al. (2004) observed a 5.9% (SD 2.4) annual atrophy rate of the hippocampus in 20 AD patients compared with 0.8% (SD 1.7) in 25 healthy elderly. In 19 AD patients, Barnes et al. (2007) reported an annual hippocampal atrophy rate of 3.4% (SD 2.2) with an average scan interval of 567 days (SD 292). In comparison, they found an atrophy rate of 0.1% (SD 0.8) in 11 control patients.

A number of groups have used semiautomatic methods to measure rates of change in hippocampal volume longitudinally. Wang et al. (2003) used a large-deformation, high-dimensional approach and reported an 8.3% (left) and 10.2% (right) volume loss in 18 very mild AD patients in a 2-year follow-up study, while the volume loss in healthy comparison subjects was 4.0% (left) and 5.5% (right) during this period of time. Barnes et al. (2004) used a hippocampal brain boundary shift integral (BBSI) and estimated an annual hippocampal volume reduction of 5.86% (SD 3.69) in 32 AD patients with a wide range of length of interval between MRI examinations. In comparison, they found a 0.2% (SD 1.06) annual rate of volume reduction in 47 comparison subjects. Using an anatomical surface-modeling approach, Thompson et al. (2004) reported annual volume loss rate of 4.9% (SD 1.8) of the left hippocampus and of 8.2% (SD −2.6) of the right hippocampus in AD as opposed to 3.8% (SD 1.6) (left) and 0.2% (SD 1.2) (right) in controls. The large difference between hemispheres might be due to the rather small samples of 12 AD patients and 14 control patients. Mungas et al. (2005) found an annual volume reduction of the hippocampus of 2.8% (SD 5.3) in 11 patients with dementia using a commercial semiautomatic software.

Overall, there is a consistent picture of several independent studies either using manual tracing of the hippocampus or different semiautomatic approaches of an increased rate of hippocampal atrophy in AD. While healthy elderly subjects show a rate of 0%–1% in annual volume loss, the reduction of hippocampal volume in AD patients is around 3%–6%.

Some groups measured the annual volume reduction of other MTL structures. The volume reduction in the entorhinal cortex has been found to progress earlier and at a slightly higher annual rate than the hippocampus in AD patients (Cardenas et al., 2003; Du et al., 2004; Ezekiel et al., 2004; Jack et al., 2004). Due to the complex and individually varying anatomy around the sulcus collateralis, however, volumetric measures of the entorhinal cortex are less stringently and reliably accessible than standardized hippocampal measures. Other groups have measured the temporal horn, showing rapid volume increases of up to 18% in AD patients per year and up to 4.7% in control patients (Thompson et al., 2004). The annual atrophy rates in AD patients depend on the disease stage. As Rusinek et al. (2004) have shown, the atrophy of MTL structures progresses faster at more advanced disease stages.

Other individual brain regions have also been examined longitudinally. Barnes et al. (2007) reported annual rates of atrophy in the cingulate gyrus of 5.9% (SD 3.5) in 19 AD patients, as compared with 0.3% (SD 1.2) in healthy comparison subjects. Several studies measured the rate of atrophy of the entire brain. Using the BBSI, Fox et al. (1996) reported an annual volume loss of 12.3 ml (range 5.8–23.6) in 11 AD patients as compared with 0.3 ml (range −1.2–1.7) in 11 age-matched control patients. In 20 AD patients, Fox et al. (2001) found an annual whole brain atrophy rate of 2.2%

(range 0.82–4.19), while 20 healthy subjects showed a rate of 0.24% (range −0.35–0.64). Very similar annual rates of volume loss have been reported in several studies (Chan et al., 2001; Fox et al., 2000; Mungas et al., 2005; O'Brien et al., 2001; Schott et al., 2005). Others reported slightly lower annual atrophy rates of around 1% in AD patients and below 0.5% in healthy comparison subjects (Fotenos et al., 2005; Whitewell et al., 2007).

A specific measure of brain tissue loss is the increase of ventricular volume. Ezekiel et al. (2004) reported an annual increase of ventricular size of 10.97% (SD 4.74) in 20 AD patients as compared with 3.34% (SD 3.77) in 22 control patients. Roughly similar results were found by Schott et al. (2005). Jack et al. (2004) reported a smaller rate of ventricular size increases. They found a rate of 4.3% (SD 3.3) in 32 slow-progressing AD patients, and of 6.4% (SD 3.7) in 33 fast-progressing AD patients compared with 1.7% (SD 0.9) in healthy subjects.

An indirect measure of cortical neuronal density is the size of the corpus callosum. Teipel et al. (2002) followed 21 AD patients over a mean of 17 months, and a group of 10 comparison subjects over 24.1 months. The authors observed annual rates of atrophy of total corpus callosum, splenium, and rostrum in AD patients of −7.7%, −12.1%, and −7.3%, respectively, and in controls of −0.9%, −1.5%, and 0.6%.

Overall, there is solid data that whole brain volume decreases with an annual rate of between 1% and 2.5% in AD and below 1% in healthy aging. In parallel to hippocampal measures, however, there is an association of an annual rate of whole brain volume reduction with disease stage. Chan et al. (2003) followed 12 AD patients from the presymptomatic to moderately severe stage. In the mild dementia stage, they observed an annual whole brain volume loss of 2.8% (95%CI: 2.32–3.29), which was accelerated by 0.32% (95%CI: 0.15–0.50) each year. Also, the ApoE-genotype influenced the rate of atrophy. Wahlund et al. (1999) reported greater rates of atrophy in ApoE4-positive AD patients than in ApoE4-negative.

Sample Size Estimation for Clinical Trials Based on Longitudinal Studies

Based on longitudinal data, several authors have provided sample size estimates for the detection of reduction rates of atrophy in clinical trials. Fox et al. (2000) estimated a sample size of 207 mild-to-moderate AD patients per arm in a 1-year treatment trial (10% drop-out per arm) to detect a 20% reduction of rate of atrophy with a power of 90% ($p < 0.05$ two-sided). Schott et al. (2005) used the BBSI method to measure ventricular and whole brain change longitudinally. The estimated group size of 165 subjects per arm for ventricular measures, and of 410 subjects per arm for whole brain measures was sufficient to detect a 20% reduction of rate of atrophy with 90% power ($p < 0.05$ two-sided) in a six-month trial. In a one-year trial, they reported the need for 141 subjects for ventricular measures and 154 for whole brain measures. Ezekiel et al. (2004) reported the following numbers needed per arm to detect a reduction of 20% rate of decline in a one-year trial with 90% power ($p > 0.05$, two-sided): ventricular BBSI – 99; cortical BBSI – 256; total BBSI – 204; entorhinal volume (manually traced) – 109; hippocampus (manually traced) – 88. Du et al. (2004) reported an estimated number of 110 patients per arm for manually traced entorhinal cortex, and of 90 for manually traced hippocampus to detect a 20% rate of reduction of atrophy again with 90% power ($p > 0.05$, two-sided). Overall, the magnitude of annual atrophy rates of the hippocampus, the entorhinal cortex, and whole brain measures (including ventricular size) in AD is large enough to

detect the effects of drugs, which slow atrophy with feasible sample sizes.

Correlation of Longitudinal MRI Findings with Clinical Variables in AD

As reported above, MRI can reliably detect the progression of brain atrophy in AD. To serve as a surrogate marker, however, this progressive atrophy has to correlate with clinically meaningful changes on the symptomatic level. In this section, we will review the data on the correlation of atrophy progression with changes in clinical variables.

Fox et al. (1999) used the BSI in 29 AD patients who were followed between six months and five years. The change in whole brain volume correlated highly with changes in the MMSE ($r = 0.80$, $p < 0.001$). Du et al. (2004) measured the hippocampus semiautomatically, and the entorhinal cortex manually in 20 AD patients. The subjects underwent MRI and neuropsychological testing on an average of 1.9 years apart. They found a correlation of change in a verbal delayed recall score with rates of entorhinal atrophy progression ($r = -0.51$, $p < 0.05$). The hippocampal atrophy rate was not correlated with change in delayed recall. When the sample was restricted to mildly impaired cases only ($n = 11$, mean MMSE: 24.6), there was a significant correlation of the entorhinal cortex atrophy rate ($r = -0.61$, $p < 0.05$) and the hippocampus ($r = -0.59$, $p < 0.05$), with change in delayed recall. Change of the MMSE, however, did not correlate with any anatomical rate of change.

Jack et al. (2004) reported a study of 64 AD patients with a clinical and an MRI follow-up of one to five years. They reported a significant correlation between the rate of change of the hippocampus ($r = 0.35$), the entorhinal cortex ($r = 0.46$), the whole brain ($r = 0.47$), and the ventricles ($r = -0.38$), with change in the MMSE. The change in the Dementia Rating Scale (DRS), the Clinical Dementia Rating (CDR) scale, and the composite score sum of boxes was only correlated significantly with the rate of whole brain volume loss ($r = 0.47$; $r = -0.45$) and ventricular size increase ($r = -0.39$; $r = 0.40$).

Teipel et al. (2002) found a correlation of atrophy rates of the corpus callosum subfield C5 as a measure of cortical neuronal density with the change in the MMSE ($r = 0.52$, $p < 0.02$) in a group of 21 AD patients covering all disease stages with an mean examination interval of 17 months (SD 8.5). In a group of 11 patients with dementia, Mungas et al. (2005) showed that memory and executive functions expressed by composite scores are associated with change in hippocampal volume, while total grey matter change is only associated with change in executive function.

In summary, there are a limited number of studies that address the association of volumetric change and change in clinical variables, like global or specific measures of cognition. These studies show that progressive clinical decline is paralleled by progressive volume loss. The correlations, however, rarely exceed $r = 0.6$. In addition to the studies reported in this section, structural MRI has been applied in clinical trails in AD. These will be outlined in the next section.

MRI in Clinical AD Trials

Structural MRI has been used to predict treatment response and to monitor effects of treatment in clinical trails in AD. First, we will review studies that used MRI markers as predictors of treatment response.

MRI as a Treatment Outcome Predictor

Csernansky et al. (2005) reported a correlation of ADAScog changes after 24 to 96 weeks of Donepezil treatment with baseline left ($r = -0.34$, $p = 0.04$) and right ($r = -0.38$, $p = 0.02$) hippocampal volumes in 37 AD patients. The finding could not be replicated by Visser et al. (2005) in 121 mild-to-moderate AD patients in a 26-week Rivastigmine trial. The authors did not find an association between treatment response and medial temporal lobe volume, nor with ApoE status. Hanyu et al. (2007) described a correlation between the thickness of the substantia innominata, which contains the nucleus basalis of Meynert as the origin of cholinergic projection to the brain, and the clinical response after 12 weeks of Donepezil treatment in 103 AD patients ($r = -0.43$, $p < 0.001$).

MRI as a Marker for Drug Effects of Brain Structure

Due to the solid evidence that MRI depicts progressive atrophy in AD, it has been integrated into some clinical drug trials to assess to effect of the drug on disease progression.

Krishnan et al. (2003) reported data from a 24-week single-center Donepezil trial in 67 patients (51 completers) with mild-to-moderate AD. They found significantly less progression of hippocampal atrophy in the Donepezil group compared with the placebo group, suggesting an effect of Donepezil on the disease itself as opposed to pure symptomatic improvement. In the placebo group, however, there was an 8.2% volume decrease in 24 weeks, which substantially exceeds the annual volume loss of roughly 2%–5% known from other AD studies. The 24-week decrease in the placebo group was 0.4%. A second independent prospective cohort study in 54 AD patients treated with Donepezil, in comparison with a historical, never-treated control group of 93 subjects, however, replicated this finding. The authors found an annual rate of atrophy in the Donepezil group of 3.82% (SD 2.84) and of 5.04% (SD 2.54) in the never-treated group, which was significantly different (Hashimoto et al., 2005). Thus, structural MRI provides evidence for a yet unexpected potential disease-modifying effect of Donepezil, which warrants further support from clinical trails.

Multicenter MRI

Due to the sample size requirements, and in order to prevent center effects, large multicenter trials are the standard for clinical AD trials. The reliability of multicenter MRI has recently been demonstrated. Ewers et al. (2006) reported a coefficient variance of 3.55% for hippocampal volume, of 5.02% for grey matter, of 4.87% for white matter, and of 4.66% for CSF in a single subject study over 11 sites. Similar reliability and validation trials are currently being conducted in the large-scale ADNI trials in the United States, Europe, Australia, and Japan.

In the context of MRI in multicenter clinical trials in AD, a very important publication originates from the milameline trial, in which the drug (milameline) did not show any treatment effect (Jack et al., 2003). The particular wealth of the imaging data of this study is related to the fact that these longitudinal data were obtained under clinical trial conditions regarding patients' inclusion criteria, neuropsychological outcomes, and multicenter design. 362 patients with mild to moderate AD were included in the MRI part of the study. Of these, 192 received the follow-up MRI investigation. One hundred and eighty-eight received the drug and 174 received placebos. The duration of the study was 52 weeks. Thirty-eight sites participated in the MRI part of the study. The overall annual volume reduction of the hippocampus in this study was 4.9% (range −15.2–0). The overall increase in temporal volume was 16.1% (range −13.1–53.5). There was no difference between the treated and the placebo group. The correlations between change in hippocampal volume and change in the ADAScog, MMSE, and GDS were not significant. However, the annual change of the temporal horn volume correlated significantly with the change in the ADAScog ($r = 0.27$, $p < 0.001$), the MMSE ($r = -0.34$, $p < 0.001$), and the GDS ($r = 0.16$, $p = 0.039$). Importantly, the volume of the hippocampus decreased in 99% of all cases, whereas the ADAScog increased only in 60.4%, and the MMSE decreased only in 66.2% of the cases. This suggests that volumetric measures are much more sensitive for the detection of disease progression in comparison with neuropsychological parameters. Based on these data, Jack et al. (2003) performed a sample size calculation for a reduction of rate of progression of 50%. They estimated a required number of subjects for a one-year trial (90% power, one-sided, t-test, $p < 0.05$) of 241 patients per arm for the MMSE, 320 patients per arm for the ADAScog, 21 patients per arm for the hippocampal volume, and 54 patients per arm for temporal horn volumes. This suggests drastically smaller sample sizes for clinical trials, if slowing of the progression of atrophy was the primary outcome. Also, this study clearly demonstrated the feasibility of multicenter MRI in clinical AD trial with an estimated variance attributable to the multicenter effects of 4.71%.

The first published multicenter MRI study of a clinical AD trial with a drug that directly aimed at disease modification presented data from the Aß active immunization trial (AN1792) Fox et al. (2005). In that study, 372 patients were enrolled, of which 288 had structural MRI scans at baseline and follow-up (mean interval: 10.9 months). The data were obtained at 17 sites. Of 231 patients with active treatment, 45 were antibody responders. These were compared with 57 patients receiving placebos. Surprisingly, antibody responders showed a significantly greater rate of whole brain atrophy (3.12%, SD 1.98) than the placebo patients (2.04%, SD 1.74) ($p = 0.007$). Also, the rate of ventricular enlargement was greater in the antibody responder group (1.10%, SD 0.75) than in the placebo group (0.48%, SD 0.40). The difference in rate of atrophy of the hippocampus was not significant. The memory composite score designed by the study group showed less decline in antibody responders than in the placebo group ($p = 0.008$). At present, there is no sufficient explanation for the increased atrophy rate paralleled by stabilization of cognitive decline in the antibody responder group. This study highlights that volumetric measures most likely reflect more than just neuronal density, and that interventions that interact with the neuropathology of the disease might accelerate shrinkage on MRI without clinical decline.

Discussion of MRI as a Candidate for a Surrogate Marker in AD

Structural MRI is the most extensively studied biomarker in AD. To be accepted as a surrogate endpoint, MRI should be related to the pathophysiological process of AD, should respond to treatment, and should predict clinical outcome.

It has been shown that MRI measures correlate with AD pathology. The progression of disease can be monitored by progression of brain atrophy. The correlation of atrophy progression with clinical progression, however, is only modest. Therefore, structural MRI might not be considered a fully sufficient surrogate marker to predict clinical outcome in 6- to 12-month clinical trials.

The progressive brain atrophy, however, is a very reliable and stable phenomenon. In contrast, cognitive and functional measures show variability in the course of the disease. This variability is related to fluctuations in cognitive functioning, different levels of cognitive reserve capacity, effects on cognition by other factors (e.g., medication, comorbidity), rater dependency of the instruments, variation of the sensitivity of cognitive tests at different disease stages, and others. Therefore, the variability in clinical measures may particularly account for the only modest association of brain volume changes and changes in cognition and functioning. In this case, brain volume changes would reflect the pathological process more directly than clinical measures. This is supported by the observation that merely all AD patients show progressive atrophy over 12 months, while only two thirds show cognitive decline (Jack et al., 2003). Therefore, the central question regarding MRI as a surrogate marker for AD treatment is the long-term prediction of clinical outcome beyond the course of standard clinical trials by rates of brain atrophy. It has been shown that greater atrophy rates are associated with faster cognitive decline (Jack et al., 2004). However, it is still unclear whether atrophy rates predict the long-term cognitive decline in AD. If so, the second question would ask whether or not drug-induced effects on the rate of atrophy predict drug-induced effects on cognitive decline. This intuitive assumption has recently been challenged by the AN1792 trial. However, if both questions could be answered positively, structural MRI could serve as a true surrogate marker in AD, since the effects of atrophy rate would then predict a clinically meaningful outcome. It would further serve the purposes of a surrogate marker to increase reliability compared with clinical measures to facilitate the shortening of clinical trials and reduce sample sizes.

Acknowledgement

Figures are derived from the paper (with kind permission from Springer Science and Business Media): Stefan J. Teipel, Thomas Meindl, Lea Grinberg, Helmut Heinsen and Harald Hampel. Novel MRI techniques in the assessment of dementia. European Journal of Nuclear Medicine and Molecular Imaging, 2008 Jan 17; [Epub ahead of print].

References

Apostolova, L. G., Lu, P. H., Rogers, S., Dutton, R. A., Hayashi KM, Toga AW et al. (2006). 3D mapping of mini-mental state examination performance in clinical and preclinical Alzheimer disease. *Alzheimer Disease and Associated Disorders*, 20: 224–231.

Archer, H. A., Edison, P., Brooks, D. J., Barnes, J., Frost, C., Yeatman, T. et al. (2006). Amyloid load and cerebral atrophy in Alzheimer's disease: An 11C-PIB positron emission tomography study. *Annals of Neurology*, 60: 145–147.

Barnes, J., Godbolt, A. K., Frost, C., Boyes, R. G., Jones, B. F., Scahill, R. I. et al. (2007). Atrophy rates of the cingulate gyrus and hippocampus in AD and FTLD. *Neurobiology of Aging*, 28: 20–8.

Barnes, J., Scahill, R. I., Boyes, R. G., Frost, C., Lewis, E. B., Rossor, C. L. et al. (2004). Differentiating AD from aging using semiautomated measurement of hippocampal atrophy rates. *Neuroimage*, 23: 574–581.

Basso, M., Yang, J., Warren, L., MacAvoy, M. G., Varma, P., Bronen, R. A. et al. (2006). Volumetry of amygdala and hippocampus and memory performance in Alzheimer's disease. *Psychiatry Research*, 146: 251–261.

Baxter, L. C., Sparks, D. L., Johnson, S. C., Lenoski, B., Lopez, J. E., Connor, D. J. et al. (2006). Relationship of cognitive measures and gray and white matter in Alzheimer's disease. *Journal of Alzheimer's Disease*, 9: 253–260.

Black, S. E., Moffat, S. D., Yu, D. C., Parker, J., Stanchev, P., and Bronskill, M. (2000). Callosal atrophy correlates with temporal lobe volume and mental status in Alzheimer's disease. *The Canadian Journal of Neurological Sciences*, 27: 204–209.

Bobinski, M., de Leon, M. J., Wegiel, J., Desanti, S., Convit, A., Saint Louis, L. A. et al. (2000). The histological validation of post mortem magnetic resonance imaging-determined hippocampal volume in Alzheimer's disease. *Neuroscience*, 95: 721–725.

Boxer, A. L., Kramer, J. H., Du, A. T., Schuff, N., Weiner, M. W., Miller, B. L. et al. (2003). Focal right inferotemporal atrophy in AD with disproportionate visual constructive impairment. *Neurology*, 61(11): 1485–1491.

Braak, H. and Braak, E. (1991). Neuropathological stageing of Alzheimer-related changes. *Acta Neuropathologica (Berlin)*, 82: 239–259.

Broich, K. (2007). Outcome measures in clinical trials on medicinal products for the treatment of dementia: A European regulatory perspective. *International Psychogeriatrics*, 19: 509–524.

Bronge, L., Bogdanovic, N., and Wahlund, L. O. (2002). Postmortem MRI and histopathology of white matter changes in Alzheimer brains. A quantitative, comparative study. *Dementia and Geriatric Cognitive Disorders*, 13: 205–212.

Buerger, K., Ewers. M., Pirttila. T., Zinkowski. R., Alafuzoff. I., Teipel. S. J. et al. (2006). CSF phosphorylated tau protein correlates with neocortical neurofibrillary pathology in Alzheimer's disease. *Brain*, 129: 30353041.

Busatto, G. F., Garrido, G. E., Almeida, O. P., Castro, C. C., Camargo, C. H., Cid, C. G. et al. (2003). A voxel-based morphometry study of temporal lobe gray matter reductions in Alzheimer's disease. *Neurobiology of Aging*, 24: 221–231.

Cahn, D. A., Sullivan, E. V., Shear, P. K., Marsh, L., Fama, R., Lim, K. O. et al. (1998). Structural MRI correlates of recognition memory in Alzheimer's disease. *Journal of the International Neuropsychological Society*, 4: 106–114.

Callen, D. J., Black, S. E., Gao, F., Caldwell, C. B., and Szalai, J. P. (2001). Beyond the hippocampus: MRI volumetry confirms widespread limbic atrophy in AD. *Neurology*, 57: 1669–1674.

Cardenas, V. A., Du, A. T., Hardin, D., Ezekiel, F., Weber, P., Jagust, W. J. et al. (2003). Comparison of methods for measuring longitudinal brain change in cognitive impairment and dementia. *Neurobiology of Aging*, 24: 537–544.

Chaim, T. M., Duran, F. L., Uchida, R. R., Perico, C. A., de Castro, C. C., and Busatto, G. F. (2007). Volumetric reduction of the corpus callosum in Alzheimer's disease in vivo as assessed with voxel-based morphometry. *Psychiatry Research*, 154: 59–68.

Chan, D., Fox, N. C., Jenkins, R., Scahill, R. I., Crum, W. R., Rossor, M. N. (2001). Rates of global and regional cerebral atrophy in AD and frontotemporal dementia. *Neurology*, 57(10): 1756–1763.

Chan, D., Janssen, J.C., Whitwell, J. L., Watt, H. C., Jenkins, R., Frost, C. et al. (2003). Change in rates of cerebral atrophy over time in early-onset Alzheimer's disease: longitudinal MRI study. *Lancet*, 362: 1121–1122.

Chen, K., Reiman, E. M., Alexander, G. E., Bandy, D., Renaut, R., Crum, W. R. et al. (2004). An automated algorithm for the computation of brain volume change from sequential MRIs using an iterative principal component analysis and its evaluation for the assessment of whole-brain atrophy rates in patients with probable Alzheimer's disease. *Neuroimage*, 22: 134–143.

Copenhaver, B. R., Rabin, L. A., Saykin, A. J., Roth, R. M., Wishart, H. A., Flashman, L. A. et al. (2006). The fornix and mammillary bodies in older adults with Alzheimer's disease, mild cognitive impairment, and cognitive complaints: a volumetric MRI study. *Psychiatry Research*, 147: 93–103.

Corder, E. H., Woodbury, M. A., Volkmann, I., Madsen, D. K., Bogdanovic, N., Winblad, B. (2000). Density profiles of Alzheimer disease regional brain pathology for the huddinge brain bank: pattern recognition emulates and expands upon Braak staging. *Exp Gerontol*, 35(6–7): 851–64. Review.

Csernansky, J. G., Hamstra, J., Wang, L., McKeel, D., Price, J. L., Gado, M. et al. (2004). Correlations between antemortem hippocampal volume and postmortem neuropathology in AD subjects. *Alzheimer Disease and Associated Disorders*, 18: 190–195.

Csernansky, J. G., Wang, L., Miller, J. P., Galvin, J. E., and Morris, J. C. (2005). Neuroanatomical predictors of response to donepezil therapy in patients with dementia. *Archives of Neurology*, 62: 1718–1722.

Davis, P. C., Gearing, M., Gray, L., Mirra, S. S., Morris, J. C., Edland, S.D. et al. (1995). The CERAD experience, Part VIII: Neuroimaging-neuropathology correlates of temporal lobe changes in Alzheimer's disease. *Neurology*, 45: 178–179.

Delacourte, A., David, J. P., Sergeant, N., Buee, L., Wattez, A., Vermersch, P. et al. (1999). The biochemical pathway of neurofibrillary degeneration in aging and Alzheimer's disease. *Neurology*, 52: 1158–1165.

Deweer, B., Lehericy, S., Pillon, B., Baulac, M., Chiras, J., Marsault, C. et al. (1995). Memory disorders in probable Alzheimer's disease: The role of hippocampal atrophy as shown with MRI. *Journal of Neurology, Neurosurgery, and Psychiatry*, 58: 590–597.

Du, A. T., Schuff, N., Kramer, J. H., Ganzer, S., Zhu, X. P., Jagust, W. J. et al. (2004). Higher atrophy rate of entorhinal cortex than hippocampus in AD. *Neurology*, 62: 422–427.

Duarte, A., Hayasaka, S., Du, A., Schuff, N., Jahng, G. H., Kramer, J. et al. (2006). Volumetric correlates of memory and executive function in normal elderly, mild cognitive impairment and Alzheimer's disease. *Neuroscience Letters*, 406: 60–65.

Ewers, M., Teipel, S. J., Dietrich, O., Schonberg, S. O., Jessen, F., and Heun, R. (2006). Multicenter assessment of reliability of cranial MRI. *Neurobiology of Aging*, 27: 1051–1059.

Ezekiel, F., Chao, L., Kornak, J., Du, A. T., Cardenas, V., Truran, D. et al. (2004). Comparisons between global and focal brain atrophy rates in normal aging and Alzheimer disease: Boundary Shift Integral versus tracing of the entorhinal cortex and hippocampus. *Alzheimer Disease and Associated Disorders*, 18: 196–201.

Fama, R., Sullivan, E. V., Shear, P. K., Cahn-Weiner, D. A., Marsh, L., Lim, K. O. et al. (2000). Structural brain correlates of verbal and nonverbal fluency measures in Alzheimer's disease. *Neuropsychology*, 14: 29–40.

Fama, R., Sullivan, E. V., Shear, P. K., Marsh, L., Yesavage, J. A., Tinklenberg, J. R. et al. (1997). Selective cortical and hippocampal volume correlates of Mattis Dementia Rating Scale in Alzheimer disease. *Archives of Neurology*, 54: 719–728.

Fleming, T. R. and DeMets, D. L. (1996). Surrogate end points in clinical trials: are we being misled? *Annals of Internal Medicine*, 125: 605–613.

Fotenos, A. F., Snyder, A. Z., Girton, L. E., Morris, J. C., and Buckner, R. L. (2005). Normative estimates of cross-sectional and longitudinal brain volume decline in aging and AD. *Neurology*, 64: 1032–1039.

Fox, N. C., Black, R. S., Gilman, S., Rossor, M. N., Griffith, S. G., Jenkins, L. et al. (2005). AN1792(QS-21)-201 Study. Effects of Abeta immunization (AN1792) on MRI measures of cerebral volume in Alzheimer disease. *Neurology*, 64: 1563–1572.

Fox, N. C., Cousens, S., Scahill, R., Harvey, R. J., Rossor, M. N. (2000). Using serial registered brain magnetic resonance imaging to measure disease progression in Alzheimer disease: power calculations and estimates of sample size to detect treatment effects. *Archives of Neurology*, 57: 339–344.

Fox, N. C., Crum, W. R., Scahill, R. I., Stevens, J. M., Janssen, J. C., and Rossor, M. N. (2001). Imaging of onset and progression of Alzheimer's disease with voxel-compression mapping of serial magnetic resonance images. *Lancet*, 358: 201–205.

Fox, N. C., Freeborough, P. A., and Rossor, M. N. (1996). Visualisation and quantification of rates of atrophy in Alzheimer's disease. *Lancet*, 348: 94–97.

Fox, N. C., Scahill, R. I., Crum, W. R., and Rossor, M. N. (1999). Correlation between rates of brain atrophy and cognitive decline in AD. *Neurology*, 52: 1687–1689.

Frisoni, G. B., Sabattoli, F., Lee, A. D., Dutton, R. A., Toga, A.W., and Thompson, P. M. (2006). In vivo neuropathology of the hippocampal formation in AD: A radial mapping MR-based study. *Neuroimage*, 32: 104–110.

Gosche, K. M., Mortimer, J. A., Smith, C. D., Markesbery, W. R., and Snowdon, D. A. (2002). Hippocampal volume as an index of Alzheimer neuropathology: Findings from the Nun Study. *Neurology*, 58: 1476–1482.

Grossman, M., McMillan, C., Moore, P., Ding, L., Glosser, G., Work, M. et al. (2004). What's in a name: voxel-based morphometric analyses of MRI and naming difficulty in Alzheimer's disease, frontotemporal dementia and corticobasal degeneration. *Brain*, 127: 628–649.

Hampel, H., Burger, K., Pruessner, J. C., Zinkowski, R., DeBernardis, J., Kerkman, D. et al. (2005). Correlation of cerebrospinal fluid levels of tau protein phosphorylated at threonine 231 with rates of hippocampal atrophy in Alzheimer disease. *Archives of Neurology*, 62: 770–773.

Hampel, H., Teipel, S. J., Alexander, G. E., Horwitz, B., Teichberg, D., Schapiro, M. B. et al. (1998). Corpus callosum atrophy is a possible indicator of region- and cell type-specific neuronal degeneration in Alzheimer disease: A magnetic resonance imaging analysis. *Archives of Neurology*, 55: 193–198.

Hampel, H., Teipel, S. J., Bayer, W., Alexander, G. E., Schwarz, R., Schapiro, M. B. et al. (2002). Age transformation of combined hippocampus and amygdala volume improves diagnostic accuracy in Alzheimer's disease. *Journal of the Neurological Sciences*, 194: 15–19.

Hanyu, H., Shimizu, S., Tanaka, Y., Hirao, K., Iwamoto, T., and Abe, K. (2007). MR features of the substantia innominata and therapeutic implications in dementias. *Neurobiology of Aging*, 28: 548–554.

Hanyu, H., Tanaka, Y., Shimizu, S., Sakurai, H., Iwamoto, T., and Abe, K. (2005). Differences in MR features of the substantia innominata between dementia with Lewy bodies and Alzheimer's disease. *Journal of Neurology*, 252: 482–484.

Hashimoto, M., Kazui, H., Matsumoto, K., Nakano, Y., Yasuda, M., and Mori, E. (2005). Does donepezil treatment slow the progression of hippocampal atrophy in patients with Alzheimer's disease? *The American Journal of Psychiatry*, 162: 676–682.

Hirata, Y., Matsuda, H., Nemoto, K., Ohnishi, T., Hirao, K., Yamashita, F. et al. (2005). Voxel-based morphometry to discriminate early Alzheimer's disease from controls. *Neuroscience Letters*, 382: 269–274.

Jack, C. R., Jr., Dickson, D. W., Parisi, J. E., Xu, Y. C., Cha, R. H., O'Brien, P. C. et al. (2002). Antemortem MRI findings correlate with hippocampal neuropathology in typical aging and dementia. *Neurology*, 58: 750–757.

Jack, C. R. Jr., Petersen, R. C., Xu, Y., O'Brien, P. C., Smith, G. E., Ivnik, R. J. et al. (2000). Rates of hippocampal atrophy correlate with change in clinical status in aging and AD. *Neurology*, 55: 484–489.

Jack, C. R. Jr., Petersen, R. C., Xu, Y., O'Brien, P. C., Smith, G. E., Ivnik, R. J. et al. (1998). Rate of medial temporal lobe atrophy in typical aging and Alzheimer's disease. *Neurology*, 51: 993–999.

Jack, C. R. Jr., Petersen, R. C., Xu, Y. C., Waring, S. C., O'Brien, P. C., Tangalos, E. G. et al. (1997). Medial temporal atrophy on MRI in normal aging and very mild Alzheimer's disease. *Neurology*, 49: 786–794.

Jack, C. R. Jr., Shiung, M. M., Gunter, J. L., O'Brien, P. C., Weigand, S. D., Knopman, D. S. et al. (2004). Comparison of different MRI brain atrophy rate measures with clinical disease progression in AD. *Neurology*, 62: 591–600.

Jack, C. R. Jr., Slomkowski, M., Gracon, S., Hoover, T. M., Felmlee, J. P., Stewart, K. et al. (2003). MRI as a biomarker of disease progression in a therapeutic trial of milameline for AD. *Neurology*, 60: 253–260.

Jagust, W. J., Zheng, L., Harvey, D. J., Mack, W. J., Vinters, H. V., Weiner, M. W. et al. (2008). Neuropathological basis of magnetic resonance images in aging and dementia. *Annals of Neurology*, 63(1): 72–80.

Jones, B. F., Barnes, J., Uylings, H. B., Fox, N. C., Frost, C., Witter, M. P. et al. (2006). Differential regional atrophy of the cingulate gyrus in Alzheimer disease: a volumetric MRI study. *Cerebral Cortex*, 16: 1701–1708.

Karas, G. B., Burton, E. J., Rombouts, S. A., van Schijndel, R. A., O'Brien, J. T., Scheltens, P. et al. (2003). A comprehensive study of gray matter loss in patients with Alzheimer's disease using optimized voxel-based morphometry. *Neuroimage*, 18: 895–907.

Kesslak, J. P., Nalcioglu, O., and Cotman, C. W. (1991). Quantification of magnetic resonance scans for hippocampal and parahippocampal atrophy in Alzheimer's disease. *Neurology*, 41: 51–54.

Kohler, S., Black, S. E., Sinden, M., Szekely, C., Kidron, D., Parker, J. L. et al. (1998). Memory impairments associated with hippocampal versus parahippocampal-gyrus atrophy: An MR volumetry study in Alzheimer's disease. *Neuropsychologia*, 36: 901–914.

Krishnan, K. R., Charles, H. C., Doraiswamy, P. M., Mintzer, J., Weisler, R., Yu, X. et al. (2003). Randomized, placebo-controlled trial of the effects of donepezil on neuronal markers and hippocampal volumes in Alzheimer's disease. *The American Journal of Psychiatry*, 160: 2003–2011.

Laakso, M. P., Lehtovirta, M., Partanen, K., Riekkinen, P. J., and Soininen, H. (2000). Hippocampus in Alzheimer's disease: A 3-year follow-up MRI study. *Biological Psychiatry*, 47: 557–561.

Laakso, M. P., Soininen, H., Partanen, K., Helkala, E. L., Hartikainen, P., Vainio, P. et al. (1995). Volumes of hippocampus, amygdala and frontal lobes in the MRI-based diagnosis of early Alzheimer's disease: Correlation with memory functions. *Journal of Neural Transmission. Parkinson's Disease and Dementia Section*, 9: 73–86.

Laakso, M. P., Soininen, H., Partanen, K., Lehtovirta, M., Hallikainen, M., Hanninen, T. et al. (1998). MRI of the hippocampus in Alzheimer's disease: sensitivity, specificity, and analysis of the incorrectly classified subjects. *Neurobiology of Aging*, 19: 23–31.

Lao, Z., Shen, D., Xue, Z., Karacali, B., Resnick, S. M., and Davatzikos, C. (2004). Morphological classification of brains via high-dimensional shape transformations and machine learning methods. *Neuroimage*, 21: 46–57.

Mauri, M., Sibilla, L., Bono, G., Carlesimo, G. A., Sinforiani, E., and Martelli, A. (1998). The role of morpho-volumetric and memory correlations in the diagnosis of early Alzheimer dementia. *Journal of Neurology*, 245: 525–530.

McKeown, M. J., Makeig, S., Brown, G. G., Jung, T. P., Kindermann, S. S., Bell, A. J. et al. (1998). Analysis of fMRI data by blind separation into independent spatial components. *Human Brain Mapping*, 6: 160–188.

Miller, M. I., Hosakere, M., Barker, A. R., Priebe, C. E., Lee, N., Ratnanather, J. T. et al. (2003). Labeled cortical mantle distance maps of the cingulate quantify differences between dementia of the Alzheimer type and healthy aging. *Proceedings of the National Academy of Sciences of the USA*, 100: 15172–15177.

Mizuno, K., Wakai, M., Takeda, A., and Sobue, G. (2000). Medial temporal atrophy and memory impairment in early stage of Alzheimer's disease: An MRI volumetric and memory assessment study. *Journal of the Neurological Sciences*, 173: 18–24.

Mori, E., Ikeda, M., Hirono, N., Kitagaki, H., Imamura, T., and Shimomura, T. (1999). Amygdalar volume and emotional memory in Alzheimer's disease. *The American Journal of Psychiatry*, 156: 216–222.

Mori, E., Yoneda, Y., Yamashita, H., Hirono, N., Ikeda, M., Yamadori, A. (1997). Medial temporal structures relate to memory impairment in Alzheimer's disease: An MRI volumetric study. *Journal of Neurology, Neurosurgery, and Psychiatry*, 63: 214–221.

Mueller, S. G., Stables, L., Du, A. T., Schuff, N., Truran, D., Cashdollar, N. et al. (2007). Measurement of hippocampal subfields and age-related changes with high resolution MRI at 4T. *Neurobiology of Aging*, 28: 719–726.

Mungas, D., Harvey, D., Reed, B. R., Jagust, W. J., DeCarli, C., Beckett, L. et al. (2005). Longitudinal volumetric MRI change and rate of cognitive decline. *Neurology*, 65: 565–571.

Murphy, D. G., DeCarli, C. D., Daly, E., Gillette, J. A., McIntosh, A. R., Haxby, J. V. et al. (1993). Volumetric magnetic resonance imaging in men with dementia of the Alzheimer type: Correlations with disease severity. *Biological Psychiatry*, 34: 612–621.

O'Brien, J. T., Paling, S., Barber, R., Williams, E. D., Ballard, C., McKeith, I. G. et al. (2001). Progressive brain atrophy on serial MRI in dementia with Lewy bodies, AD, and vascular dementia. *Neurology*, 56: 1386–1388.

Pantel, J., Schönknecht, P., Essig, M., Schröder, J. (2004). Distribution of cerebral atrophy assessed by magnetic resonance imaging reflects patterns of neuropsychological deficits in Alzheimer's dementia. *Neurosci Lett.*, 361(1–3): 17–20. PubMed PMID: 15135882.

Pennanen, C., Kivipelto, M., Tuomainen, S., Hartikainen, P., Hanninen, T., Laakso, M. P. et al. (2004). Hippocampus and entorhinal cortex in mild cognitive impairment and early AD. *Neurobiology of Aging*, 25: 303–310.

Petersen, R. C., Jack, C. R. Jr., Xu, Y. C., Waring, S. C., O'Brien, P. C., Smith, G. E. et al. (2000). Memory and MRI-based hippocampal volumes in aging and AD. *Neurology*, 54: 581–587.

Rusinek, H., Endo, Y., De Santi, S., Frid, D., Tsui, W. H., Segal, S. et al. (2004). Atrophy rate in medial temporal lobe during progression of Alzheimer disease. *Neurology*, 63: 2354–2359.

Scher, A. I., Xu, Y., Korf, E. S., White, L. R., Scheltens, P., Toga, A. W. et al. (2007). Hippocampal shape analysis in Alzheimer's disease: A population-based study. *Neuroimage*, 36: 8–18.

Schonknecht, P., Pantel, J., Hartmann, T., Werle, E., Volkmann, M., Essig, M. et al. (2003). Cerebrospinal fluid tau levels in Alzheimer's disease are elevated when compared with vascular dementia but do not correlate with measures of cerebral atrophy. *Psychiatry Research*, 120: 231–238.

Schott, J. M., Price, S. L., Frost, C., Whitwell, J. L., Rossor, M. N., Fox, N. C. (2005). Measuring atrophy in Alzheimer disease: a serial MRI study over 6 and 12 months. *Neurology*, 65: 119–124.

Schröder, J., Pantel, J., Ida, N., Essig, M., Hartmann, T., Knopp, M. V. et al. (1997). Cerebral changes and cerebrospinal fluid β-amyloid in Alzheimer's disease: a study with quantitative magnetic resonance imaging. *Mol. Psychiatry*, 2(6): 505–507.

Seab, J. P., Jagust, W. J., Wong, S. T., Roos, M. S., Reed, B. R., and Budinger, T. F. (1988). Quantitative NMR measurements of hippocampal atrophy in Alzheimer's disease. *Magnetic Resonance in Medicine*, 8: 200–208.

Sencakova, D., Graff-Radford, N. R., Willis, F. B., Lucas, J. A., Parfitt, F., Cha, R. H. et al. (2001). Hippocampal atrophy correlates with clinical features of Alzheimer disease in African Americans. *Archives of Neurology*, 58: 1593–1597.

Silbert, L. C., Quinn, J. F., Moore, M. M., Corbridge, E., Ball, M. J., Murdoch, G. et al. (2003). Changes in premorbid brain volume predict Alzheimer's disease pathology. *Neurology*, 61: 487–492.

Small, G. W., Kepe, V., Ercoli, L. M., Siddarth, P., Bookheimer, S. Y., Miller, K. J. et al. (2006). PET of brain amyloid and tau in mild cognitive impairment. *The New England Journal of Medicine*, 355: 2652–2663.

Smith, A. D. (2002). Imaging the progression of Alzheimer pathology through the brain. *Proceedings of the National Academy of Sciences of the USA*, 99: 4135–4137.

Stout, J. C., Bondi, M. W., Jernigan, T. L., Archibald, S. L., Delis, D. C., and Salmon, D. P. (1999). Regional cerebral volume loss associated with verbal learning and memory in dementia of the Alzheimer type. *Neuropsychology*, 13: 188–197.

Stout, J. C., Jernigan, T. L., Archibald, S. L., and Salmon, D. P. (1996). Association of dementia severity with cortical gray matter and abnormal white matter volumes in dementia of the Alzheimer type. *Archives of Neurology*, 53: 742–749.

Teipel, S. J., Bayer, W., Alexander, G. E., Bokde, A. L., Zebuhr, Y., Teichberg, D. et al. (2003). Regional pattern of hippocampus and corpus callosum atrophy in Alzheimer's disease in relation to dementia severity: Evidence for early neocortical degeneration. *Neurobiology of Aging*, 24: 85–94.

Teipel, S. J., Bayer, W., Alexander, G. E., Zebuhr, Y., Teichberg, D., Kulic, L. et al. (2002). Progression of corpus callosum atrophy in Alzheimer disease. *Archives of Neurology*, 59: 243–248.

Teipel, S. J., Born, C., Ewers, M., Bokde, A. L., Reiser, M. F., Moller, H. J. et al. (2007). Multivariate deformation-based analysis of brain atrophy to predict Alzheimer's disease in mild cognitive impairment. *Neuroimage*, 38: 13–24.

Teipel, S. J., Flatz, W. H., Heinsen, H., Bokde, A. L., Schoenberg, S. O., Stockel, S. et al. (2005). Measurement of basal forebrain atrophy in Alzheimer's disease using MRI. *Brain*, 128: 2626–2644.

Teipel, S. J., Meindl, T., Gringberg, L., Heinsen, H., Hampel, H. (2008). Novel MRI techniques in the assessment of dementia. *Eur J Nucl Med Mol Imaging*, 35(suppl. 1): 558–69. Review.

Teipel, S. J., Pruessner, J. C., Faltraco, F., Born, C., Rocha-Unold, M., Evans, A. et al. (2006). Comprehensive dissection of the medial temporal lobe in AD: Measurement of hippocampus, amygdala, entorhinal, perirhinal and parahippocampal cortices using MRI. *Journal of Neurology*, 253: 794–800.

Teipel, S. J., Stahl, R., Dietrich, O., Schoenberg, S. O., Perneczky, R., Bokde, A. L. et al. (2007). Multivariate network analysis of fiber tract integrity in Alzheimer's disease. *Neuroimage*, 34: 985–995.

Temple, R. (1999). Are surrogate markers adequate to assess cardiovascular disease drugs? *The Journal of the American Medical Association*, 282: 790–795.

Thomann, P. A., Wustenberg, T., Pantel, J., Essig, M., and Schroder, J. (2006). Structural changes of the corpus callosum in mild cognitive impairment and Alzheimer's disease. *Dementia and Geriatric Cognitive Disorders*, 21: 215–220.

Thompson, P. M., Hayashi, K. M., De Zubicaray, G. I., Janke, A. L., Rose, S. E., Semple, J. et al. (2004). Mapping hippocampal and ventricular change in Alzheimer disease. *Neuroimage*, 15;36(4): 1397–1398, 1754–1766.

Thompson, P. M., Mega, M. S., Woods, R. P., Zoumalan, C. I., Lindshield, C. J., Blanton, R. E. et al. (2001). Cortical change in Alzheimer's disease detected with a disease-specific population-based brain atlas. *Cerebral Cortex*, 11: 1–16.

van de Pol, L. A., Hensel, A., Barkhof, F., Gertz, H. J., Scheltens, P., and van der Flier, W. M. (2006). Hippocampal atrophy in Alzheimer disease: Age matters. *Neurology*, 66: 236–238.

van der Flier, W. M., Middelkoop, H. A., Weverling-Rijnsburger, A. W., Admiraal-Behloul, F., Bollen, E. L., Westendorp, R. G. et al. (2005). Neuropsychological correlates of MRI measures in the continuum of cognitive decline at old age. *Dementia and Geriatric Cognitive Disorders*, 20: 82–88.

Visser, P. J., Scheltens, P., Pelgrim, E., and Verhey, F. R. (2005). Dutch ENA-NL-01 Study Group. Medial temporal lobe atrophy and APOE genotype do not predict cognitive improvement upon treatment with rivastigmine in Alzheimer's disease patients. *Dementia and Geriatric Cognitive Disorders*, 19: 126–133.

Wahlund, L. O., Andersson-Lundman, G., Basun, H., Almkvist, O., Bjorksten, K. S., Saaf, J. et al. (1993). Cognitive functions and brain structures: a quantitative study of CSF volumes on Alzheimer patients and healthy control subjects. *Magnetic Resonance Imaging*, 11: 169–174.

Wahlund, L. O., Julin, P., Lannfelt, L., Lindqvist, J., and Svensson, L. (1999). Inheritance of the ApoE epsilon4 allele increases the rate of brain atrophy in dementia patients. *Dementia and Geriatric Cognitive Disorders*, 10: 262–268.

Wang, L., Miller, J. P., Gado, M. H., McKeel, D. W., Rothermich, M., and Miller, M. I. et al. (2006). Abnormalities of hippocampal surface structure in very mild dementia of the Alzheimer type. *Neuroimage*, 30: 52–60.

Wang, L., Swank, J. S., Glick, I. E., Gado, M. H., Miller, M. I., Morris, J. C. et al. (2003). Changes in hippocampal volume and shape across time distinguish dementia of the Alzheimer type from healthy aging. *Neuroimage*, 20: 667–682.

Wang, P. J., Saykin, A. J., Flashman, L. A., Wishart, H. A., Rabin, L. A., Santulli, R. B. et al. (2006). Regionally specific atrophy of the corpus callosum in AD, MCI and cognitive complaints. *Neurobiology of Aging*, 27: 1613–1617.

Whitwell, J. L., Jack, C. R. Jr., Parisi, J. E., Knopman, D. S., Boeve, B. F., Petersen, R. C. et al. (2007). Rates of cerebral atrophy differ in different degenerative pathologies. *Brain*, 130(4): 1148–1158.

Xu, Y., Jack, C.R. Jr., O'Brien, P. C., Kokmen, E., Smith, G. E., Ivnik, R. J. et al. (2000). Usefulness of MRI measures of entorhinal cortex versus hippocampus in AD. *Neurology*, 54: 1760–1767.

Zarow, C., Vinters, H. V., Ellis, W. G., Weiner, M. W., Mungas, D., White, L. et al. (2005). Correlates of hippocampal neuron number in Alzheimer's disease and ischemic vascular dementia. *Annals of Neurology*, 57: 896–903.

Brain Imaging in the Evaluation of Putative Alzheimer's Disease-Slowing, Risk-Reducing and Prevention Therapies

Eric M. Reiman and Jessica B. S. Langbaum

In this chapter, we describe the emerging role of brain imaging in evaluating the effectiveness of putative Alzheimer's disease (AD)-slowing, risk-reducing, and prevention therapies. We consider the critical need for effective AD-slowing, risk-reducing and prevention therapies, the progress now being made in the scientific discovery of promising treatments, and the reasons why brain imaging measurements and other biomarkers are needed to help evaluate them in the most rapid and rigorous way. We suggest the advantages, disadvantages, and complementary roles of structural magnetic resonance imaging (MRI), fluorodeoxyglucose positron emission tomography (FDG PET), and fibrillar amyloid-β imaging in clinical trials involving patients with probable AD, amnestic mild cognitive impairment (MCI), and cognitively normal persons at differential risk for AD. We propose the use of *multiple* brain imaging methods and other biomarker measurements in clinical trials to both help evaluate an investigational treatment's disease-slowing effects and establish their role as "surrogate endpoints" in the evaluation of other investigational AD-slowing, risk-reducing, and prevention therapies. We suggest strategies to help optimize the value and statistical power of these methods in Phase 2 and Phase 3 clinical trials, and help address a treatment's potentially confounding effects on imaging endpoints. We propose a brain imaging strategy for the rapid evaluation of putative risk-reducing and prevention therapies in cognitively normal persons at genetic risk for AD. Finally, we call on public policy makers to make the identification of effective risk-reducing and primary prevention therapies a public health priority, and we offer public policy recommendations to accelerate the evaluation of risk-reducing and prevention therapies, helping to avert what is projected to become an overwhelming public health problem.

Section 1: Progress in the Discovery of AD-Slowing, Risk-Reducing and Prevention Therapies

In this section, we suggest why brain imaging measurements and other suitable biomarkers are critically needed to evaluate the effectiveness of promising AD-slowing, risk-reducing, and primary prevention therapies. We briefly consider the enormity of the problem, the urgent need find effective AD-slowing, risk-reducing, and prevention therapies, and the substantial progress now being made in the discovery of AD-slowing, risk-reducing, and prevention treatments.

AD is the most common form of disabling memory and thinking problems in older people. It is estimated to afflict about 10% of people over age 65 and 30%–50% of those over age 85 (Evans et al., 1989; Plassman et al., 2007). Given the extraordinary toll this disorder already takes on patients and their families, the rapidly growing number and proportion of people in these older age groups (Alzheimer's Association, 2008; Hebert et al., 2001), and the financially overwhelming toll that it is projected to take on communities around the world by the time today's young adults become senior citizens (Brookmeyer, Gray, and Kawas, 1998; Ernst and Hay, 1994), there is an urgent need to find effective AD-slowing or stopping, risk-reducing, and primary prevention therapies.

We are heartened by the progress now being made in the scientific understanding of AD and the discovery of promising disease-slowing, risk-reducing, and prevention treatments. Here's why:

(a) Researchers have begun to fill in the cascade of molecular events suggested to contribute to the neuropathological and clinical features of AD (Hardy and Selkoe, 2002). Neuritic plaques are associated with the aggregation of certain amyloid-β peptides and other pathological processes; neurofibrillary tangles are associated with hyperphosphorylation of the microtubule-associated protein tau and the destabilization of microtubules; the loss of synapses and neurons, the strongest neuropathological correlate of dementia severity, is thought by many but not all researchers to be related to these processes; and other contributing processes continue to be clarified. Each molecular event suggested to contribute to the pathogenesis of AD provides a potential target for the discovery of new treatments. Indeed, an unprecedented number of industry and academic researchers have been inspired by the enormity of the problem, the growing number of afflicted and at-risk persons, and the growing number of molecular targets, to work on the discovery of promising new AD-slowing treatments.

(b) Researchers continue to characterize genetic risk factors for AD (Reiman, 2007). To date, they have identified three AD-causing genes, such that more than 200 rare mutations of the presenilin 1 (PS1) (Sherrington et al., 1995), presenilin 2 (PS2) (Rogaev et al., 1995), and amyloid precursor protein (APP) (Goate et al., 1991) genes have been linked to many of the early-onset AD cases transmitted by autosomal dominant inheritance. They have also identified a common AD-susceptibility gene, the apolipoprotein E (APOE) ε4 allele, which has been repeatedly shown to account for many cases of late-onset AD (Corder et al., 1993). Meantime, genotyping platforms have begun to permit researchers to survey the entire human genome for a rapidly increasing number of single nucleotide polymorphisms (SNPs) and copy number variations (Reiman, 2007; Reiman et al., 2007). Indeed, within the next few years, it may be possible to cost-effectively sequence all three billion base-pairs in each person's genome. While much larger subject samples and more sophisticated data analysis strategies are still needed to fulfill the promise of this rapidly developing technology, researchers now have unprecedented power to characterize the genes which, together, have been suggested to account for 60%–80% of late-onset AD risk (Gatz et al., 2006; Reiman, 2007; Reiman et al., 2007).

How can this and other genomic information help in the discovery of promising new treatments? First, the proteins produced by these and other newly discovered genes may provide additional targets at which to aim new treatments. For example, the proteins produced by the established AD-causing and susceptibility genes have already provided support for the postulated role of the amyloid-β peptide in AD pathogenesis, bolstering investment in the discovery of β-amyloid-modifying treatments. Second, AD-causing mutations have been used to develop transgenic mouse models of AD, which recapitulate many (but not all) of the neuropathological features of AD and can be used to help screen some of the treatments being considered for time-consuming and expensive clinical trials. Third, genetic risk factors could be used to identify patient subgroups with a differential response to treatment, helping to minimize attrition in the development of putative AD-slowing therapeutics (Risner et al., 2006). Fourth, the implicated genes may be used in the future to help determine which healthy people receive certain risk-reducing and prevention therapies (i.e., those individuals in whom the potential benefits outweigh the risks and cost). Finally, we have suggested that healthy people at increased genetic risk for AD can be studied in clinical trials using brain imaging endpoints, helping to identify effective risk-reducing and prevention therapies as quickly as possible (Reiman et al., 2001b).

(c) Researchers also continue to characterize nongenetic modifiers of AD risk. Suggested risk factors include older age (Kawas et al., 2000), female gender (Edland et al., 2002; Fratiglioni et al., 1997; Kawas et al., 2000; Miech et al., 2002) (which may be due to increased longevity), lower educational levels (Kawas et al., 2000; Stern et al., 1994), cardiovascular disease (Newman et al., 2005), higher mid-life blood pressure and total cholesterol levels (Kivipelto et al., 2001), insulin resistance (Akomolafe et al., 2006; Irie et al., 2008), obesity (Gustafson et al., 2003; Stewart et al., 2005), tobacco use (Debanne et al., 2007; Reitz et al., 2007), and a head injury associated with loss of consciousness (Mehta et al., 1999;

Mortimer et al., 1985). These and other suggested AD risk modifiers support the possibility that certain healthy lifestyle (Larson et al., 2006; Saczynski et al., 2006; Wang et al., 2002) and dietary interventions (Scarmeas et al., 2006), medications (Wolozin et al., 2007), and dietary supplements (Laurin et al., 2004; Zandi et al., 2004) might reduce the risk of AD.

(d) Researchers have discovered a large and growing number of investigational AD-slowing treatments (Table 20.1). Indeed, dozens of investigational AD-slowing treatments are being considered for clinical trials in the coming years. The largest number of investigational treatments includes medications, active and passive immunization therapies, and dietary supplements that target amyloid-β production, amyloid-β aggregation, or different amyloid species. If, (as many, but not all, researchers believe) amyloid-β plays a pathogenic role in AD (Hardy and Selkoe, 2002), the right amyloid-β species is targeted, and the β-amyloid-modifying treatment is implemented sufficiently early in the pathogenic cascade (possibly before the formation of plaques or the onset of symptoms) and is safe and well-tolerated, an AD-slowing or prevention therapy may have already been discovered and awaiting evaluation in clinical trials. Meantime, a smaller number of investigational treatments have been proposed to interfere with other processes thought to be involved in the pathogenic cascade. Based on studies in a triple transgenic mouse model of AD, it has been suggested by one research group that an β-amyloid-modifying treatment might be sufficient to prevent AD if initiated before the appearance of tangles, but that a combination of β-amyloid-modifying and other (e.g., tau-modifying) treatments may be needed if initiated later in the course of the illness (Oddo et al., 2004, 2006). Similar conclusions were reached in a recent amyloid-β immunization trial in aging canines (Head et al., 2008).

Considering the progress now being made in "treatment discovery," we suggest that the greatest barrier to the identification of effective AD-slowing treatments may be "treatment development"—having the means to evaluate

Table 20–1 Investigational AD-slowing Therapies

Active and Passive β-amyloid Immunization Therapies.

Amyloid-modifying Medications

   β-secretase inhibitors

   γ-secretase inhibitors

   Anti-fibrillization or deposition agents (e.g, RAGE antagonists)

   Other Amyloid-β-42 and Selective Amyloid Lowering Agents (SALAs)

Tau-phosphorylation Inhibitors

   Glycogen synthase kinase-3 inhibitors

Other neuroprotective or neurotrophic agents

Neurotransmitter modulators

Drugs based on risk factors

   Cholesterol-lowering agents

   Insulin-sensitizing agents

   Antihypertensive agents

   Antioxidants

   Anti-inflammatory agents (e.g., NSAIDs)

   Hormonal therapies

Other Nutraceuticals

these treatments in the most cost-effective, rigorous, and rapid way. The pharmaceutical industry, regulators, academic researchers, and other AD stakeholders are increasingly interested in the role that brain imaging measurements may play in helping to overcome this hurdle.

(e) Researchers have discovered an even larger and more diversified portfolio of promising AD risk-reducing and primary prevention treatments (Table 20.2). The list includes the previously noted investigational therapies that first need to be studied in a sufficient number of AD patients to determine their safety and tolerability before they are considered in primary prevention trials. It also includes a number of existing healthy lifestyle, dietary, dietary supplement, and medication interventions, many of which have been suggested to have other health-promoting effects (e.g., a reduced risk of cardiovascular disease), and have been proposed to reduce the risk of AD in epidemiological or preclinical studies. It has been noted that even a modestly effective risk-reducing treatment would have an enormous public health benefit. For instance, a treatment that delayed the onset of AD by only five years without increasing longevity would have the potential to reduce the number of AD patients by half (Brookmeyer et al., 1998; Zaven Khachaturian, personal communication).

While it is reasonable to encourage the use of safe, well-tolerated and otherwise health-promoting interventions, it is important to recognize that none of the proposed risk-reducing and prevention therapies has been established in a randomized clinical trial to reduce a person's risk of AD. If practical challenges to the evaluation of investigational AD-slowing treatments in randomized clinical trials of afflicted patients are formidable, one might find the practical challenges of the evaluation of AD risk-reducing and prevention therapies in healthy people in randomized clinical trials insurmountable. Let us not give in to a nihilistic response. In Section 5, we propose a brain imaging strategy for the cost-effective evaluation of promising AD risk-reducing and prevention therapies, and propose treatment-development strategies and public health policies to help galvanize this critical endeavor.

Table 20–2   Suggested AD Risk-reducing and Prevention Therapies

Investigational Disease-modifying Treatments

Mental Exercise

Aerobic Exercise

Vitamins A, C, E, B12, B-complex Supplements, Selenium, Folic Acid

Ginkgo Biloba Extract, other Flavonoids, other Antioxidants

Omega-3 Fatty Acids (in fish, nuts, leafy vegetables)

Curcumin (in curry)

Mediterranean Diet

Low Caloric Intake

Copper-lowering Diet, Medications

Moderate use of Wine, Alcohol; Resveratrol (in grapes, red wine)

Cholesterol-lowering Agents (e.g., statins)

Antihypertensive Agents

Insulin-sensitizing Agents

Anti-inflammatory Agents (e.g., NSAIDs)

Hormonal Therapies (but not when first administered to older women)

Section 2: Challenges in the Evaluation of Putative AD-slowing, Risk-reducing, and Prevention Therapies

As previously noted, the roadblock to identifying effective AD-slowing, risk-reducing, and primary prevention therapies may not be the discovery of promising treatments, but the means of evaluating them in the most cost-effective, productive, rapid, and rigorous way. In this section, we briefly consider some of the practical and scientific challenges involved in the clinical evaluation of these promising treatments. We will later suggest ways in which brain imaging may be help to address these challenges.

Challenge 1: Reduce the patient samples and time needed to evaluate putative AD-slowing treatments in patients with probable AD. In patients with probable AD, the evaluation of putative AD-slowing treatments in double-blind, parallel-group, placebo-controlled clinical trials requires a relatively large number of research participants and a relatively long study duration (typically about 18 months of treatment) to detect significant effects on clinical endpoints. These larger subject samples and longer study durations are needed, not just to determine whether a putative AD-slowing treatment is associated with significant clinical improvement soon after the treatment is initiated, but to determine whether it is associated with significantly less clinical decline (and, presumably, less underlying disease progression) over an extended time. Although some disease-slowing treatments could lead to an initial improvement in symptoms by enabling sick but viable neurons to recover their function, affecting other neuronal mechanisms that bolster relevant brain functions, or compensating for the disease in other ways, other disease-slowing treatments might not be associated with an initial improvement in symptoms. It is already quite difficult, time-consuming, and expensive to enroll a sufficient number of suitable probable AD patients in clinical trials. This problem will grow dramatically with the avalanche of investigational treatments anticipated to be introduced in clinical trials over the next several years, and it is likely to be compounded by the need for even larger samples and further enrollment difficulties whenever new treatments are approved, become part of the standard of care, and are permitted or required in clinical trials. In Section 4, we will discuss how brain imaging methods could be used to help reduce the number of probable AD patients and the duration of treatment needed to detect a treatment's effectiveness in clinical trials, and how they could help decide in which treatments to invest (e.g., help make "go" / "no-go" decisions) in expensive Phase 3 clinical trials.

Challenge 2: Make it practical to evaluate putative AD-slowing treatments in patients with amnestic MCI by reducing the required patient samples, study time, and funding even further. There is an increasing perception that many AD-slowing treatments may be most effective in the earliest stages of the disease—particularly, β-amyloid-modifying treatments, since amyloid-β accumulation has been suggested to be associated with the earliest disease stages, and fibrillar amyloid-β burden is not strongly correlated with dementia severity (Giannakopoulos et al., 2003; Katzman et al., 1988; Meyer-Luehmann et al., 2008). Furthermore, there is a widespread belief that treatments would have their greatest clinical and public health impact if they could avert disabling cognitive impairment (Sloane et al., 2002). With these considerations in mind, researchers are extremely interested in conducting studies in patients with amnestic MCI who have memory concerns, perform less well on memory tests than other individuals their age, but whose impairment in memory and other cognitive domains are not associated with the disabling impairment in activities of daily living needed to meet the criteria for probable AD (Petersen et al., 1999). Since a significant proportion of amnestic MCI patients already have histopathological or brain imaging evidence of fibrillar amyloid-β pathology (Forsberg et al., 2008; Kemppainen et al., 2007; Morris et al., 2001; Petersen et al., 2006: Pike et al., 2007; Small et al., 2006), and since about 10%–15% of these patients per year have been shown to clinically convert to probable AD (Morris et al., 2001; Petersen et al., 1999), they are attractive candidates for "very mild AD" (i.e., secondary prevention) clinical trials of putative AD-slowing treatments.

There are at least two reasons why it is so difficult to conduct clinical trials of putative AD-slowing treatments in amnestic MCI patients. First, these clinical trials typically require an unusually large number of amnestic MCI patients and several years to determine whether a putative AD-slowing treatment reduces rates of decline on cognitive and functional endpoints and clinical progression to probable AD. Second, since a significant minority (perhaps 30%) of those amnestic MCI patients who subsequently progress to dementia may not meet the neuropathological criteria for AD during autopsy (Jicha et al., 2006), clinical trials of treatments specifically targeting AD pathology are likely to require even more MCI participants to detect a significant AD-slowing effect. In Section 4, we will describe how brain imaging methods could be used to make it more practical for conducting clinical trials in MCI patients by reducing the number of patients and duration of treatment needed to evaluate a treatment's effectiveness, help decide those treatments in which to invest in very expensive Phase 3 clinical trials, and help select or stratify patients on the basis of their fibrillar amyloid-β pathology or estimated risk of clinical progression to probable AD.

Challenge 3: Make it possible to evaluate putative AD risk-reducing and primary prevention therapies as rapidly as possible, such that if an effective treatment exists, it can be identified without losing a generation. It currently takes too much money, too many healthy volunteers, and too many years (e.g., longer than a drug product's patent life) to evaluate the effectiveness of putative risk-reducing and prevention therapies on the basis of clinical endpoints in a randomized clinical trial. To partly address this challenge, some researchers have advocated the assessment of these treatments in patients with MCI (which could constitute an early intervention or secondary prevention study), and others have advocated for the study of elderly people, who have higher rates of conversion to MCI and AD than people at younger ages. However, some putative risk-reducing and prevention treatments (e.g., β-amyloid-modifying medication and immunization therapies) may be most effective when initiated before the onset of clinical symptoms and the neuropathology already evident at that time, and some putative risk-reducing treatments (e.g., cholesterol-reducing, anti-hypertensive, and hormone replacement therapies) may be most effective when initiated at younger ages. For instance, previous prospective observational studies reported 39%–50% lower odds of developing probable AD among hormone replacement therapy users (Kawas et al., 1997; Paganini-Hill and Henderson, 1996; Tang et al., 1996; Zandi et al., 2002). To address the potential confounds involved in observational studies, the Women's Health Initiative Memory Study (which was an ancillary part of the even larger Women's Health Initiative Study) enrolled more than 7,500 nondemented postmenopausal women in a randomized clinical trial of conjugated estrogen replacement therapy (unopposed by, or in combination with, medroxy-progesterone

depending on whether or not they had had a hysterectomy) (Craig et al, 2005; Shumaker et al., 1998). To have sufficient statistical power to detect a risk-reducing effect of treatment, the clinical trial only included women over age 65, was originally intended to last for ten years of active or placebo treatment, and used conversion to "dementia of any cause" rather than probable AD as its primary outcome measure. Although the study was discontinued early (because of a higher risk of breast cancer in those receiving combination therapy and a higher risk of stroke in those receiving unopposed estrogen therapy), the study found a surprising higher risk of all-cause dementia in the estrogen-treated group (Shumaker et al., 2003, 2004). Since the study raised the possibility that the increased risk of dementia might be related to the interaction between estrogen treatment and vascular risk factors in this older group, and since other studies raised the possibility that estrogen treatment might need to be introduced at an earlier "critical period," it would be helpful to be able to study the risk-reducing effectiveness of estrogen replacement therapy in younger women, beginning around the time of perimenopause. But such a study could require about 50,000 perimenopausal women, about 20 years of treatment, and extraordinary funding to have adequate statistical power to detect a treatment effect in a randomized clinical trial using rates of conversion to probable AD.

We need a new, rapid, rigorous and cost-effective way to study the range of putative AD risk-reducing and prevention therapies. In Section 5, we propose the use of brain imaging measurements as "surrogate endpoints" in cognitively normal persons with an increased risk of AD to accelerate the identification of effective risk-reducing and prevention therapies, and we propose a strategy to show that the effect of a treatment on these surrogate endpoints is "reasonably likely to predict a clinical benefit."

Challenge 4: Demonstrate a putative AD treatment's disease-slowing (and not just symptomatic) effectiveness, and show that a "surrogate endpoint" is reasonably likely to predict an AD-slowing treatment's clinical benefit. With the advent of investigational treatments intended not just to compensate for AD pathology but slow disease progression, regulatory agencies and pharmaceutical companies have considered the research strategies needed to distinguish between a treatment's disease-slowing (also referred to as "disease-modifying") and symptomatic effects. Why might this distinction be so important using, for instance, brain imaging or other biomarker endpoints? First, pharmaceutical companies can now use brain imaging or other biomarker measurements of a disease state or progression as surrogate endpoints in Phase 2 clinical trials to seek preliminary evidence of a treatment's disease-slowing effectiveness and thus help make strategic investment decisions about which treatments to consider in expensive multi-center clinical trials. As previously noted, these Phase 2 studies could be performed with fewer research participants and study time than would be required using traditional clinical endpoints to generate that useful information—even though regulatory agencies would not yet consider the surrogate endpoint sufficiently linked to a treatment's clinical benefit to grant marketing approval on this endpoint alone. Second, substantial evidence of both clinical improvement and disease-slowing effectiveness in Phase 3 clinical trials might be sufficient for regulatory agencies to grant marketing approval for a drug product with a disease-modifying indication. Third, brain imaging or other biomarker endpoints alone could eventually provide substantial evidence of a treatment's disease-slowing effectiveness in Phase 3 clinical trials, permitting regulatory agencies to grant marketing approval for a treatment—under "Accelerated Approval provisions" if the treatment's effect on the surrogate endpoint is "reasonably likely" to predict a clinical benefit, or under the standard approval process if the surrogate endpoint is "validated" (i.e., extremely certain) to predict a clinical benefit. As discussed below, regulatory agencies still require more substantial evidence that a treatment's effect on a surrogate endpoint is reasonably likely to predict a clinical benefit before they are willing to grant a drug product Accelerated Approval, and they will then require post-marketing studies to confirm the approved treatment's clinical benefit. Still, AD stakeholders are excited about the possibility of using brain imaging and other biomarker endpoints as surrogate endpoints to help accelerate the identification and availability of effective disease-slowing, risk-reducing, and prevention therapies.

While none of the brain imaging measurements or other biomarkers of AD pathology, progression, or risk are considered by regulatory agencies to be "validated" or even "unvalidated but reasonably likely" to predict a clinical response, the strategy to help validate them seems reasonably clear: embed as many of these brain imaging and other biomarker endpoints in clinical trials of putative AD-slowing treatments, and generate substantial evidence showing an association between the effects of one (or preferably more) treatments on the biomarker endpoints and clinical benefit. Doing so will not only assist in the evaluation of the treatment under immediate investigation, but help the entire field develop disease-slowing, risk-reducing, and prevention therapies in the most rapid and rigorous way.

Three clinical trial strategies that have been proposed to characterize a treatment's disease-slowing effectiveness include: (1) a "staggered, delayed, or randomized withdrawal" design; (2) a "staggered, delayed, or randomized start" design; and (3) use of "validated" or (unvalidated but) "reasonably likely" surrogate endpoints (Leber, 1996, 1997; Mani, 2004). Before we consider the issue of surrogate endpoints in more detail, let us consider the staggered withdrawal and staggered start strategies that are designed to evaluate a treatment's disease-slowing effectiveness using clinical endpoints.

Staggered Withdrawal Design. In the staggered withdrawal design, patients are initially randomized to active or placebo treatment and monitored under double-blind conditions for a sufficient duration, as in traditional clinical trials. While still under double-blind conditions, those patients originally assigned to active treatment are withdrawn from this treatment and assigned to placebo instead, while the patients originally randomized to placebo treatment remain on placebo. If the patients withdrawn from active treatment show an accelerated decline, causing them to approach the clinical status of patients initially treated with and maintained on placebo, the evidence would support the treatment's symptomatic (disease-compensating) effect. Conversely, if the two patient groups tend to have parallel rates of subsequent decline, such that the clinical status of the patients withdrawn from treatment will continue to be better than that of the patients initially treated with and maintained on placebo, the evidence would support the treatment's disease-modifying effect. A practical and ethical limitation of the staggered withdrawal design may include the reluctance of patients, family caregivers, and/or a clinical trial's Data and Safety Monitoring Board (DSMB) to discontinue a treatment they believe to be effective, preferring open-label extension treatment instead.

Staggered Start Design. In the staggered start design, patients are initially randomized to active or placebo treatment and monitored under double-blind conditions for a sufficient duration. While still under double-blind conditions, those patients originally assigned to placebo are then assigned to active treatment instead, while the patients originally randomized to active treatment continue to receive active treatment. If the magnitude of improvement (or attenuation in decline) in the delayed treatment group causes this group to approach the clinical status of the patient group initially assigned to and maintained on active treatment, the evidence would support the treatment's symptomatic (disease-compensating) effect. Conversely, if the two patient groups have parallel rates of decline while receiving active treatment, such that the group initially treated with placebo never reaches the clinical status of the group initially assigned and maintained on active treatment, the evidence would support the treatment's disease-modifying effect.

Staggered withdrawal and start designs offer the advantage of evaluating a putative disease-slowing effect on the basis of clinical endpoints themselves. However, there may be uncertainties about the minimum—theoretically long—duration of delay in the withdrawal or start of treatment or the minimum—theoretically large—number of participants needed to demonstrate with sufficient statistical power that the slopes of clinical change are equivalent, and the staggered withdrawal design would have the previously noted practical and ethical challenges (Aisen, 2006; Broich, 2007; Cummings, 2006; Katz, 2004; Vellas et al., 2007).

Surrogate Endpoints. Brain imaging measurement can now be used by researchers in the early detection and tracking of AD, providing useful information about AD severity, progression, and risk. Also, as previously noted, these measurements can now be used as unvalidated surrogate endpoints to provide preliminary information about a putative treatment's disease-slowing effects in early phase, proof-of-concept clinical trials. In the meantime, there is growing interest in the development and use of these and other biomarker measurements as either reasonably likely or validated surrogate endpoints, such that a treatment's effect on the biomarker is either reasonably or extremely likely to predict a clinical benefit. Before we consider this issue more fully, let us define some of the terms used in the clinical development of drug products.

The United States Food and Drug Administration (FDA) and the European Medicines Agency (EMEA) define a "clinical endpoint" as "a characteristic or variable that reflects how a patient feels, functions, or survives." (Biomarkers Definitions Working Group, 2001) To approve a treatment for the cognitive symptoms of AD, these regulatory agencies currently require substantial evidence from at least two pivotal studies (typically Phase 3 clinical trials) that the treatment is superior to placebo on "dual outcomes." Dual outcomes currently include (1) a performance-based measure of cognitive function, ideally including memory and other cognitive domains typically compromised in patients with AD, and (2) a clinician-based rating of global clinical severity, global clinical change, or the activities of daily living. These dual outcome criteria are intended to provide substantial evidence of a treatment-related improvement in core cognitive symptoms that is deemed to be clinically meaningful (Ferris and Kluger, 1997; Leber, 2002).

The most commonly used performance-based measure of cognitive function is currently the AD Assessment Scale-cognitive portion (ADAS-Cog) (Rosen et al., 1984), although it has been suggested to be suboptimal in terms of characterizing performance on some of the cognitive domains that are typically affected by AD and its lack of sensitivity to characterize cognitive change in patients with mild AD and MCI (Leber, 1996). The Neuropsychological Test Battery (NTB) (Harrison et al., 2007) was recently introduced in clinical trials in an attempt to help overcome these limitations, and other cognitive performance instruments are likely to be developed in the future. Commonly used clinician-based ratings of global clinical severity or global clinical change include the Clinical Dementia Rating (CDR) scale (Morris, 1993), the Global Deterioration Scale (GDS) (Reisberg et al., 1982), the Severe Impairment Battery (SIB) (Panisset, 1994), the AD Cooperative Study Unit Clinician's Global Impression of Change (ADCS-CGIC) (Schneider et al., 1997), and the Clinician's Interview-Based Impression of Change with Caregiver Input (CIBIC-plus) (Schneider and Olin, 1996). Commonly used clinician-based tools to assess activities of daily living include the ADCS-Activities of Daily Living inventory (ADCS-ADL) (Galasko et al., 1997) and the Disability Assessment for Dementia (DAD) (Gélinas et al., 1999). Ideally, clinical assessment tools would have high inter-rater and test-retest reliability, would be sufficiently brief and well-tolerated, would assess all of the clinically relevant symptoms and provide a single overall symptom severity score, would be applicable to a broad range of clinical disease severity and sensitive in the longitudinal assessment of clinical progression, and would include alternate forms for reliably assessing performance-based measures without significant practice effects (Ferris and Kluger, 1997; Mohs, 2000).

Regulatory agencies define a "biomarker" as "a characteristic that is objectively measured and evaluated as an indicator of normal biological processes, pathogenic processes, or pharmacologic responses to a therapeutic intervention" (Biomarkers Definitions Working Group, 2001). Currently, structural MRI and FDG PET measurements provide the best established markers of AD progression, and fibrillar amyloid-β imaging techniques now make it possible to assess amyloid plaque burden—a cardinal neuropathological feature of AD—in the living human brain. These brain imaging measurements (which can be calculated using different image-analysis techniques), other brain imaging measurements, and other nonimaging biomarker measurements (e.g., cerebral spinal fluid measures of amyloid-β_{1-42} (Fagan et al., 2006; Schoonenboom et al., 2008), total tau (Hulstaert et al., 1999), phospho-tau$_{181p}$ (Hansson et al., 2006), isoprostanes (de Leon et al., 2006; Montine et al., 2007), and protein measurements in cerebral spinal fluid, blood, or other fluids or tissues) that continue to be developed and tested have important roles to play in the early detection and tracking of AD and the evaluation of promising AD-slowing, risk-reducing, and prevention therapies—even if they do not yet fulfill criteria for reasonably likely or more fully validated surrogate endpoints.

A "surrogate endpoint" is defined as "a biomarker that is intended to substitute for a clinical endpoint. It is expected to predict clinical benefit (or lack of benefit) on the basis of epidemiologic, therapeutic, pathophysiologic, or other scientific evidence" (Biomarkers Definitions Working Group, 2001). For regulatory agencies like the FDA and EMEA to accept a biomarker as a validated surrogate endpoint, and thus to consider marketing approval based solely on the drug product's effect on the surrogate endpoint without having to invoke Accelerated Approval provisions, it must (1) be compellingly related to the pathophysiological disease process (i.e., in the causal pathway), (2) change in the predicted direction in response to treatment, and (3) fully predict the treatment's clinical response (Broich, 2007; Fleming and DeMets, 1996; Katz, 2004; Prentice, 1989). For example, regulatory agencies consider blood pressure, serum cholesterol, and intraocular pressure to be validated surrogate endpoints, and they have approved antihypertensive, cholesterol-lowering, and glaucoma treatments without requiring them to show an effect on clinical endpoints like heart attacks, stroke, or visual loss (Katz, 2004).

What would it take to fully validate a brain imaging measurement or other biomarkers as a surrogate endpoint? Ideally, clinical trials would show a strong correlation between the effect of different treatments on surrogate and acceptable clinical endpoints (e.g., a performance-based measure of cognitive function, a clinician-based rating of global clinical severity, or rates of clinical progression to MCI or AD), not just one clinical trial evaluating a single drug product, but a number of clinical trials evaluating a range of drug products (Hughes, 2002; Katz, 2004).

Recognizing the daunting nature of that task, along with the interest in making treatments more rapidly available to patients with conditions like AIDS, the FDA incorporated "Accelerated Approval provisions" into its Code of Federal Regulations in 1992. These provisions provide a more rapid mechanism for granting marketing approval for a drug product considered to be "reasonably likely" to have important benefits to patients with the most serious and life-threatening disorders, including AD, by permitting the use of unvalidated surrogate endpoints as substitutes for clinical endpoints. As noted in Subpart H of 21 CFR 314.500, "the FDA may grant marketing approval for a new drug product on the basis of adequate well-controlled clinical trials establishing that the drug product has an effect on a surrogate endpoint that is reasonably likely, based on epidemiologic, therapeutic, pathophysiologic, or other evidence, to predict clinical benefit, or on the basis of an effect on a clinical endpoint other than survival or irreversible morbidity" (Katz, 2004). A preamble to these regulations (Food and Drug Administration, 1992) made several important points about this process: (1) even though unvalidated, a treatment's effect on the surrogate endpoint must be considered "reasonably likely" to predict a clinical benefit (a criterion that has not yet been met by any of the brain imaging or other biomarker measurements for the evaluation of AD-slowing treatments); (2) the FDA will not rely on a surrogate endpoint when a clinical benefit could be demonstrated in reasonable (i.e., not excessively large or long) clinical trials; (3) the FDA will require post-marketing studies confirming the association between the surrogate endpoint, including reasonable research attempts, and supportive findings for the drug product to remain on the market.

In 1997, Congress included these provisions in Section 506(b) of the FDA Modernization Act, which permits the FDA to approve a drug product: "...upon a determination that the product has an effect on a clinical endpoint or on a surrogate endpoint that is reasonably likely to predict clinical benefit" (Katz, 2004). Once established as reasonably likely to predict a clinical benefit, surrogate endpoints could substitute for clinical endpoints in randomized clinical trials of putative AD-slowing, risk-reducing, and prevention therapies, reducing the sample size, treatment duration, and cost of conducting these studies, and giving afflicted patients and at-risk persons access to these treatments as quickly as possible.

Meantime, regulatory agencies are mindful of the uncertainties involved in interpreting the effects of different treatments on unvalidated surrogate endpoints, and regulatory experts "regularly" remind us that not all biomarkers of AD pathology or progression will prove to be valid surrogate endpoints. Indeed, they warn that the standards for surrogate marker validation are quite high, citing several examples in which seemingly well-established surrogate endpoints have failed to predict clinical benefit (Fleming and DeMets, 1996). For instance, even though higher serum total cholesterol levels are consistently associated with an increased risk of cardiovascular disease-related mortality in untreated people (and, indeed, are considered validated endpoints), all but one clinical trial has failed to show a significant relationship between the ability of treatments to lower cholesterol levels and reductions in overall mortality. Recently, a 24-month randomized clinical trial found that the previously approved combination of the cholesterol-absorption blocker ezetimibe and the cholesterol-synthesis blocking statin simvastatin was no more effective than simvastatin alone in reducing ultrasound measurements of mean carotid artery wall intima-media thickness (a surrogate endpoint of atherosclerosis used here in lieu of clinical endpoints) in patients with familial hypercholesterolemia, despite a significantly greater decrease in low-density lipoprotein (LDL) cholesterol levels (the original endpoint used to approve the combination therapy) (Kastelein et al., 2008). While this study did not include clinical endpoints, it illustrates the possibility that a drug product's effect on even a "validated" surrogate endpoint may not always predict the anticipated pathological effect or clinical benefit. Similarly, even though lower bone density is consistently associated with a higher risk of bone fractures in untreated people, some treatments have been shown to increase bone density without reducing bone fractures (e.g., by producing brittle bones). In both examples, the therapeutic agents had unintended actions independent of the disease pathway, leading to a dissociation between their effects on the biomarker and clinical endpoints.

We personally believe that the distinction between validated and unvalidated surrogate endpoints may be an artificial categorization. Rather, we believe that surrogate endpoints are more likely to exist on a continuum, reflecting the extent to which they are more or less adequately validated (but rarely certain) to predict clinical outcome. We believe that the Accelerated Approval provisions provide a prudent balance between the desire for earlier access to potentially ground-breaking treatments and the need to have as much confidence as practically possible about the treatments' effectiveness. They provide a mechanism for expediting access to those treatments judged to be "at least reasonably likely" to have a clinical benefit (i.e., what we would refer to as "adequately validated" for consideration under Accelerated Approval provisions), restricts these provisions to serious or life-threatening conditions, and requires post-marketing studies to confirm that the treatment's effect on the surrogate endpoint is associated with a clinical benefit.

In an article frequently cited by regulatory agencies, Fleming and DeMets (1996) described several reasons why otherwise promising surrogate endpoints failed to predict a clinical outcome, even when the biomarker was associated with disease risk or progression in the absence of treatment: (1) the proposed surrogate endpoint may not be in the causal pathway of the disease; (2) of several disease pathways, the intervention may influence the pathway involving the surrogate but not involving the clinical outcome; (3) the surrogate may not be in the pathway of the intervention or is insensitive to its effect; and (4) the intervention may have actions independent of the disease process (the most likely explanation for the failure of a proposed surrogate endpoint). To establish an association between surrogate and clinical endpoints, Fleming and DeMets articulated the need to establish that the surrogate endpoint is in "the only causal pathway of the disease, and the intervention's entire effect on the true clinical outcome is mediated through its effect on the surrogate" (Fleming and DeMets, 1996) (Figure 20.1).

Our take-home message is: the best way to demonstrate that the effect of different treatments on surrogate endpoints is "at least reasonably likely" to predict a clinical benefit is to embed them in clinical trials, providing direct evidence of a strong association between the surrogate and clinical endpoints in one or more

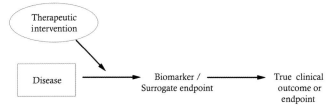

Figure 20–1 Rationale for the use of a surrogate endpoint in predicting a treatment's clinical benefit. To evaluate a treatment benefit on the basis of an adequately validated surrogate endpoint, the surrogate end point should be in the only causal pathway of the disease and fully predict the treatment's effect on the true clinical outcome. Since most biomarkers do not fulfill these criteria, we recommend embedding promising biomarkers into clinical trials to provide substantial evidence that the effects of different treatments on surrogate endpoints are "at least reasonably likely to predict the clinical outcome." Adapted from (Fleming and DeMets, 1996; Biomarkers Definitions Working Group, 2001).

trials. Given uncertainties in understanding about (a) disease mechanisms, (b) all of the known and unknown actions of the therapeutic agent, (c) the relationship between the magnitude of a treatment's effects on the surrogate and clinical endpoints, and (d) the unintended ways in which the agent might affect the surrogate endpoint or clinical outcome, we recommend humility in the use and interpretation of a treatment's effects on biomarker endpoints. We also offer the following suggestions: (1) anticipate the possibility of confounding treatment effects on biomarker measurements (e.g., effects on brain tissue volume, cerebral glucose metabolism, or amyloid-β burden independent that may not reflect clinically relevant disease progress); (2) embed as many biomarker measurements as possible in clinical trials of putative disease-slowing treatments, not just to evaluate the treatment of immediate interest, but to establish reasonably likely or valid surrogate endpoints for use by the entire field; and (3) consider other means (e.g., in the number and timing of scans) to further address potentially confounding effects of treatment on the surrogate endpoints.

Section 3: The Best Established Brain Imaging Techniques for the Evaluation of Putative AD-slowing Therapies

With the large and growing number of putative AD-slowing, risk-reducing, and prevention therapies, there is a growing interest in the role of brain imaging and other biomarker measurements in helping to evaluate these treatments in the most rapid, rigorous, cost-effective and informative way. Researchers continue to develop and test a variety of brain imaging modalities and image-analysis techniques for their potential use in the early detection and tracking of AD and the evaluation of these treatments. In this section, we briefly consider the two best-established brain imaging measurements of AD progression—FDG PET measurements of the cerebral metabolic rate for glucose (CMRgl) decline and structural MRI measurements of brain shrinkage, and new imaging techniques for the assessment of fibrillar amyloid-β burden (Figure 20.2). Since fibrillar amyloid-β imaging and the use of MRI in clinical trials of putative AD-slowing treatments is discussed more fully in Chapters 14 and 19, those imaging modalities will be discussed in less detail here than FDG PET. In Section 4, we consider ways in

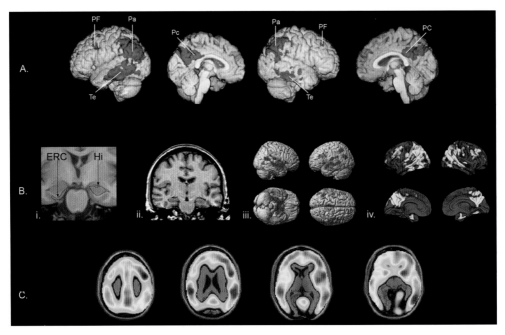

Figure 20–2   Brain imaging in the early detection and tracking of Alzheimer's disease. (a) FDG PET in the detection and tracking of AD—significantly lower CMRgl in probable AD patients than in elderly normal controls. Reprinted with permission from (Reiman et al., 1996). Copyright © 1996 Massachusetts Medical Society. All rights reserved. (b) Volumetric MRI in the detection and tracking of AD—(i) landmarks for the assessment of hippocampal and entorhinal cortex atrophy (Mike Weiner, with permission); (ii) computing whole brain atrophy (in red) from sequential MRIs (Nick Fox, with permission); (iii) significantly less gray matter in patients with probable AD than in elderly normal controls using voxel-based morphometry. Reprinted from (Baron et al., 2001). Copyright © 2001 with permission from Elsevier. All rights reserved; iv) significantly less cortical thickness in patients with probable AD than in normal controls using FreeSurfer software. Reprinted with permission from (Du et al., 2007). Copyright © 2007 Oxford University Press. All rights reserved. (c) Fibrillar amyloid imaging in the detection and tracking of AD—significantly greater PiB PET measurements of fibrillar amyloid burden in patients with probable AD than in normal controls. Statistical parametric maps generated using PiB PET images (Chris Rowe and colleagues, with permission).

which to use these imaging techniques in the evaluation of putative AD-slowing therapies, and in Section 5, we propose a strategy for the use of brain imaging in the evaluation of putative AD-risk reducing and primary prevention therapies.

FDG PET in the Early Detection and Tracking of AD

FDG PET is the functional brain imaging technique with the best-established role in the early detection and tracking of AD. In FDG PET studies, AD is associated with characteristic and progressive CMRgl reductions in the precuneus, posterior cingulate, parietal, and temporal cortex—some of which are apparent prior to the onset of dementia (Reiman et al., 1996, 2001a,b, 2004, 2005) and extend to the frontal cortex and whole brain in more severely affected patients (Alexander et al., 2002; de Leon et al., 1983; Duara et al., 1986; Foster et al., 1983; Haxby et al., 1990; Hoffman et al., 2000; Ibanez et al., 1998; Jagust et al., 1988; McGeer et al., 1990; Mega et al., 1997; Mielke et al., 1992; Minoshima et al., 1994, 1995; Silverman et al., 2001; Smith et al., 1992) (Figure 20.3). In patients with probable AD, these CMRgl reductions are correlated with dementia severity (Chase et al., 1984; Choo et al., 2007; Foster et al., 1984; Minoshima et al., 1995; Mosconi, 2005; Silverman et al., 2001; Smith et al., 1992), are progressive (Alexander et al., 2002; Haxby et al., 1990; Jagust et al., 1988; McGeer et al., 1990; Mosconi, 2005; Mosconi et al., 2008; Smith et al., 1992), predict subsequent clinical decline and the histopathological diagnosis of AD (Foster et al., 2007; Hoffman et al., 2000; Minoshima et al., 2001; Silverman et al., 2001), and may offer statistical power superior to clinical endpoints in the evaluation of putative AD-slowing treatments (Alexander et al., 2002; Chételat et al., 2005). In patients with amnestic MCI, baseline CMRgl reductions in the same locations appear to predict subsequent rates of clinical conversion to probable AD (Arnaiz et al., 2001; Drzezga et al., 2003; Drzezga et al., 2005; Minoshima et al., 1997), and may also help to predict who remains stable during the same time frames (de Leon et al., 2001; De Santi et al., 2001; Drzezga et al., 2003; Mosconi et al., 2004), thereby offering the possibility of selecting or stratifying participants in randomized clinical trials based on their estimated risk of subsequent cognitive decline and clinical conversion. Longitudinal CMRgl declines have the potential to decrease the number of MCI participants and the duration of study in randomized clinical trials of putative AD-slowing/secondary prevention therapies. In cognitively normal persons, carriers of the APOE ε4 allele have CMRgl reductions in the same brain regions as patients with AD (Reiman et al., 1996)—some of which are apparent in young adults (Reiman et al., 2004)—almost five decades before the expected median age at dementia onset; the baseline CMRgl reductions are correlated with APOE ε4 gene dose (i.e., three levels of genetic risk for AD) (Reiman et al., 2005), and appear to predict subsequent cognitive decline. Moreover, late middle-aged carriers of the APOE ε4 allele have significantly greater two-year CMRgl declines than noncarriers (Reiman et al., 2001b), which are correlated with ε4 gene dose, and raise the possibility of using FDG PET in a relatively small number of ε4 carriers to evaluate putative AD primary prevention therapies in two-year clinical trials. The AD-related CMRgl reductions could be attributable to reductions in the activity or density of

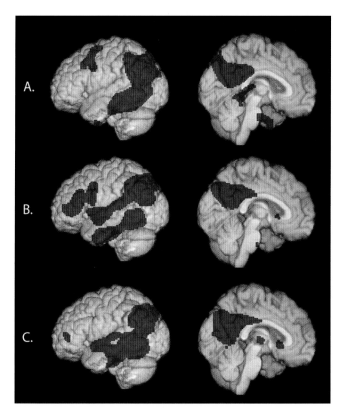

Figure 20–3 Baseline CMRgl reductions and longitudinal CMRgl declines in patients with probable AD—preliminary findings from the AD Neuroimaging Initiative (ADNI): (a) significantly lower CMRgl in 16 mildly affected probable AD patients than in 27 elderly normal controls; (b) significant six-month CMRgl declines in 78 mildly affected probable AD patients; and (c) significant 12-month CMRgl declines in 49 mildly affected probable AD patients. In each image, statistical parametric maps of significant CMRgl differences or declines ($p < 0.005$, uncorrected for multiple comparisons) are projected onto the lateral and medial surface of the left hemisphere in a spatially standardized volume-rendered MRI.

terminal neuronal fields or perisynaptic glial cells that innervate these regions (Magistretti and Pellerin, 1996; Meguro et al., 1999; Schwartz et al., 1979), mitochondrial or other metabolic dysfunctions (Liang et al., 2008; Magistretti and Pellerin, 1996; Mark et al., 1997; Mosconi et al., 2005, 2008; Piert, 1996), or a combination of these factors. They do not appear to be solely attributable to the combined effects of atrophy and partial-volume averaging (Ibanez et al., 1998).

Alzheimer's Dementia. In patients with dementia, the pattern of CMRgl reductions has been shown to predict subsequent clinical decline and the histopathological diagnosis of AD with 84%–93% sensitivity and about 73% specificity (Hoffman et al., 2000; Jagust, 2007; Silverman et al., 2001). In another study, the pattern of CMRgl reductions was found to be superior to retrospective clinical assessment in the differential diagnosis between AD and frontotemporal dementia (FTD) (Foster et al., 2007). The pattern of hypometabolism appears to mimic the atrophy observed by MRI in patients with probable AD (Chételat et al., 2008). In the United States, the Centers for Medicare and Medicaid Services (CMS) limits reimbursement for the use of PET in the differential diagnosis of AD to those patients who have evidence of dementia, have received a proper medical and laboratory evaluation, and in whom

the physician remains uncertain about the differential diagnosis of AD versus FTD.

In a longitudinal study, we and our colleagues used FDG PET to compare regional CMRgl in 14 patients with probable AD (mean Mini-Mental State Exam [MMSE] score 20) and 34 normal control participants, compute 12-month CMRgl declines in the patient group, and estimate the number of probable AD patients needed to detect a significant effect of a candidate treatment to slow down these CMRgl declines in a 12-month single-center randomized clinical trial (Alexander et al., 2002). As in other studies, the patients with probable AD had significantly lower CMRgl than the normal control participants bilaterally in regions of the posterior cingulate, parietal, temporal, and frontal cortex. During the following 12 months, quantitative CMRgl measurements (in mg/min/100g) continued to decline 6%–11% further in these regions and the whole brain. Indeed, due to the reductions in whole brain CMRgl, our effort to normalize the FDG PET images for the variation in whole brain or pontine measurements led to a slight underestimation in CMRgl declines. For this reason, we have advocated the use of a noninvasive method to transform PET images into quantitative CMRgl measurements to help optimize the power to track CMRgl declines (Chen et al., 1998).

As shown in Table 20.3a, we provided initial estimates of the number of AD patients needed per group in single-center, parallel-group randomized clinical trials of a putative AD-slowing treatment to detect 20%–50% reductions in 12-month CMRgl declines with 80% power ($p<0.01$, two-tailed, uncorrected for multiple comparisons). Based on these findings, we suggested that FDG PET could be used to evaluate putative AD-slowing treatment in 12-month Phase 2 clinical trials (or in a subset of a larger Phase 3 clinical trial) with about one-tenth the number of probable AD patients needed, using clinical ratings or neuropsychological scores as the end-point—and roughly comparable to the number of patients needed using MRI measurements of whole brain volume

Table 20–3 Originally Estimated Number of Moderate AD Patients per Group Needed to Detect AD-slowing Treatment Effects Using (a) FDG PET Measurements of Regional CMRgl or (b) MRI Measurements of Whole Brain Atrophy in a 12-month, Single-Center Randomized Clinical Trial[†]

Treatment-Related Percent Reduction

	20%	30%	40%	50%
(a) FDG PET [*]				
Frontal	85	38	22	14
Parietal	217	97	55	36
Temporal	266	119	68	44
Cingulate	343	153	87	57
(b) Structural MRI [**]				
Whole Brain Atrophy	115	51	29	18

[*] $p = 0.01$ (two-tailed), uncorrected for multiple comparisons, without adjustment for subject attrition or normal aging effects. Adapted from Alexander et al. (2002).

[**] $p = 0.05$ (two-tailed), without adjustment for subject attrition, normal aging effects, or potentially effects of amyloid-modifying treatments on brain volume unrelated to their effects on brain atrophy. Adapted from Fox et al. (2000).

[†] The estimated number of mildly affected probable AD patients per group needed to detect AD-slowing treatment effects using different FDG PET and MRI in 6-, 12-, and 24-month randomized clinical trials will be estimated using images from the ADNI.

decline (Table 20.3b) (Fox et al., 2000). However, these estimates were based on data from a relatively small number of participants from a single site. The AD Neuroimaging Initiative (ADNI), which is discussed later, is now permitting researchers to estimate the number of probable AD and amnestic MCI patients needed per group in multicenter parallel-group randomized clinical trials of putative AD-slowing treatments using FDG PET endpoints, to do so using data from a much larger number of patients than in previous studies, and to help identify the image-analysis technique with the greatest statistical power for these purposes.

Mild Cognitive Impairment. In several MCI studies, baseline CMRgl reductions in posterior cingulate, parietal, or temporal regions were significantly greater in patients who subsequently converted to probable AD than in those who remained stable during the same time interval (de Leon et al., 2001; De Santi et al., 2001; Drzezga et al., 2003; Mosconi et al., 2004, 2005, 2007) (Figure 20.4). In another preliminary study, every MCI patient with both glucose hypometabolism in a preselected posterior cingulate region-of-interest (ROI), and at least one copy of the APOE ε4 allele, subsequently converted to probable AD, whereas every MCI patient with neither of these brain imaging or genetic characteristics converted to AD during the same time interval (Drzezga et al., 2005). While this finding (and the other findings noted above) need to be confirmed in larger subject groups, it supports the possibility of capitalizing on complementary (in this case brain imaging and genetic) information to predict clinical course, histopathological diagnosis, or treatment response in future studies. Additional studies like ADNI promise to determine the extent to which baseline FDG PET measurements, other imaging measurements, other genetic and biomarker measurements, and a combination of different measurements predict subsequent rates of clinical conversion to probable AD and the histopathological diagnosis of AD.

In longitudinal studies, MCI patients who subsequently convert to probable AD have significantly greater CMRgl declines in precuneus, posterior cingulate, parietal, temporal and frontal regions than in those who remain stable during the same time interval (Drzezga et al., 2003; Mosconi et al., 2004). Our preliminary findings from ADNI are shown in Figure 20.4. As previously noted, ADNI promises to help characterize rates of regional CMRgl decline in amnestic MCI patients, determine the extent to which longitudinal CMRgl declines predict subsequent rates of clinical conversion to probable AD, estimate the number of amnestic MCI patients needed per group in a randomized multicenter clinical trials of putative AD-slowing treatments, and identify those image-analysis techniques that provide the greatest statistical power for this endeavor.

Cognitively Normal Persons. In a series of brain imaging studies, we have capitalized on the observation that an APOE ε4 gene dose (the number of ε4 alleles in a person's APOE genotype) is associated with a higher risk of late-onset AD and a slightly younger median age at the onset of dementia (Breitner, et al., 1999, 1998). Thus, we have been using FDG PET, MRI, clinical ratings, and neuropsychological tests (and most recently, PiB PET) to detect and track functional and structural brain changes in cognitively normal persons at three levels of risk for AD, including persons with two copies of the APOE ε4 allele (which is found in 2%–3% of the population and about 5% of those with a reported first-degree family history of probable AD (Corder et al., 1993)) who have an especially high risk of late-onset AD, those with one copy of the APOE ε4 allele (which is found in almost one-fourth of the population and about one-third of those with a reported first-degree

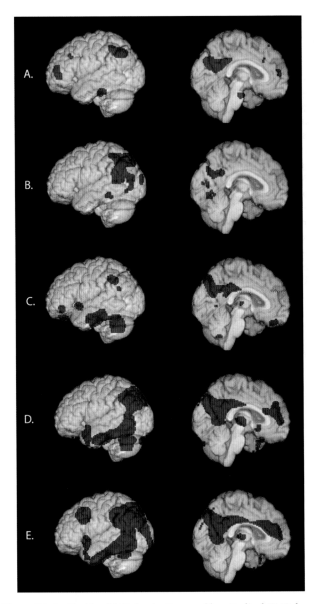

Figure 20–4 Baseline CMRgl reductions and longitudinal CMRgl declines in patients with amnestic MCI—preliminary findings from ADNI: (a) significantly lower CMRgl in 27 amnestic MCI patients than in 27 elderly normal controls; (b) significantly lower CMRgl in 14 amnestic MCI patients who subsequently progressed to probable AD than in 124 amnestic MCI patients who remained stable over the same time period; (c) significant 6-month CMRgl declines in 155 amnestic MCI patients; (d) significant 12-month CMRgl declines in 67 amnestic MCI patients; and (e) significant 18-month CMRgl declines in 55 amnestic MCI patients. In each figure, statistical parametric maps of significant CMRgl differences or declines ($p < 0.005$, uncorrected for multiple comparisons) are projected onto the lateral and medial surface of the left hemisphere in a spatially standardized volume-rendered MRI.

family history of probable AD (Corder et al., 1993), and those with no copies of the APOE ε4 allele who were individually matched for the gender, age and educational level. Our primary goal is the development of biomarkers and (ultimately) reasonably likely surrogate endpoints to evaluate putative risk-reducing and primary prevention therapies without having to study thousands of healthy participants or wait many years to compare rates of clinical conversion in a randomized clinical trial.

In a longitudinal study, we have been using FDG PET, volumetric MRI, clinical ratings, and neuropsychological tests, and most recently PiB PET every two years in cognitively normal APOE ε4 homozygotes, heterozygotes, and noncarriers who reported a first-degree family history of probable AD (to enrich our sample for ε4 heterozygotes) and were late middle-age (mean age 55), cognitively normal, and individually matched for their gender, age, and educational level at the time of their baseline visit. To date, we have made the following observations: (a) in comparison with cognitively normal noncarriers, APOE ε4 homozygote and heterozygote groups each have significantly lower CMRgl in the same posterior cingulate, precuneus, parietal, temporal, and frontal regions as patients with AD (Reiman et al., 1996, 2004); (b) the baseline CMRgl reduction in the posterior cingulate cortex provides a significantly more sensitive index of the difference between late middle-age ε4 homozygotes and noncarriers than MRI measurements of hippocampal volume—reductions in which appear to be associated with early memory decline (Reiman et al., 1998); (c) baseline CMRgl reductions in, and only in, AD-affected regions are correlated with ε4 gene dose (Reiman et al., 2005); (d) APOE ε4 heterozygotes have two-year CMRgl declines, which are significantly greater than those in the ε4 noncarriers in the previously noted and other neuropathologically relevant brain regions (Reiman et al., 2001b), whereas the ε4 noncarriers also had regional CMRgl declines (e.g., in frontal cortex) that could provide a progressive marker of normal brain aging (Reiman et al., 2001b); and (d) the two-year CMRgl declines are correlated with ε4 gene dose (Figures 20.5 and 20.6). In a related study, we found that APOE ε4 heterozygotes had significantly lower CMRgl than noncarriers in the same brain regions in young adulthood (mean age 30), almost 50 years before the possible onset of symptoms, and many years before the onset of significant AD neuropathology (Reiman et al., 2004). Based on our cross-sectional comparisons, we do not believe that the CMRgl reductions progress more rapidly between young adult and late middle-age in APOE ε4 carriers than in noncarriers, but anticipate progressive CMRgl reductions and early fibrillar amyloid-β deposition at older ages.

Based on the correlations between baseline CMRgl reductions and APOE ε4 gene doses, we proposed that FDG PET could be used as a quantitative presymptomatic "endophenotype" of AD—a biological measure more closely related to disease predisposition than the clinical syndrome itself (Gottesman and Gould, 2003)—complementing retrospective case-control studies and time-consuming prospective cohort studies in the assessment of putative genetic and nongenetic risk factors, and have begun to use it for that purpose (Reiman et al., 2001b, 2005, 2008) as well as helping to select promising risk-reducing treatments for clinical trials. Based on the two-year CMRgl declines in cognitively normal older adult ε4 heterozygotes (Figure 20.6), we estimated the number of ε4 heterozygotes needed per group in a single-center parallel-group randomized clinical trial of a putative AD-prevention treatment designed to detect 20%–50% reductions in 24-month CMRgl declines with 80% power (p < 0.01, two-tailed, uncorrected for multiple comparisons) (Reiman et al., 2001b). Thus, we suggested that FDG PET could be used to evaluate putative AD-prevention treatments in 24-month proof-of-concept trials using a fraction of the number of cognitively normal adults using clinical ratings or neuropsychological scores as the end-point, not to mention a dramatic savings in study time waiting for the participants to develop MCI or probable AD (Table 20.4).

In addition to these and other studies of cognitively normal persons at genetic risk for late-onset or early-onset AD, FDG PET studies have been used to identify characteristic and progressive

Table 20–4 Estimated Number of Late Middle-aged Cognitively Normal APOE ε4 Heterozygotes Needed to Detect Effects of an AD Risk-reducing or Prevention Therapy on FDG PET Measurements of Regional CMRgl in a 24-month Randomized Clinical Trial*

Treatment-related Reduction in Regional CMRgl Decline

	20%	30%	40%	50%
Thalamus	78	35	21	14
Parahippocampal	129	58	33	22
Cingulate	130	58	33	22
Temporal	155	70	40	27
Basal forebrain	167	75	43	29
Prefrontal	179	80	46	29

* p = 0.01 (two-tailed), uncorrected for multiple comparisons, without adjustment for subject attrition or normal aging effects. Adapted from Reiman et al. (2001b) and Reiman (2007).

Figure 20–5 Baseline CMRgl reductions and two-year CMRgl declines in cognitively normal persons at three levels of genetic risk for late-onset AD—correlations with APOE ε4 gene dose: (a) significant correlations between APOE ε4 gene dose and lower CMRgl in 160 cognitively normal late middle-aged people individually matched for their gender, age, and educational level. Reprinted with permission from (Reiman et al., 2005). Copyright © 2005 National Academy of Sciences, U.S.A. All rights reserved; and (b) significant correlations between APOE ε4 gene dose and two-year CMRgl declines in 94 cognitively normal late middle-aged people (differences between the location of maximal baseline reductions and longitudinal CMRgl declines are likely to reflect differences in the rate at which different regions decline at different ages, preclinical stages, and their interaction). In each image, statistical parametric maps of significant CMRgl differences or declines (p < 0.005, uncorrected for multiple comparisons) are projected onto the lateral and medial surface of the left hemisphere in a spatially standardized volume-rendered MRI.

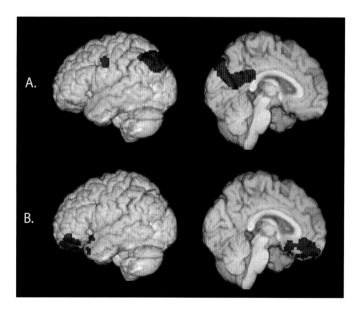

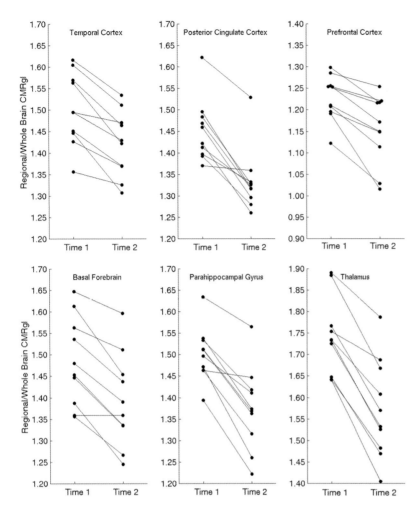

Figure 20–6 Two-year declines in regional CMRgl in cognitively normal APOE ε4 heterozygotes. These declines were significantly greater than the two-year declines in APOE ε4 noncarriers. Reprinted with permission from (Reiman et al., 2001b), Copyright © 2001 National Academy of Sciences, USA. All rights reserved.

CMRgl reductions associated with normal aging. For instance, age-related CMRgl reductions are especially prominent in the frontal cortex (De Santi et al., 1995; Martin et al., 1991), some of which begin soon after young adulthood and correspond to age-related reductions in MRI measurements of gray matter atrophy and neuropathological measurements of reduced synaptic density in other studies of normal aging. We have proposed using FDG PET and other brain imaging methods in longitudinal studies to track the progression of normal brain aging in APOE ε4 noncarriers to evaluate the effectiveness of treatments to slow down normal brain aging processes and perhaps decrease the risk of AD or other age-related brain disorders.

Structural MRI in the Early Detection and Tracking of AD

Structural MRI provides information about brain atrophy and is currently the brain imaging technique with the best-established role in the early detection and tracking of AD. These issues are reviewed in greater detail in Chapters 10, 12, and 16, and the use of structural MRI in clinical trials is discussed in Chapter 19. Patients with AD have reduced hippocampal and entorhinal cortex volumes, a corresponding increase in ventricular and sulcal volumes, and regional reductions in gray matter and cortical thickness (Figure 20.2b) (Bobinski et al., 1999; de Leon et al., 1989; Du et al., 2003; Fleisher et al., 2008; Jack et al., 1992, 1998, 2000; Juottonen et al., 1998; Rusinek et al., 1991; Visser et al., 1999). Smaller hippocampal and entorhinal cortex volumes are correlated

with dementia severity, predict subsequent clinical decline, and, although not specific for the neuropathological diagnosis of AD, are correlated with neuronal loss volumes (de Leon et al., 1989; Deweer et al., 1995; de Leon et al., 1993; Frisoni et al., 1999; Golomb et al., 1993; Jack et al., 1992, 1997, 1998; Krasuski et al., 1998; Laakso et al., 1995). In several studies, reductions in hippocampal and entorhinal cortex volume have been shown to parallel very early memory decline and herald the subsequent onset of MCI or AD (Bobinski et al., 1999; de Leon et al., 1993; Dickerson et al., 2001; Jack et al., 2004, 2005; Juottonen, 1999; Juottonen et al., 1998; Kaye et al., 1997; Killiany et al., 2002). Although MRI is indicated in the clinical evaluation of dementia (and, we suggest MCI) to exclude potentially reversible structural brain abnormalities such as tumors or subdural hematomas, and while it may provide other useful clinical information (e.g., about vascular pathology or distinctive patterns of focal atrophy), it currently lacks sufficient specificity (e.g., in hippocampal atrophy) for the clinical diagnosis of AD (Knopman et al., 2001).

Alzheimer's Dementia. In longitudinal studies, patients with AD have accelerated rates of hippocampal and entorhinal cortex atrophy, ventricular enlargement, gray matter loss and cortical thinning (Bobinski et al., 1999; de Leon et al., 1989; Du et al., 2003; Fox and Freeborough, 1997; Fox et al., 1996; Jack et al., 1992, 1998, 2000; Juottonen et al., 1998; Rusinek et al., 1991; Visser et al., 1999) (Figure 20.2b), which are likely to offer superior statistical power superior to clinical endpoints in the evaluation of putative AD-slowing treatments. In one study, rates of whole brain atrophy and ventricular enlargement (which can be computed from sequential MRIs using the originally established, semi-automated "brain boundary shift interval" or fully automated methods like "iterative principal component analysis") were better correlated with clinical decline than rates of hippocampal or entorhinal cortex atrophy, favoring the use of these particular MRI endpoints in clinical trials of putative AD-slowing treatments (Jack et al., 2005).

As shown in Table 20.3b, Fox and colleagues (Fox et al., 2000) originally estimated the number of AD patients needed per group in *single-center* parallel-group randomized clinical trials of putative AD-slowing treatment for detecting reductions in annualized rates of global brain atrophy. Their findings suggest that MRI could be used to evaluate putative AD-slowing treatment in 12-month Phase 2 clinical trials, with about one-tenth the number of probable AD patients needed using clinical ratings or neuropsychological scores as the end-point—and roughly comparable to the number of patients needed using FDG measurements of regional CMRgl decline (Table 20.3a) (Fox et al., 2000). ADNI will permit researchers to estimate the number of probable AD and amnestic MCI patients needed per group in multicenter, parallel-group, randomized clinical trials of putative AD-slowing treatments using MRI endpoints, do so using data from a much larger number of patients than in previous studies, and help identify the image-analysis technique with the greatest statistical power for this purpose.

While longitudinal studies have suggested the value of MRI and other imaging modalities in the tracking of AD and the evaluation of putative disease-slowing treatments, the Phase IIa clinical trial of the amyloid-β immunotherapy AN1792 in patients with probable AD reminds us that the use of imaging endpoints in clinical trials remains in the development phase (Fox et al., 2005). This study was terminated early due to the development of a clinically significant meningoencephalitis in 6% of the treated patients, but still permitted researchers to compare post-treatment to pretreatment MRIs with a mean interval of 11 months between scans. Antibody responders to AN1792 treatment had a significantly greater 11-month whole brain volume reduction, ventricular enlargement, and a nonsignificantly greater hippocampal volume reduction than placebo-treated patients, despite suggestive evidence of a cognitive benefit in the antibody responders—just the opposite of the predicted effect on MRI endpoints (Fox et al., 2005). Possible explanations for this seemingly paradoxical result on MRI endpoints include a treatment-related acceleration in neuronal loss, perhaps related to a subclinical meningoencephalitis in the treated patients, and which the researchers argued to be unlikely in the absence of even modestly accelerated cognitive decline; a treatment-related reduction in brain volume due to the removal of space-occupying amyloid-β plaques; and a treatment-related reduction in brain volume due to a shift in fluids from brain parenchyma to cerebrospinal fluid. For instance, it is well-known that the brain can shrink due to dehydration and steroid-induced reductions in brain tissue fluid (Mellanby and Reveley, 1982; Raskin et al., 1983; Zivadinov, 2005). As discussed in Section 4, treatments may have potentially confounding effects on MRI, FDG PET, fibrillar β-amyloid imaging, and other biomarker endpoints, making it important for researchers to anticipate and try to address these potential confounds in the design of the study and the interpretation of findings.

Mild Cognitive Impairment. Patients with amnestic MCI (and other prodromal AD syndromes) who subsequently convert to probable AD have smaller hippocampal and entorhinal cortex volumes and greater rates of hippocampal, entorhinal cortex, whole brain atrophy and ventricular enlargement, regional gray matter atrophy and cortical thinning, than those who remain stable during the same time-frame (Chételat et al., 2005; de Leon et al., 2006; Devanand et al., 2007; Jack et al., 2000, 2005; Killiany et al., 1993). Baseline MRI measurements thus offer the possibility of selecting or stratifying MCI participants in randomized clinical trials in randomized clinical trials of putative AD-slowing/secondary prevention therapies based on their estimated risk of subsequent cognitive decline and clinical conversion; and longitudinal MRI changes offer the possibility of decreasing the number of MCI participants and the duration of study in these clinical trials. Using volumetric MRI to provide secondary endpoints in a multicenter randomized clinical trial evaluating the effectiveness of vitamin E and donepezil in reducing rates of clinical progression to probable AD, patients in the active treatment groups did not differ significantly from those in the placebo groups in their annualized rates of change from baseline in hippocampal, enorhinal cortex, whole brain, or ventricular volume. These findings were consistent with the absence of significant treatment-related differences in the primary clinical endpoints (Jack et al., 2008).

Cognitively Normal Persons. MRI studies on aging reveal that with age there is greater hippocampal atrophy (de Leon et al., 1997), while the rate of ventricular volume expansion declines (Carlson et al., 2008). However, among those who subsequently develop cognitive impairment, MRI studies have noted that these individuals have greater medial temporal lobe, hippocampal, whole brain, and ventricular atrophy rates prior to declining (Carlson et al., 2008; de Leon et al., 1997; Jack et al., 2005; Rusinek et al., 2003). For those individuals at increased genetic risk for AD, with at least one copy of the APOE ε4 allele, MRI studies have noted accelerated cortical thining (Espeseth et al., 2008), lower gray matter density (Wishart et al., 2006), and accelerated brain atrophy rates (Chen et al., 2007). Gene dose is correlated with brain atrophy (Chen et al., 2007) and with a greater percent reduction in hippocampal volume in longitudinal studies (Jak et al., 2007).

Fibrillar Amyloid-β Imaging in the Early Detection and Tracking of AD

As detailed in Chapter 14, several promising PET methods have been developed for the assessment of fibrillar amyloid-β burden—a cardinal neuropathological feature of AD—in the living human brain (Cai et al., 2008; Furumoto et al., 2007; Kudo et al., 2007; Kung, 2004; Rowe et al., 2008). Researchers continue to evaluate these and other fibrillar amyloid-β imaging methods in terms of their utility for in vivo imaging, their sensitivity and specificity for fibrillar amyloid-β in animal models of AD and in living human participants, their test-retest reliability, the extent to which quantitative measurements could be confounded by alterations in radiotracer delivery, active or labeled metabolites, or competitive binding with other medications, and the best image-acquisition and image-analysis techniques to use in the effort to address different kinds of research and clinical questions. In the meantime, several of these imaging techniques have already begun to be used in the early detection and tracking of fibrillar amyloid-β burden in the living human brains of patients with AD and MCI, and cognitively normal persons at different ages, to clarify the extent to which in vivo measurements of fibrillar amyloid-β burden are related to subsequent post-mortem histopathology, to determine the extent to which the fibrillar amyloid-β burden in MCI patients predicts subsequent rates of progression to AD, and to determine the extent to which fibrillar amyloid-β burden in healthy older persons predicts subsequent rates of conversion to MCI or AD.

In addition, fibrillar amyloid-β imaging techniques are now being used to evaluate putative β-amyloid-modifying therapies in patients with AD. These studies could help determine the extent to which the putative treatments decrease fibrillar amyloid-β burden in these patients and the extent to which a treatment-related reduction in fibrillar amyloid-β predicts a better clinical outcome. Could these studies also be used to support or refute the amyloid cascade hypothesis of AD (i.e., that amyloid accumulation is in the causal pathway)? Yes and no. If a treatment-related reduction in fibrillar amyloid-β burden is shown to be associated with an improvement in clinical outcome, that finding would provide strong support for the amyloid cascade hypothesis. If, however, a treatment-related reduction in fibrillar amyloid-β burden is not found to be associated with an improvement in clinical outcome, it would beg the question: since fibrillar amyloid-β accumulates early in the course of AD, is not strongly correlated with dementia severity and has been postulated to play a relatively early role in the pathogenesis of AD, additional studies would be needed to determine if a reduction in fibrillar amyloid-β burden might be more strongly associated with an improved clinical outcome if the treatment were initiated at an earlier, perhaps even preclinical, stage of the disease. Further, since soluble amyloid-β levels are more strongly associated with neuronal loss than fibrillar amyloid-β (Lue et al., 1999; Selkoe, 2008), since certain soluble amyloid oligomers (studied in vitro but not yet directly assayed in the brain) may be especially neurotoxic (Glabe and Kayed, 2006), since some amyloid peptides may be relatively toxic and others may be relatively protective (Golde, 2007), and since some researchers have proposed that fibrillar amyloid-β might even protect neurons from the more toxic effects of soluble amyloid species (DeMattos et al., 2001), additional studies would need to assess the effects of different treatments on these soluble species. While fibrillar amyloid-β concentrations could exist in some sort of dynamic equilibrium with the concentrations of different soluble amyloid species concentrations, it is possible (but not certain) that fibrillar amyloid-β measures could provide an indirect measure of these soluble species.

It would be helpful to have other brain imaging measures of AD neuropathology, including more sensitive and specific measures of different soluble amyloid species, neurofibrillary pathology, and synaptic density. Meantime, fibrillar amyloid-β imaging techniques have extraordinary potential in the scientific understanding, early detection, and tracking of AD and in the evaluation of putative β-amyloid-modifying treatments. These techniques may also offer clinical value in the differential diagnosis of AD, providing information about the presence or absence of fibrillar amyloid-β, if they can be shown to accurately predict postmortem histopathology, rates of conversion from MCI to AD, or response to β-amyloid-modifying treatments, or if they could help guide clinical or preclinical management decisions in other meaningful ways.

To date, the most extensively validated and used imaging technique for the assessment of fibrillar amyloid-β burden utilizes PET, the ^{11}C-labeled radioligand Pittsburgh Compound B (PiB) (Klunk et al., 2004), and either semiquantitative measurements (e.g., cerebral-to-cerebellar "standardized uptake value ratios" [PiB SUVRs]) using a static image, or more quantitative measurements (e.g., cerebral-to-cerebellar PiB distribution volume ratios [PiB DVRs]) using images acquired dynamically during a longer scan. ^{11}C-PiB is now being used by a growing number of academic

sites and has been licensed to General Electric Healthcare for its potential use in diagnostic studies and clinical trials. A potential limitation of this radioligand and several others is its nonspecific binding to white matter and brainstem. Another potential limitation is its limited utility for the in vivo assessment of fibrillar amyloid-β burden in transgenic mouse models of AD using microPET, since the longitudinal assessment of fibrillar amyloid-β burden in these and other animal models could be used to help in the preclinical study of disease mechanisms and potential therapeutics. Despite these limitations, the introduction of PiB PET to the scientific community has already had an extraordinary impact on the field.

Other PET radioligands now being studied for the assessment of fibrillar amyloid-β burden, some of which are noted here. ^{18}F-FDDNP has been shown to bind fibrillar amyloid-β and neurofibrillary tangles (Small et al., 2002, 2006), and has been licensed to Siemens for its potential use in diagnostic studies and clinical trials. In comparison to PiB PET, FDDNP appears to provide significantly lower measures of fibrillar amyloid-β burden in AD cases, but greater sensitivity to the detection of subtle AD-related increases in the medial temporal lobe, perhaps reflecting neurofibrillary tangle pathology. It also binds to the pleated sheet structure of fibrillar amyloid-β at a different site than PiB PET, since this site competes with nonsteroidal antiinflammatory drugs (NSAIDs) (Agdeppa et al., 2003), raising the possibility that the use of NSAIDs could confound the interpretation of findings from diagnostic studies and clinical trials. Despite these limitations, FDDNP may prove to have complementary roles to play in some studies of AD and tauopathies. A number of ^{18}F-labeled PET amyloid-β imaging agents are also under development as described in Chapter 14, and these longer-lived radiotracers offer the potential for wider use than the short half-life ^{11}C-labeled tracers.

Alzheimer's Dementia. In patients with probable AD, PET measurements of fibrillar amyloid-β burden are especially prominent in the precuneus, parietal, temporal and frontal cortex, anterior and posterior cingulate cortex, and the striatum. Using PiB PET, regional measurements of fibrillar amyloid-β burden are highly correlated with subsequent postmortem measurements of fibrillar amyloid-β burden (Ikonomovic et al., 2008). Interestingly, they are also correlated with lower FDG PET measurements of regional CMRgl, particularly in parietal and temporal regions (Edison et al., 2007; Kemppainen et al., 2006; Klunk et al., 2004), and with MRI measurements of gray matter atrophy (Archer et al., 2006). Like neuropathological studies of patients with dementia, some imaging studies find significant correlations between clinical severity and fibrillar amyloid-β burden in some brain regions (Grimmer et al., in press), while other studies do not (Rowe et al., 2007). In a two-year follow-up study, fibrillar amyloid-β burden was correlated with dementia severity at baseline, but not at follow-up, and did not progress over time, suggesting that fibrillar amyloid-β is deposited and plateaus in the early clinical stages of AD (Engler et al., 2006). Even if fibrillar amyloid-β imaging does not turn out to provide an indicator of disease progression by the time AD patients have dementia, it still could be used to evaluate the effectiveness of treatments to reduce fibrillar amyloid burden—not unlike they way in which fibrillar amyloid-β histopathology has been used preclinically to evaluate the effectiveness of these treatments in transgenic mouse models of AD.

Mild Cognitive Impairment. In MCI patients, studies find that (on average) the mean measurement of fibrillar amyloid-β burden is intermediate between those of AD patients and normal controls. However, it has been suggested that most MCI patients have levels of fibrillar amyloid-β burden similar to either probable AD patients or normal controls, and that relatively few MCI patients have levels that are intermediate between these two groups and are likely to increase over time (Forsberg et al., 2008; Kemppainen et al., 2007; Small et al., 2006). The pattern of retention in the frontal, parietal, and temporal cortices and posterior cingulate is similar to the pattern observed in AD patients, particularly among MCI patients who convert to AD (Forsberg et al., 2008; Kemppainen et al., 2007). In one study, MCI patients with at least one APOE ε4 allele tended to have higher PiB retention (Kemppainen et al., 2007), which could reflect either an accelerated rate of fibrillar amyloid deposition in this MCI subgroup, or a higher proportion of clinically characterized MCI patients who have the neuropathological diagnosis of AD. Using FDDNP in a preliminary longitudinal study, those participants for whom there was clinical evidence of disease progression (normal to MCI or MCI to AD) had greater increases in FDDNP binding compared to stable participants (Small et al., 2006). Ongoing longitudinal PiB PET studies promise to help clarify the extent to which measures of amyloid-β burden predicts cognitive decline and development of AD.

Cognitively Normal Persons. Confirming findings from neuropathological studies, about 25% of persons over the age of 65—and even higher percentages of cognitively normal persons at older ages—have significant amyloid-β burden (Klunk et al., 2004; Mintun et al., 2006; Pike et al., 2007; Rowe et al., 2007). With the advent of imaging techniques, researchers have begun to determine the extent to which fibrillar amyloid-β burden in older normal persons predicts subsequent rates of cognitive decline and progression to MCI and AD. This imaging technique could also be used to exclude cognitively normal participants with significant amyloid-β burden in studies seeking to better characterize the cognitive, structural, and functional brain imaging changes associated with normal brain aging, independent of the potentially confounding effect of this preclinical form of AD neuropathology. In the meantime, PiB PET studies have been performed in cognitively normal young adults carrying an early-onset AD-causing gene, finding significant fibrillar amyloid-β burden years before the anticipated onset of dementia (Klunk et al., 2007), and we have begun to use PiB PET in our ongoing longitudinal study of cognitively normal late middle-aged and older persons with two copies, one copy, and no copies of the APOE ε4 allele. These studies promise to detect and track the earliest evidence of fibrillar amyloid-β deposition in persons at genetic risk for AD and hopefully permit the use of this and other complementary brain imaging measurements as surrogate endpoints for evaluating putative risk-reducing and prevention therapies in a randomized clinical trial without having to wait many years to determine whether or when the study participants progress to MCI or probable AD.

Section 4: Using Brain Imaging Methods in the Evaluation of Putative AD-slowing Therapies

In this section, we consider ways to use FDG PET, structural MRI, and fibrillar amyloid-β imaging methods in the evaluation of putative AD-slowing therapies. We consider some of the challenges in the use and interpretation of these brain imaging measurements in clinical trials. We note how ADNI will contribute to the use of these brain imaging and other biomarker and clinical measurements in multicenter clinical trials of putative AD-slowing treatments, and we propose several other strategies to help optimize the value of these imaging techniques in this endeavor.

Using Brain Imaging to Reduce the Number of Probable AD Patients and Time Needed to Evaluate Putative AD-Slowing Treatments

FDG PET and structural MRI provide information about AD progression, which can be used in patients with probable AD to evaluate the effectiveness of putative AD-slowing treatments with greater statistical power than clinical endpoints. In Phase 2 clinical trials, these imaging techniques could be used to evaluate the effectiveness of treatments for slowing down the progressive AD-related brain changes using fewer AD patients or shorter treatment durations. The proof-of-concept data could then help sponsors make strategic investment decisions about which putative AD-slowing treatments to take forward in large, time-consuming, and expensive multicenter clinical trials, using established clinical endpoints (along with the same imaging techniques in at least a subset of patients).

Fibrillar amyloid-β imaging techniques provide information about a cardinal neuropathological feature of AD. These techniques can be used to evaluate the effectiveness of putative β-amyloid-modifying treatments to reduce fibrillar amyloid-β burden, and perhaps slow the progression of amyloid-β burden if it has not already plateaued. In Phase 2 clinical trials, they would also provide information about the effectiveness of these treatments to influence a biological feature thought to be involved in AD pathogenesis, and probably do so using fewer AD patients and shorter treatment durations. The proof-of-concept data could then help sponsors make strategic investment decisions about which putative β-amyloid-modifying treatments to take forward in large, time-consuming, and expensive clinical trials using established clinical endpoints (along with the same imaging technique in at least a subset of patients).

Let us consider how to use FDG PET, structural MRI and fibrillar amyloid-β imaging in these and other clinical trials in a little more detail:

FDG PET. To date, FDG PET provides the best-established functional brain imaging of AD progression in patients with probable AD, patients with amnestic MCI, and cognitively normal APOE ε4 carriers with declines in posterior cingulate, precuneus, parietotemporal and frontal CMRgl (Chételat et al., 2003; Drzezga et al., 2003; Hoffman et al., 2000; Jagust et al., 1988; Mosconi et al., 2004; Reiman et al., 1996; Silverman et al., 2001; Small et al., 2000). For clinical trials of putative AD-slowing, risk-reducing, and prevention therapies, we recommend acquiring FDG PET measurements while participants are in the "resting state"—with eyes open or closed and directed forward, and without significant cognitive or sensory stimulation. There are two reasons for this: most longitudinal FDG PET studies of AD have been performed in the resting state, including the single-center and ongoing ADNI studies used to estimate the statistical power of this imaging technique in randomized clinical trials of putative AD-slowing treatments; and, in comparison to PET measurements acquired during the performance of a cognitive task, resting PET measurements of AD progression are more suitable for distinguishing between the effects of a disease-slowing treatment (slowing the decline in PET measurements of local neuronal activity over an extended period of time) versus a symptomatic treatment (which could be associated with increases in task-dependent measurements of local neuronal activity simply due to treatment-related improvements in task performance). Later, we suggest how the number and timing of

FDG PET scans, and the use of complementary imaging techniques, could help further distinguish a treatment's disease-slowing effects from its nondisease-related, state-dependent effects.

In clinical trials involving probable AD patients, regional FDG PET data are typically analyzed in units of PET counts after normalizing the images for the individual variation in absolute counts in the whole brain or a relatively spared region, such as the pons. Since probable AD patients have significant longitudinal CMRgl declines (in units of mg/min/100 g) in the whole brain, and even in regions that are relatively spared, we found that absolute measurements of regional CMRgl had better statistical power than normalized PET counts in characterizing AD progression and detecting AD-slowing effects (Alexander et al., 2002). Although we developed and routinely use a noninvasive technique to quantify CMRgl using dynamic PET scans and an image-derived carotid artery time-activity curve in our laboratory (Chen et al., 1998), relatively few ADNI PET sites were willing or able to implement this more time-consuming approach, suggesting that it may be more practical to analyze normalized PET counts in multicenter clinical trials. We currently recommend the FDG PET site-qualification, image-acquisition, and real-time image assessment, quality-assurance, and standardization procedures introduced by ADNI in the performance of multicenter clinical trials.

Using the declines in regional FDG PET measurements from 15 probable AD patients, we previously estimated the statistical power of FDG PET to evaluate the effectiveness of putative AD-slowing treatments in a 12-month, randomized, single-center, parallel-group, placebo-controlled clinical trial (Table 20.3a), and we suggested the testing of a putative AD-slowing treatment with approximately one-tenth the number of patients using clinical endpoints (Alexander et al., 2002). Using the declines in regional FDG PET measurements from up to 100 probable AD patients, we and our ADNI colleagues will estimate the statistical power of FDG PET to evaluate the effectiveness of putative AD-slowing treatments in 6-, 12-, and 24-month randomized, multicenter clinical trials. We and our colleagues in ADNI's PET Coordinating Center are characterizing and comparing the statistical power in tracking CMRgl declines and evaluating the effects of putative AD-slowing treatments in randomized clinical trials, thus attempting to determine the optimal image-analysis technique and regional measurements to use in these trials. We are currently using automated brain mapping algorithms (e.g., statistical parametric mapping [SPM] and stereotactic surface projection mapping), automatically defined ROIs or local maxima in predefined search regions, the number of voxels associated with significant CMRgl decline, and multivariate statistical characterization of the AD-related pattern of regional CMRgl decline.

Structural MRI. To date, the best-established structural MRI endpoints are AD-related declines in hippocampal, entorhinal cortex, and whole brain volume, an AD-related enlargement in ventricular volume, and AD-related declines in gray matter and cortical thickness (Bobinski et al., 1999; de Leon et al., 1989; Du et al., 2003, 2004; Jack et al., 1992, 1998, 2000; Juottonen et al., 1998; Rusinek et al., 1991; Visser et al., 1999). In clinical trials of putative AD-slowing, risk-reducing, and prevention therapies, we currently recommend using the same site qualification, MRI pulse sequences and orientation, quality-assurance procedures (although the value of the ADNI phantom currently remains to be clarified), and real-time image-quality assessment and control employed in ADNI randomized clinical trials. Structural MRIs now being acquired from the same ADNI participants using 1.5T and 3T systems will permit researchers to determine which of these imaging systems offers the best statistical power to track AD progression and evaluate AD-slowing treatments in randomized clinical trials using regional, whole brain, or voxel-based endpoints. Until the direct comparisons are performed, it remains possible that 3T will offer better statistical power using certain MRI endpoints (due to increased signal-to-noise), while 1.5T will offer better statistical power on other MRI endpoints (e.g., due increased susceptibility effects at higher fields on anterior temporal lobe measurements).

MRI measurements of hippocampal and entorhinal cortex volume are typically made using either labor-intensive manual methods or semi-automated methods (as in ADNI). MRI measurements of brain volume decline and ventricular enlargement are typically computed from sequential MRIs using the original semi-automated Brain Boundary Shift Integral (BBSI, as in ADNI) or using fully automated algorithms subsequently found to track AD progression with similar statistical power, such as the Iterative Principal Component Analysis (Chen et al., 2004). Researchers have previously reported comparable statistical power for tracking AD progression and evaluating the effects of putative AD-slowing treatments using MRI measurements of hippocampal, entorhinal cortex, and whole brain atrophy and ventricular enlargement (similar to PET) and much more powerful than clinical endpoints (power estimates using whole brain atrophy are shown in Table 20.3b). Based on a direct comparison of these particular measurements, it was suggested that changes in whole brain volume would be preferable to changes in hippocampal or entorhinal cortex volume as endpoints in randomized clinical trials, since those measurements can be made in a more automated fashion and were found to be more strongly associated with clinical decline in patients with probable AD (Jack et al., 2004). MRI measurements of regional gray matter atrophy are commonly made using a fully automated image-analysis strategy called "voxel-based morphometry" (VBM), typically using SPM and tissue-segmentation software. MRI measurements of decline in regional cortical thickness (i.e., "cortical thinning") are also most commonly made using a fully automated brain mapping software package (FreeSurfer). Using MRIs from up to 200 probable AD patients, researchers in ADNI's MRI Coordinating Center have begun to characterize and compare the statistical power of different MRI endpoints to evaluate the effectiveness of putative AD-slowing treatments in 6-, 12-, and (eventually) 24-month randomized, multicenter clinical trials. Again, the goal is to determine the optimal image-analysis technique and MRI measurements to use in these clinical trials.

As previously noted, the active amyloid-β immunization therapy AN1792 was associated with a seemingly paradoxical accelerated rate of whole brain volume and hippocampal volume decline in a clinical trial prematurely terminated due to serious adverse effects in some of the treated probable AD patients (Fox et al., 2005). This finding illustrates the importance of imbedding imaging endpoints in clinical trials to help confirm whether an effect on the imaging endpoint predicts a clinical outcome, and it highlights the need to anticipate and control for potentially confounding treatment effects on the imaging endpoint. Later, we suggest how the number and timing of MRIs and the use of complementary imaging techniques could help further distinguish a treatment's disease-slowing effects from its nondisease-related biological effects on MRI measurements, such as a treatment-related brain volume loss due to the shift of fluid to or from brain parenchyma, a brain volume loss due to the removal of space-occupying β-amyloid plaques, or a brain volume increase due to neuronal arborization unrelated to an effect on disease-progression. In the meantime, while we still recommend including structural MRI along with fibrillar amyloid-β imaging, we would currently recommend using FDG PET over MRI as the prioritized imaging endpoint in randomized clinical trials of putative β-amyloid-modifying treatments to minimize the potentially modality-specific confounding effects of these particular AD-slowing treatments, and thus maximize the chance that the treatment's effect on the imaging endpoint will predict a clinical benefit. We discuss our rationale for use of complementary imaging endpoints (e.g., fibrillar amyloid-β imaging, MRI and PET in the study of putative β-amyloid-modifying treatments) below.

Fibrillar Amyloid-β Imaging. Fibrillar amyloid-β imaging techniques provide an unprecedented chance to directly assess the effects of putative β-amyloid-modifying treatments on fibrillar amyloid-β burden, help bridge the gap between preclinical treatment studies in animal models of amyloid-β neuropathology and clinical trials in AD patients, and determine the extent to which reductions in the magnitude or progression of fibrillar amyloid-β burden predict clinical benefits at different presymptomatic and symptomatic stages of AD.

To date, the best-established fibrillar amyloid-β imaging technique is ^{11}C-PiB PET (Ikonomovic et al., 2008; Klunk et al., 2005). Using PiB PET (and other fibrillar amyloid-β radioligands), amyloid-β burden can be measured in voxel-based comparisons, gray matter regions of interest, or the whole brain, with the greatest differences between patient and control groups found in posterior cingulate, precuneus, parietal, and frontal cortex. As described in Chapter 14, simplified quantitative methods appear to provide reliable and valid measures of tracer uptake that are appropriate for large-scale multicenter clinical trials. Researchers continue to evaluate the optimal data analysis strategy (e.g., using some combination of manually or automatically defined gray matter ROIs or local maxima in predefined search regions) for characterizing the progression or test-retest variability of fibrillar amyloid-β measurements in probable AD patients, MCI patients, and cognitively normal persons at risk for AD—information that could be used to help inform the use of PiB PET in the evaluation of AD-slowing, risk-reducing, and primary prevention therapies.

Which fibrillar amyloid-β imaging technique should one use in a clinical trial? ^{11}C-PiB PET is the best-studied and most extensively used fibrillar amyloid-β imaging technique, but may not be available to some PET sites sufficiently close to a PiB-producing radiotracer synthesis or distribution site, potentially limiting the number of clinical sites able to participate in a multicenter study. While ^{18}F-labeled ligands have the potential to overcome this challenge, they need to be further studied—preferably in head-to-head comparisons with each other and ^{11}C-PiB—in terms of their specificity for fibrillar amyloid-β (and not, for instance, white matter), their AD case-control discrimination and test-retest variability, the accuracy of fully or simplified quantitative measurements, and the resistance of these measurements to potential confounds like competitive binding with other drugs to fibrillar amyloid-β imaging sites and any disease- or treatment-related alterations in cerebral blood flow/radiotracer delivery. Some general questions to ask in selecting the fibrillar amyloid-β technique to use in a clinical trial include:

- How well has it been studied?
- Has it been compared to the alternative fibrillar imaging techniques?

- Will it be readily available and easy to use at the relevant clinical trial sites?
- Is the radiotracer-licensing organization sufficiently supportive and committed to a clinical trial's needs and goals?

Researchers continue to determine the extent to which imaging measurements of fibrillar amyloid-β burden are progressive or stable in probable AD patients, MCI patients, and normal persons at different levels of genetic risk for AD, and its test-retest variability over different time frames. Their findings could be used to estimate the number of participants needed to evaluate the effectiveness of putative β-amyloid-modifying treatments in slowing the progression or reducing the magnitude of fibrillar amyloid-β burden. Researchers also continue to test different kinds of β-amyloid-modifying treatments in animal models of amyloid-β pathology, and they have begun to test some of these treatments in Phase 2 and Phase 3 clinical trials. Their findings could be used to estimate the time needed to observe the significant effects of treatment on fibrillar amyloid-β burden.

Using Brain Imaging Measurements to Reduce the Number of Amnestic MCI Patients and Time Needed to Evaluate Putative AD-slowing Treatments

As previously noted, it is practically difficult to conduct randomized clinical trials of putative AD-slowing treatments in patients with amnestic MCI using rates of progression to probable AD as one of the clinical endpoints, since it would require unusually large numbers of patients and a treatment duration typically exceeding three years (with associated compliance and attrition problems) (Petersen et al., 2005). For this reason, there is increasing interest in the use of brain imaging measurements as surrogate endpoints to markedly reduce the number of patients, and time needed to evaluate putative disease-slowing effects in these patients—possibly leading to an indication for "very mild AD." Indeed, ADNI has placed particular emphasis on the longitudinal study of patients with amnestic MCI for this very reason, with 400 patients being followed every six months for up to three years using volumetric MRI, half of these patients being followed with FDG PET and a smaller proportion followed with PiB PET. These and other studies around the world are poised to characterize and compare the statistical power of MRI and FDG PET measurements, and the image-analysis techniques used to track disease progression and how these longitudinal declines predict rates of subsequent cognitive decline and clinical progression to probable AD. These and other studies using PiB PET and other fibrillar amyloid-β imaging techniques will determine the extent to which imaging measurements of fibrillar amyloid-β burden are progressive or stable in amnestic MCI patients, estimate their power to detect fibrillar β-amyloid-reducing and slowing effects, and determine the extent to which baseline measurements or any longitudinal increases in fibrillar amyloid-β burden predict rates of subsequent cognitive decline and clinical progression to probable AD.

In Phase 2 clinical trials of putative AD-slowing treatments in patients with amnestic MCI, these imaging techniques can be used as surrogate endpoints to provide information about the extent to which a putative AD-slowing treatment slows the measurement of disease progression, and the extent to which putative β-amyloid-modifying treatments reduce or slow the progression of fibrillar amyloid-β deposition. The proof-of-concept data could then help sponsors make strategic investment decisions about which putative β-amyloid-modifying treatments to take forward in very large, time-consuming, and expensive clinical trials, using clinical endpoints like rates of clinical progression to probable AD along with the same imaging techniques in at least a subset of patients.

In sufficiently large and long-lasting Phase 3 clinical trials, these imaging techniques should be included along with continuous cognitive and functional endpoints (which still need to be further developed and tested), and rates of progression to probable AD. Although we think that regulatory agencies might require the trials to demonstrate that the treatment reduces rates of clinical progression to probable AD at this time, the imaging endpoints could be used to provide supportive evidence of an AD-slowing effect. More importantly, by demonstrating that the effectiveness of one or more AD-slowing treatments on the imaging endpoints predicts subsequent rates of conversion to probable AD, this information could help regulatory agencies support the use of imaging endpoints as "reasonably likely" surrogate endpoints in Phase 3 clinical trials of other putative AD-slowing treatments in the pipeline. At that point (which has not yet arrived), it would be possible to conduct Phase 3 clinical trials in fewer amnestic MCI patients and over much shorter treatment durations (i.e., without waiting for progression to AD in a sufficient number of patients to evaluate a treatment under Accelerated Approval provisions). We discuss the issue of adequately validating imaging techniques as reasonably likely surrogate endpoints later in this section.

Using Baseline Brain Imaging Measurements to Select Research Participants for Enrollment in Clinical Trials of Putative AD-slowing Treatments

In addition to using sequential brain imaging techniques to provide endpoints in clinical trials of putative AD-slowing treatments, baseline imaging measurements can be used to help select research participants for enrollment or subgroup analyses in clinical trials of putative AD-slowing treatments.

First, baseline brain imaging measurements (alone or in combination with other information) could help enrich studies for those patients most likely to show brain imaging and/or clinical evidence of AD progression during the trial. For instance, baseline FDG PET or MRI measurements could be used to select those MCI patients at highest risk for AD progression, further reducing the number of patients and duration of treatment needed to evaluate a putative AD-slowing treatment's effectiveness using imaging endpoints in Phase 2 clinical trials, clinical endpoints, or both. Second, baseline brain imaging measurements (alone or in combination with other information) could help enrich studies for those patients most likely to respond to a particular treatment. For instance, baseline PiB PET measurements could be used to select those amnestic MCI patients with significant fibrillar amyloid-β burden in a trial of a putative β-amyloid-modifying treatment. Because an estimated 30% of MCI patients who subsequently progress to dementia do not meet neuropathological criteria for AD (Jicha et al., 2006), this subject-enrichment strategy could be used to identify patients most likely to respond to a treatment specifically targeting AD pathology. Assuming that MCI patients show accelerated AD progression (Petersen et al., 1999), it could lead to an even further reduction in the number of patients and duration of treatment needed to evaluate the treatment's effectiveness using FDG PET, MRI, and clinical endpoints.

As noted, the potential advantages of using baseline images to select research participants in clinical trials include (1) identification of those individuals most likely to demonstrate a treatment effect, and (2) greater statistical power, fewer participants, less time, and less money to conduct the trial. The potential disadvantages of this or other enrichment strategies include (1) favoring inclusion of more severely afflicted patients, in whom certain treatments (e.g., β-amyloid-modifying treatments) may turn out to be less effective, (2) restricting findings (and the potential drug product indication) to only a subset of clinically characterized patients, and (3) restricting findings (and the potential drug product indication) to those patients who have been clinically evaluated using imaging as a companion diagnostic test. On the flip side, we believe the most compelling way to secure approval for an imaging agent (e.g., a fibrillar amyloid-β imaging radioligand) in the diagnosis of AD would be to show in clinical trials that baseline imaging measurements can be used to identify those individuals most likely to respond to a particular AD-slowing treatment.

Second, baseline imaging measurements (alone or in combination with other information) could be used at the time of data analysis (although the data analysis plan should be formally described before initiating the study), to investigate the differential effect of treatment in different subgroups—not knowing which of the groups might be most responsive to treatment. We refer to this strategy as "pre-analytical subgroup stratification" to distinguish it from the "pre-randomization subgroup stratification" strategy noted below. For instance, clinical trials evaluating the effectiveness of putative AD-slowing, risk-reducing, or prevention therapies in probable AD patients, amnestic MCI patients, or cognitively normal persons might not choose to exclude patients based on the presence of absence fibrillar amyloid-β pathology, but might perform secondary analyses to characterize and compare the effects of treatment in those above or below a designated level of fibrillar amyloid-β. In cognitively normal persons at genetic risk for AD, for instance, it is possible that those individuals with more fibrillar amyloid-β are preferentially responsive to a β-amyloid-modifying prevention therapy, since the treatment is targeting this pathology. But it is also possible that those individuals with less amyloid-β pathology are preferentially responsive to a β-amyloid-modifying prevention therapy, since this treatment may be most effective in the earliest preclinical stages of the disease. Advantages of this secondary analysis strategy include (1) the chance to empirically determine whether one or both subgroups are responsive to treatment, (2) the chance to generalize treatment benefits to more patients and without the aid of a companion imaging assessment if it works in the overall group, and (3) the chance to further demonstrate the value of imaging in the diagnosis of AD by showing how it can be used to guide important treatment decisions. Disadvantages include the need for (1) more participants, some of whom do not have AD, and (2) more time and more money to conduct the clinical trial than one using the enrichment strategy noted above.

Third, baseline imaging measurements (alone or in combination with other information) could be used to stratify research participants into two subgroups prior to treatment randomization (i.e., "pre-randomization subgroup stratification") to ensure having enough participants in each group to evaluate a treatment's effectiveness on imaging endpoints, clinical endpoints, or both in each of the two subgroups. This approach would offer the same advantages as those noted using the subgroup analysis strategy, and it would ensure having adequate statistical power to evaluate the putative treatment in each subgroup, even if one of the subgroups is relatively uncommon (e.g., cognitively normal persons with significant amyloid-β pathology in the evaluation of a putative prevention therapy). The main disadvantage would be the need to screen or enroll additional participants to make sure that a sufficient number of participants are enrolled in the less-common group.

Several studies have already suggested how certain MRI and FDG PET measurements could predict subsequent rates of progression to AD in patients with amnestic MCI, how FDG PET could predict subsequent rates of clinical progression and the neuropathological diagnosis of AD in patients with mild dementia somewhat better than a clinical evaluation, and the promise of fibrillar amyloid-β imaging in the assessment of this form of AD pathology (Chételat et al., 2005; Drzezga et al., 2005; Ikonomovic et al., 2008; Jack et al., 2005; Mosconi et al., 2004). Using data from the ADNI and other studies around the world, it may be possible to select the best ways in which to use baseline imaging measurements, alone or in combination with other information, to predict AD pathology and progression.

Using Brain Imaging Measurements of AD Progression and Neuropathology to Provide Substantial Evidence of a Treatment's AD-modifying Effectiveness

In Phase 2 clinical trials, FDG PET, structural MRI, and fibrillar amyloid-β imaging techniques could be used (as previously noted) to provide preliminary information about a treatment's AD-modifying effects. Fibrillar amyloid-β imaging could be used to evaluate the treatment's effects on this particular form of AD pathology, while FDG PET and MRI could provide complementary information about the treatment's effects on downstream measures of disease progression (e.g., indirect measures of synaptic and neuronal loss). In Phase 2 trials, imaging endpoints could be used for nonregulatory purposes as a surrogate for clinical endpoints, seeking to provide preliminary evidence of a treatment's AD-modifying effectiveness with fewer probable AD or MCI patients, less time, and lower costs. Alternatively, imaging endpoints could be used as a complement to clinical endpoints in patients with probable AD, seeking to provide both biological and clinical evidence of the treatment's effectiveness, and also seeking to demonstrate a strong relationship between the treatment's effects on brain imaging and clinical endpoints. This more ambitious clinical trial strategy would require more patients, time (for enrollment and possible treatment), and money to demonstrate a significant effect on clinical endpoints in a study of probable AD patients, and may be impractical in a Phase 2 clinical trial of MCI patients.

In Phase 3 clinical trials, we strongly recommend the complementary use of fibrillar amyloid-β imaging, FDG PET, structural MRI, and clinical endpoints to evaluate a putative AD-slowing treatment's effectiveness. We recommend fibrillar amyloid-β imaging to evaluate those treatments postulated to target this early form of AD pathology—FDG PET and MRI—to evaluate the effectiveness of putative β-amyloid-modifying treatments and other putative AD-slowing treatments on downstream measures of disease progression, and clinical endpoints to provide sufficient evidence of the treatment's effectiveness to merit regulatory agency approval.

The question is why would we use multiple imaging and other biomarker endpoints to evaluate the treatment's disease-slowing effectiveness. The following are several reasons for this:

- To provide converging evidence in support of a putative treatments' AD-modifying effects.
- To help overcome the possibility of imaging modality-specific confounding treatment effects (e.g., the modality-specific effects of an β-amyloid-modifying treatment on MRI measurements of brain volume unrelated to its effects on neuronal loss or the modality-specific effects of treatment on brain metabolism unrelated to synaptic loss). In hindsight, for instance, it would have been helpful to have included FDG PET measurements to evaluate an effect of the first β-amyloid immunization therapy on disease progression in the face of the treatment's unanticipated effects on MRI measurements of brain volume (Fox et al., 2005).

- To address different questions, such the treatment's effect on fibrillar amyloid-β versus its effects on downstream pathology more closely correlated with clinical severity.
- To provide the data needed to demonstrate a strong relationship between an effective treatment's effects on imaging measurements and its effects on other clinical progression, providing increasing support for the use of imaging techniques as "at least reasonably likely" surrogate endpoints in the study of other promising AD-slowing, risk-reducing, and prevention therapies.

A treatment's effects on fibrillar amyloid-β burden alone may not be sufficient to predict a clinical benefit if (a) the treatment is started too late in the pathological cascade, or (b) does not address the full range of pathogenic events (e.g., certain soluble amyloid species or other pathogenic mechanisms). Suppose one demonstrated an effect of a treatment on amyloid-β burden but failed to detect a significant clinical response in AD patients simply because the treatment was started too late in the illness. Now suppose the same treatment is shown to have an effect on fibrillar amyloid-β in MCI and is subsequently shown to predict lower rates of progression to probable AD. We are not convinced that regulatory agencies will approve this or any other β-amyloid-modifying treatment as a disease-slowing, risk-reducing, or primary prevention therapy on the basis of an amyloid-β imaging surrogate alone in the face of this conflicting evidence. Now suppose the first study included a complementary downstream measure of disease progression like FDG PET in both of these trials, and it was shown that the treatment's effect on both endpoints was needed to predict a clinical benefit. In this instance, we suggest that regulatory agencies would find the evidence from the complementary imaging endpoints more compelling as a dual surrogate outcome measure, and that the evidence would become more compelling as additional β-amyloid-modifying treatments are shown to have the same association.

In addition to using complementary imaging endpoints to help overcome potentially confounding effects of a treatment's effects on FDG PET and MRI endpoints unrelated to disease-progression, we recommend the inclusion of additional scans shortly after the treatment is initiated or discontinued (e.g., after a two- to three-month interval, or based on information about when the treatment is likely to reach a pharmokinetic and pharmacodynamic steady state) or at both of these time points. If the treatment causes an effect on the imaging endpoint (e.g, regional metabolism or brain volume) over the treatment interval, it is unlikely to be related to disease progression. If there is no significant short-term effect on the imaging endpoint, we would suggest using the baseline image as a reference image for assessment of a subsequent disease-slowing effect. If, however, there is a significant effect on the imaging endpoint, we would suggest using the first image acquired upon treatment as the reference image for assessment of a subsequent disease-slowing effect. Alternatively, one could use the pretreatment and post-discontinuation images—or all four images (at baseline, early treatment, late treatment, and discontinuation)—to minimize potentially confounding effects of treatment on the imaging endpoint. The main limitations of this strategy include uncertainties in the timing of the early initiation or discontinuation scans, and in knowing how much of the treatment effect unrelated to disease progression is addressed by this strategy.

Finally, we recommend the acquisition of preclinical information, when feasible, to help address these potential confounds. For instance, we would consider acquiring serial MRIs to examine the time course of a β-amyloid-modifying treatment's effect on brain volume in a transgenic mouse model of fibrillar amyloid-β pathology to help address the confounding effects of treatment unrelated to neuronal loss—seeking to determine how to schedule and analyze MRIs in a way that overcomes this potential confound in subsequent clinical trials. We would also consider competitive binding studies to help exclude the possibility that a putative β-amyloid-modifying treatment's effects on fibrillar amyloid-β might be attributable to competitive binding between the treatment and PET radioligand rather than on amyloid-β burden itself.

Challenges and Potential Solutions to the Use of Imaging in Clinical Trials

While brain imaging measurements offer great promise in the evaluation of putative AD-slowing, risk-reducing, and prevention therapies, there are several lingering challenges associated with their acquisition, analysis, and interpretation. Here we briefly consider some of the challenges and uncertainties and suggest several strategies to at least partly address them.

Challenge 1: Putative AD treatments could have effects on brain imaging endpoints unrelated to their effects on disease progression or pathology, which unless anticipated and properly addressed, could compromise their value as surrogate endpoints in the evaluation of AD-modifying treatments. Let us consider four examples of how a treatment could be associated with potentially confounding effects on brain imaging measurements of AD progression or pathology, and suggest strategies to at least partly address them (some of these confounds were already mentioned, but bear repeating here).

In two studies, acetylcholinesterase inhibitors—thought by most investigators to improve symptoms by bolstering cholinergic neurotransmission independent of significant AD-slowing effects—have been associated with short-term increases in regional PET measurements, perhaps possibly reflecting treatment-related increases in brain function and cognition unrelated to an effect on disease progression (Mega et al., 2001, 2005). Strategies are needed to distinguish between a treatment's purely symptomatic effects and disease-slowing effects on functional brain imaging endpoints (e.g., a compensatory increase in FDG PET measurements of neuronal activity in cognitively relevant brain regions). While not as widely recognized, we suggest that similar strategies are also needed to distinguish between a treatment's purely symptomatic effects and the disease-slowing effects on structural brain imaging endpoints (e.g., a compensatory increase in MRI measurements of gray matter density or cortical thickness related to the arborization of neurons in cognitively relevant brain regions). As previously noted, we suggest that these potential confounds could be at least partly addressed using (1) complementary brain imaging endpoints to overcome modality-specific confounding effects, and (2) additional scans shortly after the initiation or discontinuation of treatment to help distinguish a treatment's AD-slowing effects, from either of its compensatory or AD-reversing effects, and other potentially confounding treatments on imaging endpoints.

In the previously discussed (prematurely terminated) study of the first active amyloid-β immunization therapy, antibody responders had increased rates of decline in whole brain and hippocampal volume, which were not associated with cognitive decline (Fox et al., 2005). The authors attribute their findings to an unanticipated effect of β-amyloid-modifying treatment on MRI measurements unrelated to the postulated causal pathway (i.e., direct or indirect reductions in brain volume secondary to the clearance of amyloid-β plaques). Strategies are needed to use brain imaging measurements of AD-progression (in addition to fibrillar amyloid-β measurements) in the evaluation of putative β-amyloid-modifying treatments in clinical trials independent of their potentially confounding effects on brain volume. As previously noted, we suggest using (1) FDG PET to complement MRI, providing the prioritized brain imaging measurement of AD progression in the evaluation of putative β-amyloid-modifying treatments; (2) additional MRIs shortly after the initiation or discontinuation of treatment to help distinguish between a treatment's AD-slowing effects and its (probably) more immediate effects on brain volume unrelated to AD progression on MRI endpoints; and (3) MRI in preclinical studies of β-amyloid-modifying treatments in transgenic mouse models of fibrillar amyloid-β pathology to help clarify the nature and time course of this potentially confounding effect, helping to salvage MRI in the evaluation of these promising treatments.

The same investigators who developed the PET radioligand FDDNP for the evaluation of fibrillar amyloid-β and tau burden subsequently demonstrated competition between FDDNP and NSAIDs at fibrillar amyloid-β binding sites (Agdeppa et al., 2003) (the fibrillar amyloid-β binding sites for FDDNP and NSAIDs appear to be different than those for PiB). In addition to providing information about the neurobiological effects of NSAIDs, this finding provides information about the potentially confounding effect of NSAIDs on FDDNP PET measurements of fibrillar amyloid-β burden. In the absence of this important preclinical information, FDNNP PET studies could have caused researchers to interpret an NSAID treatment-related reduction in FDNNP PET measurements as evidence of this treatment's effectiveness in reducing fibrillar amyloid-β or tau burden, whether or not it actually had a fibrillar amyloid-β or tau-reducing effect. For this reason, we recommend in vitro studies to demonstrate the absence of significant competition between investigational β-amyloid-modifying treatments and the imaging radioligand at fibrillar amyloid-β binding sites prior to the use of the fibrillar amyloid-β imaging technique in clinical trials.

d) As previously noted, clinical trials of putative β-amyloid-modifying treatments in patients with probable AD might find a significant treatment-related reduction in PET measurements of fibrillar amyloid-β burden, while failing to show significant effects on clinical outcome simply because the treatment started too late for it to work. This possibility is supported by both preclinical studies (Head et al., 2008), the modest or inconsistent correlations between fibrillar amyloid-β burden and severity of cognitive impairment in patients with probable AD (Engler et al., 2006; Katzman et al., 1988), and the relatively early role amyloid-β accumulation has been postulated to play in the pathogenesis of AD (Hardy and Selkoe, 2002). As previously noted, we strongly recommend anticipating the possibility of a dissociation between an β-amyloid-modifying treatment's effects on fibrillar amyloid-β and clinical endpoints, and use complementary imaging (and other biomarker) measurements of AD progression (e.g., FDG PET) to provide information on imaging endpoints most likely to predict a clinical benefit.

Challenge 2: Optimizing the statistical power of brain imaging methods in the evaluation of β-amyloid-modifying and other putative AD-slowing treatments. We previously considered advantages, disadvantages, and complementary roles of the three best-established brain imaging modalities for the assessment of AD neuropathology and disease progression, and we encouraged the use of multiple imaging modalities to evaluate β-amyloid-modifying and other putative disease-slowing treatments in the most compelling way. We also suggested the value of acquiring FDG PET (and other functional imaging measurements) in the "resting state," independent of cognitive task performance in order to minimize potentially confounding effects of treatment on task-changes in regional CMRgl unrelated to AD progression itself. In addition, we briefly considered the data analysis strategies used to analyze these images, and noted the longitudinal data now being acquired to help determine the number of research participants and the time needed to evaluate putative AD-slowing, risk-reducing, and prevention therapies with adequate statistical power. Still, several uncertainties remain about the image-acquisition protocols, real-time quality-assurance procedures, and image-analysis techniques needed to evaluate these investigational treatments with the greatest statistical power in multicenter and single-center clinical trials.

The AD Neuroimaging Initiative. In 2004, researchers launched a 5-year, $60 million study known as the AD Neuroimaging Initiative (ADNI), with financial support from the National Institute of Health (NIH), the NIH Foundation, and interested industry partners (Mueller et al., 2005a, 2005b)—an unprecedented funding arrangement that reflects the interest of all AD stakeholders in the use of imaging and other biomarker endpoints in the evaluation of investigational AD-slowing treatments. This precedent-setting initiative is primarily intended to inform the design and performance of multicenter clinical trials seeking to evaluate putative AD-slowing treatments in patients with probable AD and MCI, and it has inspired similar initiatives in Europe, Australia, and Japan. The study is designed to: acquire serial 3T MRI, 1.5T MRI, FDG PET, and PiB PET images, CSF, blood, and urine samples (for predetermined and future biomarker measurements), neuropsychological measurements, and clinical ratings in probable AD, amnestic MCI, and elderly normal controls from 58 clinical sites with specified site qualification criteria; acquire these data, imaging phantom data, and biological specimens using carefully developed, standardized protocols (to maximize the comparability of MRI and PET images acquired on systems from different manufacturers); further ensure the comparability of brain images using centralized, real-time image quality assurance, quality control, and image prepreprocessing procedures; perform a limited number of analyses; and make all privacy-protected data and selected biological specimens publicly available for other analyses. Approximately two hundred probable AD patients, 400 MCI patients, and 200 elderly normal controls are studied using 1.5T MRI, blood and urine samples, neuropsychological tests, and clinical ratings every six months for two to three years (with modest differences in the imaging schedule and study duration depending on the subject group). Half of these participants are also studied using 3T MRI or FDG PET or both, 96 of the originally enrolled participants are now being studied using ^{11}C-PiB PET, and more than half of the participants agreed to have lumbar punctures for CSF specimens at their baseline and 12-month follow-up visits.

How will ADNI help in the design and performance of multi-center clinical trials of putative AD-slowing treatments? First, it has already developed and successfully implemented the protocols used to acquire 1.5T MRI, 3T MRI, FDG PET, and PiB PET images in a standardized way, helping to account for differences among imaging systems, and demonstrating comparability in the quality of images on most, but not all, of the imaging systems assessed. Second, it has already developed and successfully implemented the site qualification, real-time quality assurance, image pre-processing, and centralized data management procedures needed

to provide high-quality data. Third, it has demonstrated the feasibility of collecting CSF samples in a high proportion of study participants. Fourth, it has already begun to provide data and specimens for the early detection and tracking of AD. Fifth, it provides the means to evaluate promising new image analysis techniques and biomarker measurements, comparing them to existing methods and measurements in the early detection and tracking of AD. Perhaps most important, ADNI researchers have begun to characterize and directly compare different imaging methods, data analysis methods, and biomarkers in their ability to distinguish subject groups, their ability to predict rates of cognitive decline and clinical progression from MCI to probable AD, and their statistical power to evaluate putative β-amyloid-modifying and disease-slowing treatments in multicenter clinical trials. It will be less useful in estimating the statistical power of these methods to evaluate these treatments in single-center clinical trials.

In the meantime, uncertainties currently remain regarding (1) the number of probable AD or MCI patients and the time needed to evaluate β-amyloid-modifying and other putative disease-slowing patients in multicenter and single-center clinical trials; (2) the choice between 1.5T and 3T in these studies; (3) the PET and MRI image-analysis techniques with the best statistical power for detecting AD-slowing effects; (4) the extent to which fibrillar amyloid-β imaging measurements are stable or progressive; (5) the extent to which additional scans during the course of a clinical trial or prerandomization changes in brain imaging measurements will improve the statistical power to detect AD-slowing effects even further; (6) the extent to which data from different imaging techniques and other data can be used in combination to predict subsequent clinical decline, and evaluate putative AD-slowing treatments with even greater power; (7) the extent to which different imaging measurements are responsive to treatment effects; (8) the extent to which imaging system hardware changes (e.g., a new MRI head coil or imaging system change) compromise the power of AD-modifying treatment effects; and (9) studies still need to clarify the rates of change in brain imaging measurements at different clinical and preclinical stages of AD so that the correct regional measurements and statistical power estimates can be tailored to the research participants to be included in the clinical trials.

We believe that the statistical power of brain imaging measurements for tracking the progression of AD and evaluate putative AD-slowing treatments would be improved by using just one MRI system and one PET system and ensuring no hardware changes during the course of a clinical trial. We recognize practical challenges in minimizing hardware changes (especially MRI upgrades) at most academic imaging centers, and we acknowledge the possibility that some imaging measurements may be more resilient than others. Still, we have been actively exploring the means to enroll hundreds of research participants per year at a single location, conducting an entire Phase 2 clinical trial of a putative disease-slowing, risk-reducing, or prevention therapy on a single MRI system and single PET imaging system, and aiming to avoid any imaging system hardware changes during the course of the clinical trial.

Section 5: Using Brain Imaging Methods to Evaluate Putative AD Risk-Reducing and Prevention Therapies as Quickly as Possible

As previously noted, it currently takes too much money, too many healthy volunteers, and too many years to evaluate the effectiveness of putative AD risk-reducing and prevention therapies using clinical endpoints. As previously noted, we have been using FDG PET, MRI, and most recently PiB PET every two years to characterize and compare the progressive changes in regional CMRgl, brain volume, and fibrillar amyloid-β burden in initially late middle-aged, cognitively normal APOE ε4 homozygotes, heterozygotes, and noncarriers. We have shown APOE ε4 gene dose-related regional reductions in baseline CMRgl (Figure 20.5a), two-year CMRgl declines (Figure 20.5b), and two-year rates of whole brain atrophy (Chen et al., 2007). We predict that we will find APOE ε4 gene dose-related, progressive increases in fibrillar amyloid-β burden, and we predict that the baseline differences and two-year changes in these brain imaging measurements predict subsequent rates of cognitive decline and conversion to MCI and probable AD.

Also as noted, we have characterized two-year regional CMRgl declines in our cognitively normal, late middle-aged APOE ε4 heterozygotes (who represent about one-fourth of the population and about one-third of those with a reported first-degree family history of probable AD (Corder et al., 1993)) (Figure 20.6), and used these declines to estimate the number of ε4 heterozygotes needed to evaluate putative AD risk-reducing and primary prevention therapies in a two-year, randomized, parallel group, placebo-controlled trial (Table 20.4). Using FDG PET, MRI, and fibrillar amyloid-β imaging, we are planning to study at least one promising AD risk-reducing or prevention therapy every three years, with the ambitious but hopefully achievable aim of providing reasonably likely evidence of an effective risk-reducing or prevention therapy within twelve years. We have proposed the use of brain imaging measurements as surrogate endpoints to evaluate these treatments as quickly as possible in cognitively normal persons at increased genetic risk for AD (Reiman et al., 2001a, 2001b).

Here we consider those cognitively normal at-risk groups for the evaluation of putative AD risk-reducing and prevention therapies, how to handle information about the participants' risk (e.g., issue of genetic risk disclosure, as well as a strategy to support study participation without the need for genetic risk disclosure), issues to consider in the selection of a putative risk-reducing or prevention therapy for investigation, and a research strategy to help validate imaging endpoints such that a treatment's effects on the surrogate endpoints are at least reasonably likely to predict a clinical benefit. Finally, we suggest public policy changes to make the identification of effective putative AD-risk reducing and prevention therapies an urgent priority.

Which cognitively normal persons to consider in proof-of-concept primary prevention studies using brain imaging end-points?

APOE ε4 Heterozygtoes: We originally proposed the study of cognitively normal late middle-aged APOE ε4 heterozygotes (e.g., persons with the ε3/ε4 genotype) in prevention trials (using FDG PET as the primary imaging endpoint, but also including MRI, fibrillar amyloid-β imaging, and CSF biomarkers), since these individuals are widely available for study, have been characterized by us in terms of the number of participants needed to evaluate treatment effects in a two-year clinical trial, and findings from this group would be generalizable to a relatively large population of at-risk persons. The age range to include in a prevention study would depend, in part, on the treatment under investigation (e.g., about 50–65 years old for those treatments thought to be most effective in late-middle-age), and the interest in relating brain imaging changes to cognitive decline to help validate the imaging techniques at surrogate endpoints (e.g., closer to the estimated

median age of 75 at dementia onset). We would also suggest preanalytical stratification (but not pre-enrollment enrichment or stratification) on the basis of fibrillar amyloid-β burden.

APOE ε4 Homozygotes: We would also consider the study of cognitively normal late middle-aged APOE ε4 homozygotes (i.e., persons with the ε4/ε4 genotype) in prevention trials—again, using FDG PET as the primary imaging endpoint, but also including MRI, fibrillar amyloid-β imaging, and CSF biomarkers. Although these individuals are less widely available for study, and findings from their study would be generalizable to a smaller percentage of people—about 2%–3% of the population and 5% of those with a reported first-degree family history of probable AD (Corder et al., 1993)—they are at especially high genetic risk for AD. First, they might be especially suitable for the study of investigational β-amyloid-modifying and risk-reducing treatments relatively soon after the treatments have been evaluated for their safety and tolerability in Phase 3 clinical trials of probable AD patients, given the balance between uncertainties about the treatment's adverse effects and potential benefits. Second, they might be especially well-suited for relating a treatment's effects on imaging endpoints to subsequent rates of cognitively decline, and helping to validate brain imaging measurements of fibrillar AD pathology and AD progression as surrogate endpoints. Third, brain imaging data from a longitudinal study could be used to estimate the number of ε4 homozygotes to include in a two-year clinical trial. Again, the age range to include in a prevention study would depend in part on the treatment under investigation (e.g., about 50–65 years old for those treatments thought to be most effective in late middle-age) and the interest in relating brain imaging changes to cognitive decline to help validate the imaging techniques at surrogate endpoints (e.g., closer to the estimated median age of 68 at dementia onset). Again, we would suggest pre-analytical stratification (but not pre-enrollment enrichment or stratification) on the basis of fibrillar amyloid-β burden.

Early-onset AD-causing Gene Carriers: There are important humanitarian and scientific reasons to consider the study of AD-causing PS1, PS2, and APP genetic mutation carriers—who are especially high risk for early-onset AD—in prevention trials, despite the relatively small number of individuals known to have these genes. On the humanitarian side, we and other researchers who follow healthy adults at risk for early-onset AD share their sense of urgency to not only find effective AD prevention therapies before they reach the age at risk, but to give them early access to some of the most promising investigational treatments in clinical trials. We are also mindful that some of the most promising β-amyloid-modifying treatments were screened in animal models more representative of early-onset AD (a disease related to amyloid-β over-production) than late-onset AD—indeed, transgenic mice contain some of these individuals' very own mutations! But there are compelling scientific reasons as well to study this group in clinical trials of β-amyloid-modifying and other putative risk-reducing and prevention therapies. First, cognitively normal early-onset AD-causing gene carriers exhibit PiB PET evidence of amyloid-β pathology (Klunk et al., 2007), and FDG PET evidence of hypometabolism in AD-affected brain regions (Cutler et al., 1985; Kennedy, Frackowiak et al., 1995; Kennedy, Newman et al., 1995; Kennedy, Rossor, and Frackowiak, 1995; Mosconi et al., 2006), providing promising surrogate endpoints for the evaluation of putative risk-reducing and prevention therapies. Second, early-onset AD-causing gene carriers are at a certain risk for AD, and their anticipated age at dementia onset could be roughly approximated on the basis of their family history (Farrer et al., 1990; Van Duijn et al., 1991). Thus, like APOE ε4 homozygotes, early-onset AD-causing gene carriers may be especially suitable for the study of investigational β-amyloid-modifying and risk-reducing treatments relatively soon after the treatments have been evaluated for their safety and tolerability in Phase 3 clinical trials of probable AD patients, given the balance between uncertainties about the treatment's adverse effects and potential benefits. Furthermore, they may be especially well-suited for relating a treatment's effects on imaging endpoints to subsequent rates of cognitive decline, helping to validate brain imaging measurements of fibrillar AD pathology and AD progression as surrogate endpoints. As noted below, researchers could not only evaluate a putative prevention therapy's effects on surrogate endpoints, but could continue to follow participants on the basis of cognitive decline to help demonstrate that a treatment's effects on brain imaging endpoints predicts clinical (or at least early cognitive) outcome. Thus, clinical trials in early-onset AD-causing gene carriers would not only provide the basis for evaluating the treatment's effectiveness for this "orphan drug" indication, but would help validate a tool that accelerates the development of primary prevention therapies for the much larger target population of people at risk for late-onset AD. Researchers have begun to provide an infrastructure for the study of early-onset AD families, making it possible to conduct a small multicenter study in the individuals from those and other centers. We would suggest complementary studies in cognitive APOE ε4 carriers (homozygotes or heterozygotes, depending in part on the treatment) and early-onset AD-causing gene carriers, since they could provide converging evidence in support of a treatment's risk-reducing or prevention effectiveness, converging evidence to advance the use of reasonably likely surrogate endpoints, and the chance to identify any differences in treatment response related to the risk for late-onset and early onset AD (i.e., forms of AD that may be related to a problem with amyloid-β overproduction versus amyloid-β clearance, respectively). The age range to include in a prevention study could depend on the interest in relating brain imaging changes to cognitive decline to help validate the imaging techniques at surrogate endpoints (e.g., closer to the anticipated age at dementia onset) or the interest in introducing the treatment before extensive fibrillar amyloid-β pathology or perhaps even before the appearance of tangles (Head et al., 2008; Oddo et al., 2004, 2006). Again, we would suggest pre-analytical stratification (but not pre-enrollment enrichment or stratification) on the basis of fibrillar amyloid-β burden.

Nondemented Down Syndrome Patients: Although Down syndrome (Trisomy 21) patients are not cognitively normal, they are certain to develop fibrillar amyloid-β by their fourth decade of life (Beyreuther et al., 1992), a high risk of Alzheimer's dementia as they grow older (Holland et al., 2000), and reduced FDG PET measurements of regional CMRgl by the time they have dementia (Azari et al., 1994; Cutler, 1986). They have also been shown to have both reduced gray matter and increased CMRgl, perhaps reflecting compensation reductions in gray matter and an associated, perhaps compensatory, CMRgl increase in several brain regions prior to the onset of dementia (Haier, 2008; Head et al., 2003). Because an increasing number of Down syndrome patients live to beyond young adulthood to older ages (Janicki, 1999), these individuals are not only suitable candidates for future AD risk-reducing and prevention therapies, but also suitable candidates for prevention studies. Prevention studies in nondemented adults with Down syndrome would have some of the same advantages as prevention

studies in early-onset AD-causing gene carriers, given their certain risk of fibrillar amyloid-β neuropathology, as well as a larger group of research participants for inclusion in prevention studies (and another potential "orphan drug" indication). Potential disadvantages include challenges in the assessment of cognitive decline and the diagnosis of dementia in the face of pre-existing cognitive impairment (which may be relevant in the effort to help validate effects of a treatment on surrogate endpoints), and the possibility that findings in patients with this amyloid-β over-production syndrome might not generalize to people at risk for late-onset AD. The age range to include in a prevention study could depend on the interest in relating brain imaging changes to cognitive decline to help validate the imaging techniques at surrogate endpoints (e.g., closer to the anticipated age at fibrillar amyloid-β pathology and dementia onset) or the interest in introducing the treatment before extensive fibrillar amyloid-β pathology. Again, we would suggest pre-analytical stratification (but not pre-enrollment enrichment or stratification) on the basis of fibrillar amyloid-β burden.

The "oldest" old: Because the incidence of AD appears to double every 4–5 years after the age of 60 (Jorm and Jolley, 1998; Jorm, Korten, and Henderson, 1987), it may be possible to use both imaging endpoints and clinical endpoints to evaluate putative risk-reducing and primary prevention therapies in our oldest age groups (e.g., nondemented persons over the age of 85). Advantages include the large number of persons in these age groups and the potential for generalizing findings to a very large and growing population. Potential disadvantages include relatively limited information about the magnitude and course of brain imaging endpoints in this age group, the associated difficulty in estimating the number of participants needed to evaluate risk-reducing and prevention therapies with imaging endpoints with adequate statistical power in this age group, the possibility that some treatments (e.g., hormonal, antihypertensive, and cholesterol-reducing therapies) may be less effective if started at older ages, and the possibility that elderly persons might be more susceptible to the adverse effects of investigational treatments. Despite these limitations, prevention studies in elderly persons could provide valuable information about the effect of widely available treatments considered to be safe, well-tolerated, and associated with other health-promoting effects (including healthy lifestyle interventions) (DeKosky et al., 2006; Dodge et al., 2008; Kaye et al., 2008; Williamson et al., 2008; Yaffe et al., 2001). In a recently presented 42-month randomized prevention trial involving 118 cognitively normal persons 85–94 years of age, treatment with a standardized form of gingko biloba extract was associated with a slower rate of decline in MRI measurements of whole brain volume than placebo (DeKosky et al., 2006; Dodge et al., 2008; Kaye et al., 2008; Williamson et al., 2008; Yaffe et al., 2001). In other MRI analyses, the treatment did not differ significantly from placebo in the rates of hippocampal volume decline or ventricular enlargement (DeKosky et al., 2006; Dodge et al., 2008; Kaye et al., 2008; Williamson et al., 2008; Yaffe et al., 2001). In comparison with placebo using clinical endpoints from the same relatively small study, ginkgo biloba extract was not associated with significantly lower rates of memory decline or progression to MCI in the overall group, but in a secondary analysis was found to be associated with significantly lower MCI progression rates after adjusting for treatment adherence (Dodge et al., 2008). Surprisingly, the treatment was also associated with an increased rate of transient ischemic attacks and ischemic (not hemmorhagic) stroke (Dodge et al., 2008). If the much larger Ginkgo Extract Memory (GEM) and GuidAge prevention studies find that standardized ginkgo biloba extract is associated with significantly lower rates of memory decline and conversion to MCI or AD—these findings would provide initial support using MRI measurements of whole brain MRI as a surrogate endpoint in the evaluation of at least some putative AD risk-reducing and prevention therapies (DeKosky et al., 2006; Williamson et al., 2008). Since a substantial minority of elderly normal persons have significant fibrillar amyloid-β burden (Klunk et al., 2004; Mintun et al., 2006; Pike et al., 2007; Rowe et al., 2007), prevention studies could be considered using fibrillar amyloid-β imaging for pre-enrollment enrichment, pre-randomization stratification, or pre-analytical stratification. In the meantime, we recommend using other cohorts (e.g., cognitively normal APOE ε4 carriers and early-onset AD-causing gene carriers) in proof-of-concept prevention studies of those investigational treatments not yet fully evaluated for their safety and tolerability, and those treatments suggested to be most effective at younger ages.

How to Handle Information About a Research Subject's AD Risk

If the selection criteria for a primary or secondary prevention study includes information about genetic risk factors (i.e., the presence of one or two copies of the APOE ε4 allele or an early-onset AD-causing mutation) or other biomarker measurements (e.g., baseline fibrillar amyloid-β, FDG PET, or MRI measurements), what are the alternatives to dealing with the ethical and clinical implications of disclosing this information to potential research participants?

One approach would be to use a "pre-enrollment enrichment strategy," requiring participants to have the risk factor of interest for them to be enrolled in the study. This alternative would require participants to receive counseling about the risk factor and the implications of receiving information about their own suggested risk, and to provide their informed consent before they are screened. The main advantages of this approach include limiting the study of an investigational treatment with a known or uncertain chance of serious adverse effects to those individuals at highest risk for AD, and minimizing the number of research participants and time needed to evaluate a treatment's effect using imaging or clinical endpoints. Another incidental advantage, perhaps, would be motivating individuals with the newly disclosed risk factor to participate in this and future prevention studies. One disadvantage of this approach (besides limitations in the generalizability of findings) includes the potential for psychological distress from risk disclosure in the person and his or her relatives, more serious adverse effects, and even suicide. For the disclosure of APOE ε4-related genetic risk, the REVEAL trial has developed and tested a brief genetic counseling procedure that has been shown to be reasonably well-tolerated by participants, causing some individuals relatively modest psychological distress, causing others to take healthy lifestyle interventions more seriously, and not leading to significant adverse effects or even suicide (Roberts et al., 2005). For the assessment of PS1 mutations (the most common early-onset AD-causing mutations) and APOE genotype, testing is commercially available. However, most adults in families with early-onset familial AD have chosen not to be tested, and it remains possible that the disclosure of an autosomal dominant early-onset AD gene could adversely affect the psychological health of the individual and other family members (see the Alzheimer Research Forum web site, including http://www.alzforum.org/eFAD/diagenetics/essay4/essay4.asp, for a thoughtful review of the issues related to early-onset AD and genetic testing.) A related disadvantage is the possibility that some individuals concerned about their

own risk for AD might feel compelled to receive more specific and otherwise unwanted information about their own risk to participate in the prevention trials. Since most people with a family history of early-onset AD are extremely concerned about their risk but have been disinclined to receive genetic testing, it may be unreasonably coercive for these particular people to require them to be tested and informed about the presence or absence of an autosomal dominant AD gene for them to be included in a clinical trial. For this reason, we would suggest a "pre-randomization stratification strategy" and no risk disclosure requirement for clinical trials involving persons from early-onset AD families instead.

When pre-enrollment enrichment and the disclosure of risk information is not a reasonable option for the evaluation of investigational treatments with established or uncertain adverse effects that would preclude their use in healthy people at relatively low risk for AD (e.g., an investigational β-amyloid-modifying treatment thought to be safe and well tolerated but evaluated for its safety and tolerability in only several hundred probable AD patients), we would recommend the use of a pre-randomization strategy and no risk disclosure requirement. Using this approach, research participants would be informed that the study would include a roughly equal number of participants with and without the risk factor of interest and that risk disclosure would not be required. Eligible participants would be stratified into three groups prior to double-blind randomization and treatment, including the at-risk group randomized to active treatment, the at-risk group randomized to placebo treatment, and the low-risk group also assigned to placebo.

As previously noted, a "pre-randomization stratification strategy" could also be used to stratify patients on the basis of the risk factor before randomizing each of the two stratified groups to active-treatment or placebo. In one example, one could stratify participants on the basis of fibrillar amyloid-β imaging measurements, making it possible to evaluate the effects of a putative treatment independently in participants with higher or lower levels of fibrillar amyloid-β burden. In another example, one could stratify APOE ε4 carriers and noncarriers, making it possible to eliminate the need to disclose genetic information, enroll only half of the participants one would find in the general population to enroll a sufficient number of APOE ε4 carriers, and permit independent assessment of a putative AD risk-reducing treatment's effects on imaging endpoints related to AD in the ε4 carriers and its effects on imaging endpoints related to normal aging in the ε4 noncarriers.

Finally, one could use a "pre-analytical stratification strategy," selecting participants and randomizing them to treatment irrespective of the risk factors of interest—but ensuring that the number of participants permits an analysis of treatment effects in the at-risk groups with adequate statistical power. Then, in addition to the overall analysis, secondary analyses could characterize and compare the effects of treatments on those at higher and lower risk levels. This strategy would require more participants to enroll the targeted number of at-risk persons, recognizing that the largest group will typically be comprised of persons at lower risk for AD. This strategy may be most suitable for the study of treatments already established to be safe, well-tolerated and heath-promoting, and it could provide information about a treatment's effect on imaging endpoints in both the high-risk and larger low-risk groups.

Selecting a Treatment for Evaluation in Primary Prevention Studies

As previously noted, a large and growing portfolio of promising investigational AD-slowing treatments, marketed medications, dietary supplements, and lifestyle interventions has been suggested to reduce the risk or even prevent AD. Here, we briefly consider some issues related to the selection of treatments in prevention studies using imaging endpoints in persons with an increased genetic risk of AD.

We suggest using our proposed strategy for the evaluation of investigational AD-slowing treatments in cognitively normal persons at increased genetic risk for AD using imaging endpoints right after they have been adequately evaluated for their safety and tolerability in probable AD patients. Indeed, we would suggest studying many of these investigational treatments in these primary prevention studies whether or not there is substantial evidence of an AD-slowing effectiveness in patients with more advanced neuropathology.

We also suggest using brain imaging endpoints to evaluate putative risk-reducing and prevention therapies already thought to be safe and well-tolerated in research participants that exhibit increased genetic risk for AD, or participants at both higher and lower risk for AD, depending in part on the availability of funding. When it comes to the evaluation of health-promoting lifestyle interventions that are suggested to decrease the risk of AD, one could consider the evaluation of an individual treatment or a combination of treatments. Evidence to support the effectiveness of an individual treatment (e.g., aerobic exercise or a cholesterol-lowering treatment) on imaging endpoints could then be used to galvanize interest and support for a larger study of that particular intervention, and also promote study of the treatment's underlying AD risk-reducing mechanisms. Alternatively, a combination of treatments (e.g., a combination of healthy lifestyle interventions) might increase the chance of detecting an effect on imaging endpoints and galvanize interest and support for larger studies of each of the component interventions and their underlying mechanisms of action. While positive findings from this "kitchen sink" approach would beg questions about underlying disease mechanisms and the differential effects of each particular treatment on slowing the brain changes associated with AD risk, normal aging, and their interaction, they could be used to help galvanize the entire field of AD prevention (and cognitive aging) research.

Validating Surrogate Endpoints for the Evaluation of AD Risk-reducing and Prevention Therapies

Here, we suggest what it takes to provide substantial evidence that an effect of putative AD risk-reducing and prevention therapies on surrogate endpoints is reasonably likely to predict the treatments' clinical benefit. First, we suggest embedding potentially complementary brain imaging measurements and nonimaging biomarkers in all clinical trials of putative AD-slowing treatments, and acquiring biological specimens for the future assessment of newly suggested biomarkers. If one could demonstrate that the postulated effects of one (or preferably more) disease-slowing treatments on these biomarker endpoints predicts clinical benefit in probable AD patients, and that the effects on these biomarker endpoints predict cognitive decline and subsequent rates of progression to probable AD in patients with amnestic MCI, that would provide supportive evidence that similar effects of risk-reducing and prevention therapies on the biomarker measurements are reasonably likely to predict their clinical benefit. As previously noted, we would strongly recommend the use of complementary brain imaging endpoints to anticipate and overcome potentially confounding effects of treatment on imaging endpoints while building the arsenal of sufficiently well-validated surrogate endpoints for their use in prevention studies.

Second, we recommend performing clinical trials of promising risk-reducing and primary prevention therapies using similar brain imaging and nonimaging biomarker endpoints, acquiring biological specimens for future use, and starting to conduct parallel studies of the range of promising treatments starting now. We also recommend incorporating strategies to demonstrate that the postulated effects of one or more risk-reducing or prevention therapies on these biomarker endpoints predicts subsequent rates of cognitive decline and, if necessary, rates of conversion to MCI and probable AD. For instance, one could evaluate putative AD risk-reducing and prevention therapies in cognitively normal APOE ε4 and/or early-onset AD-causing gene carriers every three years—one year for enrollment, and two years for treatment. If the treatment does not have the predicted effect on the imaging endpoints, the study's DSMB could recommend trial termination and (with a few exceptions) the participants would be eligible for another prevention study. If, however, the treatment is found to have the postulated effect on surrogate imaging endpoints, the trial would continue to determine whether the treatment-related effects on the surrogate endpoint predicted significant treatment-related differences in rates of cognitive decline or (if needed to provide more substantial evidence) progression to MCI or AD. Ideally, the DSMB would discontinue the clinical trials based on substantial evidence of treatment-related differences in cognitive decline, open-label extension treatment would restore the function compromised by viable neurons in the placebo group, and everyone in the trial would benefit from the AD risk-reducing effects of treatment. Most important, we suggest that this strategy would permit the identification and use of effective AD risk-reducing and prevention therapies as quickly as possible.

Public Policy Recommendations

We have suggested what researchers can do to accelerate the evaluation of promising AD risk-reducing and prevention therapies. Here, we offer public policy recommendations to help find effective treatments as quickly as possible (Reiman, 2008).

1 Encourage pharmaceutical companies to include complementary brain imaging measurements and other biological markers of AD pathology and progression in clinical trials of every promising AD-slowing treatment. As in ADNI, the federal government, regulatory agencies, and pharmaceutical companies should band together to provide the surrogate endpoints needed to evaluate promising treatments in the most rigorous, rapid, and cost-effective way. If regulatory agencies are confident that a treatment's effect on these biological markers predicts a good clinical outcome in affected patients, they are more likely to approve risk-reducing or prevention therapies on the basis of its biological effects alone without waiting many years to see if healthy research participants develop disabling symptoms.

2 Give pharmaceutical companies a compelling financial incentive to evaluate promising risk-reducing and prevention therapies. Offering to extend a drug's patent has promoted the development of effective treatments for rare disorders. Imagine what it could do to promote the identification of an effective AD prevention therapy.

3 Provide the federal funding needed to evaluate the risk-reducing effects of currently available medications, dietary supplements, and otherwise healthy lifestyle interventions for which there is no patent incentive for industry to do so (other

than investigational AD-slowing treatments—most of the suggested AD risk-reducing treatments fall into this category).

4 Make the scientific understanding, treatment, and prevention of AD a national priority before it is too late. With a dramatic increase in funding, and the right strategic focus, the scientific community has an extraordinary chance to avert a looming crisis.

Conclusions

In this chapter, we noted the urgent need to find effective treatments to stop and end AD. We briefly reviewed scientific progress in the discovery of promising AD-slowing treatments, risk-reducing, and prevention therapies, including the large and growing number of promising treatments that remain as studies. We suggested that the roadblock to the identification of effective treatments may not be treatment discovery but treatment development—having the means to evaluate these treatments in the most rapid and rigorous way. We considered three of the best established brain imaging measurements for the assessment of AD progression and pathology, and their critically important emerging role in the evaluation of AD-slowing treatments. We identified some of the challenges in their use, some of the strategies to address, and the reasons to embed complementary imaging techniques in clinical trials of every promising AD-slowing treatment. Finally, we proposed how brain imaging techniques could be used to help find effective treatments (AD risk-reducing and prevention therapies) without having to lose a generation.

In 1961, President Kennedy called on this nation to send a man to the moon and return him safely to earth before the end of the decade—and with fewer scientific resources to address that challenge than are now available to address the challenge of AD, the nation completed the job ahead of schedule. We are keenly aware of the stakes, the opportunities, and the challenges at hand. Let us work together to find effective treatments for stopping and ending Alzheimer's disease without losing another generation, and let us take the steps needed to complete the job ahead of schedule.

Acknowledgements

The authors thank their colleagues from the Banner Alzheimer's Institute, the Arizona Alzheimer's Consortium, and the AD Neuroimaging Initiative, and they gratefully acknowledge NIH grants R01 MH057899, R01 AG031581, P30 AG19610 and U01 AG024904, the Alzheimer's Association and the State of Arizona, which contributed to some of the findings described in this chapter.

References

Agdeppa, E. D., Kepe, V., Petri, A., Satyamurthy, N., Liu, J., Huang, S. C. et al. (2003). In vitro detection of (S)-naproxen and ibuprofen binding to plaques in the Alzheimer's brain using the positron emission tomography molecular imaging probe 2-(1-[6-[(2-[(18)F]fluoroethyl)(methyl)amino]-2-naphthyl]ethylidene)malono nitrile. *Neuroscience*, 117: 723–730.

Aisen, P. S. (2006). Commentary on "Challenges to demonstrating disease-modifying effects in Alzheimer's disease clinical trials". *Alzheimer's and Dementia*, 2: 272–274.

Akomolafe, A., Beiser, A., Meigs, J. B., Au, R., Green, R. C., Farrer, L. A. et al. (2006). Diabetes mellitus and risk of developing Alzheimer disease: Results from the Framingham Study. *Archives of Neurology*, 63: 1551–1555.

Alexander, G. E., Chen, K., Pietrini, P., Rapoport, S. I., and Reiman, E. M. (2002). Longitudinal PET evaluation of cerebral metabolic decline in dementia: A potential outcome measure in Alzheimer's disease treatment studies. *The American Journal of Psychiatry*, 159: 738–745.

Alzheimer's Association (2008). 2008 Alzheimer's disease facts and figures. *Alzheimer's and Dementia*, 4: 110–133.

Archer, H. A., Edison, P., Brooks, D. J., Barnes, J., Frost, C., Yeatman, T. et al. (2006). Amyloid load and cerebral atrophy in Alzheimer's disease: an 11C-PIB positron emission tomography study. *Annals of Neurology*, 60: 145–147.

Arnaiz, E., Jelic, V., Almkvist, O., Wahlund, L. O., Winblad, B., Valind, S. et al. (2001). Impaired cerebral glucose metabolism and cognitive functioning predict deterioration in mild cognitive impairment. *Neuroreport*, 12: 851–855.

Azari, N. P., Pettigrew, K. D., Pietrini, P., Horwitz, B., and Schapiro, M. B. (1994). Detection of an Alzheimer disease pattern of cerebral metabolism in Down syndrome. *Dementia*, 5: 69–78.

Baron, J. C., Chételat, G., Desgranges, B., Perchey, G., Landeau, B., de la Sayette, V. et al. (2001). In vivo mapping of gray matter loss with voxel-based morphometry in mild Alzheimer's desease. *Neuroimage*, 14: 298–309.

Beyreuther, K., Dyrks, T., Hilbich, C., Monning, U., Konig, G., Multhaup, G. et al. (1992). Amyloid precursor protein (APP) and beta A4 amyloid in Alzheimer's disease and Down syndrome. *Progress In Clinical and Biological Research*, 379: 159–182.

Biomarkers Definitions Working Group (2001). Biomarkers and surrogate endpoints: preferred definitions and conceptual framework. *Clinical Pharmacology and Therapeutics*, 69: 89–95.

Bobinski, M., de Leon, M. J., Convit, A., De Santi, S., Wegiel, J., Tarshish, C. Y. et al. (1999). MRI of entorhinal cortex in mild Alzheimer's disease. *Lancet*, 353: 38–40.

Breitner, J. C., Jarvik, G. P., Plassman, B. L., Saunders, A. M., and Welsh, K. A. (1998). Risk of Alzheimer disease with the epsilon4 allele for apolipoprotein E in a population-based study of men aged 62–73 years. *Alzheimer Disease and Associated Disorders*, 12: 40–44.

Breitner, J. C., Wyse, B. W., Anthony, J. C., Welsh-Bohmer, K. A., Steffens, D. C., Norton, M. C. et al. (1999). APOE-e4 count predicts age when prevalence of AD increases, then declines: The Cache County Study. *Neurology*, 53: 321–331.

Broich, K. (2007). Outcome measures in clinical trials on medicinal products for the treatment of dementia: A European regulatory perspective. *International Psychogeriatrics*, 19: 509–524.

Brookmeyer, R., Gray, S., and Kawas, C. (1998). Projections of Alzheimer's disease in the United States and the public health impact of delaying disease onset. *American Journal of Public Health*, 88: 1337–1342.

Cai, L., Liow, J. S., Zoghbi, S. S., Cuevas, J., Baetas, C., Hong, J. et al. (2008). Synthesis and evaluation of N-Methyl and S-Methyl 11C-Labeled 6-Methylthio-2-(4'-N,N-dimethylamino)phenylimidazo[1,2-a]pyridines as radioligands for imaging beta-amyloid plaques in Alzheimer's disease. *Journal of Medicinal Chemistry*, 51: 148–158.

Carlson, N. E., Moore, M. M., Dame, A., Howieson, D., Silbert, L. C., Quinn, J. F. et al. (2008). Trajectories of brain loss in aging and the development of cognitive impairment. *Neurology*, 70: 828–833.

Chase, T. N., Foster, N. L., Fedio, P., Brooks, R., Mansi, L., and Di Chiro, G. (1984). Regional cortical dysfunction in Alzheimer's disease as determined by positron emission tomography. *Annals of Neurology*, 15(Suppl.): S170–S174.

Chen, K., Bandy, D., Reiman, E., Huang, S. C., Lawson, M., Feng, D. et al. (1998). Noninvasive quantification of the cerebral metabolic rate for glucose using positron emission tomography, 18F-fluoro-2-deoxyglucose, the Patlak method, and an image-derived input function. *Journal of Cerebral Blood Flow and Metabolism*, 18: 716–723.

Chen, K., Reiman, E. M., Alexander, G. E., Bandy, D., Renaut, R., Crum, W. R. et al. (2004). An automated algorithm for the computation of brain volume change from sequential MRIs using an iterative principal component analysis and its evaluation for the assessment of whole-brain atrophy rates in patients with probable Alzheimer's disease. *Neuroimage*, 22: 134–143.

Chen, K., Reiman, E. M., Alexander, G. E., Caselli, R. J., Gerkin, R., Bandy, D. et al. (2007). Correlations between apolipoprotein E e4 gene dose and whole brain atrophy rates. *The American Journal of Psychiatry*, 164: 916–921.

Chételat, G., Desgranges, B., de la Sayette, V., Viader, F., Eustache, F., and Baron, J. C. (2003). Mild cognitive impairment: Can FDG-PET predict who is to rapidly convert to Alzheimer's disease? *Neurology*, 60: 1374–1377.

Chételat, G., Desgranges, B., Landeau, B., Mézenge, F., Poline, J. B., de la Sayette, V. et al. (2008). Direct voxel-based comparison between grey matter hypometabolism and atrophy in Alzheimer's disease. *Brain*, 131: 60–71.

Chételat, G., Eustache, F., Viader, F., de la Sayette, V., Pélerin, A., Mézenge, F. et al. (2005). FDG-PET measurement is more accurate than neuropsychological assessments to predict global cognitive deterioration in patients with mild cognitive impairment. *Neurocase*, 11: 14–25.

Chételat, G., Landeau, B., Eustache, F., Mézenge, F., Viader, F., de la Sayette, V. et al. (2005). Using voxel-based morphometry to map the structural changes associated with rapid conversion in MCI: a longitudinal MRI study. *Neuroimage*, 27: 934–946.

Choo, I. H., Lee, D. Y., Youn, J. C., Jhoo, J. H., Kim, K. W., Lee, D. S. et al. (2007). Topographic patterns of brain functional impairment progression according to clinical severity staging in 116 Alzheimer disease patients: FDG-PET study. *Alzheimer Disease and Associated Disorders*, 21: 77–84.

Corder, E. H., Saunders, A. M., Strittmatter, W. J., Schmechel, D. E., Gaskell, P. C., Small, G. W. et al. (1993). Gene dose of apolipoprotein E type 4 allele and the risk of Alzheimer's disease in late onset families. *Science*, 261: 921–923.

Craig, M. C., Maki, P. M., and Murphy, D. G. (2005). The Women's Health Initiative Memory Study: Findings and implications for treatment. *Lancet Neurology*, 4: 190–194.

Cummings, J. L. (2006). Challenges to demonstrating disease-modifying effects in Alzheimer's disease clinical trials. *Alzheimer's and Dementia*, 2: 263–271.

Cutler, N. R. (1986). Cerebral metabolism as measured with positron emission tomography (PET) and [18F] 2-deoxy-D-glucose: healthy aging, Alzheimer's disease and Down syndrome. *Progress In Neuropsychopharmacology and Biological Psychiatry*, 10: 309–321.

Cutler, N. R., Haxby, J. V., Duara, R., Grady, C. L., Moore, A. M., Parisi, J. E. et al. (1985). Brain metabolism as measured with positron emission tomography: Serial assessment in a patient with familial Alzheimer's disease. *Neurology*, 35: 1556–1561.

de Leon, M. J., Convit, A., Wolf, O. T., Tarshish, C. Y., De Santi, S., Rusinek, H. et al. (2001). Prediction of cognitive decline in normal elderly subjects with 2-[(18)F]fluoro-2-deoxy-D-glucose/poitron-emission tomography (FDG/PET). *Proceedings of the National Academy of Sciences of the USA*, 98: 10966–10971.

de Leon, M. J., DeSanti, S., Zinkowski, R., Mehta, P. D., Pratico, D., Segal, S. et al. (2006). Longitudinal CSF and MRI biomarkers improve the diagnosis of mild cognitive impairment. *Neurobiology of Aging*, 27: 394–401.

de Leon, M. J., Ferris, S. H., George, A. E., Reisberg, B., Christman, D. R., Kricheff, I. I. et al. (1983). Computed tomography and positron emission transaxial tomography evaluations of normal aging and Alzheimer's disease. *Journal of Cerebral Blood Flow and Metabolism*, 3: 391–394.

de Leon, M. J., George, A. E., Golomb, J, Tarshish, C., Convit, A., Kluger, A. et al. (1997). Frequency of hippocampal formation atrophy in normal aging and Alzheimer's disease. *Neurobiology of Aging*, 18: 1–11.

de Leon, M. J., George, A. E., Stylopoulos, L. A., Smith, G., and Miller, D. C. (1989). Early marker for Alzheimer's disease: the atrophic hippocampus. *Lancet*, 2: 672–673.

de Leon, M. J., Golomb, J., George, A. E., Convit, A., Tarshish, C. Y., McRae, T. et al. (1993). The radiologic prediction of Alzheimer disease: The atrophic hippocampal formation. *American Journal of Neuroradiology*, 14: 897–906.

De Santi, S., de Leon, M. J., Rusinek, H., Convit, A., Tarshish, C. Y., Roche, A. et al. (2001). Hippocampal formation glucose metabolism and volume losses in MCI and AD. *Neurobiology of Aging*, 22: 529–539.

De Santi, S., de Leon, M. J., Convit, A., Tarshish, C., Rusinek, H., Tsui, W. H. et al. (1995). Age-related changes in brain: II. Positron emission tomography of frontal and temporal lobe glucose metabolism in normal subjects. *The Psychiatric Quarterly*, 66: 357–370.

Debanne, S. M., Bielefeld, R. A., Cheruvu, V. K., Fritsch, T., and Rowland, D. Y. (2007). Alzheimer's disease and smoking: Bias in cohort studies. *Journal of Alzheimers Disease*, 11: 313–321.

DeKosky, S. T., Fitzpatrick, A., Ives, D. G., Saxton, J., Williamson, J., Lopez, O. L. et al. (2006). The Ginkgo Evaluation of Memory (GEM) study: design and baseline data of a randomized trial of Ginkgo biloba extract in prevention of dementia. *Contemporary Clinical Trials*, 27: 238–253.

DeMattos, R. B., Bales, K. R., Cummins, D. J., Dodart, J. C., Paul, S. M., and Holtzman, D. M. (2001). Peripheral anti-A beta antibody alters CNS and plasma A beta clearance and decreases brain A beta burden in a mouse model of Alzheimer's disease. *Proceedings of the National Academy of Sciences of the USA*, 98: 8850–8855.

Devanand, D. P., Pradhaban, G., Liu, X., Khandji, A., De Santi, S., Segal, S. et al. (2007). Hippocampal and entorhinal atrophy in mild cognitive impairment: Prediction of Alzheimer disease. *Neurology*, 68: 828–836.

Deweer, B., Lehericy, S., Pillon, B., Baulac, M., Chiras, J., Marsault, C. et al. (1995). Memory disorders in probable Alzheimer's disease: The role of hippocampal atrophy as shown with MRI. *Journal of Neurology, Neurosurgery, and Psychiatry*, 58: 590–597.

Dickerson, B. C., Goncharova, I., Sullivan, M. P., Forchetti, C., Wilson, R. S., Bennett, D. A. et al. (2001). MRI-derived entorhinal and hippocampal atrophy in incipient and very mild Alzheimer's disease. *Neurobiology of Aging*, 22: 747–754.

Dodge, H. H., Zitzelberger, T., Oken, B. S., Howieson, D., and Kaye, J. (2008). A randomized placebo-controlled trial of ginkgo biloba for the prevention of cognitive decline. *Neurology*, 70: 1809–1817.

Drzezga, A., Grimmer, T., Riemenschneider, M., Lautenschlager, N., Siebner, H., Alexopoulus, P. et al. (2005). Prediction of individual clinical outcome in MCI by means of genetic assessment and (18)F-FDG PET. *Journal of Nuclear Medicine*, 46: 1625–1632.

Drzezga, A., Lautenschlager, N., Siebner, H., Riemenschneider, M., Willoch, F., Minoshima, S. et al. (2003). Cerebral metabolic changes accompanying conversion of mild cognitive impairment into Alzheimer's disease: A PET follow-up study. *European Journal of Nuclear Medicine and Molecular Imaging*, 30: 1104–1113.

Du, A. T., Schuff, N., Kramer, J. H., Ganzer, S., Zhu, X. P., Jagust, W. J. et al. (2004). Higher atrophy rate of entorhinal cortex than hippocampus in AD. *Neurology*, 62: 422–427.

Du, A. T., Schuff, N., Kramer, J. H., Rosen, H. J., Gorno-Tempini, M. L., Rankin, K. et al. (2007). Different regional patterns of cortical thinning in Alzheimer's disease and frontotemporal dementia. *Brain*, 130: 1159–1166.

Du, A. T., Schuff, N., Zhu, X. P., Jagust, W. J., Miller, B. L., Reed, B. R. et al. (2003). Atrophy rates of entorhinal cortex in AD and normal aging. *Neurology*, 60: 481–486.

Duara, R., Grady, C. L., Haxby, J. V., Sundaram, M., Cutler, N.R., Heston, L. et al. (1986). Positron emission tomography in Alzheimer's disease. *Neurology*, 36: 879–887.

Edison, P., Archer, H. A., Hinz, R., Hammers, A., Pavese, N., Tai, Y. F. et al. (2007). Amyloid, hypometabolism, and cognition in Alzheimer disease: An [11C]PIB and [18F]FDG PET study. *Neurology*, 68: 501–508.

Edland, S. D., Rocca, W. A., Petersen, R. C., Cha, R. H., and Kokmen, E. (2002). Dementia and Alzheimer disease incidence rates do not vary by sex in Rochester, Minnesota. *Archives of Neurology*, 59: 1589–1593.

Engler, H., Forsberg, A., Almkvist, O., Blomquist, G., Larsson, E., Savitcheva, I. et al. (2006). Two-year follow-up of amyloid deposition in patients with Alzheimer's disease. *Brain*, 129: 2856–2866.

Ernst, R. L. and Hay, J. W. (1994). The US economic and social costs of Alzheimer's disease revisited. *American Journal of Public Health*, 84: 1261–1264.

Espeseth, T., Westlye, L. T., Fjell, A. M., Walhovd, K. B., Rootwelt, H., and Reinvang, I. (2008). Accelerated age-related cortical thinning in healthy carriers of apolipoprotein E epsilon 4. *Neurobiology of Aging*, 29: 329–340.

Evans, D. A., Funkenstein, H. H., Albert, M. S., Scherr, P. A., Cook, N. R., Chown, M. J. et al. (1989). Prevalence of Alzheimer's disease in a community population of older persons. Higher than previously reported. *The Journal of the American Medical Association*, 262: 2551–2556.

Fagan, A. M., Mintun, M. A., Mach, R. H., Lee, S. Y., Dence, C. S., Shah, A. R. et al. (2006). Inverse relation between in vivo amyloid imaging load and cerebrospinal fluid Ab42 in humans. *Annals of Neurology*, 59: 512–519.

Farrer, L. A., Myers, R. H., Cupples, L. A., St George-Hyslop, P. H., Bird, T. D., Rossor, M. N. et al. (1990). Transmission and age-at-onset patterns in familial Alzheimer's disease: evidence for heterogeneity. *Neurology*, 40: 395–403.

Ferris, S. H. and Kluger, A. (1997). Assessing cognition in Alzheimer disease research. *Alzheimer Disease and Associated Disorders*, 11: 45–49.

Fleisher, A. S., Sun, S., Taylor, C., Ward, C. P., Gamst, A. C., Petersen, R. C. et al. (2008). Volumetric MRI vs clinical predictors of Alzheimer disease in mild cognitive impairment. *Neurology*, 70: 191–199.

Fleming, T. R. and DeMets, D. L. (1996). Surrogate end points in clinical trials: Are we being misled? *Annals of Internal Medicine*, 125: 605–613.

Food and Drug Administration (1992). New drug, antibiotic, and biological drug product regulations; accelerated approval—FDA. Final rule. *Federal Register*, 57: 58942–58960.

Forsberg, A., Engler, H., Almkvist, O., Blomquist, G., Hagman, G., Wall, A. et al. (2008). PET imaging of amyloid deposition in patients with mild cognitive impairment. *Neurobiology of Aging*, 29: 1456–1465.

Foster, N. L., Chase, T. N., Fedio, P., Patronas, N. J., Brooks, R. A., and Di Chiro, G. (1983). Alzheimer's disease: Focal cortical changes shown by positron emission tomography. *Neurology*, 33: 961–965.

Foster, N. L., Chase, T. N., Mansi, L., Brooks, R., Fedio, P., Patronas, N. J. et al. (1984). Cortical abnormalities in Alzheimer's disease. *Annals of Neurology*, 16: 649–654.

Foster, N. L., Heidebrink, J. L., Clark, C. M., Jagust, W. J., Arnold, S. E., Barbas, N. R. et al. (2007). FDG-PET improves accuracy in distinguishing frontotemporal dementia and Alzheimer's disease. *Brain*, 130: 2616–2635.

Fox, N. C., Black, R. S., Gilman, S., Rossor, M. N., Griffith, S. G., Jenkins, L. et al. (2005). Effects of Ab immunization (AN1792) on MRI measures of cerebral volume in Alzheimer disease. *Neurology*, 64: 1563–1572.

Fox, N. C., Cousens, S., Scahill, R., Harvey, R. J., and Rossor, M. N. (2000). Using serial registered brain magnetic resonance imaging to measure disease progression in Alzheimer disease: power calculations and estimates of sample size to detect treatment effects. *Archives of Neurology*, 57: 339–344.

Fox, N. C. and Freeborough, P. A. (1997). Brain atrophy progression measured from registered serial MRI: Validation and application to Alzheimer's disease. *Journal of Magnetic Resonance Imaging*, 7: 1069–1075.

Fox, N. C., Warrington, E. K., Freeborough, P. A., Hartikainen, P., Kennedy, A. M., Stevens, J. M. et al. (1996). Presymptomatic hippocampal atrophy in Alzheimer's disease. A longitudinal MRI study. *Brain*, 119: 2001–2007.

Fratiglioni, L., Viitanen, M., Von, S. E., Tontodonati, V., Herlitz, A., and Winblad, B. (1997). Very old women at highest risk of dementia and Alzheimer's disease: Incidence data from the Kungsholmen Project, Stockholm. *Neurology*, 48: 132–138.

Frisoni, G. B., Laakso, M. P., Beltramello, A., Geroldi, C., Bianchetti, A., Soininen, H. et al. (1999). Hippocampal and entorhinal cortex atrophy in frontotemporal dementia and Alzheimer's disease. *Neurology*, 52: 91–100.

Furumoto, S., Okamura, N., Iwata, R., Yanai, K., Arai, H., and Kudo, Y. (2007). Recent advances in the development of amyloid imaging agents. *Current Topics in Medicinal Chemistry*, 7: 1773–1789.

Galasko, D., Bennett, D., Sano, M., Ernesto, C., Thomas, R., Grundman, M. et al. (1997). An inventory to assess activities of daily living for clinical trials in Alzheimer's disease. The Alzheimer's Disease Cooperative Study. *Alzheimer Disease and Associated Disorders*, 11 (Suppl. 2): S33–S39.

Gatz, M., Reynolds, C. A., Fratiglioni, L., Johansson, B., Mortimer, J. A., Berg, S. et al. (2006). Role of genes and environments for explaining Alzheimer disease. *Archives of General Psychiatry*, 63: 168–174.

Gélinas, I., Gauthier, L., McIntyre, M., and Gauthier, S. (1999). Development of a functional measure for persons with Alzheimer's disease: The disability assessment for dementia. *The American Journal of Occupational Therapy*, 53: 471–481.

Giannakopoulos, P., Herrmann, F. R., Bussiere, T., Bouras, C., Kovari, E., Perl, D. P. et al. (2003). Tangle and neuron numbers, but not amyloid load, predict cognitive status in Alzheimer's disease. *Neurology*, 60: 1495–1500.

Glabe, C. G. and Kayed, R. (2006). Common structure and toxic function of amyloid oligomers implies a common mechanism of pathogenesis. *Neurology*, 66: S74–S78.

Goate, A., Chartier-Harlin, M. C., Mullan, M., Brown, J., Crawford, F., Fidani, L. et al. (1991). Segregation of a missense mutation in the amyloid precursor protein gene with familial Alzheimer's disease. *Nature*, 349: 704–706.

Golde, T. E. (2007). The pathogenesis of Alzheimer's disease and the role of Ab42. *CNS Spectrums*, 12: 4–6.

Golomb, J., de Leon, M. J., Kluger, A., George, A. E., Tarshish, C., and Ferris, S. H. (1993). Hippocampal atrophy in normal aging. An association with recent memory impairment. *Archives of Neurology*, 50: 967–973.

Gottesman, I. I. and Gould, T. D. (2003). The endophenotype concept in psychiatry: etymology and strategic intentions. *The American Journal of Psychiatry*, 160: 636–645.

Grimmer, T., Henriksen, G., Wester, H., Förstl, H., Klunk, W. E., Mathis, C. A. et al. (in press). Clinical severity of Alzheimer's disease is associated with PIB uptake in PET. *Neurobiology of Aging*.

Gustafson, D., Rothenberg, E., Blennow, K., Steen, B., and Skoog, I. (2003). An 18-year follow-up of overweight and risk of Alzheimer disease. *Archives of Internal Medicine*, 163: 1524–1528.

Haier, R. J., Head, K., Head, E., and Lott, I. T. (2008). Neuroimaging of individuals with Down's syndrome at-risk for dementia: evidence for possible compensatory events. *Neuroimage*, 39: 1324–1332.

Hansson, O., Zetterberg, H., Buchhave, P., Londos, E., Blennow, K., and Minthon, L. (2006). Association between CSF biomarkers and incipient Alzheimer's disease in patients with mild cognitive impairment: A follow-up study. *Lancet Neurology*, 5: 228–234.

Hardy, J. and Selkoe, D. J. (2002). The amyloid hypothesis of Alzheimer's disease: progress and problems on the road to therapeutics. *Science*, 297: 353–356.

Harrison, J., Minassian, S. L., Jenkins, L., Black, R. S., Koller, M., and Grundman, M. (2007). A neuropsychological test battery for use in Alzheimer disease clinical trials. *Archives of Neurology*, 64: 1323–1329.

Haxby, J. V., Grady, C. L., Koss, E., Horwitz, B., Heston, L., Schapiro, M. et al. (1990). Longitudinal study of cerebral metabolic asymmetries and associated neuropsychological patterns in early dementia of the Alzheimer type. *Archives of Neurology*, 47: 753–760.

Head, E., Lott, I. T., Hof, P. R., Bouras, C., Su, J. H., Kim, R. et al. (2003). Parallel compensatory and pathological events associated with tau pathology in middle aged individuals with Down syndrome. *Journal of Neuropathology And Experimental Neurology*, 62: 917–926.

Head, E., Pop, V., Vasilevko, V., Hill, M., Saing, T., Sarsoza, F. et al. (2008). A two-year dtudy with fibrillar beta-amyloid (Abeta) immunization in aged canines: effects on cognitive function and brain A{beta}. *Journal of Neuroscience*, 28: 3555–3566.

Hebert, L. E., Beckett, L. A., Scherr, P. A., and Evans, D. A. (2001). Annual incidence of Alzheimer disease in the United States projected to the years 2000 through 2050. *Alzheimer Disease and Associated Disorders*, 15: 169–173.

Hoffman, J. M., Welsh-Bohmer, K. A., Hanson, M., Crain, B., Hulette, C., Earl, N. et al. (2000). FDG PET imaging in patients with pathologically verified dementia. *Journal of Nuclear Medicine*, 41: 1920–1928.

Holland, A. J., Hon, J., Huppert, F. A., and Stevens, F. (2000). Incidence and course of dementia in people with Down's syndrome: Findings from a population-based study. *Journal of Intellectual Disability Research*, 44 (Pt 2): 138–146.

Hughes, M. D. (2002). Evaluating surrogate endpoints. *Controlled Clinical Trials*, 23: 703–707.

Hulstaert, F., Blennow, K., Ivanoiu, A., Schoonderwaldt, H. C., Riemenschneider, M., De Deyn, P. P. et al. (1999). Improved discrimination of AD patients using beta-amyloid(1–42) and tau levels in CSF. *Neurology*, 52: 1555–1562.

Ibanez, V., Pietrini, P., Alexander, G. E., Furey, M. L., Teichberg, D., Rajapakse, J. C. et al. (1998). Regional glucose metabolic abnormalities are not the result of atrophy in Alzheimer's disease. *Neurology*, 50: 1585–1593.

Ikonomovic, M. D., Klunk, W. E., Abrahamson, E. E., Mathis, C. A., Price, J. C., Tsopelas, N. D. et al. (2008). Post-mortem correlates of in vivo PiB-PET amyloid imaging in a typical case of Alzheimer's disease. *Brain*, 131: 1630–1645.

Irie, F., Fitzpatrick, A. L., Lopez, O. L., Kuller, L. H., Peila, R., Newman, A. B. et al. (2008). Enhanced risk for Alzheimer disease in Persons with Type 2 Diabetes and APOE e4: The Cardiovascular Health Study Cognition Study. *Archives of Neurology*, 65: 89–93.

Jack, C. R., Jr., Petersen, R. C., Grundman, M., Jin, S., Gamst, A., Ward, C. P. et al. (2008). Longitudinal MRI findings from the vitamin E and donepezil treatment study for MCI. *Neurobiology of Aging*, 29: 1285–1295.

Jack, C. R., Jr., Petersen, R. C., O'Brien, P. C., and Tangalos, E. G. (1992). MR-based hippocampal volumetry in the diagnosis of Alzheimer's disease. *Neurology*, 42: 183–188.

Jack, C. R., Jr., Petersen, R. C., Xu, Y., O'Brien, P. C., Smith, G. E., Ivnik, R. J. et al. (2000). Rates of hippocampal atrophy correlate with change in clinical status in aging and AD. *Neurology*, 55: 484–489.

Jack, C. R., Jr., Petersen, R. C., Xu, Y., O'Brien, P. C., Smith, G. E., Ivnik, R. J. et al. (1998). Rate of medial temporal lobe atrophy in typical aging and Alzheimer's disease. *Neurology*, 51: 993–999.

Jack, C. R., Jr., Petersen, R. C., Xu, Y. C., Waring, S. C., O'Brien, P. C., Tangalos, E. G. et al. (1997). Medial temporal atrophy on MRI in normal aging and very mild Alzheimer's disease. *Neurology*, 49: 786–794.

Jack, C. R., Jr., Shiung, M. M., Gunter, J. L., O'Brien, P. C., Weigand, S. D., Knopman, D. S. et al. (2004). Comparison of different MRI brain atrophy rate measures with clinical disease progression in AD. *Neurology*, 62: 591–600.

Jack, C. R., Jr., Shiung, M. M., Weigand, S. D., O'Brien, P. C., Gunter, J. L., Boeve, B. F. et al. (2005). Brain atrophy rates predict subsequent clinical conversion in normal elderly and amnestic MCI. *Neurology*, 65: 1227–1231.

Jagust, W., Reed, B., Mungas, D., Ellis, W., and DeCarli, C. (2007). What does fluorodeoxyglucose PET imaging add to a clinical diagnosis of dementia? *Neurology*, 69: 871–877.

Jagust, W. J., Friedland, R. P., Budinger, T. F., Koss, E., and Ober, B. (1988). Longitudinal studies of regional cerebral metabolism in Alzheimer's disease. *Neurology*, 38: 909–912.

Jak, A. J., Houston, W. S., Nagel, B. J., Corey-Bloom, J., and Bondi, M. W. (2007). Differential cross-sectional and longitudinal impact of APOE genotype on hippocampal volumes in nondemented older adults. *Dementia Geriatric Cognitive Disorders*, 23: 382–389.

Janicki, M. P., Dalton, A. J., Henderson, C. M., and Davidson, P. W. (1999). Mortality and morbidity among older adults with intellectual disability: health services considerations. *Disability and Rehabilitation*, 21: 284–294.

Jicha, G. A., Parisi, J. E., Dickson, D. W., Johnson, K., Cha, R., Ivnik, R. J. et al. (2006). Neuropathologic outcome of mild cognitive impairment following progression to clinical dementia. *Archives of Neurology*, 63: 674–681.

Jorm, A. F. and Jolley, D. (1998). The incidence of dementia: A meta-analysis. *Neurology*, 51: 728–733.

Jorm, A. F., Korten, A. E., and Henderson, A. S. (1987). The prevalence of dementia: a quantitative integration of the literature. *Acta Psychiatria Scandinavica*, 76: 465–479.

Juottonen, K., Laakso, M. P., Insausti, R., Lehtovirta, M., Pitkanen, A., Partanen, K. et al. (1998). Volumes of the entorhinal and perirhinal cortices in Alzheimer's disease. *Neurobiology of Aging*, 19: 15–22.

Juottonen, K., Laakso, M. P., Partanen, K., and Soininen, H. (1999). Comparative MR analysis of the entorhinal cortex and hippocampus in diagnosing Alzheimer disease. *American Journal of Neuroradiology*, 20, 139–144.

Kastelein, J. J., Akdim, F., Stroes, E. S., Zwinderman, A. H., Bots, M. L., Stalenhoef, A. F. et al. (2008). Simvastatin with or without Ezetimibe in Familial Hypercholesterolemia. *The New England Journal of Medicine*, 358: 1431–1443.

Katz, R. (2004). Biomarkers and surrogate markers: An FDA perspective. *NeuroRx*, 1: 189–195.

Katzman, R., Terry, R., DeTeresa, R., Brown, T., Davies, P., Fuld, P. et al. (1988). Clinical, pathological, and neurochemical changes in dementia: A subgroup with preserved mental status and numerous neocortical plaques. *Annals of Neurology*, 23: 138–144.

Kawas, C., Gray, S., Brookmeyer, R., Fozard, J., and Zonderman, A. (2000). Age-specific incidence rates of Alzheimer's disease: The Baltimore Longitudinal Study of Aging. *Neurology*, 54: 2072–2077.

Kawas, C., Resnick, S., Morrison, A., Brookmeyer, R., Corrada, M., Zonderman, A. et al. (1997). A prospective study of estrogen replacement therapy and the risk of developing Alzheimer's disease: the Baltimore Longitudinal Study of Aging [published erratum appears in Neurology 1998 Aug;51(2): 654]. *Neurology*, 48: 1517–1521.

Kaye, J. A., Dodge. H., Zitzelberger, T., Moore, M., and Oken, B. (2008). MRI evidence for a disease modifying effect of ginko bioloba extract in a dementia prevention trial. *Alzheimer's and Dementia*, 4: T772.

Kaye, J. A., Swihart, T., Howieson, D., Dame, A., Moore, M. M., Karnos, T. et al. (1997). Volume loss of the hippocampus and temporal lobe in healthy elderly persons destined to develop dementia. *Neurology*, 48: 1297–1304.

Kemppainen, N. M., Aalto, S., Wilson, I. A., Nagren, K., Helin, S., Bruck, A. et al. (2006). Voxel-based analysis of PET amyloid ligand [11C]PIB uptake in Alzheimer disease. *Neurology*, 67: 1575–1580.

Kemppainen, N. M., Aalto, S., Wilson, I. A., Nagren, K., Helin, S., Bruck, A. et al. (2007). PET amyloid ligand [11C]PIB uptake is increased in mild cognitive impairment. *Neurology*, 68: 1603–1606.

Kennedy, A. M., Frackowiak, R. S., Newman, S. K., Bloomfield, P. M., Seaward, J., Roques, P. et al. (1995). Deficits in cerebral glucose metabolism demonstrated by positron emission tomography in individuals at risk of familial Alzheimer's disease. *Neuroscience Letters*, 186: 17–20.

Kennedy, A. M., Newman, S. K., Frackowiak, R. S., Cunningham, V. J., Roques, P., Stevens, J. et al. (1995). Chromosome 14 linked familial Alzheimer's disease. A clinico-pathological study of a single pedigree. *Brain*, 118: 185–205.

Kennedy, A. M., Rossor, M. N., and Frackowiak, R. S. (1995). Positron emission tomography in familial Alzheimer disease. *Alzheimer Disease and Associated Disorders*, 9: 17–20.

Killiany, R. J., Hyman, B. T., Gomez-Isla, T., Moss, M. B., Kikinis, R., Jolesz, F. et al. (2002). MRI measures of entorhinal cortex vs hippocampus in preclinical AD. *Neurology*, 58: 1188–1196.

Killiany, R. J., Moss, M. B., Albert, M. S., Sandor, T., Tieman, J., and Jolesz, F. (1993). Temporal lobe regions on magnetic resonance imaging identify patients with early Alzheimer's disease. *Archives of Neurology*, 50: 949–954.

Kivipelto, M., Helkala, E. L., Laakso, M. P., Hanninen, T., Hallikainen, M., Alhainen, K. et al. (2001). Midlife vascular risk factors and Alzheimer's disease in later life: longitudinal, population based study. *British Medical Journal*, 322: 1447–1451.

Klunk, W. E., Engler, H., Nordberg, A., Wang, Y., Blomqvist, G., Holt, D. P. et al. (2004). Imaging brain amyloid in Alzheimer's disease with Pittsburgh Compound-B. *Annals of Neurology*, 55: 306–319.

Klunk, W. E., Lopresti, B. J., Ikonomovic, M. D., Lefterov, I. M., Koldamova, R. P., Abrahamson, E. E. et al. (2005). Binding of the positron emission tomography tracer Pittsburgh compound-B reflects the amount of amyloid-beta in Alzheimer's disease brain but not in transgenic mouse brain. *Journal of Neuroscience*, 25: 10598–10606.

Klunk, W. E., Price, J. C., Mathis, C. A., Tsopelas, N. D., Lopresti, B. J., Ziolko, S. K. et al. (2007). Amyloid deposition begins in the striatum of presenilin-1 mutation carriers from two unrelated pedigrees. *Journal of Neuroscience*, 27: 6174–6184.

Knopman, D. S., DeKosky, S. T., Cummings, J. L., Chui, H., Corey-Bloom, J., Relkin, N. et al. (2001). Practice parameter: diagnosis of dementia (an evidence-based review). Report of the Quality Standards Subcommittee of the American Academy of Neurology. *Neurology*, 56: 1143–1153.

Krasuski, J. S., Alexander, G. E., Horwitz, B., Daly, E. M., Murphy, D. G., Rapoport, S. I. et al. (1998). Volumes of medial temporal lobe structures in patients with Alzheimer's disease and mild cognitive impairment (and in healthy controls). *Biological Psychiatry*, 43: 60–68.

Kudo, Y., Okamura, N., Furumoto, S., Tashiro, M., Furukawa, K., Maruyama, M. et al. (2007). 2-(2-[2-Dimethylaminothiazol-5-yl]ethenyl)-6- (2-[fluoro]ethoxy)benzoxazole: a novel PET agent for in vivo detection of dense amyloid plaques in Alzheimer's disease patients. *The Journal of Nuclear Medicine*, 48: 553–561.

Kung, M. P., Hou, C., Zhuang, Z. P., Skovronsky, D., and Kung, H. F. (2004). Binding of two potential imaging agents targeting amyloid plaques in postmortem brain tissues of patients with Alzheimer's disease. *Brain Research*, 1025: 98–105.

Laakso, M. P., Soininen, H., Partanen, K., Helkala, E. L., Hartikainen, P., Vainio, P. et al. (1995). Volumes of hippocampus, amygdala and frontal lobes in the MRI-based diagnosis of early Alzheimer's disease: correlation with memory functions. *Journal of Neural Transmission Parkinson's Disease And Dementia Section*, 9: 73–86.

Larson, E. B., Wang, L., Bowen, J. D., McCormick, W. C., Teri, L., Crane, P. et al. (2006). Exercise is associated with reduced risk for incident dementia among persons 65 years of age and older. *Annals of Internal Medicine*, 144: 73–81.

Laurin, D., Masaki, K. H., Foley, D. J., White, L. R., and Launer, L. J. (2004). Midlife dietary intake of antioxidants and risk of late–life incident dementia: The Honolulu-Asia Aging Study. *American Journal of Epidemiology*, 159: 959–967.

Leber, P. (1996). Observations and suggestions on antidementia drug development. *Alzheimer Disease and Associated Disorders*, 10(Suppl. 1): 31–35.

Leber, P. (1997). Slowing the progression of Alzheimer disease: Methodologic issues. *Alzheimer Disease and Associated Disorders*, 11(Suppl. 5): S10–S21.

Leber, P. (2002). Criteria used by drug regulatory authorities. In N. Qizilbash, L. Schneider, H. Chui, P. Tariot, H. Brodaty, J. Kaye, and T. Erkinjuntti (eds.), *Evidence-Based Dementia Practice* (pp. 376–387). Oxford, UK: Blackwell Science.

Liang, W. S., Reiman, E. M., Valla, J., Dunckley, T., Beach, T. G., Grover, A. et al. (2008). Alzheimer's disease is associated with reduced expression of energy metabolism genes in posterior cingulate neurons. *Proceedings of the National Academy of Sciences of the USA*, 105: 4441–4446.

Lue, L. F., Kuo, Y. M., Roher, A. E., Brachova, L., Shen, Y., Sue, L. et al. (1999). Soluble amyloid beta peptide concentration as a predictor of synaptic change in Alzheimer's disease. *American Journal of Pathology*, 155: 853–862.

Magistretti, P. J. and Pellerin, L. (1996). Cellular bases of brain energy metabolism and their relevance to functional brain imaging: Evidence for a prominent role of astrocytes. *Cerebral Cortex*, 6: 50–61.

Mani, R. B. (2004). The evaluation of disease modifying therapies in Alzheimer's disease: A regulatory viewpoint. *Statistics in Medicine*, 23: 305–314.

Mark, R. J., Pang, Z., Geddes, J. W., Uchida, K., and Mattson, M. P. (1997). Amyloid beta-peptide impairs glucose transport in hippocampal and cortical neurons: involvement of membrane lipid peroxidation. *Journal of Neuroscience*, 17: 1046–1054.

Martin, A. J., Friston, K. J., Colebatch, J. G., and Frackowiak, R. S. (1991). Decreases in regional cerebral blood flow with normal aging. *Journal of Cerebral Blood Flow Metabolism*, 11: 684–689.

McGeer, E. G., Peppard, R. P., McGeer, P. L., Tuokko, H., Crockett, D., Parks, R. et al. (1990). 18Fluorodeoxyglucose positron emission tomography studies in presumed Alzheimer cases, including 13 serial scans. *The Canadian Journal of Neurological Science*, 17: 1–11.

Mega, M. S., Chen, S. S., Thompson, P. M., Woods, R. P., Karaca, T. J., Tiwari, A. et al. (1997). Mapping histology to metabolism: Coregistration of stained whole-brain sections to premortem PET in Alzheimer's disease. *Neuroimage*, 5: 147–153.

Mega, M. S., Cummings, J. L., O'Connor, S. M., Dinov, I. D., Reback, E., Felix, J. et al. (2001). Cognitive and metabolic responses to metrifonate therapy in Alzheimer disease. *Neuropsychiatry Neuropsychology and Behavioral Neurology*, 14: 63–68.

Mega, M. S., Dinov, I. D., Porter, V., Chow, G., Reback, E., Davoodi, P. et al. (2005). Metabolic patterns associated with the clinical response to galantamine therapy: A fludeoxyglucose f 18 positron emission tomographic study. *Archives of Neurology*, 62: 721–728.

Meguro, K., Blaizot, X., Kondoh, Y., Le Mestric, C., Baron, J. C., and Chavoix, C. (1999). Neocortical and hippocampal glucose hypometabolism following neurotoxic lesions of the entorhinal and perirhinal cortices in the non-human primate as shown by PET. Implications for Alzheimer's disease. *Brain*, 122: 1519–1531.

Mehta, K. M., Ott, A., Kalmijn, S., Slooter, A. J., Van Duijn, C. M., Hofman, A. et al. (1999). Head trauma and risk of dementia and Alzheimer's disease: the Rotterdam study. *Neurology*, 53: 1959–1962.

Mellanby, A. R. and Reveley, M. A. (1982). Effects of acute dehydration on computerized tomographic assessment of cerebral density and ventricular volume. *Lancet*, 2: 874.

Meyer-Luehmann, M., Spires-Jones, T. L., Prada, C., Garcia-Alloza, M., de Calignon, A., Rozkalne, A. et al. (2008). Rapid appearance and local toxicity of amyloid-ß plaques in a mouse model of Alzheimer's disease. *Nature*, 451: 720–724.

Miech, R. A., Breitner, J. C., Zandi, P. P., Khachaturian, A. S., Anthony, J. C., and Mayer, L. (2002). Incidence of AD may decline in the early 90s for men, later for women: The Cache County study. *Neurology*, 58: 209–218.

Mielke, R., Herholz, K., Grond, M., Kessler, J., and Heiss, W. D. (1992). Differences of regional cerebral glucose metabolism between presenile and senile dementia of Alzheimer type. *Neurobiology of Aging*, 13: 93–98.

Minoshima, S., Foster, N. L., and Kuhl, D. E. (1994). Posterior cingulate cortex in Alzheimer's disease. *Lancet*, 344: 895.

Minoshima, S., Foster, N. L., Sima, A. A., Frey, K. A., Albin, R. L., and Kuhl, D. E. (2001). Alzheimer's disease versus dementia with Lewy bodies: Cerebral metabolic distinction with autopsy confirmation. *Annals of Neurology*, 50: 358–365.

Minoshima, S., Frey, K. A., Koeppe, R. A., Foster, N. L., and Kuhl, D. E. (1995). A diagnostic approach in Alzheimer's disease using three-dimensional stereotactic surface projections of fluorine-18-FDG PET. *Journal of Nuclear Medicine*, 36: 1238–1248.

Minoshima, S., Giordani, B., Berent, S., Frey, K. A., Foster, N. L., and Kuhl, D. E. (1997). Metabolic reduction in the posterior cingulate cortex in very early Alzheimer's disease. *Annals of Neurology*, 42: 85–94.

Mintun, M. A., Larossa, G. N., Sheline, Y. I., Dence, C. S., Lee, S. Y., Mach, R. H. et al. (2006). [11C]PIB in a nondemented population: Potential antecedent marker of Alzheimer disease. *Neurology*, 67: 446–452.

Mohs, R. C. (2000). Neuropsychological assessment of patients with Alzheimer's disease. Psychopharmacology—the fourth generation of Progress [On-line]. Available: http://www.acnp.org/g4/GN401000133/Default.htm

Montine, T. J., Quinn, J., Kaye, J., and Morrow, J. D. (2007). F(2)-isoprostanes as biomarkers of late-onset Alzheimer's disease. *Journal of Molecular Neuroscience*, 33: 114–119.

Morris, J. C. (1993). The Clinical Dementia Rating (CDR): Current version and scoring rules. *Neurology*, 43: 2412–2414.

Morris, J. C., Storandt, M., Miller, J. P., McKeel, D. W., Price, J. L., Rubin, E. H. et al. (2001). Mild cognitive impairment represents early-stage Alzheimer disease. *Archives of Neurology*, 58: 397–405.

Mortimer, J. A., French, L. R., Hutton, J. T., and Schuman, L. M. (1985). Head injury as a risk factor for Alzheimer's disease. *Neurology*, 35: 264–267.

Mosconi, L. (2005). Brain glucose metabolism in the early and specific diagnosis of Alzheimer's disease. FDG-PET studies in MCI and AD. *European Journal of Nuclear Medicine and Molecular Imaging*, 32: 486–510.

Mosconi, L., De Santi, S., Li, J., Tsui, W. H., Li, Y., Boppana, M. et al. (2008). Hippocampal hypometabolism predicts cognitive decline from normal aging. *Neurobiology of Aging*, 29: 676–692.

Mosconi, L., Perani, D., Sorbi, S., Herholz, K., Nacmias, B., Holthoff, V. et al. (2004). MCI conversion to dementia and the APOE genotype: A prediction study with FDG-PET. *Neurology*, 63: 2332–2340.

Mosconi, L., Sorbi, S., de Leon, M. J., Li, Y., Nacmias, B., Myoung, P. S. et al. (2006). Hypometabolism exceeds atrophy in presymptomatic early-onset familial Alzheimer's disease. *The Journal of Nuclear Medicine*, 47: 1778–1786.

Mosconi, L., Tsui, W. H., De Santi, S., Li, J., Rusinek, H., Convit, A. et al. (2005). Reduced hippocampal metabolism in MCI and AD: Automated FDG-PET image analysis. *Neurology*, 64: 1860–1867.

Mosconi, L., Tsui, W. H., Pupi, A., De Santi, S., Drzezga, A., Minoshima, S. et al. (2007). (18)F-FDG PET database of longitudinally confirmed healthy elderly individuals improves detection of mild cognitive impairment and Alzheimer's disease. *Journal of Nuclear Medicine*, 48: 1129–1134.

Mueller, S. G., Weiner, M. W., Thal, L. J., Petersen, R. C., Jack, C., Jagust, W. et al. (2005a). The Alzheimer's disease neuroimaging initiative. *Neuroimaging Clinics of North America*, 15: 869–877, xi–xii.

Mueller, S. G., Weiner, M. W., Thal, L. J., Petersen, R. C., Jack, C. R., Jagust, W. et al. (2005b). Ways toward an early diagnosis in Alzheimer's disease: the Alzheimer's Disease Neuroimaging Initiative (ADNI). *Alzheimers and Dementia*, 1: 55–66.

Newman, A. B., Fitzpatrick, A. L., Lopez, O., Jackson, S., Lyketsos, C., Jagust, W. et al. (2005). Dementia and Alzheimer's disease incidence in relationship to cardiovascular disease in the Cardiovascular Health Study cohort. *Journal of the American Geriatrics Society*, 53: 1101–1107.

Oddo, S., Billings, L., Kesslak, J. P., Cribbs, D. H., and LaFerla, F. M. (2004). Abeta immunotherapy leads to clearance of early, but not late, hyperphosphorylated tau aggregates via the proteasome. *Neuron*, 43: 321–332.

Oddo, S., Vasilevko, V., Caccamo, A., Kitazawa, M., Cribbs, D. H., and LaFerla, F. M. (2006). Reduction of soluble Aß and tau, but not soluble Aß alone, ameliorates cognitive decline in transgenic mice with plaques and tangles. *Journal of Biological Chemistry*, 281: 39413–39423.

Paganini-Hill, A. and Henderson, V. W. (1996). Estrogen replacement therapy and risk of Alzheimer disease. *Archives of Internal Medicine*, 156: 2213–2217.

Panisset, M., Roudier, M., Saxton, J., and Boller, F. (1994). Severe impairment battery. A neuropsychological test for severely demented patients. *Archives of Neurology*, 51: 41–45.

Petersen, R. C., Parisi, J. E., Dickson, D. W., Johnson, K. A., Knopman, D. S., Boeve, B. F. et al. (2006). Neuropathologic features of amnestic mild cognitive impairment. *Archives of Neurology*, 63: 665–672.

Petersen, R. C., Smith, G. E., Waring, S. C., Ivnik, R. J., Tangalos, E. G., and Kokmen, E. (1999). Mild cognitive impairment: clinical characterization and outcome. *Archives of Neurology*, 56: 303–308.

Petersen, R. C., Thomas, R. G., Grundman, M., Bennett, D., Doody, R., Ferris, S. et al. (2005). Vitamin E and donepezil for the treatment of mild cognitive impairment. *The New England Journal of Medicine*, 352: 2379–2388.

Piert, M., Koeppe, R. A., Giordani, B., Berent, S., and Kuhl, D. E. (1996). Diminished glucose transport and phosphorylation in Alzheimer's disease determined by dynamic FDG-PET. *Journal of Nuclear Medicine*, 37: 201–208.

Pike, K. E., Savage, G., Villemagne, V. L., Ng, S., Moss, S. A., Maruff, P. et al. (2007). b-amyloid imaging and memory in non-demented individuals: evidence for preclinical Alzheimer's disease. *Brain*, 130: 2837–2844.

Plassman, B. L., Langa, K. M., Fisher, G. G., Heeringa, S. G., Weir, D. R., Ofstedal, M. B. et al. (2007). Prevalence of dementia in the United States: the aging, demographics, and memory study. *Neuroepidemiology*, 29: 125–132.

Prentice, R. L. (1989). Surrogate endpoints in clinical trials: Definition and operational criteria. *Statistics In Medicine*, 8: 431–440.

Raskin, R. J., Schnapf, D. J., and Mehlman, I. (1983). Corticosteroid hormonal influence on cranial computerized tomography: observations in the Rhesus monkey. *Journal of Rheumatology*, 10: 977–980.

Reiman, E. M. (2007). Linking brain imaging and genomics in the study of Alzheimer's disease and aging. *Annals of the New York Academy of Sciences*, 1097: 94–113.

Reiman, E. M. (2008). Give priority to fighting Alzheimer's. Arizona Republic, B5.

Reiman, E. M., Caselli, R. J., Alexander, G. E., and Chen, K. (2001a). Tracking the decline in cerebral glucose metablolism in persons and laboratory animals at genetic risk for Alzheimer's disease. *Clinical Neuroscience Research*, 1: 194–206.

Reiman, E. M., Caselli, R. J., Chen, K., Alexander, G. E., Bandy, D., and Frost, J. (2001b). Declining brain activity in cognitively normal apolipoprotein E ε4 heterozygotes: A foundation for using positron emission tomography to efficiently test treatments to prevent Alzheimer's disease. *Proceedings of the National Academy of Sciences of the USA*, 98: 3334–3339.

Reiman, E. M., Caselli, R. J., Yun, L. S., Chen, K., Bandy, D., Minoshima, S. et al. (1996). Preclinical evidence of Alzheimer's disease in persons homozygous for the ε4 allele for apolipoprotein E. *The New England Journal of Medicine*, 334: 752–758.

Reiman, E. M., Chen, K., Alexander, G. E., Caselli, R. J., Bandy, D., Osborne, D. et al. (2004). Functional brain abnormalities in young adults at genetic risk for late-onset Alzheimer's dementia. *Proceedings of the National Academy of Sciences of the USA*, 101: 284–289.

Reiman, E. M., Chen, K., Alexander, G. E., Caselli, R. J., Bandy, D., Osborne, D. et al. (2005). Correlations between apolipoprotein E ε4 gene dose and brain-imaging measurements of regional hypometabolism. *Proceedings of the National Academy of Sciences of the USA*, 102: 8299–8302.

Reiman, E. M., Chen, K., Caselli, R. J., Alexander, G. E., Bandy, D., Adamson, J. L. et al. (2008). Cholesterol-related genetic risk scores are associated with hypometabolism in Alzheimer's-affected brain regions. *Neuroimage*, 40: 1214–1221.

Reiman, E. M., Uecker, A., Caselli, R. J., Lewis, S., Bandy, D., de Leon, M. J. et al. (1998). Hippocampal volumes in cognitively normal persons at genetic risk for Alzheimer's disease. *Annals of Neurology*, 44: 288–291.

Reiman, E. M., Webster, J. A., Myers, A. J., Hardy, J., Dunckley, T., Zismann, V. L. et al. (2007). GAB2 alleles modify Alzheimer's risk in APOE ε4 carriers. *Neuron*, 54: 713–720.

Reisberg, B., Ferris, S. H., de Leon, M. J., and Crook, T. (1982). The Global Deterioration Scale for assessment of primary degenerative dementia. *The American Journal of Psychiatry*, 139: 1136–1139.

Reitz, C., den, H. T., Van, D. C., Hofman, A., and Breteler, M. M. (2007). Relation between smoking and risk of dementia and Alzheimer disease: The Rotterdam Study. *Neurology*, 69: 998–1005.

Risner, M. E., Saunders, A. M., Altman, J. F., Ormandy, G. C., Craft, S., Foley, I. M. et al. (2006). Efficacy of rosiglitazone in a genetically defined population with mild-to-moderate Alzheimer's disease. *The Pharmacogenomics Journal*, 6: 246–254.

Roberts, J. S., Cupples, L. A., Relkin, N. R., Whitehouse, P. J., and Green, R. C. (2005). Genetic risk assessment for adult children of people with Alzheimer's disease: The Risk Evaluation and Education for Alzheimer's Disease (REVEAL) study. *Journal of Geriatric Psychiatry and Neurology*, 18: 250–255.

Rogaev, E. I., Sherrington, R., Rogaeva, E. A., Levesque, G., Ikeda, M., Liang, Y. et al. (1995). Familial Alzheimer's disease in kindreds with missense mutations in a gene on chromosome 1 related to the Alzheimer's disease type 3 gene. *Nature*, 376: 775–778.

Rosen, W. G., Mohs, R. C., and Davis, K. L. (1984). A new rating scale for Alzheimer's disease. *The American Journal of Psychiatry*, 141: 1356–1364.

Rowe, C. C., Ackerman, U., Browne, W., Mulligan, R., Pike, K. L., O'Keefe, G. et al. (2008). Imaging of amyloid beta in Alzheimer's disease with (18)F-BAY94-9172, a novel PET tracer: proof of mechanism. *Lancet Neurology*, 7: 129–135.

Rowe, C. C., Ng, S., Ackermann, U., Gong, S. J., Pike, K., Savage, G. et al. (2007). Imaging beta-amyloid burden in aging and dementia. *Neurology*, 68: 1718–1725.

Rusinek, H., de Leon, M. J., George, A. E., Stylopoulos, L. A., Chandra, R., Smith, G. et al. (1991). Alzheimer disease: Measuring loss of cerebral gray matter with MR imaging. *Radiology*, 178: 109–114.

Rusinek, H., De Santi, S., Frid, D., Tsui, W. H., Tarshish, C. Y., Convit, A. et al. (2003). Regional brain atrophy rate predicts future cognitive decline: 6-year longitudinal MR imaging study of normal aging. *Radiology*, 229: 691–696.

Saczynski, J. S., Pfeifer, L. A., Masaki, K., Korf, E. S., Laurin, D., White, L. et al. (2006). The effect of social engagement on incident dementia: The Honolulu-Asia Aging Study. *American Journal of Epidemiology*, 163: 433–440.

Scarmeas, N., Stern, Y., Mayeux, R., and Luchsinger, J. A. (2006). Mediterranean diet, Alzheimer disease, and vascular mediation. *Archives of Neurology*, 63: 1709–1717.

Schneider, L. S. and Olin, J. T. (1996). Clinical global impressions in Alzheimer's clinical trials. *International Psychogeriatrics*, 8: 277–288.

Schneider, L. S., Olin, J. T., Doody, R. S., Clark, C. M., Morris, J. C., Reisberg, B. et al. (1997). Validity and reliability of the Alzheimer's disease cooperative study-clinical global impression of change. The Alzheimer's disease cooperative study. *Alzheimer Disease and Associated Disorders*, 11 (Suppl 2): S22–S32.

Schoonenboom, N. S., van der Flier, W. M., Blankenstein, M. A., Bouwman, F. H., Van Kamp, G. J., Barkhof, F. et al. (2008). CSF and MRI markers independently contribute to the diagnosis of Alzheimer's disease. *Neurobiology of Aging*, 29: 669–675.

Schwartz, W. J., Smith, C. B., Davidsen, L., Savaki, H., Sokoloff, L., Mata, M. et al. (1979). Metabolic mapping of functional activity in the hypothalamo-neurohypophysial system of the rat. *Science*, 205: 723–725.

Selkoe, D. J. (2008). Soluble oligomers of the amyloid beta-protein impair synaptic plasticity and behavior. *Behavioural Brain Research*, 192: 106–113.

Sherrington, R., Rogaev, E. I., Liang, Y., Rogaeva, E. A., Levesque, G., Ikeda, M. et al. (1995). Cloning of a gene bearing missense mutations in early-onset familial Alzheimer's disease. *Nature*, 375: 754–760.

Shumaker, S. A., Legault, C., Kuller, L., Rapp, S. R., Thal, L., Lane, D. S. et al. (2004). Conjugated equine estrogens and incidence of probable dementia and mild cognitive impairment in postmenopausal women: Women's Health Initiative Memory Study. *The Journal of the American Medical Association*, 291: 2947–2958.

Shumaker, S. A., Legault, C., Rapp, S. R., Thal, L., Wallace, R. B., Ockene, J. K. et al. (2003). Estrogen plus progestin and the incidence of dementia and mild cognitive impairment in postmenopausal women: The Women's Health Initiative Memory Study: a randomized controlled trial. *The Journal of the American Medical Association*, 289: 2651–2662.

Shumaker, S. A., Reboussin, B. A., Espeland, M. A., Rapp, S. R., McBee, W. L., Dailey, M. et al. (1998). The Women's Health Initiative Memory Study (WHIMS): A trial of the effect of estrogen therapy in preventing and slowing the progression of dementia. *Controlled Clinical Trials*, 19: 604–621.

Silverman, D. H., Small, G. W., Chang, C. Y., Lu, C. S., Kung De Aburto, M. A., Chen, W. et al. (2001). Positron emission tomography in evaluation of dementia: Regional brain metabolism and long-term outcome. *The Journal of the American Medical Association*, 286: 2120–2127.

Sloane, P. D., Zimmerman, S., Suchindran, C., Reed, P., Wang, L., Boustani, M. et al. (2002). The public health impact of Alzheimer's disease, 2000–2050: Potential implication of treatment advances. *Annual Review of Public Health*, 23: 213–231.

Small, G. W., Agdeppa, E. D., Kepe, V., Satyamurthy, N., Huang, S. C., and Barrio, J. R. (2002). In vivo brain imaging of tangle burden in humans. *Journal of Molecular Neuroscience*, 19: 323–327.

Small, G. W., Ercoli, L. M., Silverman, D. H., Huang, S. C., Komo, S., Bookheimer, S. Y. et al. (2000). Cerebral metabolic and cognitive decline in persons at genetic risk for Alzheimer's disease. *Proceedings of the National Academy of Sciences of the USA*, 97: 6037–6042.

Small, G. W., Kepe, V., Ercoli, L. M., Siddarth, P., Bookheimer, S. Y., Miller, K. J. et al. (2006). PET of brain amyloid and tau in mild cognitive impairment. *The New England Journal of Medicine*, 355: 2652–2663.

Smith, G. S., de Leon, M. J., George, A. E., Kluger, A., Volkow, N. D., McRae, T. et al. (1992). Topography of cross-sectional and longitudinal glucose metabolic deficits in Alzheimer's disease. Pathophysiologic implications. *Archives of Neurology*, 49: 1142–1150.

Stern, Y., Gurland, B., Tatemichi, T. K., Tang, M. X., Wilder, D., and Mayeux, R. (1994). Influence of education and occupation on the incidence of Alzheimer's disease. *The Journal of the American Medical Association*, 271: 1004–1010.

Stewart, R., Masaki, K., Xue, Q. L., Peila, R., Petrovitch, H., White, L. R. et al. (2005). A 32-year prospective study of change in body weight and incident dementia: the Honolulu-Asia Aging Study. *Archives of Neurology*, 62: 55–60.

Tang, M. X., Jacobs, D., Stern, Y., Marder, K., Schofield, P., Gurland, B. et al. (1996). Effect of oestrogen during menopause on risk and age at onset of Alzheimer's disease. *Lancet*, 348: 429–432.

Van Duijn, C. M., Van, B. C., Hardy, J. A., Goate, A. M., Rossor, M. N., Vandenberghe, A. et al. (1991). Evidence for allelic heterogeneity in familial early-onset Alzheimer's disease. *British Journal of Psychiatry*, 158: 471–474.

Vellas, B., Andrieu, S., Sampaio, C., and Wilcock, G. (2007). Disease-modifying trials in Alzheimer's disease: A European task force consensus. *Lancet Neurology*, 6: 56–62.

Visser, P. J., Scheltens, P., Verhey, F. R., Schmand, B., Launer, L. J., Jolles, J. et al. (1999). Medial temporal lobe atrophy and memory dysfunction as predictors for dementia in subjects with mild cognitive impairment. *Journal of Neurology*, 246: 477–485.

Wang, H. X., Karp, A., Winblad, B., and Fratiglioni, L. (2002). Late-life engagement in social and leisure activities is associated with a decreased risk of dementia: a longitudinal study from the Kungsholmen project. *American Journal of Epidemiology*, 155: 1081–1087.

Williamson, J. D., Vellas, B., Furberg, C., Nahin, R., and DeKosky, S. T. (2008). Comparison of the design differences between the Ginkgo Evaluation of Memory study and the GuidAge study. *The Journal of Nutrition, Health and Aging*, 12: 73S–79S.

Wishart, H. A., Saykin, A. J., McAllister, T. W., Rabin, L. A., McDonald, B. C., Flashman, L. A. et al. (2006). Regional brain atrophy in cognitively intact adults with a single APOE e4 allele. *Neurology*, 67: 1221–1224.

Wolozin, B., Wang, S. W., Li, N. C., Lee, A., Lee, T. A., and Kazis, L. E. (2007). Simvastatin is associated with a reduced incidence of dementia and Parkinson's disease. *BMC Medicine*, 5: 1–28.

Yaffe, K., Barnes, D., Nevitt, M., Lui, L. Y., and Covinsky, K. (2001). A prospective study of physical activity and cognitive decline in elderly women: women who walk. *Archives of Intern Medicine*, 161: 1703–1708.

Zandi, P. P., Anthony, J. C., Khachaturian, A. S., Stone, S. V., Gustafson, D., Tschanz, J. T. et al. (2004). Reduced risk of Alzheimer disease in users of antioxidant vitamin supplements: The Cache County Study. *Archives of Neurology*, 61: 82–88.

Zandi, P. P., Carlson, M. C., Plassman, B. L., Welsh-Bohmer, K. A., Mayer, L. S., Steffens, D. C. et al. (2002). Hormone replacement therapy and incidence of Alzheimer disease in older women: The Cache County Study. *The Journal of the American Medical Association*, 288: 2123–2129.

Zivadinov, R. (2005). Steroids and brain atrophy in multiple sclerosis. *Journal of the Neurological Science*, 233: 73–81.

21

Databasing the Aging Brain

John Darrell Van Horn and Arthur W. Toga

Introduction

Over 150 years ago, the incredible case of Phineas Gage began what may be considered as the modern era of the localization of brain function (Haas, 2001). In this famous event, damage to the frontal lobe produced profound changes in personality and cognitive function. Nearly a decade later, the examination by Paul Broca of aphasic patients with damage to the left inferior frontal areas solidified the notion that function could be linked to specific areas of cortical tissue (Cowie, 2000). Then, in 1901, Dr. Alois Alzheimer (a German psychiatrist) identified the first case of what became known as Alzheimer's disease in a 50 year-old patient (Auguste D.) and followed her to her death in 1906, when he first reported the case (Goedert and Ghetti, 2007). Since that time, a principle goal of neuroscience has been to identify the specific brain locations for the unique functional components of complex thought, and how these functions might be altered in response to an injury or as the result of disease. With the emergence of brain imaging as the primary tool for the examination of the brain in vivo during cognitive task performance over the past 20 years, the mapping of cognitive function has given rise to an explosion of functional data collection and an ever-widening interest in understanding brain processes from fields beyond traditional neuroscience (e.g., economics, philosophy, social science, etc.). This intense effort and flood of data has emphasized the realization that there is considerable individual variation in brain size and shape that must be accounted for in the processing of brain imaging data and the assignment of functional activation. Evaluation and comparison of brain imaging data with respect to and against well-defined anatomical references is now a critical element in the localization of essential cognitive functions in nearly all functional imaging investigations.

Openly Available Atlases of the Brain

An increasing number and variety of brain atlases for humans, as well as other species, are being made openly available online for the neuroscience community to use as authoritative references for inclusion in data-processing pipelines, or for the display of results. These include probabilistic anatomical atlases (Mazziotta et al., 1995; Toga et al., 2001; Toga et al., 2006), white matter fiber atlases (Wakana et al., 2004), and cortical surface atlases (Van Essen, 2005). A brief listing of several is provided in Table 21.1.

Considerable interest has emerged concerning the notion of databasing the results of and the raw data from studies of human neuroimaging (Fox and Lancaster, 2002; Toga, 2002; Van Horn et al., 2004). Databases can provide a wealth of structural and functional data obtained from across a range of subjects or patient groups. Study result summaries based upon spatial atlases can be viewed collectively to permit inference across diverse samples. For example, data from a large database of functional MRI studies was mined to explore the differences between young, older, and dementia subjects. Prominent coactivation of the hippocampus, detected in all groups, implied that the so-called default-mode network (Raichle and Gusnard, 2002) may be closely involved with episodic memory processing. The dementia patients showed decreased resting-state activity in the posterior cingulate and hippocampus, however, suggesting that disrupted connectivity between these two regions accounts for the posterior cingulate hypometabolism commonly detected in positron emission tomography studies of early dementia (Greicius et al., 2004). The use of databases can and will continue to be an important resource for examining functional and structural activity, and structure in aging populations and diseases associated with older individuals. Standardized databases and accompanying atlases of the normal aging process would be a highly desirable resource for the community.

Data Repositories Related to Diseases Associated with Aging

The National Institute of Health policy on data sharing has recognized that "data sharing is essential for expedited translation of research results into knowledge, products, and procedures to improve human health" (http://grants.nih.gov/grants/policy/data_sharing/data_sharing_guidance.htm). The contribution of data to neuroimaging archives has become increasingly important for assimilating the information that can lead to new knowledge. To that end, the National Institute on Aging (NIA) has funded the National Alzheimer's Coordinating Center (NACC; http://www.alz.washington.edu/) to maintain a database of demographic, clinical, and pathological data collected by the 29 NIA-funded Alzheimer's disease research centers (ADRCs). ADRC researchers have worked to translate research advances into improved diagnosis and care for Alzheimer's disease (AD) patients while, at the same time, focusing on the program's long-term goal—finding a way to cure and possibly prevent AD. Although each center has its own unique area of emphasis, a common goal of the ADRCs is to enhance research on AD by providing a network for sharing new ideas as well as research results. Collaborative studies draw upon

Table 21–1 A list of several notable neuroimaging brain atlas resources.

Name	URL(s)	Comment
The Whole Brain Atlas	http://www.med.harvard.edu/AANLIB/home.html	Human brain atlas including images from post-mortem serial sections and MRI. Includes aging brain images.
The Allen Brain Atlas	http://www.alleninstitute.org/ http://www.brain-map.org/	Atlas of gene expression in the mouse.
The Human Brain Atlas	http://www.msu.edu/%7ebrains/brains/human/index.html	Stained sections of human brain.
Brainmaps.org	http://brainmaps.org/	Scanned images of serial sections of both primate and non-primate brains.
The Mouse Brain Library	http://www.mbl.org/	High-resolution images and databases of brains from many genetically characterized strains of mice.
The fMRI Data Center (fMRIDC)	http://www.fmridc.org/	Complete fMRI data sets from published studies of cognitive function.
Comparative Mammalian Brain Collections	http://www.brainmuseum.org/	Photos of whole brain and serial sections from a range of primate brains.
White Matter Atlas	http://www.dtiatlas.org/	Human brain white matter maps obtained from diffusion tensor imaging (DTI).
ICBM/LONI Probabilistic Atlas Series	http://www.loni.ucla.edu/Atlases	Human brain atlases based upon probabilistic metrics of regional location.
Surface Data Management System (SuMs) Atlases	http://sumsdb.wustl.edu:8081/sums/humanpalsmore.do	Standardized brain surface models with links to associated functional data.

the expertise of scientists from many different disciplines. Some ADCs have satellite facilities that offer diagnostic and treatment services and research opportunities in underserved, rural, and minority communities. The National Alzheimer's Coordinating Center (NACC) at the University of Washington coordinates data collection and fosters collaborative research among ADRCs. Additionally, the National Cell Repository for Alzheimers Disease maintains a database of family histories and medical records and provides genetic researchers with cell lines and/or DNA samples. Several of the ADRCs also conduct neuroimaging investigations, but some of these data may not necessarily be widely available to researchers outside of each individual center. Many of the ADRCs have specific neuroimaging cores and are acquiring MRI, PET, fMRI, and/or DTI data on subjects who are participating at their centers. The ability to safely pool and share these data among the ADRCs, and with external investigators studying AD, prediction and progression would be a positive development in cooperative research. Many of the ADRCs are also participating in the AD Neuroimaging Initiative (ADNI), in which imaging data is pooled and shared with the scientific community. The NACC database is made available to qualified research scientists.

The highly successful NIA ADNI program was established to increase knowledge of the mechanisms of AD through the use of neuroimaging, thereby informing the development of treatment strategies aimed at slowing down or preventing neuronal death. ADNI has been instrumental in helping to identify clinical, neuroimaging, and biomarker outcome measures, as well as longitudinal changes and the prediction of disease transitions. In particular, this has included neurodegeneration—the clinically and pathologically heterogeneous disease entity associated with slowly progressive neuronal loss in different anatomical and functional systems of the brain. Owing to increasing knowledge about the mechanisms leading to neurodegeneration as a result of ADNI, the development of treatments able to modify the neurodegenerative process will be easier. While more research is clearly needed to determine the continued value of newer neuroimaging modalities (i.e., diffusion, perfusion, and functional MRI and MR spectroscopy) for clinical trials with neuroprotective drugs, the ADNI project can be considered a highly successful first step in large-scale neuroimaging and the sharing of that information with a larger community studying the efficacy of leading-edge treatment.

The Laboratory of Neuro Imaging (LONI) has notably been serving as a central repository for single- and multisite neuroimaging research studies for a number of years (Toga, 2002), participating in both ARDC and ADNI initiatives. More than 24 000 medical images for over a dozen major research projects are currently managed within the LONI Image Data Archive (IDA). LONI has established robust procedures in key areas for storing, managing, and protecting medical image data, which include:

- A strict set of rules that are used to govern the control and distribution of data

- A user's access level, which determines the features and functions available and may be set by the study investigator using the integrated user access management interface

- The IDA system, which tracks dissemination of data in a HIPAA compliant manner, logging all uploads, downloads, edits, and deletions

- Study investigators who may perform queries across the clinical and imaging data, and browse, update, and organize the data

- An integrated image viewer that allows the image data to be visually inspected

Users may form data collections and download the data locally or pass the collections to the LONI pipeline processing environment.

Brain Atlases as an Emergent Property of Databases

Brain atlases (Figure 21.1) can now incorporate data describing multiple aspects of brain structure or function—like the LONI IDA—at different scales from different subjects, at different times, yielding a truly integrative and comprehensive description of this organ during health and disease (Roland and Zilles, 1994; Toga and Thompson, 2001). The complexity and variability of brain structure, especially in the gyral patterns of the human cortex, present challenges in creating standardized brain atlases that reflect the anatomy of a population (Toga and Thompson, 2002). Based on well-characterized subject groups, age-specific atlases can potentially contain thousands of structure models, composite maps, average templates, and visualizations of structural variability, asymmetry, and group-specific differences. They correlate the structural, metabolic, molecular, and histologic hallmarks of the disease (Narr et al., 2000; Thompson et al., 2002). Figure 21.2 shows an example of a typical registration against the ICBM40 average brain atlas. Rather than simply arithmetically averaging information from multiple subjects and sources, new mathematical strategies can be introduced to resolve group-specific features not apparent in individual scans (Davatzikos, 1996). High-dimensional elastic mappings, based on covariant partial differential equations, are developed to encode patterns of cortical variation (Davatzikos, 1997; Thompson et al., 2000; Weaver et al., 1998). In the resulting brain atlas, age-stratified features and regional asymmetries emerge that are not apparent in individual anatomies. The resulting probabilistic atlas spaces can be used to identify patterns of altered structure and function, and can guide algorithms for knowledge-based image analysis, automated image labeling, tissue classification, data mining, and functional image analysis. These integrative approaches have provided significant motivation for human brain-mapping initiatives, and have important applications in health and the understanding of how the brain changes through normal aging.

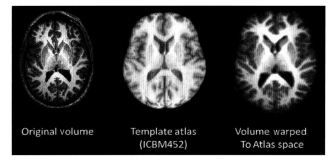

Figure 21–2 Basic warping of data obtained during imaging experiments has become the *de facto* first step for many data-processing workflows involving both normal and patient samples. Affine and nonlinear approaches for warping anatomical image volumes (**a**) to standardized spaces (**b**) have been developed, each having certain advantages and disadvantages in terms of accuracy or computational load. However, the warping of patient data to "normal" template atlases may lead to improper conclusions concerning the localization of brain activity, the degree of alteration under voxel-based morphometry in patients when contrasted against normative samples, and other confounds.

Methods for Brain Atlas Construction

Creating atlases relies on the accumulation and compilation of many image sets, along with appropriate registration and warping strategies, indexing schemes, and nomenclature systems. Here lies the importance of databases as the source of data for structural and functional atlas construction. The processing of multimodal brain images in the context of an atlas enables a more meaningful interpretation (e.g. as depicted in Figure 21.1). The complexity and variability of human brain (as well as other species) across subjects is so great that reliance on atlases is essential to effectively manipulate, analyze, interpret, and render brain data (Figure 21.3). Central to these tasks is the construction of averages, templates, and models to describe how the brain and its component parts are organized. Design of appropriate reference systems for human

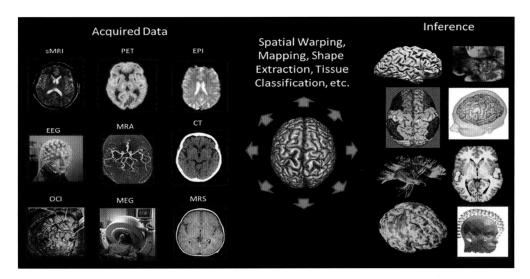

Figure 21–1 A variety of neuroimaging methods permit the acquisition of brain data over time and space with a range of resolution granularity. Moreover, variation across individuals and how this changes over the lifespan must be accounted for in statistical examination of the data. Mapping these data to known spatial coordinate systems enables highly accurate inference concerning the brain's structural change over time, between populations, or in terms of localizing functional change. Atlases denoting this variation after spatial warping, the characterization of shape, 3D distortion, etc., will be essential in describing structural and functional alteration associated with normal aging as well as in disease.

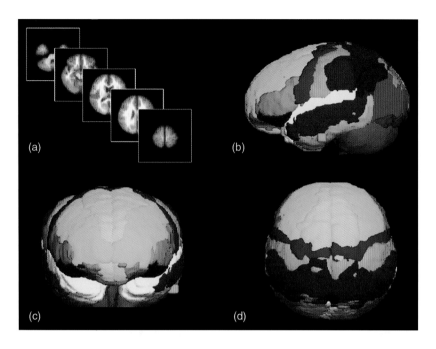

Figure 21–3 Averaged normal subjects (**a**) against an atlas space permits automated extraction of "average" brain regions using sophisticated voxel position and intensity-sorting algorithms (**b–d**).

brain data presents considerable challenges, since these systems must capture how brain structure and function vary in large populations, across age and gender, in different disease states, across imaging modalities, and even across species. Let us introduce several noteworthy approaches here.

Basic Image Registration: Image registration is central to many of the challenges in brain imaging today (Gholipour et al., 2007) and is routinely applied in studies of normal—as well as patient—samples. Initially developed as an image processing subspecialty to geometrically transform one image to match another (e.g., Figure 21.2), image registration using openly available software packages (e.g., AIR, FSL, etc) permits spatial averaging and the creation of population-based atlases. Basic volume registration now has a vast range of applications, including: methods developed for automated image labeling and pathology detection in individuals or groups (Woods et al., 1998); Registration algorithms can encode patterns of anatomical variability in large human populations, and can use this information to create disease-specific, population-based brain atlases (Woods et al., 1998); while they may also fuse information from multiple imaging devices to correlate different measures of brain structure and function. Finally, registration algorithms can serve as a basic measure for patterns of structural change during brain development, tumor growth, or degenerative disease processes (Woods, 2003).

Geodesic Averaging of Brain Shape: The goal in geodesic approaches has been to promote variational methods for anatomical averaging that operate within the space of the underlying image registration problem (Avants and Gee, 2004). This approach is effective when using the large deformation viscous framework, where linear averaging might not be appropriate. The theory behind it is similar to registration-based techniques, but with single-image forces replaced by the average forces from multiple sources. These group forces drive an average transport ordinary differential equation, allowing one to estimate the geodesic that moves an image toward the mean shape configuration. This model provides large deformation atlases that are optimal with respect to the shape manifold, as defined by the data and the image registration assumptions. These procedures generate refined average representations of highly variable anatomy from distinct populations. For instance, the population statistics show a significant

doubling of the relative prefrontal lobe size in humans, as compared to chimpanzees (Avants et al., 2006).

Shape and Pattern Theory: Of particular relevance in dealing with brain sub-structures are methods used to define a mean shape in such a way that departures from this mean shape can be treated as a linear process (Rohlfing and Maurer, 2007). Linearization of the pathology detection problem, by constructing various shape manifolds and their associated tangent spaces, allows the use of conventional statistical procedures and linear decomposition of departures from the mean to characterize shape change. These approaches have been applied to detect structural anomalies in schizophrenia by identification of statistical differences in the mean shape of brain structures (Corouge et al., 2004; Narr et al., 2007; Thompson et al., 2000).

Encoding Brain Variation: Measuring and accounting for the considerable variability in brain shape across human populations necessitates realistically complex mathematical strategies to encode comprehensive information on structural variability. Particularly relevant is three-dimensional (3D) statistical information on group-specific patterns of variation and how these patterns are altered through disease. This information can be represented so that it can be exploited by expert diagnostic systems, whose goal is to detect subtle or diffuse structural alterations in disease. Strategies for detecting structural anomalies can leverage information in anatomical databases by invoking encoded knowledge on the variations in geometry and the location of neuroanatomical regions and critical functional interfaces, especially at the cortex.

Density-Based Atlases: Initial approaches to population-based atlasing concentrated on generating "average" representations of anatomy through the "intensity pooling" of multiple MRI scans. This involves large numbers of MRI scans that are each linearly transformed into stereotaxic space, intensity-normalized, and averaged on a voxel-by-voxel basis, producing an average-intensity MRI dataset. The average brains that result have large areas, especially at the cortex, where individual structures are blurry due to spatial variability in the population. While this blurring limits their usefulness as a quantitative tool, the templates can be used as targets for the automated registration and mapping of MR and coregistered functional data into stereotaxic space.

Label-Based Atlases: In label-based approaches, large ensembles of brain data are labeled or "segmented" by a human operator into subvolumes after mapping individual datasets into stereotaxic space. A probability map is then constructed for each segmented structure by determining the proportion of subjects assigned a given anatomical label at each voxel position in stereotactic space. The prior information that these probability maps provide on the location of various tissue classes in stereotactic space has been useful in designing automated tissue classifiers and approaches to correct radio frequency and intensity inhomogeneities in MR scans. Statistical data on anatomical labels and tissue types normally found at given positions in stereotactic space provide a vital independent source of information to guide and inform mathematical algorithms that analyze neuroanatomical data in stereotactic space (e.g., Figure 21.3).

Deformation Atlases: When applied to two different 3D brain scans, a nonlinear registration, or warping algorithm, calculates a deformation map that matches up brain structures in one scan with their counterparts in the other. The deformation map indicates 3D patterns of anatomical differences between the two subjects. In probabilistic atlases based on deformation maps, statistical properties of these deformation maps are encoded locally to determine the magnitude and directional biases of anatomical variation. Encoding of local variation can then be used to assess the severity of structural variants outside of the normal range, which may be a

sign of disease. A major goal in designing this type of pathology detection system is to recognize that both the magnitude and local directional biases of structural variability in the brain may be different at every single anatomical point. Such atlases are not only cortically-based, but can also be done, for instance, on substructures and cerebellum (for instance, see Diedrichsen, 2006).

Disease-specific Atlases: Disease-specific atlases are designed to reflect the unique anatomy and physiology of a particular clinical subpopulation. Based on well-characterized patient groups, these atlases contain thousands of structure models, as well as composite maps, average templates, and visualizations of structural variability, asymmetry, and group-specific differences. Figure 21.4 provides an example of atlas construction utilizing $N = 400$ patient structural volumes drawn from the ADNI database. Such atlases act as a quantitative framework that correlates the structural, metabolic, molecular, and histological hallmarks of the disease. Because they retain information on group anatomical variability, disease-specific atlases are a type of probabilistic atlas specialized to represent a particular clinical group. The resulting atlases can identify patterns of altered structure or function, and can guide algorithms for knowledge-based image analysis, automated image labeling, tissue classification, and functional image analysis.

Genetic Atlases: Inclusion of genetic data in an atlas makes it possible to go beyond simply describing the effects of a disease on the brain, to investigating its fundamental causes. This allows the

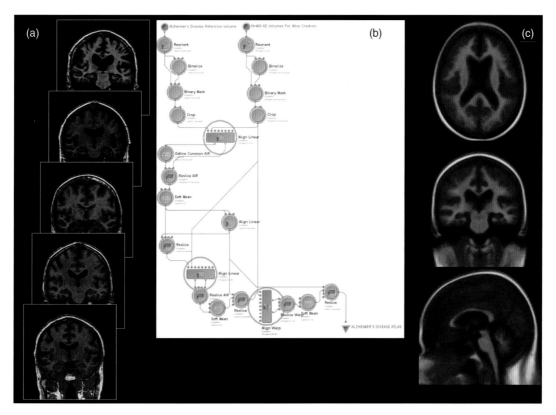

Figure 21–4 $N = 400$ Alzheimer's disease subjects were drawn from the ADNI database housed at LONI/UCLA, of which examples of five are shown here (**a**). These data were systematically submitted to the LONI grid computer cluster via the use of a purpose-built LONI Pipeline workflow (**b**), comprised of a heterogeneous collection of processing modules from commonly available software packages (e.g., AIR, FSL, and related toolsets). The data were spatially reoriented, warped against an Alzheimer's disease subject reference volume, a common realignment solution was identified (and so on) to produce a disease-specific Alzheimer's atlas volume (**c**) against which individual variability may be assessed or used for specific studies underway at other laboratories. The workflow does not contain any operations against a "normal" brain atlas. The processing of this number of subjects required approximately 50 minutes using the LONI Pipeline and LINUX computational grid.

direct mapping of genetic influences on brain structure, and lets us quantify heritability for different features of the brain. Familial, twin, and genetic linkage studies have recently begun to expand the atlas concept to tie together genetic and imaging studies of disease (Thompson et al., 2002; Toga and Thompson, 2005). Atlases that contain genetic brain maps and a means to analyze them can help screen relatives for inherited disease. They also offer a framework for mining large imaging databases for risk genes and quantitative trait loci, as well as genetic and environmental triggers of disease.

Age and Developmental Stratification: The brain changes remarkably in its size and complexity over the lifespan. There is considerable need to account for the age of particular populations in the context of brain maturation and the development of age-stratified normal brain atlas spaces (Toga et al., 2006). People who are mildly cognitively impaired, for instance, are at a fivefold increased risk of imminent conversion to dementia, and present specific structural brain changes that are predictive of imminent disease onset (Apostolova and Thompson, 2007; Apostolova et al., 2007). Language impairment in AD patients is also correlated with cortical atrophy in the left temporal and parietal lobes, bilateral frontal lobes, and right temporal pole (Apostolova et al., 2008). However, characterizing such change presents particular computational challenges. The fitting of brain anatomy to a single template of undetermined age specification may lead to errors in inference about brain morphometry or function because of an inappropriate underlying template. Alternative approaches can also be fruitful and metrics such as shape (Scher et al., 2007), cortical thickness mapping, tensor-based morphometry (TBM) may be better suited for shedding light on the neuroscience of aging and brain degeneration in AD and mild cognitive impairment (MCI) (Thompson et al., 2007).

Brain Atlas Updating, Error Correction, and Revision

Mapping of any variety is an ongoing process of determining accurate spatial position for content appropriate to that mapping's purpose. Because previous content in a map changes, or as new information is obtained, these maps need to be updated, corrected, and/or modified to reflect these changes in knowledge and the importance of what is being conveyed. For instance, the information contained in aeronautical charts in the United States is republished approximately every 3 months to (in part) reflect changes in the Earth's magnetic field isogonic declination lines that point toward the magnetic North Pole. These field lines vary across North America, from approximately −19 in the Western United States through to nearly +20 in the East, and must be taken into account when locating the direction of the true North Pole when charting a navigational course. However, the Earth's magnetic field has been drifting slowly westward, moving roughly 0.1 degrees per year. Failure to periodically update published maps that incorporate this shift in magnetic declination, as well as other information concerning changes in the Earth's topographical features—the construction of tall buildings in urban areas, alterations in air traffic routing, errors in earlier revisions, etc.—could result in pilots or computers making substantial navigational errors due to improper compass and course directional settings.

Errors often appear in maps resulting from the information that was used to create them. Landmarks of note may be mislocated and place names misspelled or mistranslated. Alternative representations of shape can be well-intentioned, but may not prove

favorable. Oronce Finé (1494–1555), for example, was a French mathematician and cartographer who, in attempting to rectify new discoveries from travelers such as Marco Polo and others with existing information, mapped the surface of the Earth to the shape of a heart in 1536. Other maps may be entirely wrong—for instance, considering California as an island lying to the southeast of the main North American continent. Still others require revision as new information is gained or sufficient change has made an earlier version unreliable, despite being generally accurate. For instance, a modern map of the city of Los Angeles, California may retain the geographic features to that of a similar map from the turn of the 20th Century, but will clearly show the extent of urban growth and civil alteration that has occurred since that time.

This would also be true for brain mapping atlases where previous inaccuracies must be addressed, additional data included, or data from other modalities considered. Cytoarchitectonic maps from the classical period of describing brain anatomy have been noted as failing to incorporate sulcal pattern, showing variation in cell orientation, and being presented as idealized versions of brain structure (see Toga et al., 2006, for review). However, even modern approaches, using multimodal methods, large databases, and sophisticated computer methods, are not immune from introducing errors. Electronic versions of the atlas of Talairach and Tournoux (Talairach and Tournoux, 1988), including the Talairach Daemon (http://ric.uthscsa.edu/projects/talairachdaemon.html) and the official versions published by Thieme, have been found to contain a discrepant region of the precentral gyrus on axial slice +35 mm that extends far forward into the frontal lobe. This area is anatomically incorrect and internally inconsistent within the digital atlas software applications that employ multiplanar cross-referencing tools (Maldjian et al., 2004). This may likely be a case of simple mislabeling, but other forms of atlas warping are known to result in distortions that must be predicated in context with the accurate interpretation of location. As new data are included in large-scale archives, and novel techniques are developed to inform atlases that are open to scrutiny by researchers with ongoing updates and corrections, these representations become most widely valuable.

The Role of Databases for Functional Inference

Without reference to known geometries or atlas spaces, functional localization is not strictly possible at the population level. For instance, fMRI studies of human cognition analyzed using the Statistical Parametric Mapping (SPM) software package rely on the MNI atlas as the basis for within-group and between-group statistical comparisons. Typically, each subject's high resolution anatomical image is warped to the MNI multisubject T1 whole-brain template using nonlinear and affine methods. This transformation is then applied to the collection of linearly aligned functional MRI or PET images. Once data are transformed into the MNI atlas space, statistical modeling and comparisons may be undertaken. Areas of "activation" or statistically significant signal change may then be referred back into the space of Talairach and Tournoux using a simple matrix transformation. This mapping localizes the regions of activity to the known reference and accompanying Brodmann's areas. Other software packages, such as FSL and Brain Voyager, perform a similar process.

Continued improvement and enhancement of extant atlases, such as the Talairach atlas (Nowinski, 2005), the several iterations of the MNI atlas, and those of the ICBM probabilistic atlas, provide greater accuracy with respect to functional data and hence, localization power. Modification of Talairach landmarks, for example, can enable more rapid calculation of spatial transformations, thereby providing flexibility for specific applications. In stereotactic and functional neurosurgery, the internal intercommissural distance is the most suitable for providing a high accuracy for subcortical structures (Nowinski, 2001).

Data Mining

The process of data mining is an increasingly important analytic process designed to explore data in a search of consistent patterns and/or systematic relationships between variables (Goutte et al., 2001), and then to validate the findings by applying the detected patterns to new subsets of data (Sidtis et al., 2003). The ultimate goal of data mining in brain research is prediction—and predictive data mining is the most common type of data mining, and one that has the most direct application for new experimentation (Fox et al., 1998). The process of data mining typically consists of three stages:

Exploration: This stage frequently starts with data preparation, involving conditioning of the data, atlas transformations, selecting subsets of scan volumes or functional MR time series, and—in the case of data sets with large numbers of variables in its experimental design—performing some preliminary feature selection operations to find a minimal set of predictor variables.

Model Construction and Validation: This stage involves considering various processing frameworks or mathematical models and choosing the best one based on their predictive performance (i.e., explaining the variability in question, reducing bias, and producing stable results across samples). Workflow tools like the LONI Pipeline can be important at this stage for constructing competing models, applying them to the same data set, and then comparing their performance to choose the best or most efficient approach (Rex et al., 2004). Such techniques in bioinformatics, often considered the core of predictive data mining, include voting, averaging, boosting, stacking, and machine-learning (see Saeys et al., 2007), and similar approaches have been considered for neuroimaging (Strother et al., 2004).

Deployment: The final stage involves applying the selected model as the most superior among those assessed in the previous stage and applying it to new data to generate predictions or estimates of the expected outcome (Chen et al., 2006; Hansen et al., 2001; Lange et al., 1999; Strother et al., 1995).

The concept of data mining for brain imaging data has become increasingly popular as a knowledge extraction tool, where it is expected to reveal aspects of the data not readily observed in standard statistical treatment that can guide decisions in conditions of limited certainty (Lancaster et al., 2005). An important difference in the focus and purpose between data mining and more traditional exploratory data analysis is that data mining is more oriented towards applications than the basic nature of the underlying phenomena. That is, data mining is relatively less concerned with identifying the specific relationships between the involved variables *per se*, but rather the focus is on producing a solution that can generate useful predictions. Therefore, data-mining approaches can involve "black box" means of exploration or

knowledge discovery. For neuroimaging, however, these often include such techniques as discriminant analysis (Carlson et al., 2003) or Bayesian frameworks (Friston et al., 2002).

Data mining and meta-analytic approaches in aging research can be driven by specific database queries against those databases, or can draw from published studies to create ad-hoc databases of study parameters. Examples of each have involved examinations of MR spectroscopy, systematic NAA, choline, and creatine alterations with age (Haga et al., 2007); differences in rCBF response to faces in the elderly compared to young controls (Grady, 2002); structural and functional changes in Alzheimer's disease (Zakzanis et al., 2003); and fronto-temporal degeneration with age (Schroeter et al., 2007). These meta-analyses exploring the various influences of aging on brain structure and function—drawn from databases and from the literature of activation loci—enhance the original studies from which they were drawn and make testable predictions that can lead to new empirical assessment.

Discussion

The evolution of brain databases and resulting atlases has seen tremendous advances. Databases continue to become rich resources for both published and unpublished raw, processed, and results data. They can now accommodate observations from multiple modalities and from populations of subjects collected at different laboratories. The probabilistic atlasing systems described here show promise for identifying patterns of structural, functional, and molecular variation from across the contents of large-image databases, for pathology detection in individuals and groups, and for determining the effects of age, gender, handedness, and other demographic or genetic factors on brain structures in space and time. Integrating these observations to enable statistical comparison has already provided a deeper understanding of the relationship between brain structure and function. Importantly, the utility of an atlas depends on appropriate coordinate systems, registration, and deformation methods that allow the statistical combination of multiple observations in an agreed on, but expandable, digital reference framework. In this section, we highlight sources of data that will have an increasingly important role in integrative brain atlases: molecular architectonics, and DTI. Once stored in a population-based atlas, information from these techniques can help to interpret more conventional functional and structural brain maps by integrating them with data on molecular content, physiology, and fiber connections—a development that can help to formulate and test new types of neuroscientific models. A goal of systems neuroscience is to establish brain systems that underlie cognitive processes and the factors that influence them. DTI data on fiber connectivity, stored in an atlas coordinate system, can offer a rigorous computational basis to test how identifiable anatomical systems (i.e., visual, limbic, or corticothalamic pathways) interact. This atlas information can be invoked as regions of interest that are incorporated into the statistical design of functional brain-mapping studies (i.e., with fMRI or electroencephalography), even when underlying fiber connections are not evident in the data being collected for a particular study. Molecular architectonic mapping also provides a complementary perspective in which known neurotransmitter and receptor pathways—the physiology and molecular features of which are now well understood—can be associated with the functional subdivisions of the cortex identified with tomographic imaging. For example, an fMRI study of inhibitory cognitive processes in mild cognitive impairment might be informed by other modalities of data on limbic-prefrontal connectivity (from DTI), or on cortical monoamine receptor distributions (from architectonic mapping). In each of these contexts, the coordinate system of the atlas and the transformations that equate different modality data in the same reference frame provide the means to build and test systems-level models of cognition or disease, incorporating data from traditionally separate domains of neuroscience.

As brain databases begin to incorporate data from thousands of subjects, new questions in basic and clinical neuroscience can be addressed that were previously out of reach. For example, quantitative genetic studies are underway to link functional, structural, and connectivity information with variations in candidate genetic polymorphisms that could influence them. As polygenic disorders involve the interaction of multiple genetic variations, each with a small effect on the overall phenotype, digital atlases provide the ideal setting to mine large numbers of images computationally with hybrid techniques from computational anatomy and quantitative genetics (such as linkage and association studies in which a statistic is computed at each voxel location in the brain).

Should atlases be constructed specific to different age groups or different age-related diseases? Numerous other papers (Toga et al., 2006; Van Essen, 2002) have come to this conclusion and many population-based atlases have emerged in response to this need (Mazziotta et al., 2001). But the same logic can be carried to the next level by creating many different population-based atlases, each specific to the group demographics, disease, age, or other characteristics of the subjects being studied. These provide not only population statistics within the map, but they arguably better represent the morphological signature of that particular cohort. What must be included in all analyses are confidence statistics on where the activity takes place. Whether this entails a statistic on probability, percentile, or another metric may depend on the experimental design and other factors. Adoption of a single normal atlas—even a probabilistic version—for all subject studies provides the nominal capability for easier comparisons, but in doing so fails to adequately measure the nuances within or between each group (Figure 21.5). It therefore seems that it might be

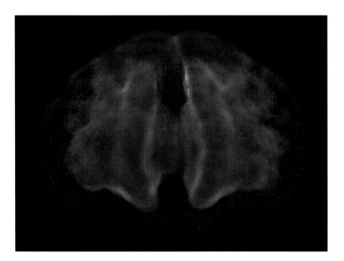

Figure 21–5 Variability in brain structure leads directly to the consideration of probabilistic localization of brain structure and function. The figure represents the structural probability obtained from across $N = 10$ normal subjects. Classification likelihood estimates can measure the membership of subjects against the atlas space, wherein low a posteriori probabilities will indicate significant statistical deviation indicative of structural change due to aging or age-related disease.

prudent to avoid dependency on a single modality, or single group representation, for every study (see also Devlin and Poldrack, *NeuroImage*, for critique and commentary). Any given imaging experiment will be better served by mapping to a population-based atlas that closely resembles the cohort under study. We suggest that population atlases for groups such as Alzheimer's (Mega et al., 2005; Thompson et al., 2007), schizophrenia (Cannon et al., 2006; Yoon et al., 2005), pediatric populations (Jelacic et al., 2006; Wilke et al., 2002), autism (Joshi et al., 2004), and even decades of life (Mazziotta et al., 2001) should be utilized, as appropriate, for the subject group (for examples, see Figure 21.6).

Large-scale databases and the next generation of population-based atlases will provide the necessary statistical power to identify demographic, genetic, and environmental factors that influence therapeutic response. These will be essential in the study of normal and abnormal human brain aging. Most important of all, brain databases are now being enriched with data from newer technologies, such as DTI, NIRS, and modern high-resolution imaging methods. These efforts are yielding whole new avenues of research into the functional organization of the brain, and how this is altered as we age, that will be of interest not just to specialists in neuroimaging, but to all basic and clinical neuroscientists.

Summary

Relating functional importance to structural location in the brain has been among the greatest challenges to neuroscientists since descriptions of brain injury patients in the 1800s. The characterization of the brain architecture responsible for producing human thought received a boost in momentum with the emergence of in vivo functional and structural neuroimaging technology over the past two decades. What became abundantly clear from technological advances such as MRI was that individual variability in cortical gyrification, as well as the pattern of blood flow-related activity measured using fMRI and PET made it difficult to directly compare across subjects without spatially accommodating brain size and shape. This particular challenge has spawned its own unique subdiscipline within neuroscience that now involves the collective efforts of neuroscientists, mathematicians, and computer scientists to database and produce common brain atlas spaces against which the locations of activity may be accurately referenced. In particular, the enormous diversity of brain maps and imaging methods has spurred the development of population-based digital brain atlases. However, the construction of databases and brain atlases are in themselves dynamic processes subject to first passes, false starts, gross inaccuracies, new adaptations, and the incorporation of new or updated information. In this chapter, we examine these processes and what they mean for making inferences about brain function based upon imperfect standard atlases. We review recent developments in brain databases and computational methods that have greatly expanded our ability to analyze brain structure and function. Drawn from extensive archives, these atlases encapsulate information on how the brain varies across age and gender, across time, in health and disease, and in large human populations. We discuss group patterns of cortical organization, asymmetry, and disease-specific trends that can be resolved from intersubject atlases that may not be apparent in individual brain maps. Finally, we describe the creation of four-dimensional (4D) maps that store information on the dynamics of brain change in development and disease. In summary, large-scale archives of primary neuroimaging

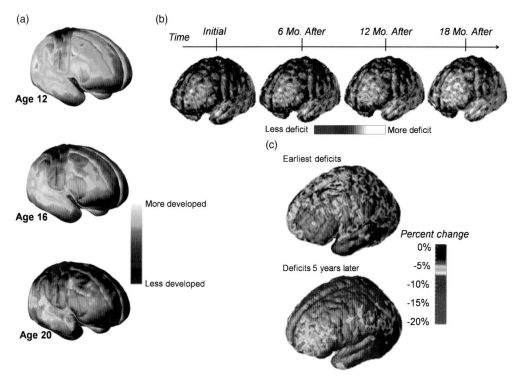

Figure 21–6 Consideration of specific population-based averages provides references against which (**a**) brain maturation, and (**b**) age-related diseases such as Alzheimer's, rapidly progress over time, and (**c**) the tracking of structural deficits in mental illnesses such as schizophrenia.

data show considerable promise in encompassing fundamental patterns of structural and functional variation in human populations, and how atlases can be used to highlight neurological features dependent upon demographic, genetic, cognitive, and clinical parameters.

References

Apostolova, L. G., Akopyan, G. G. et al. (2007). Structural correlates of apathy in Alzheimer's disease. *Dementia and Geriatric Cognitive Disorders*, 24(2): 91–97.

Apostolova, L. G., Lu, P. et al. (2008). 3D mapping of language networks in clinical and pre-clinical Alzheimer's disease. *Brain and Language*, 104(1): 33–41.

Apostolova, L. G. and Thompson, P. M. (2007). Brain mapping as a tool to study neurodegeneration. *Neurotherapeutics*, 4(3): 387–400.

Avants, B. and Gee, J. C. (2004). Geodesic estimation for large deformation anatomical shape averaging and interpolation. *Neuroimage*, 23(Suppl 1): S139–S150.

Avants, B. B., Schoenemann, P. T., and Gee, J. C. (2006). Lagrangian frame diffeomorphic image registration: morphometric comparison of human and chimpanzee cortex. *Medical Image Analysis*, 10(3): 397–412.

Cannon, T. D., Thompson, P. M. et al. (2006). Mapping heritability and molecular genetic associations with cortical features using probabilistic brain atlases: methods and applications to schizophrenia. *Neuroinformatics*, 4(1): 5–19.

Carlson, T. A., Schrater, P., and He, S. (2003). Patterns of activity in the categorical representations of objects. *Journal of Cognitive Neuroscience*, 15(5): 704–717.

Chen, X., Pereira, F., Lee, W., Strother, S., and Mitchell, T. (2006). Exploring predictive and reproducible modeling with the single-subject FIAC dataset. *Human Brain Mapping*, 27(5): 452–461.

Corouge, I., Dojat, M., and Barillot, C. (2004). Statistical shape modeling of low level visual area borders. *Medical Image Analysis*, 8(3): 353–360.

Cowie, S. E. (2000). A place in history: Paul Broca and cerebral localization. *Journal of Investigative Surgery*, 13(6): 297–298.

Davatzikos, C. (1996). Spatial normalization of 3D brain images using deformable models. *Journal of Computer-Assisted Tomography*, 20(4): 656–665.

Davatzikos, C. (1997). Spatial transformation and registration of brain images using elastically deformable models. *Computer Vision and Image Understanding*, 66(2): 207–222.

Diedrichsen, J. (2006). A spatially unbiased atlas template of the human cerebellum. *Neuroimage*, 33(1): 127–138.

Fox, P. and Lancaster, J. (2002). Mapping context and content: the BrainMap model. *Nature Reviews Neuroscience*, 3(April): 319–321.

Fox, P. T., Parsons, L. M., and Lancaster, J. L. (1998). Beyond the single study: function/location metanalysis in cognitive neuroimaging. *Current Opinion in Neurobiology*, 8(2): 178–187.

Friston, K. J., Glaser, D. E. et al. (2002). Classical and Bayesian inference in neuroimaging: applications. *Neuroimage*, 16(2): 484–512.

Gholipour, A., Kehtarnavaz, N., Briggs, R., Devous, M., and Gopinath, K. (2007). Brain functional localization: a survey of image registration techniques. *IEEE Transactions on Medical Imaging*, 26(4): 427–451.

Goedert, M. and Ghetti, B. (2007). Alois Alzheimer: his life and times. *Brain Pathology*, 17(1): 57–62.

Goutte, C., Hansen, L. K., Liptrot, M. G., and Rostrup, E. (2001). Feature-space clustering for fMRI meta-analysis. *Human Brain Mapping*, 13: 165–183.

Grady, C. L. (2002). Age-related differences in face processing: A meta-analysis of three functional neuroimaging experiments. *Canadian Journal of Experimental Psychology*, 56(3): 208–220.

Greicius, M. D., Srivastava, G., Reiss, A. L., and Menon, V. (2004). Default-mode network activity distinguishes Alzheimer's disease from healthy aging: evidence from functional MRI. *Proceedings of the National Academy of Sciences of the USA*, 101(13): 4637–4642.

Haas, L. F. (2001). Phineas Gage and the science of brain localisation. *Journal of Neurology, Neurosurgery, and Psychiatry*, 71(6): 761.

Haga, K. K., Khor, Y. P., Farrall, A., and Wardlaw, J. M. (2007). A systematic review of brain metabolite changes, measured with (1)H magnetic resonance spectroscopy, in healthy aging. *Neurobiology of Aging*, 30(3): 353–363.

Hansen, L. K., Nielsen, F. A., Strother, S. C., and Lange, N. (2001). Consensus inference in neuroimaging. *Neuroimage*, 13(6 Pt. 1): 1212–1218.

Jelacic, S., de Regt, D., and Weinberger, E. (2006). Interactive digital MR atlas of the pediatric brain. *Radiographics*, 26(2): 497–501.

Joshi, S., Davis, B., Jomier, M., and Gerig, G. (2004). Unbiased diffeomorphic atlas construction for computational anatomy. *Neuroimage*, 23(Suppl. 1): S151–S160.

Lancaster, J. L., Laird, A. R., Fox, P. M., Glahn, D. E., and Fox, P. T. (2005). Automated analysis of meta-analysis networks. *Human Brain Mapping*, 25(1): 174–184.

Lange, N., Strother, S. C. et al. (1999). Plurality and resemblance in fMRI data analysis. *Neuroimage*, 10(3 Pt. 1): 282–303.

Maldjian, J. A., Laurienti, P. J., and Burdette, J. H. (2004). Precentral gyrus discrepancy in electronic versions of the Talairach atlas. *Neuroimage*, 21(1): 450–455.

Mazziotta, J., Toga, A. et al. (2001). A four-dimensional probabilistic atlas of the human brain. *Journal of the American Medical Informatics Association*, 8(5): 401–430.

Mazziotta, J. C., Toga, A. W., Evans, A. C., Fox, P. T., and Lancaster, J. L. (1995). Digital brain atlases. *Trends in Neurosciences*, 18(5): 210–211.

Mega, M. S., Dinov, I. D. et al. (2005). Automated brain tissue assessment in the elderly and demented population: Construction and validation of a sub-volume probabilistic brain atlas. *Neuroimage*, 26(4): 1009–1018.

Narr, K. L., Bilder, R. M. et al. (2007). Asymmetries of cortical shape: effects of handedness, sex and schizophrenia. *Neuroimage*, 34(3): 939–948.

Narr, K. L., Thompson, P. M. et al. (2000). Mapping morphology of the corpus callosum in schizophrenia. *Cerebral Cortex*, 10(1): 40–49.

Nowinski, W. L. (2001). Modified Talairach landmarks. *Acta Neurochirurgica (Wien)*, 143(10): 1045–1057.

Nowinski, W. L. (2005). The cerefy brain atlases: continuous enhancement of the electronic talairach-tournoux brain atlas. *Neuroinformatics*, 3(4): 293–300.

Raichle, M. E. and Gusnard, D. A. (2002). Appraising the brain's energy budget. *Proceedings of the National Academy of Sciences of the USA*, 99(16): 10237–10239.

Rex, D. E., Shattuck, D. W. et al. (2004). A meta-algorithm for brain extraction in MRI. *Neuroimage*, 23(2): 625–637.

Rohlfing, T. and Maurer, C. R. Jr. (2007). Shape-based averaging. *IEEE Transactions on Image Processing*, 16(1): 153–161.

Roland, P. E. and Zilles, K. (1994). Brain atlases—a new research tool. *Trends in Neurosciences*, 17(11): 458–467.

Saeys, Y., Inza, I., and Larranaga, P. (2007). A review of feature selection techniques in bioinformatics. *Bioinformatics*, 23(19): 2507–2517.

Scher, A. I., Xu, Y. et al. (2007). Hippocampal shape analysis in Alzheimer's disease: a population-based study. *Neuroimage*, 36(1): 8–18.

Schroeter, M. L., Raczka, K., Neumann, J., and Yves von Cramon, Dl. (2007). Towards a nosology for frontotemporal lobar degenerations-a meta-analysis involving 267 subjects. *Neuroimage*, 36(3): 497–510.

Sidtis, J. J., Strother, S. C., and Rottenberg, D. A. (2003). Predicting performance from functional imaging data: methods matter. *Neuroimage*, 20(2): 615–624.

Strother, S., La Conte, S. et al. (2004). Optimizing the fMRI data-processing pipeline using prediction and reproducibility performance metrics: I. A preliminary group analysis. *Neuroimage*, 23(Suppl. 1): S196–S207.

Strother, S. C., Kanno, I., and Rottenberg, D. A. (1995). Principal component analysis, variance partitioning, and "Functional Connectivity". *Journal of Cerebral Blood Flow and Metabolism*, 15: 353–360.

Talairach, J. and Tournoux, P. (1988). *Co-Planar Stereotactic Atlas of the Human Brain*. New York: Tieme.

Thompson, P., Cannon, T. D., and Toga, A. W. (2002). Mapping genetic influences on human brain structure. *Annals of Medicine*, 34(7–8): 523–536.

Thompson, P. M., Giedd, J. N. et al. (2000). Growth patterns in the developing brain detected by using continuum mechanical tensor maps. *Nature*, 404(6774): 190–193.

Thompson, P. M., Hayashi, K. M. et al. (2007). Tracking Alzheimer's disease. *Annals of the New York Academy of Sciences*, 1097: 183–214.

Thompson, P. M., Woods, R. P., Mega, M. S., and Toga, A. W. (2000). Mathematical/computational challenges in creating deformable and probabilistic atlases of the human brain. *Human Brain Mapping*, 9(2): 81–92.

Toga, A. W. (2002). Imaging databases and neuroscience. *Neuroscientist*, 8(5): 423–436.

Toga, A. W. and Thompson, P. M. (2001). Maps of the brain. *The Anatomical Record*, 265(2): 37–53.

Toga, A. W. and Thompson, P. M. (2002). New approaches in brain morphometry. The *American Journal of Geriatric Psychiatry*, 10(1): 13–23.

Toga, A. W. and Thompson, P. M. (2005). Genetics of brain structure and intelligence. *Annual Review of Neuroscience*, 28: 1–23.

Toga, A. W., Thompson, P. M., Mega, M. S., Narr, K. L., and Blanton, R. E. (2001). Probabilistic approaches for atlasing normal and disease-specific brain variability. *Anatomy and Embryology (Berlin)*, 204(4): 267–282.

Toga, A. W., Thompson, P. M., Mori, S., Amunts, K., and Zilles, K. (2006). Towards multimodal atlases of the human brain. *Nature Reviews. Neuroscience*, 7(12): 952–966.

Toga, A. W., Thompson, P. M., and Sowell, E. R. (2006). Mapping brain maturation. *Trends in Neurosciences*, 29(3): 148–159.

Van Essen, D. C. (2002). Windows on the brain: The emerging role of atlases and databases in neuroscience. *Current Opinion in Neurobiology*, 12(5): 574–579.

Van Essen, D. C. (2005). A Population-Average, Landmark- and Surface-based (PALS) atlas of human cerebral cortex. *Neuroimage*, 28(3): 635–662.

Van Horn, J. D., Grafton, S. T., Rockmore, D., and Gazzaniga, M. S. (2004). Sharing neuroimaging studies of human cognition. *Nature Neuroscience*, 7(5): 473–481.

Wakana, S., Jiang, H., Nagae-Poetscher, L. M., van Zijl, P. C., and Mori, S. (2004). Fiber tract-based atlas of human white matter anatomy. *Radiology*, 230(1): 77–87.

Weaver, J. B., Healy, D. M. Jr., Periaswamy, S., and Kostelec, P. J. (1998). Elastic image registration using correlations. *Journal of Digital Imaging*, 11(3 Suppl. 1): 59–65.

Wilke, M., Schmithorst, V. J., and Holland, S. K. (2002). Assessment of spatial normalization of whole-brain magnetic resonance images in children. *Human Brain Mapping*, 17(1): 48–60.

Woods, R. P. (2003). Characterizing volume and surface deformations in an atlas framework: theory, applications, and implementation. *Neuroimage*, 18(3): 769–788.

Woods, R. P., Grafton, S. T., Holmes, C. J., Cherry, S. R., and Mazziotta, J. C. (1998). Automated image registration: I. General methods and intrasubject, intramodality validation. *Journal of Computer-Assisted Tomography*, 22(1): 139–152.

Woods, R. P., Grafton, S. T., Watson, J. D., Sicotte, N. L., and Mazziotta, J. C. (1998). Automated image registration: II. Intersubject validation of linear and nonlinear models. *Journal of Computer Assisted Tomography*, 22(1): 153–165.

Yoon, U., Lee, J. M. et al. (2005). Quantitative analysis of group-specific brain tissue probability map for schizophrenic patients. *Neuroimage*, 26(2): 502–512.

Zakzanis, K. K., Graham, S. J., and Campbell, Z. (2003). A meta-analysis of structural and functional brain imaging in dementia of the Alzheimer's type: a neuroimaging profile. *Neuropsychology Review*, 13(1): 1–18.

Index

Note: The locators with "*f*" and "*t*" denotes a figure or a table in that page.